www.harcourt-internat

Bringing you products from all Harcourt
companies including Baillière Tindall, Churchill Livingstone,
Mosby and W.B. Saunders

- ▶ **Browse** for latest information on new books, journals and electronic products

- ▶ **Search** for information on over 20 000 published titles with full product information including tables of contents and sample chapters

- ▶ **Keep up to date** with our extensive publishing programme in your field by registering with **eAlert** or requesting postal updates

- ▶ **Secure online ordering** with prompt delivery, as well as full contact details to order by phone, fax or post

- ▶ **News** of special features and promotions

If you are based in the following countries, please visit the country-specific site to receive full details of product availability and local ordering information

USA: www.harcourthealth.com

Canada: www.harcourtcanada.com

Australia: www.harcourt.com.au

✣ Baillière Tindall   ⬥ CHURCHILL LIVINGSTONE   ℳ Mosby   W.B. SAUNDERS

Human Physiology

Commissioning Editors: Ellen Green, Laurence Hunter
Project Development Manager: Barbara Simmons
Designer: Sarah Russell
Page make-up: Kate Walshaw
Project Controller: Nancy Arnott

Human Physiology

Andrew Davies BSc PhD
Professor of Physiology
University of Glamorgan
Pontyprydd
Mid Glamorgan, UK

Asa G. H. Blakeley BM BS DPhil
Late Professor of Human Physiology and Pro-Vice-Chancellor
University of Leicester
Leicester, UK

Cecil Kidd BSc PhD FIBiol FRSA
Professor Emeritus of Physiology
University of Aberdeen
Aberdeen, UK

Consulting Editor
J. G. McGeown MB BCh BSc PhD
Senior Lecturer in Physiology
Queen's University
Belfast, UK

Illustrated by **bounford.com and Ian Ramsden**

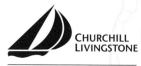
CHURCHILL LIVINGSTONE

EDINBURGH LONDON NEW YORK PHILADELPHIA ST LOUIS SYDNEY AND TORONTO 2001

CHURCHILL LIVINGSTONE
An imprint of Harcourt Publishers Limited

First published 2001

ISBN 0443 045593
International Student Edition 0443 046549

British Library Cataloguing in Publication Data
A catalogue record for this book is available from the British Library

Library of Congress Cataloging in Publication Data
A catalog record for this book is available from the Library of Congress

Medical knowledge is constantly changing. As new information becomes available, changes in treatment, procedures, equipment and the use of drugs become necessary. The editors/authors/contributors and the publishers have, as far as it is possible, taken care to ensure that the information given in this text is accurate and up to date. However, readers are strongly advised to confirm that the information, especially with regard to drug usage, complies with the latest legislation and standards of practice.

The
publisher's
policy is to use
**paper manufactured
from sustainable forests**

Printed in Spain

Preface

Human Physiology is an important component of the education of all students of medicine and the allied health professions such as nursing, physical therapy, dentistry, intensive care, pharmacy and nutrition. It is also a significant contributor to many degree programmes in the biomedical sciences, including physiology, pharmacology, neuroscience, sports science, pathology and other medical and biomedical sciences. Our aim in writing this book has been to present a core of human physiology that is appropriate for students reading about the subject for the first time and can also be used as a reference source in future studies.

In the UK, the USA and elsewhere, new curricula have been developed that emphasize a problem-solving approach. Much of the didactic component of these courses has been removed: in some courses, completely so. Either way, students need an accurate base of factual knowledge and understanding in order to undertake problem-solving successfully. We have, therefore, attempted to provide a distillate of those fundamental aspects of human physiology that underpin a broader knowledge base and are useful for under-standing and analysing clinical and biomedical scientific problems.

In addition to providing core physiology, we have introduced many features that should make learning and teaching from this book easier and more enjoyable. They include the following:

Applied Physiology chapters

As the title implies, the primary focus of the book is human and mammalian physiology. Our account starts at the molecular and cellular levels and moves systematically through the various body systems. In recognition of the fact that all of these systems in practice operate in an integrated way, we conclude each section with an Applied Physiology chapter that is devoted to integrative topics such as exercise, temperature regulation, stroke, shock, etc. These chapters emphasise the important overall 'wholeness' of the physiological mechanisms in the body and the ways they interact.

Basic Science boxes

Experience shows that students' understanding of physiology can be greatly improved by reminding them of basic physical or biological principles. In the Basic Science boxes we provide brief and simple explanations of aspects of physics or chemistry, concentrating in particular on areas where students are known to encounter difficulties.

Clinical Examples

Throughout the book, the clinical relevance of basic physiology is highlighted through the use of Clinical Examples. These sections are introduced as appropriate within the chapters and demonstrate clearly the application of physiological knowledge to clinical situations.

Examples include respiratory disease, motor disorders and spasticity, and glomerulo-nephritis.

Recent Advances boxes

Recent Advances boxes are placed at appropriate points in each section. They highlight areas where knowledge is advancing rapidly and may have important implications for the future. As well as providing a brief introduction, they emphasise the fact that physiology is not a static discipline and that the limits of physiological knowledge are constantly developing and expanding. These boxes also provide material for students who wish to explore physiology further.

Summary boxes

To focus students' attention on the essential points of a topic, we have included frequent Summary boxes. These are intended to aid learning and assist in preparation for examinations.

Multiple Choice questions

Each section of the book ends with MCQs and explanatory answers. These can be used to test understanding, prepare for exams, or simply to reinforce learning.

Preparation of a major textbook takes a considerable amount of time and effort, and it would not have been possible without the contributions and help of our friends. Any errors of content are our own, and we would welcome having them brought to our attention.

AD
CK

Dedication

Human Physiology is dedicated to Professor Asa Blakeley, who first conceived the idea for this book but, tragically, did not live to see it completed. We hope it has realized his original vision.

Acknowledgements

We are very grateful to our colleagues who made essential scientific contributions to this book's contents – they are listed separately. We would like to single out for special mention Dr J.G. McGeown, Consulting Editor, who read and commented on the manuscript and also contributed the MCQ sections, and his colleague in Belfast, Professor William Wallace, who contributed substantially to the clinical application sections. Dr Catherine Bright also contributed clinical examples and provided general support. Professor John Hampton, Professor John Norman and Dr M.A. Radcliffe also helped in the early stages of the project. Dr Margaret Jones, consultant radiologist at Llandough Hospital in Cardiff, provided excellent radiographic images at short notice.

Many other friends and colleagues have given generously of their advice and specialist knowledge without recognition, and to them we are equally grateful.

Finally, our thanks also go to the team at Harcourt Health Sciences, Barbara Simmons, Ellen Green and Laurence Hunter, who have faithfully and enthusiastically supported this project from the first. Sue Beasley deserves a particular mention and thanks for the style and precision, as well as encyclopaedic knowledge, that she brought to the task of editing the final manuscript.

AD
CK

Contributors

Tony Ashton BSc(Hons) PhD
Senior Lecturer
School of Applied Sciences
University of Glamorgan
Pontyprydd, UK

Applied physiology: Good diet

Catherine Bright MB BCh BSc PhD MRCPsych
Consultant Psychiatrist
NHS, Wales

Clinical examples

Janice M. Marshall DSc PhD BSc F Med Sci
Professor of Physiology
University of Birmingham Medical School
Birmingham, UK

The renal system

J.G. McGeown MB B Ch BSc PhD
Senior Lecturer in Physiology
Department of Physiology
Queen's University
Belfast, UK

Consulting Editor
Multiple choice questions and answers

Peter N. McWilliam BSc PhD
Professor
School of Healthcare Studies
University of Leeds
Leeds, UK

Preliminary chapters for
The cardiovascular system

Carl Moores BSc MB ChB FRCA
Consultant Anaesthetist
Royal Infirmary of Edinburgh
Edinburgh, UK

Applied physiology: Congenital defects in the neonate

Stewart Petersen MA PhD
Head of Medical Education
Leicester Warwick Medical School
Leicester, UK

The gastrointestinal system
Applied physiology: Temperature regulation

Kathleen Rayfield BSc PhD MBA
Senior Lecturer in Physiology
School of Healthcare Studies
University of Leeds
Leeds, UK

The endocrine system *and*
The reproductive system and
neonatal physiology

Jon Scott BSc PhD
Director of Biological Sciences
Senior Lecturer in Physiology
Department of Pre-Clinical Sciences
University of Leicester
Leicester, UK

Chapters in Neurological communication and
control *and* Special senses and higher functions

William F.M. Wallace BSc MD FRCP FRCA
Professor of Applied Physiology
School of Biomedical Science
Faculty of Medicine
Queen's University
Belfast, UK

Applied physiology:
Ageing and the special senses

Applied physiology:
Chronic obstructive pulmonary disease

Applied physiology: Renal failure

Clinical examples

Contents

8 The renal system

9 The gastrointestinal system

10 The reproductive system and neonatal physiology

The cell and its membrane

1

Introduction

We begin this physiology book by defining physiology as:

> the science of the normal functions and phenomena of living things.

Of the few words in that definition 'living' is the most difficult to define. Rather than attempt a daunting philosophical discussion so early in our explanation of our science, we satisfy ourselves, and we hope our readers, by describing in this section some current ideas of the origin and evolution of the phenomenon that most of us would say we recognize as life. In this section the overriding attribute of living organisms, the ability to control and stabilize the environment within themselves, is emphasized.

The control systems that give living organisms their stability would be powerless against changes in the surroundings if the individual components of the organism, its cells, were not protected from the environment by an envelope whose permeability can itself be controlled. This envelope is the cell membrane. Moreover, the specialized structures that make up the organelles within each cell are themselves separated from the general cytoplasm which forms the body of a cell by membranes which contribute to their function, and we see in this section how movement of substances across cell membranes controls the composition of the fluid contents of the cell and its fluid surroundings.

In trying to understand so complicated a system as a living organism it is common to reduce it to its component parts, in this case cells. A common property of living cells is their excitability, which is the production of an active response to a stimulus from the environment. Perhaps the most dramatic expression of excitability of cells is the electrical phenomenon known as the action potential, seen in nerves and muscles and important in the control of whole systems of the body described in subsequent sections. We do not leave the subject of the cell and its membranes, however, without touching upon other methods of controlling and signalling to cells through cell junctions and receptors evolved to accept the controlling messages.

Section overview

This section outlines:

- A definition of life
- The origin and evolution of life
- The elements of control systems
- The structure of lipid membranes
- Differences in intracellular and extracellular environments
- Water movement across cell membranes and osmosis
- Transmembrane diffusion
- Active transport
- Transepithelial movements
- The composition of intracellular and extracellular fluids
- The membrane permeability of excitable cells
- Membrane potentials and action potentials
- Conduction of nerve impulses
- Cell-to-cell signalling
- Receptor types.

Life

The Oxford English Dictionary defines physiology as: 'the science of the normal functions and phenomena of living things'.

This definition itself requires a definition of life, and that is a considerable scientific task.

Defining life

The defining attributes of living things, growth, reproduction, repair and adaptation to varied conditions, ultimately arise from two properties:

- the ability to self-duplicate
- the presence of discrete change (mutation).

That is to say living things reproduce themselves but with mutations, some of which persist from generation to generation.

The great mathematician John von Neumann in 1948 provided a theoretical analysis of the properties of life which can be used to define it. It is fascinating in this computerized and automated age that von Neumann's analysis allows for certain automated non-biological systems, as well as organisms, to be described as alive if they:

A. collect raw materials and convert them into an output specified by a 'written' instruction
B. contain a duplicator which accepts this instruction and copies it
C. have a controller which, when given an instruction, first passes the instruction to

3

B for duplication, then to A for action, passes a copy of the instruction to the 'progeny' (the output of A) and keeps a copy for itself

D. possess the written instruction.

The interesting part of von Neumann's argument is that it is not based on exclusively biological systems (an automated factory might fulfil the criteria) and every organism larger than a virus fulfils all the criteria. In these living organisms the categories A–D are as follows:

A. the organelles known as ribosomes
B. the enzymes RNA and DNA polymerase
C. the repressor and the de-repressor controlling molecules involved in cell reproduction
D. the genetic message written in DNA.

These philosophical considerations lead us to question if a virus is in fact alive, and whether life is as easy to define as we might first suppose.

The origin of life

It is generally agreed that life in the generally understood meaning of the word has not always existed on earth, although it is not universally agreed that the picture obtained from the fossil record of all life evolving from small single-celled beings is correct.

Astronomical and geological evidence is that the earth condensed out of interstellar material in a process beginning 4.5 billion years ago, and by 3.8 billion years ago it was the sphere it is today. Then for half a billion years it seems the earth was without life of any kind, or if it existed it left no record we can discern.

For some 30 years, scientists have been speculating as to what conditions might have existed on the lifeless earth to give rise to proteins which form the catalysts of life and the nucleic acids (DNA and RNA) that embody the instructions for the synthesis of proteins.

The materials required for the construction of the chemical basis of life have been known

for some time. Indeed, Charles Darwin in a letter to Hooker, written in February 1871, observed: 'If we could conceive in some warm little pond, with all sorts of ammonia and phosphoric salts, light, heat, electricity etc. present, that a protein compound was chemically formed ready to undergo still more complex changes …'. These protein compounds, speculated Darwin, formed the physical basis of life.

The same Charles Darwin, with others, pointed out that once established, the development of life into the forms we see today depended on *evolution* and that evolution depended on *the survival of the fittest* and competition for resources in a population.

Molecular evolution

Before life appeared, the process of evolution applied only to the formation of complex molecules from simpler ones (see Basic Science 1.1.1). The elements hydrogen and carbon form long-chain compounds, hydrocarbons, that are amongst the most stable of large molecules. They can also include oxygen and nitrogen within their structures. In this period of evolution, fitness equated with stability, and therefore complex 'organic' structures began to accumulate. The atmosphere of the earth at this time was devoid of molecular oxygen. This further allowed these complex molecules to remain intact for long periods. At some stage of evolution, associations of these complex moieties generated life (Fig. 1.1.1).

Our most dramatic evidence for early life lies in the geological record where there is a clear distinction between the Cambrian rocks, which carry a multitude of visible fossils of burgeoning life, and the apparently lifeless older Precambrian rocks. Microscopic investigation reveals, however, that Precambrian times were not lifeless, although the earliest life forms encountered consisted only of tiny anaerobic prokaryotic (without a nucleus) cells. From these prokaryotes evolved, 2.5 billion years ago, photosynthesizing cyanobacteria probably producing oxygen as a 'weapon', highly toxic to their anaerobic competitors. Next evolved the eukaryotes (cells with a nucleus) whose cellular architecture is the pattern of our own. It is remarkable to note how long it took eukaryotes to evolve (more than 3 billion years after the formation of the earth) when it took less than 1 billion years for life itself to evolve from a sterile world.

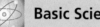

Basic Science 1.1.1

The origins of complex biological molecules

Assuming that life evolved from inorganic material, we can expect the conditions under which that took place to have been very different from those we see around us today. If that were not so, we would expect to see life still being spontaneously created.

Much speculation has taken place about what conditions were like when life was first formed, but there is general agreement that for the fragile molecules which form the building blocks of living material to survive long enough to evolve into more complex forms there must have been little or none of the highly reactive oxygen we see in abundance in the atmosphere and bound in the rocks today. It is this atmospheric oxygen, released into the atmosphere by early living organisms that succeeded in harnessing the energy of sunlight, which terminated conditions that made the original appearance of life possible.

Scientists have reproduced the conditions that they think existed on the primitive earth, with mixtures of hydrogen, water, methane and ammonia heated in flasks irradiated with ultraviolet light, and through which sparks of electricity are passed (Fig. BS1.1.1).

In view of the difference in volume between these experimental flasks, holding a litre or two, and the volume of the whole of the primeval sea, it is perhaps surprising that it seems to have taken life as long as a billion years to appear, when in less than a week the building blocks of biological macromolecules, in the form of

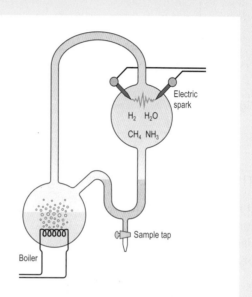

Fig. BS1.1.1 A model of conditions on the primitive earth.

aldehydes, carboxylic acids and amino acids were appearing in the flasks. The next step in chemical evolution was the formation of proteins, for which the presence of 20 amino acids is enough. For the formation of that other essential component of life, nucleic acids, sugars can be built up from formaldehyde, and purines and pyrimidines from, for example, diaminomaleonitrile. Thus, the primeval sea could easily contain the chemical constituents of life, although their assembly into the first cell-membrane-enclosed 'protobiont' or perhaps 'naked gene' – and which came first– is another more contentious story.

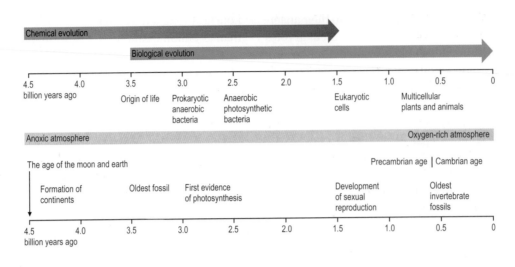

Fig. 1.1.1 Stages in the evolution of life.

The properties of living things

It is not easy to define life unambiguously and, for our purpose, it is perhaps best to simply describe those common properties of living organisms that allow us to recognize them.

- Living organisms isolate themselves from their environment with an envelope (membrane) and maintain within that envelope a well-controlled microenvironment in which the chemical processes of the organism can proceed. We call these basic units of life cells.
- Living organisms maintain themselves by energy-consuming processes which we call metabolism.
- Living cells propagate themselves by division of the cell into two daughter cells each of which contains all the features of the parent cell.
- The replication process is not exact and the small differences introduced are acted upon by selective pressures to produce darwinian evolution into more and more complex and successful forms of life.
- From a physiologist's point of view the most conspicuous feature of living organisms is

that all the processes of life are controlled. Indeed, physiology is the study of these control processes.

Control processes operate at all levels in complex multicellular organisms. Their effects are evident at the level of the enzyme, for example end-product inhibition of an enzyme system such as that synthesizing the autonomic neurotransmitter noradrenaline (see Ch. 3.2). At a whole animal level, complex control processes manage the reproductive cycles in both men and women (see Ch. 10.1).

It is the honing of control processes by natural selection that leads to the development of more successful species.

Evolution of the species

The fittest increase in numbers whilst the less fit decline. How should we define fitness? In common parlance the Olympic athlete is fitter than the couch potato. Although in competition in the athlete's chosen event this may seem self-evident, in terms of evolution the athlete may well be less fit – physical training reduces the fertility of both men and women and also brings with it much degenerative disease. So extreme performance of one function is not enough for evolutionary success. Indeed, the only unchallengeable definition of evolutionary fitness is almost a circular one – it is that fitness leads to preferential survival.

The complexity of the factors that lead to better evolutionary fitness can perhaps be hinted at by considering the predator–prey relationships of the wolf, which has common ancestry with our domesticated dogs. Wolves chase their prey, which are typically large herbivores; therefore running ability is obviously important. By selective breeding, man has produced breeds of running dogs that can easily outstrip a wolf. Why has natural selection not developed this potential in the wolf? One has only to look at a greyhound to realize that speed has been achieved by making the animal light and fragile looking. So in the wolf, speed is only developed to the point where brute strength is not compromised. One might say that the wolf is fast enough but no faster. This process of development is one of optimization – the benefits and cost of any development are weighed one against the other and fitness is the approach to the balance between cost and benefit that leads to the best chance of survival.*

You will find that this process of optimization occurs at many levels in physiology. In Chapter 6.3 you will find that the amount of red cells in the blood is determined by the need to minimize the work needed to transport O_2 and CO_2 around the body. More red cells mean that less volume of blood must be pumped to transport a given amount of the gases, but the

Summary

Life

- A definition of physiology requires a definition of life.
- Physiology is the science of the normal functions and phenomena of living things.
- Life is characterized by self-duplication and discrete change (mutation).
- The most conspicuous characteristic of living things is that their processes are controlled.
- Biological evolution on earth was preceded by molecular evolution.

viscosity of the blood is increased. If the work to transport a given amount of oxygen is plotted against the haematocrit (the fraction of the blood volume occupied by the red cells) it passes through a minimum (an optimum situation) close to the value found in normal individuals. If the same is done for individuals living at high altitude, where oxygen partial pressures in the air are low, the haematocrit is seen to move to a higher but still optimum value.

Control systems

The elements of a control system

Physiology is a study of the systems that control the processes of life. We are all familiar with simple control mechanisms that we use in everyday life. We like the inside environment of our houses to be maintained at a comfortable temperature – in temperate climates we control it by the manipulation of some heating device. The simplest is a free-standing electrical heater which we can switch on and off. On a cold day we switch on the heater, and experience will suggest that if it is very cold outside this will be at its highest setting.

---

* The competition between predator and prey, where chase is involved, is usually settled by the relative abilities of the two to manage the heat burden generated by running. The dog manages this particularly well by having a close association between the main arteries and veins in the neck that acts as a countercurrent heat exchanger, confining the heat to the body of the dog. It also ensures that the blood perfusing the brain is preferentially cooled by blood returning from the tongue, a major heat-losing organ.

How effective is this system? Indeed how would you assess its effectiveness? Perhaps the first question might be: 'Is my room heated to a comfortable temperature on the coldest days of the year?' Put in a simpler manner: 'Is the heater powerful enough?' A second question might be: 'Does the system keep the room temperature within the range of temperatures that I find comfortable?' If the sun shines into the room, does the room become too hot? If the day gets colder, does the room feel cold? With this simple system you will have to manually alter the heater output to keep comfortable. The jargon for such a system is an open loop system (Fig. 1.1.2).

The obvious faults in the simple system described are addressed in most modern central heating systems by including a thermostat – a temperature-controlled switch – in the system. The occupant sets the desired room temperature of the thermostat. If the room is cooler than this, the heat is turned on. If the room is warmer, the heat is turned off. Heat supply is inversely (negatively) related to the difference between the temperature of the room and the temperature set.

Such a system, where the effect of the output is measured and used to control the amount of output, is called a feedback-controlled system. It is a closed loop system. Because of the negative relationship between the difference between the achieved and the set temperature, it is called a **negative-feedback** system (Fig. 1.1.3).

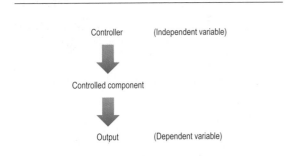

Fig. 1.1.2 Open loop control. An open loop control system is one in which the controlled component alters its behaviour or output in direct conformity with instructions from a controller that is uninfluenced by the output of the controlled component. An example of such a system might be a janitor sitting in the warm boiler-house of a college altering the output of his boilers at his whim and independently of the feelings of the occupants of the building.

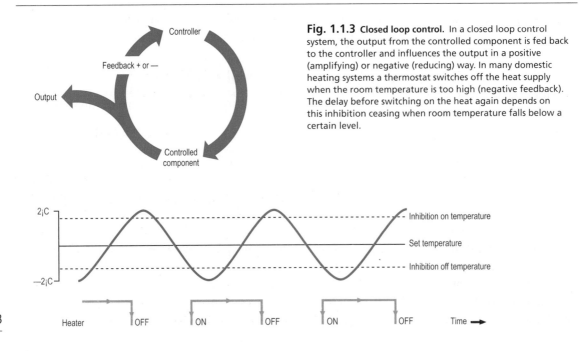

Fig. 1.1.3 Closed loop control. In a closed loop control system, the output from the controlled component is fed back to the controller and influences the output in a positive (amplifying) or negative (reducing) way. In many domestic heating systems a thermostat switches off the heat supply when the room temperature is too high (negative feedback). The delay before switching on the heat again depends on this inhibition ceasing when room temperature falls below a certain level.

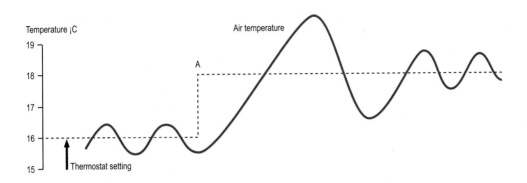

Fig. 1.1.4 Inertia in control systems. Changes in temperature in a room where the thermostat is fixed to a wall of high thermal inertia. At A, the thermostat is reset to a higher temperature. The heaters quickly raise the air in the room to that temperature but the wall responds more slowly causing overshoots of decreasing amplitude until the new set point is reached. It should be noted that the temperatures set on the thermostat represent mean temperatures around which the actual room temperature oscillates.

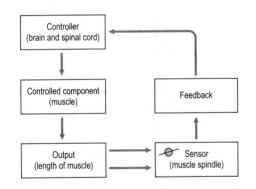

Fig. 1.1.5 Muscle feedback. The position of a limb, or movement of a limb, is controlled by the brain setting the length of the muscles around the joints of the limb. To do this in a regulated and purposeful way the brain must 'know' the lengths of these muscles, which it interprets as position. This information is provided by feedback from sensors (muscle spindles) in the muscles themselves.

How do we assess the effectiveness of this more complex control system? As with the first system we want to know that it will cope with the coldest weather. 'How powerful is it?' Secondly, does it maintain the room temperature within a comfortable range in face of varying outside temperatures? 'How precise is it?'

Another question might also be asked. 'What is the response of the system to a change in the setting of the thermostat by the room's occupants?' Suppose you change the setting of your room thermostat from 16°C to 18°C. The speed at which the new temperature is reached largely depends on the power of the heaters and the size of the room. The way in which the final temperature is reached depends on a number of factors. To choose but one, control systems are said to have 'inertia'. In the present case this might be the thermal inertia of the wall on which the thermostat is situated. This means that the thermostat may not warm up as rapidly as the room air and there will be considerable overshoot while the new set temperature is reached. These oscillations are generated by a negative-feedback system which includes a time delay in the feedback circuit (Fig. 1.1.4).

Can one ask similar questions of a biological system?

At a microscopic level, the cell creates within its membrane-bound cytoplasm a microenvironment kept at a constant composition to allow the processes of the cell to proceed unaffected by the medium in which the cell is placed. At a whole animal level, the questions asked about the heating system can be best illustrated by considering the control of movement by the skeletal muscle system (Fig. 1.1.5).

How powerful is a particular set of muscles?

This is a question whose answer can easily be understood in terms of the maximum force that they can generate.

How precisely can a given position be maintained?

Experience will tell you that this varies from muscle to muscle. The extraocular muscles that control the fixation point of the eye can hold the gaze constant to within a tiny limit; look at a small distant object intently – no change in fixation will be detectable by you. On the other hand, hold out your arm and point at the same object with one finger – your point of aim will dance obviously around your intended mark. If you were to try this with your leg and toe, the errors would be even worse.

How does the system respond to a sudden change in the set point?

In the case of the control of eye movement, once again changing from one point of fixation to another does not produce any overshoot that you can detect. On the other hand, changing the aim of the pointing finger will produce obvious overshoot and oscillation about the point of aim.

The beautiful control of eye movement is the result of complex feedback control mechanisms and their critical damping by means of the vitreous humour (see Ch. 4.1).

Are oscillations always a bad thing? – another kind of feedback

You will see in the diagram of the closed loop control system (Fig. 1.1.3) that the feedback to the controller can be negative (reducing), which we have discussed, or positive (amplifying).

Positive feedback is used extensively in physiology as a means of generating rhythms

and rapidly switching systems on or off. Rhythms and switching are an essential part of life.

For positive feedback to be useful, however, it is essential that there is a mechanism to terminate it; otherwise the system 'runs away' and can eventually produce damage. An example of this 'run-away' is the howl produced when a microphone is placed too close to the speakers of an amplified system. A whisper is picked up by the microphone, amplified, passed out of the speakers as a shout which is picked up by the microphone, amplified, passed out of the speakers and so on (Fig. 1.1.6).

This type of feedback sounds as if it is a dangerous nuisance but it forms the trigger for many important events in your life, including the beating of your heart. Your heart beats because the voltage between the inside and outside of the heart cell changes with a rhythm of about 1 Hz throughout life.

This electrical rhythm triggers the contraction of the heart. The membrane of heart cells is slightly permeable to ions and they trickle in. This causes the membrane voltage to creep towards zero volts. At a certain voltage just below zero, called the *threshold*, specific channels in the membrane are opened by the voltage and even more ions are allowed in, accelerating the fall in voltage. This process is positive feedback and has to be terminated or no rhythm will be generated. The membrane will simply stay locked at one extreme of voltage and the heart will cease to beat. The positive feedback is terminated by the inlet channels of the membrane closing and others opening to allow ions out of the cell.

The smallest structures in the body in which feedback mechanisms can be seen to be operating to maintain a constant environment are the individual cell organelles, and the whole process of maintaining a constant internal environment is called **homeostasis**.

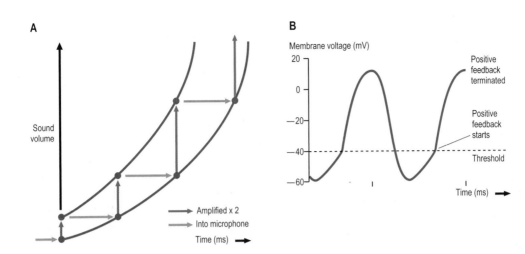

Fig. 1.1.6 Positive feedback. A. How positive feedback produces 'howl' when the microphone of an amplified system is placed too close to the speakers. A sound picked up by the microphone is amplified (in this case a modest ×2), comes out of the speakers as a louder sound to be picked up by the microphone, is amplified – and so on. **B.** In the case of heart muscle, positive feedback at threshold voltage triggers the contraction of the heart. Positive feedback is frequently seen in physiology being used to bring about such 'all-or-nothing' events.

Summary

Control systems

- Much of physiology is the study of control systems that operate in living things.
- Control systems can be 'open loop' where there is no feedback or 'closed loop' where the output of the system feeds back and influences the controller.
- The feedback of the output on the controller can be negative, which reduces changes in output, or positive, which amplifies changes.

- The precision with which a variable is controlled depends on the power and speed of response of the controller, the sensitivity of the sensor and the 'inertia' of the system.
- Positive feedback is frequently used in physiology to produce rhythmic activity and trigger events.
- To be useful, positive feedback systems must include a mechanism to terminate the effect.

The cell membrane

1.2

Cell structure

Animal cells share a common basic structure (Figs 1.2.1 and 1.2.2). The cell components (its **cytoplasm** and nucleus) are enclosed in a continuous cell membrane or **plasmalemma**. This membrane is a barrier between the cell and its environment, across which all communication takes place. It is selectively permeable and contains transport mechanisms. This membrane allows the cell to keep the composition of its interior relatively constant in the face of changes in its environment. The cell must also communicate across its membrane with its environment. Both these functions are carried out by proteins within the membrane.

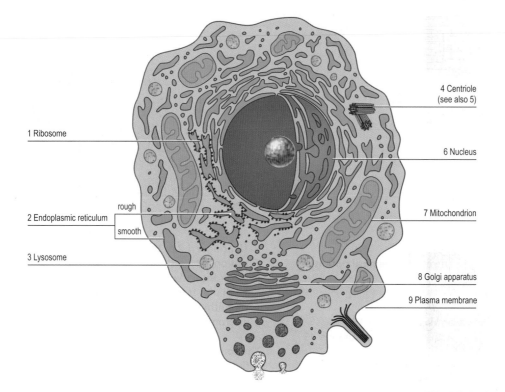

4 Centriole
(see also 5)

1 Ribosome

6 Nucleus

2 Endoplasmic reticulum — rough
— smooth

7 Mitochondrion

3 Lysosome

8 Golgi apparatus

9 Plasma membrane

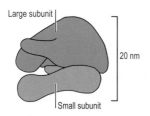

Large subunit

20 nm

Small subunit

1 Ribosome. Almost all the RNA in cells is found in ribosomes, which catalyse protein synthesis. They are not bounded by a membrane and are very numerous – several hundred per cell.

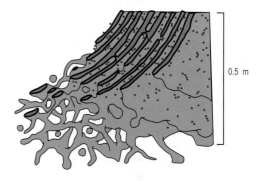

0.5 m

2 Endoplasmic reticulum. Continuous with the outer membrane of the nuclear envelope, the endoplasmic reticulum can be rough – owing to its outer face being studded with ribosomes engaged in protein synthesis – or smooth, when it is involved in lipid metabolism.

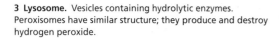

0.5 m

3 Lysosome. Vesicles containing hydrolytic enzymes. Peroxisomes have similar structure; they produce and destroy hydrogen peroxide.

Fig. 1.2.1 A typical animal cell and its organelles.
$1\ \mu m$ (micron, micrometre; 10^{-6} m) $= 1000$ nm (10^{-9} m)
$= 10\ 000$ Å (10^{-10} m).

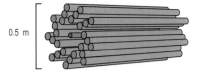

0.5 m

4 Centriole. Two centrioles make up a centrosome to which the cell's cytoskeleton of microtubules is attached.

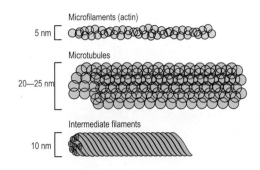

Microfilaments (actin)

5 nm

Microtubules

20—25 nm

Intermediate filaments

10 nm

Chromatin　Nucleolus

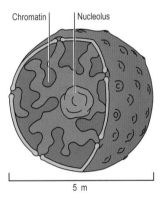

5 m

6 Nucleus. All the chromosomal DNA of a cell is held in the nucleus in chromatin fibres. The nucleolus assembles the cell's ribosomes and communicates with the cell's cytoplasm through pores in the double-layered nuclear envelope.

5 Cytoskeleton. Makes up the framework that gives an animal cell its shape and provides the basis for movement.

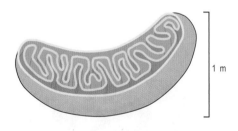

1 m

7 Mitochondrion. The power plant of animal cells. The matrix contains enzymes which begin the process of producing ATP by the oxidation of food. The final stages of the process take place at the inner membrane.

Arriving

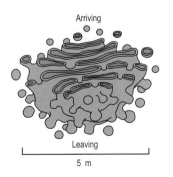

Leaving

5 m

8 Golgi apparatus. A number of flattened sacs which receive vesicles from the endoplasmic reticulum, modify, sort and package their contents and secrete it to other organelles.

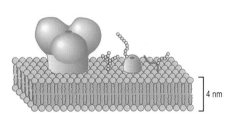

4 nm

9 Plasma membrane. A lipid bilayer 40 Å thick, which acts as a two-dimensional fluid in which protein structures are embedded and act as pumps and channels.

A

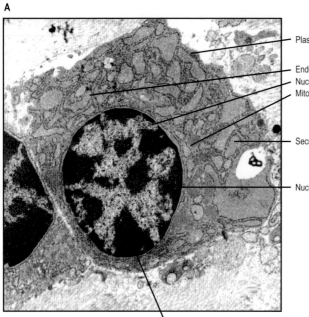

Plasmalemma

Endoplasmic reticulum
Nuclear pore
Mitochondrion

Secretory vesicles

Nuclear membrane

Condensed chromatin

B

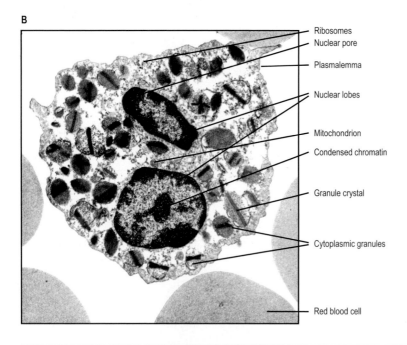

Ribosomes
Nuclear pore

Plasmalemma

Nuclear lobes

Mitochondrion

Condensed chromatin

Granule crystal

Cytoplasmic granules

Red blood cell

Fig. 1.2.2 Electron micrograph of a white blood cell. **A.** Plasma cell. **B.** Eosinophil. (Images courtesy of Dr MJ Birtles, Massey University, New Zealand.)

Basic Science 1.2.1

The electrochemical potential of ions

A mass suspended on a spring, charge separated on a capacitor, and a charged battery all have the potential to do work if they are allowed to discharge down the energy gradients created and in doing so reduce the potential difference between their two states (Fig. BS1.2.1).

The potential difference (μ) of an ion species results from its concentration gradient and electrical gradient across a separating membrane.

The potential (μ_x) of an ion, X, in solution, related to its concentration, is proportional to ln[X], the natural log of the ion's concentration.

$$(\mu_x) \propto \ln[X].$$

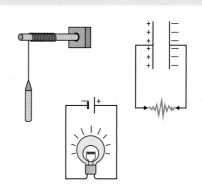

Fig. BS1.2.1 Potential energy.

The potential difference between two solutions a and b of different concentrations is therefore:

$$(\mu_x)_{conc} \propto \ln[X_{higher}] - \ln[X_{lower}].$$

Remember that $\ln a - \ln b = \ln(a/b)$. Therefore:

$$(\mu_x)_{conc} \propto \ln \frac{[X_a]}{[X_b]}.$$

Note that it is the ratio of the concentrations that is important.

The constant of proportionality is RT, the gas constant times absolute temperature:

$$(\mu_x)_{conc} = RT \times \ln \frac{[X_a]}{[X_b]}.$$

An ion in solution also has potential related to its charge. This potential depends upon the voltage gradient ($E_a - E_b$), the charge on the ion, and its valency, z:

$$(\mu_x)_{elect} \propto z(E_a - E_b).$$

The constant of proportionality is F, the Faraday constant:

$$(\mu_x)_{elect} = zF(E_a - E_b).$$

The total potential, the sum of the two, is called its electrochemical potential:

$$(\mu_x)_{electrochemical} = (\mu_x)_{conc} + (\mu_x)_{elect}$$

$$= RT \times \ln \frac{[X_a]}{[X_b]} + zF(E_a - E_b).$$

The unit of μ_x is energy/mole. R is the gas constant and T the absolute temperature. [X] and E are the concentration of X and the electrical potential in the two compartments a and b. z is the valency of the ion and F is Faraday's constant (electric charge per mole of a univalent ion).

Lipid membranes

Most cellular structures are made up of lipid membranes, thin bimolecular sheets of phospholipid and protein in approximately equal quantities. Phospholipids have a polar head and a non-polar tail and, if placed in water, spontaneously arrange themselves into mono- or bimolecular layers. The proteins found in biological membranes tend to be globular and have hydrophobic amino acid side-chains that can act as contacts with lipids. Membranes formed from these components are held together by weak non-covalent bonds. They are fluid sheets and the proteins in the membrane are free to move about within the membrane (Fig. 1.2.1).

The cell membrane or plasmalemma

The cell membrane separates the cell from its environment. Proteins included in the cell membrane control its permeability to water and polar solutes, and pump ions. They control the exchanges of substances between the cell and its environment. Other proteins in the plasmalemma are involved as receivers and transmitters of information. They act as cell surface receptors that 'taste' the environment and signal the presence of important agents to the cell. They also facilitate the release of chemical signals into its environment.

The outer surface of the cell membrane has carbohydrates in it. These carbohydrates are covalently bound to lipid or protein to form glycoproteins. Glycoproteins are important in cell–cell attachment and for organ assembly. Membrane carbohydrates are also responsible for blood-type antigenicity of cell surfaces. These latter aspects of plasmalemma function, communication, will be dealt with in Section 3.

The function of the plasmalemma as a barrier between the cytoplasm and the environment of the cell, across which water and ions must pass, will now be considered.

Summary

Cell membrane

- To survive and control its internal environment, the cell must be separated from its surroundings.
- Animal cell components (cytoplasm and nucleus) are surrounded by a membrane (plasmalemma).

- The plasmalemma is a bimolecular sheet of lipids and proteins in about equal quantities.
- The lipids have hydrophobic and hydrophilic ends.
- Proteins and glycoproteins in the membrane form receptors and transmitters of substances, control entry and exit to and from the cell and form cell–cell attachments.

Basic Science 1.2.2

Artificial lipid membranes

It is possible to make artificial membranes that mimic many of the properties of cell membranes. So-called 'black membranes' form as a bimolecular layer when a soap bubble is blown to bursting point. They are opaque (black) because of their thinness which approaches the wavelength of visible light. Similar membranes can be constructed across small holes in partitions separating two aqueous solutions (Fig. BS1.2.2A). Being made solely of lipid they are impermeable to water and polar substances but are freely permeable to lipid-soluble substances including CO_2 and O_2.

Artificial channels (ionophores)

Selective permeability can be given to a black membrane by including in it molecules called **ionophores**. Some antibiotics have this property. The inclusion of these ionophores in a membrane selectively allows some ions to move through. Valinomycin is a large cyclic molecule rather like a doughnut (Fig. BS1.2.2B). This fits into the membrane, creating a water-filled pore just large enough to admit hydrated K^+ (radius 2.32 Å) but not hydrated Na^+ (radius 2.76 Å). Valinomycin increases the permeability of black membranes to K^+ by several orders of magnitude without much effect on the movement of Na^+. Another antibiotic, alamethicin, effectively inserts tiny pores, water-filled channels, into the membrane and increases the permeability of the membrane to water-soluble substances in a non-selective fashion.

A

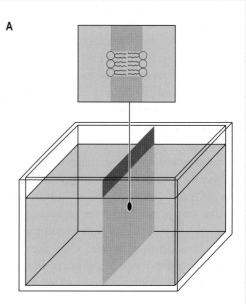

B

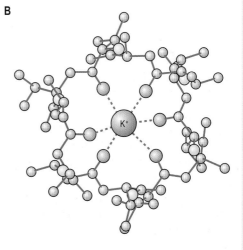

Fig. BS1.2.2 A. A black membrane. **B.** The valinomycin ionophore.

Intracellular and extracellular environments

Water is a unique solvent. Its abundance on Earth allowed life as we know it to evolve. It is a relatively stable molecule and, because of its aggregation into super-molecules (Fig. 1.2.3), it is a liquid over a higher and wider range of temperatures than might be expected from its molecular weight. Its ability to form clusters with a high dielectric constant around charged molecules allows polar solutes to ionize and enter into solution. Hydration (the addition of water molecules) of many macromolecules is also of great significance for living matter.

Life probably evolved in an environment much like our present-day sea in its composition, containing a large amount of soluble salts, particularly sodium chloride. One means by which the independence of primitive life forms from their environment was achieved was the formation of cellular organisms. Self-replication was facilitated by isolating the process from the environment by enclosing the self-replicating macromolecules in a semipermeable membrane.

The construction of 'the cell' has two important consequences:

1. The presence of macromolecules will lower the water potential within the cells, which are thus required to control their internal water potential (an **osmotic** problem).
2. Biologically important macromolecules are largely anionic at neutral pH, thereby causing an uneven charge distribution to be generated across the membrane (an **electrochemical** equilibrium).

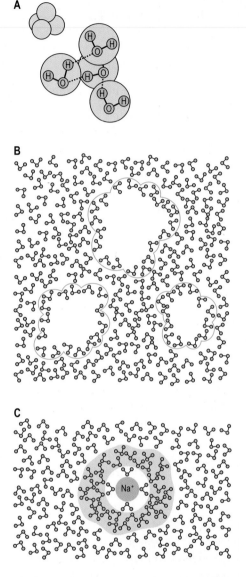

Fig. 1.2.3 The structure of water. Water has more of a structure than could be expected for a liquid. **A.** In ice its molecules form tetrahedrons. **B.** Even in its liquid form, its molecules form aggregates or clusters. **C.** Many molecules form 'hydration shells' in water and this increases their effective size and reduces their ability to penetrate pores in the cell membrane.

Water movement across cell membranes

Most mammalian cell membranes allow water to move across freely. This is possible because lipid membranes have significant *free volume* within their structure, caused by kinking in the CH_2 chains of the lipids. These kinks, and the associated free volume, diffuse within the membrane. The water permeability of biological membranes is about three times greater than that of the crystalline phase of lipid. It is important to understand the factors that control water movement into and out of the cell.

Osmotic pressure

If two aqueous solutions of different concentrations are separated by a membrane permeable only to the solvent, the water potential being lower in the compartment with the higher solute concentration, water will diffuse across the membrane until its potential is equalized. This might occur either when the concentration of the solute became equal on both sides of the membrane or if water potential at the membrane were equalized by raising the hydrostatic pressure of the compartment containing the higher concentration of solute and thus with the lower water potential (Fig. 1.2.4).

The hydrostatic pressure required to prevent the movement of solvent into a solution across a semipermeable membrane separating it from pure solvent is called its **osmotic pressure** and is related to the amount of solute in solution in a manner very similar to the way the pressure of a given mass of gas can be calculated using the **gas laws** (see Basic Science 1.2.3). As in the case of gases, it is the number of particles present that determines the pressure, be these particles molecules or ions, and a weak acid or base will exert an osmotic pressure which depends upon its degree of ionization and thus upon the pH of the solution.

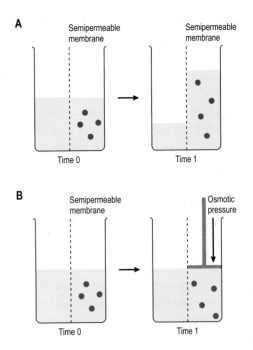

Fig. 1.2.4 Osmosis. A. Water moves from a dilute to a concentrated solution through a semipermeable membrane. **B.** This movement can be stopped by applying pressure to the concentrated solution. The pressure required to just stop the movement from pure water into a solution is called the osmotic pressure of that solution.

 Basic Science 1.2.3

Osmotic effects

Particles of a solute in a solution behave very like gas molecules in a container. Just as in a gas, where the pressure (P) is proportional to the concentration of molecules bombarding the walls of its container ($P = (RT)/V$; where R is a constant, T is the absolute temperature and V is the volume):

$$\text{Osmotic Pressure} \propto \text{Concentration of active particles}$$

and 1 gram mol (or ion) in 22.4 litres of solvent at 0°C exerts 1 atmosphere of pressure.

The **osmolarity** of a solution is the concentration of osmotically active particles and is expressed as osmol/l.

Basic Science (Continued)

The confusingly similar measure of osmotic potential, **osmolality**, which is the number of osmotically active particles in unit mass of water (osmol/kgH$_2$O) is more commonly used as it does not involve assumptions about volume, which changes with temperature and is not easy to measure in tissues (in cells some 75% of their volume is water). The effective osmotic potential will only be correctly predicted from a calculation of osmolality in an **ideal solution**, one that is infinitely dilute. The **osmotic coefficient** (*g*) is a correction factor for the interaction between the solute molecules in more concentrated solutions. It is always less than unity and for NaCl at concentrations found in extracellular fluid it is approximately 0.9.

The osmotic pressure developed across a membrane between two solutions of different osmotic potential is dependent on the properties of the membrane. An ideal semipermeable membrane is only permeable to the solvent (in biology, water) and totally impermeable to the solute in question. Real membranes are never

so selective. The degree of selectivity for any solute is described as its **reflexion coefficient** (*σ*) at the membrane, and for a totally impermeant solute is 1.

The **tonicity** of a solution (*π*) is the osmotic pressure produced by a solution across a membrane separating it from plasma. The terms **iso-**, **hypo-** and **hypertonic** describe solutions whose osmotic potential across biological membranes is the same as, less or greater than that of plasma.

That part of the osmotic pressure potential of a solution that is due to the presence of larger molecules like proteins is called the **oncotic** or **colloid osmotic pressure** as opposed to the **crystalloid osmotic pressure** due to the presence of smaller molecules.

If a difference in osmolality (Δ_{osm}) is present across a membrane, the difference in osmotic pressure ($\Delta\pi$) is calculated from van't Hoff's relationship:

$$\Delta\pi = \sigma \times R \times T \times (\Delta_{osm} \times g).$$

Cell volume regulation

The presence of macromolecules themselves within the cell contributes very little to the osmolarity of the cell contents because, despite their large size, each only counts as one molecule in the calculation of osmotic pressure. They are important because they carry many electrical charges, and therefore attract many other ions that put the cell in jeopardy of osmotic swelling as water moves down its potential gradient from the medium into the cell. The solution is either to pump water out of the cell

or to restore the water potential within the cell by exclusion of an extracellular ion from it. Mammals use the second mechanism. The cell membrane is only very slightly permeable to sodium and there is a powerful sodium extrusion pump that lowers the internal sodium concentration. It is continuously active to cope with membrane leaks of sodium back into the cell (see Fig. BS1.2.3).

The result of this is that the compositions of the intracellular fluid and extracellular fluid differ greatly.

Basic Science 1.2.4

Equilibria across membranes

The Gibbs–Donnan equilibrium

In electrostatics, unlikes attract and neutralize each other. Therefore positive charges are attracted to negative and vice versa.

The presence within cells of large charged molecules (mainly proteins) which cannot cross the cell membrane produces several important effects. These large molecules are mainly anions (negatively charged). The major diffusible ions are K^+ and Cl^- because the membrane of most cells is quite impermeable to Na^+ for most of the time (but see Action potential, p. 44) and any Na^+ that gets in is pumped out again.

The negative protein charge 'draws' the cation K^+ to it, increasing its concentration within the cell. But ions diffuse from regions of high concentration to regions of low concentration. This diffusion out of the cell is resisted by the inward 'pull' of the charge on the protein.

A dynamic equilibrium is reached when the rate of attraction into the cell is exactly balanced by the rate of diffusion out. At this point the negative charge on the protein is not completely neutralized by the K^+ and so a potential difference exists across the cell membrane, with the inside being negative (Fig. BS1.2.3).

The two processes of diffusion and generation of an electrical potential difference are inextricable entwined. Diffusion out of the cell by K^+ tends to leave negative charge on the protein 'uncovered'; this negative charge opposes diffusion of K^+ out of the cell.

The movement of charge required to produce a substantial potential difference across the cell membrane is small. For example, only 1 in every 10 000 potassium ions in the average mammalian cell needs to move from inside to outside the membrane to generate a potential difference of 100 mV.

The potential difference across a cell membrane is also reflected in the distribution of diffusible anions, mainly Cl^-. The negative potential within the cell (the negative charges on the protein) makes the interior less attractive to negatively charged ions and they are more concentrated outside.

The reciprocal distribution of diffusible cations and anions in electrochemical equilibrium is called the Gibbs–Donnan equilibrium, and in mammalian cells where K^+ and Cl^- are the major diffusible ions:

$$\frac{[K^+]_{in}}{[K^+]_{out}} = \frac{[Cl^-]_{out}}{[Cl^-]_{in}}.$$

The Nernst equation and equilibrium potential

Since K^+ and Cl^- are in equilibrium across the membrane, the tendency for them to move down their concentration gradients must be exactly matched by another gradient, their electrical gradient (see above).

At equilibrium their concentration potential $(\mu_x)_{conc}$ is equal in magnitude and opposite in sign to their electrical potential $(\mu_x)_{elect}$:

$$RT \times \ln \frac{[X_a]}{[X_b]} + zF(E_a - E_b) = 0$$

$$E_a - E_b = \frac{-RT}{zF} \times \ln \frac{[X_a]}{[X_b]}.$$

This is the Nernst equation and computes the equilibrium electrical potential (often referred to simply as '**equilibrium potential**') for any ion species. The sign is opposite for anions and cations since z is positive for cations and negative for anions.

Logs to the base 10 are more familiar to you than natural logs ($\ln X = 2.303 \log X$).

Basic Science *(Continued)*

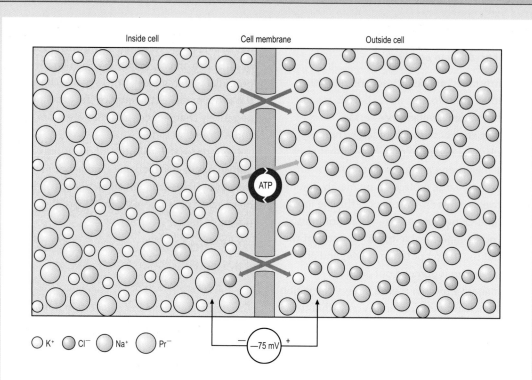

Fig. BS1.2.4 The Gibbs–Donnan equilibrium. This figure shows how the presence of negatively charged protein inside the cell, but too large to get out through the pores in the membrane, affects diffusible ions (mainly K^+ and Cl^-), which, because of the negative charge, distribute themselves either side of the cell membrane as shown with the K^+ being attracted into the cell by the protein's charge but forced out by its high concentration inside (the reverse being true for Cl^-). The numbers of 'ions' shown represents their concentration in a living cell. The sodium pump which ejects the few sodium ions that manage to penetrate the membrane is powered by adenosine triphosphate (ATP). The membrane potential of –75 mV exists because the negative charge on the protein is not completely neutralized by the K^+.

It is useful to evaluate $2.303 \times (RT)/F$. Its value is close to 60 mV at 30°C. The Nernst equation then becomes:

$$E_a - E_b = \frac{-60 \text{ mV}}{z} \times \log \frac{[X_a]}{[X_b]}.$$

For a monovalent cation ($z = 1$), it is:

$$E_a - E_b = -60 \text{ mV} \times \log \frac{[X_a]}{[X_b]}.$$

that is, 60 mV for a 10-fold concentration ratio.

The steady state achieved with several permeant ions

In real cells more than one ion species has to be thought of. The steady-state membrane potential achieved with several ion species diffusing towards their individual equilibria will clearly depend upon the relative amounts of charge being carried by any ion at that time, i.e. their relative contributions to the current across the cell membrane. This current for any ion can be calculated by Ohm's law:

$$\text{Current} = \frac{\text{Driving voltage}}{\text{Resistance}}$$

or   = Driving voltage
          × Membrane conductance

(where: Conductance = 1/Resistance and is determined for a particular type of ion by the permeability of the membrane to that ion).

The current for an ion will therefore be greater if the membrane potential is far from its equilibrium potential and if the membrane is more permeable to it.

The steady-state voltage across a membrane separating two solutions containing only two ions to which it is permeable will therefore be closest to the equilibrium potential of the most permeant ion. If the permeability of the membrane to one of the ions can be switched between a high and a low conductance, then the membrane voltage will be switched between two values, one closer to that ion's equilibrium than the other (see Table 1.2.1).

The way in which several ions contribute to the potential across a membrane as a function of their concentrations and relative permeabilities is described by the Goldman equation (Equation 1.2.1). In this, as in the Nernst equation (Basic Science 1.2.4, p. 23), E is the membrane potential, RT and F are constants and ln is the natural log.

The brackets ( ) and [ ] represent the permeability and concentration of the ions.

Diffusion kinetics

Thermal agitation causes molecules to move randomly within a solution. This process is called diffusion. The mean square displacement of particles ($\bar{x}^2$) from their start point can be shown to increase with time (Basic Science 1.2.5). Large molecules move more slowly than small ones and are slowed in a viscous medium.

$$E = \frac{RT}{F} \times \ln \frac{(PK)[K^+]_{\text{outside}} + (PNa)[Na^+]_{\text{outside}} + (PCl)[Cl^-]_{\text{inside}}}{(PK)[K^+]_{\text{inside}} + (PNa)[Na^+]_{\text{inside}} + (PCl)[Cl^-]_{\text{outside}}}$$

Equation 1.2.1

Table 1.2.1 Lipid membrane permeability and equilibrium potential for water and three common ions. The resting membrane potential of a cell is closest to the equilibrium potential of the ions to which its membrane is most permeable. The increased permeability to sodium when an action potential passes along a nerve largely explains the value of an action potential voltage

	Permeability (cm/s)	Equilibrium potential (voltage inside cell)
Water	1.2×10^{-2}	—
Cl⁻	1.1×10^{-10}	−70 mV
K⁺	6.0×10^{-11}	−80 mV
Na⁺	1.0×10^{-12}	+50 mV

Basic Science 1.2.5

The mean square displacement of particles, $\bar{x}^2$

$$\bar{x}^2 \propto \text{time (t)}$$

and

$$\propto \frac{1}{\text{Molecular size}}$$

and

$$\propto \frac{1}{\text{Viscosity}}.$$

Using a constant of proportionality, the diffusion coefficient (D), we can say that the velocity of thermal agitation is proportional to

absolute temperature (T). The drag on the molecule as it moves will be greater if the molecule is large (the molecular radius (r) is proportional to the cube root of the molecular weight (MW)) and is in a medium of high viscosity.

$$D \propto \frac{T}{r \times \text{Viscosity}}$$

or

$$D \propto \frac{T}{\sqrt[3]{MW} \times \text{Viscosity}}$$

$\therefore$

$$\bar{x}^2 \propto \frac{T}{\sqrt[3]{MW} \times \text{Viscosity}} \times t.$$

For biologically important molecules in an aqueous medium at 30°C an average movement of 1 μm will be achieved in about 1 ms. The time required to cover longer distances grows by a square law: 100 μm will be moved in about 10 s, while 1 cm will require about 1 day (Fig. 1.2.5).

The limits imposed by diffusion limit the size of cells and created the need for the development of intracellular transport mechanisms in large

cells and a circulation or active stirring of intercellular fluid even in small multicellular organisms. The distance between cells and perfused capillaries in active mammalian tissues is some 30 μm. Diffusion of small molecules like CO_2 and O_2 is therefore sufficiently rapid for their efficient exchange between tissue and the blood.

Summary

Water and ions

- Water is the major constituent of our bodies and has several unique and important properties.
- Water is a unique solvent of high dielectric constant.
- Water forms 'super-molecules' and clusters of molecules round charged particles.

- The concentration of molecules inside cells lowers the water potential there.
- Water moves from regions of high to regions of low water potential – osmosis.
- Movement of ions across the cell membrane depends on the membrane's permeability to them and the voltage difference across it.

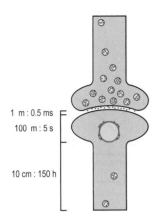

1 m : 0.5 ms
100 m : 5 s
10 cm : 150 h

Fig 1.2.5 A synapse. Diffusion of substances across gaps (synapses) in the nervous system illustrates the time-course of diffusion over biological distances. The transmitter substance is across the gap in 0.5 ms (0.0005 s), takes 5 s to penetrate 100 µm into the cell body and almost a week to diffuse 10 cm along the axon.

Transmembrane movement

Diffusion across a permeable membrane containing fluid-filled channels obeys the same rules as diffusion in solutions and is described by Fick's first law of diffusion:

Net flux $\propto$ −grad C

(grad C is proportional to the concentration difference between the two solutions).

This law describes the flux of a substance across a boundary separating two solutions of different concentration.

The flux of a substance is the rate of its flow across the membrane and the net flux is the difference between the fluxes in either direction across the membrane. Net flux is *down* the concentration gradient, hence the minus sign in the above proportionality.

When the boundary is a biological membrane the constant of proportionality includes the free diffusion coefficient, D:

Net flux $\propto$ −$D \times$ grad C.

For many substances their permeability through cell membranes can be predicted from their oil–water partition coefficient. It may be assumed that they pass through the lipid part of the membrane by dissolving in it. Water and many small water-soluble uncharged molecules pass across the membrane more easily than is predicted by their lipid solubility. Their passage is either through channels in the membrane formed by proteins or through the 'free space' in the membrane (see p. 20).

Ions, being insoluble in lipids, do not permeate cell membranes easily unless specific channels are inserted into the membrane. Special carrier mechanisms are also found that aid the movement of larger uncharged water-soluble species. The following mechanisms of transmembrane movement are illustrated in Figure 1.2.6.

Simple diffusion

Where a substance moves across the membrane in simple solution in water or lipid, Fick's law is obeyed and at any temperature the rate of diffusion is proportional to the concentration gradient across the membrane. This is called *simple diffusion*. The process is only weakly affected by temperature and the rate is simply related to the concentration gradient. It does not saturate.

Carrier-mediated (facilitated) diffusion

Substances that cannot cross the membrane by simple diffusion may have their movement *facilitated* by attachment to a carrier molecule. If the substance moves across the membrane attached to such a mobile carrier, then the amount of the carrier present within the membrane and its mobility will limit the maximum rate of the whole transport process. The process is more temperature sensitive than simple diffusion.

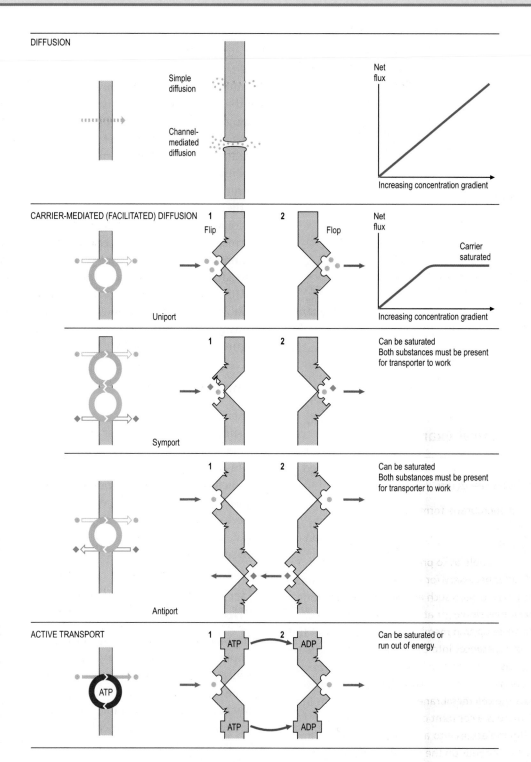

DIFFUSION

Simple diffusion

Channel-mediated diffusion

Net flux

Increasing concentration gradient

CARRIER-MEDIATED (FACILITATED) DIFFUSION

1 Flip

2 Flop

Net flux

Carrier saturated

Increasing concentration gradient

Uniport

1

2

Can be saturated
Both substances must be present for transporter to work

Symport

1

2

Can be saturated
Both substances must be present for transporter to work

Antiport

ACTIVE TRANSPORT

ATP

1 ATP

2 ADP

ATP

ADP

Can be saturated or run out of energy

Fig. 1.2.6 Membrane carrier mechanisms. This figure shows, on the left, the conventions used in this book to represent the various ways in which materials cross the cell membrane. Highly diagrammatic representation of the conformational changes of the carrier mechanisms involved is shown in the middle column, and the way in which carrier mechanisms can be saturated is shown on the right.

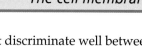

Increasing the concentration gradient across the membrane will only increase the rate of diffusion until the carrier is saturated. Raising the concentration gradient further will not increase flux. The transport process will be *saturable*. These processes are described by Michaelis–Menton kinetics (first developed to describe enzyme kinetics).

Selective permeability

Water-filled pores can exhibit some sieve-like selectivity towards the ions that can pass through. The selection is based upon the size of the ion or the shell of water molecules that surround it (hydration shell).

The existence of individual carriers in a membrane leads to greater selectivity in the movement of ions across the membrane. This selectivity varies from carrier to carrier.

Some carriers do not discriminate well between related species.

If more than one species is able to be carried, then they will compete for the carrier and each will reduce the amount of carrier free to carry the other. This is described as *competitive inhibition*. This inhibition will be limited to those species able to use that carrier.

Exchange diffusion

Carrier-mediated permeation explains an important phenomenon, **exchange diffusion**. This is the rapid exchange of permeant species across a membrane even when the species is in equilibrium and the net flux is zero. This is revealed when tracer amounts of labelled molecules are added to one compartment – there is a rapid initial movement of the label into the other compartment in *exchange* for unlabelled material.

Clinical Example

Lipid-soluble drugs

The cell membrane forms the barrier which makes it possible for the cell to exist in its watery surroundings. This barrier must not, however, be so impermeable as to prevent the passage of molecules necessary for the cell's existence. In specialized organs such as the lungs, intestine and kidney, single, or at the most a few, layers of cells make up thin membranes which allow the flux of substances into or out of the body. Many drugs also act inside cells rather than at their surface and these chemicals must gain access across the cell membrane.

If there is a constant concentration gradient driving molecules into a cell, access to the cell's interior depends on the nature of the molecule entering and the nature of the cell membrane.

For the purpose of considering the access of molecules to a cell, the membrane can be roughly described as a lipid layer containing water-filled pores and carrier molecules. Because a large percentage of the cell membrane is undifferentiated lipid, and because many drug molecules are too large to traverse the pores in the membrane, lipid solubility is an important factor determining their access to the cell's interior. Another way of expressing lipid solubility is as partition coefficient between lipid (the cell membrane) and water (the cell's surroundings). Lipid solubility is a major determinant of the pharmacokinetics of a drug and determines, for example, its rate of absorption from the gut and penetration of many tissues.

Active transport powered by concentration gradients

(see Primary active transport, below)

The presence of a carrier system within a membrane allows transport mechanisms to use energy to move a species up its concentration gradient. Various simple schemes can do this. In all, the rule is that for any given substance to be transported against its energy gradient net movement will *only* take place if at least an equivalent amount of energy is released by the movement of another species down its concentration gradient.

Countertransport occurs when a carrier is able to convey more than one species but at the same site each will compete with the other for the carrier. If one of the species, A, is evenly distributed across the membrane but the other, B, is in a higher concentration on one side of the membrane, the competition by B for the carrier against A will be greatest where B's concentration is higher. A will therefore move in the opposite direction to B.

If the carrier is only able to transport if occupied by two substances A and B simultaneously then **cotransport** occurs. If A and B must bind at the same side of the membrane then it is described as a **symport** and the net movement of the two substances is in the same direction (Fig. 1.2.7). If they must bind on opposite sides of the membrane then it is known as an **antiport** which will cause net movement of the two in opposite directions.

Active transport powered by phosphorylation (primary active transport)

Metabolic energy can be used directly to do work moving substances up their concentration gradients. An example of this is the sodium pump. The pumping of sodium out of the cell is linked to the pumping of potassium into the cell. The action of this pump keeps the cytoplasmic sodium concentration low.

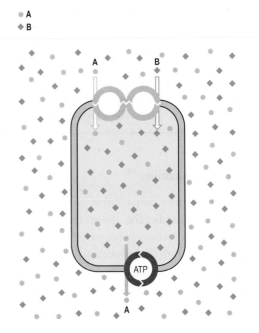

● A
◆ B

Fig. 1.2.7 Powering transport mechanisms. By actively pumping ions (frequently Na^+) out of its interior, a cell creates a concentration gradient whose potential energy can be used to drive mechanisms that transport other substances – something like a water wheel powered from a pond filled by an electric pump. Ion A is actively pumped out of the cell, creating a gradient which powers the cotransporter (in this case a symport) which brings ion B into the cell.

The sodium pump is a membrane protein. It is an ATPase and by splitting ATP it is alternately phosphorylated and dephosphorylated. This causes its conformation to change between the E_1 form and the E_2 form. The E_1, phosphorylated, form has a high affinity for Na^+ and a low affinity for K^+, with the binding sites on the cytoplasmic surface of the cell membrane. The E_2 form has its binding sites facing out and has high affinity for K^+ and low affinity for Na^+. The presence of Na^+ inside the cell and K^+ outside thus stimulates the splitting of ATP and the exchange of the two ions across the membrane.

The exchange ratio of Na^+ to K^+ is not 1:1; rather some three Na^+ are pumped out for two K^+ moving in. The action of the pump is not therefore electrically neutral. The importance of this charge movement is often overestimated.

It is not responsible for the resting membrane potential. The resting membrane potential of cells is caused by the concentration gradients for K^+ and Na^+ across the membrane that are maintained by membrane impermeability to Na^+ and the activity of the sodium pump.

The metabolic cost of the Na^+ pump is high. The work to be done, ΔG, in moving 1 mole of a substance (C) from a medium of low concentration $[C_{low}]$ to a higher $[C_{high}]$ is:

$$\Delta G = RT \times \ln \frac{[C_{high}]}{[C_{low}]}.$$

The sodium pump as an energy source

The sodium pump is responsible for a large part of the resting oxygen consumption of cells, and the sodium gradient it generates is used to power many other cellular transport processes. It can be thought of as charging an energy store that can be tapped by others.

This store can be tapped in several ways but all involve allowing Na^+ to run down the gradient created by the sodium pump and using the potential energy so released to do work on some other component of the system (Fig. 1.2.8). This coupling can be achieved by a symport or antiport system.

It is important to remember that evolution generally adapts an existing mechanism to carry out any newly required function. The sodium pump pumps sodium *out* of cells. Where material is to be moved across an epithelium and this movement involves sodium pumping, it will occur at the pole of the cell where sodium moves out of the cell. Where sodium moves from the lumen of a hollow viscus, the pump will be on the interstitial pole of the cell. Where sodium secretion into the lumen occurs, the pump will be active on the luminal pole of the cell.

The transmembrane movement of lipid-soluble molecules

Lipid-soluble molecules dissolve in, and move freely across, the lipid bilayer of cell membranes.

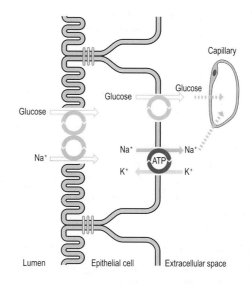

Fig. 1.2.8 The transport of glucose into the body from the gut lumen. This is an example of the potential energy of a concentration gradient being used to power cotransport. In this case the active transport of sodium out of the epithelial cell produces a gradient which powers transport of glucose into the cell. From there, carrier-mediated diffusion facilitates its movement into the extracellular space and capillaries. Cotransport of glucose is unique to the cells of the gut and kidney. Other cells rely on carrier-mediated diffusion alone. Movement into and out of the capillary lumen is augmented by diffusion through pores in its wall.

CO_2 and O_2 move easily out of and into cells by diffusion. Small organic molecules also pass unhindered across membranes unless they are acids or bases when their ionization renders them lipid insoluble.

The distribution of weak acids and bases across cell membranes is therefore much affected by the pH of the cell and its environment. The pH of the two compartments may be different.

Ion trapping occurs when a pH difference exists across a membrane which causes a weak acid or base to be much more ionized on one side. Since only the unionized form crosses the membrane and will equilibrate, the total amount of the substance (ionized + unionized) will be greatest on the side where ionization is greatest (Fig. 1.2.9).

31

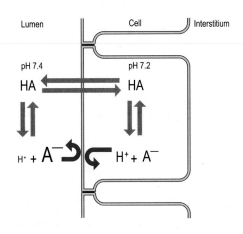

Fig 1.2.9 Ion trapping. The total concentration of a weak acid or base on either side of the cell membrane depends on the pH at these two sites if only the unionized form can cross the membrane. The total concentration of the substance is the sum of the ionized concentration $[H^+] + [A^-]$ + the unionized concentration $[HA]$. Because HA can cross the membrane, its concentration will be the same on both sides (any difference evens out by diffusion) so any differences in total concentration must be due to different concentrations of the ionized part $[A^-]$. H^+ does not count as part of the molecule because it is present in both aqueous solutions, inside and outside the membrane. H^+ *does* count in its effect on the ionization of HA, however. Inside the cell high H^+ concentration (low pH) prevents the ionization of HA and so reduces its concentration within the cell.

Ion trapping is very important in the absorption of some drugs. For example, aspirin is a weak acid and therefore prevented from ionizing in the stomach. The concentration of unionized aspirin (HA) on either side of the stomach wall is therefore about the same at equilibrium. The amount of ionized aspirin (A^-) that can exist in the less acid plasma outside the stomach, however, is 6000 times greater than can exist in the stomach. The final sum is therefore:

	Stomach	Plasma
Unionized	1	1
Ionized	1	6000
TOTAL	2	6001

Of course these levels do not exist because the plasma moving round the circulation washes

Basic Science 1.2.6

Ion trapping

Consider a cell with an internal pH of 7.0 bathed in a medium of pH 7.4 containing a weak acid HA.

$$pH = pK_a + \log \frac{[A^-]}{[HA]}$$

(see Henderson–Hasselbalch equation, p. 686)

or

$$pK_a = pH - \log \frac{[A^-]}{[HA]}.$$

Therefore:

$$pH_{inside} - \log \frac{[A^-_{inside}]}{[HA_{inside}]} = pH_{outside} - \log \frac{[A^-_{outside}]}{[HA_{outside}]}$$

or

$$pH_{inside} - pH_{outside} = \log \frac{[A^-_{inside}]}{[HA_{inside}]} - \log \frac{[A^-_{outside}]}{[HA_{outside}]}.$$

Since HA is in equilibrium across the membrane (it is lipid soluble):

$$HA_{inside} = HA_{outside}$$

and

$$pH_{inside} - pH_{outside} = \log [A^-_{inside}] - \log [A^-_{outside}]$$

or

$$pH_{inside} - pH_{outside} = \log \frac{[A^-_{inside}]}{[A^-_{outside}]}.$$

In the example, the pH difference was –0.4 log units, or a 2.5-fold difference with more of the anion outside the cell.

the aspirin away. In this case, ion trapping is acting as a pump of aspirin into the blood. A mathematical treatment of this phenomenon is given in Basic Science 1.2.6.

Filtration

Filtration is an important process that allows selective movement of substances down a gradient across membrane barriers. The gradient is a hydrostatic or osmotic pressure difference. If a pressure difference occurs across a barrier permeable to water (for example across a blood capillary wall), fluid will be forced across the barrier. The composition of that fluid, the filtrate, will be determined by the properties of the barrier. The basis of the selection is the size of the particles in solution. The barrier behaves as a molecular sieve, allowing small molecules to pass but retaining those larger than the sieve size. In the case of the blood capillary, all molecules smaller than plasma albumin, a protein, pass through pores between the endothelium cells lining the capillary. Any small species that binds to the proteins (protein-binding) will be retained within the capillary along with the protein.

Endocytosis and exocytosis

Large molecules like proteins cannot pass across biological membranes. Their movement into and out of cells involves the processes of endocytosis and exocytosis (Fig. 1.2.10).

In **endocytosis** a bulk material, solid or liquid (pinocytosis), is captured by the cell throwing out a curtain of cell membrane which encloses it; and the captured mass is taken into the cell in a membrane-enclosed vesicle. Endocytosis can be bulk phase – where there is little discrimination about what is picked up – or receptor-mediated as shown in Figure 1.2.10A where the substance to be absorbed (the ligand) binds to the receptor and the whole diffuses to a 'coated pit'. The pit, coated mainly with the protein clathrin, invaginates to form a vesicle which looses its receptors and clathrin back to the cell membrane.

In **exocytosis** large protein molecules for secretion by the cell are synthesized by rough endoplasmic reticulum and encapsulated in membrane to form vesicles. These secretory granules migrate to the cell boundary, where they fuse with the cell membrane. The point of fusion in some sites (neuroendocrine cells) involves special proteins, **synapsins**, which allow the secretion to be controlled by Ca^{2+}. The membrane of the vesicle is added to the cell membrane, increasing its area. Substantial amounts of membrane may be subtracted from or added to the cell surface by the process of endo- and exocytosis. White blood cells (macrophages) recycle their whole surface in half an hour as a result of endocytosis.

Exocytosis is not simply the reverse of endocytosis and can itself be divided into two types – the constitutive secretory or default pathway which takes place in all cells (Fig. 1.2.10B), and the regulated secretory pathway in which selected proteins from the Golgi apparatus are stored in vesicles until a signal stimulates their secretion (Fig. 1.2.10C). The movement of the vesicles in exocytosis is along microtubule 'tracks'.

Both endocytosis and exocytosis are energy-dependent processes.

Intracellular transport (axonal transport)

Within the cells, vesicles and other structures are moved bodily around the cell by special transport proteins. This is most obvious in the case of nerve cells whose axons may be more than a metre long and whose terminals are thus far from the nucleus. Axonal transport of vesicles along the axon occurs both to and from the nucleus. That toward the nucleus is conventionally referred to as **retrograde**, and that away from the nucleus as **anterograde** (Fig. 1.2.11).

The transport process occurs along the cytoplasmic microtubules composed of several proteins including tubulin. These microtubules are polarized with a positive end away from the nucleus. The vesicles are coated with several proteins that associate with tubulin.

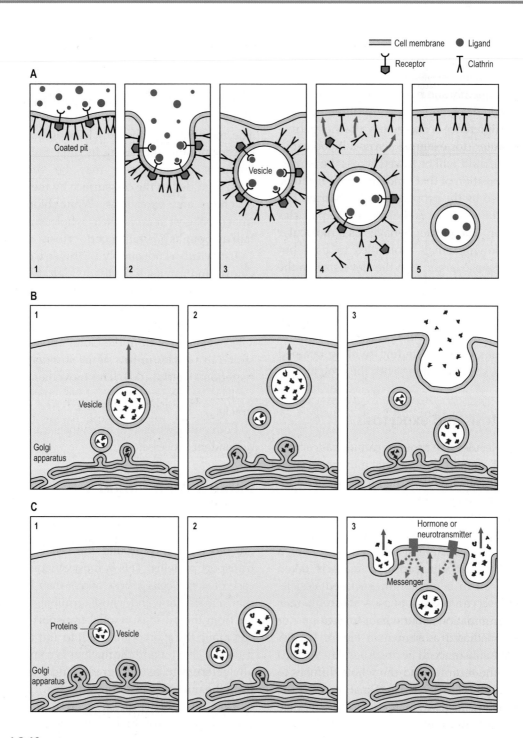

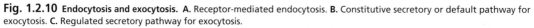

Fig. 1.2.10 Endocytosis and exocytosis. A. Receptor-mediated endocytosis. **B.** Constitutive secretory or default pathway for exocytosis. **C.** Regulated secretory pathway for exocytosis.

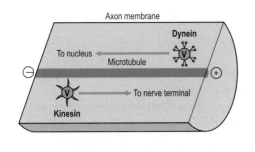

Fig. 1.2.11 Microtubules. Movement of membrane-bound organelles within a cell involves microtubules, which anchor themselves between other cellular structures and have polarity, with the + end away from the nucleus. The motor proteins that provide the motive force to move organelles along the microtubule tracks are themselves polarized: dyneins move toward the cell body while kinesins move to the periphery. This process is most dramatically seen in the axon of nerve cells which may be up to 1 metre long.

These 'microtubule-associated proteins' (MAPs) include **kinesin** and **dynein**. Minute latex beads coated with one of these proteins will, in the presence of ATP, move along microtubules. If the coating is of kinesin, the bead moves toward the positive end of the tubule; if dynein, away from it. A vesicle coated with kinesin in a nerve axon would therefore be transported to the terminal of a nerve, one coated with dynein to the cell body. It may be that all vesicles are coated by both types of MAP but that only one is active depending upon the history of the vesicle. Since all proteins are made in the cell body, dyneins must first be carried to the periphery in an inactive form before they can begin their journey back to the cell centre.

Transepithelial movement of ions and macromolecules

We have considered the passive and active movement of substances between the cytoplasm and the surrounding medium across cell membranes. The mechanisms involved are also responsible for the transepithelial movement of many substances between different compartments in the body.

The most common membrane pump is that transporting Na^+ out of the cell, the Na^+/K^+-stimulated ATPase. This pump is a common component of many important epithelial transport processes in the kidney (see p. 734) and the gut (see p. 817). The result of its action is to create an Na^+ gradient across the cell membrane down which Na^+ will diffuse into the cell if it is allowed to do so, powering transepithelial transport of useful substances from hollow structures like the gut into the body.

Consider the cells forming the lining of a hollow structure. A mechanism to move glucose might be constructed as follows:

- The cells forming the lining are joined together in a manner that does not allow movement through the junction.
- The Na^+ pump situated on the abluminal membrane of the epithelial cells moves Na^+ out of the cell into the body, keeping the cell $[Na^+]$ low.
- Na^+ diffuses down its concentration gradient from within the structure, moving through the adluminal membrane by means of a carrier that also binds glucose (a symport; see p. 30).
- Glucose is thus driven up its concentration gradient out of the lumen of the structure. This raises the glucose concentration within the cell.
- The glucose then diffuses down the concentration gradient thus established across the abluminal epithelial cell membrane into the body (see Fig. 1.2.8).

You will find other ways of linking Na^+ pumping to the movement of other molecules in subsequent chapters.

⚡ Summary

Transmembrane movement

- Movement (flux) of a substance across cell membranes can be of several types.
- Simple diffusion takes place in the water or lipid of the membrane and obeys Fick's law.
- Carrier-mediated (facilitated) diffusion only takes place down a concentration gradient, like simple diffusion, but uses a carrier molecule which facilitates the process but can be saturated.
- Simple diffusion and carrier-mediated diffusion can show selective permeability.

- Active transport is movement of a substance up its concentration gradient.
- Active transport requires energy – this can come from movement of another substance *down* its concentration gradient or from the energy in phosphorylated molecules (primary active transport).
- Endocytosis and exocytosis move very large molecules across cell membranes in vesicles.
- These processes of selective movement across epithelia determine the composition of body fluids.

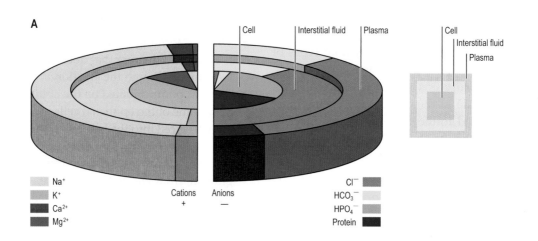

A

Cell | Interstitial fluid | Plasma

Cell | Interstitial fluid | Plasma

- Na⁺
- K⁺
- Ca²⁺
- Mg²⁺

Cations +   Anions −

Cl⁻
HCO₃⁻
HPO₄⁻
Protein

B

Lactic acid | Uric acid / Creatinine / Bilirubin / Bile salts

Urea

Glucose

Neutral fat

Cholesterol

Phospholipids

Fig. 1.2.12 Constituents of body fluid. The constituents of fluids must be in electrical equilibrium, that is, the number of positive charges must equal the number of negative charges. However, because the membrane of cells is selectively permeable to certain dissolved substances the compositions of intra- and extracellular fluid are quite different and, because of this, a voltage develops across the membrane. **A.** The importance of protein as an impermeate anion inside the cell. **B.** The composition of non-electrolytes in the extracellular fluid. Because the molecules of proteins and non-electrolytes are so large they only exert 5% of the osmotic pressure of plasma while making up 90% of the weight of dissolved constituents.

The composition of intracellular and extracellular fluids

Extracellular fluid, like sea water, is predominantly a solution of NaCl. The other major component is KCl but in only one-fiftieth the concentration of the NaCl (Fig. 1.2.12).

In intracellular fluid the ratio of Na^+ to K^+ is reversed, K^+ being the principal cation. Negatively charged protein provides the anion complement together with a little Cl^-. The ratio of $[Cl^-_{inside}] : [Cl^-_{outside}]$ is about $1 : 50$, similar to that for $[K^+_{outside}] : [K^+_{inside}]$.

Since the cell membrane is permeable to water, the concentration of osmotically active particles must be equal on either side of the membrane. On both sides of the membrane, anion and cation numbers must balance to preserve electroneutrality. The osmotic potential of multivalent ions is less for a given charge than for a monovalent ion. In the extracellular fluid there are more multivalent cations than multivalent anions. In the intracellular fluid the reverse is true and the presence of polyvalent intracellular anions (macromolecules like proteins or DNA) allows a smaller number of anions to maintain electroneutrality within the cell. The sum of osmotically active particles on either side of the membrane must be equal. Thus the total concentration of cations inside the cell exceeds that outside the cell by some 20%. Similarly the presence of protein in the plasma means that although it is in osmotic equilibrium with the *interstitial* fluid (see Ch. 6.5) the concentration of anions is greater in the plasma.

Cell excitability

The action potential

A common property of living matter is its **excitability**. Excitability is the ability to produce an active **response** to a **stimulus** from the environment. Electrical excitability, where the response, the **action potential**, is electrical, is common to both plants and animals. We live in what will in future be called the electronic age. The 20th century saw our ability to measure minute electrical events grow. It is not surprising that we have thus achieved a minute grasp of the physiology of electrically excitable cells.

The student should not be upset by the excess of 'facts' available on this subject. The action potential is simple and is easily understood.

The student should understand that in electrically excitable cells:

- An electrical potential difference, the membrane potential, results from the differing ionic compositions of the inside and outside of the cell.
- Its value is determined by the relative permeabilities of the cell membrane to the different ions present.
- The permeability of the membrane to ions can be changed by altering the membrane potential.
- The action potential is simply a series of membrane-potential-induced changes in the permeability of the membrane to individual ions.

39

- These changes in membrane permeability allow ions to flow down their electrochemical gradients, causing the membrane potential to change.

This sequence is not mysterious and is capable of logical understanding.

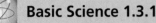

Basic Science 1.3.1

Circuits for alternating currents

Electrical circuits are made up of parts called components (Fig. BS1.3.1). These can be passive – they do not change the current passing through them or the voltage applied to them; they simply act as resistors to the flow of current or as capacitors holding a fixed amount of electricity within themselves. Some components are called active – they do something to the current or voltage applied to them. Amplifiers, as their name suggests, amplify a voltage applied to them, and the transistor which forms the basis of integrated circuits used in computers, behaves in different ways depending on the voltage applied to it.

There are also two kinds of current. Direct current (DC) is provided by cells or batteries or by rectifiers which change the second kind of current we will deal with (AC) into direct current. In a simple direct current circuit, when the battery is connected and things have settled down there is no further change in the amount of current flowing through the circuit.

With alternating current (AC) (the current you get from the mains), however, things are more complicated. The voltages and therefore currents in the circuit swing backward and forward, maybe in a simple sinusoidal way (like the mains), in a 'sawtooth' way or like an action potential for example (Fig. BS1.3.2). This makes things more difficult to calculate than with direct current.

All circuits have resistance and capacitance in them no matter how small. This is true for biological circuits such as the cell membrane as well as circuits made out of metal.

In designing circuits we want to know how long it is going to take for such a circuit to 'settle down', that is, to reach a stable state.

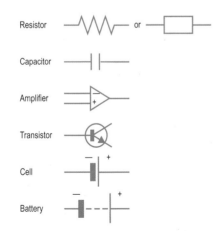

Fig. BS1.3.1 Symbols for components of electrical circuits.

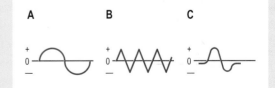

Fig. BS1.3.2 Voltage changes in an AC circuit. **A.** Sinusoidal wave. **B.** Sawtooth wave. **C.** Action potential.

Basic Science *(Continued)*

Take the case of a capacitor we are going to charge with electricity from a battery through a resistance (Fig. BS1.3.3).

If we measure the voltage across the capacitor, you will intuitively understand that the time for everything to settle down when the switch is closed depends on the rate at which the resistor lets electricity through to the capacitor and how big the capacitor is (how much electricity it can hold). The higher the resistance and the bigger the capacitor the longer it is going to take to 'fill up'. The voltage across the capacitor rises as shown in Figure BS1.3.4.

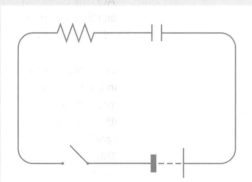

Fig. BS1.3.3 Charging a capacitor.

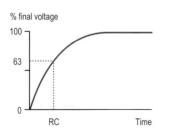

Fig. BS1.3.4 Voltage across a charging capacitor. *R* = resistance; *C* = capacitance; *RC* = *T* = the time constant.

We do not measure the time to completely fill the capacitor. The curve describing the filling is an exponential and all exponentials are described by a formula containing the constant *e* = 2.72. The reciprocal of this constant = 1/2.72 = 0.37 and so, for reasons relating to the shape of the curve, and to compare one curve with another, we measure the time for the voltage and current to reach within 37% of their final value. This is called the **time constant** of the circuit and for a circuit containing resistance (*R*) and capacitance (*C*) the time constant is:

$$T = R \times C.$$

Things become much more difficult to calculate if alternating current had been used to charge the capacitor. If the current was alternating at a high enough frequency, the capacitor would not have time to 'fill' before the direction of current would change and it would begin to empty, so the frequency of the current would be important.

There is one more component which is important in understanding simple passive circuits, that is the inductance. Inductance is particularly the property of coils of wire. A coil builds up a magnetic field when a current flows through it; this field tends to resist changes in the current once it has been established. It resists the increase of current in a circuit when the switch is closed and the reduction of current when the switch is opened. So it also imposes its influence on the time constant of a circuit. This property of inductance is frequently, and confusingly, called impedance which as we will see has a more general application.

The term **impedance** which can be used to describe the property of coils is also used to describe the overall resistance of a circuit to alternating current. The units of impedance are the same as those of resistance to direct current,

Basic Science *(Continued)*

ohms (Ω). But when we come to calculate the impedance (Z) of a circuit containing resistance (R), impedance (L) and capacitance (C) which is connected to an alternating voltage, we have to introduce the frequency (f) at which the voltage is alternating:

$$Z = \sqrt{R^2 + (2\pi fL - 1/_2\pi fC)^2} \text{ ohms.}$$

The changes in voltage applied to the circuit may have the simple smooth 'sine wave' shape of the voltage we get out of the mains electricity supply or they may have the jagged and rapidly changing shape of potentials found in the nervous system which cause physiologists much trouble in the design of their electrical recording equipment.

Membrane permeability of excitable cells

The membranes of excitable cells have ion channels that allow ions to diffuse selectively across. These ion channels can be opened and closed. In this section we shall be concentrating on those that can be controlled by variations in the voltage across the membrane, voltage-gated ion channels. In later sections of this book, ion channels will be described that are controlled by receptors for chemical messengers, hormones and neurotransmitters, or by mechanical or other stimuli.

The cell membrane is some 40 Å thick and a potential difference of about 80 mV exists across it at rest. The voltage gradient across the membrane is therefore:

$$\frac{80 \times 10^{-3}}{40 \times 10^{-10}}$$

or 2×10^7 V/m, 20 MV/m (megavolts per metre).

To put this into perspective, the voltage gradient between the conducting cables and the metal frame of the pylons of the National Electricity Grid is 100 kV, 200 times less.

During an action potential this can be reversed to as much as −10 MV/m. As membrane proteins contain many groups capable of ionization, it is not surprising that this huge reversal of field can change their conformation and properties dramatically.

Ion channels, which are membrane-spanning proteins, can exist in several states. In their active state they can be open or closed. When open, they allow the admitted ions to diffuse down their concentration gradient. The larger the opening voltage, usually depolarization from the resting membrane potential, the greater the proportion of time they are in the open state. The membrane permeability for the ion passing through any class of channel will therefore be related to the membrane potential.

These gating effects of voltage are very rapid and transient. Slower and more persistent effects of voltage can change the state of channels, switching them between an active and an inactive state. The mechanism of inactivation is distinct from that which opens and closes the channel, but clearly overrides it. The mechanism of the Na^+ action potential, as you will see later (p. 45), is that depolarization rapidly *opens* Na^+ channels and then *inactivates* them, effectively shutting them for some time (Fig. 1.3.1).

Membrane potential

At rest, the membrane is only slightly permeable to ions. Most of that permeability is to K^+ and Cl^-. It is almost impermeable to Na^+.

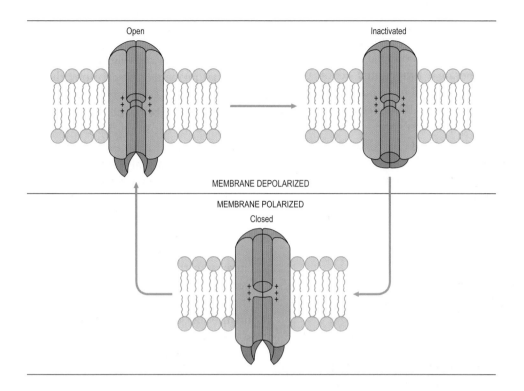

Open

Inactivated

MEMBRANE DEPOLARIZED

MEMBRANE POLARIZED

Closed

Fig. 1.3.1 Ion channel gating. The channels which allow ions through the cell membrane are specific to particular ions. One of these types of channel can exist in three states depending on the membrane potential, and is therefore known as a voltage-gated ion channel. An example is the voltage-gated Na^+ channel.

When the membrane is polarized (the inside is highly negative to the outside) this type of channel shows a strong tendency to be closed. In this 'closed' state the positively charged central section in some way blocks the passage of Na^+. When the membrane is depolarized (the inside voltage is close to or even positive in respect to the outside) these channels can be 'open', which is a rather precarious state, or 'inactivated', which is much more stable. The opening of Na^+ channels is what depolarizes the membrane, and depolarization is what opens the channels, so you can see that the cell could be stuck in a state of depolarization. What saves it from this fate is that after a certain time 'open' channels are 'inactivated' by a part of their structure, 'the inactivating particle', blocking the channel irrespective of the state of depolarization and it stays that way for a short time.

Because the membrane is permeable to more than one ion species, the resting membrane potential will not be exactly at any individual equilibrium potential (see Basic Science 1.2.4, p. 23). But it will be described by the Goldman equation for all permeant ions as seen earlier (p. 25). Currents will flow through each type of ion channel and tend to drive the membrane potential towards the equilibrium potential for that ion. The greater the permeability of the membrane for any ion species the closer will be the membrane potential be to its equilibrium. A large current will swamp a smaller. The K^+ and Cl^- diffuse down any electrochemical gradient that exists, tending to extinguish it. As a result, the membrane potential is held at –70 to –80 mV, close to the equilibrium potential (the potential at which the concentration and electrical gradients are equal and opposite) of these ions. The small Na^+ permeability results in the membrane potential being at a level a little positive to the K^+/Cl^- equilibrium potential.

Generator potentials

Generator potentials are *graded local* depolarizations of the membrane potential of excitable cells that may generate a **propagated** action potential. They are produced in sensory receptors by a variety of stimuli. The **adequate stimulus** (that specific for the receptor) – deformation of a touch receptor for example – might increase the conductance of the membrane to an ion species like Na^+ whose equilibrium potential is more positive than the resting potential, or decrease the conductance of the membrane to an ion like K^+ whose equilibrium potential is more negative than the resting potential.

Summary

Membrane potential

- There is a potential difference across the membrane of cells (the membrane potential) in which the interior of the cell is negative to the surrounding fluid.
- Membrane potential results from different ionic concentrations inside and outside the cell.
- Membrane potential is determined by those ions to which the membrane is most permeable.
- Permeability to different kinds of ions changes.
- Movement of the membrane potential away from 0 V is called hyperpolarization; movement towards or past 0 V (the inside becomes positive) is called depolarization.
- Permeability of the membrane to ions is changed by opening and closing of 'gated' channels in the membrane.
- Generator potentials are graded depolarizations of the membrane of a receptor produced by an adequate stimulus.

The constituents of the action potential

The action potential (Fig. 1.3.2) is a depolarization that propagates itself along the membrane of an excitable cell, conducting the excitation throughout the cell. The depolarization is produced by an explosive inrush of Na^+ or Ca^{2+}. This section will refer to the Na^+ action potential found with only small variations in all nerves and skeletal muscle.

The action potential is described as an 'all-or-none' event – a stimulus is either too small to excite the cell or, if large enough, evokes a single response that is not further increased by increasing the size of the stimulus. In sensory nerves, information about the magnitude of the stimulus is conveyed by increasing the *number*, not the size, of the action potentials evoked. The series of events that are the action potential will now be explained.

Threshold

The stimulus for the action potential is a brief depolarization of the nerve membrane. If stimuli of increasing intensities are applied to an excitable cell, below a certain level no action potential will be generated but an action potential will be generated by all stimuli above that level. This is called the **threshold** (Fig. 1.3.3). The stimulus might be produced by a sensory receptor, an action potential in nearby parts of the cell or from an electrical current applied experimentally. Current flowing into the cell lowers the membrane potential towards zero. There are two immediate effects:

1. The difference between the membrane potential and the K^+ equilibrium potential increases – more K^+ flows out of the cell. This tends to repolarize the cell.
2. The voltage-controlled Na^+ channels are opened allowing Na^+ to flow down its gradient into the cell. This tends to produce further depolarization.

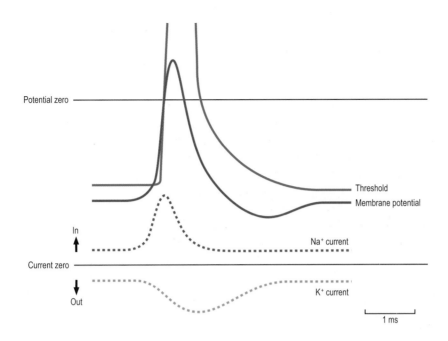

Fig. 1.3.2 **The action potential.** The changes in membrane potential that make up the action potential in nerves and muscles result from changes in conductance of the cell membrane to Na⁺ and K⁺. These changes in conductance result from opening, closing and inactivation of channels in the cell membrane specific to each type of ion. Many voltage-sensitive Na⁺ channels open when the membrane voltage reaches threshold, which produces the upstroke of the action potential. These channels spontaneously become inactivated, and gated K⁺ channels open to form the downstroke. Inactivated Na⁺ channels have a much higher threshold for opening than closed channels and this causes a nerve to be refractory when many of its Na⁺ channels are inactivated rather than simply closed. Na⁺ channels operate about 10 times faster than K⁺ channels.

The result is determined by the relative sizes of these two effects. With small depolarizations the effect on the K⁺ current is larger than that on the Na⁺ channels and the outward K⁺ current exceeds the inward Na⁺ current. When the stimulus ends, the membrane repolarizes itself. If the stimulus is bigger, the effect on the Na⁺ current exceeds that on the K⁺ current and the inward Na⁺ current exceeds the outward K⁺ current, leading to more depolarization. The smallest level of depolarization that has this effect is the threshold.

The upstroke of the action potential

Above the threshold, depolarization leads to more depolarization. This is *positive feedback*. The membrane potential keeps on falling towards zero, opening more and more Na⁺ channels.

The membrane potential becomes dominated by the Na⁺ current and moves rapidly towards the Na⁺ equilibrium potential. These are the immediate effects of the depolarization and occur in tens of microseconds.

The downstroke of the action potential

Depolarization also has slower effects on the Na⁺ and K⁺ channels, which take place over the next millisecond or so. At this time the K⁺ channels are opened but the Na⁺ channels are inactivated. Inward Na⁺ current ceases and the increased outward K⁺ current repolarizes the membrane. The membrane potential is then close to the original resting level but the membrane is not in its original state. More K⁺ channels are open and the Na⁺ channels are inactivated.

45

Change of membrane potential (mV)

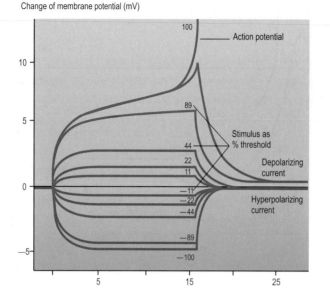

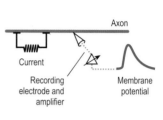

Fig. 1.3.3 **Subthreshold stimulation.** If current is passed into or taken out of a nerve axon at a rate that does not raise the membrane potential to threshold, the membrane becomes hyperpolarized or depolarized as shown. Because the flow of current into the anode of a pair of stimulating extracellular electrodes is in such a direction as to hyperpolarize the membrane it becomes less sensitive to stimulation in this region.

After-potentials

In many excitable cells the depolarizing phase of the action potential is followed by an after-potential. This is due to the Na^+ and K^+ channels not having returned to their previous states. The after-potential can be either a hyper- or a hypopolarization. If the K^+ channels recover slowly, then the membrane potential will be more negative than its normal resting value for a time after the action potential.

The refractory period

For a short time after an action potential, the excitability of the cell is lower than normal. It is **refractory** to further stimuli. Because the Na^+ channels are inactivated by the action potential, a second stimulus given within a few milliseconds of a previous action potential will not

be able to open the inactivated Na^+ channels and will not therefore trigger an action potential. The membrane is said to be in its **absolute refractory period**. The lingering effects of depolarization on the Na^+ and K^+ channels decay over the next few milliseconds. As the Na^+ channels reactivate, they become able to respond to a depolarization by opening, but until full recovery from inactivation occurs, a larger than normal stimulus will be needed to evoke an action potential. The membrane is said to be in its **relative refractory period**. During the relative refractory period the threshold is higher than normal. As the Na^+ and K^+ channels return to their resting state, Na^+ channels becoming active and K^+ channels closing, the membrane potential returns to normal, the threshold falls toward its resting level, and the cell becomes normally excitable again.

Summary

Action potential

- Action potentials are the 'language' of the nervous system and the trigger of muscle contraction; they pass along nerves and are transmitted from nerve to nerve and nerve to muscle.
- An action potential is a self-propagating (spreading) depolarization of the membrane.
- It is an 'all-or-none' event.
- It is very brief (ms) produced by an inrush of Na^+ (nerves) or Ca^{2+} (heart and smooth muscle).
- Depolarization of an excitable cell membrane to *threshold* triggers an action potential which spontaneously propagates.
- The upstroke of an action potential results from Na^+ gates in the membrane opening and Na^+ rushing in.
- The downstroke results from the Na^+ gates closing, K^+ gates opening and K^+ rushing out.
- After an action potential has occurred, it is impossible for the nerve to produce another for a short time (absolutely refractory) and difficult to provoke another for a longer time (relatively refractory).

Spontaneously active cells

Nerve and muscle cells are normally inactive unless stimulated. Their threshold is normally at a *less* negative level than the resting membrane potential. Some cells, like those of heart muscle, beat spontaneously. The difference between normally silent and spontaneously active cells is simply that in spontaneously active cells the threshold is *more* negative than the resting membrane potential. This relates to the relative numbers and rates of recovery from inactivation of the Na^+ and K^+ channels.

After the action potential in many spontaneously active cells, the K^+ channels are open and the Na^+ channels are inactivated. The return to the resting membrane potential allows most of the K^+ channels to close and the Na^+ channels to become active. The membrane potential slowly depolarizes, moving away from the K^+ equilibrium potential as the K^+ channels close. This depolarization is called the **pacemaker potential** and leads to the opening of the now active Na^+ channels, causing more depolarization, and the upsweep of the next action potential begins.

Variations in membrane stability

In the stable cell, the number of K^+ channels remaining open is sufficient to keep the membrane sufficiently polarized to prevent regenerative opening of the Na^+ channels.

Stable cells can therefore become unstable if either fewer K^+ channels are available or more Na^+ channels are open. More Na^+ channels would be open at a given membrane potential if either there is less inactivation or the relationship between their opening and the membrane potential changes so that more Na^+ channels are opened at any given level of depolarization. Drugs like veratridine activate the Na^+ channels and initially cause the cell to become hyperexcitable; but eventually the membrane becomes permanently depolarized and inexcitable.

Conversely, spontaneously active cells can be stabilized if fewer Na^+ channels open upon membrane depolarization. Local anaesthetics and some antiarrhythmic drugs block the Na^+ channels and increase the amount of depolarization needed to cause regenerative opening of Na^+ channels. They are collectively known as membrane stabilizers.

Ca²⁺ and excitability

The most important regulator of cell excitability is the extracellular Ca^{2+} concentration. Free Ca^{2+} concentrations in the extracellular fluid are closely regulated by hormones from the parathyroid gland. This is important because of the many important roles that calcium has in the body. In excitable cells, Ca^{2+} in the extracellular fluid reduces the opening effect that depolarization has upon Na^+ channels and by so doing stabilizes the membrane. Low extracellular Ca^{2+} concentrations leave the Na^+ channels more sensitive to depolarization, moving the threshold negative to the normal resting membrane potential and leading to spontaneous action potentials in what was normally a stable membrane.

Parathyroid tetany, the hyperexcitability of motor nerves to skeletal muscle that occurs if the parathyroid gland is accidentally removed during surgery, is due to the resulting low blood Ca^{2+}.

Excitation caused by hyperpolarization

Excitable cells are usually stimulated by membrane currents that depolarize the cell. However, hyperpolarizing currents can be excitatory. Inactivation of Na^+ channels can be reduced by hyperpolarizing the cell. More Na^+ channels will be open at any given membrane potential. Thus, if an external polarizing current passing into a cell is suddenly removed, an Na^+ current will flow into the cell, taking the membrane potential to a less negative value than the normal resting potential. Because more Na^+ channels are in their active state, the threshold will be lower. If the altered resting membrane potential is above the altered threshold, an action potential will occur.

Strength–duration curve (Fig. 1.3.4)

An electrical stimulus used to excite cells is conventionally given in the form of a brief square wave pulse whose polarity is such that it depolarizes the cell. Such a pulse can be easily

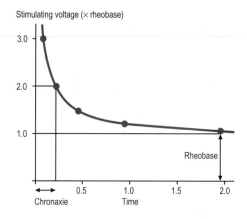

Fig. 1.3.4 The strength–duration curve. The cell membrane is 'leaky' to current. If current is injected into an excitable cell in an attempt to depolarize it and cause an action potential, the injection must be at least as fast as the current leaks away if the membrane potential is to be changed. The voltage that just produces this situation is called a rheobase. The time needed for a voltage of 2 × rheobase to trigger a cell is called chronaxie and is a measure of the excitability of the cell. The strength–duration curve expresses the fact that attempting to change the membrane potential from its resting value to threshold is like trying to fill a leaky bucket, the time to fill is inversely related to the rate at which you pour in water.

described by stating its strength and duration. Because depolarization not only opens Na^+ channels (rapidly) but also inactivates them (slowly), the relationship between the strength and duration of stimuli in a particular situation is complex. An early observation in neurophysiology was that for any nerve there was a minimum strength of stimulus below which the current could be continued indefinitely without excitation occurring. This was called **rheobase**. The time needed for a stimulus given at twice rheobase to trigger an action potential, **chronaxie**, is useful as a measure of excitability. Greater excitability goes with a shorter chronaxie.

In general, nerves are more excitable than muscle, myelinated nerves more than non-myelinated nerves, and striated muscle is more excitable than smooth muscle. Within these groups the higher the conduction velocity of the action potential (see p. 54) the greater the excitability.

The practical importance of this is that when a stimulus is applied to a tissue containing several elements whose excitabilities vary, some degree of selective stimulation can be achieved by using stimuli of appropriate form. For instance, if a stimulus of duration less than 1 ms is applied to a blood vessel, which contains smooth muscle innervated by non-myelinated nerves, the difference between the strength of stimulus required to stimulate smooth muscle directly and that required to stimulate the nerves is large. The nerves are very much more sensitive than the smooth muscle. This makes the selective stimulation of the nerves easy. It is also possible to stimulate the very sensitive fast sensory fibres in peripheral nerves and yet not excite the less sensitive smaller unmyelinated fibres. This is very useful in the relief of pain (see p. 272).

Clinical Example

Local anaesthetics

That pain is transmitted by nerves has long been recognized and, even before that time, attempts were made to block pain by cooling painful tissue, which interferes with nerve conduction. Many kinds of compounds block conduction and therefore pain, but they permanently damage nerve cells. The great advantage of local anaesthetics is that their blocking action is reversible. When applied in appropriate concentrations they block all types of nerve fibre, sensory, central and motor. The action of local anaesthetics is to block sodium channels in the nerve cell membrane and this action is utilized in the *Class I* antidysrhythmic drugs, some of which are local anaesthetics, to reduce excitability in non-pacemaker regions of the heart.

Local anaesthetics act non-specifically on membranes as surface-active agents, as do volatile anaesthetics, but the major effect of most is to block voltage-dependent Na^+ conducting channels. This they do in a most convoluted manner which puzzled pharmacologists for many years. Local anaesthetics can exist in ionized and non-ionized form at or near the pH of body tissue. They must be in the non-ionized form to penetrate nerve sheaths and axonal membranes, but it is the cationic form that is active and this is only active from *inside* the nerve membrane. So, applied to the outside of a nerve axon, a local anaesthetic is useless; it must first penetrate, for which it must be non-ionized, then it must ionize to be active from the inside of the membrane.

From inside the nerve, local anaesthetics block by dissolving in the membrane and by entering the Na^+ channels they block. Thus the more often a channel is open the more it is likely to be blocked. This 'use-dependent blocking' together with the fact that small diameter nerve fibres are more readily blocked than large is of considerable scientific interest but of little clinical importance.

Of more importance are the unwanted effects of local anaesthetics on other systems of the body when they escape from their site of application. Paradoxically, they cause stimulation of the central nervous system (probably by blocking inhibitory regions) which can progress to convulsions. Greater doses in the central nervous system produce depression, most seriously respiratory depression.

In the cardiovascular system, local anaesthetics depress the activity of the myocardium by the mechanism already described for antidysrhythmics and cause vasodilatation, which combined with the cardiac effects can produce a fatal fall in blood pressure.

If a depolarizing stimulus of less than rheobase intensity has a long duration, then the Na⁺ channels will be inactivated without the generation of an action potential and the cell will become refractory. Easily excitable cells are also most easily affected by this **anodal block**. This is the basis of a technique that allows the selective stimulation of the less excitable elements in a mixed population of excitable cells. A subthreshold depolarizing stimulus is given immediately preceding a suprathreshold stimulus for the less sensitive elements. Adjustment of their relative strengths will ensure that the more excitable cells are not stimulated by the second stimulus in spite of its being above the normal threshold of all the elements.

The role of the Na⁺ pump in the action potential

During the action potential, Na⁺ flows into the cell and K⁺ flows out. The amounts involved are small. A single action potential will not change the intracellular composition measurably. Several hundred action potentials could be supported by the ion gradients normally present. The rundown of these gradients is normally prevented by the action of the Na⁺ pump (see p. 30) which pumps the Na⁺ out of the cell in exchange for K⁺.

Ca²⁺ action potential

Ca²⁺, like Na⁺, is present in the cytoplasm at much lower concentrations than in the extracellular fluid. In heart and smooth muscle cells the upstroke of the action potentials is not generated by the inflow of Na⁺ alone. In smooth muscle, voltage-gated Ca²⁺ channels fulfil the role played by Na⁺ channels described above. In the heart, both Na⁺ channels and Ca²⁺ channels are gated by depolarization. The response of the Na⁺ channels is rapid and is responsible for the initial upstroke of the action potential, but a slower opening of Ca²⁺ channels results in a maintained plateau of depolarization after this initial spike (Fig. 1.3.5).

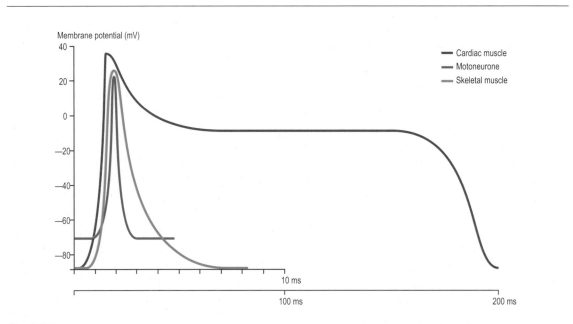

Fig. 1.3.5 Action potentials. Action potentials in different cell types have different properties. Note the different time-courses of the motoneurone and cardiac muscle action potential. However, whatever the shape and size, it is propagated unchanged through the length of the muscle or nerve.

Summary

Membrane stability

- Physical characteristics of excitable cell membranes determine their permeability and therefore electrical stability.
- Cardiac muscle has a leaky membrane which allows the potential to drift towards and eventually reach threshold.
- Pharmacological manipulation of the number of channels open in the membrane affects its stability.
- Extracellular Ca^{2+} is the most important physiological regulator of stability.
- The amount of electricity required to trigger an action potential is a product of the stimulating voltage and the time it is applied – the strength–duration curve.
- The amount of Na^+ entry in one action potential is very small and rapidly removed by the membrane Na^+ pump.

Conduction of the nerve impulse

The role of the action potential, which is a local event in excitable cells, is to generate an electrical signal which is **conducted** along the surface of excitable cells as a command or message, a piece of information. The type of information carried (warmth, pain, etc.) is identified by recognizing the identity of the cells carrying the signal. Warmth is felt if a warm receptor is stimulated by any means. The magnitude of the message is indicated by the frequency of the action potentials. The role of the action potential in nerves is to conduct the information over long distances. In other cells, like muscle, a rapidly conducted action potential ensures that the whole contractile mechanism of a cell is activated at once. In nerves, when the message reaches the terminals, the information is **transmitted** to adjacent cells by the release of **neurotransmitters**. These neurotransmitters may excite an action potential in these cells or an intracellular chemical messenger, a **second messenger**, may be released, triggering a biochemical response in the receiving cell.

Action potentials in nerves

Nerves are specially developed to allow rapid conduction of the action potential over long distances.

You will be familiar with several ways by which electrical signals are conducted from one place to another. When you make a telephone call, the electrical signal is conducted to its destination along wires for at least the first and last parts of its journey. The National Grid conducts electricity from the power stations to your home along overhead wires. The problem is that the conductors used are not perfect. A perfect signal conductor would allow the signal to pass along it without loss. Such a perfect conductor would present no impedance (see Basic Science 1.3.1) to the signal's passage and would not allow any of it to leak away to the environment. All real conductors have some impedance, and losses occur along their path. You will be familiar with the crackle of electricity jumping the insulators on a power pylon on a damp day.

The problem faced by both these electrical systems also affects nerves. Like signal cables, they are conductors; their cytoplasm is surrounded by an insulator, the cell membrane. The resistance of cytoplasm is high; the cell membrane leaks – a far from ideal situation. In the telephone system, the losses are made up by repeater amplifiers boosting the signal at several points along its way. In the nerve, the action potential excites further action potentials as the signal is conducted along the nerve, boosting the signal continually throughout its journey.

1

Passive spread of excitation

The spread of the electrical signal down the nerve from one end to another involves the passive spread of the signal down the axon and the active propagation of the signal by the action-potential-generating sites. If a small current is injected into a nerve whose action-potential-generating mechanism has been destroyed, a resulting voltage change can be recorded from within the nerve. The signal is greatest at the point of current injection and gets smaller the further one moves away from it. The signal leaks away to the outside medium through the leaky membrane. The more leaky the nerve, the more the signal decays with distance. The signal fades out in an exponential manner with distance. The distance over which the signal is reduced to $1/e$ (37%) of its original size is called the **length** (or **space**) **constant**. In large nerve fibres the length constant is only 2–3 mm. Thus if the nerve were depolarized to zero, at a point 1 cm away the depolarization would be less than 5% of the resting membrane potential. (The length constant of electrical telephone cable is measured not in millimetres but in miles.)

The length constant of nerves increases with fibre diameter, which reduces the internal resistance, and is further increased if the leakiness of the membrane is reduced.

Active propagation of action potentials

The dramatic changes in the nerve membrane potential that make up an action potential are of no use in transmitting information if they do not move, and transmission of information is the business of the nervous system.

It is clear that passive spread of an action potential is insufficient to carry it over any useful distance – the voltage drops dramatically with distance. To achieve communication over the metre or so between your foot and spinal cord, for example, the action potential must be regenerated as it travels along, if it is going to survive.

We have seen that the voltage changes which make up the action potential are produced by a flow of charge (flow of charge is electrical current), and if we consider what is happening at one point on a nerve while the action potential occurs we would find that this current is divided into two parts:

1. that part used to change the membrane potential at that point and produce the characteristic action potential, and
2. that part that travels along the nerve 'neutralizing' the negative charge inside the membrane and so allowing the membrane potential to reach threshold. This part causes the action potential to be propagated along the nerve.

At the peak of the action potential, the entire current (due to Na^+ influx) is travelling along the nerve. This Na^+ current must be large enough to be divided into the two parts mentioned above and still be able to change the membrane potential and travel along the nerve. We might ask why this rolling loop does not reach the end of the nerve and 'rebound' back along the path it has just taken, just like a ball rebounds when rolled against a wall. The reason is that the sodium gates in the membrane that open to allow the Na^+ current necessary for propagation are inactivated for some time after the action potential has passed (see The refractory period, p. 46). So the action potential cannot pass that way again until the gates have had time to convert back to their closed state.

Myelin and glia (Fig. 1.3.6)

Nerve cells have long axons and dendrites. Parts of the cell can thus be more than 1 m from the cell body. Nerves are always associated with support cells called glia in the central nervous system (CNS) and Schwann cells in peripheral nerves. Besides supporting the metabolic function of nerves, these cells reduce the leakiness of the nerve membrane by wrapping layers of their cell membrane around the axons of some nerves, forming an insulator called **myelin**. This greatly reduces the rate of decay of any signal with distance from its origin: the length constant is increased.

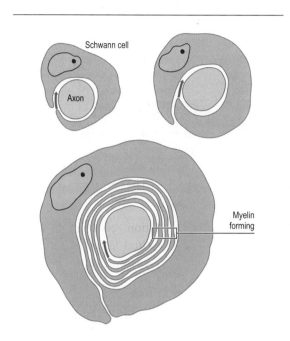

Fig. 1.3.6 Myelination. This transverse section of an axon shows how a Schwann cell sends out a 'tongue' of myelin-rich membrane to wrap round and insulate the axon. This roll of insulation is interrupted at regular intervals along the axon at the nodes of Ranvier.

In these myelinated nerves, action potentials are not generated at all points along the nerve but only at gaps in the myelin (nodes) where the nerve membrane is not covered. This is called **saltatory** (leaping) conduction (Fig. 1.3.7).

Compound action potentials

The activity of nerves and muscle can be monitored by placing recording electrodes close alongside the tissue. What is seen is the sum of the activity of the population of cells. The signal detected is of very small voltage compared with that recorded by electrodes inserted within the cell. This extracellularly recorded signal is contributed to by all the active fibres in the nerve at the recording site. If the nerve bundle is stimulated electrically at a point, the activity recorded at some distance from the point of stimulation is called a **compound action potential** (Fig. 1.3.8).

The form of the signal recorded is much affected by the position of the recording electrodes with relation to the active cells. If the nerve bundle is made up of only one type of nerve and the recording is made with bipolar electrodes (two electrodes connected to an

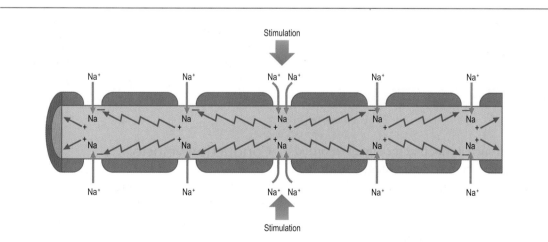

Fig. 1.3.7 Saltatory conduction. Propagation of an action potential in an unmyelinated nerve involves the opening and closing of ion channels. This is a biological process and therefore slow compared to the physical conduction of electricity in a wire. In saltatory conduction there is physical conduction along the myelinated section of the axon from node to node where the action potential is regenerated at each one. This speeds up transmission along the nerve.

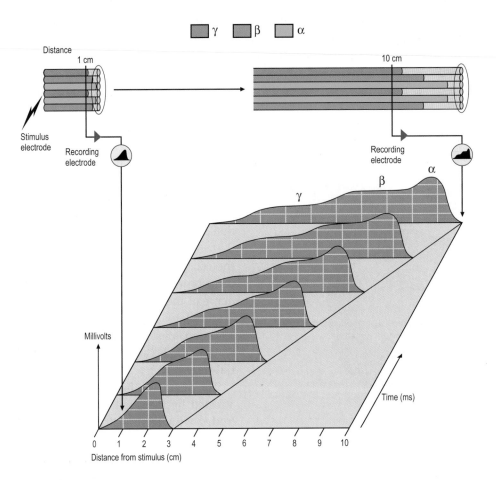

Fig. 1.3.8 The compound action potential. Nerve bundles are made up of axons of different diameters, and diameter determines speed of conduction. This speed is measured by placing a stimulating electrode on a nerve with a recording electrode a known distance away and measuring the time it takes an action potential to cover the distance.

The action potential that arrives at the recording electrode is not the same shape as one recorded from a single axon or a nerve bundle made up of axons of all the same diameter. Because of differences in conduction velocity, action potentials in large-diameter fibres arrive before those in small, and so the greater distance of recording from the stimulating electrodes the greater the time for the action potentials to arrive and the more spread out they will be. This is like runners in a marathon race who start together, are very close together after the first few metres, but are well spread out at the end.

amplifier in such a way that the signal recorded is the difference between the voltages on the two electrodes), the recorded signal as the action potentials pass both the electrodes is diphasic, the signal having first a negative-going then a positive-going component. If the action potentials pass only one of the electrodes the signal will have only one, negative-going, component (Fig. 1.3.9).

Conduction velocity

If the nerve bundle is made up of several groups of fibres of different size or contains myelinated and unmyelinated fibres, the fibres will conduct excitation at different speeds. In a bundle containing two or more groups of fibres, the **compound action potential** will contain signals that can be attributed to the activity of each group.

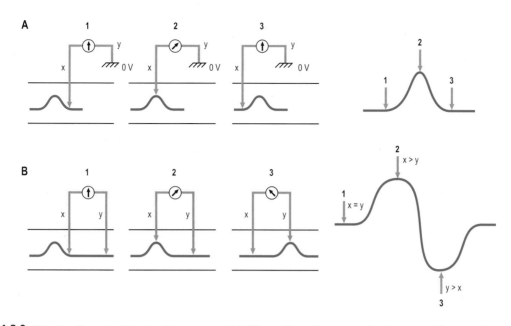

Fig. 1.3.9 Diphasic action potentials. A voltage or potential difference has to be measured against some reference value. One electrode is placed at the site whose voltage is required to be known and the other at the reference site (frequently earth). If this is done with a single axon, or a group of axons of the same type, a **monophasic action potential** is recorded. **A.** One electrode, x, placed on the nerve records the voltage as the action potential passes by with respect to earth which is always zero. **B.** If both electrodes are placed on the nerve, a **diphasic action potential** is recorded. While electrode y is at the resting membrane potential, the potential at x rises as the action potential passes by (points 1 to 2), as in the monophasic case, but as the action potential passes y, the potential at x is now lower than at y and there is a reversal of the signal (point 3).

If the compound action potential is recorded at two sites along the nerve, the speed with which the excitation moves along the nerves – the conduction velocities of its different components – can be measured (see Fig. 1.3.8).

The fastest mammalian nerves are large myelinated fibres conducting at some 100 m/s. The smallest myelinated fibres conduct at some 10 m/s and unmyelinated fibres conduct at about 1 m/s.

 Summary

Conduction of the impulse

- Characteristics of a nerve and its surroundings determine how it conducts action potentials.
- Action potentials are self-regenerating as they pass along a nerve.
- Without regeneration, an action potential falls to 37% of its original value at a distance called the space constant of that nerve (2–3 mm for a large nerve).

- Myelination of nerves insulates them and greatly increases the space constant.
- In saltatory conduction the action potential 'jumps' from node to node.
- Conduction velocity is increased by myelination and/or increased nerve diameter.
- A nerve bundle made up of fibres of different diameters shows a compound action potential because of their different conduction velocities.

Recent Advances

Receptors for autonomic neurotransmitters and the new biology

Modern DNA technology has permitted new insights into the structures and mechanisms of autonomic neurotransmitter receptors. The close dependence of biological activity of agents upon chemical structure led Clark, in the 1930s, to write 'the most interesting feature of drug action is the extraordinary specificity of the action of drugs and the manner in which slight changes in chemical constitution alter their actions'. This observed specificity led to studies of the structure–activity relationships of agonists and antagonists. The observation that many specific agents had effects on intracellular metabolism, but only if applied to the outer surface of cells, suggested the existence of 'drug receptors' – structures embedded in the membranes of cells, with recognition sites on the outer surface and an intracellular part that conveys a unitary stimulus to the effector apparatus of the cell. The receptors were assumed to be proteins.

The study of the relationships between the structure of receptor-active substances, and their specificity of effect, suggested that different receptors had different shapes. In the case of the acetylcholine receptor, study of the size of bismethonium compounds was particularly revealing. A series of these bases containing two methonium bases separated by carbon chains of different length, has effects on acetylcholine receptors that depend on the length of the hydrocarbon chain. The ganglionic nicotinic receptors are sensitive to hexamethonium, in which the two methonium groups are separated by a 6-carbon chain. Those of the skeletal neuromuscular junction are not sensitive to hexamethonium, but they do react with decamethonium, in which the separating chain has 10 carbon atoms. Muscarinic receptors are

relatively insensitive to these compounds. These observations suggested the existence of at least three distinct acetylcholine receptors.

Structures were suggested for two nicotinic receptors, each of which had, in addition to a site that reacted with acetylcholine nitrogen, a second site capable of binding another methonium group but separated from the first by different distances. Each was optimally fitted by different members of the bismethonium series, which thus exhibited effects selective for one type.

Although advances were made in the understanding of the events triggered by these cell surface receptors, until recently the receptor remained a 'black box'. However, the situation has now changed dramatically with the application of techniques based upon our greatly increased understanding of the biology of DNA. The ability to sequence DNA allows us to determine the amino acid sequences of the coded protein. Expression of DNA in foreign host cells is also possible. These advances have led to identification of the primary sequences of several receptor proteins, including those of the adrenoceptors and muscarinic cholinoceptors. The new technology has allowed a consideration of receptor (rather than drug) structure–activity relationships, and has permitted a new approach in the search for new drugs.

The cloning of receptor genes or their cDNAs has revealed structures that have much in common with each other. Some regions of members of the same family of receptors have as much as half of their amino acid sequences in common, and even receptors for different transmitters – adrenoceptors and cholinoceptors – share one-fifth of their structure.

The function of these receptors requires that they span the membrane of the cell. It is possible to identify, from their amino acid sequences,

Recent Advances *(Continued)*

those parts of the protein that are hydrophobic and thus likely to be embedded in the lipid membrane of the cell. Hydrophilic regions will be more likely to extend into the aqueous media on either surface of the membrane. All the protein structures identified for the adrenoceptor and cholinoceptor families have a common feature: they have seven hydrophobic segments of a size able to span the membrane. It is these segments that share the most amino acid sequences across groups, the similarity being greatest between members of similar pharmacological types of receptor.

To explain the specific sensitivities and effects of drug action, attempts have been made using DNA technology to ascribe function to specific parts of the revealed protein structure. It is possible to modify, add or delete segments of the receptor gene and to study the effects of such

changes on the function of the receptor when it has been expressed in a cell. One powerful approach of this kind has been the production of chimeric genes, genes with large pieces replaced by components taken from a different receptor gene.

Both α_2 and β_2 receptors are activated by adrenaline with high affinity but have very different second messenger mechanisms: the α_2 receptor inhibits adenyl cyclase, but the β_2 receptor activates the enzyme. Chimeras were produced that associated one receptor agonist selectively with the effector system of the other (Fig. RA1.3.1). When such chimeras were expressed on oocytes, it was shown that the determinants were located in just two of the membrane-spanning portions of the receptor protein. One of the chimeras, made up of the main part of the β_2 receptor with just one of the

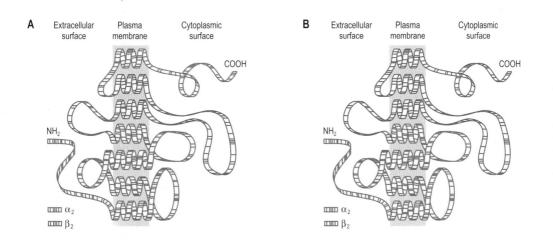

Fig. RA1.3.1 An illustration of two chimeral receptors made up of components of α_2 and β_2 adrenoceptors.
Those parts of the new receptors that are from the α_2 receptor are blue and those from the β_2 receptors are red. Chimera **(A)** has the binding properties of an α_2 receptor but unlike the natural form activates adenyl cyclase. Chimera **(B)** has β_2 binding characteristics and, like the natural β receptor, also activates adenyl cyclase.

Recent Advances *(Continued)*

end membrane-spanning segments replaced by that from the α_2 receptor, had an α_2 antagonist binding profile but activated adenyl cyclase.

A most exciting aspect of these advances had been the possibility of the development of better new drugs. The more specific and localized the effect of a drug, the less likely it is to produce unwanted side-effects that might limit its usefulness. In the past, selectivity has been improved by the study of the structure–activity relationships of existing drugs.

However, though this approach has achieved much, it has had to rely too much on serendipity. The definition of the primary structure of these receptors opens up the possibility of the rational design of selective new agonists and antagonists. The study of receptor genes has revealed the existence of subtypes of receptors whose existence had not been suspected previously. There are now known to be at least five subtypes of the muscarinic receptors and two α_2 adrenoceptors.

Cell-to-cell signalling

Intercellular communication

A multicellular organism consists of many individual cells integrated into a whole. The prime requirement for this integration is communication between the cells. Cells in close proximity affect each other in a number of ways. At the simplest level physical contact between cells will allow force to be transmitted from one cell to its neighbours. The composition of the cells' shared environment will be modified as a result of their basic metabolic activity; nutrients are removed and metabolic products accumulate. Thus one cell might alter the metabolic activity of another in a variety of ways. Cells have also developed special forms of communication that permit specific and detailed information to be passed between them.

Nerve cells communicate with each other over short distances by releasing specific chemicals, transmitters, for which the recipient nerve possesses sensitive receptor molecules (see p. 61). The spread of the message is strictly limited to the intended target cell by the dilution of the transmitter as it diffuses away from the site of release. Only the nearest cell receives a high concentration of the transmitter. In some situations, inactivation mechanisms exist which also serve to limit the spread of the transmitter.

Chemical messengers can also act over large distances within the body. Hormones are released into the bloodstream by the endocrine glands and are transported throughout the body. The concentration seen by the target cells is lower than the local concentrations reached by neurotransmitters. Nevertheless, hormonal effects are limited to a specific target population of cells because the receptors for hormones are not only more sensitive than those for neurotransmitters but are also highly selective. Small differences in the structure of a hormone molecule can alter its effectiveness drastically.

Cell–cell junctions

Cells are physically attached to their neighbours to maintain the structure of the body and transmit information.

They are attached to each other in a variety of ways. Some cells insert processes like tongues into adjacent cells creating an irregular border between the cells and making a physical attachment between the two. In other cells, although the surface of adjacent cells is smooth, they approach each other closely and the 200 Å gap between them is filled with glycoproteins from the cell coats which may have an adhesive effect.

There are also obviously specialized structural links between cells. These are called junctions. There are three main types of junction: tight, gap and adherens (Fig. 1.4.1).

Tight junctions are found between cells lining a space, where a seal must be created to control the permeability of the lining. The important feature of this type of junction is that two outer lamellae of the lipid bilayer cell membranes are fused together to form a three-layered structure. Their appearance on an electron micrograph is of five lines, three dark and two light. Such tight junctions are found in the lining of the tubule of the kidney and of the gastrointestinal tract where movement of water and solutes must be controlled. Tight junctions also prevent proteins in the cell membrane from migrating from one site to another.

Gap junctions (also known as nexi) are found where excitation is passed electrically

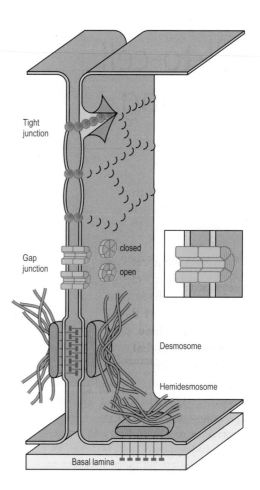

Fig. 1.4.1 Cell junctions. The three main types of junctions between cells are:

- Tight junctions where protein from each adjacent plasma membrane forms continuous strands across the intercellular space. Epithelial cells alter their tight junctions to allow the passage of materials, and the protein strands which make up the junction also serve to localize membrane enzyme systems to particular regions of the cell.

- Gap junctions provide electrical and chemical coupling between cells which can be controlled by the opening or closing of the junction. This connection is important for cell-to-cell signalling, particularly in controlling development of the embryo.

- Desmosomes are adherens-type junctions which exist as 'mirror image' structures. Cytoplasmic keratin filaments are attached to a 'reinforcing' plaque close to each cell membrane. Each plaque extends proteins through its cell membrane to the proteins from the opposite plaque. Hemidesmosomes are 'half desmosomes' in which the transmembrane proteins are embedded in the basal lamina.

from cell to cell. The membranes of the two cells approach each other to within 20 Å. The outer lamellae do not fuse, so an electron micrograph shows seven lines, four dark and three light, in such a junction. The gap between the two membranes is crossed by structures that are embedded in the abutting cells and penetrate into the cytoplasm of the cells. These structures function as pores connecting the two cells. Gap junctions are found between the muscle cells of the heart and of the gut. In both situations, the muscles form a functional electrical syncytium, behaving as a single cell and being excited as a unit.

The **adherens** type of junction is one in which the abutting cells are separated totally and do not approach closer than 200 Å but the adhesion of the cells is very good. If separated, the tearing occurs at the junction. The important feature of these junctions, also known as **desmosomes**, is that the cytoplasmic side of the adhering membranes is much thickened by structures forming a plaque. Tonofilaments, intracellular structural elements, loop into the plaque concentrating any force into it. Desmosomes are found in many places where structural integrity of soft tissue is required and are found in large number in the deeper layers of the skin.

Summary

Cell junctions

- Cell junctions attach cells to each other, determine the permeability of membranes and allow direct cell-to-cell communication.
- Tight junctions control the movement of water and solutes between cells which line hollow structures.
- Gap junctions link cells electrically.
- Adherens junctions form physical 'welds' between cells.

Receptors

Cells, by their metabolic activity, alter the composition of the interstitial fluid in which they are bathed. These changes affect their immediate neighbours. They also release chemicals designed to transmit specific messages. These can convey information to the next cell, as in the case of the neurotransmitters, or to cells far distant in the body when hormones are conveyed in the circulating blood from endocrine gland to target cell.

Specialized structures, receptors, on the target cells recognize the chemical message and decode it into biochemical instructions to the relevant effector mechanism.

The concept of the cell surface receptor was originally proposed by Langley at the end of the 19th century and he suggested that the effects of drugs might be governed by the laws of mass action. These ideas became the basis of our understanding of drug action after their extensive development by Clark in the 1920s.

The important properties of these cell-surface receptors are that they confer on the cell a very selective and sensitive transduction mechanism that allows the cell to respond to chemical messages from other cells in the organism.

Receptors can be very specific in their ability to distinguish between molecules with only small structural differences. For example, acetylcholine receptors will respond to that substance when it is present at concentrations down to 10^{-6} M but choline is 1000 times less potent. This selectivity allows acetylcholine's action to be rapidly terminated after hydrolysis by the enzyme acetylcholinesterase, because the product of hydrolysis, choline, does not stimulate.

The sensitivity of these receptors is illustrated by the fact that a biological assay system for acetylcholine has been developed which will detect 10^{-15} mole of the substance. Such an assay system is called a bioassay. The selectivity and sensitivity of these bioassays was the basis of many advances in physiology in the 20th century.

The term 'receptor' in the context of the cell membrane is best reserved for structures which have a regulatory role when combined with specific molecules known as **ligands**. Ligands that activate receptors are called **agonists** and those that prevent this effect **antagonists**.

Clinical Example

Insulin

A dramatic example of the action of receptors in the cell membrane is seen in the case of insulin deficiency and diabetes.

Diabetes mellitus is a disease characterized by the production of copious amounts of glucose-containing urine. In diabetes high levels of glucose build up in the blood. It is filtered in such large amounts into the kidney tubules that it overwhelms the resorptive mechanisms and 'overflows' into the urine.

Diabetes mellitus presents in two forms:

- insulin-dependent diabetes mellitus (IDDM; Type I)
- non-insulin-dependent diabetes mellitus (NIDDM; Type II).

Type I is due to a deficiency of insulin production, Type II to a partial deficiency plus a resistance of the tissues to the action of insulin.

It may seem strange that the absence of a hormone should cause an excess of a substance but the effect of insulin is to remove glucose, and fats and proteins, from the blood into the tissues. It does this by acting as a ligand on a receptor in the cell membrane. Strangely enough, only about 10% of the insulin receptors of a cell need to be occupied to produce the maximum effect.

Although there is one type of insulin receptor, which spans the cell membrane, there are several immediate metabolic effects and long-term actions which include effects on cell replication.

Insulin is a protein and was the first protein to have its structure fully determined. This was done by Frederick Sanger in 1955, for which he received the Nobel Prize.

Some patients with diabetes can control their condition with special diets and drugs (sulphonylureas) which stimulate the limited insulin secretion of the patient and reduce the tissue resistance to the action of existing insulin. Other patients, as we have already noted, are absolutely dependent on an external supply of insulin.

Because it is a protein, insulin cannot be taken orally – it would be digested. If it has to be given, it must therefore be given by injection. The sources of human insulin available are pig insulin, which is chemically modified into the human form by changing the amino acid alanine into threonine and by genetically modifying the bacterium *Escherichia coli* to produce proinsulin, which is then enzymatically cleaved to form insulin.

Normal individuals have a background secretion of insulin on which is superimposed sharp increases after meals. Many of the problems of the diabetic life are associated with the difficulty of mimicking this pattern by injection.

Receptor classification

The most sensible classification for receptors of physiological importance is that based upon the identity of the chemical to which they evolved to respond. Receptors for a single substance may not, however, be homogeneous throughout the body. Variations between receptors can sometimes be revealed by their differing sensitivities to foreign substances, i.e. drugs. Acetylcholine receptors involved in the control of skeletal muscle are stimulated by nicotine, whereas those on the smooth muscle of gut respond to muscarine. The muscarinic receptors are not a single group but have been further separated into at least five subgroups.

Receptors classified according to their agonist sensitivity are named accordingly. Cholinoceptors are stimulated by acetylcholine-like compounds. Adrenoceptors are stimulated by adrenaline and related catecholamines. An older usage describes these receptors as cholinergic and adrenergic. The suffix -ergic is, however, best reserved to describe the nerves that release a given transmitter. Thus cholinergic nerves release acetylcholine.

Another sensible classification of receptors is based upon the signal transduction mechanisms activated by the stimulated receptor. Such a classification has three divisions (Fig. 1.4.2):

- receptors linked to and controlling ion channels in the cell membrane
- receptors linked to so-called G-proteins
- receptors linked to enzymes.

Clinical Example

Myasthenia gravis (grave weakness)

An example of dysfunction of receptors is the acquired autoimmune condition myasthenia gravis. It is characterized by weakness and fatigue in the proximal limb and ocular muscles. It occurs in 1 in 25 000 of the population, with a prevalence in women twice that in men.

The command for a muscle to contract comes in the form of acetylcholine released from the end of motor nerves (see Ch. 3.5, p. 210). This acetylcholine activates receptors in the muscle membrane and then is destroyed by cholinesterases. If there are no receptors on the muscle to accept the acetylcholine, the muscle will not contract. That is what happens in myasthenia gravis.

The myasthenic patient has produced antibodies to his own acetylcholine receptors.

These antibodies do not so much interfere with the function of the receptors as identify them for early breakdown by muscle enzyme systems. There are therefore fewer receptors to stimulate.

One effective course of treatment is to give the patient anticholinesterase drugs. These block the destruction of acetylcholine and so there is more acetylcholine to stimulate the fewer receptors.

Because this is an immune disease, removal of the thymus (an important part of the immune system) often produces relief.

The immune response can also be damped down by immunosuppressant drugs such as corticosteroids, which are used when the response to anticholinesterases is disappointing and bring relief in 75% of cases.

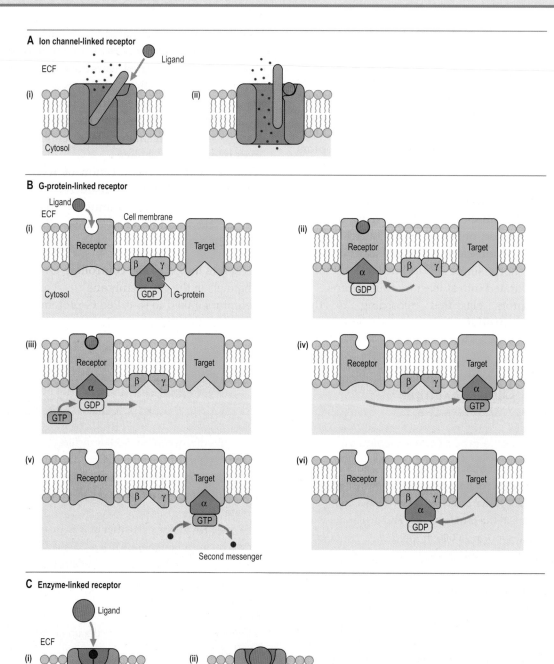

Fig. 1.4.2 Three types of cell-membrane-situated receptors. One way of classifying cell-membrane-situated receptors is based on the mechanisms activated by the binding of the receptor-specific molecule (ligand) to the receptor. The effects of activating **(A)** ion channel-linked, **(B)** G-protein-linked and **(C)** enzyme-linked receptors are shown. An important feature of these different mechanisms is the amplifying effect common to them all. A single molecule of ligand activates systems that admit or activate many molecules controlled by the receptor.

Receptors linked to ion channels

These are conceptually the simplest. The receptor is part of a membrane ion channel. Binding of an agonist to the receptor controls the opening and closing of the channel (Fig. 1.4.2A). The response can be fast, reaching a peak in a few milliseconds and being over almost as rapidly. It may be amplified by the generation of an action potential by the cell.

Receptors linked to ion channels are found in nerve and muscle. Nicotinic acetylcholine receptors are found in skeletal muscle and on neurones. Neuronal glutamate, glycine, 5-hydroxytryptamine (5-HT) and γ-aminobutyric acid (GABA) receptors are abundant in the CNS. So far, the only receptors of this type established as being present on autonomically innervated effectors are some of those sensitive to purines, the P_{2x}-purinoceptors. The simplest gate the influx of Ca^{2+}. Intracellular free Ca^{2+} controls many important cell processes.

Receptors coupled to G-proteins

A large family of receptors are coupled to a guanine nucleotide (GDP, guanine diphosphate, or GTP, guanine triphosphate) binding protein, or G-protein, which couples to and controls an enzyme. The activation of this enzyme may lead to the release of an intracellular diffusible moiety, or second messenger such as cAMP (cyclic 3′,5′-adenosine monophosphate) or inositol 1,4,5-trisphosphate (IP_3). Some G-proteins directly regulate ion channels. The effects of these receptors are slower than those linked directly to ion channels and their time-course is measured in seconds.

G-protein regulatory cycle

One model for the role of the G-protein in the transduction process between the stimulated receptor and the effect in the cell is as follows:

- The receptor, G-protein and target enzyme are present in the membrane as separate mobile moieties.

- The G-protein is an oligomer made up of three subunits, α, β and γ.
- The α-subunit can bind either GDP or GTP.
- GTP binding to the α-subunit of the G-protein causes the α-subunit–GTP complex to separate from the β- and γ-subunits.
- The free α-subunit slowly hydrolyses the bound GTP to GDP restoring its own affinity for the β- and γ-subunits. (GDP remains bound to the α-subunit.)
- The oligomer reforms.
- In this idling state, this splitting of GTP is slow because GDP only slowly dissociates from the oligomer and this limits the rate of the above reactions.
- If an agonist binds to the receptor, the resulting complex can bind to G-protein (Fig. 1.4.2B(i) and (ii)).
- Binding of an agonist–receptor complex to G-protein reduces its affinity for GDP, allowing GDP to dissociate more rapidly (Fig. 1.4.2B(iii)).
- GTP binds to the vacated α-subunit.
- The effect is to raise the concentration of free α-subunit–GTP complexes in the membrane.
- The α-subunit–GTP complexes are the activators of the effector enzyme.
- They are free to diffuse within the membrane and thus are able to activate membrane-bound enzymes leading to an effect (Fig. 1.4.2B(iv–vi)).

The signal, the presence of agonist bound to the receptor, is amplified at two stages in this process. When GTP is bound to the G-protein its affinity for the agonist–receptor complex is reduced, allowing the complex to activate more G-proteins. Also, the long life of the α-subunit–GTP complex allows it to activate many effector enzyme molecules.

The effector enzyme activated by this system can be one of several important enzymes, including adenylate cyclase, producing substances called second messengers.

Effects of second messengers

Ca^{2+} is a very common second messenger. Intracellular free Ca^{2+} is normally held at a very low level, $<10^{-7}$ M, by cell membrane pumps that transport it out of the cell and by the endoplasmic reticulum that actively binds Ca^{2+}. Transient increases in intracellular free Ca^{2+} are used to control contractile proteins that allow both smooth and striated muscle to contract (see p. 94). Exocytotic release of hormones and neurotransmitters is triggered by the binding of Ca^{2+} to synapsin (see p. 163). Many other intracellular processes are Ca^{2+} dependent. Intracellular Ca^{2+} can itself be regulated by the second messenger IP_3, which binds to a receptor on the endoplasmic reticulum and releases Ca^{2+} from stores.

The role of cAMP as a second messenger was discovered in the 1950s. cAMP is involved in many control mechanisms at many cellular levels. It acts by activation of various protein kinases – enzymes that phosphorylate other inactive cellular enzymes, thereby activating them. Such kinases control lipolysis, glycogen synthesis and breakdown, and thus the energy metabolism of the whole organism.

Receptors coupled directly to enzymes

Receptors can also be directly linked to an effector enzyme (Fig. 1.4.2C). Atrial natriuretic peptide (ANP) is typical of peptide messengers in that it activates such a receptor. The ANP receptor and the membrane enzyme guanylate cyclase are parts of a single protein. The effects of receptors like these have time-courses measured in minutes.

Intracellular steroid hormone receptors

There are also intracellular receptors that respond to agonists that, because of their lipophilic nature, are able to pass through the cell membranes.

Summary

Receptors

- Specialized areas on the cell surface, receptors, receive chemical messages from the surroundings.
- Receptors are stimulated by agonists and inhibited by antagonists.
- Among the many types of receptors are those linked to ion channels in the membrane and those linked to G-proteins.
- Receptor activation may produce an effect or it may cause a second messenger to be produced which produces the effect.
- Receptors for steroid hormones are not on the cell membrane but in its nucleus.

Steroid hormone receptors within the nucleus of the cell control mRNA synthesis and through this protein synthesis. The proteins produced may be structural or enzymatic and the effects of these receptors are long-lasting and slow in onset. The time-course of their effects is measured in hours.

Trophic effects

Cells interact with their neighbours in many important though unspectacular ways to maintain the integrity of the body. A cut heals, leaving little trace of the wound. A broken bone restores its original shape. In all repair and maintenance processes cells react with their neighbours cooperatively. The mechanisms of this cooperation are poorly understood.

Several examples of this cooperation could be given which suggest that the organization (and certainly the reorganization after damage) of the nervous system is not rigidly laid down by genetic programming. Neurones are left to 'make their own arrangements' much more than was previously imagined. For example, when a nerve cell is damaged, not only does it degenerate but frequently neurones with which it was in contact suffer. The damaged neurone appeared to have been providing *trophic factors* to its neighbours as if to sustain the relationship they had established.

Another example is provided by frog muscle fibres, which only have one motor nerve attached to them. If other motor axons are placed close to the muscle fibre, they are ignored. If, however, the original motor nerve is cut, the muscle will form a new partnership with a new nerve. It seems that the muscle releases *nerve growth factors* to bring about the introduction.

Summary

Trophic effects

- Trophic factors are important methods of intercellular communication which coordinate cell activity, particularly in growth and repair.
- Embryological organization depends to a large extent on trophic effects.
- Nerve growth factors which coordinate repair and re-innervation of muscles are examples of trophic factors.

Clinical Example

Cholera

In this chapter we have touched on the beautifully adapted mechanisms of cell-to-cell signalling which control the activities of cells. We can sometimes take over this control pharmacologically where necessary for therapeutic purposes. However, in the disease cholera, we see what happens when 'a maniac takes over the controls'.

Cholera is caused by the flagellate bacillus *Vibrio cholerae* of the family Spirillaceae. In the 19th and early 20th centuries six pandemics originating in the Bengal basin ravaged the world. The rapid onset of the disease with vomiting and diarrhoea causes rapid dehydration and hypovolaemic shock which killed 30% of those infected within 2–3 days and imbued cholera with an apocalyptic reputation.

Cholera is heralded by sudden onset of effortless vomiting and profuse 'rice water' stools, so called because of their watery colourless appearance flecked with mucus and their distinctive fishy sweet odour. It is this dehydrating diarrhoea which can cause death in 12–24 hours.

Transmission of cholera is by the faecal–oral route when bacilli are ingested in contaminated food or water. It appears that the amount needed to cause infection is very small.

Hypochlorhydria (lack of hydrochloric acid in the stomach) facilitates survival of the bacilli into the small intestine where they exert their effect. There is no inflammation of the mucosa and no invasion of the intestinal wall. There is a massive outpouring of isotonic fluid by the gut mucosal cells under the influence of a potent exotoxin called enterotoxin which is produced by the bacilli.

The exotoxin causes persistent activation of a G-protein (G_s) which activates the adenylate cyclase system that causes secretion. This usually normal system has been hijacked by the exotoxin. Nor will the 'maniac' relinquish the controls; it is bound irreversibly to the receptors to exert its effect for 24–48 hours, which is the life span of the intestinal cells.

Clinical Example *(Continued)*

Although the disease can present dramatically, treatment is simple and effective. Oral rehydration using a glucose–electrolyte solution reduces mortality to less than 1%. Intravenous rehydration may be required in severely dehydrated patients and antibiotic treatment with tetracycline helps to eradicate the infection.

Good hygiene and sanitary living conditions are the best preventive measures.

Circadian rhythms – clocks within cells

What are circadian rhythms, and why do they exist?

Our ability to control our environment, at the touch of a switch to turn night to day with an electric light, to make the winter into summer with central heating in our homes, makes us forget that all organisms have evolved to fill the ecological niche in which they should naturally find themselves.

This evolution began some four thousand million years ago when we would have found conditions much more difficult than they are today. In those Precambrian times conditions alternated between freezing cold and scorching ultraviolet radiation in about a 24-hour cycle as the earth rotated. It was to the advantage of the organisms that existed then to be able to time their activities to avoid this destructive radiation, and so evolved inborn clocks.

Today, we can see rhythm generation in all living organisms. This might be related to specific internal rhythms, such as heartbeat or respiration, or to environmental cycles: annual; lunar-monthly; tidal; or **circadian**, which means about a day (*circa* – about; *dies* – day).

Many of us know people who have what is known in rural areas as a 'head clock'. They can wake up in the morning at a time they decided before going to sleep and can tell accurately what length of time has passed without consulting a watch. This remarkable ability implies either a particular sensitivity to some highly regulated external event that other mortals are unaware of, or some kind of internal clock which marks off the passage of time. There is still considerable debate at a high scientific level as to what contribution unconscious sensitivity to external events, such as changes in the earth's magnetic field, play in the rhythms we see in all individuals, but it seems certain now that rhythm generation on a daily, monthly, or yearly timescale exists within us.

There is a variety of evidence for internal clocks. It is very easy to recognize rhythm in our daily lives. We all seem to have a special time of day when we are at our best. Some people are 'morning people', some 'evening people' (there seem to be few 'afternoon people'). These rhythms can be detected in more objective ways. Thus reaction time (alertness), body temperature and secretion of hormones follow a daily measurable pattern (Fig. 1.5.1).

More socially orientated experimenters have investigated the rate at which individuals metabolize alcohol at different times of day. We have in our liver, enzyme

systems to remove the small amounts of alcohol produced by fermentation in our gut. Imbibed alcohol is dealt with by the same system. In an experiment in which volunteers consumed equal portions of whisky at fairly regular intervals throughout 24 hours, it was found that it was metabolized almost 25% more rapidly between 2 p.m. and midnight than during the rest of the day (Fig. 1.5.2). Less pleasantly, perception of pain, in the form of stimulation of dental nerves, also shows a diurnal rhythm. It is unfortunate that the increasing sensitivity shown by this curve coincides with the afternoon, a time when many of us will visit the dentist.

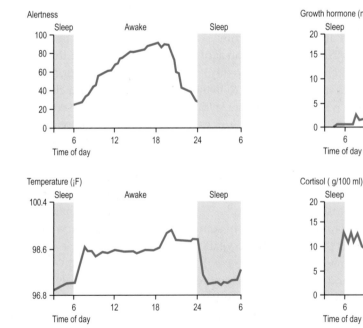

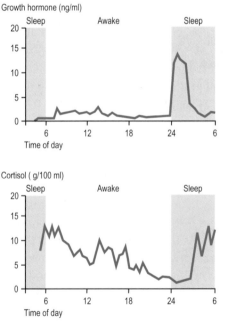

Fig. 1.5.1 Diurnal rhythms measured in a subject over a 24-hour period.

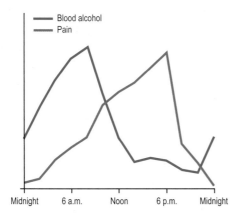

Fig. 1.5.2 **The daily rhythm in the metabolism of alcohol (red line) and the sensitivity of teeth to a painful stimulus (blue line).** (Redrawn from data of Wilson R, Newman E, Newman H 1956 Journal of Applied Physiology 8: 556–558 and Jones A, Frees J 1937 Deutsche Medizinische Wochenschrift 63: 962–963 respectively.)

Under normal circumstances these rhythms are locked to our 24-hour daily lives. It is very easy to argue that it is the events of the day that are imposing these rhythms – an increase in temperature, for example, being brought about by the onset of physical activity. Many ingenious experiments have been carried out to test this theory and one, which will be well understood by anyone who has suffered from jet-lag, involved honey-bees. The bees were accustomed to feed at 8 p.m. local time at their home in Paris. One night, while the bees were resting in their hive, the hive was transported to New York. The next day and for several days following, the bees continued to feed as if in Paris, i.e. at 1 a.m. in the morning New York time – a totally inappropriate time.

What is equally important as this demonstration of an internal clock is the fact that left in New York the bees would eventually adapt to a normal New York feeding time. In other words, something to do with the earth's geophysical 24-hour period would eventually impose itself on them.

Other experiments have been designed to remove the effect of the earth's rotation and its associated apparent movement of the sun, moon and stars. One of the most ingenious was carried out at the South Pole where a turntable was set up exactly over the pole and caused to rotate one revolution every 24 hours against the rotation of the earth; effectively standing still while the earth rotated underneath it. Hamsters, fruit-flies, beans and fungi

placed on the table continued to show a daily rhythm to their lives.

Experiments with human beings have frequently involved isolating them in underground caves or bunkers without any measure of the passage of time or contact with the normal world. The subjects could eat and sleep when they wished. Under these circumstances the subjects' internal clocks can 'run free' and it becomes evident that the majority of subjects have an internal clock which gives them the impression of a day greater than 24 hours, sometimes up to 28 hours, while a minority of subjects have a subjective day of less than 24 hours. Understandably, when the 'long day' subjects are asked to estimate the passage of an hour they guess a time interval longer than an actual hour – their clocks run slower than reality. The opposite is true for the 'short day' subjects. While living in the normal world, provided with the clues to tell them what was appropriate activity, the subjects lived a normal life. This synchronization with the rotating earth is called *entrainment*.

Isolated subjects who develop days longer than 24 hours eat less frequently. It might be expected that they would eat more at each meal to keep up their caloric intake or that they would lose weight. In fact neither of these things

71

happens but the subjects become less active, using less energy in a day.

Heart rate

The average heart rate of young adults is said by most physiology books to be about 70 beats/minute. If we measure heart rate at hourly intervals over 24 hours, we find that even with the subject completely at rest the rate is modulated, being greatest during the day. This rhythm is very easily attributed to such factors as alertness, temperature or any variety of external cues. However, in the totally unnatural environment of a space capsule in low orbit round the earth where 'days' last 80–130 minutes and not more than one-third of each orbit is spent in the earth's shadow, the 24-hour rhythm persists, being disturbed only (not surprisingly) during launch and re-entry.

The heart of the developing human fetus begins to beat about 4 weeks after conception. At this stage it is almost invisible to the human eye. Although the mother's heart displays the normal daily cycle, the heart of her fetus beats regularly at about 133/minute. Only about 1 month after birth does rhythm begin to appear, when the night-time rate begins to fall.

Hearts isolated from the body can be kept alive for long periods of time. Not only do these hearts show the circadian rhythm of their rate of beat, but if the heart is exposed to enzymes which cause it to break up into its individual cells, these cells themselves continue to pulse with a rate which has a circadian rhythm.

Sleep

Sleep is a marker that defines the limits of our days. We usually have one main sleep episode during a circadian cycle of whatever length. This usually coincides with the daily fall in body temperature to its minimum (see Fig. 1.5.1). Apart from the main sleep episode, we often take naps during our waking period and these are most often associated with the maximum point in the temperature cycle. Naps have the same structure of rapid eye movement sleep (REM) and non-REM sleep as the main sleep episode and do not affect the duration of the main episode. In the bunker-living, free-running individuals already described, the duration of naps was found to be positively related to the duration of the waking period that contained them, i.e. people who developed long wake periods took long naps.

We will see later that all cells of the body and even single-celled organisms have the property of circadian rhythms. In mammals, however, an anatomical structure has been identified as the site of the circadian oscillator.

This is a small group of cells appropriately close to the optic chiasma called the suprachiasmatic nucleus (SCN). There is a pathway from the retina to the SCN which provides the input to enable its rhythms to be entrained by light, and several output pathways to produce the SCN's effects (Fig. 1.5.3).

Animals with lesions in this region of their brain are arrhythmic in their activity, showing no clear cycle. Transplantation of fetal SCN cells into their brain restores rhythmicity. Some animals have a special *tau* (τ) mutation of their genetic material which shortens their cycle. If cells from these are used, then the recipient adopts the shortened cycle of the donor.

Sleep itself is divided into REM and non-REM phases. Levels of activity in neurones using different transmitters is different in wakefulness and the two types of sleep. In the shift from waking through non-REM to REM sleep there is a progressive decrease in aminergic activity and an increase in cholinergic activity in the brain. It may be by modulating this activity that the SCN modulates the sleep–wake pattern.

The close proximity of the optic chiasma, and the anatomical pathways linking it to the optic tract provides a basis for explaining entrainment

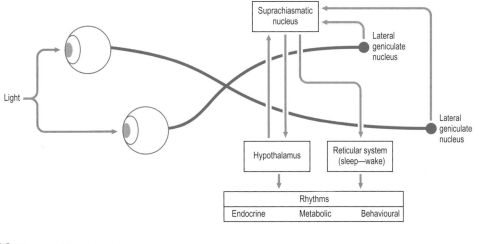

Fig. 1.5.3 The suprachiasmatic nucleus.

by light. Moderate variations in ambient temperature also have substantial effects on circadian rhythms, particularly in hibernating animals.

Depression

Clinically depressed patients classically report that their moods vary during each day in a very constant way. They also report sleep disturbances including early morning wakening. Aside from these daily cycles, their illness frequently has a seasonal recurrence at particular times of the year. This seasonal affective disorder (SAD) is characterized by depressive episodes in autumn and winter alternating with hypomania in spring and summer. These psychological symptoms are accompanied by physiological symptoms including fatigue, increased sleep times, food cravings and weight gain. A number of therapies linked to human circadian rhythms appear to be effective in some of these cases. Sleep deprivation is used with some depressed patients and can dramatically shift them from depressed to hypomanic in a few hours.

Because it was discovered that human melatonin secretion by the pineal gland could be suppressed by sunshine or bright artificial light it was thought that this was the mechanism of SAD. However melatonin given at different times of day or blocked by drugs does not affect the condition. Nevertheless, brief (3-hour) exposures to bright light are now routinely used to treat SAD, and these exposures would produce a change in circadian rhythm of about 3 hours if all else were kept constant. The most recent hypothesis regarding SAD is that the retina of these patients has an abnormal sensitivity to light.

The idea that affective disorders involve disorder of circadian rhythm receives support from the results of experiments involving the effect of antidepressant drugs on circadian rhythms, which were found to be modified in amplitude and duration in a wide variety of organisms. The prime site of action of these drugs seems to be the SCN but many act at more than one site. In particular, they all modify retinal sensitivity and many act on the visual pathway to the SCN.

Shift work

Many people in industrial, police and medical employment often work on a 24-hour shift system, with duties being confined to night or day. In an attempt at fairness employers usually routinely alternate their employees between the night and day shift. Beginning one of these shifts after working the other is the equivalent of being transported half-way round the world as far as circadian rhythms are concerned and generally brings general disruption to the employee's life. After a sufficient number of cycles, the new rhythms will impose themselves and all will be well. This will not happen if, as in a normal working week, the worker takes 2 days off at the weekend and rejoins the normal daytime world, only to return to the night-shift on the following Monday.

One way of dealing with this situation is to do away with the weekend and work all the night-work required in a month, say, at one sitting; so there will be only two phase changes each month. As the performance of individuals is undoubtedly worse at the times of these changes, it is definitely worthwhile taking this into account in situations where people's lives may be at risk.

Birth and death

The Victorian passion for accurate recording enables us to see that the two cardinal events of life, birth and death, are also subject to the circadian clock. Old hospital and local records from Victorian times to the present day establish without a doubt modes of time for birth and death. The onset of labour as signified by the beginning of painful contractions or the rupture of fetal membranes occurs most usually between 1 a.m. and 7 a.m. in the case of live births. It is interesting that in stillbirth the rhythm is greatly altered, with a much broader peak occurring about midday. Mortality too has its time documented in the records with the most common time of death being at 6 a.m.

Tissue and cell rhythms

The physiological rhythms measured in whole organisms must of course be the result of rhythms in tissues and, ultimately, cells. The rhythms of heart rate frequency have been mentioned as existing in isolated heart cells and many overt rhythms are due to the rhythmic output of hormones from endocrine organs controlled by the hypothalamus, which is in close anatomical association with the suprachiasmatic nucleus.

The rhythmic change in frequency of beating of the isolated cells of the heart leads us to the important question of whether we can suppose that these rhythms are the rule in most if not all cells, i.e. does every cell have a clock? Do these rhythms depend on the rhythms of individual cells or is there a 'circuit' of cells in tissues, all of which are necessary for the rhythm to be established, just as there are several components in your electronic watch, all of which are necessary for it to run?

The consensus of opinion is that all eukaryotic cells (cells with a nucleus and multiple chromosomes) have clocks of one kind or another. Prokaryotes (single-celled organisms, bacteria for example, which do not have a nucleus and only a single chromosome) appear to possess no circadian rhythms. This may be because their life span is frequently less than 24 hours and so such rhythms would be irrelevant. Even the simplest eukaryotes, protozoa and unicellular algae, have circadian rhythms and one of them, *Euglena*, has been extensively studied for its rhythmic cell division and rate of movement.

Almost 200 years ago it was realized that the rate of division of the cells of plants had a daily cycle imposed on it even when the plants were kept under constant conditions. 60 years ago the same circadian rhythm of cell division was first observed in human tissue by the ingenious plan of collecting the foreskins of boys circumcized at different hours of the day. Those removed during the afternoon and evening contained cells which were dividing most rapidly.

More scientifically rigorous, if less dramatic, are the observations of the nuclei of cells cultured under constant conditions from the salivary glands of fruit-flies. The nuclei swell and shrink in a clear pattern with two peaks per 24 hours. Equally interestingly, individual cells get out of phase with their neighbours, which tells us that there is no need for a 'circuit' of cells to produce a timing mechanism. Each cell has its own clock, even if some run slightly slower than others. The swelling and shrinking of the nucleus of these cells is a visible expression of the rate of synthesis of mRNA and proteins. We are now getting close to the molecular basis of circadian rhythms.

One of the surprising but extremely important observations to come out of the last 20 years of molecular biology is that, in general, all cells tend to do the same things in the same way. This means that the observations on cellular clocks in humble fungi probably apply to the most sophisticated human beings. Such observations have identified at least seven genetic loci on chromosomes in fungi which are important for constructing or running cellular clocks. These have been identified as single alleles, and mutations of these cause changes in the periodicity of the clock. The *per* gene of the fruit-fly *Drosophila* has its products widely distributed in the fly's brain, particularly in neurones which appear to control rhythmic activity. The fly's *per* gene is similar to the human ARNT sequence that translocates specific cellular receptors and it may be that these two genetic sequences both serve the same function in these two very different organisms.

It seems then that the genetic code not only regulates the activity of cells and eventually organisms in terms of control in response to changing external conditions; but the code also imposes a rhythm of its own, whose beat was set into single cells at the very dawn of life on earth.

Further reading

Alberts B, Bray D, Lewis J, Raff M, Roberts K, Watson J 1994 *Molecular biology of the cell*, 3rd edn. Garland Publishing, New York.

A truly outstanding textbook, up to date and readable. Encyclopaedic in its coverage and spanning many disciplines. If you have to have a textbook of cell biology, this is the one.

Aldridge S 1996 *The thread of life: the story of genes and genetic engineering*. Cambridge University Press, Cambridge.

A monograph on the subject of DNA. Pleasantly didactic with emphasis on the practical importance of the new genetics.

Bernal J D, Synge A 1976 *The origin of life*. Oxford Biology Readers, Oxford University Press, Oxford.

A very brief and didactic introduction to the origins of life, which makes very comfortable reading.

Carpenter R H S 1996 *Neurophysiology*, 3rd edn. Arnold, London.

A very readable undergraduate textbook which comes with an interactive teaching computer program.

Cooper G M 1997 *The cell: a molecular approach*, 2nd edn. Sinauer Associates Incorporated, Sunderland, USA

An accessible introduction to current cell biology, less intimidating than many other textbooks on the subject.

Fillenz M 1990 *Noradrenergic neurons*. Cambridge University Press, Cambridge.

A monograph covering the development of our understanding of noradrenergic mechanisms.

Fox R F 1988 *Energy and the evolution of life*. W H Freeman, Basingstoke.

Innovative suggestions on the origins of life for the more advanced student with an interest in physics and chemistry.

Leaky R E 1986 *The Illustrated Origin of Species by Charles Darwin*. Abridged and introduced by R E Leaky. Faber & Faber, London.

This annotation and illustration of Darwin's classical work makes it accessible to all students interested in evolution.

Scientific American 1978 *Evolution*. W H Freeman, San Francisco.

Chapters 3 and 4 of this volume provide a very readable account of the origins of life at a level suitable for first year undergraduates.

Smith J M, Szathmary E 1997 *The major transitions in evolution*. Oxford University Press, Oxford.

One of the few books at this level to address the origins of life and the great transitions of evolution – the first eukaryotic cells, sexual reproduction, the appearance of multicellular organisms.

Stjarne L, Msghina M, Stjarne E 1990 *Upstream regulation of the release probability in sympathetic nerve varicosities*. Neuroscience 36: 571–587.

Contentious aspects of the regulation of the local control of sympathin release are reviewed in a stimulating manner.

Watson J D 1968 (reissued 1997) *The double helix*. Weidenfeld & Nicholson, London.

A wonderful personal account of the discovery of a fundamental building block in our understanding of nature. Most interesting if only for its description of a scientific community now passed.

Questions

Answer true or false to the following statements:

1.1

In a homeostatic control system:

A. There is a detector sensitive to the controlled variable.
B. Positive feedback is important.
C. The measured value of the controlled variable is compared with a reference value.
D. The controlled variable tends to oscillate around a mean value known as the set point.
E. Open loop control systems are frequently involved.

1.2

The plasmalemma:

A. Consists of a bilayer of phospholipids.
B. Is readily permeable to ionic substances.
C. Contains glycoproteins.
D. Is readily permeable to water.
E. Makes use of facilitated diffusion to maintain ionic gradients between the cytoplasm and the extracellular fluid.

1.3

With regard to osmosis across the plasmalemma:

A. Water moves up its potential gradient.
B. Cells will swell in hypotonic solutions.
C. The osmolality of a solution dictates its tonicity.
D. Proteins are the most important osmotically active solutes in the extracellular fluid.
E. Increased intracellular hydrostatic pressure would help to oppose osmotic swelling.

1.4

G-proteins:

A. Diffuse into the cell cytoplasm when activated.
B. Bind to GDP when activated by agonist–receptor complexes.
C. Consist of three main subunits.
D. May activate membrane-bound enzymes, leading to second messenger production.
E. Split off the α-subunit when active.

1.5

Depolarization:

A. In response to an electrical stimulus will be slower in cells with long time constants.
B. Refers to an increase in membrane potential.
C. During an action potential is caused by opening of voltage-activated ion channels.
D. Is associated with an increased membrane permeability to Na^+ in nerves and striated muscle.
E. Will close voltage-gated Na^+ channels.

1.6

Action potentials:

A. Are graded electrical events.
B. Are conducted over the surface of excitable cells.
C. Are produced by sub-threshold stimuli.
D. Inhibit further stimulation during or immediately after the action potential.
E. Are associated with a repolarization phase caused by outward movement of Cl^- ions.

(Answers overleaf →)

1.7

In excitable cells:

A. The conduction velocity is increased as the space constant increases.

B. Hypocalcaemia promotes spontaneous firing of action potentials.

C. The resting membrane potential is largely dictated by the Na^+ concentration gradient across the membrane.

D. GTP-energized ion pumps are used to maintain the transmembrane ion gradients.

E. Unidirectional propagation of the action potential is possible because of the refractory period.

1.8

With regard to junctions between cells:

A. Tight junctions help limit epithelial permeability.

B. Gap junctions are regions where cells are more widely spaced than normal.

C. Electrical syncytia depend on ion channels which connect the cytoplasm of adjacent cells.

D. Nexi show up as five lines in electron micrographs because the outer coats of the lipid membrane are fused.

E. Desmosomes promote the transmission of tension from cell to cell.

1.9

Membrane-bound receptors:

A. Bind to agonists according to the law of mass action.

B. May be structurally integrated into ligand-gated ion channels.

C. For acetylcholine may be classified as muscarinic or nicotinic.

D. Consist largely of carbohydrate.

E. Are frequently linked to G-proteins.

1.10

Second messengers:

A. Often activate specific kinases inside the cell.

B. Are usually manufactured by cytoplasmic enzymes.

C. Allow for amplification of an extracellular signal.

D. Include the cyclic nucleotides which are degraded by phosphatase enzymes.

E. Include Ca^{2+} which can be released from intracellular stores.

Answers

1.1

A. True.

B. False. Homeostasis requires negative feedback.

C. True. This occurs in the comparator or integrator and the reference value is known as the set point.

D. True. This oscillation is sometimes referred to as hunting. The size of the oscillation depends on both the inertia of the detectors and the amplification or gain of the output.

E. False. Homeostasis requires feedback, i.e. a closed loop control system.

1.2

A. True. The phospholipid molecules have both a hydrophilic region – the glycerol/phosphate segment of the phospholipid – and a hydrophobic region – the hydrocarbon chains of the fatty acids.

B. False. The lipid in the plasmalemma makes it permeable to lipid-soluble substances but relatively impermeable to ions which can only pass readily through the water-filled pores of ion channels or attached to carrier proteins.

C. True.

D. True. Water is small enough to diffuse through the free-space between the fatty acid hydrocarbon chains of the phospholipids.

E. False. Diffusion, whether simple or facilitated, always tends to reduce concentration gradients. Active transport is required to pump ions uphill against their concentration gradient, e.g. via the Na^+/K^+-ATPase pump.

1.3

A. False. Water moves down its potential gradient from regions of low solute concentration to regions of high solute concentration.

B. True. This is almost a definition of hypotonicity; since hypotonic solutions have less osmotic effect at the plasmalemma than normal extracellular fluid, water enters the cell, causing swelling.

C. False. Osmolality only depends on the number of particles per kg of solvent, whereas tonicity also depends on how easily the solute permeates the plasmalemma. An urea solution with the same osmolality as plasma is extremely hypotonic, causing almost immediate cell lysis, because urea diffuses readily across the plasmalemma and so has very little osmotic action. In other words, osmotic activity can only occur at a semipermeable membrane, i.e. one which allows the solvent but not the solute to permeate.

D. False. The total concentration, and therefore the osmotic effect, of protein molecules is about 1/300th of that of osmotically active ions, particularly Na^+ and Cl^-.

E. True. Hydrostatic pressure will help oppose osmotic absorption of water by the cell. With hypotonic solutions, water entry to the cell increases both the intracellular hydrostatic pressure and the intracellular water potential by dilution. Both effects tend to limit further water entry, and a new steady state may be reached at increased cell volume. If the extracellular solution is too hypotonic, however, mechanical stretch causes rupture, or lysis, of the plasmalemma.

1.4

A. False. They diffuse away from the receptor but remain in the membrane.

B. False. The α-subunit binds GTP when activated.

C. True. There are α-, β- and γ-subunits.

D. True.

E. True. The α-subunit bound to GTP splits off from the β- and γ-subunits when activated.

79

1.5

A. **True.** The time constant is a measure of how long it takes to charge up the membrane capacitance.

B. **False.** Depolarization refers to any change in membrane potential in the positive direction. By convention this is regarded as a decrease in membrane potential because the absolute size of the potential is reduced. This differs from standard mathematical practice which regards less negative values as larger.

C. **True.** Na^+ or Ca^{2+} channels open.

D. **True.** This is because of the opening of Na^+ channels.

E. **True.** This is inactivation; depolarization first activates but then inactivates Na^+ channels.

1.6

A. **False.** They are all-or-nothing responses.

B. **True.**

C. **False.** Threshold or supra-threshold stimuli produce action potentials.

D. **True.** The refractory period; this may be absolute or relative.

E. **False.** Repolarization is usually caused by an outward K^+ current.

1.7

A. **True.** This happens, for example, in myelinated nerves.

B. **True.** Normal levels of extracellular Ca^{2+} partially inhibit voltage-activated channels, preventing inappropriate spontaneous action potentials in nerves and skeletal muscle.

C. **False.** K^+ is the most important ion, because the resting permeability to K^+ is much higher than that to Na^+.

D. **False.** The pumps use ATP as an energy source.

E. **True.** This prevents previously excited membrane from being immediately re-excited.

1.8

A. **True.** They are particularly important in the gastrointestinal tract and the renal tubules.

B. **False.** These are regions where channels called connexons provide cytoplasmic continuity between cells.

C. **True.** This is one important function of gap junctions, e.g. in the heart.

D. **False.** A nexus is another name for a gap junction in which the bilipid layers of the cell membranes never come into contact with each other.

E. **True.** These structures form cell-to-cell links in adherens-type junctions.

1.9

A. **True.**

B. **True.** The best-understood example of this is the nicotinic receptor for acetylcholine at skeletal neuromuscular junctions.

C. **True.** The classification is based on their pharmacological agonist specificity.

D. **False.** They consist of protein.

E. **True.**

1.10

A. **True.** For example, cAMP activates protein kinase A.

B. **False.** The relevant synthetic enzymes are usually bound to the membrane.

C. **True.** This is one of their benefits.

D. **False.** They are degraded by phosphodiesterases; phosphatases remove phosphate groups from proteins.

E. **True.** Stores of Ca^{2+} are located particularly in the endoplasmic reticulum or the sarcoplasmic reticulum.

Muscle

2

Introduction

Muscle is perhaps the most conspicuous part of our bodies, making up about half of our adult mass. The muscles we see as fleshing out the structure of our bodies are attached to our skeletons and represent only one of three types. Two of these, the skeletal and cardiac muscles, appear striped when viewed under the microscope because of the regular arrangements of the proteins (actin and myosin) which make up their contractile mechanisms. They are therefore referred to as striated muscle. The skeletal muscles which cause movement of our body about its joints are attached to the skeleton by tough connecting structures called tendons. Skeletal muscles are under our conscious control and are therefore sometimes alternatively referred to as voluntary muscle. This type of muscle, because in part it represents a large fraction of our mass, accounts for a quarter of our oxygen consumption at rest; this oxygen usage can increase 20 times during vigorous exercise. The cells which make up skeletal muscle are called fibres because of their extremely elongated shape. Muscle fibres have the power to shorten to an amazing degree. Shortening is brought about by the molecules of their cells sliding between each other. When a whole skeletal muscle shortens, not all its fibres necessarily participate. A whole skeletal muscle is made up of groups of fibres called motor units, each commanded by a single motoneurone; as the demand for tension is increased, more and more of the members of this 'team' are recruited. It is common experience that our voluntary muscle can fatigue, although different muscle fibres have different abilities to resist fatigue.

Cardiac muscle on the other hand has built-in protection against fatigue, although even it can be worked beyond its considerable powers of endurance. Uniquely situated in the heart, it is important that all the cells of this muscle type act in unison. To ensure this synchronization, all cardiac muscle cells are in electrical contact with each other and contract spontaneously, independently of motor nerves, although nerves of the autonomic system influence the rhythm of this contraction.

The third type of muscle found in our bodies is smooth muscle, so called because its contractile structures, although the same as those found in skeletal and cardiac muscle, are not arranged in a regular way and so do not form striations. Smooth muscle is inconspicuous because it is largely restricted to internal organs but is important because these organs include arteries, veins, the urinary bladder and gut. Smooth muscle exhibits properties which make it well suited to form the walls of these hollow organs and its activity is in many cases spontaneous but modulated by hormonal and neural control.

Section overview

This section outlines:

- The three basic muscle types, their origins, development and differences

- The division of a voluntary muscle into its parts by connective tissue

- The structure of the myofilaments of actin and myosin which interdigitate to give striated muscle its striped appearance

- How Ca^{2+} controls contraction and how contraction is released

- Sliding filament theory and how this depends on crossbridge formation

- Details of crossbridge cycling powered by ATP

- Triggering of contraction by excitation–contraction coupling

- Elastic properties of muscle, which exist even when it is not contracting

- Isotonic and isometric contractions which can be pre- or afterloaded

- The energetics of contraction and how an O_2 debt develops

- Two major types of voluntary muscle, slow-twitch and fast-twitch

- Training effects and heat production

- The consequences of less organized smooth muscle general structure on its microscopic appearance and contractile properties

- Differences in innervation of the two types of smooth muscle

- How excitation and inhibition of smooth muscle differs from that of voluntary muscle

- The contractile mechanisms and mechanical properties of smooth muscle.

Cardiac muscle is dealt with in detail in Section 6.

Origin and types

Introduction

Movement is a universal characteristic of living material and may have evolved from the changing shape shown by some enzyme and protein molecules when they are involved in energy exchanges, usually linked to ATP.

Movement of this type – at a cellular level – drives the slow migration of the elements of the mitotic spindle in cell division, and displays several characteristics of the more rapid movements of the structures within muscles.

Muscle is a tissue with a very ancient history. The anaerobic biochemical pathways used by our muscles when the energy demands on them exceed their oxygen supply are probably the same as those used by cells over 3500 million years ago, before oxygen became a constituent of the earth's atmosphere. The humble and ancient amoeba extended its pseudopodia through primeval seas using the same body chemicals and energy sources that activate your fingers to turn these pages. Even the primitive ciliated organisms of prehistory caused their cilia to beat by mechanisms which can claim lineage with the basic mechanism that slides one filament of our muscles over another, causing them to contract (the protein involved in the cilium, dynein, is slightly different from that in our muscles but the principle is the same).

Basic Science 2.1.1

Muscle forces

Muscles are involved in producing forces, and consequently produce stress and strain within themselves and their tendons.

Force (L. *fortis* – strong). Force is an ambiguous concept, the meaning of which everyone understands but few can define. We can do worse than use one of the Oxford English Dictionary's definitions: 'an agency or influence that produces or tends to produce a change in the motion of a moving body, or produces motion or stress in a stationary body'.

When an external force is applied to a body it either moves or, if it is standing on a surface, say, and the applied force cannot produce movement, a reactionary force is generated such that the body is distorted by the two forces. In this case, the body's molecules are displaced from their rest positions. They tend to return to their original position and this tendency accounts for the **elasticity** of a body.

Stress is a measure of the cause of a deformation, and is defined by:

$$\text{Stress} = \frac{\text{Force}}{\text{Area}}.$$

The unit of stress is the pascal (Pa) or the newton per square metre (N/m^2): $1\ Pa = 1\ N/m^2$.

Thus the stress on a muscle depends not only on the force it is producing but also on its cross-sectional area.

Strain is a measure of the extent of deformation, and is defined by:

$$\text{Strain} = \frac{\text{Change in dimension (length say)}}{\text{Original dimension}}.$$

Muscles make up about half of the body mass and account for a large but extremely variable fraction of the body's metabolism (25% at rest). Skeletal muscle can alter its metabolic rate more than any other tissue, increasing its activity to more than 20 times its rest level. The demands for oxygen and nutrients and the need to remove metabolites and heat increase in step with this change in activity, and vigorous muscular activity is accompanied by increased activity in those organs which service the muscle's requirements.

Types of muscle

Muscle exists in three basic types:

- skeletal (voluntary) ⎫
- cardiac (heart)   ⎬ striated
- smooth (involuntary) ⎭ unstriated.

Development

All three types show their common origin in the embryo where mesodermal cells called **myoblasts** form **somites**, the origins of **skeletal muscles** (except those of parts of the head and limbs), and cells which, early in development, migrate to form the smooth and cardiac muscles of the body.

From the fifth to the eighth week of human embryonic development, muscles differentiate into their mature shapes and positions in the body. The paired somites (Fig. 2.1.1), which develop into the majority of skeletal muscles, are made up of distinct layers which form very different parts of the embryo. The **dermatome** (Gr. skin slice) develops into connective tissue, including the dermis of the skin. The **sclerotome** (Gr. hard slice) migrates to spaces around the developing spinal cord where it forms connective tissue.

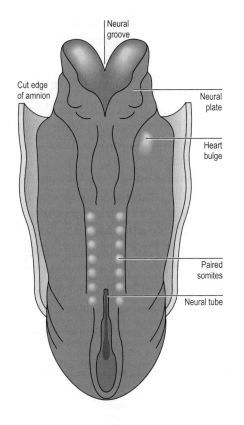

Neural
groove

Cut edge
of amnion

Neural
plate

Heart
bulge

Paired
somites

Neural tube

Fig. 2.1.1 Dorsal view of 21-day-old embryo. The paired somites are seen on either side of the neural tube.

The **myotome** (Gr. muscle slice) or middle layer of each somite is made up of cells which come to lie parallel with the long axis of the embryo and eventually differentiate into the majority of the skeletal muscles of the body. Some of the muscles of the anterior part of the body, however, are derived from branchial (gill) arch cells.

Like the two other types of muscle, **smooth muscle** develops from the middle layer of the three-layered early embryo (the mesoderm). Rather than forming paired somites like skeletal muscle, or developing at a single site like **cardiac muscle**, the primitive mesodermal cells of smooth muscle migrate to the linings of the developing digestive, vascular, respiratory, urinary and reproductive organs; and to the millions of individual sites in the skin where

they will make up the arrector pili muscles associated with single hairs.

Cardiac muscle develops very early, probably because the embryonic circulatory system is called upon even before the third week after fertilization to fulfil the nutritional and respiratory needs of the embryo. A tube of endocardium becomes covered with muscular myocardium and twisted into an S shape which by the fourth week can be seen to be dividing into functional segments.

We can see that even at this early age the muscles of our body are set along very different paths from their common mesodermal origin toward their final varied functions. Nevertheless, the prime function of muscle of any type, contraction, depends on a common 'sliding filament' mechanism, even though smooth muscle shows ingenious adaptations which enable it to be 'latched' or locked in a contracted state to save energy. This common sliding filament mechanism is built up in different ways to provide the varied structural basis of varied function. Thus in smooth muscle there is no practical limit to the distance the filaments can slide relative to each other and this gives smooth muscle its superior extensibility compared with skeletal or cardiac muscle. This difference is clearly seen in the way regularly repeated molecular structures of the sliding filaments give skeletal and cardiac muscle their striated appearance while smooth muscle structure has, until recently, eluded definition because, in part, of its irregular nature.

Innervation

The innervation of the types of muscle found in our bodies reflects the differences in the muscle fibres themselves. Skeletal muscle, utilized for immediate and rapid action or postural maintenance, is innervated by large-diameter motor nerves which can rapidly recruit more and more fibres to provide the force required. Smooth muscle on the other hand shows a degree of automatic contraction in response to stretch of the hollow organs it surrounds, and can also respond to activity in both branches of the autonomic nervous system, hormones in the blood, and intrinsic slow waves of membrane depolarization and repolarization. Cardiac muscle shows the extreme case of this independence from innervation and sets its own rate of contraction and relaxation that makes up the cardiac rhythm, although this is modified extensively by autonomic nerves.

Subdivisions

The three major types of muscle can themselves be subdivided:

- skeletal muscle into white, fast-twitch muscles and red, slow-twitch muscles

suitable for prolonged and steady contraction (although most human muscles are a mixture of both)
- smooth muscles into 'single-unit' (unitary), where large numbers of cells are united to form a sheet or mass, and 'multi-unit' where each fibre operates independently, usually in response to its individual innervation
- cardiac muscle into contractile cells that make up the atria and ventricles, and cells that conduct electrical impulses in the heart; the latter have lost most of their contractile ability, but are muscle cells nevertheless.

A comparison of some of the properties of types of muscles is made in Table 2.1.1.

Table 2.1.1 Differences between muscle types

Alternative names	Skeletal Voluntary Striated	Cardiac Heart	Smooth Visceral Unstriated
General structure	Bundles of cells with some connective tissue	Syncytium with little connective tissue	Sheet of cells or individual cells in connective tissue
Connection	Both ends to bones	To itself to form cavity	To itself to form cavity or tube
Cell size	10–100 µm diameter Very long (cms)	10–20 µm diameter 50–100 µm long forming a syncytium	2–5 µm diameter 100 µm long
Nuclei	Many per cell	One per cell	One per cell
Intracellular filaments	Regularly organized parallel to long axis of cell	Regularly organized parallel to long axis of cell	Run in many directions
Filament attachment	Intracellular Z-disk	Intracellular Z-disk	Dense bodies and dense bands
Mechanical connection of cells	In parallel. Can function independently	Connected end to end and in parallel. Function as a unit	Mechanically linked, all bear same stress
Innervation	Motor fibres	Autonomic	Autonomic
Effect of innervation on contraction	Contraction totally dependent on innervation	Innervation modifies contraction	Innervation initiates or modifies contraction

Table 2.1.1 *(continued)*

Alternative names	Skeletal Voluntary Striated	Cardiac Heart	Smooth Visceral Unstriated
Neuromuscular junction	Motor endplate	Free nerve terminals	Free nerve terminals and varicosities
Electrical activity	Stereotype brief action potential	Stereotype sustained action potential	Slow changes in membrane potential and action potentials
Excitation–contraction coupling	Troponin	Troponin	Calmodulin
Source of Ca^{2+} for contraction	Sarcoplasmic reticulum	Sarcoplasmic reticulum and extracellular fluid	Mainly ECF
Speed of contraction	Voluntarily controlled, fast or slow	Autonomically controlled, fast or slow	Generally slow
Metabolic cost of contraction	High	High	Low

Summary

Differences and similarities between muscle types

- Muscle exists in three types – skeletal, cardiac (both striated) and smooth (unstriated).
- All types originate from the embryonic mesoderm.
- All muscular contraction depends on a common 'sliding filament' mechanism.

- The muscle types show clear differences in the way their cells are connected, their innervation, type of electrical activity and speed of contraction.
- The three major types can be further subdivided in terms of their metabolic, electrical and mechanical properties.

Striated muscle

2.2

Introduction

Skeletal and cardiac muscles are striated because the orderly arrangement of the contractile proteins **actin** and **myosin** which make up the majority of their bulk gives them a striped (striated) appearance of light and dark bands. We will first consider skeletal muscle (sometimes called voluntary muscle because it is usually consciously activated). Cardiac muscle is dealt with in detail in Section 6 in the context of the structure and function of the heart.

The parts of a muscle

A skeletal muscle is made up of very many individual multinucleate muscle cells or **fibres**, so called because of their elongated shape (Fig. 2.2.1). These are composed of the functional units of striated muscle, the **myofibrils**, which in turn consist of the contractile mechanisms of muscle, interacting myosin and actin filaments.

The individual muscle cells are held together by fibrous connective tissue, **fascia**.

The connective tissue which covers the whole skeletal muscle is **epimysium**. That which separates the muscle fibres into bundles (fasciculi) is **perimysium** and that which covers individual muscle fibres (single muscle cells) is **endomysium**. These connective tissues are continued beyond the body of the muscle, gradually blending into a **tendon** which attaches the

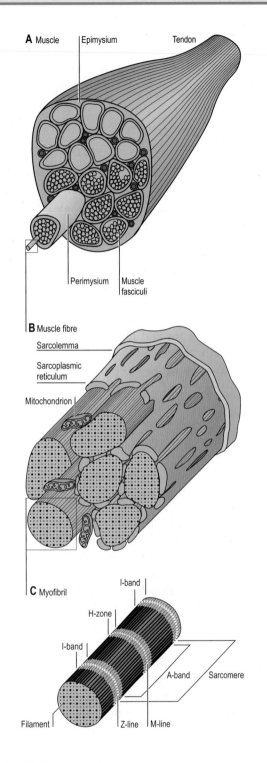

Fig. 2.2.1 The parts of a muscle. The component parts of a voluntary muscle, from the functional units (myofibrils) to the epimysium which contains the whole muscle and is continuous with the tendons of origin and insertion. **A.** Muscle. **B.** Muscle fibre (cell). **C.** Myofibril.

skeletal muscle to bone or cartilage. Tendons which are in the form of thin sheets are called **aponeuroses**. The tendon attaching a muscle to a stationary part of the body, the body trunk for example, is called the **origin**. The more mobile tendon is the **insertion** and is usually distal.

The arrangement of the cells in a skeletal muscle is ideally suited to producing a controlled, graded response to order. The cells are enormously long and all are parallel to each other. Each cell is part of a motor unit consisting of those cells activated by a single motoneurone. A muscle is made up of many motor units. Thus the force exerted by an individual muscle is determined by the number of motor units activated and the intensity of that activation.

Skeletal muscles almost invariably come in opposing pairs. A skeletal muscle cannot return to its rest length of its own accord after

Summary

Structure of striated muscle

- A striated muscle is made up of fasciculi made up of fibres made up of fibrils made up of filaments.
- Muscle fibres (muscle cells) are bound together by connective tissue endomysium, the fasciculus so formed is covered by perimysium and the bundle of fasciculi which makes up a muscle is covered by epimysium.
- A striated muscle cell contains many nuclei.
- The connective tissue covering the contractile elements of a muscle blend together to form the proximal tendon of origin and the more distal and mobile tendon of insertion.
- Skeletal muscles usually come in opposing pairs because a muscle cannot return to its rest length of its own accord and must therefore be stretched.

contracting, but must depend on an opposing muscle or gravity to stretch it. Similarly, smooth and cardiac muscle in the walls of hollow organs rely on internal pressure to stretch them back to their rest length after contracting.

Skeletal muscles (Fig. 2.2.2) are often described, rather fancifully, in terms of their shape, as, for example, pennate (feather-like) or digastric (two stomachs).

Fine structure of a muscle

Functional units

The major characteristic of skeletal muscle is its ability to produce tension and shorten in a controlled fashion. This graded response results from activation of increasing numbers of functional units (motor units) within the whole muscle.

The cells of skeletal muscle are very long (see Fig. 2.2.1), often extending the whole length of small muscles (although several end-to-end are required to extend the length of most muscles), and very thin, 10–100 μm in diameter. The muscle cell is multinucleated with sometimes as many as several hundred nuclei in a single fibre. Large muscles contain large-diameter fibres while small muscles contain small-diameter fibres. The diameters of all fibres in a particular muscle are about the same. All these cells lie parallel with the long axis of the muscle.

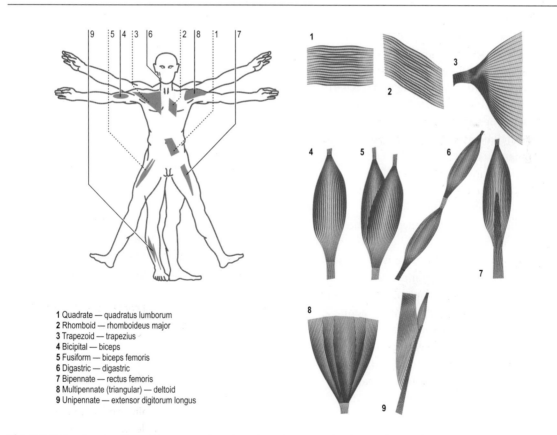

1 Quadrate — quadratus lumborum
2 Rhomboid — rhomboideus major
3 Trapezoid — trapezius
4 Bicipital — biceps
5 Fusiform — biceps femoris
6 Digastric — digastric
7 Bipennate — rectus femoris
8 Multipennate (triangular) — deltoid
9 Unipennate — extensor digitorum longus

Fig. 2.2.2 Muscle types. The architecture, and naming, of muscle types, is closely related to the function of the muscle. A strap muscle, for example, has all its fascicles running parallel to the long axis of the muscle. Pennate (feather-like) muscles have many short fascicles set at an angle to a tendon which extends the whole length of the muscle. Circular muscles, which do not attach to a tendon, are a rather rare form of voluntary muscle and include the orbicularis oris which encircles the mouth, the orbicularis oculi which surrounds the eye and the muscles of the external anal sphincter.

Duchenne muscular dystrophy

The muscular dystrophies are a group of
inherited diseases which usually affect skeletal
but occasionally cardiac muscle. The Duchenne
form affects only boys and the locus of the
defect has been identified on the Xp21 region
of the X chromosome. It occurs in 1 in 3000
boys, both as a result of inheritance and, in
1 out of 3 cases, as a result of spontaneous
mutation. The sister of an affected individual
has a 50% chance of carrying the defective
gene and a 70% chance of having raised
creatine phosphokinase levels in her blood,
a fact used in diagnosis. Accurate carrier and
prenatal diagnosis can be made using cDNA
probes that are co-inherited with the
dystrophic locus on the gene.

The result of this defect is the absence of
dystrophin, a rod-shaped protein that is part
of the muscle cytoskeleton. Muscle biopsy
shows disorder of the cytostructure of the
cells with some fibres becoming hypertrophic
and others atrophic. There is fibre necrosis
and replacement of fibres by fat. The
deposition of large amounts of fat and
connective tissue gives this disease the
alternative name of pseudohypertrophic
muscular paralysis.

The condition is usually obvious by the age
of 5 with the boy showing great weakness, so
much so that he has to 'climb up his legs with
his hands' to stand upright (Gower's sign).
There is no cure. The boy is usually severely
disabled by the age of 10 with the
myocardium becoming affected and he
seldom survives beyond his teens. Death
commonly results from involvement of the
respiratory muscles.

Within each cell are thick and thin **myofilaments** which are the physical basis of muscle contraction. The cytoplasm surrounding the myofilaments is the **sarcoplasm**. The muscle cell, and therefore the myofilaments within it, is divided at very regular intervals along its length into **sarcomeres**. The sarcomeres are separated by Z-disks which segment the muscle cell into compartments, somewhat like a tube train is divided into compartments. In longitudinal histological sections, these disks are cut through and appear as **Z-lines**. To the Z-lines are attached thin actin myofilaments held in strict hexagonal array (Fig. 2.2.3). The **I-band** (seen as a light band in a micrograph of striated

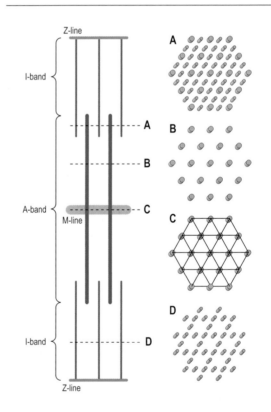

Fig. 2.2.3 Structure of a sarcomere. Longitudinal (left) and cross-sectional (right) diagrams showing the arrangement of actin (thin) and myosin (thick) filaments. The light and dark bands of a sarcomere, extending between two Z-lines, are the result of the presence of:

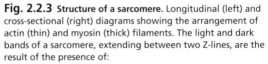

- actin filaments only (I-band; section D)
- actin and myosin filaments (A-band; section A)
- myosin filaments only (H-zone; section B).

muscle) extends from either side of the Z-line to the beginning of the thick myosin myofilaments which make up the **A-band**. The width of the I-band and the light **H-zone** in the centre of the sarcomere (see Fig. 2.2.1C) depend on the state of contraction of the muscle. A disk of delicate filaments, the **M-line**, in the middle of the H-zone holds the myosin myofilaments in position, each surrounded, outside the H-zone, by six actin filaments.

Structure of the myofilaments

The actin filaments which stretch from the Z-lines consist of two helical strands of **F-actin**, each made up of approximately 200 units of globular **G-actin**. The whole is like two strands of a bead necklace twined together (Fig. 2.2.4A). On each of the 'beads' is a site where myosin can bind during contraction. Laid along the grooves between the two actin strands and

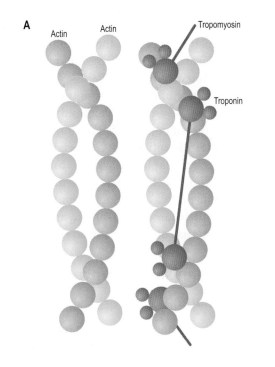

A Actin Actin Tropomyosin

Troponin

Fig. 2.2.4 Filaments.

A. The actin 'thin filament' consists of a 1 μm long double-stranded helix of F-actin made up of molecules of G-actin with strands of tropomyosin stretched between troponin complexes covering units of 7G-actin molecules. Ca^{2+} interacts with the troponin complex to alter the configuration of tropomyosin and allow the bridging of actin and myosin.

B. The myosin 'thick filament' is 1.5 μm long and 15 nm diameter. It is made up of about 200 myosin molecules shaped like golf clubs with double heads. (i) Each myosin molecule consists of a tail of two coiled peptide chains of 'light meromyosin' and a head of two units of 'heavy meromyosin' and four light chains which exert regulatory functions. The ATPase activity of the molecule appears to be concentrated in the head. (ii) The myosin molecules are set in the filament with their tails toward the centre so that the heads are concentrated towards two ends leaving the centre portion bare. (iii) It is suggested that there are two 'hinges' in the molecule, one where the light and heavy meromyosin of the tail meet and one below the head. The light meromyosin of the tail is thought to be fixed to the body of the thick filament and the heavy component of the tail can tilt out to allow the head to engage the actin filament.

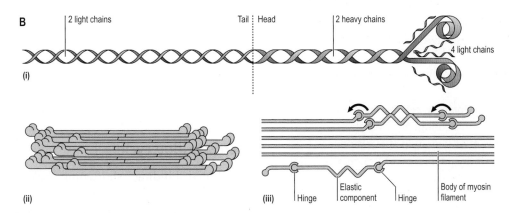

B 2 light chains Tail : Head 2 heavy chains 4 light chains

(i)

(ii) (iii) Hinge Elastic component Hinge Body of myosin filament

93

governing their binding to myosin are two strands made up of **tropomyosin**, a long molecule stretching along seven G-actin 'beads', and alternating with molecules of **troponin**, which has affinities for actin, tropomyosin, and calcium.

The tropomyosin is like a cable slung between pylons of troponin, which govern the cable's position and are themselves, in turn, controlled by Ca²⁺ concentration.

The myosin filaments that make up the A-band of a sarcomere, each surrounded by six actin filaments, are of a very different structure. They consist of approximately 100 myosin molecules, each shaped like a golf club with a double head. About 50 molecules have their 'heads' pointing in one direction, and 50 point in the other (Fig. 2.2.4B(ii)). The 'head' of the molecule is hinged and the shaft is capable of shortening. ATPase in the heads can release energy from ATP and cause the head to bind to the active site on an actin molecule. This

connection is called a **crossbridge**. Because the myosin heads are all concentrated at the two ends of the filament, the centre cannot form crossbridges and makes up the central part of the H-zone of the sarcomere.

Cell membrane systems – the supply of Ca²⁺

Packed between the myofibrils are numerous mitochondria and glycogen granules as might be found in many other types of active cell. However, muscle cells have a unique arrangement of regular invaginations of the sarcolemma which project into the fibre and wrap round the sarcomeres where the actin and myosin filaments overlap. Being continuous with the exterior of the cell, these **transverse** or **T-tubules** contain extracellular fluid. Near the T-tubules, the smooth endoplasmic reticulum, the **sarcoplasmic reticulum**, a specialized part of the intracellular network of tubules, is enlarged to form **terminal cisternae** which actively transport calcium ions from the sarcoplasm into their lumen. A T-tubule and its two adjacent cisternae are called a **triad** (Fig. 2.2.5).

The mechanism of contraction

Sliding filaments

When muscles shorten, the filaments of actin and myosin which make up a sarcomere do not shorten; rather they slide past each other like the fingers of two hands interdigitating. Actin and myosin molecules bind strongly to each other both in vitro and in vivo. In muscle this binding of myosin heads to the actin chain must be cyclical and involve many repeated shortenings of the myosin shaft to make up the substantial contraction of a whole active muscle.

The crossbridge cycle

The repeated binding, shortening, releasing and re-binding of crossbridges is something like a man climbing hand-over-hand up a rope

Summary

Structure of striated cells

- The cytoplasm of a muscle cell is called sarcoplasm and contains long, thick and thin myofilaments parallel with the long axis of the cell.
- The overlapping of these filaments gives voluntary muscle its striped appearance.
- The structures between two Z-lines make up a sarcomere.
- Myofilaments are thick (myosin) or thin (actin).
- The interaction between thick and thin filaments which brings about contraction is the result of formation of crossbridges – a result of the interaction of troponin and Ca²⁺.

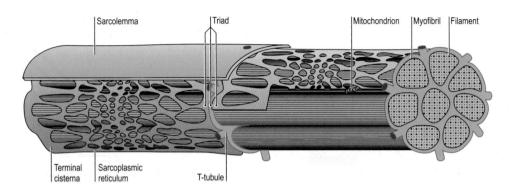

Fig. 2.2.5 **Triads.** The tubular system of a sarcomere consists of an intracellular sarcoplasmic reticulum which is made up of branching longitudinal tubes which enlarge into terminal cisternae where they abut the extracellular transverse, T-tubule system at the A-band–I-band junction. During contraction the junction moves in relation to the triads.

(Fig. 2.2.6). Recent research suggests that the myosin filaments rotate as they interact with the six actin filaments that surround them and bond with alternate myofilaments. So it may be more like a man climbing up six ropes but grasping only three.

In this **sliding filament theory** of muscle contraction, crossbridges are formed asynchronously so that some are 'gripping' while others are 'changing their grip'. This enables tension to be sustained. Myosin heads, which form crossbridges, only occur at the ends of the myosin filaments. This explains the fall off of tension with length on either side of a maximum value when a muscle is stimulated (Fig. 2.2.7).

Overstretching muscle does not allow the optimum number of crossbridges to make contact (Fig. 2.2.7(a)). Below the optimal length, crossbridges on the myosin are covered by actin filaments 'going the wrong way' (Fig. 2.2.7(b)), and eventually the myosin filament extends the whole length of the sarcomere (Fig. 2.2.7(c)), and can go no further.

The activity of the actomyosin crossbridges which bind actin filaments to myosin represents the fundamental process converting chemical energy into contraction by muscle. Each crossbridge has essential structural features which are involved in the contraction cycle. These

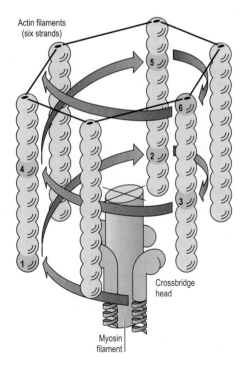

Fig. 2.2.6 **A myosin head 'climbing' its six actin filaments.** The myosin crossbridge binds with alternate actin filaments of the six that surround its myosin filament. The crossbridges on the myosin come in pairs at 180° to each other (like a nail driven right through a rod of wood), at 14.3-nm intervals along the filament, and with each pair turned through 120°. Therefore, in a straight line along the myosin filament, crossbridges occur directly underneath each other at every third interval ($3 \times 14.3 = 42.9$ nm).

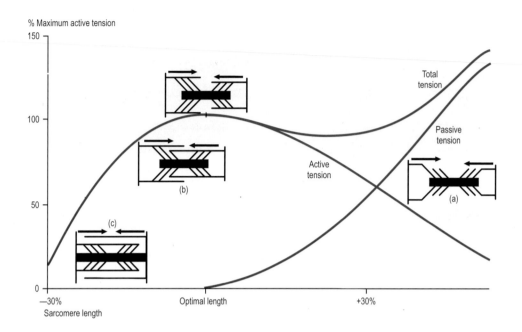

Fig. 2.2.7 **Length/tension of skeletal muscle.** The passive (due to stretching of elastic elements), active (due to contraction of sarcomeres alone) and total (sum of passive + active) tension in a skeletal muscle in relation to the optimal length for active tension production. The submaximal tension of the active curve on either side of the optimal length is due at (a) to the sarcomeres being so stretched that the filaments do not overlap and crossbridges cannot form, (b) the filaments overlapping to such a degree that crossbridges at the ends of the myosin filaments meet actin filaments 'coming in the wrong direction', (c) the myosin filament stretching from end to end of the sarcomere.

include a double head of myosin which contains the ATPase activity of the crossbridge and the potential to bind strongly to actin while at the same time rotating hinge-like relative to the crossbridge shaft (Fig. 2.2.8).

The shaft itself also has a 'hinge' where it joins the myosin filament, and elastic properties which can store energy when put under tension by rotation of the crossbridge head. X-ray diffraction studies demonstrate that the crossbridges form a spiral along the myosin filament with an interval of 14.3 nm between bridges. This interval is so tiny it will be clear that each bridge will have to 'pull itself along' the actin filament many times to produce any significant shortening of the whole muscle. The cyclic nature of this 'hand-over-hand' activity is probably as follows, and shown in Figure 2.2.8.

In resting muscle the crossbridge lies parallel to the myosin filament with its head perpendicular to it and not attached to the actin filament (1 in the cycle).

When contraction is triggered by release of Ca^{2+} from the sarcoplasmic reticulum (see below) the actin filament can accept the myosin head, which swings out to bind with it (2 in the cycle).

After attachment, the head tilts (3) using the energy stored in the myosin–ATP complex of the head. This is the power stroke of the crossbridge which stretches its elastic component to provide the energy to drag the actin filament along (4). ADP and P are released at this time which means that the head is primed to accept another ATP molecule which will cause it to detach (5).

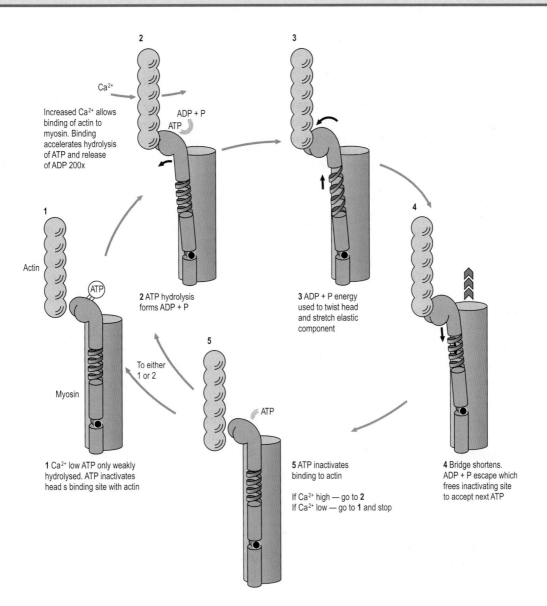

Fig. 2.2.8 The crossbridge cycle and the reactions which provide its energy.

Step 1. When Ca^{2+} concentration is low (less than 10^{-7} M), ATP in the crossbridge head is only weakly hydrolysed. The binding site on the actin filament is also blocked, so only weak, if any, crossbridges are formed.

Step 2. Elevated levels of Ca^{2+} allow the binding of the crossbridge head to the actin filament. Actin is a cofactor for myosin ATPase, increasing the rate-limiting step for hydrolysis and increasing by 200 times the release of ADP and P. Liberation of P binds the crossbridge more tightly.

Step 3. Energy from the hydrolysis of ATP causes the head of the crossbridge to twist, which stretches the elastic component of the shaft.

Step 4. The elastic component retracts drawing the actin filament along – this is the shortening step. ADP and P escape from the head, freeing the site for another molecule of ATP.

Step 5. The arrival of a new molecule of ATP in the crossbridge head releases its binding from the actin filament. Things can now go one of two ways. If Ca^{2+} is abundant, binding sites are still exposed on the actin and the cycle continues with attachment at a new binding site. If Ca^{2+} has been reabsorbed into the sarcoplasmic reticulum, the ATP is not fully hydrolysed and inhibits strong binding.

The cycle will continue until Ca^{2+} is removed by control systems which bring about relaxation or until ATP is exhausted and the muscle goes into **rigor**, as in **rigor mortis** of death when a large percentage of crossbridges remain attached to the actin filaments. ATP therefore acts at two points in the process of contraction:

1. it provides energy for contraction, and
2. it detaches the crossbridge from actin to allow the attachment–contraction–detachment cycle to be repeated. This is known as a plasticizing effect.

The energetics of a crossbridge cycling is outlined in Figure 2.2.8. The absolute permissive role of Ca^{2+} in allowing crossbridge formation is being questioned. It is now thought that up to 25% of the myosin heads maintain a weak binding even during relaxation and the block of crossbridge formation in the absence of Ca^{2+} is not as complete as was once supposed.

Summary

Initiation of striated muscle contraction

- Within a sarcomere, transverse T-tubules are sandwiched between terminal cisternae to form triads which control calcium levels in the sarcoplasm.
- Increased Ca^{2+} levels in the sarcoplasm initiate muscle contraction.
- Contraction is brought about by the sliding of actin and myosin filaments over each other.
- Sliding of filaments is brought about by the cyclic formation, shortening and release of crossbridges.
- Crossbridge formation is powered by the hydrolysis of ATP.

Triggering and types of contraction

Triggering contraction

The mechanism by which an action potential produced in the sarcolemma at the neuromuscular junction (see Section 3) triggers contraction of a muscle is called **excitation–contraction coupling**.

The interaction of Ca^{2+} with troponin, which holds tropomyosin in place, covering the binding sites for myosin crossbridges on actin, is central to this process.

When a muscle fibre is at rest, the sarcoplasmic reticulum pumps Ca^{2+} out of the sarcoplasm into the cisternae where most of it is stored by binding reversibly to a protein, **calsequestrin**. Ca^{2+} in the sarcoplasm is reduced to $0.1 \, \mu mol/l$, which is below the level which influences troponin orientation. To initiate contraction, a muscle action potential initiated by a motor nerve spreads rapidly over the sarcolemma and into the transverse tubules, opening Ca^{2+} channels in the membrane.

Ca^{2+} floods out of the cisternae into the sarcoplasm, raising the concentration to more than $10 \, \mu mol/l$, saturating binding sites on troponin. Activating these sites on troponin molecules causes them to allow the tropomyosin molecules strung between them to penetrate deeper into the groove between the two actin chains. This exposes sites which allow the myosin crossbridges to bond more strongly with the actin and begin the contraction cycle. The contraction will be maintained as long as the level of Ca^{2+} is high. The duration of a **twitch** (see Fig. 2.2.9) produced by a single action potential therefore depends on the rate at which the sarcoplasmic reticulum can pump Ca^{2+} back into the terminal cisternae. Fast-twitch fibres achieve this deactivation in 10 ms; slow-twitch fibres may take 50 ms. Human muscles are not made up exclusively of one or the other type of fibre but of different proportions of the two. The properties of the two major skeletal muscle types are listed in Table 2.2.1. Type II fibres can be further divided into Types IIa and IIb, where IIa fibres are more similar to Type I fibres.

Resting tension

Even when the contractile elements of a muscle have not been activated, it still exerts tension when stretched. This means that it has passive elastic properties and these are thought to be both in **series** and in **parallel** with the contractile elements (Fig. 2.2.10). Although the tendons and connective tissue of a whole muscle form obvious sites of elasticity in series with the contractile elements, it has now been shown that

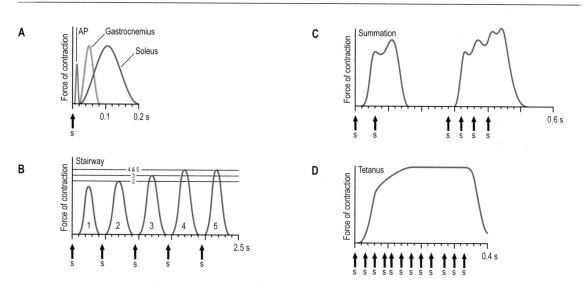

Fig. 2.2.9 Muscle stimulation at different frequencies. A. Single twitches of relatively fast (gastrocnemius) and slow muscles resulting from a stimulus (S) which produces a single action potential (AP). **B.** A stairway of increasing force of contraction resulting from repeated stimulation, at a frequency too low to produce summation, of a muscle which has been resting for some time. Eventually a plateau of force is reached (action potential is not shown). **C.** Summation of single twitches produced by stimuli applied at too great a rate to allow the muscles to completely relax between contractions. **D.** Tetanus where high rates of stimulation produce complete fusion of contractions.

Table 2.2.1 Comparison of skeletal muscle types			
	Type I	**Type IIa**	**Type IIb**
Alternative names	Slow, oxidative (red)	Fast, oxidative (red)	Fast, glycolytic (white)
Fibre diameter (diffusion distance)	Intermediate	Small	Large
Oxidative capacity (capillary density, mitochondria, myoglobin)	High	Very high	Low
Twitch duration	Long	Short	Short
Motor unit size	Small	Intermediate	Large
Recruitment order	Early	Intermediate	Late
Resistance to fatigue	Best	Intermediate	Worse

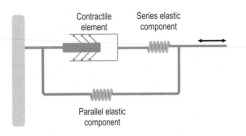

Fig. 2.2.10 A physical model of the components of skeletal muscle. The model shows the contractile element made up of actin and myosin and the elastic components which explain the behaviour of a whole muscle. Although the elastic components are shown outside the contractile element, a substantial proportion of both resides within the contractile mechanism.

even single skeletal muscle fibres have elasticity; which may reside in the 'hinges' or elastic components of the crossbridges themselves. The parallel component of muscle elasticity can, to a large extent, be attributed to the sarcolemma. There is, however, an additional intracellular contribution made by the highly elastic protein **titin** (tubulin), which forms a network around the actin and myosin filaments and probably contributes to the high resting tension at long sarcomere lengths when crossbridge formation is not possible (Fig. 2.2.7).

Isometric and isotonic contractions

Stimulation of a motoneurone results, after a **latent period** while excitation–contraction coupling is achieved, in contraction of a group of muscle fibres. The structure – motoneurone plus the muscle fibres it activates – is a **motor unit**.

Muscle fibres are only innervated by one motoneurone; so, while many (or few depending on the muscle) fibres can be innervated by one motoneurone, a muscle fibre can only have one motoneurone. Thus the total force developed by a skeletal muscle depends on:

- **Summation** of individual twitches which takes place when a second stimulus follows on a first stimulus before all the Ca^{2+}

released has been resequestered and the sliding filaments have returned to their original position (Fig. 2.2.9).
- **Recruitment** when more and more motor units become active, recruiting more and more fibres. Those units associated with small numbers of fibres are recruited first. This means that we can apply a force with our muscles in a graded fashion, starting off gently and building up the tension. Also, muscles performing delicate precise movements are made up of motor units with small numbers of muscle fibres; muscles performing crude, powerful movements have motor units with many muscle fibres. The muscles of the eye have units of about 10 fibres. The muscles of the leg have units of several hundred.

Summation of twitches ultimately results in a **tetanus**, which is the normal type of contraction we use to lift and hold a weight (Fig. 2.2.9). To contract in this way a muscle must:

- respond to high levels of Ca^{2+} with sustained crossbridge formation
- have single twitches which last longer than a muscle action potential (so that action potentials can arrive at a rate that ensures that the Ca^{2+} concentration is maintained by repeated release).

When a muscle attempts to contract against an immovable load it is said to undergo an **isometric** (constant length) contraction in which **tension** in the muscle increases. If a muscle is already supporting a weight before it contracts, the weight, and therefore the tension in the muscle, does not increase with the contraction, which is **isotonic** (constant tension), but the muscle shortens.

If skeletal muscle which has been resting for some time is activated by a rapid but subtetanic series of stimulations, the successive contractions produced increase in amplitude until a steady-state is reached. In other words, the steady-state is not reached with the first stimulation. This is

Contracture

This term is used clinically to describe sustained shortening of a muscle (or other tissue such as a burn or scar). In the context of muscle, the important difference between contrac*ture* and a sustained (tetanic) contrac*tion* is the absence of action potentials in the muscle sarcolemma.

In normal muscle contraction, a single suprathreshold stimulus of the motor nerve generates an action potential which is transmitted to the muscle and generates a muscle action potential. This spreads rapidly over the sarcolemma, initiating contraction, which follows at a much slower rate.

This excitation–contraction coupling depends on the release of Ca^{2+} and is terminated by the removal of Ca^{2+} back to its storage sites within the muscle. If this removal does not take place, a sustained contracture results.

The contracture is the result of some pathology short-circuiting the normal excitation–contraction mechanism. Muscle action potentials may be present or absent but they are irrelevant because the contraction mechanism is now being controlled further down the chain of command.

Contractures are seen in a variety of conditions including McArdle's disease (see below), muscular dystrophy and malignant hyperthermia. If the underlying pathology can be reversed they disappear.

called the '**staircase**' phenomenon. If the rate of stimulation is suddenly decreased, the amplitude of contraction decreases with successive stimulations until the second steady-state is reached. The staircase phenomenon is best, and was first, observed in cardiac muscle, and is thought to be due to the distribution of Ca^{2+} within the cell changing with changes in stimulus frequency.

High levels of Ca^{2+} persisting after tetanic stimulation of a muscle also explain the exaggerated single twitch displayed by fast muscles after a period of tetanus; and pharmacological agents which promote the release, or prevent the uptake, of Ca^{2+} can produce a state of prolonged contraction in the absence of action potentials, known as **contracture**.

Preload and afterload

When a muscle is stimulated directly or via its motor nerve, there is a delay or **latent period** before tension begins to develop. This is only in part due to the time taken up by excitation–contraction coupling. The rest of the time is taken in stretching elastic elements of the muscle in series with the contractile elements. By loading or stretching the muscle in different ways, the nature of the contractile process and the part played by elastic tissue have been investigated.

A **preloaded** muscle is stretched by the weight it supports even before it begins to contract (Fig. 2.2.11). The latent period before it begins to lift (or attempts to lift) the weight is largely due to the time taken by excitation–contraction coupling and is fairly constant. Because the overall time from stimulation to the end of contraction is constant, the duration of the mechanical process of contraction is also constant. The distance shortened by the muscle, however, depends on the load being lifted.

When a muscle is **afterloaded**, the elastic tissue in series with the contractile portion is

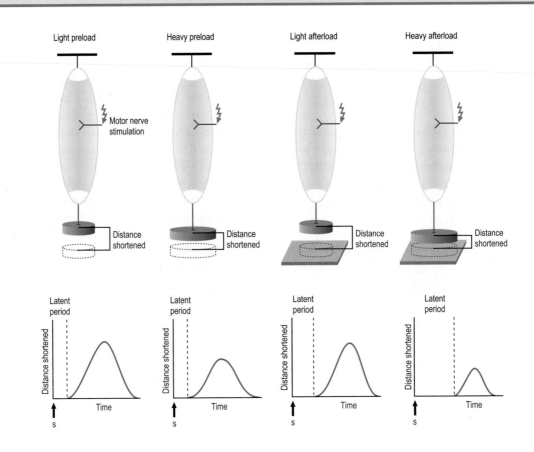

Fig. 2.2.11 Preloading and afterloading: the effects on muscle shortening and latency in response to a single stimulation. Increasing preload does not affect latent period and slightly reduces the distance shortened. Increasing afterload increases the latent period and reduces the distance shortened.

slack. (The load is supported in such a way as to be closer to the muscle than its resting length.) When an afterloaded muscle contracts it must first take up this slack and then put sufficient tension in the elastic element to lift the load before any shortening of the whole muscle is seen. Because the latent period now incorporates the time taken to stretch the elastic component to a tension that will lift the load, latent period is now proportional to the afterload. This encroaches on the total time for the twitch and so the duration of the mechanical shortening and the distance shortened both depend on the afterload on the muscle (Fig. 2.2.11).

The relationship between passive, active and total tension of a muscle in relation to its length can, in part, be explained in terms of its active component and the elastic component in series with it (Fig. 2.2.7). It now seems that the interdigitation of the actin and myosin filaments is inadequate to explain the rising phase of the total tension curve, and that Ca^{2+} sensitivity of the actin filaments, which is influenced by muscle length, is involved.

![icon] **Summary**

The build-up of tension in a striated muscle

- Excitation–contraction coupling involves an action potential spreading from the neuromuscular junction releasing Ca^{2+} from the cisternae of the sarcoplasmic reticulum.
- Ca^{2+} in the sarcoplasm promotes the movement of tropomyosin to expose binding sites which form contractile crossbridges between the actin and the myosin.
- The duration of a single muscle twitch is largely determined by the rate at which Ca^{2+} can be removed from the sarcoplasm.
- Single twitches can summate, ultimately resulting in a tetanus.

- Muscles have elastic components in series and parallel with their contractile components. These produce a passive tension on stretching.
- The functional unit of a muscle is a motor unit. These are recruited sequentially as a muscle increases its tension.
- Attempted contraction against an immovable load is called isometric contraction. Contraction which produces constant tension by moving a constant load is called isotonic.
- A muscle is preloaded when its load produces tension even before it begins to contract.
- A muscle is afterloaded when it must contract before it begins to lift its load.

Muscle energetics and oxygen debt

The source of energy used for all the molecular activities of resting or active muscle is ATP. The majority of this is used to:

- drive the Na^+/K^+ pump which maintains ionic gradients across the sarcolemma
- resequester the Ca^{2+} into the cisternae
- power contraction.

Of course, in an active muscle, contraction is the major user of ATP. The production of ATP can be the result of **anaerobic** respiration (without oxygen), which breaks glucose down into ATP and lactic acid, or **aerobic** respiration (with oxygen) when ATP, carbon dioxide and water are formed. Aerobic respiration is much more efficient than anaerobic, producing 38 molecules of ATP from each glucose molecule, compared to anaerobic respiration's 2. However, anaerobic respiration more rapidly supplies ATP, especially when oxygen, and therefore aerobic metabolism, is limited.

A major problem for muscles follows the immediate demand for energy during the first few seconds of exercise, after which the normal resting levels of ATP would be exhausted. To help avoid this, a second immediate reserve of energy exists in the form of **creatine phosphate**, which can donate phosphate to ADP to form ATP, becoming itself creatine. When a muscle is at rest, the excess ATP present favours the formation of creatine phosphate. In a resting muscle, glucose is stored as **glycogen** and in such a muscle, or one undergoing sustained moderate exercise, aerobic respiration synthesizes ATP from glucose or more usually **fatty acids**. During intense exercise, anaerobic respiration and the breakdown of creatine phosphate provide energy for a brief period (10–20 s), limited by the depletion of creatine phosphate and glucose and the build-up of lactic acid, which diffuses out of the muscle cell to allow anaerobic respiration to proceed for a little longer. Some of the lactic acid that enters the blood is re-synthesized to glucose by an energy-requiring pathway in the liver. This glucose can then be

McArdle's disease

McArdle's is a rare autosomal recessive glycogen storage disease. Unlike most of these diseases which manifest themselves very early in life, McArdle's presents in adults.

Glycogen can be made to a limited extent by all cells but the major manufacturers and users are liver and muscle. Glycogen is broken down in normal muscle by muscle phosphorylase to provide energy after the short-term fuels, ATP and creatine phosphate, have been used up. The end-product of this energy source is lactic acid. Patients with McArdle's disease specifically lack the muscle phosphorylase enzyme and so the effects of losing this glycogen energy source are restricted to the skeletal muscle system.

These effects, as could be predicted, are fatigue and painful muscle cramps. The absence of phosphorylase means that lactic acid is not produced and tests for this disease include demonstrated absence of lactic acid by nuclear magnetic resonance, absence of lactic acid in the venous blood after anaerobic exercise or absence of phosphorylase in a muscle biopsy. High glucose or fructose diets have been reported to produce some improvement but patients usually have to modify their lifestyles to avoid the symptoms.

reused by the muscles that produced the lactic acid. This is the **Cori cycle**.

It was once thought that the elevated oxygen consumption after exercise – used to repay what is called the **oxygen debt** – was the result of the activity of the Cori cycle after the end of exercise. It now appears that much of the oxygen consumption after exercise is due not to the lactic acid Cori cycle but to changes in circulation, body temperature and hormone levels persisting after the end of exercise (Fig. 2.2.12).

Fibre types and training

The capability of some muscles to contract quickly but become quickly fatigued and other muscles to resist fatigue but contract slowly depends on the fibre types that make them up.

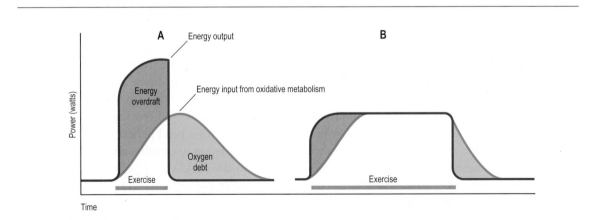

Fig. 2.2.12 Oxygen debt. A. The development of an 'oxygen debt' when fast glycolytic fibres generate a brief intense burst of energy which 'overdraws' on metabolic reserves. Oxygen consumption remains elevated until the debt is repaid. **B.** The timecourse of events when slow oxidative fibres alone are activated.

Muscle fibres are generally defined as being slow-twitch or fast-twitch.

Slow-twitch muscle fibres are relatively small in diameter, well-supplied with blood vessels and mitochondria and more resistant to fatigue than fast-twitch fibres. Aerobic metabolism provides their source of ATP and this form of metabolism is supported by **myoglobin** which acts as a small store of oxygen when the blood supply is cut off during muscle contraction. It is myoglobin that gives muscles in chicken legs their red colour. This muscle has a different function from that of the white muscle of the chicken's breast which is made up of fast-twitch fibres.

Fast-twitch muscle fibres are adapted for rapid contraction but this can only be sustained for a short time. Their speed of contraction is associated with the high speed at which their crossbridges can form, release and re-form. Fast-twitch fibres are less well supplied with blood vessels and mitochondria than are slow fibres but they contain large amounts of glycogen and rely heavily on anaerobic metabolism to provide ATP.

Slow- and fast-twitch fibres are sometimes called Type I and Type II respectively. Some people further divide Type II into Types IIb and IIa, the latter of which is intermediate between Type I and Type IIb (see Table 2.2.1).

Exercise and fatigue

Unlike the muscles of other animals, which can be made up exclusively of fast or slow fibres, human muscles usually contain fast and slow fibres in different proportions. For example, postural muscles contain mainly slow fibres while arm muscles are mainly fast. Exercise cannot change one type of fibre into the other, nor can it change the number of fibres in a muscle. Exercise increases the size of individual muscle fibres by increasing the number of myofibrils and sarcomeres within the fibre. Aerobic or anaerobic exercise preferentially trains those fibres that preferentially use one or other form of respiration, that is, slow or fast fibres respectively.

Training produces a greater improvement in muscular performance than might be expected from the increase produced in muscle size. This is due to an increase in the number of motor units that the nervous system can recruit simultaneously and an improvement in the number of capillaries perfusing the muscle.

Increase in bulk and strength of muscles has been the goal of many individuals. To increase strength by training, the most important factor appears to be to produce loads that are almost maximal for the muscle being trained. It does not seem to matter how you do this and a regimen of only 10 contractions per day, if strictly observed, will produce a significant increase in strength.

Not surprisingly, there is a highly significant difference in the percentage of muscle in the limbs of men and women. The forearms of young men contain 72% muscle while those of young women contain 60%. It is tempting to attribute this difference to the male sex hormone testosterone; and anabolic steroids which mimic its action can help to restore muscle mass to people who have become emaciated. However, it seems that the only advantage of such drugs in a healthy individual is to enable him or her to endure the damage of a punishing training schedule. Reviews of scientific studies of the effects of anabolic steroids suggest that benefits to healthy individuals are minimal, with the weight and muscle girth gains obtained probably being due to retention of water and salt. The dangerous side-effects of taking these drugs are clearly not worth the theoretical gains obtained (see Recent Advances box, p. 107).

Fatigue is a phenomenon that everyone has experienced. The discomfort or even pain associated with fatigue usually terminates exercise before the ability of muscles to contract is compromised. The basis of the discomfort of fatigue involves many factors including changes in pH and lowering of blood glucose. Although the output of neurotransmitter (acetylcholine) at the neuromuscular junction may be reduced, the function of the central nervous system motor pathways is not impaired. Only highly trained or highly motivated (frightened?) individuals will endure the discomfort of exercise to the point where actual physiological motor unit fatigue takes place. Such fatigue results from the inability of metabolic and contractile processes of the muscle fibres to function. The limited reserves of a muscle, and its dependence on a blood supply, are demonstrated by the almost complete fatigue of a muscle within 60 s of its blood supply, and therefore nutrient and particularly oxygen supply, being cut off. Interruption of blood supply occurs completely during maximal contraction of most muscles and to a lesser extent at lower tensions.

In experimental investigation of the development of fatigue, this circulatory component can be eliminated by exhausting the muscle by a series of brief tetani produced by electrical stimulation of its motor nerve. In the interval between contractions, perfusion returns to normal. In such an experiment involving a muscle made of a mixture of Type I and Type II fibres (most human muscles) tension falls rapidly with successive stimulation to a level that can be sustained for a long time.

This fatigue is due to rapid failure of the fast Type II fibres (Fig. 2.2.13) accompanied by glycogen and creatine phosphate depletion and accumulation of lactic acid.

Since the development of fatigue occurs before the ATP pool is much reduced, attention has been turned to other effects of acidosis on the energetics and mechanisms of contraction. Intracellular pH in muscle falls from about 7.1 at rest to about 6.5 at fatigue with a parallel fall in maximum force production. The increase in H^+, in particular, interferes directly with in vitro muscle contraction. The relevance of these changes to in vivo human fatigue is not clear since data from humans demonstrate that maximal muscle force is not necessarily reduced during acidotic conditions.

During recovery from exercise, muscle blood flow and oxygen consumption are elevated for some time. There is an oxygen debt which is related to the amount of energy used in the exercise in excess of that provided by oxidative metabolism (Fig. 2.2.12). Oxygen debt occurs even at low levels of exercise because slow oxidative muscle fibres consume considerable ATP before oxidative metabolism can increase ATP production. The debt is, of course,

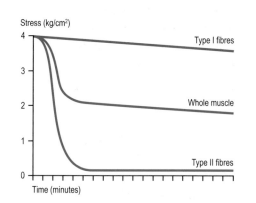

Fig. 2.2.13 Fatigue of Type I and Type II fibres. Development of fatigue in a skeletal muscle made up of Type I and Type II fibres as a result of brief tetanic stimulations at 1-second intervals. The Type I fibres maintain their normal response, the Type II fibres rapidly fatigue.

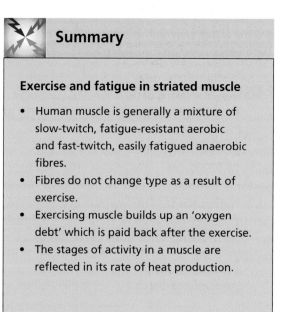

Summary

Exercise and fatigue in striated muscle

- Human muscle is generally a mixture of slow-twitch, fatigue-resistant aerobic and fast-twitch, easily fatigued anaerobic fibres.
- Fibres do not change type as a result of exercise.
- Exercising muscle builds up an 'oxygen debt' which is paid back after the exercise.
- The stages of activity in a muscle are reflected in its rate of heat production.

much greater in strenuous exercise when fast glycolytic fibres are in action.

Heat production

The metabolic activity involved in contraction recovery and the repayment of the oxygen debt is reflected by the rate of heat production by a muscle. Depriving a resting muscle of oxygen reduces its rate of heat production by about half, indicating that half its resting heat production is aerobic. When oxygen is resupplied there is additional heat production corresponding to the metabolism involved in repaying the 'oxygen debt'.

Isometric tetanic contraction is preceded by a burst of **initial heat** production and the sustained contraction is accompanied by the production of **maintenance heat**. After the contraction has ceased, heat production is elevated above resting level as **recovery heat**, which is related to the delayed oxidative metabolism of the oxygen debt. Part of the initial heat is related to the release of calcium from the sarcoplasmic reticulum to initiate contraction and is called **activation heat**. The production of heat by muscle contraction is necessary to maintain body temperature. During shivering, heat production from this source can increase up to five times.

Recent Advances

Anabolic steroids – bottled muscle

There is no doubt that for male and female athletes, anabolic steroids can increase muscle bulk and body weight. However, increases in strength are restricted to those who also undertake a regular training regimen. The long-term side-effects of steroid use are severe and can include early death from cardiovascular disease, sterility, masculinization in women and fetal effects. Perhaps the most sinister aspect of these effects is the delay of decades that occurs between the taking of large doses of steroids in youth and the full impact of the induced pathological changes in middle age.

Since time immemorial the waning of men's sexual and physical power has been associated with testicular failure, and many gruesome and unsuccessful remedies involving the testes of animals have been devised to reverse the process.

The active agent of the testes, testosterone, was first synthesized in 1935 and shown to have both androgenic actions, maintaining primary and secondary sexual characteristics, and anabolic

actions which are mainly due to stimulation of protein synthesis, particularly in skeletal muscle.

Testosterone is a C-19 steroid hormone (Fig. RA2.2.1) derived from cholesterol. Men produce about 8 mg/day, 95% from the testes, 5% from the adrenal cortex. After puberty, plasma testosterone levels are approximately 60 μg/l in men and 3 μg/l in women, in whom the adrenal cortex and ovary are the major sources of production. Like most steroid hormones, testosterone acts on the nucleus of cells to activate the synthesis of proteins, which may be enzymes or structural proteins.

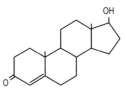

Fig. RA2.2.1 Structure of testosterone.

Recent Advances *(Continued)*

The clinical use of anabolic steroids is based on their mimicking the effects of testosterone.

They are used as replacement therapy in men and to stimulate sexual development. They combat breast tumours in postmenopausal women. The major clinical application with relevance to their use in sport is their use from the early 1940s to aid muscle regeneration after surgery, in debilitating disorders and in treating the emaciated victims from concentration camps. It is probably the publication of the results of such treatment that promoted the first use of anabolic steroids in attempts to increase muscle strength in athletes. It is clear from the results of these attempts that anabolic steroids alone will not increase strength, and that the increase in weight and muscle bulk in non-exercising healthy individuals is due to water and electrolyte retention. It is only in maximally exercising individuals that the positive, strength-enhancing effects of anabolic steroids are seen.

If such improvements are restricted to continuous hard-training regimes, why is it that so many more general claims are made for steroids? It may be that steroids make athletes 'feel better' by making them more competitive and aggressive; also, anabolic steroids improve the reparative powers of muscles, allowing more intense exercise to take place, thus stimulating muscle growth.

This effect on muscle healing is not without considerable costs. Of these the most significant to athletes are cardiovascular – since exercise imposes particular strain on the cardiovascular system – and hepatic – since anabolic steroids are suspected hepatic carcinogens in the doses taken by athletes.

Steroids increase the rate of atherosclerosis in arteries and arterioles. It is thought to be the effects of testosterone that cause the greater incidence of coronary heart disease in men compared to women. Anabolic steroids decrease the concentration of high-density lipoproteins

(HDL) which appear to protect against atherosclerosis. It has been suggested that a reduction of 10% in blood HDL increases the chance of coronary heart disease by 25%. In athletes taking anabolic steroids, HDL commonly falls by 20%.

The retention of salt and water by steroid users, which produces gains in body weight and muscle circumference but not in strength, also increases the blood volume and workload on the heart. This is a basis for potentially fatal hypertension in athletes on anabolic steroids.

Tumour formation, particularly in the liver and kidney of athletes taking steroids, has now been firmly established, together with significant changes in liver biochemistry in 80% of these otherwise healthy athletes. This may also be associated with a type of hepatitis in which hepatic tissue degenerates and is replaced by blood-filled spaces. Some of the most dramatic effects of anabolic steroids are, as one might expect, on the reproductive system. During administration, sperm counts fall by 73% with a 30% decrease in the number of mobile sperm. Much clinical data suggest that steroids produce irreversible atrophy of testicular tissue.

Because of their lower circulating levels of testosterone, the effects of a specific dose of anabolic steroids on women athletes is greater than in men, with concomitantly greater risks of side-effects including acne, facial hair, deepening of the voice and menstrual irregularities.

With more and more sophisticated methods of detecting steroid abuse becoming available, rogue athletes or their coaches are turning to other substances to improve performance. One of the most sinister of these is human growth hormone (hGH) and there is suspicion that unscrupulous individuals have been giving hGH to prepubertal children of athletic promise in the hope of producing a group of super-athletic giants.

Smooth muscle

23

Introduction

General structure and specific variations

Smooth muscle is widely distributed throughout the body and is particularly associated with hollow internal organs, the pupil of the eye, the skin (attached to hair), and glands. Unlike skeletal muscle, which develops from paired segmental somites in the embryo, smooth muscle develops from mesodermal cells which *migrate* to their final sites in the walls of hollow organs and even to the myriad of sites that finally make up the tiny arrector pili muscles associated with individual hairs.

The wide variety of structures containing smooth muscle reflects the more varied functions of this type compared with striated or cardiac muscle. Although many organs contain smooth muscle with properties appropriate to its function, it is a universal fact that smooth muscle cells are smaller (1/20th the diameter) than striated muscle cells, being from 20–200 μm long and 5–10 μm in diameter.

The absence of striations within the cells and the less organized arrangement of the fibres give this type of muscle its 'smooth' appearance under the microscope. That these fibres differ from striated muscle is demonstrated by their slower, more energy-efficient contraction. Unlike striated muscle, each cell of smooth muscle contains only one nucleus situated near the centre

Fig. 2.3.1 The microscopic structure of a smooth muscle fibre.

A

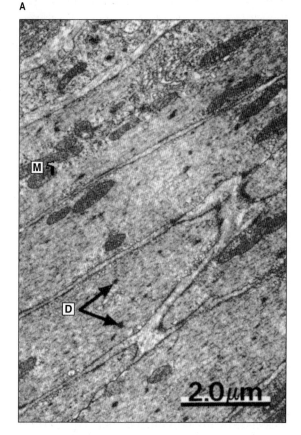

A. Myosin and actin criss-cross through the cytoplasm of each cell, forming the thick and thin filaments respectively. The irregular arrangement of these filaments results in an absence of the regular striations seen in voluntary muscle. The dense bodies (D) may provide anchoring points against which the filaments pull. When attached to the membrane they form bands called attachment junctions between cells (see Figure 2.3.2). (From Young B, Heath J W 2000. *Wheater's Functional Histology*, 4th edn. Churchill Livingstone, Edinburgh.)

B. High-power transverse section showing: (T) a halo of thin filaments (7 nm diameter) surrounding a thick (15 nm diameter) filament. Intermediate thickness filaments (IF; 10 nm diameter) join the dense bodies (DB). (Courtesy of Dr Andrew P Somlyo, University of Virginia, USA)

C. The probable arrangement of fibres and dense bodies in a smooth muscle cell. The dense bodies (DB) provide anchor points for the thin filaments (S) and intermediate filaments (IF), somewhat like the Z-lines in striated muscle. When these bodies are attached to the plasma membrane (PM), they are known as dense bands (D) and may form physical links between cells. The intermediate filaments may assist in transmitting the force produced by the interaction between the thick (T) and thin filaments to the dense regions of the cell.

C

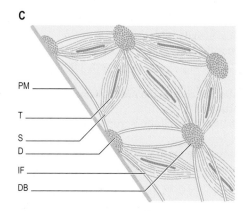

PM

T

S

D

IF

DB

B

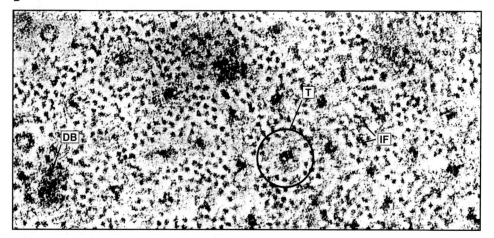

of the fibre, its widest point. Although the contents of the fibres are similar to those of striated muscle, actin, myosin, tropomyosin (troponin is absent), the actin and myosin myofilaments within the myofibrils are very thin and there are slight differences in chemical composition compared to striated muscle. The internal structures of a sarcoplasmic reticulum are sometimes poorly developed, and the T-tube system is absent.

Unique structures found in smooth muscle fibres are the **dense bodies** (Fig. 2.3.1) or, where they are fixed to the plasma membrane, dense bands (so called because they are electron dense to the beam of the electron microscope). These are made of α-actinin and represent condensations of actinin on the actin filaments in the fibre. The dense bodies are made up of the same material as the Z-disks in striated muscle and may serve the same function of providing an anchor against which the actin–myosin mechanism can pull. The dense bands on the membrane are attached to microfibrils which extend out of the cell and anchor on collagen fibres in the surrounding connective tissue, thus binding together all the individual cells in the sheet of muscle.

Scattered among the actin filaments with their dense bodies are thick myosin filaments, 2.5 times the diameter of the thin actin filaments but only about 1/12th in number. Although it contains less myosin, a smooth muscle can generate as much tension as a striated muscle of the same cross-sectional area.

Although the sarcoplasmic reticulum in many smooth muscle fibres consists only of tubules restricted to the periphery of the cells, where their membrane is invaginated into many dimples called **caveolae** (Fig. 2.3.2), the sarcoplasmic reticulum in others is as extensive as in striated muscle. The responses of smooth muscle depend on the influx of Ca^{2+}. Because smooth muscle cells are small, diffusion distances are short, and this coupled with the relatively slow speed of events in their contraction and relaxation allows the sarcolemma and the extracellular space to play the roles of the termi-

nal cisternae and T-tubules in striated muscle in regulating intracellular Ca^{2+}.

Because smooth muscle is arranged in sheets in the walls of a variety of hollow organs, rather than being connected to two bones, there is a greater variety of orientation of the fibres. For example, the sheets of fibres in the small intestine are arranged at right angles to each other so that segmentation and shortening of the gut are brought about by the circular and longitudinal layers respectively.

Hollow organs in which regulation of pressure or expulsion of contents is their function have smooth muscles arranged in their walls in a more random fashion. This is the case for the bladder and uterus. The diameter of conducting channels such as the bronchi and arteries is effectively controlled by smooth muscle arranged in circular layers.

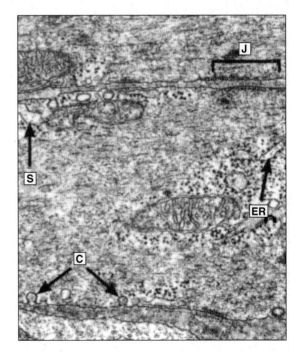

Fig. 2.3.2 The plasma membrane and endomembrane system of smooth muscle. Invaginations of the cell membrane, caveolae (C) may be involved in pinocytosis and frequently appear in association with poorly developed tubular structures (S) and endoplasmic reticulum (ER). An attachment junction (J) between cells is seen in this micrograph. (From Young B, Heath J W 2000. *Wheater's Functional Histology*, 4th edn. Churchill Livingstone, Edinburgh.)

Smooth muscle types

The arrangement of smooth muscle within an organ is largely determined by the function it serves, and, on the basis of its arrangement into single bodies or bundles, it is often classified as single-unit or multi-unit type.

Single-unit smooth muscle

This is sometimes called visceral smooth muscle because it surrounds the hollow organs of the body – the stomach, intestines, urinary bladder, uterus and some blood vessels. This type of muscle is arranged in large sheets of fibres (Fig. 2.3.3A).

Visceral smooth muscle exhibits many **gap junctions** (Fig. 2.3.4) between the cells which allow action potentials to pass from cell to cell producing a steady wave of contraction that travels through the whole sheet of muscle as if it were a single unit. The smooth muscle fibre that receives the stimulus from a nerve that initiates the contraction that is then passed on to adjacent fibres is called the **pacemaker**. In addition to this stimulated form of contraction, which is found for example in the bladder, visceral smooth muscle often shows two types of automatic activity:

- **Autorhythmic activity** is found in the digestive tract, and the rhythmicity is modulated by nervous activity.
- **Tonic activity** causes the muscle to remain in a constant state of tonus or partial contraction until deliberately relaxed. This tonus is found in the sphincters which regulate the movement of food through the digestive tract. Tonus relaxation also prevents a permanent stretching of organs such as the stomach and bladder, which regularly undergo large changes in volume. In such organs, passive increase or decrease of volume produces only transitory changes in tension of their walls, which is restored to normal by changes in tonus of the single-unit smooth muscle they contain.

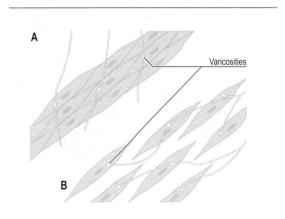

A

Varicosities

B

Fig. 2.3.3 **Types of smooth muscle. A.** Single-unit or visceral in which few fibres are innervated and impulses for contraction pass from cell to cell via gap junctions. **B.** Multi-unit in which every fibre is individually innervated.

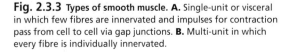

✕ Summary

Smooth muscle structure and types

- Smooth muscle cells are smaller (20–200 μm by 5–10 μm) than striated muscle cells.
- They only have one nucleus per cell.
- They appear 'smooth' because there is no regular arrangement of their fibres as in striated muscle.
- Dense bodies may serve the same anchoring function as Z-disks in striated muscle.
- Caveolae on smooth muscle cell membrane regulate the influx of Ca^{2+} which initiates contraction.
- Single-unit (visceral) smooth muscle has gap junctions in its cell membrane which are involved in passing the signal for contraction from cell to cell, promoting autorhythmicity and tonic contraction.
- Multi-unit smooth muscle lacks gap junctions, is less autorhythmic than single-unit muscle and mainly contracts in response to nerves or hormones.

Multi-unit smooth muscle (Fig. 2.3.3B)

This is made up of individual fibres not connected by gap junctions, which can be stimulated by separate autonomic motor nerves. Multi-unit muscle is much less autorhythmic than single-unit and generally only contracts when stimulated by nerves or hormones. It is found in the ciliary muscles of the eye, and in its iris where rapid adjustments are necessary. This type of smooth muscle is found in sheets in the walls of blood vessels or as small bundles or single cells as in the capsule of the spleen.

A

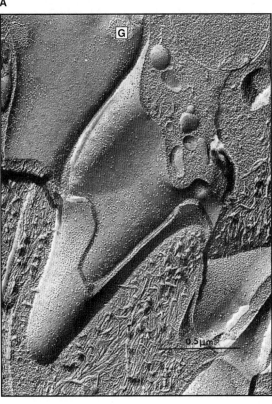

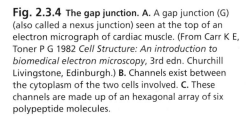

Fig. 2.3.4 The gap junction. **A.** A gap junction (G) (also called a nexus junction) seen at the top of an electron micrograph of cardiac muscle. (From Carr K E, Toner P G 1982 *Cell Structure: An introduction to biomedical electron microscopy*, 3rd edn. Churchill Livingstone, Edinburgh.) **B.** Channels exist between the cytoplasm of the two cells involved. **C.** These channels are made up of an hexagonal array of six polypeptide molecules.

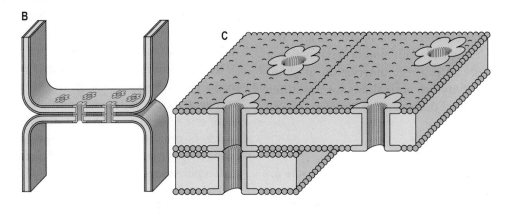

Activation of smooth muscle

Innervation

One of the most important characteristics of many groups of smooth muscle is their property of autorhythmic contractions in the absence of direct neural stimulation. This property is modified by sympathetic and parasympathetic nerves. Unlike striated muscle, smooth muscle cells are not organized into motor units. The autonomic nerves which initiate or modify their activity pass from fibre to fibre forming swellings, varicosities, on the cell surface. These varicosities show little specialization of either their pre- or postjunctional membranes. The gap between nerve and muscle can be from 20–200 nm and the density of innervation varies from a junction on almost every muscle cell in the vas deferens to a sparse innervation in the uterus where excitation spreads from cell to cell via intercellular connections. The dual innervation of smooth muscle by the sympathetic and parasympathetic autonomic systems allows for an increase or decrease in the largely intrinsic activity of the muscle. Thus parasympathetic activity generally increases strength of contraction whereas sympathetic activity, which can have what are known as α- or β-type effects, generally excites or inhibits respectively.

The ability to modify the activity of smooth muscle by interfering pharmacologically with these α- and β-type effects is of considerable importance in the treatment of diseases such as hypertension, where the object of treatment is to reduce arterial blood pressure by relaxing smooth muscle in the walls of arteries and arterioles. Although smooth muscle can function in the absence of extrinsic innervation, it shows supersensitivity to normal neurotransmitters after a period of denervation.

Electrical activity

The electrical properties of smooth muscle are much less uniform than those of striated muscle, reflecting its more diverse properties and functions. Its resting membrane potential can range from −50 to −60 mV compared to −85 mV in striated muscle, although both are probably generated by the same mechanisms. Unlike striated muscle, smooth muscle contracts in response to both action potentials and slow changes in resting membrane potential. The sensitivity to each type of stimulus depends on the type of smooth muscle. **Single-unit smooth muscle** (found in many viscera) generates action potentials (Fig. 2.3.5A) which spread through the muscle via gap junctions. The response is not all-or-none as in skeletal muscle; a series of action potentials usually results in a slow sustained contraction. Slow changes in the resting membrane potential due to spontaneous changes in the muscle membrane permeability to, or pumping of, Na^+ and Ca^{2+} also cause bursts of action potentials which in turn cause contraction (Fig. 2.3.5B).

The slow waves themselves do not cause contraction in this type of smooth muscle. However, a type of depolarization intermediate between slow waves and action potential, and very similar to a cardiac action potential, does occur – **action potential with plateau** (Fig. 2.3.5C). This plateau, which can last for up to 1 second, accounts for the prolonged contraction seen in smooth muscles of the uterus and certain blood vessels.

The cell membrane of a single-unit smooth muscle is depolarized by stretching. This, combined with the normal slow waves of depolarization, sets up a series of action potentials causing the muscle to contract. This kind of activity is most clearly seen in the gut in response to distension by food.

In **multi-unit smooth muscle** (found in many blood vessels) electrical activity is not propagated from cell to cell and the characteristic of this type of muscle is to develop tension which is proportional to the degree of membrane depolarization even in the absence of action potentials (Fig. 2.3.5D).

The absence of action potentials in multi-unit smooth muscle may be related to the small size

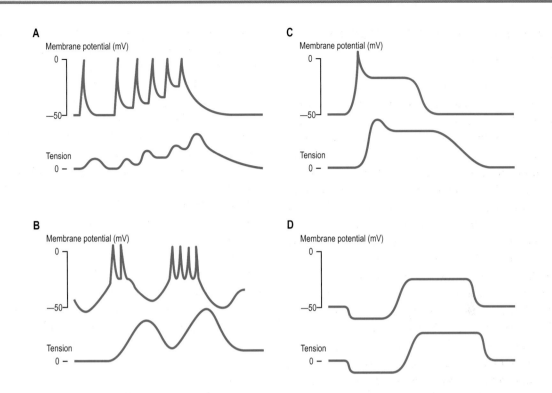

Fig. 2.3.5 **The relationship between membrane potential and tension in types of smooth muscle. A.** Action potentials characteristic of single-unit smooth muscles produce single or summated twitches. **B.** Slow changes in the resting membrane potential can trigger action potentials which produce changes in tension. This behaviour is typical of self-excitatory smooth muscle of the gut. **C.** Action potentials with plateaux occur in the smooth muscle of the uterus and some vascular smooth muscle and result in prolonged contractions. **D.** Depolarization without action potentials takes place in smooth muscle fibres too small to generate action potentials – such as are found in the iris of the eye. These waves of depolarization cause muscle contraction even in the absence of action potentials.

of its cells, 50 or more need to be depolarizing simultaneously before a self-propagating action potential can be recorded. This absence of action potentials does not prevent the muscle from functioning, usually in response to acetylcholine or noradrenaline secreted by nerves of the autonomic nervous system. These transmitters cause a local depolarization on the cell membrane which spreads 'electrotonically' over the whole fibre, bringing about a contraction. It might seem surprising that multi-unit smooth muscle, with its absence of conventional brief action potentials is generally found where a rapid contraction is required, the iris and ciliary muscles of the eye for example, sites where the properties of ubiquitous smooth muscle approach those of its striated relative.

Summary

Innervation and electrical activity in smooth muscle

- Smooth muscle can be autorhythmic and is not organized into motor units.
- Activity can be initiated and/or modulated by autonomic nerves passing from muscle fibre to fibre.
- Unlike single-unit smooth muscle, multi-unit muscle activity is not propagated via junctions, and tension is proportional to membrane potential.

The smooth muscle neuromuscular junction

The connection between the two previous topics, 'Innervation' and 'Electrical activity' in smooth muscles, is at the neuromuscular junction. Here chemicals released by nerves alter the electrical properties of the muscle cells to initiate, increase or decrease the likelihood of, or inhibit contraction. This is an altogether more varied response than that found in striated muscle where the activity of the neuromuscular junction is directed towards one end – a muscle action potential producing muscle contraction.

Factors which influence the neural control of smooth muscle include:

- the types of innervation and the transmitters released
- the receptors of the neurotransmitters on the muscle cell membrane
- the anatomical arrangement of the nerves in relation to the muscle fibres.

We have already seen that the innervation of smooth muscle by the autonomic nervous system can be divided into visceral (single-unit) or multi-unit types. These two main types can be supplied by three categories of nerve:

- extrinsic innervation – from the autonomic nervous system, which in turn can be mainly sympathetic (arteries), parasympathetic (ciliary muscles) or both (gut)
- intrinsic innervation – in self-contained plexuses within the smooth muscle itself (particularly in the gut)
- afferent sensory neurones – which, while not strictly having a direct effect on smooth muscle cells, set up reflex activation of motoneurones that do.

The importance of the innervation of smooth muscle is illustrated by the fact that the innervation of gut smooth muscle alone contains more nerve cells than the skeletal motor system. That much of this innervation is intrinsic is demonstrated by the continued peristalsis of gut

taken out of the body, whereas a skeletal muscle with its nerve supply interrupted is flaccid.

The autonomic nerve fibres that innervate smooth muscle are usually restricted to the surface of the muscle sheet. The neurones do not have branching ends with motor endplates typical of skeletal muscle motor nerves but rather there are bulges, **varicosities**, at intervals along the nerve. At these points the covering layer of Schwann cells is absent to allow the free diffusion of transmitter substances released from vesicles within the varicosities. The process of release of the transmitter is similar to that in skeletal muscle and in some cases, called **contact junctions**, in multi-unit smooth muscle, the gap between nerve and muscle is as small (20–30 µm). This proximity reduces the latent period of smooth muscles innervated in this fashion to that of skeletal muscle. Where the distance for diffusion is greater, in **diffuse junctions**, the delay is, of course, longer, producing an average total contraction time of about 2 seconds, 30 times that of the average striated muscle, but with a range of 0.2–30 seconds.

The transmitter substances released by the autonomic nerves serving smooth muscle are also more varied than the ubiquitous acetylcholine released by motor nerves of skeletal muscle. Acetylcholine and noradrenaline are the transmitters released to smooth muscle; they are *never* both manufactured by the same nerve (Dale's principle), although some autonomic nerves release more than one transmitter. Both these transmitters can have either excitatory or inhibitory effects on smooth muscle, and which effect dominates is determined by the type of receptor present in a particular muscle. Some examples of this diversity of response of different smooth muscle sites to the same substances are given in Table 2.3.1.

This diversity is due to the variety of excitatory and inhibitory receptors found on the cell membrane of smooth muscle. These receptors also respond to substances circulating in the blood or released locally in the tissues to open channels in the cell membrane.

Table 2.3.1 The effect of sympathetic and parasympathetic nerve stimulation on various tissues (adapted from Rang H P, Dale M M, Ritter J M 1999 *Pharmacology*, 4th edn. Churchill Livingstone, Edinburgh)

Organ	Receptor type	Sympathetic	Parasympathetic
Heart			
SA node	β_1	Rate ↑	Rate ↓
Atrial muscle	β_1	Force ↑	Force ↓
AV node	β_1	Automaticity ↑	Conduction velocity ↓
			AV block
Ventricular muscle	β_1	Automaticity ↑	No effect
		Force ↑	
Blood vessels			
Arterioles			
Coronary	α	Constriction	
Muscle	β_2	Dilatation	No effect
Viscera			
Skin	α	Constriction	No effect
Brain			
Erectile tissue	α	Constriction	Dilatation
Salivary gland			
Veins	α	Constriction	No effect
	β_2	Dilatation	
Viscera			
Bronchi			
Smooth muscle	β_2	No sympathetic innervation, but dilated by circulating adrenaline	Constriction
Glands		No effect	Secretion
GI tract			
Smooth muscle	α_2, β_2	Motility ↓	Motility ↑
Sphincters	α_2, β_2	Constriction	Dilatation
Glands		No effect	Secretion
Uterus			
pregnant	α	Contraction	Variable
non-pregnant	β_2	Relaxation	
Male sex organs	α	Ejaculation	Erection
Eye			
Pupil	α	Dilatation	Constriction
Ciliary muscle	β	Relaxation (slight)	Contraction
Skin			
Sweat glands	α	Secretion (mainly cholinergic)	No effect
Pilomotor	α	Piloerection	No effect
Salivary glands	α, β	Secretion	Secretion
Lacrimal glands		No effect	Secretion
Kidney	β_2	Renin secretion	No effect
Liver	α, β_2	Glycogenolysis Gluconeogenesis	No effect

Summary

Smooth muscle junctions and hormones

- The smooth muscle neuromuscular junction is more varied in structure than that found in striated muscle.
- Varicosities on the autonomic nerves serving smooth muscles act as the junction, releasing a variety of neurotransmitters.
- Excitatory or inhibitory receptors on the muscle cell membrane respond to neurotransmitters and substances in the extracellular fluid.

Local tissue factors and hormones

Smooth muscle responds rapidly to changes in the interstitial fluid surrounding it. This provides an efficient local homeostatic mechanism responding to changes in the respiratory gases, pH, ions and temperature. Many hormones, carried by the circulation, affect smooth muscle contraction. These include adrenaline, angiotensin, oxytocin, antidiuretic hormone (vasopressin), histamine and 5-hydroxytryptamine. As with the neurotransmitters noradrenaline and acetylcholine, the effects of these hormones may be excitatory or inhibitory. The mechanism of excitation can be dealt with separately from that of contraction.

Excitation of contractile mechanisms and their properties

Mechanisms of excitation or inhibition of smooth muscles

The final common pathway which leads to contraction of smooth muscle (or other muscle) cells is a rise in intracellular calcium concentration. Depolarization of the cell membrane,

with or without action potentials, can be caused by the opening of Na^+ and Ca^{2+} channels; the influx of Ca^{2+} causes depolarization and increases intracellular $[Ca^{2+}]$ as a primary effect (Fig. 2.3.6). Many of these types of channels respond to membrane receptor activation and are called '**receptor-operated**'. Calcium channels which open in response to depolarization of the membrane are said to be **voltage gated**; others are independent of depolarization; and yet other receptors activate **phospholipase C**, which, by a series of steps, releases Ca^{2+} from the sarcoplasmic reticulum, which increases intracellular Ca^{2+} without any flux across the cell membrane.

However, most of the Ca^{2+} involved in contraction of most smooth muscle comes from the extracellular fluid and so, when extracellular $[Ca^{2+}]$ is reduced, so is smooth muscle contraction (like cardiac muscle but unlike skeletal muscle). Removal of this influx of Ca^{2+} is necessary for relaxation and most of this is done by membrane pumps. Like many other things about smooth muscle, these are slower than the pumps of striated muscle sarcoplasmic reticulum.

Recapture of Ca^{2+} by the smooth muscle sarcoplasmic reticulum is an active process driven by ATP and modulated by receptor activity. The fall in $[Ca^{2+}]$ that results brings about relaxation. Relaxation of smooth muscle can also be brought about by the inactivation of an enzyme MLCK (myosin light-chain kinase), an essential component in the contraction process. The β effects of the sympathetic system largely act in this way (Fig. 2.3.6B).

The contractile mechanism of smooth muscle

Perhaps because of its more leisurely rate of contraction than striated muscle and less dramatic action than cardiac muscle, smooth muscle is often accorded a more primitive status. Quite the opposite is true; there is no equivalent

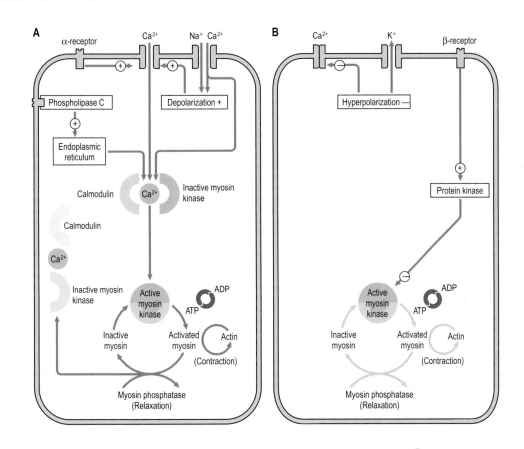

Fig. 2.3.6 Receptor activation on smooth muscle. **A.** Initiation and **B.** inhibition of smooth muscle contraction by receptor activation. Only a few of the routes by which receptor activation can increase intracellular Ca^{2+} (the final common pathway to active myosin kinase) are shown. There are also many forms of protein kinase which inhibit the activation of myosin kinase, sometimes called myosin light-chain kinase.

of vertebrate smooth muscle in the primitive phyla. Nevertheless, this inferior status is reflected in the lack of information available about the contractile apparatus of smooth muscle. The functional equivalent of the sarcomere in striated muscle is not yet defined and may be the thick and thin filaments stretching between two dense bodies (see Fig. 2.3.1).

The proportions of the components of the contractile mechanism of striated muscle are different in smooth muscle. The regulatory protein troponin is absent and there is twice as much actin and tropomyosin. Myosin, on the other hand, is only one-quarter as plentiful as

in striated muscle, which is explained by the paucity of thick filaments.

The actin and myosin from smooth or striated muscle interact in the same way when extracted from the body and mixed in vitro. The initiation of this interaction is caused by an increase in the concentration of Ca^{2+}. We have seen that in smooth muscle this can result from changes in membrane permeability produced by stretching, spontaneous electrical activity, neurotransmitters, hormones and changes in the extracellular fluid composition. In striated muscle, contraction is regulated by the interaction of Ca^{2+} with the protein troponin which regulates actin–myosin crossbridge formation. This regulatory role is taken over in smooth muscle by an entirely different protein, **calmodulin**. This protein binds with Ca^{2+} to form a complex which, in turn, binds with an enzyme **myosin (light-chain) kinase** (Fig. 2.3.6) and, by phosphorylation, activates the myosin heads which form the crossbridges between actin and myosin. The energy for this phosphorylation comes from ATP, which is degraded to ADP.

You will remember from the section on striated muscle that the myosin molecule 'head' which forms a crossbridge has four light chains attached to it as well as the two heavy chains which attach it to the myosin filament. One of the light chains is a **regulatory chain** and, when phosphorylated by the myosin kinase–Ca^{2+}–calmodulin complex, the bridge goes through the attachment–shortening–release cycle described for striated muscle, which brings about contraction of the filament.

These final steps of attachment and shortening of the crossbridges are identical to those found in striated muscle in which the process of contraction is brought to an end by the removal of Ca^{2+}, allowing troponin to resume its inhibitory role. In smooth muscle there is no troponin and so while removal of Ca^{2+} reverses most of the process of contraction, it does not detach phosphate from the myosin molecule head, which consequently remains attached to the actin filament.

To bring about this removal, and relaxation of the muscle, requires a further enzyme, **myosin phosphatase**, and the rate of smooth muscle relaxation depends on the concentration of this enzyme.

This tendency of the filaments of smooth muscle to 'hang on' even when activating Ca^{2+} levels have fallen is quite different from the behaviour of striated muscle, which quickly 'lets go' once the motor nerve activity has ceased and Ca^{2+} has been rapidly reabsorbed into the extensive sarcoplasmic reticulum. This

property of smooth muscle is sometimes called a 'latch' mechanism. Because of this, the activation of smooth muscle, by nerves for example, can be reduced and yet the muscle will maintain its force of contraction. The energy to sustain this latched contraction is only 1/100th of that required to sustain a similar effort in striated muscle in which only a very slight latch effect can be seen. By this mechanism, smooth muscle can sustain a contraction for hours with little expenditure of energy or stimulation from nerves.

Even the rate at which crossbridges are formed and released is different in smooth muscle, being up to 300 times slower than in striated muscle. As part of this effect, the time a crossbridge spends joining the actin and myosin filament together is increased; and as it is this which determines the force of contraction we can see why the maximum force of contraction per cm^2 cross-section for smooth muscle is of the order of 6 kg and that for striated muscle 4 kg.

Only one molecule of ATP is used to form and release one crossbridge. This slow rate of cycle in smooth muscle brings with it economies of energy usage (without loss of power, as seen above). This is very important in terms of those organs of the body that must maintain contraction at all times.

The immediate energy supply for contraction in smooth muscle comes from ATP, as is the case with striated muscle. Unlike striated muscle, there is no energy reserve in the form of creatine phosphate. The characteristically slower speed of shortening of smooth muscle offsets this to some extent by spreading out the demand for ATP. Smooth muscle also uses a wider variety of fats and carbohydrates as substrates for the production of ATP. However, smooth muscles are poorly adapted to anaerobic metabolism; they do not develop an oxygen debt and, in the absence of an adequate supply, quickly fatigue.

Summary

Excitation, inhibition and contraction

- Smooth muscle (like striated) contracts in response to an increase in intracellular Ca^{2+}.
- Depolarization of the cell membrane is caused by opening of Na^+ and Ca^{2+} channels.
- Channels can be receptor gated or voltage gated.
- Receptors can activate phospholipase C to release Ca^{2+} from the sarcoplasmic reticulum.
- Smooth muscle cells contain twice as much actin and tropomyosin and only a quarter as much myosin as striated muscle.

- Troponin is absent and its regulatory role is taken over by calmodulin.
- Smooth muscle myosin tends to 'hang on' to actin even when Ca^{2+} levels fall.
- Myosin phosphatase brings about crossbridge release, and the rate of relaxation of smooth muscle depends on its concentration.
- Crossbridges form more slowly and efficiently in smooth than in striated muscle.
- Smooth muscles have poor energy reserves and under anaerobic conditions fatigue quickly.

Mechanical properties of smooth muscles

A variety of innervation, sensitivity, biochemistry and arrangement within a connective tissue matrix of variable composition endows smooth muscle with a much greater variety of mechanical properties than the more stereotyped striated and cardiac muscles. These properties have, of course, evolved to fit the role carried out by the particular muscle. The smooth muscles of the iris of the eye do not have properties that would be useful in the stomach, and vice versa. The diversity of properties found in smooth muscle is not even restricted to its properties of contraction. Its relationship with its surrounding connective tissue is more intimate than previously supposed. If smooth muscle cells, with all the characteristics of normal contractile muscle, are isolated and placed in tissue culture, they lose their contractile characteristics of myosin and actin filaments and develop an extensive endoplasmic reticulum

and Golgi apparatus. These structures then proceed to make collagen and elastin (constituents of the whole muscle matrix) and lay them down outside the cells. It is almost as if the isolated cells are building a complete new muscle. This idea is reinforced by the observation that after laying down a certain amount of matrix, the cells regain their actin and myosin filaments, as if preparing to take up their contractile activity once more.

Smooth muscle can shorten to a much smaller fraction of its relaxed length than striated muscle (to one-third and two-thirds of their rest lengths respectively). This is a very useful property when smooth muscle has to reduce the lumen of a tube to zero, as in the case of sphincters in the gut or bladder, or in precapillary sphincters in the circulation. An important adjunct to the significant contraction of sphincter muscle in providing a 'watertight' seal is that the tissue underlying the muscle is incompressible and forms a 'bung' in the lumen of the tube of smooth muscle (Fig. 2.3.7).

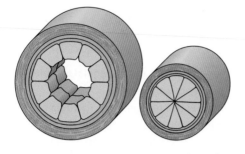

Fig. 2.3.7 Smooth muscle 'plugging' of sphincters. Smooth muscle can contract to a much smaller percentage of its rest length than can skeletal muscle. This is a useful property in the formation of sphincters where compression of tissue beneath a ring of smooth muscle in sustained contraction forms a watertight 'plug'.

This ability to contract to a smaller fraction of its rest length than can striated muscle is probably due to smooth muscle having longer actin filaments over which the myosin filaments can move.

It is common knowledge that exercise increases the size of skeletal muscle. This increase is almost exclusively due to an increase in the size of the individual cells, with only a fraction of a per cent of the increase due to increase in cell number. Smooth muscle cells, on the other hand, retain the ability to proliferate as well as increase in size in response to exercise.

Summary

Mechanical properties of smooth muscle

- Smooth muscle types show a greater variety of mechanical properties than striated muscles.
- Smooth muscles shorten to a much smaller fraction of their relaxed length than striated muscle.
- Unlike striated muscle, smooth muscle can proliferate as a result of training.

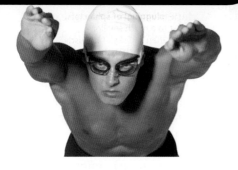

Exercise

Introduction

It seems to be generally agreed that this is the most sedentary age in history for most people in the western world. We are constantly chided by the media (usually at the prompting of manufacturers of sports equipment or sporting organizations) to take more exercise for our own good. The power used in carrying out a number of different activities is shown in Table 2.4.1. Like most campaigns by some to change the behaviour of others, these exhortations deserve closer examination before being swallowed whole.

Table 2.4.1 Power used by activities

Activity	Energy expenditure (watts)
Sleeping	86
Sitting	120
Housework	175
Walking	350
Marathon running	1000
Sprinting	4000

Most comparisons of the working lives of today seem to be made with those which are within oral history; grandparents and great-grandparents tell how they endured the excesses of the late Industrial Revolution when many types of work were not only long and physically demanding but took place under conditions which were harmful, uncomfortable, or often frankly dangerous. Undoubtedly conditions of work have become less physically arduous, but the Industrial Revolution in the late 18th and early 19th century was a very brief, if cataclysmic, period in social evolution. Taking even a slightly longer view, we see that the medieval peasant, with his working day circumscribed by the hours of daylight and a calendar punctuated by many feast and 'holy-days', may have worked fewer hours a year and under less stressful conditions than his modern counterpart who wishes to sustain the lifestyle the advertising agencies advise him is appropriate. Women, liberated from domestic drudgery, are now expected to find gainful employment outside the home. And, of course, peer pressure to conform with what is an acceptable appearance is as important in determining our activities as any wish to improve our health.

Victorians aspiring to be gentlefolk protected their skin from the tanning effects of sunlight to show that they did not labour in the open air. Today, their equivalents risk the most virulent types of skin cancer under ultraviolet lamps to give the impression that they can afford winter holidays in the High-Alps.

Rubens' voluptuous models, who demonstrated a clear ability to be well fed in a time in which people starved, would be considered pathologically obese in these days when a thin body flaunts the financial resources to provide an ideal diet and plenty of free time to spend at the exercise machines (*O tempora, O mores!*).

The effects of exercise on the body

Exercise is perhaps the best example of integration of the systems of the body, because most, if not all, are involved when one exercises. Of all the systems of the body that are changed by exercise, the musculoskeletal system is perhaps the most obvious and the one most usually intended to be changed. It may be that the participant in exercise wishes to lose fat (frequently euphemistically referred to as 'weight'), but it is the musculoskeletal system that is frequently used, in part, to achieve that end.

What does exercise do to skeletal muscle?

The effects on skeletal muscle depend on the type of exercise undertaken. There are as many exercise regimens as there are coaches willing to teach them, but they all fall somewhere between two extremes aimed at improving strength or endurance.

- In exercise to improve *endurance*, light loads are moved continuously for long periods of time, as in long-distance running.
- In exercise to improve *strength*, heavy loads, even straining against immovable objects, are briefly applied a small number of times.

The effects on the skeletal muscles and the other systems of the body of these two types of regimen are very different, but before we can describe the different *types* of exercise we need a measure of *how much* exercise an individual is doing. At rest, we metabolically 'burn' the substrate of foodstuff to provide the energy to sustain us at a fairly low rate. When we exercise we consume substrate and oxygen at increasing rates with increasing levels of exercise up to the maximum level we can sustain for just a few seconds. We are then using oxygen at our maximum rate. This is called our $\dot{V}O_{2max}$ and against this we usually measure the level at which we are working.

Endurance training

This type of training is frequently undertaken to improve general 'fitness' and its global effect on all the systems of the body makes it ideal for that purpose.

During endurance training, the workload must be sufficiently light (and usually isotonic; see p. 100) to enable it to be sustained for the long periods necessary to improve endurance. A subject might start at a work rate which produces an oxygen consumption of less than $50\% \dot{V}O_{2max}$ working up slowly to $80\% \dot{V}O_{2max}$ or higher.

Metabolism of the exercising muscles during endurance training must be mainly aerobic (p. 103) or it could not be sustained. The changes that take place in the other systems of the body as a result of this type of exercise are necessary to support this increased metabolism. The slow muscle fibres (p. 105) are mainly affected by endurance training, although there is little obvious change in the muscle mass or appearance of the fibres under the microscope. The changes which take place within the muscle itself are mainly an increase in the number of mitochondria, which generate ATP (p. 103), and an increase in the density of capillaries that provide oxygen to enable the mitochondria to do this. This increase in mitochondria and capillaries results from low oxygen partial pressure (it also occurs at altitude), an increase in blood flow and a build-up of metabolites. The decrease in partial pressure of oxygen is of course a result of increased oxygen consumption. Endurance training improves performance in activities such as walking, cycling, running and swimming over appreciable distances.

Strength training

Unlike endurance training, strength training is specific to the muscles being trained, and the general effects on the other systems of the body, although present, are less marked. Anyone who has suffered a broken limb which is immobilized by a cast may have experienced the results of abstaining from strength training, which manifests itself as weakness and atrophy of the immobilized muscles. These deleterious effects can very simply be counteracted by a small number of powerful contractions a few times a day, which in the case of a broken limb must of course not impose stress on the healing bone.

Strength training involves lifting weights which must be at least 50% of the muscle's maximum capacity or straining to an equivalent muscle tension against an immovable object (an isometric contraction; see p. 100). These exercises need only be performed a remarkably few times to achieve significant improvements in strength. Programmes involving 10 repetitions three times per week are not uncommon. If more than 10 repetitions can be performed, the muscle is not loaded sufficiently to obtain maximum effect; and if the set of 10 contractions is repeated more than three times per week, there is insufficient time for the muscle to recover from the injury which is almost inevitable in this type of training. The remarkable specificity of this type of exercise to the muscle being trained extends to the type and range of movement which is used. The muscle will be strongest over the range of movement for which it has been trained and, if trained by slow movements, will show significant improvements in strength at those speeds only.

Strength training results in muscle fibre hypertrophy; the fibres become thicker and stronger by laying down more protein in the form of the contractile mechanism in each fibre. The contractile mechanism of the muscle does not become stronger at the molecular level, there are just more contractile proteins in each fibre, and strength bears a very close relationship to the cross-sectional area of a muscle. As is the case with endurance training, specific muscle fibre types, the fast fibres, are trained in strength training. Adult muscle fibres do not normally divide and so training does not occur by producing more fast fibres, although there is some evidence that intermediate or even slow fibres begin to take on the properties of fast fibres with strength training. Testosterone, the male sex hormone, improves the response to strength training, and so men respond better to this type of training than do women. It is debatable whether this is a direct effect on the response of fast fibres to exercise, an improvement in their ability to repair, or the individual's increased ability to tolerate damage resulting from excess loads as well as a psychological effect improving motivation (see Recent Advances: Anabolic steroids – bottled muscle, p. 107). Activities associated with strength training include weightlifting, wrestling, shot-putting and isometric exercises where the load does not move against the muscle effort and there is consequently no muscle shortening.

A moderated form of strength training is of particular interest to a specific group of patients – postmenopausal women. Many of these women lose bone mass because of the decline in female hormones. It has been demonstrated that applying loads to the skeleton, as in exercise, slows down this loss.

These two types of exercise training for strength or endurance represent the extremes of the range on which most sports lie. They have different effects on the different physiological systems of the body, and the effects on the cardiovascular system are a good example of this.

The cardiovascular system

Together with the skeletal muscle system, the cardiovascular system shows the most dramatic changes in response to exercise training, and, of the two types, endurance training has the more profound effects. We have already remarked on the increase in capillary density that takes place in trained skeletal muscle, but training

also affects cardiac muscle. In a similar way to skeletal muscle, cardiac muscle responds to increased levels of exercise by hypertrophy and the ability to contract more strongly, emptying the ventricle more quickly and completely during systole. The response to endurance training is, however, very different from the response to strength training.

Endurance training results in an increased filling pressure of the venous return, as a result of the pumping action of the muscles and the imposed increased cardiac output, so the heart is *preloaded* (see p. 526) and the left ventricle increases in size without much increase in wall thickness (Fig. 2.4.1). In strength training just the opposite occurs with the left ventricle remaining the same volume but the wall

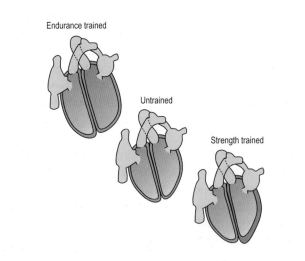
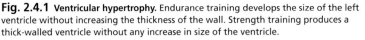

Fig. 2.4.1 Ventricular hypertrophy. Endurance training develops the size of the left ventricle without increasing the thickness of the wall. Strength training produces a thick-walled ventricle without any increase in size of the ventricle.

increasing in thickness. There is a suggestion that this increase in wall thickness increases the risk of heart disease by increasing the distances for diffusion of oxygen to the centre of the wall. Endurance-trained hearts on the other hand are enlarged to produce an increased stroke volume which means a slower rate is required to produce any given cardiac output. The resting heart rate of some endurance athletes falls below 40 per minute, some sustaining 'ventricular pauses' between beats of more than 2 s. These people are at risk of block of the cardiac conducting system, 'heart block'(see p. 526) and in several cases pacemakers have been implanted to relieve this life-threatening condition.

Regular endurance training reduces resting blood pressure. In normal individuals, systolic blood pressure rises during exercise while diastolic pressure is unchanged or may even fall slightly. Because moderate hypertensives have no greater increases in blood pressure on exercise than normals they may use the beneficial effects of training to improve their condition.

With endurance training comes a change to the blood which seem to have a protective effect on the results of sustained exercise – plasma volume increases by up to 15%. This is accompanied by a smaller increase in the number of red corpuscles and so the blood appears to be slightly anaemic, which one would assume to be a bad thing. However this 'thin' blood is less viscous than normal and therefore easier for the heart to pump. Also, when athletes lose water during sweating, the blood becomes more concentrated, returning viscosity to normal values; so reduced viscosity and increased plasma volume before sustained exercise begins assists trained athletes in maintaining the high cardiac output they require during exercise.

Training for strength presents an entirely different cardiovascular picture where brief intervals of intense activity are interposed between long periods of rest. There is never the overall high rate of oxygen consumption required to provide training of the cardiovascular system. Even worse, the brief intense increases in blood pressure produced by maximal muscle contraction produces hypertrophy of the left ventricle, which does not increase in size as in endurance training. The ventricle wall can become thickened to such an extent that its stroke volume is reduced below that of an untrained individual.

The respiratory system

At rest, an individual might take a breath of 500 ml every 5 seconds, a minute ventilation of 6 litres per minute. During exercise, each breath may increase to more than 3 litres at an interval of less than 2 seconds. Thus the respiratory system can increase its performance 25 times compared to the heart's more modest fivefold increase in cardiac output on exercise.

The energy cost of breathing is very low, even during heavy exercise, less than half that used by the heart. It seems that breathing or the transfer of oxygen from the air into the blood does not limit even the most extreme forms of exercise in healthy individuals. There appears to be plenty of reserve in the performance of the respiratory system and perhaps because of this it has not been possible to prove that training improves the functions of the lungs. Other systems limit our exercise before we can reach the limits of our respiratory system. However, recent experiments in which subjects train their respiratory muscles by breathing against resistances show that these muscles can improve their performance as measured by such dynamic tests as FEV_1 (see p. 668). This training is probably of most use to individuals suffering from lung diseases such as asthma rather than athletes and normal individuals. This form of training must be highly specific to the muscles concerned because, although people who have had the respiratory disadvantage of living at high altitude for many generations have lung volumes 30% greater than those living at sea level, a sojourn of a mere lifetime at altitude does not improve respiratory performance.

Water and salts and heat

Homiothermy, maintenance of a constant internal temperature, confers the advantage of stabilizing the rate of the chemical reactions which make up metabolism. To maintain a constant internal temperature we must strike a balance between the heat produced and lost by our bodies.

When we exercise hard we produce more than 10 times more heat than at rest and we visibly sweat; this is most obvious in hot surroundings. Sweating is a most efficient way of losing heat and depends on the high latent heat of vaporization of water (2300 kilojoules per litre). Theoretically we could lose all the heat produced by our resting metabolism by evaporating 4 litres of sweat per day. This is clearly not feasible, particularly during exercise, and we also lose heat by convection, conduction and, to a lesser extent, radiation.

The passive mechanisms of losing heat come into play first during exercise. Flow of blood to the skin increases and therefore skin temperature. Heat is more readily lost to the environment. However, as skin temperature rises there is less transfer of heat from blood to skin and the blood is not cooled so efficiently. The temperature of the skin must therefore be controlled by increasing convective and evaporative losses. The excess heat produced by hard physical work of the type that could be sustained for about 30 minutes is nicely balanced by the heat removed by evaporation at the maximum rate of sweating of the average individual of about 1 litre per hour.

Blood flow to the skin and the production of sweat is under the control of the hypothalamus and modification of this control is the basis of most acclimatization to exercise under hot conditions. Acclimatization improves the cooling mechanisms of the body and improves the individual's tolerance of raised body temperature. The maximum flow of blood to the skin is increased, but this is limited by the demands of other tissues for blood, and sweat production is modified. The acclimatized individual begins to sweat sooner after the start of exercise, produces more sweat by having more active sweat glands which are more sensitive than normal and produces sweat with a lower salt content, thus conserving salt and volume of the blood.

Conservation of volume is an important issue in sustained exercise such as the marathon. Water for sweat is initially extracted from the plasma, which in turn draws water from interstitial fluid, so 1 litre of sweat is made up of about equal amounts of water from plasma and water from the interstitial fluid (with of course the salt lost in sweat). An important part of the conservation of body water is carried out by the kidney producing concentrated urine by reabsorbing water under the stimulation of antidiuretic hormone (ADH; see p. 762). Exercise stimulates the release of this hormone and thus the retention of water. Loss of about 2 litres of plasma volume as sweat or otherwise will result in cardiovascular collapse (shock). This does not occur during exercise because when plasma volume drops sufficiently to affect cardiac output the ability to exercise drops as well, a natural brake preventing damage. If the athlete is sufficiently foolish, sometimes called 'well motivated', he will continue to exercise despite this dehydration; the body now diverts blood from the skin to maintain cardiac output and of course there is an explosive temperature rise which terminates his efforts. Rehydration normally takes place by absorption of water from the gut.

The gut

Energy for exercise and water and salt to replace sweat come from food and drink processed by the gut. As far as water replacement is concerned, the position is simple; water is absorbed best from dilute solutions. This issue has been clouded by manufacturers of 'isotonic' drinks which are claimed to enhance performance. If these drinks do as they claim, and some seem to at least in part, it is by the addition of carbohydrate in the form of large sugar polymers which provide carbohydrate but do not exert much osmotic effect to prevent the absorption of water. In this context, endurance athletes should beware of consuming sugar immediately before competing as this will promote the secretion of insulin which depresses blood glucose; however, exercise itself has the opposite effect (see below). Exercise imposes increased demands on almost all components of the diet and requires that the gut is able to absorb them in adequate amounts. To support strength training one should have about 1 g of protein per kg of body weight per day. Most European diets contain about 90 g per day, which is adequate, but in poor countries development of strength is limited by dietary factors.

The nervous and endocrine systems

All the systems that have been mentioned in relation to exercise are influenced by the nervous system:

- the central nervous system in terms of motor performance
- the autonomic nervous system in terms of control of the cardiovascular system and increasing levels of circulating catecholamines (adrenaline and noradrenaline) and cortisol.

An immediate increase in blood levels of catecholamines is seen at the beginning of exercise. This is due to sympathetic nervous system activity. This and the activity of the sympathetic system on the liver mobilize stored lipid and glycogen. Noradrenaline stimulates glycogen breakdown in muscles.

Within a few minutes of the start of exercise, ACTH-controlled levels of cortisol begin to rise. Cortisol increases the resistance to physical stress and has a permissive role on the effects of adrenaline and noradrenaline, its presence being required for them to be fully effective. Increased sympathetic activity to the pancreas during exercise stimulates glucagon secretion, which aids adrenaline and cortisol in releasing energy, and inhibits insulin release. This reduction in insulin means that the permeability of muscle fibres to glucose would be reduced just when they need glucose most. Evolution has dealt with this problem by causing exercise to increase the number of insulin receptors present on muscle fibres, to 'make the most' of the insulin molecules available. This effect of exercise can be used by diabetics to reduce the amount of insulin they have to inject.

In training for specific exercises, like training to play the piano, movements are learned by the motor systems of our brain and become more fluent. An interesting effect of exercise is the increased production of endorphins by the brain. The release of these *end*ogenous *m*orphines' within the brain is enhanced by exercise and they produce morphine-like euphoria as well as reducing the awareness of pain. They may be responsible for 'runner's high', a pleasant state of mind that occurs about half an hour into quite strenuous exercise and lasts for several hours. Unfortunately this state is followed a few days after the exercise by withdrawal symptoms in which the 'addict' feels anxious and depressed and has to take another bout of exercise.

Exercise, by the endorphin mechanism or some other, has been shown to improve mood; and exercise has been successfully prescribed for mildly depressed patients and found to be as effective as some drug treatments. Endorphins released during exercise suppress the sensation of pain and modulate the effects of other hormones. Endorphin effects are so powerful that they can obliterate the warning signs during prolonged exercise and allow marathon runners, for example, to continue until they collapse. This is obviously a dangerous situation which leads us to ask again if exercise is in fact a good thing.

Is exercise a good thing?

We have seen that pure strength training restricts its effects very largely to the muscles being trained. It is difficult to identify any benefit in this type of training other than a cosmetic one and perhaps a reduction in the incidence of damage due to overload of the muscles and joints.

Endurance training on the other hand has a wider spectrum of effects, particularly on the cardiovascular system. Experiments have shown that exercise makes hearts more vascular, with the number and diameter of their coronary arteries increased. Exercise also reduces blood cholesterol and low-density lipoprotein, important components of atherosclerotic plaque. If atherosclerosis does occur and one artery becomes blocked in the trained heart, there are more than normal 'in reserve' to supply the affected region. More and more patients are being given exercise as therapy after a heart attack and many become fitter than they were before their attack. However, any such programme, for patients or used prophylactically, should be initiated with caution. It is well known that endurance athletes of all ages do die of heart attacks. A heroic fitness programme intemperately entered into, particularly by the middle-aged, may cause the heart attack it was intended to prevent.

High blood pressure (hypertension) is frequently used to identify those at risk from cardiovascular disease. The association is well proven in populations, but it is still difficult to identify which individual members of a population will develop pathology as a result of their high blood pressure. The problem facing the heart of the hypertensive patient is easy to visualize, with the heart pumping against a 'brick wall' of increased peripheral resistance. Increasing systolic pressure, as in exercise, would seem to be (literally) the last thing to do. However, it is quite clear now that the systolic pressure of mild to moderate hypertensives increases to values equivalent to those found in exercising normal subjects and they too enjoy the benefits of the reduced diastolic pressure of exercise. After exercise, blood pressure is reduced for several hours in these patients, giving their hearts a period of respite.

Whatever the mechanism is, many studies have shown that people who remain fit have prolonged lives. Mortality of fit people between 60 and 70 is one-third of that of the unfit. This figure should not be simply attributed to exercise. People who take exercise are usually interested in their diet and lifestyle and make conscious efforts to improve the possibility of extending their active life. It may be that by exercise these people provide themselves with a functional reserve in the systems trained by exercise which they can call upon if they do become ill. There seems no doubt therefore that a *judicious* exercise regimen can improve the chances of an extended active life.

Further reading

Bagshaw C R 1992 *Muscle contraction*, 2nd edn. Chapman & Hall, London.

A clearly written little book by a biochemist who brings together information from many disciplines at a level between general textbooks and specialist reviews. Sufficiently modern for the sections on technical development and molecular genetics to still be relevant. Useful for students undertaking an honours degree in physiology.

Bülbring E (ed) 1981 *Smooth muscle: an assessment of current knowledge.* Edward Arnold, London.

Although the material in this compilation is no longer 'current', it is a fascinating presentation of the work of the great names in muscle physiology at that time, edited by one of the leaders in the field. Of interest to the advanced student.

Jones D A, Round J M 1990 *Skeletal muscle in health and disease.* Manchester University Press, Manchester.

A very readable and concise book for undergraduates covering the physiology of skeletal muscle, then training and the problems of fatigue, pain, damage and muscle disease. A breadth of subjects not usually found between the same covers.

Junquiera L C, Carneiro J, Kelly R O 1995 *Basic histology,* 9th edn. Appleton & Lange, Maidenhead.

Chapter 10 illustrates much of what is known of the structure of muscle.

Katz B 1970 *Nerve, muscle, and synapse.* McGraw-Hill, London.

One of the best undergraduate textbooks on this subject at its time. Still most readable and fascinating to have one of the leaders of the field 'chatting' to you about what they had been doing about the subject.

Kingston B 1996 *Understanding muscle.* Nelson Thornes, Cheltenham.

A novel book of tasks to encourage the interactive learning of the functional anatomy of the major muscles. Great fun and an excellent book for undergraduate medical students and others who are encouraged to carry out the tasks (and perhaps drawings) on themselves and their friends.

Mottram D R (ed) 1995 *Drugs in sport,* 2nd edn. Spon, London.

The bad news for anyone contemplating enhancing his or her sporting performance with drugs.

Perry S V 1996 *Molecular mechanisms in striated muscle.* Cambridge University Press, Cambridge.

An excellent, readable book on the molecular basis of muscle contraction suitable for honours degree students.

Walsh E G 1992 *Muscles, masses and motion.* Cambridge University Press, Cambridge.

A most interesting book which is at the same time scholarly and readable and concentrates on the control of movement. Can be read by all levels for information and entertainment.

Questions

Answer true or false to the following statements:

During contraction of striated muscle:
A. The length of both A- and I-bands decreases.
B. The force generated depends on the initial sarcomere length.
C. ATP is broken down by the myosin ATPase during the power stroke, i.e. as the myosin crossbridge is pulling on the actin.
D. ATP binding by myosin causes it to detach from actin.
E. Crossbridge formation is promoted by an elevation of sarcoplasmic $[Ca^{2+}]$.

2.1

Skeletal and smooth muscle:
A. Are controlled by different types of nerve.
B. Differ in that only skeletal muscle contains Z-disks.
C. Both make use of troponin to regulate contraction.
D. Both rely on nerves to initiate contraction.
E. Can both produce sustained contraction at low energy cost.

2.5

Excitation–contraction coupling:
A. Depends on Ca^{2+} binding to tropomyosin in skeletal muscle.
B. Depends on Ca^{2+} binding to calmodulin in smooth muscle.
C. Links changes in membrane potential to changes in mechanical state.
D. Can lead to fused tetany in skeletal muscle because the sarcoplasmic $[Ca^{2+}]$ stays elevated for some time after the repolarization of the action potential.
E. Produces shorter twitches in Type I than in Type II skeletal muscle fibres.

2.2

In skeletal muscle:
A. Individual muscle fibres are covered by a connective tissue sheet known as the epimysium.
B. Muscle fibres are usually arranged in series.
C. Muscle fibres are multinucleate.
D. Each motor unit is innervated by several motoneurones.
E. Muscle fibres are made up of myofibrils which contain the myofilaments.

2.6

Skeletal muscle metabolism:
A. Uses glucose as its main energy source under resting conditions.
B. Produces large reductions in ATP levels during contractile activity.
C. Is mainly aerobic in Type I (slow-twitch) fibres.
D. Produces lactic acid at high workloads.
E. Is likely to be mainly aerobic in fibres which contain a high density of mitochondria.

2.3

In striated muscle:
A. The thick myofilaments are attached to the Z-disks.
B. The T-tubules act as a Ca^{2+} store.
C. A sarcomere extends from one Z-disk to the next.
D. The length of the thin myofilaments can be calculated from the width of the I-band.
E. The length of the thick myofilaments can be calculated from the width of the A-band.

2.7

Skeletal muscle contraction in humans:

A. Is usually isometric during normal activity.
B. Usually involves a mixture of fast- and slow-twitch fibres.
C. Is an important source of heat in the body.
D. Promotes hypertrophy of the contracting fibres.
E. Can lead to an oxygen debt, part of which is due to anaerobic production of lactic acid.

2.8

Smooth muscle:

A. Of the visceral type, functions as an electrical syncytium because of the presence of gap junctions.
B. Has a lower myosin content than skeletal muscle and so can contract less forcefully.
C. Contains dense bodies which are attached to myosin molecules.
D. Can transmit force from one cell to the other via dense bands on the cell membrane.
E. Is made up of mononucleate fibres.

2.9

Smooth muscle contraction:

A. May be stimulated by muscle stretch.
B. Requires a much slower rate of ATP breakdown than striated muscle contraction.
C. Can be stimulated by humoral agents which activate phospholipase **C.**
D. Can be regulated by sympathetic and parasympathetic nerves.
E. Is rapid in comparison with striated muscle.

2.10

Excitation–contraction coupling in smooth muscle:

A. Is always dependent on Ca^{2+} release from intracellular stores.
B. Depends on phosphorylation of actin.
C. Is terminated by a phosphatase enzyme.
D. Following a rise in sarcoplasmic Ca^{2+} can lead to a maintained contraction even after sarcoplasmic Ca^{2+} levels have fallen again.
E. Requires troponin.

Answers

2.1

A. **True.** Somatic nerves control skeletal muscle, whereas autonomic nerves control smooth muscle.

B. **True.**

C. **False.** Troponin is central to excitation–contraction coupling in skeletal muscle but is absent from smooth muscle.

D. **False.** Skeletal muscle relies on nervous stimulation but many smooth muscles are spontaneously active, with the nerves modulating contraction.

E. **False.** This is a feature of smooth rather than skeletal muscle.

2.2

A. **False.** Endomysium surrounds individual muscle fibres; epimysium covers an entire muscle.

B. **False.** Muscle fibres are in parallel in most skeletal muscles.

C. **True.**

D. **False.** A motor unit consists of a single motoneurone and the fibres it innervates.

E. **True.**

2.3

A. **False.** Thick myofilaments are connected by the M-line or disk, thin myofilaments connect to the Z-disk.

B. **False.** The sarcoplasmic reticulum is the Ca^{2+} store.

C. **True.** This is the contractile subunit of the muscle fibres.

D. **False.** Thin myofilaments extend beyond the I-band because they interdigitate with the thick myofilaments in the A-band region.

E. **True.** The A-band is caused by the thick myofilaments.

2.4

A. **False.** Only I-band decreases in length.

B. **True.** This is reflected in the length–tension relationship for the whole muscle and relates to changes in the amount of myofilament overlap with changing length.

C. **False.** ATP breakdown is linked with repositioning of the detached myosin head prior to attachment at a new position on the actin; this stores energy within the myosin molecule. The power stroke, which pulls the actin along, is associated with release of ADP and phosphate from the myosin.

D. **True.** ATP depletion after death prevents this, causing rigor mortis.

E. **True.** This is a crucial step in excitation–contraction coupling.

2.5

A. **False.** Ca^{2+} binds to troponin, which in turn moves the tropomyosin to allow myosin and actin to bind.

B. **True.** There is no troponin in smooth muscle.

C. **True.** This is what the term means.

D. **True.** This results in a contraction which is longer than the electrical event which stimulated it, so further action potentials can be fired before the fibre has had time to relax.

E. **False.** Type I fibres are slow-twitch fibres.

2.6

A. **False.** Fatty acids are mainly used at rest, but use of glucose is greatly increased during exercise.

B. **False.** ATP levels only drop a little because creatine phosphate is used to rapidly replenish the ATP levels.

C. **True.** Anaerobic metabolism is more a feature of Type II, particularly Type IIb, fast-twitch fibres.

D. **True.** Lactic acid is produced as a result of anaerobic glycolysis.

E. **True.** Mitochondria are the site of oxidative phosphorylation during aerobic metabolism.

2.7

A. **False.** Normal contractions are usually neither isometric nor isotonic, since both muscle length and tension change.

B. **True.** Most human muscles contain both types of fibre.

C. **True.** This is used to maintain body temperature in cold conditions, e.g. through shivering.

D. **True.** This explains the exercise-induced increase in muscle size; the number of fibres does not increase.

E. **True.** Oxygen is used to manufacture glucose from lactic acid in the liver via the Cori cycle; this is probably only one cause of the oxygen debt, however.

2.8

A. **True.** Gap junctions in single-unit or visceral smooth muscle allow electrical signals to spread from cell to cell.

B. **False.** The myosin content is reduced in smooth muscle, but the contractile force per unit cross-section is similar to or greater than that in skeletal muscle.

C. **False.** They are attached to the actin.

D. **True.** Dense bands are connected to extracellular connective tissue by microfibrils.

E. **True.** This is unlike skeletal muscle, which is multinucleate.

2.9

A. **True.** This is possibly due to opening of stretch-activated membrane channels.

B. **True.** This allows contraction to be maintained at lower energy cost.

C. **True.** Phospholipase C leads to production of inositol 1,4,5-trisphosphate (IP_3) which releases Ca^{2+} from intracellular stores in smooth muscle.

D. **True.** The response depends on the transmitter and the receptors present.

E. **False.** It tends to be slow because of the slow rate of ATP breakdown.

2.10

A. **False.** Ca^{2+} entry across the sarcolemma from the extracellular space is important too.

B. **False.** It is myosin which is phosphorylated by the MLCK (myosin light-chain kinase) enzyme, which is activated by Ca^{2+}-calmodulin.

C. **True.** This myosin (light-chain) phosphatase reverses the effect of MLCK.

D. **True.** This is referred to as the latch state.

E. **False.** The troponin–tropomyosin system does not play a role in smooth muscle.

Neurological communication and control

3

Introduction

In the first two sections of this book we have
dealt with the excitability of living cells
(the way they respond to specific changes in
the environment) and the way in which they
use this excitability to control each other by
cell-to-cell signalling. These two properties are
basic to the process of homeostasis, which in
turn is fundamental to existence. The whole
purpose of a plant or animal's existence is to
ensure the continuation of its genetic material
in as many successful progeny as possible, and
only with the coming of humanity has any
other reason for existence become valid.
Existence depends on successful homeostasis.
Success at homeostasis depends on control,
and control depends on communication.

The mechanisms of control are laid down in
the genetic material within each cell. These
mechanisms operate at a molecular level
within individual cells. This control within a
cell or between cells of the same type is called
autocrine regulation. **Paracrine** regulation
involves substances released by cells to control
cells of a different type within range of
immediate diffusion. **Endocrine** regulation
involves substances, hormones, released so far
from their target that they depend on some
transport mechanism (a circulation) to carry
the message. **Neurocrines** (neurotransmitters
and neuromodulators) on the other hand are
released by neurones in the immediate vicinity
of their target cells, but only as a result of a
distant command. All these control mechanisms
depend on the diffusion of fairly large
molecules and so when diffusional distances
become larger than the dimensions of a cell the
times involved become considerable. In a
single-celled organism such as an amoeba, its
tiny size and leisurely lifestyle make these time
constraints acceptable, because diffusion over
small distances is rapid. When an organism
grows in size, however, even to the size of the
hardly visible hydra comprising a few hundred
cells, diffusion alone is not enough. In
multicellular organisms part of regulation is
taken over by neurocrine chemicals released
close to target cells, but in this case the release
is itself controlled by messages transmitted at a
very high speed over considerable distances in
what we know as nerves.

This common denominator of chemical
control exists in the apparently very different
regulating systems in our bodies. The
important difference between our nervous and
the endocrine systems is one of time rather
than mechanism. A voluntary movement of
our eyes is completed in a fraction of a second,
over and done with and a new movement
undertaken. But for the one-third of our life we

spend asleep this voluntary control is in abeyance. The slow movements of the gut digesting a meal, are modulated minute by minute by activity in the autonomic (vegetative) nervous system. When digestion is complete, autonomic activity in the gut subsides for hours on end. The control of the levels of glucose in our blood by the endocrine system begins before we are born and continues without halt for the rest of our waking and sleeping lives. You can see then that the communication and control systems of our body have more in common than might be supposed. We will deal first with the more rapid of our communication and control systems – the nervous system.

Section overview

This section covers:

- The autonomic nervous system as a model for peripheral neurotransmission
- The special features of the sympathetic and parasympathetic divisions of the autonomic system
- The synthesis, release and termination of neurotransmitters
- The special structures and functions of the neuromuscular junction that ensure transmission
- The postjunctional response of the muscle
- Drugs used to block and enhance neuromuscular transmission
- How inhibitory and excitatory postsynaptic potentials summate to determine if an action potential takes place
- How summation can be spatial or temporal
- Long-term potentiation as a basis for learning and memory
- The variety of central neurotransmitters
- Motor unit structure and muscle type
- Stretch and tendon reflexes as spinal control of muscles and control of movement by the brain
- The mechanisms that transduce physical energy into neural activity and the paths this takes to the cerebral cortex
- How pain is generated at nociceptors, and how their afferent activity is gated and modified by descending pathways.

The nervous system: a general introduction

Role of the nervous system

Our perceptions of the world around us, the feelings these perceptions generate and the actions we take as a result of these all depend on a rapid and complex flow of information within the nervous system. The incoming information is transduced from different forms of physical and chemical energy on entering, and the commands issued to structures are transduced into chemical transmitters on leaving the nervous system.

Within the nervous system the currency of this information is the action potential, which we have seen is generated by the membrane of excitable cells briefly becoming permeable to specific ions. The rapid transmission of information over long distances in the form of action potentials makes high-speed control possible.

The action potential is essentially stereotyped and it is difficult to associate the richness of our sensations and the freedom of our actions with such an unvarying entity. The secret lies in the enormous variety of pathways that exist for action potentials among the 10 billion neurones that make up our central nervous system.

We have only begun to understand the central nervous connections that make up our communication with reality, but we have been able to map out in some detail the incoming sensory and outgoing motor nervous systems that make contact with the world around and within us.

Evolution never favours wasteful systems and to use a high-speed system to control a

141

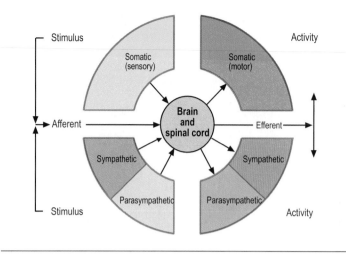

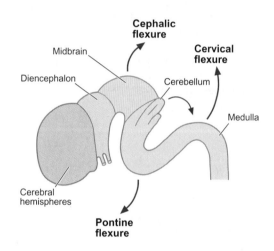

Fig. 3.1.1 **Organization of the nervous system.** Showing the flow of information from the sensory somatic and autonomic peripheral nervous system (PNS) to the central nervous system (CNS) and motor commands flowing to the autonomic and somatic motor systems. Afferent flow = toward the CNS; efferent flow = away from the CNS.

mechanism that does not require very rapid responses would be wasteful. Many of the sustained and slower responses of our bodies are therefore controlled by the endocrine system which, like the nervous system, ultimately relies on chemical command. The endocrine system is considered in Section 5.

Origin and outline of the nervous system

In learning physiology, a knowledge of structure always helps the understanding of function and nowhere more so than in the nervous system.

The human nervous system is divided into the **central** nervous system (brain and spinal cord) and the **peripheral** nervous system, which is itself divided into the **somatic** system, with sensory (**afferent**) and motor (**efferent**) components, and the **autonomic** system, which is divided into afferent and efferent sympathetic and parasympathetic parts (Fig. 3.1.1).

The brain and spinal cord can present an anatomical picture of intimidating complexity. Fortunately, a robust understanding of its functions, particularly at a clinical level, does not require a detailed knowledge of all its internal connections.

Much of the difficulty with the anatomy of the brain in particular results from it folding over on itself during development.

Fig. 3.1.2 **The flexures of the developing brain.** Regions are labelled with the names of the adult structures which will develop.

In the early embryonic disc a long streak of ectoderm forms a midline neural plate from which the nervous system will be formed. The edges of the plate lift up and fuse to form a tube. This tube is segmented, and our 31 pairs of spinal nerves that develop from these segments bear witness to the segmental nature of our primitive ancestors. At the anterior end of the embryonic neural tube the process of cephalization vastly expands the amount of neural material present and, as if to compress it into the smallest space possible, folds the tube over on itself (Fig. 3.1.2).

A

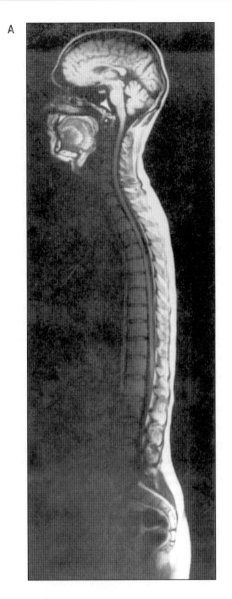

B

Cerebrum

Diencephalon and
basal ganglia

Brainstem

Midbrain

Pons

Medulla

Cerebellum

Spinal cord

Rostral
(Superior)

Ventral
(Anterior)

Dorsal
(Posterior)

(Inferior)
Caudal

Fig. 3.1.3 The central nervous system as (A) a midsagittal
MRI and (B) a diagram labelling major parts. (Image (A)
Courtesy of Philips Medical Systems)

In the human embryo 12 pairs of segmental
nerves, the cranial nerves, arise at the cephalic
end of the neural tube and in the adult are compressed into about 10 cm of brain, compared to
the whole remaining length of the spinal cord
being occupied by only 31 pairs of segmental
spinal nerves. In the embryo the sides of the
forebrain develop into two outgrowths, the

cerebral hemispheres, which cover the original
forebrain, which becomes the diencephalon
(the between brain) situated between these two
hemispheres. Development and reorganization
goes forward at an amazing rate, and with a
complexity which defies human understanding,
let alone emulation, to arrive at the structure
imaged in Figure 3.1.3.

Naming of parts of the nervous system

Central and peripheral somatic systems

Between the enveloping **cerebral hemispheres** of the human brain and the spinal cord are the **diencephalon**, which includes everything with the name 'thalamus' (thalamus, hypothalamus, epithalamus, subthalamus), the **basal ganglia** (the cordate nucleus, the globus pallidus, the putamen, claustrum and amygdala), the **midbrain**, the **cerebellum** (= little brain), the **pons** (= bridge), and the **medulla** (= marrow). These structures are functionally joined together and to the spinal cord by bundles of neurones called pathways. When found within the CNS, such a bundle may also be known as a tract, fasciculus, peduncle or lemniscus. Outside the CNS these bundles are simply known as nerves; which

demonstrates a major problem with neuro-anatomy – too many names for the same thing. For our purposes, the structure of the central nervous system can be reduced to the barest outline shown in Figure 3.1.4 on which the pathways in which we are interested can be traced.

This outline, functionally useful though it is, needs to be related to a few anatomical landmarks, many of which are obscured in human beings by the huge overgrowth of the *cerebrum* which is characteristic of our species. In relation to species differences, there is a matter of orientation that can cause confusion and arises from the human upright stance. The horizontal axis of quadrupeds becomes a vertical axis (Fig. 3.1.5) and dorsal–ventral, rostral–caudal becomes superior–inferior, anterior–posterior.

The cerebrum consists of a cortex of grey matter, made up largely of cell bodies, and deeper white matter, made up of nerve axons. It is divided into two hemispheres by the *median longitudinal fissure*. Deep fissures and shallow *sulci* (singular – sulcus) divide the surface of each hemisphere into large *lobes* and smaller convolutions called *gyri* (singular – gyrus; Fig. 3.1.6). Parts of these lobes have been given numbers (the Brodmann system) to more accurately relate structure to function. Cutting the brain in half along the median fissure

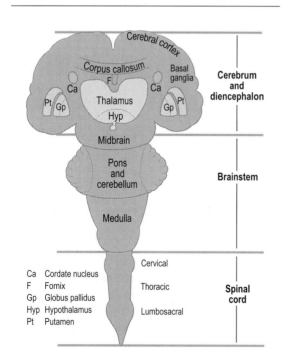

Fig. 3.1.4 Highly schematic outline of the anatomical organization of the central nervous system.

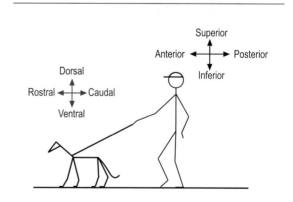

Fig. 3.1.5 Anatomical orientation with the upright stance. In terms of anatomical equivalence, what is ventral in the dog is anterior in man and what is dorsal in the dog is posterior in man.

(Fig. 3.1.7) reveals how great the division of the two cerebral hemispheres is, because only the most innermost structures stretch across the midline, starting with the *corpus callosum* – the major connection between the two cerebral hemispheres.

The structures labelled in our outline (Fig. 3.1.4) can be seen in relation to the other

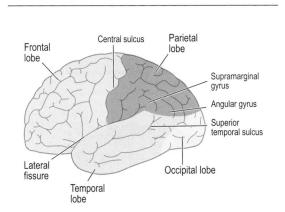

Fig. 3.1.6 **Surface anatomy of the cerebral hemispheres.** Deep fissures and shallow sulci divide the surface into large lobes and smaller gyri.

parts of the head and also the 3rd and 4th *ventricles* – spaces filled with cerebrospinal fluid, which is secreted by the walls of the ventricles and escapes from the 4th ventricle via *foramina* to fill the subarachnoid space between the brain and the arachnoid layer, the middle of the three coverings between the brain and the skull. Ventricles 1 and 2 are the two lateral spaces which connect with the 3rd ventricle.

The *cerebellum*, posterior and inferior to the cerebral hemispheres, consists of a central *vermis* and two *lateral hemispheres*. It connects with the rest of the brain via three *peduncles* on each side. Finally, the *pons* forms a bridge between the higher parts of the brain and the *medulla oblongata*, identified by its bilateral swellings, *pyramids*, which contain fibres crossing over from one side to the other in their journey to and from the spinal cord.

In a fetus of up to 3 months the spinal cord extends the whole length of the vertebral canal in which it lies. Because the vertebral canal grows much more than the cord, the cord in adults ends at the first lumbar vertebra. The 31 segments of the cord each give rise to a pair of spinal nerves comprising an anterior motor and posterior sensory root (Fig. 3.1.8). The relationship between white and grey matter in the

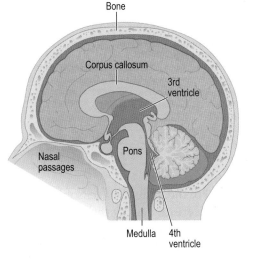

Fig. 3.1.7 **Sagittal view of the brain cut along the median fissure.**

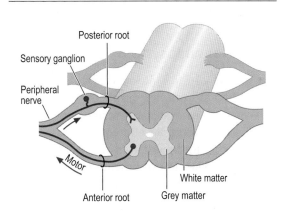

Fig. 3.1.8 **Spinal cord cross-section.** The afferent and efferent components of a segmental spinal nerve are shown.

![Summary icon] **Summary**

Structure of the nervous system

- This comprises central, peripheral somatic and peripheral autonomic nervous systems.
- The somatic system is made up of afferent (sensory) and efferent (motor) parts.
- The nervous system is formed from embryonic ectoderm.
- Cerebral hemispheres overlie most of the brain.

- Human upright stance means a different orientation from that of quadrupeds is sometimes used to describe human neural structures.
- Afferent and efferent nerves run in clearly defined tracts in both sides of the spinal cord.
- Some tracts in the cord cross over to the other side before reaching the brain.

spinal cord is the reverse of that seen in the brain because the majority of cell bodies in the cord are found at its core. Although the nerve tracts in the spinal cord synapse and cross from one side to the other (decussate) in complicated ways, they, like buses, are generally helpfully named by their origins and destinations; thus *corticospinal* tracts start from the cortex and run to the spine while *spinothalamic* tracts run from the spine to the thalamus. However, it would be impossible for anatomists to totally eschew classical allusion and the *fasciculus gracilis* and *cuneatus* refer to graceful and wedge-shaped little bundles of ascending fibres respectively (Fig. 3.1.9).

The autonomic system

The anatomy of the *autonomic nervous system* is very different from the peripheral somatic sensory and motor systems described so far. It is usually considered an efferent system serving all but the motor innervation of skeletal muscle. However, there are arguments that it should include the afferent (sensory) fibres which run with its efferent neurones. The *enteric nervous system*, whose cells lie in the plexuses of the gut, is part of the autonomic system and is capable

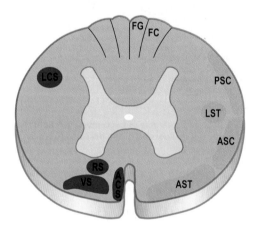

Fig. 3.1.9 Principal tracts in the spinal cord. Ascending tracts are on the right, descending on the left: FG = fasciculus gracilis; FC = fasciculus cuneatus; ASC = anterior spinocerebellar; PSC = posterior spinocerebellar; LST = lateral spinothalamic; AST = anterior spinothalamic; LCS = lateral corticospinal; RS = reticulospinal; VS = vestibulospinal; ACS = anterior corticospinal.

of control of the motor and sensory activities of the gut independently of the autonomic input which modulates it. Unlike the somatic motor system, in which a single motoneurone extends from the central nervous system to a muscle, the peripheral autonomic nervous pathways are

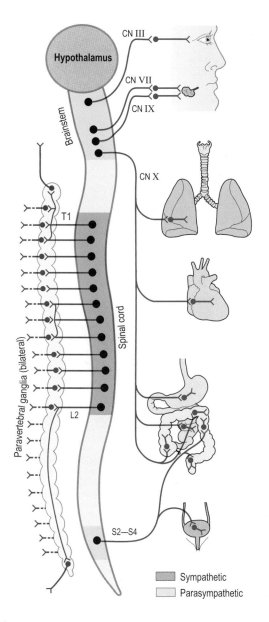

Summary

The autonomic nervous system

- This comprises the sympathetic, parasympathetic and, in some classifications, the enteric systems.
- It is a two-neurone system with the preganglionic cell body within the CNS.
- Sympathetic outflow leaves the CNS in segmental thoracic and lumbar roots.
- Parasympathetic outflow is in cranial nerves and the sacral region.
- The sympathetic system forms a chain of ganglia either side of the spine.
- The parasympathetic system forms ganglia close to or on the organ innervated.

Fig. 3.1.10 Schematic view of the autonomic nervous system. The sympathetic system is on the left and the parasympathetic on the right.

made up of a preganglionic and postganglionic neurones. The arrangement of the ganglia where these two synapse is one way of differentiating between *sympathetic* and *parasympathetic* divisions of the autonomic system. The parasympathetic outflow from the central nervous system is via cranial nerves and the sacral region of the spinal cord. Parasympathetic ganglia are found near or on their target organs (Fig. 3.1.10). Sympathetic outflow is segmental from the thoracic and lumbar regions of the spinal cord and its ganglia mainly form two chains, one either side of the vertebral column, and from these long postganglionic fibres innervate the target organs.

The peripheral autonomic system

Introduction

In describing the nervous system, it is usual to divide it into somatic and autonomic systems on the basis of apparent differences in function. The somatic nervous system provides voluntary motor control of skeletal muscle, whereas the autonomic nervous system provides an involuntary control of the internal environment and the viscera. However, this is not to say that the two systems are entirely separate and independent of one another. True, we have voluntary control over the movements of our limbs, but while I may flex my wrist at will, can I control individual muscles such as flexor carpi radialis in isolation? Just as the activity of this muscle is an inseparable part of the control of the wrist during voluntary movement, so is the control of the blood supply of the active skeletal muscle by the autonomic nervous system. Similarly, accommodation of the eye during voluntary examination of the print of this text cannot be distinguished from the act of fixation of vision, even though the first is 'autonomic' and the latter 'voluntary'. The real difference between autonomic and voluntary systems is mainly that you are aware of controlling skeletal muscle through the latter (Fig. 3.2.1). However, once the basis of the division is understood, such mental compartmentalization of the nervous system can help understanding.

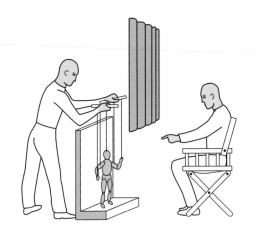

Fig. 3.2.1 A rehearsal at a puppet theatre. The director (conscious awareness) reports to the puppeteer (unconscious learnt skills) on his success in following the play's stage directions (the intended action). The information available to each is different and each contributes to the final result in a complementary manner. In the final production (the learnt action) the director has to remain in the wings.

 Basic Science 3.2.1

Diffusion

The process of diffusion is of immense importance to the operation of many physiological systems; not least the nervous system in which information is passed from one nerve cell to the next by movement of chemicals across the gap between them by a process known as diffusion.

At temperatures above absolute zero (–273°C) molecules are in constant thermal motion and vibration. A microscopic particle in a liquid undergoes about 10^{15} collisions per second with these moving molecules and if small enough to be moved but large enough to be seen under the microscope will be seen to undergo a continuous and continual chaotic 'random walk' as a result of this battering. This is sometimes called brownian motion. The molecular movements which bring about this motion of a visible particle suspended in a solution are of course invisible but equally chaotic and random. This random movement is called diffusion. It causes a net movement from regions of high to low concentration which will eventually obliterate any differences in concentration in the solution involved.

Because the movement of a molecule or ion undergoing diffusion is random it could move in any direction within a theoretical sphere surrounding it at each step in its 'random walk'. This enables us to calculate that the time to reach equilibrium of concentration by diffusion is proportional to the square of the distance over which diffusion takes place. This means that diffusion over a few microns takes seconds while diffusion over centimetres takes days. This time constraint is the reason most metabolically active cells cannot be much bigger than 20 μ diameter or more than about the same distance from a capillary.

The rate of diffusion of a substance in solution through a 'window' in space (see Fig. BS3.2.1) is defined by the Fick equation:

$$dv/dt = -D \times A(dc/dx)$$

where dv/dt is the rate of diffusion in molecules per second (that the movement is down the

Basic Science *(Continued)*

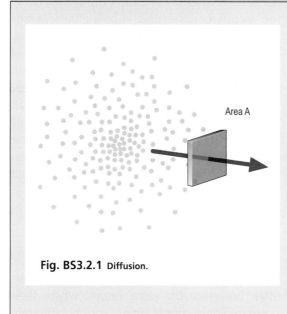

Area A

Fig. BS3.2.1 Diffusion.

concentration gradient is shown by the negative sign), *A* is the area of the 'window', (*dc/dx*) is the concentration gradient and *D* is the diffusion coefficient, which can be interpreted as the ease of movement of the molecule within the solution.

The diffusion coefficient of a molecule depends on a number of factors: its shape, whether it is carrying a charge, the nature of the solvent through which it is moving and very importantly the square root of its molecular weight so that small molecules diffuse much more easily than large ones. Thus water molecules diffuse 10 times more easily than sucrose (MW 340) and 40 times more easily than haemoglobin (MW 64 500) in aqueous solution.

When we need to consider the diffusion of substances across the lipid membranes of cells, things become even more complicated. The viscosity of cell membranes is about 1000 times greater than that of water, and the importance of the partition coefficient of the substance between the surrounding water and the membrane (the partition coefficient is the ratio of the concentrations of the substance dissolving in water and the membrane at equilibrium) is such that the ease of diffusion of water through cell membranes is 10^8 times greater than that of sucrose.

Structure and function

At the turn of the century, the English physiologist, Langley, subdivided the peripheral autonomic nervous system into three parts, using anatomical criteria. The subdivisions were **sympathetic** and **parasympathetic** (both of which are motor) and **visceral afferent sensory fibres**. Only in the 1970s was the enteric system – the peripheral extension of the autonomic nervous system to the gastrointestinal tract – accepted as an entity capable of some independent function.

The final common pathway of each of the two autonomic motor systems – sympathetic and parasympathetic – comprises two sets of motoneurones in sequence. The cell bodies of the preganglionic neurones lie in the brainstem and spinal cord; their axons make synaptic connection with postganglionic neurones. The cell bodies of these postganglionic neurones lie outside the CNS, frequently forming swellings (ganglia) on the nerves.

Efferent (motor) outflows: sympathetic and parasympathetic divisions

The location of the cell bodies of the preganglionic fibres is the basis of the anatomical subclassification of the peripheral autonomic nervous system. Motoneurones in the lateral horn of the grey matter of the thoracic and upper lumbar regions of the spinal cord form the preganglionic sympathetic division (the **thoracolumbar outflow**). Motor cells in cranial nerve nuclei III, VII, IX and X and in the grey matter of the sacral part of the spinal cord form the preganglionic components of the parasympathetic division (the **craniosacral outflow**).

Sympathetic preganglionic fibres pass via ventral roots and white rami communicantes to the sympathetic chain, where they synapse with postganglionic fibres in the prevertebral and paravertebral ganglia. The adrenaline-secreting cells of the adrenal medulla (chromaffin cells) have the same embryological origin as sympathetic postganglionic cells, and are innervated directly by sympathetic preganglionic nerves.

Parasympathetic preganglionic fibres pass directly to the destination organs, and the synapse between pre- and postganglionic fibres lies close to or within the innervated tissue. The parasympathetic postganglionic fibres are shorter than sympathetic postganglionic axons.

The preganglionic fibres of both divisions are of small diameter, (about 3 μm), many being myelinated B fibres conducting impulses at about 5–15 m/s. The postganglionic fibres are unmyelinated C fibres, 1 μm in diameter and conducting at about 1 m/s.

Figure 3.2.2 shows the destinations of autonomic fibres. The sympathetic system is distributed widely throughout the body, innervating the viscera, heart, lungs, gastrointestinal tract and most glands. Sympathetic fibres innervate the smooth muscle of most blood vessels.

The parasympathetic system has a specific, restricted distribution. Thus, the IIIrd cranial nerve innervates the eye, the VIIth cranial nerve the lacrimal, nasal and submaxillary glands and the IXth nerve the parotid salivary gland. The innervation to the thoracic and abdominal tissues is largely derived from the vagus (Xth cranial nerve), which supplies the heart, lungs, oesophagus and stomach, small intestine, gall bladder, pancreas and upper urethra. Pelvic sacral parasympathetic fibres form the pelvic nerves, which leave the sacral plexus to innervate the colon, rectum, external genitalia and bladder.

Effects of parasympathetic and sympathetic activation

The sympathetic and parasympathetic divisions often innervate the same organ, where their postganglionic fibres may supply different tissues (e.g. smooth muscle or secretory cells) or the same tissue (e.g. cardiac pacemaker cells); other tissues may be innervated by only a single division.

Table 3.2.1 shows the effects of increased activation of parasympathetic and sympathetic nerve fibres, together with the receptors involved. From this, it can be seen that the actions on tissues are diverse and are frequently opposite (though not invariably so). For example, both sympathetic and parasympathetic (vagal) efferent fibres innervate the cells of the heart that control the rate of beating (SA node). The effects of their activity are opposite, in that the vagal fibres induce a slowing of the heart rate while sympathetic fibres evoke an increase in heart rate. Changes in heart rate (chronotropic effects) are controlled by simultaneous but reciprocal changes in impulse activity within the two divisions.

The two divisions also have opposing effects on the vigour of contraction of heart muscle (inotropic effects). Cardiac ventricular muscle

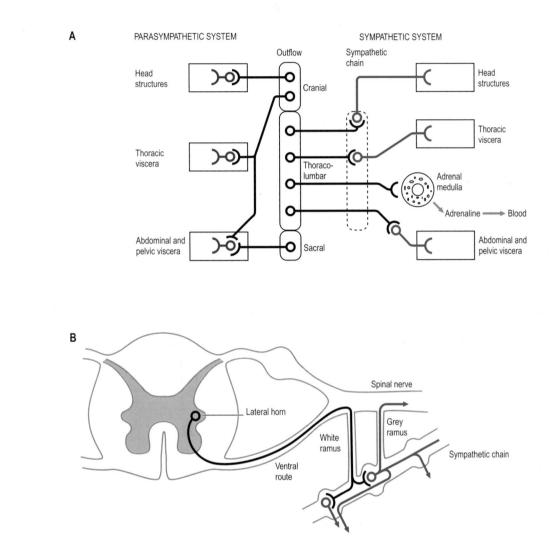

Fig. 3.2.2 The sympathetic and parasympathetic motor outflows from the central nervous system. A. The parasympathetic outflow comes from two sources – the cranial and sacral outflows. The sympathetic outflow comes from the thoracic and upper lumbar regions of the spinal cord and includes innervation of an endocrine gland, the adrenal medulla. **B.** The source of the sympathetic preganglionic fibres in the lateral horn of the cord.

fibres are supplied by sympathetic fibres whose activity increases their vigour of contraction (positive inotropic action); vagal fibres do not supply ventricular muscle, although they do influence (negatively) the vigour of contraction of atrial muscle. In the eye, the two divisions again act reciprocally, on different sets of opposing muscles, when controlling pupil diameter.

Table 3.2.1 Effects of parasympathetic and sympathetic nerve activation

Organ/system	Tissue	Sympathetic response	Sympathetic receptor	Parasympathetic response*
Eye	Pupil (dilator muscle)	Contraction	α	—
	Pupil (sphincter muscle)	—		Contraction
	Ciliary muscle	Relaxation (slight)	β	Contraction
Exocrine glands	Salivary glands	Mucus secretion (slight)	α	Serous secretion
	Tear glands	—		Secretion
	Gastric and pancreatic glands	Decreased secretion or no effect	α	Enzyme secretion
	Sweat glands	Secretion	Cholinergic	—
Gastrointestinal tract	Longitudinal and circular smooth muscles	Decreased motility	α and β	Increased motility
	Sphincters	Contraction	α	Relaxation
Heart	Pacemaker	Increased rate (+ve chronotropy)	β	Decreased rate (−ve chronotropy)
	Muscle	Increased force of contraction (+ve inotropy)	β	Decreased force (−ve inotropy, atrium only)
Arteries and arterioles	Of skin, mucosa	Contraction	α	—
	Of muscle	Contraction	α	—
		Dilatation	β	—
		Dilatation	Cholinergic	—
Veins	Most	Contraction	α	—
Spleen		Contraction	α	—
Urinary bladder	Detrusor muscle	Relaxation	β	Contraction
	Trigone	Contraction	α	—
Trachea and bronchi	Smooth muscle	Relaxation	β	Contraction
Piloerector muscles		Contraction	α	—
Genital organs	Seminal vesicles	Contraction	α	—
	Vas deferens	Contraction	α	—
	Uterus	Contraction	β	—
		Relaxation (variable)	β	—
	Blood vessels of penis and clitoris	—		Dilatation
	Arteries and veins	Constriction	α	—

* All parasympathetic responses result from muscarinic receptor activation.

Physiological range of impulse activity

In both sympathetic and parasympathetic divisions, the number of action potentials passing down the fibres depends upon the activity of the central nervous system and will frequently be modified by peripheral reflex inputs. While an increase in efferent impulse traffic induces an increased response, the overall frequency remains low and a plateau is quickly reached where further increases induce little enhancement of response.

Figure 3.2.3 shows the relationship between impulse frequency in sympathetic efferent fibres and the increase in resistance to blood flow evoked by contraction of the smooth muscle of small blood vessels. The range of effective response is produced by between <1 and 10 impulses/s. Frequencies higher than this produce relatively smaller effects. Similar frequency–response relationships are found in the parasympathetic system.

A second important characteristic of both motor divisions is the frequent, though not invariable, presence of tone. It is important to distinguish between '**neurogenic**' tone due to neural traffic and '**myogenic**' tone which is an inherent property of some smooth muscle.

Neurogenic tone is a maintained low frequency of nerve impulses under 'resting' conditions. For example, at rest, impulse activity in vagal nerves causes a tonic slowing of the heart rate in man to 65–75 beats/min, so that when the effects of the vagal nerves are blocked it rises to some 120 beats/min. Such vagal tone is particularly obvious in athletes and young people. Similarly, a partial constriction of arteries and arterioles (vascular tone) induced by activity in sympathetic efferent nerve fibres contributes to the maintenance of arterial blood pressure. The presence of tonic activity in autonomic nerve fibres enables an increase or decrease in, say, heart rate to occur simply as a result of an increase or decrease in tonic impulse activity in a single set of nerve fibres.

The importance of neurogenic tone is vividly illustrated by the catastrophic fall in arterial blood pressure, owing to the profound fall in the peripheral resistance, when ganglionic transmission to sympathetic efferent fibres innervating vascular smooth muscle is blocked throughout the body by the ganglion-blocking agent, hexamethonium (see Clinical Example: Hexamethonium man).

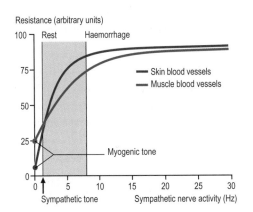

Fig. 3.2.3 The relationship between the frequency of action potentials in sympathetic fibres and the response of an effector. Both myogenic and neuronal tonic activity are indicated, together with that elicited by stress (haemorrhage). Note that the relationship is different for blood vessels of skin and muscle. The shaded area indicates the range of normal sympathetic control (see text for details).

Clinical Example

Hexamethonium man

W D M Paton, in 1954, vividly described the effects of a dose of hexamethonium, which blocks transmission in sympathetic and parasympathetic ganglia, in what has since been known as 'hexamethonium man' (Fig. CE3.2.1):

He is a pink-complexioned person, except when he has stood in a queue for a long time, when he may get pale and faint. His handshake is warm and dry. He is a placid and relaxed companion; for instance he may laugh but he can't cry because tears cannot come. Your rudest story will not make him blush, and the most unpleasant circumstances will fail to make him turn pale. His collars and socks stay very clean and sweet. He wears corsets and may, if you meet him out, be rather fidgety (corsets to compress his splanchnic vascular pool, fidgety to keep the venous return going from his legs). He dislikes speaking much unless helped by something to moisten his dry mouth and throat. He is long-sighted and easily blinded by bright light. The redness of his eyeballs may suggest irregular habits and in fact his head is rather weak. But he always behaves like a gentleman and never belches or hiccups. He tends to get cold and keeps well wrapped up. But his health is good; he does not have chilblains and those diseases of modern civilisation, hypertension and peptic ulcer, pass him by. He gets thin because his appetite is modest; he never feels hunger pains and his stomach never rumbles. He gets rather constipated so that his intake of liquid paraffin is high. As old age comes on, he will suffer from retention of urine and impotence, but frequency, precipitancy and strangury will not worry him. One is uncertain how he will end, but perhaps, if he is not careful, by eating less and less and getting colder and colder he will sink into a symptomless, hypoglycaemic coma and die, as was proposed for the universe, a sort of entropy death.

From this vivid picture we can see the result of giving hexamethonium to an animal or a man depends primarily on the pattern and intensity of the autonomic tone prevailing. This is partly because no effect can be seen if an inactive pathway is blocked, and partly because the more intense the activity at the ganglionic synapse, the more sensitive proportionately it becomes to a block. Ganglion-blocking agents therefore tend to pick out the most active autonomic processes.

Several illustrations of this arise in the action on the blood pressure. With a supine, normal

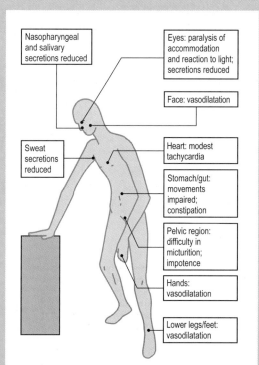

Nasopharyngeal and salivary secretions reduced

Eyes: paralysis of accommodation and reaction to light; secretions reduced

Face: vasodilatation

Sweat secretions reduced

Heart: modest tachycardia

Stomach/gut: movements impaired; constipation

Pelvic region: difficulty in micturition; impotence

Hands: vasodilatation

Lower legs/feet: vasodilatation

Fig. CE3.2.1 Hexamethonium man. This man has been given an effective dose of the ganglion-blocking agent hexamethonium, which has effectively removed all his sympathetic tone and abolished any parasympathetic responses. He is in a parlous state!

Clinical Example *(Continued)*

patient this action may be quite slight; but if he is tilted or stands up, or is dehydrated, or has lost blood, or is pyrexial, or has a labile neurogenic hypertension, or has lost extracellular fluid by the action of a diuretic – all conditions which lead to an increase in vasomotor sympathetic tone – the hypotension produced by ganglionic block is considerably increased. The hypotensive effect, therefore, varies according to the circumstances, as well as from patient to patient.

Other circulatory effects include vasodilatation of the skin of the feet and lower parts of the legs, and of the hands and face, with usually a modest tachycardia due to vagal block. Cardiac output and renal blood flow are not reduced unless a severe hypotension is produced by postural adjustment. The skin becomes warm and heat is lost from the body, so that the body temperature may fall by 1–2°C and shivering develops, despite relatively warm extremities. Cardiovascular reflexes, such as the response to painful stimuli, or the 'overshoot' in blood pressure after a Valsalva manoeuvre, are weakened or abolished. The effect of infused noradrenaline may be augmented, since the reflexes limiting the rise in blood pressure

(including a reflex bradycardia) are paralysed on the effector side.

Paralysis of the sympathetic pathways may also have less obvious consequences. For instance, ganglionic block may both intensify the hypoglycaemic effect of insulin and diminish the autonomic signs of hypoglycaemia.

Block of parasympathetic pathways also occurs. In the eye there is a paralysis of accommodation and of the pupil's reaction to light; the intraocular pressure usually falls, probably because of the accompanying hypotension. Secretions are reduced not only in the eye but throughout the body, including sweat, salivary and nasopharyngeal secretion, and that of the stomach and alimentary tract. Movements of the stomach and gut are impaired, since the ganglion plexuses which mediate peristaltic reflexes are blocked. As a result, delay in stomach emptying and constipation may develop. Sometimes, with continued administration, ileus may be produced, but diarrhoea is also seen. Paralysis of the pelvic outflow may lead to difficulty in micturition or to impotence.

One can thus see why hexamethonium did not become a popular antihypertensive agent, in spite of its potent blood pressure-lowering effects.

Visceral afferent fibres

Visceral afferent fibres originate from sensors (receptors) in the internal organs. They constitute a high proportion of the fibres in the vagus (80%) and splanchnic nerves (50%), whose cell bodies are in the nodose ganglia (inferior and superior vagal ganglia) and spinal ganglia (spinal afferents) respectively. Afferent fibres from the carotid area, which contains receptors sensitive to arterial pressure (baroreceptors) or

chemical changes in arterial blood (chemoreceptors), pass in the glossopharyngeal nerve (IXth). Afferent fibres from the pelvic organs pass directly to the spinal cord. Some visceral afferent fibres sense pressure (baroreceptors), volume (bladder receptors) or shear forces (small intestine); others are chemosensory, e.g. arterial chemoreceptors sensing the P_{O_2}, P_{CO_2} and pH of arterial blood, or glucoreceptors in intestinal mucosa. Such receptors are frequently involved in the neural and hormonal control of visceral functions through negative feedback circuits involving the brainstem and spinal cord. One group of visceral afferent fibres, nociceptors, are excited by stimuli which elicit sensations of visceral pain, e.g. strong stretch or contraction of the gastrointestinal tract or urinary bladder. These fibres pass into the spinal cord with the sympathetic nerves as spinal afferent fibres. Such 'painful' sensations are not normally encoded by vagal visceral afferent fibres.

Summary

The autonomic system

- The somatic nervous system provides voluntary motor control of skeletal muscles. The autonomic nervous system involuntarily controls the viscera and internal environment.
- The peripheral autonomic nervous system is subdivided into sympathetic and parasympathetic motor systems and a visceral afferent sensory division.
- Sympathetic preganglionic fibres synapse close to the spinal cord. Parasympathetic preganglionic fibres pass directly to their destination organs. Parasympathetic postganglionic fibres are much shorter than sympathetic postganglionic fibres.
- The effects of the sympathetic and parasympathetic systems are frequently (but not invariably) opposite.
- In both autonomic motor systems there is a persistent low-frequency background activity (tone). A modest increase in frequency produces maximum effect.
- Visceral afferent fibres from internal sensory receptors synapse in the brainstem and spinal cord to produce homeostatic reflexes or the sensation of pain.

The specific role of visceral afferent fibres and functions in which they are involved are discussed elsewhere.

Autonomic neuroeffector mechanisms

Research into autonomic neuroeffector mechanisms is developing rapidly. This section is concerned with the classical neurotransmitters **acetylcholine** (ACh) and **noradrenaline** (NA) – the study of which has suggested a common basic mechanism of neurotransmitter release, modified according to the specialized function of the particular nerve. Other, non-classical potential neurotransmitters are discussed later in the chapter.

The identification of autonomic transmitters

Acetylcholine and noradrenaline have been identified as important transmitters in the autonomic nervous system and are referred to as the 'classical transmitters'. Much work has been carried out to identify other possible neurotransmitters of widely differing forms. There is general agreement that, for a substance to be convincingly accepted as a transmitter agent, it should satisfy at least the following criteria:

- The putative neurotransmitter must be shown to be released from the nerve by physiological mechanisms and its action mimicked at appropriate concentrations by an externally applied substance.
- Receptors capable of inducing the physiological actions must be present at the effector cells.
- Adequate mechanisms for synthesizing, transporting and releasing the transmitter have to be present in the nerve terminal and shown to be capable of operating under physiological conditions.
- Adequate mechanisms for destruction and/or inactivation of the putative

neurotransmitters must be present at the terminal or immediately adjacent in the effector tissues.

Because of the complexity surrounding many synapses, particularly those in the central nervous system (CNS), only tentative identification of their neurotransmitters has been possible following satisfaction of only one or two criteria.

The structure of the autonomic neuroeffector junction

Unmyelinated autonomic nerves release neurotransmitter from a series of varicose expansions of the axon situated every few microns along the terminal. These 'boutons' are 'en passant' contacts where the nerve is very close to the membrane of the effector cells. Each axon branches several times, forming an autonomic ground plexus. This structure can be visualized under a light microscope, when the fluorescent properties of several neurotransmitter derivatives can be exploited to make the nerve terminals visible (Fig. 3.2.4).

The association between the autonomic nerve and effector cells varies. In some situations, three to eight axons are grouped into a bundle by a Schwann cell and release transmitter from a position remote (110–200 nm) from the effector cell. The response is then widely distributed and slow in both onset and decay. Other axons form close contacts with effector cells, separated from them by a gap of only 20 nm; this allows localized fast electrical responses in the effector cell. Close contacts are found, for example, in

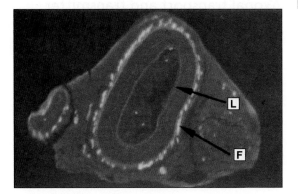

Fig. 3.2.4 Autonomic neurotransmitters. Noradrenaline, the postganglionic neurotransmitter of the sympathetic nervous system becomes fluorescent when treated with formalin. This figure shows the distribution of noradrenergic nerve endings in the outer layer (F) and elastic lamina (L) of an artery. (From Young B, Heath J W 2000. *Wheater's Functional Histology*, 4th edn. Churchill Livingstone, Edinburgh.)

the vas deferens, while the smooth muscle in the gastrointestinal tract and blood vessels is influenced by more remote release sites. In blood vessels, sympathetic fibres rarely penetrate the full depth of the smooth muscle in the tunica media, but are restricted to the outer medioadventitial border.

Within varicosities, the transmitter is stored within **vesicles**. These have been classified according to their size and the presence of an electron-dense core. Deductions can be made as to the transmitter stored from the appearance of the vesicle. Immunohistochemical tests have identified the transmitter contents of several vesicle populations (Table 3.2.2). While the categorization thus produced may be an oversimplification, it is useful.

Table 3.2.2 The characteristics and contents of synaptic vesicles

Appearance	Name	Size (nm)	Core	Contents
Large granular (LGV)	P-type	60–100	Yes	Peptides and 5-hydroxytryptamine
Small granular (SGV)	a-type	30–60	Yes	Noradrenaline
Small clear (SCV)	c-type	20–60	No	Acetylcholine

Axonal transport and transmitter synthesis

Cellular proteins are synthesized in the Golgi apparatus in the nerve cell body. The structural proteins and enzyme systems of the nerve terminal are transported down the axon as vesicles. It was thought at one time that neurotransmitter arrived in the terminal solely by this means, but it is now regarded as important only in the case of the peptide neurotransmitters. Non-peptide transmitters are synthesized largely in the terminal where they are to be released.

Release of transmitter

The arrival of an action potential at the release site triggers calcium-dependent release of transmitter, probably via exocytosis (Fig. 3.2.5). The vesicle contents are expelled by fusion of the vesicle with the axonal membrane and its eversion to the outside of the cell. This was first suggested by the observation that large protein molecules, which cannot cross an intact membrane, are released with smaller neurotransmitters. Cytoplasmic enzymes, such as lactate dehydrogenase, are not released. The demonstration of vesicles in the early stages of this process, in nerves stimulated at the moment of fixation, confirmed this view (Fig. 3.2.6).

Exocytosis, which is the expulsion of the contents of an intracellular vesicle from a cell and which involves the fusion of the vesicle

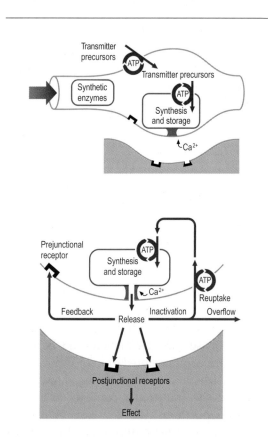

Fig. 3.2.5 The basic steps of neurotransmission. Synthetic enzymes (proteins) are transported from the cell body. At the release site (the varicosity) neurotransmitter precursors from the interstitial fluid are transported into the cell where transmitter is synthesized and then stored in vesicles. An action potential causes an inrush of Ca^{2+}, thereby triggering the release of transmitter from vesicles bound to the varicosity membrane. The effector is activated by the interaction of the neurotransmitter with specific membrane receptors. Other receptors on the nerve may also be activated by the transmitter and modulate subsequent release. Released neurotransmitter is inactivated by diffusion away from the receptors, by enzymatic destruction or by recapture by the nerve. Recaptured transmitters are taken back into the vesicle and reused.

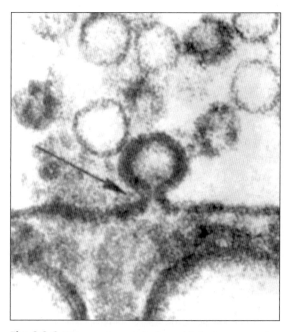

Fig. 3.2.6 Electron micrograph of a vesicle in the process of discharging its contents during the process of neurosecretion.

membrane with the wall membrane, eventually resulting in the incorporation of the vesicle membrane into the wall membrane, is an important part of neurosecretion. Exocytosis, which differs according to the site and specialization of the process, permits fast, brief, local communication between cells. All exocytosis appears to be dependent on the presence of Ca^{2+} and may be regulated by controlling intracellular Ca^{2+} concentrations. In the case of all large molecules, activation of several intracellular enzyme systems leads to exocytosis after a delay which may be measured in seconds. The process can continue for minutes.

However, neurosecretion (which involves relatively small molecules) is both rapid and brief. The synaptic delay (the interval between the arrival of the nerve action potential and the first detectable postjunctional effect) in mammalian nerves is a fraction of a millisecond, and the duration of the effects of the transmitter is also short, a few milliseconds. In order to achieve such rapid changes of state, a membrane macromolecule must be altered. One of the most rapidly acting protein kinases, phosphorylase β kinase, will phosphorylate 15 mmol of substrate/min per mg of enzyme, or 1 substrate molecule/catalytic subunit each 12 ms. This is rapid enough for most secretory mechanisms but not for the release of fast neurotransmitters. Such a rapid mechanism might be operated by the induction of a conformational change of a macromolecule. The current suggestion is that a change occurs in a preformed **fusion pore** which has already bound the vesicle to the membrane. The site may involve special binding proteins present at defined places in the vesicle and in the membrane.

The trigger for change in conformation of the pore protein is the inflow of Ca^{2+} ions caused by the axonal action potential. The high local concentration of Ca^{2+} thus achieved at the membrane would decay rapidly enough by simple diffusion into the bulk of the axonal cytoplasm to explain the short period of release initiated by each action potential.

Neuronal exocytosis is also unusual in that the vesicular membrane is not permanently incorporated into the cell membrane, but is somehow recaptured for reuse by the cell as a new vesicle.

Transmitter within nerve fibres is divided into several compartments or pools which differ in their availability for release. During intense activity, it is the newly synthesized transmitter that is most immediately available.

Quantal content of the release process

The vesicle is probably the **quantum**, or least unit of currency, of the transmission process. In contrast to the skeletal neuromuscular junction, where quantal release by each action potential is measured in hundreds, at the autonomic neuroeffector junction each action potential releases only a few quanta from each release site.

Presynaptic control of release

The release of transmitter may be controlled by substances in the interstitial fluid. The membranes of nerve terminals contain receptors which are activated by transmitters and other substances. Receptor activation can modulate the amount of transmitter being liberated through variation in the resting membrane potential, or mechanisms which involve second messengers.

The control of circulation of the blood through active tissues is one role of the autonomic nervous system. One of the factors relevant to the control of the perfusion of a tissue by the circulation is its current metabolic needs. Active tissues use O_2 and produce CO_2. Tissue hypoxia, hypercapnia or low pH all depress the release of neurotransmitters. This will reduce the effective sympathetic vasomotor tone of active tissues and tend to increase their perfusion. The effect of this local modulation varies. The innervation of some tissues is more susceptible than are others. For example, vasomotor fibres to skeletal muscle, where local and reflex control are important, are much more susceptible than those to the skin, whose circulation must be dominated by the CNS and the demands for thermoregulation.

Autonomic effector mechanisms

Autonomic neurotransmitters produce their effects by action upon specific receptors: **nicotinic** and **muscarinic** acetylcholine receptors and **α** and **β adrenoceptors**. Activation of these receptors may cause changes in membrane permeability or induce enzyme-mediated second messenger formation in effector cells.

Second messenger systems

The responses triggered in effector cells by the action of neurotransmitters depend finally upon the modification of target cell metabolism. This is brought about by changes in the activation of enzymes mediated by protein kinases and free Ca^{2+} levels.

Changes in intracellular free Ca^{2+} have long been recognized as second messengers involved in the contraction of muscles and neurosecretion. Cellular free Ca^{2+} levels may rise following receptor activation either through an effect of the receptor upon Ca^{2+} channels in the cell membrane, or via a second messenger which may release intracellular Ca^{2+}.

Two other important second messenger systems involve **cyclic AMP** (cAMP) and derivatives of the membrane constituent phosphoinositide diphosphate. The receptor-activated enzyme adenylyl cyclase forms cAMP from ATP. Cyclic AMP diffuses within the cell and activates protein kinases, under whose influence other cellular enzymes are activated by phosphorylation, leading to the cell's response (Fig. 3.2.7).

Phosphoinositide-based second messenger systems involve the receptor activation of the enzyme phospholipase C. This yields two metabolites, **inositol trisphosphate** and **diacylglycerol**, two independent second messengers. Diacyglycerol acts within the membrane, activating kinases which control membrane ion channels, while inositol trisphosphate causes the release of Ca^{2+} from intracellular stores.

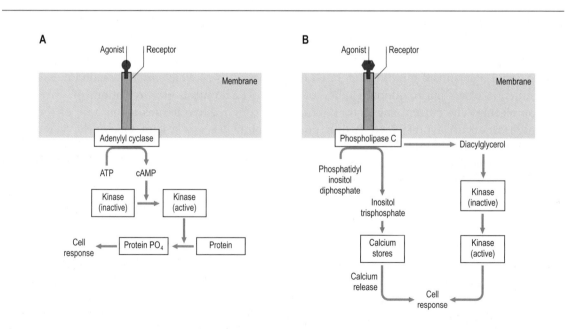

Fig. 3.2.7 Two second messenger mechanisms found in the autonomic nervous system. The effector response results from the formation of the second messengers cAMP (**A**) and inositol trisphosphate or diacylglycerol (**B**).

Termination of effect

The effect of the released transmitter may be terminated in one of several ways. The most important mechanism is simple diffusion of the transmitter away from its site of release. This process, unless impeded, rapidly lowers the local concentration to below an effective level. Additionally, there may be enzymatic destruction of the transmitter or its reuptake by the nerves that released it. The result of both of

Summary

Neurotransmitters

- The classical neurotransmitters of the parasympathetic and sympathetic systems are acetylcholine and noradrenaline respectively.
- The equivalent in the autonomic system of the neuromuscular junction of striated muscle is 'varicosities' set at intervals along the nerve terminal.
- The varicosities (sometimes called boutons) are much more variable in structure than neuromuscular junctions.
- Arrival of an action potential at a release site triggers Ca^{2+}-dependent transmitter release by exocytosis.
- Release and subsequent removal of neurotransmitter is over in a few milliseconds.
- Autonomic neurotransmitters act upon specific nicotinic and muscarinic acetylcholine receptors and α and β adrenoceptors.
- The effects of released transmitter are terminated by diffusion away from the receptor site, enzymatic destruction of neurotransmitter and reuptake by the presynaptic terminal.

these active processes may be to reuse all or part of the transmitter molecule.

Cholinergic mechanisms

Acetylcholine (ACh) is released by preganglionic nerve fibres of both sympathetic and parasympathetic divisions of the autonomic nervous system and by postganglionic nerves of the parasympathetic division (Fig. 3.2.8). The sympathetic innervation of sweat glands is also cholinergic.

Acetylcholine synthesis (Fig. 3.2.9)

Acetylcholine is synthesized in the nerve terminals. Acetyl-coenzyme A (AcCoA) is manufactured in mitochondria and the acetyl group transferred to choline through action of the enzyme choline acetyl transferase or choline acetylase (ChAT). ChAT is synthesized in the cell body and transported by axoplasmic flow to the nerve endings. Choline is accumulated in the terminals by active uptake from interstitial fluid. This uptake is an important rate-limiting step in ACh synthesis. Much of the choline released by breakdown of released ACh (see below) is taken up again by the terminals and recycled (see Fig. 3.2.11).

Acetylcholine storage and release

Following synthesis, ACh is stored in vesicles in the terminals; each vesicle contains approximately 10^4 ACh molecules, which are released as a single packet (quantum).

The arrival of an action potential in the presynaptic axon terminal causes an influx of Ca^{2+} which causes release of ACh from vesicles already bound to the inner surface of the nerve cell membrane by a protein link (the protein may be synapsin) into the space between the nerve terminal and the effector tissues (Fig. 3.2.10). Mobilization of unbound vesicles towards the presynaptic membrane replaces those released.

163

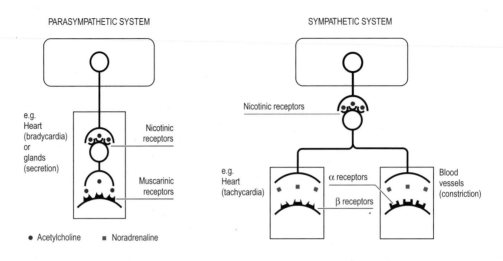

PARASYMPATHETIC SYSTEM

e.g.
Heart
(bradycardia)
or
glands
(secretion)

Nicotinic
receptors

Muscarinic
receptors

● Acetylcholine ■ Noradrenaline

SYMPATHETIC SYSTEM

Nicotinic receptors

e.g.
Heart
(tachycardia)

α receptors

β receptors

Blood
vessels
(constriction)

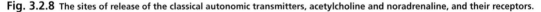

Fig. 3.2.8 The sites of release of the classical autonomic transmitters, acetylcholine and noradrenaline, and their receptors.

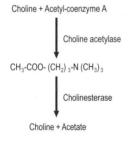

Choline + Acetyl-coenzyme A

Choline acetylase

$CH_3\text{-}COO\text{-}(CH_2)_3\text{-}N(CH_3)_3$

Cholinesterase

Choline + Acetate

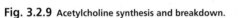

Fig. 3.2.9 Acetylcholine synthesis and breakdown.

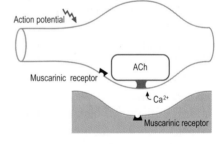

Action potential

Muscarinic receptor

ACh

Ca^{2+}

Muscarinic receptor

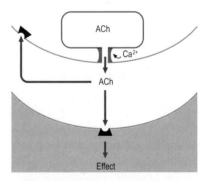

ACh

Ca^{2+}

ACh

Effect

Receptors

The effects of ACh on tissues are the result of an action of the neurotransmitter upon a **receptor** present in the membrane of the effector cells. Several types of ACh receptors have been characterized by their sensitivity to agonists (which mimic the action of ACh) or antagonists (which specifically block the action of ACh).

Some acetylcholine receptors are most easily activated by agonist molecules, such as nicotine

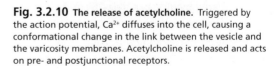

Fig. 3.2.10 The release of acetylcholine. Triggered by the action potential, Ca^{2+} diffuses into the cell, causing a conformational change in the link between the vesicle and the varicosity membranes. Acetylcholine is released and acts on pre- and postjunctional receptors.

(**nicotinic receptors**); others are more sensitive to muscarine (**muscarinic receptors**). Selective antagonists also exist. Atropine selectively blocks muscarinic receptors, and quaternary ammonium bases, such as hexamethonium or decamethonium, selectively block nicotinic receptors. Recent work has suggested that there are also other types of ACh receptor and further developments can be expected.

Nicotinic receptors are found on the post-ganglionic side of synapses between the pre-ganglionic and postganglionic fibres of both parasympathetic and sympathetic divisions. The cholinergic link between postganglionic fibres of the parasympathetic division and the effector tissues operates via a muscarinic receptor (see Fig. 3.2.8).

Acetylcholine inactivation

At cholinergic junctions, high concentrations of the enzyme **acetylcholinesterase** (or choline-sterase) are present. This enzyme rapidly hydrolyses acetylcholine and is important in its inactivation (Fig. 3.2.11).

Noradrenergic mechanisms

Noradrenaline is a most important sympathetic transmitter.

Noradrenaline synthesis

Noradrenaline is synthesized from the amino acid tyrosine by the Blaschko pathway (Fig. 3.2.12). A hydroxyl group is added to the aromatic ring of tyrosine, forming DOPA (3,4-dihydroxyphenylalanine). This is decar-boxylated to the amine, dopamine, which in turn is hydroxylated in the β-position to nor-adrenaline. The enzymes involved have names that are simply descriptive of their function.

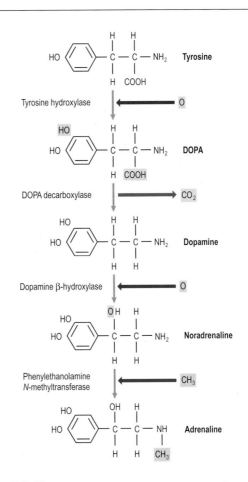

Fig. 3.2.12 **The Blaschko pathway for the synthesis of noradrenaline and adrenaline.**

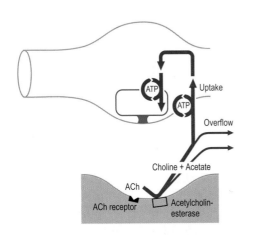

Fig. 3.2.11 **The inactivation of acetylcholine.**
Acetylcholinesterase splits the transmitter, releasing choline which is then recaptured by the nerve and reused in the vesicle to form more acetylcholine.

The conversion of tyrosine to DOPA is the rate-limiting step in catecholamine synthesis. Tyrosine hydroxylase undergoes end-product inhibition by noradrenaline, thus controlling synthesis according to the release of transmitter and the consequent depletion of the nerve ending store. The other enzymes are not saturated by the substrates, and other suitable substrates presented to them can be taken into the pathway and eventually lead to the production of 'false transmitters' in the nerve which can be released when the nerve is active. Introduction of α-methyl DOPA into the pathway leads to the accumulation of α-methyl noradrenaline in the nerves. This strategy has therapeutic implications.

Noradrenaline release

Noradrenaline is stored in synaptic vesicles together with ATP and some proteins, including dopamine β-hydroxylase (Fig. 3.2.13). Each vesicle contains several thousand molecules of noradrenaline.

An action potential traversing the varicosity causes an influx of Ca^{2+} and the subsequent release of noradrenaline along with the ATP and protein stored in the vesicle. Ca^{2+} influx initiates exocytosis by inducing a conformational change in the protein, synapsin, which bonds the vesicles to the membrane of the varicosity. Each action potential induces the release of only a few quanta (vesicles). The mean quantal content of release by an individual release site is less than 1. Release is intermittent with many action potentials failing to release transmitter from a given varicosity.

Noradrenergic receptors on effector cells

The pharmacologist Ahlquist (1948) divided the effector receptors to catecholamines into two major types, α and β, on the basis of their agonist sensitivities. Noradrenaline stimulates α receptors at lower concentrations than are

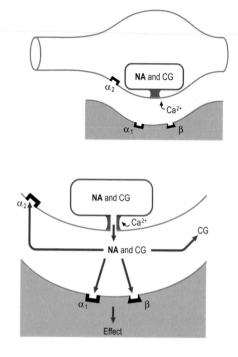

Fig. 3.2.13 The release and effects of noradrenaline. Triggered by the action potential, Ca^{2+} diffuses into the cell causing a conformational change in the link between the vesicle and the varicosity membranes. Noradrenaline (NA) is released together with several vesicle proteins collectively known as chromogranins (CG). The noradrenaline acts on the pre- and postjunctional receptors.

needed to stimulate β receptors. Adrenaline is equipotent at both sites. More recently, both α and β receptors have been divided into two subtypes – $α_1$ and $α_2$, and $β_1$ and $β_2$. Further subdivision of these types is to be expected.

Presynaptic noradrenergic receptors

Once released from the nerve, noradrenaline acts on the effector organ to initiate a response. In addition, it may act on receptors on the motor fibres themselves, modulating subsequent release of transmitter by these fibres. Noradrenergic nerve release sites have $α_2$ adrenoceptors, which, when activated, depress subsequent release. This mechanism could form the basis of a negative-feedback control of release by individual release sites. It is more likely, however, that transmitter released by one site acts on nearby sites to modulate their activity. Such a mechanism would evenly distribute the stimulus to the effector cells. A fibre in an active region would be more depressed by noradrenaline released by its neighbours than one in an inactive region. Noradrenergic nerves also have receptors for several other putative transmitters, including acetylcholine and adenosine. The possibilities for complex interaction between autonomic nerves and the tissues have not yet been fully investigated.

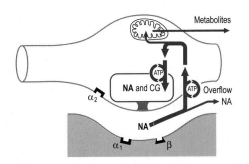

Fig. 3.2.14 Overflow, active reuptake, reuse and enzymatic degradation in noradrenaline (NA) inactivation.

The fate of the released noradrenaline
(Fig. 3.2.14)

The action of released noradrenaline is terminated by its active uptake by the releasing fibres, or its dispersion by diffusion. Recapture by the nerves accounts for the major part of the released transmitter and involves an energy-dependent, carrier-mediated transport process named **uptake-1**. A less selective, less avid, facilitated diffusion of noradrenaline takes place into smooth muscle; this process is called **uptake-2**. Noradrenaline recaptured by uptake-1 is concentrated by a vesicle uptake mechanism and can be subsequently reused by the nerve. This reuse is necessary for the maintenance of noradrenaline stores. Without reuse, the synthetic capability of the Blaschko pathway is not sufficient to maintain the nerve-ending stores, even during the resting tonic activity of the sympathetic nerves. Thus, blocking uptake-1 not only prolongs transmitter action, but also leads to a rundown of both noradrenaline stores and release.

As with the synthetic pathway, the uptake processes for noradrenaline can concentrate related compounds, which leads to interference with the function of the nerve. This is mitigated by the presence in the mitochondria of the nerve of an enzyme, monoamine oxidase

(MAO). Although noradrenaline is a substrate for this enzyme, other amines are attacked more avidly. Originally, MAO was thought to have a role in terminating transmitter action (by analogy with acetylcholinesterase). However, it is clear from its intraneuronal location in the mitochondria, that this function is not possible. In the fibre terminal, MAO removes false transmitter precursors like tyramine, which enter into the nerve via uptake-1. Tyramine, an amine found in several foods, is an indirectly acting sympathomimetic – it displaces noradrenaline from the vesicle stores, causing it to leak out of the nerve in a calcium-independent manner. This effect is normally prevented by the destruction of any intracellular tyramine by MAO.

Another enzyme, catechol-*O*-methyl transferase (COMT), located extraneuronally, can attack noradrenaline. Circulating catecholamines are metabolized sequentially by COMT and MAO, with formation of several inactive products.

The development of fluorescent derivatives of catecholamines led to the description of many noradrenaline-containing nerves, and confirmed the belief that noradrenaline was the principal sympathetic transmitter. The existence of postganglionic sympathetic nerve fibres which released acetylcholine and induced sweat gland secretion or dilated skeletal muscle blood vessels was accepted as an exception to the rule.

Non-adrenergic, non-cholinergic (NANC) mechanisms

A fascinating recent development in physiology is that concerned with new neurotransmitters. New insights into the physiology of the classical transmitters are still appearing, and new unconventional transmitters, such as amino acids (e.g. GABA) and peptides (e.g. VIP, substance P) have been demonstrated. Their roles have not yet been fully elucidated. This new research is in an exciting phase and new developments are likely to occur rapidly. Drugs that affect **NANC** transmission are proving to be important in psychopharmacology (see Clinical Examples: Anxiety disorders, p. 191; and Schizophrenia, p. 195).

While the evidence for existence and release of noradrenaline is unchallenged, it is now clear that the situation is more complex than was previously thought. Firstly, in some tissues, other amines such as 5-hydroxytryptamine or dopamine are released: **5-hydroxytryptamine** (5-HT or serotonin) has been demonstrated in interneurones of the enteric nervous system and the brain. Secondly, immunological techniques have led to the identification of many peptides in nerve endings. These peptides are familiar elsewhere in the body as hormones, e.g. cholecystokinin (CCK). The list is lengthening, and includes somatostatin, encephalins, substance P, vasoactive intestinal peptide (VIP) and neuropeptide Y (NPY). The purine derivatives, ATP and ADP, are now firmly established as neurotransmitters.

The mechanism for inactivation and destruction of peptide transmitters appears to be slow, involving proteolytic enzymes. Peptides act over a longer time-course, and they may have a role in modifying the sensitivity of the postsynaptic effector tissues to the action of classical transmitters (neuromodulation).

Co-transmission and co-release

For some of the new transmitters, an association with 'classical' transmitters can be demonstrated. Thus, VIP and calcitonin gene-related peptide (CGRP) are co-located with acetylcholine in postganglionic parasympathetic terminals, and NPY is co-located with noradrenaline in sympathetic terminals. It is likely that they may be co-released (Fig. 3.2.15). Stimulation of many mixed nerves releases more than one active substance. This may be due to the presence of a mixed population of nerve fibres in the tissue (the simultaneous stimulation of sensory nerves and their effect is often boldly ignored in these experiments) or to the release of a number of active agents by a single nerve. A nerve fibre might release more than one transmitter simultaneously in several different ways (Fig. 3.2.15). Several transmitters may be stored in the same vesicle and released together in unvarying proportions (co-transmission). Alternatively, a nerve ending may contain different transmitters located in separate vesicles (co-release) which may then be released either together or independently depending on the state of the nerve.

The vesicles that contain noradrenaline and adrenaline in the adrenal medulla also contain proteins, the chromogranins (see Fig. 3.2.13) and ATP. Both the chromogranins and ATP are released with noradrenaline. In some tissues, part of the postjunctional response is due to the action of ATP. But since the release of ATP and noradrenaline can be separated, it seems likely that separate purinergic nerves release ATP. The significance of the granular ATP for transmission is not clear.

It is unlikely that any nerve liberates only one molecular species; nonetheless, rigorous testing of any claim for a particular co-transmission is necessary.

Co-transmission

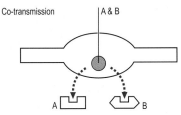

Co-release

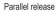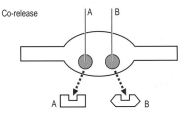

Parallel release

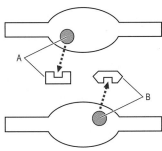

Fig. 3.2.15 Co-transmission, co-release and parallel release of transmitters A and B. A and B may be stored together in the same vesicle, in separate vesicles in the same nerve, or in separately activatable nerves.

Summary

Transmitter release

- Acetylcholine (ACh) is released by the preganglionic terminals of both sympathetic and parasympathetic autonomic nerves and postganglionic parasympathetic nerves.
- ACh is synthesized in the nerve terminals by the acetylation of choline actively taken up from interstitial fluid in a process of recycling.
- Each vesicle (quantum) of ACh contains about 10^4 molecules.
- Noradrenaline is synthesized from tyrosine.
- Released noradrenaline modulates release of noradrenaline from nearby fibres.
- The majority of released noradrenaline is recaptured by the releasing nerves by a process known as uptake-1.
- Non-adrenergic, non-cholinergic (NANC) neurotransmitters including many amino acids and peptides seem to exert a more long-term effect, modifying the action of classic neurotransmitters.
- More than one transmitter may be released at a site by the process of co-transmission, co-release and/or parallel release.

The variety of mechanisms in the sympathetic neuroeffector junction is not unexpected when its range of function is considered. In different tissues sympathetic nerves perform very different functions. Those innervating the arterioles of a skeletal muscle maintain a constant high level of activity, or tone, remitted only occasionally, in modern man at least, during exercise, when local metabolism will alter their rate of transmitter release. At the other extreme, the sympathetic innervation of the vas deferens is only occasionally stressed, and may not need to respond to local conditions.

Recent Advances

Non-synaptic transmission

It was once thought that the nervous system was a single entity functioning as a whole. The idea that the nervous system was made up of discrete units (neurones) whose functional contact with others of their kind was via gaps (synapses) whose properties largely governed the functioning of the system was something of an intellectual novelty when it was first proposed at the end of Queen Victoria's reign.

Evidence quickly accrued that the nervous system is in fact a circuit of neurones broken by synapses across which chemical transmitters are quantally released. As in many other cases in science, ideas have come full circle and there are now a number of investigators involved in demonstrating that there is also a more general release of transmitters from non-synaptic sites, and that these transmitters diffuse over relatively large distances to distant targets, or to the nearest synapse, to provide a background of transmitter to whole volumes of the nervous system.

In the gut, administration of noradrenaline or activation of noradrenergic neurones inhibits acetylcholine release from neighbouring cholinergic nerves without there being any synaptic connection involved. Blockade of α_2 adrenoceptors on the other hand results in increased cholinergic transmission from neurones which have no synaptic connection with adrenergic fibres. These findings imply a functional connection between these neurones. Other substances, including nitric oxide (NO) and carbon monoxide (CO), have been implicated as transmitters in these non-synaptic interactions.

The presynaptic equivalent

It has been known for some time that postganglionic neurones in the autonomic nervous system have swellings (varicosities) at intervals along their length; these are sometimes called *boutons-en-passant*. They can be considered as non-directional synapses, specialized to ensure a widespread effect of transmitter. The adrenal cortex, for example, in addition to being under the control of the pituitary gland, appears to be under direct local neural modulation. Adrenergic nerve endings lie in close proximity to the zona cells without making synaptic contact and influence steroid secretion. Recent studies suggest that this type of transmission is more common in the CNS than was previously supposed. The nerve varicosities can be considered as unspecialized equivalents of the highly specialized presynaptic region of the neuromuscular junction and account for about 20% of the innervation of the cerebral cortex.

The hippocampus is very rich in noradrenergic varicose axons and the majority of these varicosities (2 million per mm^3) do not form synapses. This sort of density means that, on average, each varicosity is surrounded by a volume of about 500 μm^3 of extracellular space. The concentration of transmitter in that space will of course depend not only on the number of varicosities but on their rate of release. These two factors provide the equivalent of spatial and temporal summation at conventional synapses.

Release of transmitter from non-synaptic sites can be vesicular (which is extracellular calcium $[Ca^{2+}]_o$ dependent) and cytoplasmic (non-$[Ca^{2+}]_o$ dependent). This type of release

Recent Advances *(Continued)*

from the neuromuscular junction has been calculated to be greater than that due to spontaneous miniature endplate potentials. It has been suggested that synaptic transmission should be considered as rapid 'digital' transmission, while non-synaptic activity should be considered as an 'analogue' modulation of the sensitivity of the system.

The transmitters

In addition to the conventional transmitters that have been associated with non-synaptic transmission, nitric oxide (NO) and carbon monoxide (CO) have received particular attention. These substances are released as gases and, with a half-life of several seconds,

NO generated at a single varicosity should be able to exert an effect in a sphere of 300 µm, which is a large volume compared to the synaptic gap. The persistence of NO and its diffusivity mean it can diffuse over 100 µm in 5 s, which fits it very well for the role of a non-synaptic transmitter where interactions could be expected to occur on a time-scale of seconds or minutes and over distances of hundreds of micrometers.

If non-synaptic transmission proves to have significance in the central nervous system, then it will also have therapeutic implications for the drug treatment of psychiatric disorders. Non-synaptic chemical communication may provide an additional level of versatility and plasticity to the 'hard-wired' synaptic circuitry of the brain.

The neuromuscular junction

Introduction

For the voluntary system of muscles in our body to function in a controlled way there must be a reliable chain of command from the higher motor centres in the brain to the muscles themselves.

This chain is made up of many neurones and, finally, muscles. Transmission between nerve and muscle is via the skeletal **neuromuscular junction** (NMJ), a highly specialized neurotransmission system. Its only role is to maintain one-to-one transmission of impulses of excitation from an α-motoneurone to the muscle fibres it innervates. This transmission must be reliable and stereotyped to allow the CNS to assume a predictable response to any centrally generated programme of activity – an action potential in a motor nerve must result in an action potential in the muscle innervated. The muscle action potential then initiates the muscle contraction. To maintain this one-to-one relationship – one neural action potential produces one muscle action potential – the NMJ has evolved to minimize the effects of influences that at other junctions in the nervous system vary the postjunctional response. These influences include:

- activity-related facilitation and fatigue of transmitter release
- local modulation of release in response to anoxia or the products of metabolism.

173

The second category is of obvious importance in active skeletal muscle where activity causes high oxygen use and metabolite production. The robust nature of neuromuscular transmission is clearly demonstrated in a rhythmically contracting muscle in which unmodified transmission persists in the face of local modulation which powerfully affects the sympathetic innervation of the blood vessels supplying the muscle.

The function of the neuromuscular junction can be likened to that of a detonator in a bomb, when a tiny pulse of electricity (the nerve action potential) must absolutely reliably trigger a response in a much more massive system (the muscle). The key to this function lies in the structure of the junction.

Structure (Fig. 3.3.1)

Near the neuromuscular junction, the motoneurone loses its myelin sheath and divides into fine terminal branches. The actual junction

A

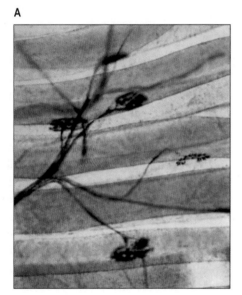

Fig. 3.3.1 Neuromuscular junction.
(A) A micrograph of neuronal axons branching as they contact a skeletal muscle. (From Young B, Heath J W 2000 *Wheater's Functional Histology*, 4th edn. Churchill Livingstone, Edinburgh.)
(B) The structure of the junction is shown diagrammatically.

B

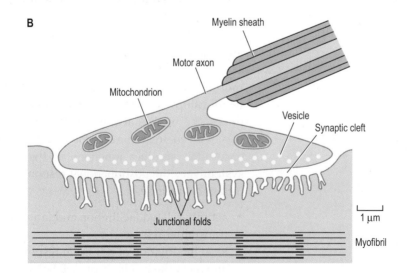

in skeletal muscle is between these fine un-myelinated branches and single muscle fibres. Originally it was thought that contact between nerve and muscle at a 'gap junction' allowed uninterrupted transmission of an electrical impulse; however, the resolution of the electron microscope has revealed a gap about 500 Å (50 nm) wide. The axon terminals of this region spread out and give the neuromuscular junctions its alternative name – the **endplate** (although the term 'endplate' is now usually used to refer to the postjunctional muscle membrane). The special features of the regions on either side of the gap in the endplate are induced by their close physical proximity to each other. The developmental mechanisms that produce these features are known as trophic effects.

As the nerve terminals approach the muscle they lose their myelin sheath, although a Schwann cell may overlie the axon. Within the cytoplasm of the terminal are seen electron-translucent (clear) vesicles which contain the neurotransmitter substance acetylcholine. The vesicles are most numerous close to the cell membrane where it in turn is closest to the muscle.

The endplate region of the muscle forms a trough in which the nerve terminal lies. The walls of this trough are thrown into complex folds, the outer surface of which is covered by acetylcholine receptors and acetylcholinesterase which destroys acetylcholine. The receptors are concentrated on the crests of the folds opposite the clusters of vesicles in the nerve terminal. The esterase is more uniformly distributed through the endplate. If the motor nerve supplying a motor fibre dies, the features of an endplate on the surface of the muscle fibre disappear. The acetylcholine receptor density at the site of the old endplate decreases and receptors appear on the rest of the muscle. If re-innervation occurs this change is reversed. Thus, normally, acetylcholine is only active on the muscle membrane at the neuromuscular junction and there only on the external surface;

Summary

Structure of the NMJ

- The neuromuscular junction is a highly-specialized neurotransmission system between motor nerve and muscle.
- Its role is reliable one-to-one translation of motoneurone action potentials into muscle action potentials.
- The essential structural features of the neuromuscular junction are spreading motor axon terminals containing vesicles, a gap of 50 nm and a much-folded muscle cell membrane below the terminals.

acetylcholine injected into the interior of the muscle fibre, even at the neuromuscular junction, fails to produce any effect.

The endplate is a unique synaptic structure. Some other junctions between elements of the nervous system show some evidence of specialization but nowhere else is the density of synaptic vesicles, receptors and inactivating enzyme systems so great. The function of these structures can be discovered by measuring endplate potentials.

Endplate potentials

The function of the neuromuscular junction is to enable the tiny currents that constitute an action potential in a relatively small motor nerve to reliably bring about contraction of a relatively massive muscle.

To excite a muscle to contract, its membrane potential must be lowered some 40 mV from −90 to about −50 mV. It can be calculated that if all the current of an action potential in a motoneurone were passed to the muscle fibre it innervates, it could produce a potential change of only 1–2 mV. The electrical situation is, however, much worse because of the gap between nerve and muscle, which would reduce the potential change at the muscle fibre membrane to less than 1 pV. This problem of electrical 'mismatching' renders the possibility of direct electrical excitation extremely unlikely. Nevertheless, electrical activity can be detected on both sides of the neuromuscular junction in the following experiment (Fig. 3.3.2).

If an electrode is placed on the surface of a neuromuscular junction, the change in voltage at the surface as a result of current flow in either the motor nerve or muscle can be recorded. An action potential is experimentally triggered in the nerve by an electrical signal which produces an artefact (A). After an interval, while the action potential travels down the nerve the action potential is detected at the electrode (B). Some 0.5 to 0.75 ms later the massive muscle fibre action potential occurs (at C).

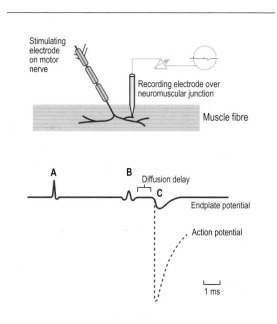

Fig. 3.3.2 Surface recording at a neuromuscular junction.
The change of voltage is of the opposite sign to that seen when the recording electrode is intracellular, and an endplate potential is only seen when the much larger action potential that usually obscures it is blocked.

This experiment demonstrates that there is a delay between the arrival of the action potential at the nerve terminal and the development of the muscle action potential. Further evidence for the independence of these two events is the fact that the muscle event can be selectively suppressed by bathing the nerve and muscle with a solution low in Ca^{2+} or high in Mg^{2+} or containing a drug called curare. Experiments such as this present evidence for electrical discontinuity at the junction. The electrical activity of the nerve has come to an end, and some non-electrical process has intervened to trigger the more massive electrical activity of the muscle.

That the intermediate process of transmission between nerve and muscle is chemical, and that it is sufficient to allow the minute energies of a nerve action potential to cause an action potential in a muscle fibre was demonstrated by Sir Henry Dale and his collaborators who showed that acetylcholine is released by motoneurones, and that this substance is a potent stimulant of skeletal muscle contraction. Dale laid down general 'laws' which can be applied to any substance that is a candidate for the role of chemical transmitter. These are described in detail on page 194 and can be summarized as follows:

1. The substance must be released from a presynaptic site.
2. It must act at a postsynaptic site.
3. The amount released must be sufficient to initiate postsynaptic activity.
4. Mechanisms must be present for its destruction.

Acetylcholine at the neuromuscular junction fulfils these criteria.

Acetylcholine synthesis, storage and release

Acetylcholine is synthesized in the nerve terminal from choline and acetyl-coenzyme A (AcCoA) by the enzyme choline acetyl transferase. AcCoA is produced by the nerve cell but choline has to be captured from the extracellular fluid and transported into the cell by a choline transport system capable of transporting choline up its electrochemical gradient. Much of the choline comes from the hydrolysis of previously released acetylcholine by acetylcholinesterase. This reuse of costly transmitter is a feature of many other neurotransmitter systems, and pharmacological interference with the process is therapeutically used in a number of psychoactive drug therapies.

Acetylcholine is concentrated and stored in synaptic vesicles found in the nerve terminals. Each vesicle stores approximately 10^4 molecules. These loaded vesicles are released as the basic quanta, or packets, of the transmission process. The amount of acetylcholine released during motor nerve stimulation has been estimated to be a few million molecules per action potential per endplate. At rest, single packets are released at random intervals at a rate of about 1 per second. This spontaneous release causes small, 0.4 mV, depolarizations of the muscle membrane of the endplate called **miniature endplate potentials**. There is evidence that a non-quantal release also occurs as a sort of diffusional trickle. This release is not large and its importance is not understood.

When an action potential arrives at the nerve terminal of the neuromuscular junction, a synchronized release of several hundred vesicles occurs. At most other junctions (synapses) in the nervous system only a few quanta are released by a single action potential.

The sudden precipitate release of vesicles is caused by the depolarization of the nerve terminal opening Ca^{2+} channels in the membrane, which allows Ca^{2+} to flood in. Acetylcholine release is by the process of exocytosis where the vesicles fuse with the nerve cell membrane forming an opening through which the acetylcholine is ejected into the extracellular space (Fig. 3.3.3).

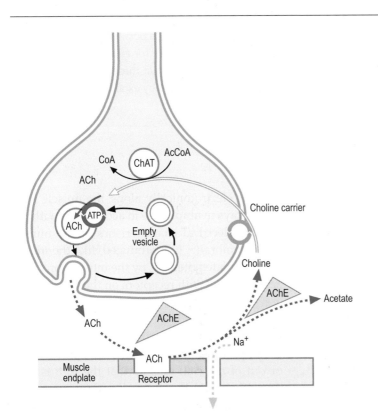

Fig. 3.3.3 Neuromuscular junction release and recycling of transmitter substance. Acetylcholine (ACh) is synthesized in nerve terminals by the acetylation of choline by the enzyme choline acetyl transferase (ChAT), which uses acetyl-coenzyme A (AcCoA) as a source of acetyl groups and choline from the hydrolysis of 'used' acetylcholine by cholinesterase. Formed acetylcholine is stored in vesicles at high concentration by active transport and is released into the junction cleft by exocytosis triggered by the arrival of an action potential in the motor nerve. About two-thirds of the released acetylcholine survives the diffusional journey across the gap to trigger receptor-operated channels in the muscle membrane. It remains on the receptor for about 2 ms and is then released to suffer the fate of the acetylcholine that did not successfully make the journey – hydrolysis by acetylcholinesterase (AChE) before it has time to interact with a second receptor site. About half of the choline formed in this way is recaptured by the nerve terminals to make more acetylcholine.

Clinical Example

Denervation

The motoneurone of the neuromuscular junction releases acetylcholine, which activates receptors on the muscle fibre directly below the nerve ending. Application of acetylcholine to other regions of the muscle, and even injection into the fibre, normally produce no effect. An interesting exception to this is that some time after the motor nerve to a muscle has been cut the whole muscle becomes sensitive to acetylcholine. This is called *denervation hypersensitivity* and is due to a spread of acetylcholine receptors all over the fibre. If a new axon now grows toward the muscle fibre this sensitivity disappears, and the original pattern of receptors (only below the nerve ending) reappears.

It seems that nerve cells, via their synapses, not only transmit information but by trophic agents control the structure of cells on which they impinge. Another example of these trophic effects is seen in a technique much used by anatomists to follow the path of axons through the central nervous system. In this technique the axon of a nerve is cut close to the cell body, the axon distal to the injury dies off (just as your arm would die if cut off your body) and the anatomists follow this 'wallerian degeneration' to map out the pathways they love to trace. What is interesting in this context is that the next neurone in the chain, separated from the dying axon by the synaptic gap, also degenerates. The dead axon was not only sending information to the next neurone but supporting it with trophic agents as well.

Another form of control exists. A motoneurone will jealously prevent the muscle fibre it innervates from making contact with a second motoneurone, but if that neurone dies the faithless muscle fibre will immediately allow another neurone to make contact.

These findings have implications for the physical basis of memory, but what is even more exciting, they present the possibility that the brain may be responsible for arranging its own neuronal connections, that these are not fixed and may be determined by experience.

The postjunctional response

The rapid release of relatively large amounts of acetylcholine into the narrow cleft between nerve and muscle produces a depolarization of the muscle fibre localized to the endplate. This depolarization of the membrane beneath the nerve terminals must be distinguished from the muscle action potential it produces. It is called an **endplate potential** (EPP), has a rise time of 1–2 ms and, unlike an action potential which has the same amplitude at all points on a nerve or muscle, the EPP can be of varying amplitude, spreads electrotonically along the muscle fibre and decays in amplitude in accordance with the passive electrical characteristics of the muscle fibre membrane. It is produced, like the miniature endplate potential, by the interaction of the acetylcholine with receptors on the muscle. The acetylcholine receptor forms an ion channel across the membrane. The reversal potential of this mechanism (the artificially imposed membrane potential at which ions do not flow into or out of the cell) tells us that the EPP is produced by an influx of small cations, predominantly Na^+. There are more than 10^7 receptors on each endplate and the channels associated with them are normally closed. When they open, for about 1 ms, they admit small, positively charged ions into the cell. It is important to remember that although the EPP can be of variable amplitude, once it reaches the threshold of the muscle membrane, it triggers a stereotypical self-propagating muscle action potential (a detonator either triggers a bomb or it does not; when it does, the bomb goes off in a very stereotypical way).

The depolarizing current produced by the release of hundreds of quanta of acetylcholine when a nerve action potential reaches its terminals is more than sufficient to cause the initiation of an action potential in the muscle membrane surrounding the endplate. The EPP can be reduced by 75% and still trigger a muscle action potential. There is thus a large safety factor in the transmission process at the skeletal neuromuscular junction. This safety factor exists because of the exceptionally large release of acetylcholine by the nerve into a very narrow gap and because of the high sensitivity of the endplate related to the density of receptors. This reduces the possibility of transmission failure due to fatigue of the nerve terminal or desensitization of the muscle endplate region. As the muscle action potential spreads over the muscle fibre, it invades the T-tubules and releases Ca^{2+} from the sarcoplasmic reticulum into the sarcoplasm, and the muscle contracts.

Transmitter inactivation

The most important route of inactivation of acetylcholine in the neuromuscular junction is by hydrolysis by **acetylcholinesterase** (Fig. 3.3.3). In most synapses diffusion of the transmitter from its site of release is sufficiently rapid to reduce the local concentration by several orders of magnitude in a millisecond. At the skeletal neuromuscular junction the high density of receptors retaining the transmitter delays this diffusion. Each acetylcholine–receptor interaction holds the transmitter

Summary

Function of the NMJ

- The essential biochemical features are vesicles containing acetylcholine and a synaptic gap containing an abundance of acetylcholinesterase which hydrolyses acetylcholine.
- Neuronal action potentials release acetylcholine which diffuses across the gap.
- Acetylcholine depolarizes the muscle membrane and produces an endplate potential (EPP).
- If it reaches threshold, the EPP produces a muscle action potential and subsequent contraction.
- After depolarizing the muscle membrane, the acetylcholine is hydrolysed by acetylcholinesterase to choline and acetic acid.
- Choline is reabsorbed by the nerve and recirculated.

molecule for about 1 ms. The efficiency of acetylcholinesterase is such that the half-life of the transmitter in the junction is about 1 ms. Few transmitter molecules make more than one interaction with a receptor before they are destroyed. The importance of this can be seen if acetylcholinesterase is blocked with an anticholinesterase such as neostigmine when the endplate potential is prolonged and a single nerve action potential can lead to repetitive muscle action potentials.

Drugs and the neuromuscular junction (see also Clinical Example, p. 181)

Theoretically, it is possible to interfere with neuromuscular transmission at pre- or post-synaptic sites. Presynaptic pharmacology seems to be confined to the research laboratory or to the realms of toxicology. Transmission can be halted by substances that block the uptake of choline or transport of acetylcholine into synaptic vesicles. Even more dramatically, acetylcholine release can be inhibited by neurotoxins such as botulinum toxin, produced by *Clostridium botulinum* under anaerobic conditions in badly preserved food; and α-bungarotoxin contained in cobra venom. These incredibly potent and extremely unpleasant substances are thought to inactivate the actin which brings about the exocytosis of acetylcholine vesicles from the presynaptic nerves.

Drugs that affect the postsynaptic membrane are of great importance in surgery where surgeons like to have their patients' muscles very relaxed. This can be achieved by deepening the level of anaesthesia or, more safely and effectively, by blocking neuromuscular transmission. Drugs that are used for this are described as either non-depolarizing or depolarizing according to their mode of action.

Non-depolarizing agents like *d*-tubocurarine bind to the acetylcholine receptor but do not open the receptor-gated ion channels in the muscle membrane. They bind to the receptor but do not stimulate it. By binding to the receptor they deny access to it by the acetylcholine molecules and thus reduce their effect. Reducing the effect of acetylcholine reduces the size of the endplate potential that a nerve impulse produces; when this fails to reach the threshold for initiation of the muscle action potential, the muscle stops contracting.

Increasing the amount of acetylcholine produced or preventing its breakdown increases its concentration and the number of receptor interactions. It will also displace the blocking molecules; transmission will be restored and the paralysis reversed.

Depolarizing agents like suxamethonium or decamethonium on the other hand have structures which closely resemble acetylcholine; they bind to the acetylcholine receptor and open the receptor-gated ion channel. Although of similar structure to acetylcholine, they are not broken down by acetylcholinesterase and so persist for some time. Their first effect is to mimic the effects of acetylcholine. The muscles twitch. The persistent depolarization of the endplate leads to inactivation of the voltage-gated Na^+ channels in the muscle membrane around the endplate. This blocks the initiation of muscle action potentials by endplate potentials and the muscle stops contracting. Increasing the amount of acetylcholine only intensifies the block. The action of suxamethonium is brief because it is hydrolysed by a plasma esterase. Some individuals do not have this enzyme and in them the action of suxamethonium is long-lasting. The action of non-depolarizing blockers can be usefully reversed by drugs that block acetylcholinesterase and thus prolong the action of acetylcholine. In therapeutic doses anticholinesterases do not cause a build-up of acetylcholine. They simply prolong its action and allow the more slowly rising endplate potential to reach the threshold for a muscle action potential and subsequent contraction.

Summary

Drugs and the NMJ

- Neuromuscular-blocking drugs block choline uptake or acetylcholine release or, clinically more importantly, depolarize the postsynaptic muscle fibre or block access of acetylcholine to it and prevent depolarization.
- Non-depolarizing block is reversed by anticholinesterases. Depolarizing block is intensified by them.

Clinical Example

Neuromuscular blocking drugs

Increased muscle tone is a disadvantage during surgery; it increases metabolic demands and in many cases interferes with the procedures. However, the manipulations involved in surgery in many cases increase muscle tone. Although general anaesthetics reduce muscle tone, the level of anaesthesia required to produce this effect to any significant degree is dangerously deep, and drugs which specifically block transmission at the neuromuscular junction are extensively used by anaesthetists to reduce the amount of general anaesthetic required to produce the desired level of relaxation. These drugs act either by blocking the transmitter (ACh) at the neuromuscular junction – these are known as non-depolarizing blockers – or by depolarizing the neuromuscular junction and rendering it insensitive to further stimulation.

Non-depolarizing agents

Non-depolarizing drugs are exemplified by curare, which is a mixture of alkaloids found in South American plants used by natives of that continent as a poison on their arrows. The dramatic effects of these substances were naturally noted by the first Europeans to come in contact with them (either personally or by observation) and their origins and antiquity have given rise to some strange names in our pharmacopoeia. Thus tubocurarine is so called because the natives originally stored it in bamboo tubes, while C-toxiferine was stored in calabashes (gourds). Difficulties in obtaining sufficient quantities of these naturally occurring substances led to the synthesis of their modern equivalents, the most important including gallamine, atracurium,

pancuronium and vecuronium. These drugs compete with acetylcholine for the receptors of the muscle endplate.

Because the neuromuscular junction has such a large safety margin, with acetylcholine being produced in quantities 10 times greater than are needed to ensure a muscle contraction, 90% of the receptors on the muscle must be blocked before contraction fails. Because muscle fibres are blocked in an 'all or nothing' manner, muscles with different-size motor units are paralysed at different concentrations of these drugs. Extrinsic eye muscles are paralysed first; respiratory muscles are paralysed last and are the first to recover.

Drugs are rarely perfectly specific in their actions, and we find that these drugs exert a blocking action at the sympathetic ganglia and thus cause an unwanted fall in blood pressure. They are strongly basic and cause a release of histamine from mast cells. This can be dangerous to asthmatic patients where the histamine may cause bronchoconstriction.

The actions of non-depolarizing blockers are reversed by any procedure that increases the concentration of acetylcholine at the neuromuscular junction. In particular, anticholinesterase drugs, which protect acetylcholine from hydrolysis, increase the life of molecules of acetylcholine and increase the chances of them finding an unoccupied receptor. Neostigmine is administered for this purpose, usually with atropine to block the muscarinic effects of accumulating acetylcholine. The use of neostigmine to reverse the effect of non-depolarizing blockers is another example of the many pharmacological balancing acts that are carried out clinically. In the absence of the blocker, anticholinesterases would cause unpleasant muscle twitches (fasciculation).

Clinical Example *(Continued)*

Depolarizing agents

The other major type of muscle relaxant that exerts its effect at the neuromuscular junction is the depolarizing blocking agents. Paradoxically these substances depolarize the muscle membrane and this results in the fasciculation which precedes a block. One might expect a drug which produces depolarization of the muscle endplate to produce a sustained contraction but the initial depolarization, which produces a twitch, is followed by sustained electrical insensitivity of the endplate, which can no longer produce an action potential in the muscle. The initial twitching of muscles causes considerable postoperative muscle pain.

Perhaps the most important characteristic of blocking agents used in surgery is their duration of action. Excessive persistence, particularly in effects on the respiratory muscles, is a serious disadvantage during recovery from surgery when a patient needs to ventilate the lungs effectively. Suxamethonium, perhaps the only significantly used depolarizing blocker, normally acts for about 5 minutes and so is popular for brief procedures such as electroconvulsive therapy.

Another difficulty with depolarizing agents is that they are removed by renal and hepatic action, which in patients may be impaired. An ingenious solution to this problem has been the development of atracurium, a depolarizing blocker which is stable under the acid conditions in which it is stored but breaks down rapidly at plasma pH. The patient is kept paralysed by an infusion of the drug, the effects of which rapidly wear off when the infusion is stopped.

A rare but dangerous condition known as malignant hyperpyrexia can develop with the use of suxamethonium. There is widespread muscle rigidity and hyperpyrexia due to an unidentified congenital muscle membrane defect. Mortality is as high as 65%. The muscle spasm is usually treated with dantrolene, which blocks muscle contraction by inhibiting Ca^{2+} release from the sarcoplasmic reticulum.

Central neurotransmission

3.4

Introduction: the neurone as an analogue computer

The clearest evidence we can obtain that an individual's central nervous system is functioning is that some appropriate response can be elicited if a stimulus is applied. To allow this, the sensory system must detect the stimulus, and the central nervous system must recognize the stimulus and construct a suitable output to the effectors. I see John – I recognize John – I say, 'Hello John'. All these activities require much neuronal activity. We will discuss what is meant by seeing and recognizing in Chapter 4.1. The complexity of the brain is so large that we cannot yet hope to understand its workings completely. We have come to understand the basic element from which it is made up, the neurone or nerve cell. Each neurone behaves as a small analogue computer. An analogue computer is one in which the magnitude of any input or output is proportional to the size of the entity being represented – 1 volt represents something larger than that represented by 0.5 volts. This contrasts with a digital machine in which size is represented numerically – 1000 represents something greater than that represented by 0111. Although the input of neurones is treated by the neurone in an analogue fashion, the output is a series of 'all-or-none' pulses whose frequency represents the strength of the output.

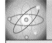

The transmission system must be such that the pattern of activity evoked (for example by seeing John) must be constant from day to day and year to year, and must also allow controlled modification when something is learnt. The susceptibility of **neurotransmission** to modification by local environment, by anoxia and the build-up of the products of metabolism, is high. This is exploited by the peripheral nervous system to optimize blood supply to active tissues (see Ch. 6.4) and is so important that the control of the local environment of the brain is the prime responsibility of the circulation and respiration of the individual (see Ch. 6.7). If this fails, as when the heart stops, unconsciousness comes on within seconds. Neurones are still active but the pattern of activity is garbled and meaningless.

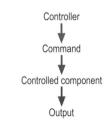

Basic Science 3.4.1

Control theory – feedback

Physiology is the study of homeostasis, which is the control of the internal environment of the body. The control systems that operate in the body are subject to the same rules that govern control systems in other situations, in engineering, chemical production or domestic heating.

Control systems consist essentially of a *controller* (the independent variable) which governs the *controlled component* (the dependent variable). Two major types of control system exist, one a development of the other.

Open loop control (Fig. BS3.4.1) is where the controller sends its signal to the controlled component, which alters its output in strict 'obedience'. Such systems are sometimes called 'deterministic' or 'non-stochastic'.

Closed loop control (Fig. BS3.4.2) is where the output of the controlled component influences the controller. Control is now mutual with controlled and controller influencing each other in an interdependent way.

It is difficult to predict the behaviour of closed loop systems and they are sometimes called 'stochastic' (i.e. a guess). The most general description of such systems differentiates between negative and positive feedback influence of the output of the controlled component on the controller.

In *negative feedback*, the output of the controlled component acts in an opposite sense on the signal from the controller. Thus in a central heating system, excessive output by the boiler feeds back to the controller (room thermostat), which reduces its signal to the boiler.

For example, in the body excess thyroid hormone in the blood feeds back to the

Controller

↓

Command

↓

Controlled component

↓

Output

Fig. BS3.4.1 Open loop control.

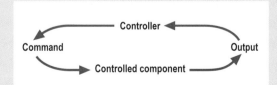

Fig. BS3.4.2 Closed loop control.

Basic Science *(Continued)*

controller (pituitary gland), which reduces its signal (make thyroid hormone) to the thyroid gland.

It should not be thought that negative feedback is used exclusively in a homeostatic way in biological systems. It is also used as a method of generating rhythmic patterns, as in the changes of oestrogen levels in the menstrual cycle (see p. 901).

A more uncommon type of feedback is *positive feedback*, in which the output of the controlled component acts in the same sense on the signal from the controller. Increase in output feeds back to the controller, encouraging it if you like to produce more signal which says more output.

An example of positive feedback from the physical world is the 'howl' produced when a microphone is placed too close to the speaker of an amplifier system. A tiny sound (the output) is picked up by the microphone (controller), which sends a tiny electrical signal to the controlled component (amplifier and speaker), which outputs a large sound, which feeds back into the microphone, which sends a large signal to the amplifier speaker which outputs a very large sound and so on.

Provided an independent system for limiting the excursions of the output and returning things to normal exists, positive feedback can be used to produce intense peaks or pulses of signal or rapidly bring about an important event. Positive feedback brings about ovulation, the propagation of the nerve action potential and the rapid formation of a blood clot.

The neurone – its basic elements

We have mentioned neurones as the cellular basis of the autonomic nervous system (Ch. 3.2) to introduce the concepts of neurotransmission. We must now look at neurones in more detail.

The basic structure of the neurone is a cell body that can be divided into the **axon hillock** and the **soma** (Fig. 3.4.1). Long processes arise from both parts of the cell body. A single **axon** arises from the axon hillock and may extend, in very large animals, for several metres before branching and forming a terminal arborization. The axon may be myelinated. Many **dendrites** arise from the cell body. They are short, not more than a centimetre or so long, and are not myelinated. The axon terminals form synapses (junctions) with other neurones. They release a **neurotransmitter** that affects the activity of the next cell. The axon conveys action potentials from the axon hillock to the terminals.

The axon hillock of this little computer produces an output, a train of action potentials, whose frequency is proportional to the depolarization of its membrane. The signal is frequency modulated.

This depolarization is due to the action of transmitters upon the soma and dendrites of the cell. Some input synapses are excitatory and generate a depolarization of the hillock and some are inhibitory and tend to polarize the membrane. The position of the terminal determines the magnitude of the effect any input will have. Synapses on the soma will have a larger effect than those along the dendrites that are remote and whose signal must pass by electrotonic conduction (passive current flow) along the dendrite.

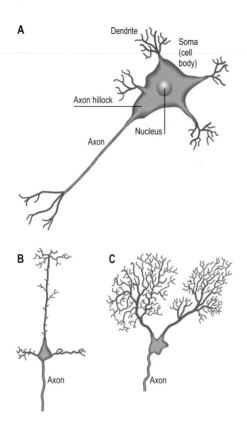

A

Dendrite

Soma
(cell
body)

Axon hillock

Nucleus

Axon

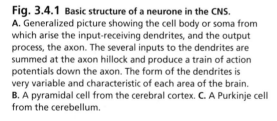

B

Axon

C

Axon

Fig. 3.4.1 Basic structure of a neurone in the CNS.
A. Generalized picture showing the cell body or soma from which arise the input-receiving dendrites, and the output process, the axon. The several inputs to the dendrites are summed at the axon hillock and produce a train of action potentials down the axon. The form of the dendrites is very variable and characteristic of each area of the brain. **B.** A pyramidal cell from the cerebral cortex. **C.** A Purkinje cell from the cerebellum.

Density of dendrites and axons

Each neurone in the central nervous system receives input (via synaptic boutons) from many other neurones. The number varies but some neurones in the frontal cortex receive input from several thousand others. Axons from most cells must thus have numerous terminal branches, called terminal arborizations. This allows for complex interactions between many sources of information. The magnitude of the effect on any cell of a single input varies. Only in a few instances is input from one neurone alone able to produce output from the next. In the case of the Renshaw cell in the spinal cord, which forms a potent negative feedback loop controlling the motoneurone pool, a single input from one motoneurone is followed by a train of action potentials in the Renshaw cell.

Signal coding

Any signalling system has to contain information about both the intensity and the quality of the signal. There are two basic coding methods used by the brain:

- Intensity is coded both by frequency of action potentials and by their postsynaptic effect on arrival at their destination. Both of these can be reprogrammed by previous activity as in learning (see Ch. 4.5).
- The quality of any input, light, sound, etc., is coded for by the identity of the particular active neurones. The same sensation is always carried by the same neurones; they form **labelled lines**.

Summary

The neurone

- The basic structure of the neurone is a cell body divided into the soma with many dendrites and an axon hillock from which a single long axon arises.
- The unit of information in the nervous system is the action potential. This is of constant size for a particular neurone and passes away from the cell body, along the axon to cross a gap (synapse) to the dendrites or soma of the next neurone.
- Intensity and quality of sensation are signalled by the frequency of action potentials and the specific neurones in which they are travelling, respectively.

Excitation and inhibition

Excitatory inputs to a neurone cause a brief depolarization of the cell, which spreads **electrotonically** to the axon hillock. The effect produced is called an **excitatory postsynaptic potential** (EPSP). Single presynaptic bouton activity will produce only a small depolarization, 1–2 mV, which will not by itself produce an action potential in the postsynaptic cell.

Inhibitory inputs to a neurone cause a brief hyperpolarization of the cell which spreads electrotonically to the axon hillock. This is called an **inhibitory postsynaptic potential** (IPSP). EPSPs and IPSPs add at the axon hillock. The net change in potential determines the output from the neurone (Fig. 3.4.2).

Summation of EPSPs and IPSPs

The summation of the input currents at the axon hillock is described by two terms:

- **spatial summation** when two separate inputs to the cell add at the axon hillock
- **temporal summation** when later inputs add on to the remnant of the response from previous inputs from the same or a different bouton (Fig. 3.4.3).

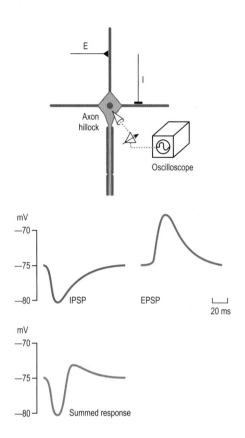

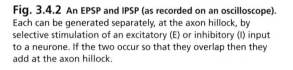

Fig. 3.4.2 An EPSP and IPSP (as recorded on an oscilloscope). Each can be generated separately, at the axon hillock, by selective stimulation of an excitatory (E) or inhibitory (I) input to a neurone. If the two occur so that they overlap then they add at the axon hillock.

Physiological changes in transmitter release

Trains of action potentials in a terminal bouton can also result in a changing postsynaptic response because of changing transmitter release. **Facilitation** is the process whereby the transmitter release rises, often by many-fold, during the first few action potentials of a train. Facilitation only lasts fractions of a second. **Post-tetanic potentiation** (PTP) is the process whereby the transmitter release from trains of stimuli is increased after a previous high-frequency burst of action potentials in the nerve. PTP is longer-lasting than facilitation, persisting for minutes.

Both these effects on transmitter release are the result of an increase in the quantal content of the release and reflect an increase in the probability of release of vesicles bound to the presynaptic membrane and an increase in the number so bound (transmitter mobilization). An increase in the level of free intracellular Ca^{2+} is an important cause of both these effects.

Continuous activity in a synaptic input will eventually cause a decrease in the postjunctional response. This is called fade or fatigue. There is a reduced individual quantal content of the release and fewer quanta are released. Recovery takes place within seconds when transmitter mobilization restores the transmitter pool from which release occurs.

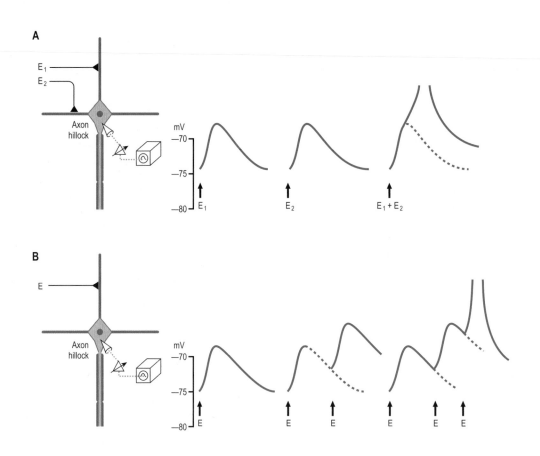

Fig. 3.4.3 Summation of responses (as recorded on an oscilloscope). This occurs, at the axon hillock, because either (**A**) responses from different inputs coincide (spatial summation) or (**B**) responses from a single input occur at a rate high enough for successive responses to overlap and produce temporal summation.

The release of transmitter can also be modified by synapses on presynaptic nerve terminals (presynaptic inhibition, see below and Fig. 3.4.4). So far, mainly inhibitory effects of this kind have been described.

Effects of anoxia and hypercapnia

It is obvious to anyone who has experienced or witnesses a faint that consciousness is dependent upon the continuous adequate perfusion of the brain's vasculature. An individual with a damaged circulation, who experiences postural hypotension, loses consciousness within seconds of moving from a lying to a standing posture. This is due to the fall in local O_2 tension and a consequent reduction in the release of central neurotransmitters garbling the information flow.

CO_2 is a general anaesthetic and if it is not removed adequately, consciousness is first impaired and then lost. Excessive CO_2 removal by hyperventilation causes a fall in free Ca^{2+} levels which changes both the excitability of neurones and their ability to release transmitter (see p. 184). This also alters consciousness.

These presynaptic activities alter the release of transmitter by the terminal on which they are acting and this selectively modifies the input to the neurone it innervates. **Presynaptic inhibition** is more common than facilitation.

Presynaptic inhibition and facilitation probably produce their effects by modifying the levels of intracellular free Ca^{2+} in the presynaptic nerve terminal. This may be brought about by direct control of voltage-dependent Ca^{2+} channels or indirectly by the modification of the membrane potential by actions on other channels.

The important difference between the effects of pre- and postsynaptic mechanisms upon the activity of the controlled neurone is that, whilst presynaptic mechanisms are input selective, postsynaptic mechanisms affect the response to all inputs to the cell.

Habituation/sensitization

Like all receptors, those in the CNS respond to changes in the maintained level of stimulation. Their number increases after an absence of stimulation and decreases if a high level of stimulation is maintained. This leads to **sensitization** and **habituation** or desensitization of the postsynaptic response respectively. Habituation is particularly important in the development of tolerance to opioids. Opium abusers can tolerate doses of the drug that would be fatal to the naive individual.

Post-tetanic effects

Post-tetanic potentiation (PTP) occurs in many synapses. After a burst of high-frequency activity in a synaptic input, the postjunctional effect of a single action potential in that input is enhanced. This effect is related to the inability of the Ca^{2+} transporters of the nerve terminal to immediately remove all the Ca^{2+} that moved into the terminal during the period of activity. Whilst the intracellular free Ca^{2+} remains elevated, transmitter release also remains elevated

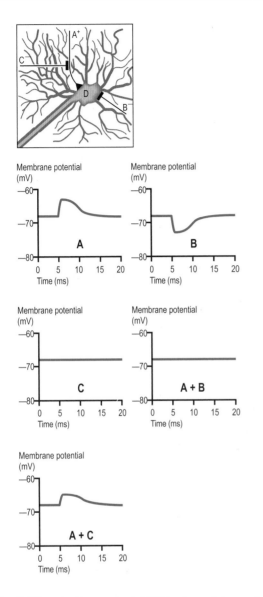

Fig. 3.4.4 **Pre- and postsynaptic inhibition by excitatory and inhibitory inputs to a motoneurone.** In the top diagram A represents an excitatory input, B an inhibitory input and C a presynaptic inhibitory input acting on terminal A to reduce its effect on the motoneurone, D. The motoneurone's output, i.e. whether it fires an action potential or not, depends on the balance between the excitatory and inhibitory inputs.

Presynaptic inhibition

Nerve endings make contact not only with the cell bodies and dendrites of neurones but also with the terminal regions of their output axons.

because the number of quanta released per action potential is raised. Thus the effect is upon the probability of quantal release.

Ca^{2+} affects several steps in the process of transmitter release, and transmitter mobilization may also be important. Before release, transmitter-containing vesicles must move from the central part of the axon terminal to the membrane and bind to it via **synapsin**. This process is also Ca^{2+} dependent.

After periods of repetitive activity, transmitter release may also be depressed. This is associated with a reduction in the quantal effect on the postjunctional neurone and is related to a fall in the amount of transmitter in individual presynaptic vesicles. This is due to a failure of transmitter synthesis to keep up with the loss.

Both these processes occur simultaneously and the net effect of repetitive activity is determined by the balance of their effects. With shorter periods of activity, potentiation is often the outcome; and with more sustained activity, depression.

Long-term potentiation

Post-tetanic potentiation usually decays in minutes. In some synapses, for example in the hippocampus, a more persistent process has been observed in which potentiation is maintained for days. This **long-term potentiation** (LTP) may be the basis of memory and learning. The mechanism of LTP in the hippocampus is probably related to the influx of Ca^{2+} through a glutamate receptor-controlled channel. The channel is both receptor controlled and voltage dependent. It will only open if both the agonist is present and the dendritic spine is depolarized. Depolarization is produced by glutamate acting on its AMPA receptor (named after its agonist α-amino-3-hydroxy-5-methyl-isoxazole) to produce an EPSP, whilst at the same time glutamate is acting on its NMDA (*N*-methyl D-aspartate) receptor subtype to gate the Ca^{2+} channel. Ca^{2+} rises in the cell, leading to the

changes that are the basis of the persistent potentiation. One of these processes may be the release, by the dendrite, of a retrograde messenger, perhaps nitric oxide.

Learning and memory

Memory formation is a very complex process. It can be divided into short-term memory and long-term memory. The hippocampus is critical for the memory of events of the recent past (minutes and hours). Long-term memory (>> 1 day) is probably located in the association and limbic cortices.

Short-term memory seems to rely on neuronal circuit activity to retain a trace of the stored event. Deep general anaesthesia or electroconvulsive shock therapy is associated with a period of retrograde amnesia, since it disrupts normal synaptic activity. Long-term memory involves biochemical and structural reorganization of the synaptic structure of the brain and can be interfered with by agents that block protein synthesis.

The transfer of information from short-term to long-term storage is enabled by cholinergic mechanisms and disruption of cholinergic connections may be the cause of the early memory loss in Alzheimer's disease.

Central neurotransmitters

Central neurotransmitters are many and their mechanisms of action various. Many act to gate ion channels, others additionally modify the metabolism of the postsynaptic cell. Ion channels can be gated directly by the binding of the transmitter to the channel changing the molecules configuration and opening it. In other cases the receptor is not directly attached to the channel but acts indirectly via a G-protein which either is itself directly coupled to the channel or activates an enzyme that produces a second messenger which then acts on the channel.

Fast responses

The transmitters that produce fast responses are amino acids. Glutamate is the main transmitter involved in the production of fast EPSPs. Its receptors control a directly gated channel which is selectively permeable to Na^+ and K^+.

Fast IPSPs are produced by the action of glycine or GABA on directly gated channel that are selectively permeable to Cl^-.

Slower responses

Slower, neuromodulatory, responses usually involve a G-protein coupling. The catecholamines, adrenaline, noradrenaline and dopamine together with histamine and 5-HT (serotonin) act via a G-protein directly coupled to a channel to produce slower responses.

A large and growing group of neurotransmitters, the neuropeptides, produce slow or neuromodulatory responses via the production of second messengers.

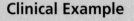

Clinical Example

Anxiety disorders

Anxiety disorders are very common; they are characterized by persistent generalized anxiety not related to any particular circumstance (once called 'free floating anxiety'). They occur in up to 4% of the general population at some time in their lives.

Anxiety is more common in females than in males and the average age of onset is in the 20s and 30s. The state of anxiety can be well understood by considering its roots in Latin, *anxietos* – a painful mind, and Greek, *anxo* – to squeeze.

The physiology of anxiety

Anxiety is a normal phenomenon in the presence of danger and has evolved as a strategy to alert the organism to threats to its well-being. In physiological terms it was first described by Cannon (the originator of the term homeostasis) as the 'fight or flight reaction'. During this state the sympathetic nervous system is provoked into sustained and enhanced activity which readies the organism for life-preserving activity.

Mass discharge of the sympathetic system causes a number of physiological and metabolic changes. An increased cardiac output is selectively directed to the muscles, whose increased metabolism is sustained by increased levels of blood glucose brought about by muscle glycolysis. Subjects report increased mental activity and a sense of being able to sustain increased physical activity.

Emotional states can activate the sympathetic system as well as physical stress. For example, extreme anger or fear, emotions which like others arise in the hypothalamus, activates the reticular formation and hence the sympathetic system to a state ready for 'fight or flight'. For animals, which is chosen depends on the particular situation, and the same was true of our primitive ancestors.

Present-day humans encounter situations that call for an actual fight or flight less frequently than situations which provoke anxiety. In these situations, abnormally high levels of sympathetic activity, more suited to the primitive condition, are associated with anxiety disorders.

Appropriate anxiety is normal; it is abnormal when it is out of proportion to the threat, when

Clinical Example *(Continued)*

it persists long after the threat has vanished or indeed is triggered by a situation generally thought to be harmless.

In animals and man moderate anxiety improves mentation. However, the relationship between performance and anxiety is described by what is sometimes known as the Yerks–Dodson law which can be represented graphically (Fig. CE3.4.1).

Some anxiety improves performance but higher levels impair it. A good example of the Yerks–Dodson phenomenon is seen in students preparing for examinations. Low levels of anxiety 8 weeks before the examination motivate the student to start revision. However, 2 days before the examination, high levels of anxiety prevent some people from learning.

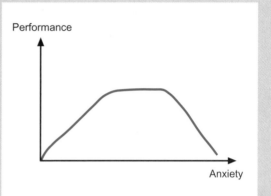

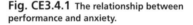

Fig. CE3.4.1 The relationship between performance and anxiety.

The symptoms of anxiety

There are several psychological and physiological symptoms of anxiety and for clinical anxiety to be diagnosed a number must be present at the same time.

The mood of anxiety is one of apprehension or the expectation that there is some, frequently undefined, impending danger. The patient is in a state of tense alertness scanning the environment for signs of danger. The parallel between this picture and one of a prey animal in the vicinity of a predator is irresistible. There is a physiological increase in muscle tone and the patient may become visibly restless. Another common manifestation of anxiety is the symptom of breathlessness, which may provoke hyperventilation resulting in hypocapnia and hypocalcaemia. This results in feelings of dizziness, paraesthesia and, if serum calcium falls by more than about 33%, carpopedal spasm due to the hypocalcaemia causing increased

excitability of the peripheral nerves. The hypocapnia of hyperventilation can be most simply relieved by calming the patient, encouraging slow regular breathing and if possible getting the patient to rebreathe air from a paper bag to retain carbon dioxide.

Other common symptoms of anxiety include sweating, palpitations, tachycardia, diarrhoea and increased frequency of urination, all of which have their physiological basis in increased discharge of the sympathetic system. In addition to fearfulness, the patient may describe psychological symptoms of insomnia, exaggerated responses to being startled, a sense of unreality and increased irritability.

Treatment of anxiety disorders

Patients have often suffered for several years before they present with symptoms of anxiety. Treatment is therefore frequently not straightforward as the patient may have grossly modified his life to avoid situations that trigger attacks.

Clinical Example *(Continued)*

There may be therapeutic behavioural changes which can be made, for example to reorganize a pressured work schedule. Education to reduce the fear of palpitations and tachycardia often helps. Relaxation and anxiety management training are widely employed to reduce symptoms. If behavioural and cognitive approaches fail, pharmacological treatment can be used with varying success.

Benzodiazepines

These are probably the most commonly used anxiolytics, although fears of dependency developing have limited their use. Benzodiazepines act at γ-aminobutyric acid (GABA) receptors to potentiate their action. GABA is found throughout the brain as an inhibitory transmitter (see Clinical Example: Motor disorders and spasticity, p. 208). The fact that benzodiazepines modulate GABA activity suggests that there might be an endogenous ligand which might naturally act at the benzodiazepine receptor. Benzodiazepines are rapidly absorbed from the gut and eliminated by conjugation in the liver. Reduced hepatic function with age mandates care in their use with the elderly. Benzodiazepines act as sedatives and anticonvulsants (see Clinical Example: Epilepsy, p. 239). Their most serious side-effects include dependence and tolerance.

Tricyclic antidepressants and SSRIs *(selective serotonin reuptake inhibitors)*

Depression is often seen with anxiety. These drugs, used in depression, have significant anxiolytic effects though the relationship between the two effects remains unclear. Their physiological action is to selectively inhibit the reuptake of serotonin (5-hydroxytryptamine, 5-HT) and noradrenaline by presynaptic neurones in the brain.

β-blockers

β-adrenoceptor antagonists such as propranolol can be used in the treatment of anxiety. Work with musicians anxious before a performance suggests that it is the reduction of tremor, which presumably acts as a feedback signal of anxiety, rather than any effect on the emotional component that produces the beneficial effect. Side-effects limit the usefulness of these drugs in anxiety.

Buspirone

Serotonin-containing neurones in parts of the raphe nucleus appear to be involved in the types of behavioural activity seen in anxiety. Buspirone is an antagonist at 5-HT_{1A} receptors and exerts powerful anxiolytic actions. These effects are very slow to develop, taking up to 3 weeks, which suggests that their action is indirect rather than a straightforward pharmacological block at receptor sites.

Most patients who have anxiety disorders will benefit from a combined pharmacological and psychological approach. Progress depends on the type of anxiety disorder but in many cases the condition is troublesome to treat, presenting as it often does in the chronic phase of the disorder.

Criteria for identification of central transmitters

In order for a substance to be convincingly accepted as a transmitter agent in the peripheral nervous system it is usual to test this claim against the criteria we have already mentioned:

- The putative transmitter must be shown to be released from the nerve by physiological mechanisms and its action mimicked at appropriate concentrations by externally applied substance.
- Receptors capable of inducing the physiological actions must be present at the effector cells.
- Adequate mechanisms for synthesizing, transporting and releasing the agent have to be present in the nerve terminal and shown to be capable of operating under physiological conditions.
- Adequate mechanisms for destruction and/or inactivation of the putative transmitters must be present at the terminal or immediately adjacent in the effector tissues.

The application of these tests to the CNS in a strict manner is not easy. By using multi-barrelled microelectrodes to record from central neurones and to apply putative transmitters to them, it is possible to identify receptors on individual neurones. Pharmacological comparisons can then be made between the responses to these agents and the responses to synaptic inputs to the cell to identify the transmitter responsible for them. The first two criteria can therefore be tested.

Testing the last two criteria, where adequacy is an important element, is less easy. It is not possible to do this except on the basis of studies of transmitter turnover in quite large pieces of brain. Even if these are circumscribed nuclei, they will contain a very large number of different neurones with different transmitter systems. Estimating the range of the normal activity in any given type of nerve terminal is not possible with any precision.

The list of accepted central neurotransmitters is growing rapidly. A full review would not be useful but some important members of the group are considered below.

Acetylcholine

Acetylcholine was the first transmitter to be identified with certainty in the CNS. Dale's principle, that if a transmitter is released from one terminal of an axon it will be released from all other terminals of the same axon, suggested that the collaterals of the α-motoneurones that innervate the Renshaw cell (see Ch. 3.6) would release acetylcholine as did their branches that form the skeletal neuromuscular junction. In the CNS many of the receptors for acetylcholine are of the nicotinic type as in the neuromuscular junction, though with a slightly different subunit structure.

Amines

Dopamine is a very important transmitter in the brain. In Parkinson's disease degeneration of dopaminergic neurones of the substantia nigra leads to hypokinesia, rigidity and tremor. It is thought that cholinergic neurones of the corpus striatum, which receive an inhibitory innervation from the nigral dopaminergic neurones, become hyperactive. Parkinson's disease has been treated by muscarinic antagonists, which reduce the effects of this hyperactivity, and by dopaminomimetics, which replace the effects of the lost dopamine.

The action of amine transmitters is terminated, in part, by enzyme systems that destroy the transmitter molecule. For example, mono-amine oxidases in mitochondria degrade amines. Monoamine oxidase inhibitors (MAOIs) are used therapeutically to block this system; they increase the level of transmitter and improve mood in depressed patients.

Amino acids

It may seem surprising that several common amino acids incorporated in the general metabolism of cells can also act as highly specific neurotransmitters, e.g. aspartate, glycine, glutamate. Gamma-aminobutyric acid is synthesized from glutamate and is found in high concentrations widely distributed in the central nervous system. These substances must be stored and used separately from the general metabolic amino acids when they are used as transmitters.

Opioid peptides

The pentapeptide enkephalins are found widely distributed in the CNS with a high concentration in the substantia gelatinosa of the spinal cord. The substantia gelatinosa is the site of the first synapse in the sensory pathway involving pain. The receptors for the enkephalins are stimulated by morphine and similar analgesics which may modulate our perception of pain here (see Ch. 3.10).

Serotonin and noradrenaline

These two central neurotransmitters have attracted much interest lately because their release and reuptake can now be modified by new types of drugs that are used to treat psychiatric disorders (see Clinical Examples: Anxiety disorders, p. 191; Schizophrenia, see below).

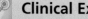

Summary

Synaptic transmission

- Excitatory or inhibitory action potential activity can summate postsynaptically as EPSP or IPSP.
- Transmission at a synapse can also be affected presynaptically, usually as inhibition.
- Persistent or absent activity at a synapse leads to habituation or sensitization.
- Memory can be divided into long- and short-term memory which have different anatomical sites in the brain and physiological bases.
- There are many putative central neurotransmitters, which must meet at least four well-established criteria to be accepted.

Clinical Example

Schizophrenia

Schizophrenia is a major mental illness which occurs equally in men and women in all cultures. The lifetime risk of developing the disorder is approximately 1%. It is a disease believed to be caused by both genetic and environmental factors. Schizophrenia may have an acute or insidious onset in the late teens or early twenties for males and normally later in females.

Typically the illness occurs as acute episodes of hallucinations, and delusional disorganized thinking (positive symptoms) against a background of negative symptoms characterized by paucity of expressive gesture and language. Both these features are accompanied by social decline, loss of interpersonal relationships and loss of self-care. There may be a failure to achieve the expected level of interpersonal, academic or occupational achievement.

Clinical Example *(Continued)*

Schizophrenia is largely misunderstood by the general public who often associate the disease with a 'split personality'.

The brain in schizophrenia

There is evidence of underlying organic pathology in some schizophrenia sufferers. A major finding is that the lateral ventricles are enlarged and there is a resultant reduction in the grey matter of the temporal lobe. The hippocampus and associated areas are most affected and there is a general reduction of brain tissue of about 5%. There is some evidence that the left side of the brain is more affected than the right. It is likely that the negative symptoms are most marked in patients with more pronounced neurophysiological changes.

Some studies have indicated an increase in basal ganglia volume but this was probably due to the effect of antipsychotic medication. In addition to the anatomical abnormalities of a shrivelled brain there are functional abnormalities.

Functional magnetic resonance imaging has demonstrated abnormalities of regional blood flow in the brains of schizophrenics; increases in the left frontal and temporal regions and Broca's area are associated with the experience of auditory hallucinations. Because Broca's area is involved with the production of words, it has been suggested that these patients are misinterpreting their own inner speech.

In addition to perceptual difficulties, schizophrenic patients perform poorly in cognitive tests of their frontal lobe function such as verbal fluency tests. There appears to be a general association between decreased frontal lobe activity and negative symptoms.

In general, patients with schizophrenia suffer from abnormalities in function of the brain areas associated with interpretation of sensory material and the regulation of mental activity.

Neurotransmitter abnormalities

Dopamine

Before the introduction of chlorpromazine, a phenothiazine drug, in the 1950s the treatment of schizophrenia was very limited. Chlorpromazine and other neuroleptic drugs were found to act as dopamine antagonists, and in its simplest form the dopamine hypothesis postulated that the corticolimbic and nigrostriatal dopaminergic system was overactive in patients with schizophrenia. Neuroleptics are effective in the treatment of agitation or excitement of whatever cause, in acute confusional states, mania and other forms of psychosis as well as schizophrenia. They have a general sedative effect. Interference with dopaminergic systems may explain their unwanted extrapyramidal parkinsonian effects. The major antipsychotic effects are thought to occur at the corticolimbic site whereas the side-effects appear to be centred on the nigrostriatal tracts.

As with other neurotransmitters, the original single receptor type for dopamine has been subdivided as populations with slightly different properties are discovered. Early evidence for the site of action of antipsychotics was based on their affinity for D_2 receptors but modern antipsychotics have D_3 and D_4 preferences (clozapine and D_4 for example).

Administration of amphetamine, which releases dopamine, leads to exacerbation of schizophrenic symptoms. Post-mortem studies show increased D_2 receptor density in the basal ganglia of schizophrenic patients. Arguments

Clinical Example *(Continued)*

against the dopamine hypothesis are that there is a poor correlation between dopamine blockade and clinical response to antipsychotic drugs and, despite early block of dopamine receptors, there is a late onset of clinical effect (3–4 weeks). There is also no elevation of CSF levels of dopamine metabolites in untreated schizophrenic patients.

Serotonin (5-hydroxytryptamine, 5-HT)

The role of 5-HT in schizophrenia has become clearer with the introduction of atypical neuroleptics which have less widespread dopaminergic antagonistic activity and therefore less difficult side-effects. Some of the more modern drugs bind specifically to limbic and cerebral sites and so reduce the side-effects associated with nigrostriatal binding. Many atypical antipsychotics have specific 5-HT$_2$ receptor antagonist activity. Evidence for the basis of this antipsychotic effect comes from research into LSD (lysergic acid diethylamide), which can induce psychotic symptoms in normal people and has a similar molecular structure to 5-HT.

Glutamate and aspartate

The two major excitatory amino acids in the CNS are glutamate and aspartate, which inhibit dopamine release. Glutamate and aspartate are agonists at the NMDA (*N*-methyl-D-aspartate) receptor site. Psychotomimetic drugs such as phencyclidine and ketamine, which bind to this site, have been found to produce both positive and negative symptoms in volunteers. Post-mortem analysis of schizophrenic brains shows a reduction in glutamate receptors, although this may reflect neuronal loss.

In the pharmacological treatment of schizophrenia atypical neuroleptics have become more popular than typical neuroleptics because of their fewer side-effects. Most atypical drugs have specific dopamine and 5-HT receptor antagonist activity.

Prognosis in schizophrenia

The disease tends to run a prolonged course. Acute relapse can occur years after remission. Progress is largely dependent on initial presentation. Progress is better in females than males when the onset is sudden with florid psychotic features (e.g. hallucinations and delusions). A major cause of death is suicide with a rate of about 10% occurring early in the disease and mainly in males. Progress is improved by early recognition of the disease and early antipsychotic medication.

The motor system: peripheral/spinal organization

Introduction

The ability to move oneself wholly or in part in a controlled manner is an essential requirement for life. If breathing fails and with it ventilation of the lungs, death follows in minutes. One's ability to cope with the stresses of modern life is severely reduced by any accident or disease which impairs motor control. Full function requires that the central nervous system is intact and that the musculoskeletal system is connected to it by peripheral nerves. Local damage to parts of these systems produces specific pattern of defects that has allowed function to be ascribed to the parts of the central nervous system and is an aid to diagnosis.

The effects of damage become more subtle and kaleidoscopic the higher up the system they are located. Cutting a peripheral nerve simply paralyses the muscles it innervates. Damage to the spinal cord which completely destroys both motor and sensory nerves has a similar effect. Lesions higher in the system have more complex effects.

The motoneurones of the cord are connected to the motor cortex by the **pyramidal** (corticospinal tract). If this tract is damaged by a haemorrhage, say, then initially the patient has a flaccid paralysis of the affected muscles, but later the affected limbs often become stiff or spastic. This is because the lesion causing the damage is often located in the internal capsule and damages another motor outflow tract, the extrapyramidal system. The increase in tone after capsular damage is due to the removal of the inhibitory pathways of the extrapyramidal system.

The **extrapyramidal** system reaches the cord after synapsing several times, importantly in the **basal ganglia** and midbrain nuclei. Damage to the basal ganglia can lead to excessive inappropriate movements. Athetosis (writhing), ballismus (flinging) and chorea (restless movement) are all part of the clinical picture of degeneration of the extrapyramidal system.

Some very specific losses have powerful effects. Lesions of the dopamine-containing neurones of the basal ganglia lead to the shaking palsy, Parkinson's disease.

The **cerebellum** is important in the coordination of movement. Cerebellar deficits lead to poor coordination and also affect muscle tone. In any movement there may be errors in the rate, range and force achieved, and there will be a marked intention tremor.

The surface of the cerebral cortex is organized into a patchwork with function being localized into discrete areas. The **motor cortex** is situated immediately anterior to the central sulcus and on it the various parts of the body are projected. Damage to the hand area of the motor cortex will lead to paralysis of the hand to the extent that voluntary movement is not possible, though the hand may take part in balancing movements. The motor control of

Basic Science 3.5.1

Stress and strain

Movement of the limbs and objects propelled by our limbs and even the movement of whole individuals' bodies is controlled by muscles and nerves and can be described by Newton's laws of motion. We will meet these laws in more detail later when we discuss the motion of the fluid in our inner ears which gives us our sense of balance. In the context of muscles stimulated by nerves to contract, all we need to know at present is that they generate **force**, and force can only be easily visualized by its effect on the acceleration of a body or on the elasticity of a body. Newton's laws tell us that the greater the force that is applied to a movable object the more rapidly it will be accelerated. If the object does not move, the force will distort the object no matter how minutely. Thus, if you lean on the Great Pyramid of Cheops you do not move it but you do distort it, if ever so slightly.

Our voluntary muscles apply their force through the tendons that attach them to our bones, and it is here that an understanding of the physics of the situation is important, as tendons can be pulled apart by too great a force.

The units of force are newtons (N). Force applied over an area is called **pressure** when it causes compression and so pressure depends on both the magnitude of the force and the area over which it is applied. It has the units of force per unit area (N/m^2). When force causes stretching, as in pulling a rope or tendon, it is said to produce tension or **stress**, which has the same units as pressure.

Because you need a large force (and therefore tension in your muscles) to bring about rapid accelerations, athletes 'warm-up' their muscles before undertaking violent exercise. They believe that this will protect their muscles and tendons against tearing under the large stresses they are going to produce. There is some doubt about whether this is so.

speech is located in a centre in the inferior frontal gyrus (Broca's speech centre). If this is damaged, although the muscles involved in speech can be used for other movements, they cannot be used for sound formation.

Components of the motor system

Nerve fibres going to and coming from the CNS have been classified in two ways, both based on their diameter and therefore conduction velocity. These classifications will be referred to several times in subsequent chapters and are outlined in Table 3.5.1, which will repay perusal before reading further.

The skeletal muscle fibres receive their motor innervation from α-**motoneurones** (also referred to as lower motoneurones), which have their cell bodies in the ventral horn of the spinal cord or in the cranial nerve motor nuclei. Their axons project peripherally. These α-motoneurones are the final common path to the muscles, of

control signals originating in the spinal and supraspinal systems. Important supraspinal systems include the brainstem, basal ganglia, cerebellum and cerebral cortex (Fig. 3.5.1).

The motor system at work

During many movements, great reliance is placed on learnt motor programs which set the basic pattern of the movement. During development the child learns, with many tumbles, the programs for walking and running. Once learnt, these movements only rarely require conscious control. Similarly, when learning to ride a bicycle, the rider has to concentrate hard on maintaining balance. Once the program has been learnt, it becomes automatic and no longer requires conscious intervention. Learning motor programs and their subsequent execution is largely a function of the cerebellum.

The motor system is highly dependent on a continuous flow of sensory information to

---

Table 3.5.1 The major classifications of nerve fibres

Class	Myelination	Conduction velocity (m/s)	Diameter (μm)	Function
I (a & b)	+	70–120	12–20	Afferent from muscle spindles and tendon organs
II	+	25–70	4–12	Afferent from muscle spindles, touch and pressure
III	+	3–30	1–4	Afferent from cold and pain receptors
Aα	+	50–120	8–20	Efferent to extrafusal muscle fibres
Aβ	+	30–70	5–12	Efferent to intra- and extrafusal fibres, skin afferents
Aγ	+	10–50	2–8	Efferent to intrafusal muscle fibres
Aδ	+	3–30	1–5	Afferent pain, cold
B	+	5–15	1–3	Preganglionic autonomic
C (sometimes called IV)	–	<2	<1	Postganglionic autonomic, visceral and somatic afferents for pain and temperature sensation

Much of the confusion in fibre classification arises because there are two systems (I, II, III, IV and A, B, C) describing the same thing – the diameter and conduction velocity of the population of nerve fibres which extends from thick myelinated fibres at one extreme (group I or Aα or even simply α) to thin unmyelinated at the other extreme (group IV or C fibres). The major difference is that one focuses, but not exclusively, on afferent and the other on efferent fibres. The student should remember that although the group I, II, II, IV system is usually used for muscle afferents and the Aα–δ, B, C system for motor nerves and skin afferents, both systems are based on fibre diameter and conduction velocity and are as equivalent as measuring length in millimetres or inches.

A

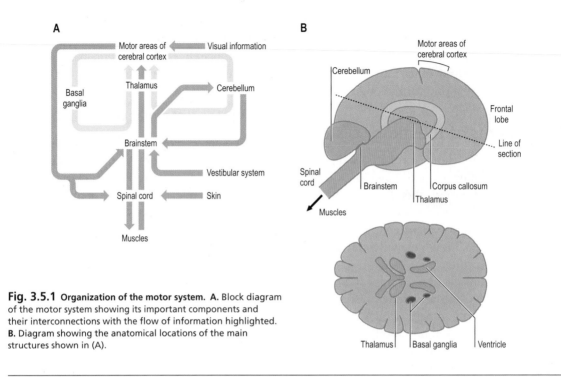

B

Fig. 3.5.1 Organization of the motor system. A. Block diagram of the motor system showing its important components and their interconnections with the flow of information highlighted. **B.** Diagram showing the anatomical locations of the main structures shown in (A).

monitor the movement during its execution, and to correct for any errors. This sensory information comes from many sources. Information is provided by exteroceptors, such as the eyes, which supply the brain with information about the position of the target with respect to the body, and proprioceptors which relay information regarding the angles of the joints and the contractile forces and movements of the muscles.

The ability to correct for errors during movements is clearly of great importance but it has limitations: detection of the error and the transmission of that information to the appropriate region of the central nervous system take time and therefore correction of fast movements is strictly limited. The most rapid feedback control mechanism is the spinal reflex (see p. 218). Even the fastest of these reflexes involves two neurones and a delay of tens of milliseconds. This primitive and rather crude mechanism is limited in its usefulness and in man is overshadowed by visual reflexes that involve much

computing of information, and therefore delay, before they can be applied to the motor system.

Peripheral and spinal organization of the muscle system

The motor unit

The fundamental unit of muscle control is the **motor unit**. A motor unit is a single α-motoneurone and the group of skeletal muscle fibres that it innervates. Each skeletal muscle fibre is innervated by only one α-motoneurone but each α-motoneurone will innervate a number of muscle fibres, the muscle fibres within a given motor unit being called the muscle unit (Fig. 3.5.2).

Within the muscle, the muscle fibres of each motor unit are widely distributed so that a cross-sectional view of the muscle, in which fibres of a single motor unit are picked out, reveals the fibres of a given unit scattered as a

A

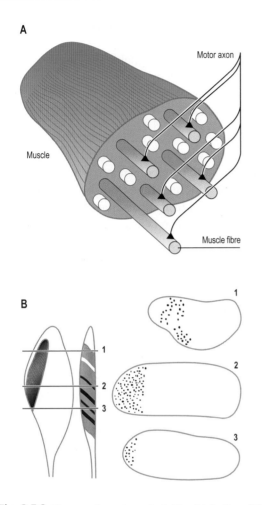

Motor axon

Muscle

Muscle fibre

B

1

1

2

2

3

3

Fig. 3.5.2 Diagram of a motor unit. A. The distribution of the muscle fibres of a single motor unit. Repeatedly stimulating a single α-motoneurone repeatedly contracts only the muscle fibres it controls and depletes them of their energy source – glycogen. If the muscle is then stained to show up glycogen, the fibres that make up the stimulated motor unit can be identified by their lack of glycogen. **B.** An example of where such fibres of a single motoneurone might be found at three levels in a muscle.

Neurotransmission at the skeletal neuromuscular junction

Transmission between the α-motoneurone and the innervated muscle fibres is specialized to ensure that it is maintained even when the system is severely stressed by the local oxygen lack and carbon dioxide build-up that occur during maintained heavy muscular effort (see p. 106). An action potential in the nerve releases hundreds of vesicles of acetylcholine which act on a very sensitive postjunctional membrane, the muscle endplate, to produce a local depolarization. This potential, the endplate potential, is normally many times greater than the minimum required to evoke an action potential in the muscle fibre. The process has a high safety factor which ensures that it takes place. The endplate potential is brief because of the presence of acetylcholinesterase on the endplate which rapidly hydrolyses the released transmitter. A single action potential in the motoneurone will give rise to a single, synchronous twitch contraction of all the muscles fibres of the unit.

This 1:1 transmission can fail in myasthenia gravis, an autoimmune disease (see Clinical Example, p. 63). In this disease there is a reduction in the number of acetylcholine receptors in the postjunctional membrane. As a result, the endplate potential is reduced, abolishing the safety factor of transmission and leading to fatigue or failure of the contractions during any sustained effort. The neuromuscular junction is described in more detail in Chapter 3.3.

The muscle unit represents the smallest contractile element available to the CNS. The size of the motor units in different muscles varies with their function. The ratio between the number of α-motoneurones and the total number of skeletal muscle fibres is termed the **innervation ratio**. The innervation ratio is small (i.e. the number of muscle fibres per unit is small) in muscles like the extraocular muscles that are involved in fine, smooth movements. Muscles like the glutei, generating powerful but coarser

mosaic amongst the fibres of many other units (see Fig. 3.5.2). This has the effect of distributing the demands made on the muscle circulation by the activity of the units evenly through the muscle. This distribution also has important implications for the unit's interactions with the tendon organs that monitor muscle tension (p. 212).

Table 3.5.2 Numbers of motor units and muscle fibres per unit for various skeletal muscles

Muscle	No. of units	No. of muscle fibres per unit
Eye muscle	1740	13
Hand	98	110
Upper arm	774	210
Lower leg	580	1720

movements, have a large number of muscle fibres per unit (Table 3.5.2). In the limbs, the innervation ratio tends to decrease from the proximal to the distal parts of the limbs.

During ageing there is a progressive loss of neurones, including α-motoneurones, owing to cell death. When a motoneurone dies, the denervated muscle fibres release trophic factors that stimulate neighbouring motoneurone terminals to sprout and re-innervate them. Thus there is a progressive increase in the innervation ratio, which contributes to deterioration of fine control with ageing. This is particularly noticeable in the small muscles of the hand.

Motor unit classification

The motor units making up each skeletal muscle may be characterized according to their contractile and histochemical properties. It is worth reminding ourselves of the types of skeletal muscle that exist, and their properties, because these have a bearing on the way they are recruited. Classification according to contractile force and rates of fatigue is the basis of three groupings (see also Section 2):

- Type I – slow (S) units which have slow speeds of contraction, generate small amounts of force but are extremely resistant to fatigue
- Type IIA – fast, fatigue-resistant (FR) units which produce more force and contract

more rapidly whilst also being relatively resistant to fatigue
- Type IIB – fast, fatiguable (FF) units which contract more rapidly and generate large amounts of force but also fatigue very quickly.

The speed of contraction of the unit and its fatiguability are functions of the enzyme complement and metabolism of its muscle fibres. Fibres of different types can be visualized by histochemical techniques that stain for the specific enzymes. The fast-contracting fibres of the FF and FR units (type IIB and IIA fibres, respectively) are rich in myosin ATPase compared with the slowly contracting fibres of the S units (type I fibres). This enables them to break down the ATP more rapidly and to contract faster. The fatiguable muscle fibres have few mitochondria, a glycolytic metabolism, and relatively few capillaries, so that a muscle rich in FF units appears white. Conversely, the fatigue-resistant fibres of the S units have an oxidative metabolism, large numbers of mitochondria and a rich blood supply, so that the muscle appears red. The properties of the motor-unit types are summarized in Table 3.5.3.

The muscles fibres of each motor unit are homogeneous for physiological and histochemical properties. Most muscles comprise a mix of the three types of motor unit but the proportions vary according to the function of the muscle. Thus the soleus muscle, which is used for maintenance of posture during standing and therefore is active for long periods of time, consists almost exclusively of slow units. In contrast, the gastrocnemius muscles, which are particularly active during running and jumping, have a higher proportion of FR and FF units.

The unit mix of a muscle is also determined by the use to which it has been put. Exercise training is important for determining the properties of skeletal muscles. For example, endurance training, such as long-distance running, leads to an increase in vascularization and

Table 3.5.3 Classification and properties of motor units in skeletal muscle

	Physiological type		
	Slow (S)	**Fast, fatigue resistant (FR)**	**Fast, fatiguable (FF)**
Histochemical profile	Slow, oxidative	Fast, oxidative–glycolytic	Fast, glycolytic
Fibre type	I	IIA	IIB
Contraction speed	Slow	Fast	Fast
Contractile strength	Weak	Intermediate	Strong
Fatiguability	Fatigue resistant	Fatigue resistant	Easily fatigued
Capillary supply	Rich	Rich	Sparse
Fibre diameter	Small	Medium–small	Large

the density of mitochondria, thereby increasing the resistance to fatigue without there being any marked increase in total muscle strength. Training regimes for explosive exercise such as weightlifting, lead to a substantial hypertrophy of the FF units, giving extra strength and muscle bulk without great increase in endurance. It is important therefore for athletes to realize that fitness for one activity may not transfer to another and that the type of training must be tailored to the required activity.

Recruitment and discharge rates of motor units

The contractile force produced by a muscle is controlled by varying the number of motor units that are active and their rate of discharge. Under normal conditions these two variables are controlled so as to produce a smooth output of force.

The cell bodies of the α-motoneurones vary in size in accordance with their physiological type: thus the type S units have the smallest cell bodies, the FF units the largest. During a graded contraction, there is normally a specific order of recruitment of the units such that the smallest cells start to discharge first and the largest last. This is referred to as the **size principle**. Thus when small forces are required of

the muscle, the only units active are the weak, slowly contracting type S units, which are also the most resistant to fatigue. The FF units are only activated when large amounts of force are required (Fig. 3.5.3).

During controlled movements at low force levels, the force increase due to recruitment of a motor unit is very small because only the type S and FR units will be active and therefore very fine control is possible. It is much harder to exert fine control when the force output is approaching maximum levels (control is achieved by different strategies, such as co-activation of the antagonist muscles).

Figure 3.5.3 illustrates the pattern of motor unit recruitment during activity of the medial gastrocnemius muscle. When standing, only the type S units are recruited and they represent about 25% of the motor-unit pool but only generate 5% of the total force. During walking and slow running, there is a progressive recruitment of the FR units in addition. At maximum FR activation, approximately 50% of the pool is active but the muscle is still only generating 20% of its total force. During fast running, the FF units start to be recruited but there is only maximal recruitment during jumping.

Force is controlled not only by varying unit recruitment but also by varying the firing rate of the units. The contractile force generated by a

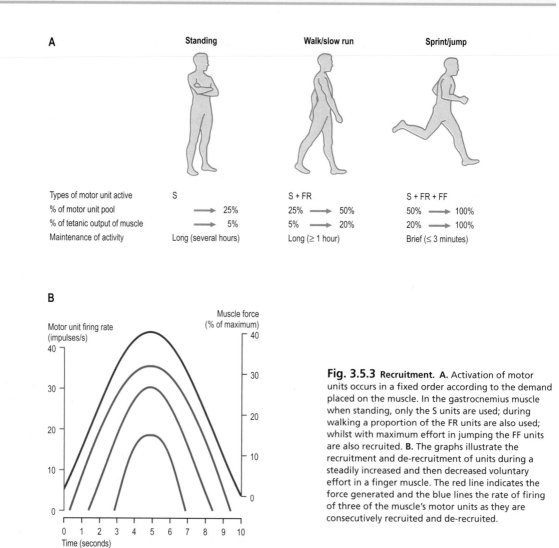

Types of motor unit active: S | S + FR | S + FR + FF
% of motor unit pool: → 25% | 25% → 50% | 50% → 100%
% of tetanic output of muscle: → 5% | 5% → 20% | 20% → 100%
Maintenance of activity: Long (several hours) | Long (≥ 1 hour) | Brief (≤ 3 minutes)

Fig. 3.5.3 Recruitment. A. Activation of motor units occurs in a fixed order according to the demand placed on the muscle. In the gastrocnemius muscle when standing, only the S units are used; during walking a proportion of the FR units are also used; whilst with maximum effort in jumping the FF units are also recruited. **B.** The graphs illustrate the recruitment and de-recruitment of units during a steadily increased and then decreased voluntary effort in a finger muscle. The red line indicates the force generated and the blue lines the rate of firing of three of the muscle's motor units as they are consecutively recruited and de-recruited.

motor unit is dependent on its rate of stimulation. For most units, during a steady contraction, the minimum firing rate for recruited units is about 5–8 Hz. This rises to a maximum of about 40 Hz. Units occasionally discharge at higher frequencies but then only for very brief periods.

During a gradually increasing contraction of the whole muscle, the first units start to discharge and increase their firing rates. At certain, individual force thresholds, new units are recruited and, in turn, progressively increase their firing rates (Fig. 3.5.3B) and so on. As the force output from the muscle is reduced, the pattern is reversed so that the units that were the last to be recruited will be the first to stop firing and the last units discharging will be the smallest S units. Note that during muscle contractions at less than maximum force many of the active units will be contracting. Although

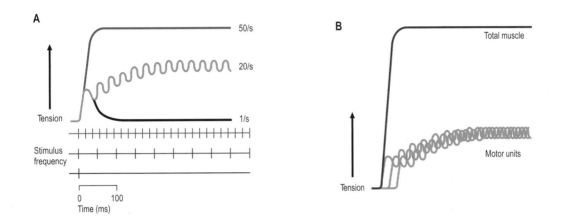

Fig. 3.5.4 **Smoothing of muscle tension.** **A.** Activation of an individual motor unit at different frequencies. If the rate of activation is high enough there is summation of force. At 20 Hz stimulation an unfused tetanic contraction is produced, at 50 Hz the contraction is fused (the effect of individual stimuli is not apparent). **B.** In the case of voluntary contractions many motor units fire at much less than the fusion frequency but because their activity is not synchronized the tension generated by the muscle is smoothed.

the tension profile of each unit is uneven, the overall force output from the muscle remains smooth because the activity of the units is unsynchronized (Fig. 3.5.4B). During fatigue, fear or in certain disease states such as Parkinson's disease, synchronous activity may occur, giving rise to a marked muscle tremor.

The constant practice of fine movement results in a reduction in the tremor, implying that desynchronization can be learnt.

Summary

Motor units

- A motor unit is the spinal α-motoneurone and the muscle fibres it innervates. The motoneurone is the final common pathway of command to the muscle unit.
- Axons of motoneurones leave the spinal cord via the ventral roots.
- Motor units are connected to the motor cortex of the brain (the highest level of the motor system) by the pyramidal (corticospinal) tracts.

- Motor units can be classified physiologically as slow, fast, fatigue resistant or fast fatiguable.
- Slow units produce the least tension and are recruited first; fast fatiguable units are only recruited when high levels of force are required.
- Regulation of contractile force is achieved by varying (i) the rate of discharge of each α-motoneurone and (ii) the number of motor units active.

Clinical Example

Motor disorders and spasticity

When you consider the complexity of the motor system there is little wonder at the potential for dysfunction. A command for movement may be corrupted anywhere in its path from the motor cortex to the skeletal muscle that brings it about. Specific clinical defects of movement such as parkinsonism and epilepsy are dealt with elsewhere, but there are a variety of conditions that involve an increase in muscle tone that is disabling and painful. This hypertonia, usually accompanied by an increased resistance to stretching, is called spasticity and may result from birth injury, trauma to the spinal cord, cerebrovascular disease or the local irritation of arthritis. This spasticity can be treated with drugs that act at different points in the motor chain.

Benzodiazepine tranquillizers are mainly used to reduce anxiety and produce sedation. They do, however, have a significant muscle relaxant effect and in high enough doses are anticonvulsants. Their relaxant effect is particularly useful in patients whose anxiety produces painful muscle tension. The action is at spinal and supraspinal levels where they depress polysynaptic transmission in an interesting if somewhat complex way. Benzodiazepines bind (and can therefore be supposed to act) most strongly at the cerebral cortex, less in the brainstem and spinal cord and hardly at all in other tissue. The specific binding site is one of the family of GABA receptors that produce the increase in chloride permeability which is the basis of GABA's inhibitory effect as a naturally occurring neurotransmitter. Benzodiazepines do not bind at the same site as GABA but on the same receptor, where they in some way increase its affinity for GABA and consequently the opening of chloride channels in nerve membranes (see Fig. CE3.5.1).

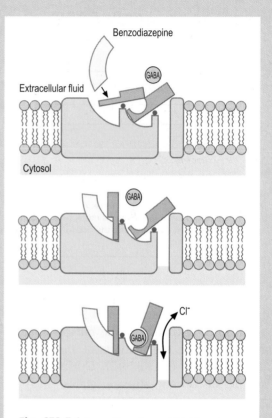

Fig. CE3.5.1 Benzodiazepine and GABA receptors.

Benzodiazepines are usually given by mouth but can be given intravenously when rapid action is required as when controlling an epileptic fit.

The inhibitory effects of the neurotransmitter GABA imbue it with potentially potent therapeutic effects. Much work has therefore gone into modifying its molecule to assist its penetration of the blood–brain barrier. One of the many substances produced during this work is baclofen which acts on a different subset of GABA receptors than do the benzodiazepines. Baclofen appears to act by reducing excessive γ-motoneurone activity and because of this action is used to treat the spasticity of multiple sclerosis. Its inability to

Clinical Example *(Continued)*

relieve spasticity of cerebral origin demonstrates that its site of action is the spinal cord.

The rationale of stimulating inhibitory pathways to reduce excessive muscle tone (as in the case of benzodiazepines and GABA) is also utilized in treatment with the drug tizanidine. This is an α_2 agonist which inhibits supraspinal and spinal polysynaptic reflexes. It has the great advantage of reducing excessive tone without reducing the patient's muscular strength.

The drugs carisoprodol and methocarbamol are of the same chemical family and cause selective inhibition of polysynaptic excitation of motoneurones. Thus the polysynaptic flexor reflex is inhibited while the tendon jerk reflex is unaffected. It has been suggested that this distinction between poly- and monosynaptic pathways is the result of the drug altering the refractory period of neurones. The monosynaptic pathway would carry a single synchronous burst of activity which would be less affected than the trains of action potentials in the polysynaptic pathway.

An alternative, entirely peripheral, method of reducing muscle tone is demonstrated by the drug dantrolene which acts directly on the sarcoplasmic reticulum to impair the Ca^{2+} release that is essential for the initiation of contraction. Dantrolene is much less effective in preventing contraction of cardiac and smooth muscle because these utilize external Ca^{2+} for their contraction rather than that stored in their sarcoplasmic reticulum.

One of the most dramatic pharmacological muscle relaxants must be the toxin of the microorganism *Clostridium botulinum*. This is one of the most toxic substances known. The organism lives in soil and its spores can contaminate food and survive heating to 100°C. Unlike the toxins of most bacteria, *C. botulinum* toxin is active by mouth. It has two very unpleasant actions:

- agglutination of red blood cells
- prevention of transmission at peripheral cholinergic junctions, a property which is used as a muscle relaxant.

Poisoning by *C. botulinum* is called *botulism* and the overall mortality is of the order of 70%. Death results from paralysis of the respiratory muscles with consequent suffocation. The action of the toxin is to bind to presynaptic nerve membranes where it inactivates actin, a protein involved in the exocytosis of acetylcholine transmitter. The binding is so powerful that antitoxin administration is no use once the symptoms appear and the effects persist for weeks, until the affected regions of membrane are replaced in the normal process of membrane turnover. This powerful binding means that the toxin does not spread and enables it to be used therapeutically by close local injection to treat blepharospasm (a persistent and disabling eyelid spasm), hemifacial spasm and equinus due to spasticity in cerebral palsy. The persistent action of botulinum toxin is useful in these conditions but as one would imagine its use is highly specialized.

A few other substances such as β-bungarotoxin inhibit release of acetylcholine at the neuromuscular junction but this constituent of cobra venom understandably has little clinical application. The majority of neuromuscular blockers of clinical importance exert their effect at the next step in the chain from brain to muscle – the postsynaptic muscle membrane. These clinically useful drugs exert their action by blocking muscle receptors to acetylcholine or persistently depolarizing them. Their major use is not in the treatment of spasticity but in surgery because their actions are usefully brief. They are described in Chapter 3.3 in the context of the neuromuscular junction, which is where they act.

Spinal cord distribution of motoneurones

The α-motoneurones have large cell bodies (up to 100 μm in diameter) which are located in the ventral horn of the spinal cord and in the nuclei of cranial motor nerves in the brainstem which supply skeletal muscles. The α-motoneurones innervating a given muscle (the **motoneurone pool** of the muscle) are grouped together in longitudinal columns which may extend over several segments of the cord.

Within the ventral horn, the motoneurone pools of the muscles of the axis of the body, the muscles concerned with posture and trunk movements, are located medially, while the limb muscles are represented more laterally with the distal muscles having their pools in the most dorsolateral part of the horn. Furthermore, the cell bodies of the motoneurones innervating the flexor muscles tend to lie dorsally to those of the extensor muscles (Fig. 3.5.5).

The α-motoneurone as a final common path

The α-motoneurone is a summing device whose output is dependent on the balance of the excitatory and inhibitory inputs to it and the level of excitability of the neurone at the time. The effect of any individual synaptic input depends upon its magnitude and upon the input impedance of the postsynaptic cell. The EPSPs evoked by single synaptic inputs tend to be largest in the small motoneurones of the type S units and smallest, and therefore least effective, in larger FF motoneurones. This variation is related to the way in which the synaptic inputs are arranged on the postsynaptic cell.

A typical α-motoneurone can be regarded as having four functional components: the cell body, dendrites (Fig. 3.5.6), an axon hillock and the axon itself.

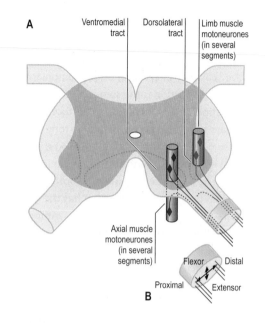

Fig. 3.5.5 Distribution of motoneurones. Within the spinal cord the motoneurones are arranged in functional groups. **A.** Motoneurones of individual muscles are innervated by several spinal segments of the cord in columns running axially within the cord. **B.** Medial groups control the muscles of the spine. Lateral groups innervate the other muscles, with the most distal muscles being innervated by the most lateral neurones. The motoneurones of flexor muscles lie dorsal to those of the extensors.

The dendrites arise from the cell body and branch (arborize) extensively. They make numerous synaptic connections with axon terminals. The cell body itself also receives synaptic inputs. The cell body at the axon hillock gives rise to a single, large-diameter myelinated axon.

In the cord the axon leaves the ventral horn, passing through the ventral white matter and entering the ventral root, from where it becomes part of one of the mixed spinal nerves and courses to the periphery. On leaving the ventral horn, the axons may give rise to a branch, termed a recurrent collateral, which re-enters the grey matter and synapses with inhibitory interneurones, called **Renshaw cells** (see p. 220).

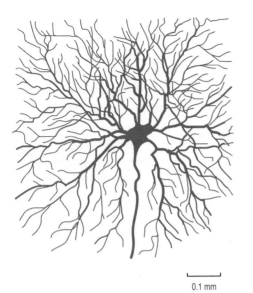

0.1 mm

Fig. 3.5.6 The dendrite tree of a single α-motoneurone from the spinal cord visualized by staining with horseradish peroxide (HRP). The motoneurone gives rise to a single large-diameter myelinated axon which runs to a muscle.

Synaptic integration

The synaptic inputs to a neurone are both inhibitory and excitatory. Each neurone can be regarded as a pre-programmed analogue computer that sums these inputs, both excitatory and inhibitory, and generates an output related to their sum. Although the inputs to a neurone are summed in an 'analogue' way, the output is a series of 'all-or-none' pulses (action potentials) whose frequency represents the strength of the output.

The axon hillock is the region of the neurone where the action potentials are generated and it is here that the integration of the inputs occurs. Even large synaptic inputs to the dendrites do not fire action potentials in the dendrites but produce synaptic currents that spread passively from the dendrites to the cell body and the axon hillock. They spread by cable conduction, decreasing in amplitude as they pass along the length of the dendrite. Inputs close to the cell body will not be significantly attenuated by this process. Thus synapses at the ends of dendrites, far removed from the cell body, will tend to produce a smaller depolarization of the axon hillock compared with a similar input close to or on the soma itself. The synaptic inputs are therefore weighted in terms of their effect.

The depolarization of the axon hillock is dependent on the sum of the individual currents, and this represents both a spatial and temporal summation of the synaptic events on that neurone, as in other parts of the CNS (see p. 187).

Another form of inhibition important in regulating the discharge rates of α-motoneurones is **presynaptic inhibition**. In this case an axon synapses with the pre-terminal region of another axon which is directly synapsing with the α-motoneurone (see p. 174). The effect of this axon-on-axon synapse is to reduce the release of neurotransmitter by the terminal. An important difference between presynaptic inhibition and inhibition (or facilitation) directed to the dendrites or some other part of the postsynaptic cell is that presynaptic inhibition has the effect of selectively controlling one input to the motoneurone without affecting the excitability of the motoneurone directly. The activity of the motoneurone will only be changed by the presynaptic input if the terminal involved is active (see Fig. 3.4.4, p. 189).

The α-motoneurone is the last point at which other neurones within the CNS can act on the motor impulse to the muscle. This important fact is emphasized by it sometimes being referred to as '**the final common pathway**'.

Summary

α-motoneurones

- They are located in the ventral horn of the spinal cord and in cranial motor nerves.
- Those innervating one muscle are found in several segments of the spinal cord.
- Innervation of trunk and limbs and flexor and extensor muscles is topographically arranged in the ventral roots of the spinal cord.

- As the final common pathway out of the CNS, α-motoneurones are the last place a motor command can be modified by the CNS.
- The motoneurone frequently gives off a recurrent collateral branch which returns to the spinal cord to synapse with inhibitory Renshaw cells.

Motor control: receptors and reflexes

3.6

Introduction

The control of skeletal muscle by the central nervous system is a complex affair. In this chapter we will describe some simple elements of this control, the peripheral receptors and the reflexes built upon them.

A reflex response can be described as an automatic response to a sensory stimulus – dust on the eye makes you blink. These programmed responses are the elements with which complex behaviour is built up. They may be included in a response unmodified or after appropriate tuning by the higher centres of the CNS. One of the simplest reflexes is the muscle stretch reflex which involves only two neurones. Stretching a muscle receptor, the muscle spindle, leads to activity in the fibres of that muscle which opposes the stretch. This negative feedback reflex is important in the control of movement and is tested by physicians as the tendon jerk when they wish to test the functional state of the spinal cord.

The most striking feature of the stretch reflex is that its sensitivity to the length of the muscle is determined by the CNS. Spinal efferents, γ-motoneurones, adjust the range of lengths over which the muscle spindle responds. This permits:

- a very sensitive receptor of finite and small dynamic range (the range of movement within which changes in length produce

213

changes in receptor output) to report usefully over a large range of movement

- the possibility that movement of the muscle might be initiated by resetting the response of the muscle spindle.

In bringing about a controlled movement, the CNS runs one of its learnt motor programs evoking a pattern of muscle activity that is predicted to achieve the intended movement. The actual movement produced is compared with that intended and any error corrected by adjusting the motor output. The movement is monitored by several systems: visual, joint position sensors and the stretch reflex. The stretch reflex is, perhaps, most important in compensating for unexpected resistance to movement, for example picking up a suitcase full of books when expecting it to be empty.

Muscle receptors

Control of skeletal muscle contraction is strongly dependent on the sensory feedback coming from the receptors within the muscles. Skeletal muscles contain two types of highly specialized proprioceptors specifically concerned with movement, the **tendon organ** and the **muscle spindle**. The tendon organ responds mainly to muscle tension generated by active contraction. The muscle spindle is a stretch receptor which is particularly sensitive to lengthening of the muscle.

The density of tendon organs and muscle spindles in a given skeletal muscle is, like the innervation ratio (p. 203), a function of the location and function of that muscle. The muscles of the hand, which are small and are used to execute fine movements, have a high density of receptors, whereas the thigh muscles have lower densities.

The tendon organ

The tendon organ is a relatively simple receptor organ located at the junction between the

muscle fibres and the tendon. Tendon organs are less numerous than muscle spindles. Their numbers are highest in muscles producing fine movements. The body of the tendon organ is made up of strands of collagen which branch and join together in a complex lattice enclosed within a fibrous capsule. The organ is innervated by a single nerve ending of a group Ib afferent (see Table 3.5.1). The nerve forms spray-like endings around and amongst the collagen (Fig. 3.6.1). At the tendinous end, the collagen strands merge onto the tissue of the tendon; at the muscle end a group of 10–20

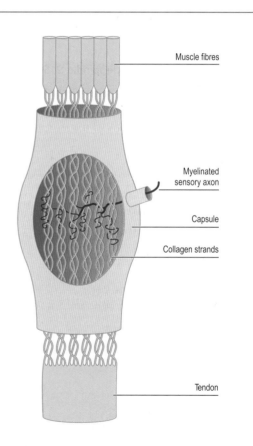

Fig. 3.6.1 Structure of the tendon organ. The sensory nerve endings, classified on the basis of their axons' conduction velocity as group Ib afferents, intertwine the collagenous insertions of several motor units. The fibres and terminals are encapsulated in gelatinous material. The fibres are compressed and twisted when the collagen fibres are tensed as the muscle generates force, causing them to discharge a volley of action potentials.

skeletal muscle fibres insert into the organ, fusing with the strands of collagen.

The tendon organ is extremely sensitive to tension generated by the several muscle fibres inserted into it (Fig. 3.6.2). The skeletal muscle fibres comprising each motor unit (those muscle fibres innervated by a single common α-motoneurone) are distributed at random throughout a wide cross-section of the muscle (p. 90). In any group of 10–20 muscle fibres attached to a single tendon organ, not more than one or two of the fibres will belong to the same motor unit. The tendon organ thus monitors the contractile activity of a number of motor units. The distribution of the tendon organs is such that every motor unit will be monitored by at least one tendon organ and thus the combined activity of all the Ib afferent axons provides a picture of the overall tension development by the muscle.

The muscle spindle

The muscle spindle is a very complex sense organ. It is about 10 μm in length and is composed of a bundle of small, highly specialized muscle fibres. These are called the **intrafusal** (within the spindle) **muscle fibres**. In their central region, the intrafusal fibres have few or no myofibrils (contractile elements). This space is packed with nuclei. The intrafusal muscle fibres are divided into two types on the basis of their size and the organization of their nuclei:

- **nuclear bag** fibres (usually two per spindle) have a central region that is relatively large with the nuclei clustered together
- **nuclear chain** fibres (4–10 per spindle) are smaller and have a single row of nuclei in their more slender central region.

In both types of intrafusal fibre, the nuclei are scarce on either side of the central region and the intrafusal muscle fibres are contractile.

The innervation of the muscle spindle

Sensory nerves

The muscle spindle is richly innervated with both sensory and motor axons. In the central, nucleated region, the intrafusal fibres are innervated by a large-diameter, group Ia afferent axon. The Ia axon forms characteristic annulospiral endings around each of the intrafusal muscle fibres (Fig. 3.6.3). These are called primary endings. Each spindle may also be innervated by from zero to five secondary endings formed by smaller-diameter group II afferent axons. Secondary endings are found mainly on the nuclear chain fibres.

Motor nerves

The contractile ends of the intrafusal fibres are innervated by spinal motor nerves. This innervation is by two groups of efferent axons: the γ-motoneurones, which have small-diameter axons and only innervate the intrafusal muscle

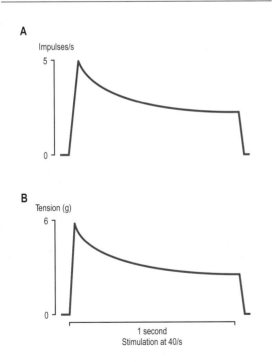

Fig. 3.6.2 Tension and afferent output from a muscle tendon organ. The motor nerve of the muscle, held at fixed length, is stimulated for 1 second at 40 Hz. In the short term the organ discharge frequency (**A**) follows the tension developed (**B**).

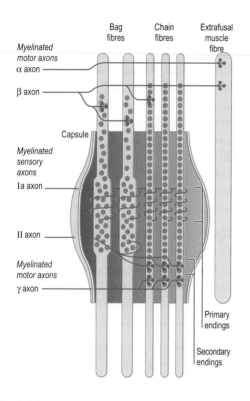

Fig. 3.6.3 The muscle spindle showing, diagrammatically, the intra- and extrafusal muscle fibres and their motor and sensory innervations.

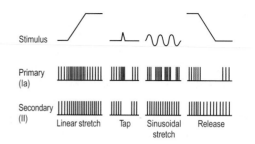

Fig. 3.6.4 Responses of primary and secondary spindle afferents to various forms of stretch of muscle, showing adaptation (after Mathews P B C 1964 Muscle spindles and their motor control. *Physiological Reviews* 44: 219–288).

the sensory endings around them. This distortion opens stretch-sensitive channels in the nerve terminal membranes and leads to a receptor potential and an increase in the rate of action potential discharge in the afferent axon.

As with all mechanoreceptors, adaptation occurs – the response to a maintained change in length disappears with time. The two types of sensory endings of the muscle spindle are both slowly adapting but adapt at different rates.

The responses of the two types to passive movements of the muscle are illustrated in Figure 3.6.4. The primary ending shows a response during the stretch, the dynamic component, which is related to the velocity of the stretch. After the stretch has finished, the afferent discharge declines to a level related to the new muscle length. This is called the static component. When the muscle is held stretched, the firing rate is dependent on the new length of the muscle. The primary endings are thus showing a high degree of adaptation. The response of the secondary ending shows little or no dynamic component and is closely related to muscle length throughout. The secondary ending shows much less adaptation than the primary ending.

The role of motor innervation of the muscle spindle

Contraction of the ends of the intrafusal fibres stretches their central nuclear region. The motor

fibres and the β-motoneurones which are like the α-motoneurones that innervate the **extrafusal** (outside the spindle) muscle fibres in that they have large diameter axons. They not only innervate the extrafusal muscle fibres but also give off a branch that innervates the intrafusal muscle fibres. Contraction of the ends of the intrafusal muscle fibres stretches their non-contractile nucleated middle regions.

Afferent responses from the muscle spindle

The muscle spindle lies in parallel with the skeletal muscle fibres and merges, at each end, with the connective tissue of the muscle. When the muscle is stretched the spindle is stretched. The stretching of the intrafusal fibres distorts innervation of the spindle therefore changes the relationship between the total length of the muscle spindle and the sensory discharge of the afferents. These effects can also modify the adaptation of the response. The β- and γ-motoneurones are divided into two types, termed static and dynamic, according to their effects on the stretch response.

- The dynamic motoneurones increase the dynamic sensitivity of the endings, the rapidly adapting component of the response, so that they become much more sensitive to the velocity and changes in velocity of a movement.
- The static motoneurones increase the static sensitivity of the endings, the slowly adapting component of the response.

The CNS can thus control both the magnitude and character of the response of the spindle afferents to movement.

When the muscle shortens passively, the primary endings usually fall silent. During shortening due to muscle contraction, however, the intrafusal fibres almost always contract with the extrafusal fibres. The motor innervation of the spindle, the β- and γ-motoneurones will increase their discharge at a rate similar to that of the α-motoneurone pool whose output drives the extrafusal fibres. The γ-motoneurones are also activated by a process called α–γ **coactivation**. As a result, the contraction of the intrafusal muscle fibres takes up the slack in the spindle produced by muscle shortening and so the terminals of the sensory endings remain stretched and continue to discharge. The CNS can interpret the afferent signal by reference to the spindle efferent drive it is providing at the time. The muscle spindle discharge is interpreted, at the conscious level, as movement of the appropriate joint rather than a sense of actual muscle length. This has been demonstrated by pulling on the tendons of exposed muscles in human subjects: the subjects report movement of the appropriate joint even if the joint itself has been prevented from moving.

Other proprioceptors

As well as the muscle spindles and tendon organs, a number of other receptors contribute to the sensory feedback during movement. The ligaments and capsules of the joints contain receptors that respond to joint movement. Individual receptors often have a limited range of response, with the ranges of different receptors overlapping; thus the position of the joint may be signalled by which of the receptors are discharging, a mechanism termed **range fractionation**.

Some free-ending afferents within the muscles respond to the compressive forces generated during muscle contraction. There is also evidence that receptors in the skin respond to the deformation of the skin during movement and that this also provides an important source of sensory feedback, particularly in the hands and feet. While standing or when picking up a delicate object like an egg, information about pressure on the skin allows precise control of the forces on the egg or the balance of the body.

Summary

Muscle receptors

- Muscle spindles and tendon organs monitor, respectively, length and tension of muscles.
- Muscle receptor reflexes provide a very rapid and flexible system for controlling movement.
- The intrafusal fibres of a muscle spindle are in parallel with the extrafusal fibres of the main muscle.
- Activation of the intrafusal fibres changes the sensitivity of the spindle.
- Proprioceptors in ligaments, joints and, particularly, the skin contribute to sensory feedback and control during movement.

Spinal reflexes

A reflex response is a highly stereotyped automatic response to a specific stimulus. In common parlance a 'knee-jerk' response is an immediate unthinking response to provocation. The spinal reflexes affecting skeletal muscles, typified by the knee-jerk, represent the simplest sets of motor behaviour. Because of their reproducibility and relative simplicity, these reflexes have formed a starting point for studies of sensorimotor integration. The spinal reflexes comprise five elements:

1. a sensory receptor (e.g. the muscle spindle)
2. an afferent pathway to the spinal cord
3. synaptic connections, via interneurones or directly, onto
4. an efferent pathway which is usually the motoneurone, and
5. an effector, usually skeletal muscle.

These elements are usually arranged to form a negative-feedback circuit as shown in Figure 3.6.5 for the knee-jerk' reflex. An exception to this is the bite reflex of mastication which includes an initial positive feedback.

The stretch reflex (Fig. 3.6.6)

The simplest neuronal circuit of all is that of the stretch reflex (also known as the myotatic reflex) since this pathway only involves two neurones, the afferent Ia from the muscle spindle and the α-motoneurones that form the efferent output, with a single synapse linking the ascending and descending paths. It is a monosynaptic reflex. The best-known stretch reflex, the knee-jerk reflex, is elicited by tapping the patella tendon, which tilts the patella, thus

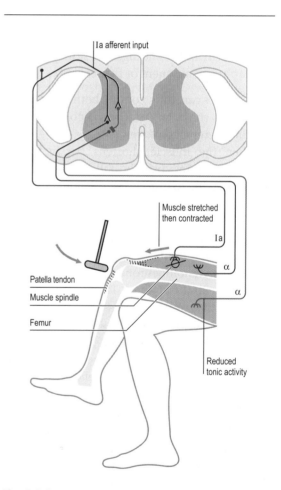

Fig. 3.6.6 **Basic elements of the spinal stretch reflex showing their arrangements and their function in the stretch reflex.** The patella hammer strikes the tendon, stretching the belly of the muscle and the muscle spindles in it. A **monosynaptic** reflex causes the stretched muscle, an extensor, to contract. A **disynaptic** reflex, reciprocal inhibition, inhibits flexor activity. The knee jerks into extension.

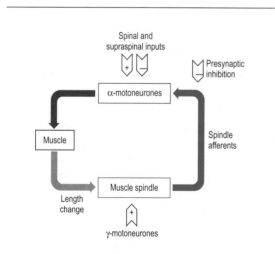

Fig. 3.6.5 **The neuronal circuit of the myotatic (stretch) reflex.** The strength of the reflex can be modified by γ-motoneurone effects on intrafusal muscle fibres, by presynaptic inhibition of α-motoneurones by tendon organs and by spinal and supraspinal inhibition or facilitation.

producing a brisk stretch of the quadriceps femoris muscle. This stretch elicits a burst of impulses in the Ia afferents of the quadriceps muscle spindles. On reaching the cord, this volley of excitatory impulses to the α-motoneurones evokes in them a burst of action potentials causing the muscle to contract. The whole process from the tendon tap to the start of the contraction takes about 25 ms. This response time of the reflex varies depending on the length of the afferent and efferent pathways. The delay in the spinal synapse is less than 1 ms.

The reflex arc is therefore a potent negative-feedback pathway which acts to control muscle length, the muscle contraction acting to restore the original length of the muscle. Tendon jerks are all artificial and do not give a good representation of the physiological role of the stretch reflex. In particular, their massive overshoot and their pendular nature are clearly not features that make them obviously useful components of a control system. The significance of the tendon jerk to clinicians is that it tests the integrity of the system and the excitability of the spinal cord.

Stretch reflexes are particularly important in the extensor muscles, and one of the major roles of these reflexes is in the maintenance of posture. The reflex is responsible for maintaining a steady contraction in response to the stretching of the muscle as it supports the posture against the force of gravity. When holding a steady posture, there will be maintained activity of the type S (see p. 204) motor units in the contracting muscles. Contraction of the intrafusal muscle fibres will maintain the discharge of the spindle afferents at the set length of the muscle. Disturbance of the postural position will lead to muscle stretch and the reflex response thereby leads to rapid restoration of the required position.

The stretch reflex is also involved in the regulation of muscle contraction during active movements (p. 221).

The stretch reflex, like the other spinal reflexes, is modified by the higher centres of the CNS during activation. The amplitude of the reflex is controlled by a number of factors acting at different points in the pathway. The sensitivity of the muscle spindle itself may be controlled by variations in the level of γ-motoneurone discharge; the efficacy of the synaptic connections onto the α-motoneurones may be altered by presynaptic inhibition (p. 189), and the excitability of the α-motoneurones may be controlled by other excitatory or inhibitory inputs. The nervous system thereby regulates the strength of the reflex according to the requirements of the current motor activity. This is demonstrated by the reinforcement of the knee-jerk that is produced if the subject grasps the hands together in front of the body and pulls hard.

The stretch reflex is also built upon by higher centres. The spinal stretch reflex in hand muscles is followed by a second reflex response about 20–30 ms later called the **long-loop reflex**. This is also a stretch reflex but is mediated by the motor cortex (p. 225) and involves several synapses. This long-loop reflex has a significant role in the muscles controlling the hand. The size of the response is very variable according to the activity being performed, allowing a relatively rapid but flexible response of the hand to mechanical disturbances during movements.

Reciprocal inhibition

The stretching of a muscle produces effects in other muscles.

The afferents from the muscle spindle branch profusely within the spinal cord, making connections not only with the α-motoneurones of the same muscle but also with those of its synergists and with interneurones that synapse with the α-motoneurones innervating the antagonistic muscles (Fig. 3.6.6). When one muscle of a limb is stretched and a stretch reflex is evoked, the limb will be supported by other muscles and there will be reciprocal inhibition of antagonist muscles. Thus reflex-induced contraction is not opposed by ongoing contraction in the antagonists.

Inverse myotatic reflex (tendon reflex)

Just as the stretch reflex controls the length of muscles, the inverse myotatic reflex controls the tension developed by them. The sensory input to the inverse myotatic reflex comes, via the Ib afferent neurones, from the tendon organs which are stimulated by the development of tension in the tendon (Fig. 3.6.7). These afferent fibres make synaptic connections with inhibitory interneurones in the cord which in turn synapse with the α-motoneurones of the muscle from which they came (hence the alternative name of this reflex – autogenic inhibition) and its agonists. This again is an example of a negative-feedback reflex. This reflex is of greater importance in extensor than in flexor muscles and serves two purposes: it prevents muscles from developing damaging tensions and it maintains constant tension in a muscle regardless of its length.

Recurrent inhibition

Another autogenic inhibitory mechanism is recurrent inhibition. Axons of the α-motoneurones leaving the ventral horn give rise to a collateral branch which goes back into the horn (i.e. is recurrent) and synapses with an inhibitory interneurone called the Renshaw cell (Fig. 3.6.8). The Renshaw cells make synaptic connections with the α-motoneurones innervating the same muscle and to a lesser extent other agonist muscles. This has the effect of spreading the excitation more evenly throughout the motor units within a muscle.

All of the pathways so far described form **segmental reflexes**, where the neurones involved only make synaptic connections with other neurones within the same spinal segment. Some reflex pathways involve several spinal segments, an example being the flexion reflex.

Flexion reflex

The flexion, or withdrawal, reflex (Fig. 3.6.9) is evoked by a noxious stimulus to the distal parts of a limb. Standing on a pin causes contraction of the flexor muscles around all the joints of the leg, withdrawing the limb from the source of the pain. The contraction of the flexors is accompanied by relaxation of the extensor muscles of that leg to aid the withdrawal. As experience shows, the more painful the stimulus, the more violent is the withdrawal and the more muscles are involved. With increasing stimulus strength, the effects spread to involve more spinal segments and more powerful excitation of the flexor muscles. The afferent axons

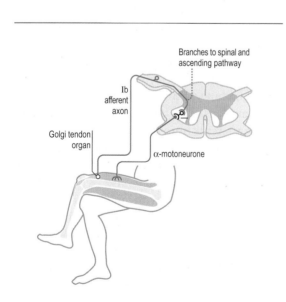

Fig. 3.6.7 The myotatic reflex. The Golgi tendon organ, via a Ib afferent nerve, stimulates an inhibitory interneurone acting on the motoneurone of the muscle attached to the tendon.

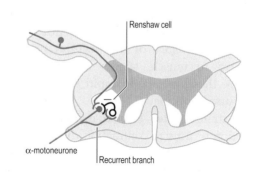

Fig. 3.6.8 Renshaw inhibition of an α-motoneurone.

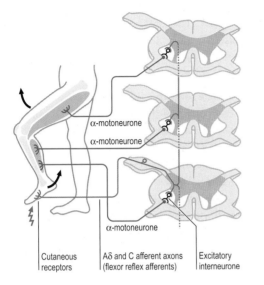

| Cutaneous receptors | Aδ and C afferent axons (flexor reflex afferents) | Excitatory interneurone |

Fig. 3.6.9 The flexion (withdrawal) reflex to noxious stimuli.

mediating this reflex are termed the **flexor reflex afferents** (FRA) and are predominantly high-threshold cutaneous, joint and muscle afferents that innervate nociceptors.

The flexion reflex may be accompanied by the **crossed extensor reflex** which contracts extensors and relaxes the flexor muscles of the contralateral limb. This reflex provides a postural adjustment to compensate for removal of the injured limb from the ground. In man the crossed extensor reflex is confined to the legs.

Reflex control of movement

The sensory feedback from the joints and muscles is used in a number of reflexes that control movement at the spinal level. Most of these reflexes include negative-feedback loops and play a key role in the regulation of posture and locomotion.

The stretch reflex is important in the maintenance of posture (see p. 231) but is active during all movements, especially where the execution is slow and deliberate (i.e. not a ballistic or throwing movement).

Indeed, muscle movements can be initiated by a change in the motor output to the muscle spindle, via the γ-efferents, rather than by activity in the α-motoneurones. If the muscle spindle length is changed by its motor innervation this will, through the stretch reflex, cause the extrafusal muscle fibre length to follow or track the spindle length. If the γ drive to the spindle is increased the ends of the spindle will contract, stretching the nucleated mid-portion. A reflex contraction of the extrafusal fibres will shorten the muscle, returning the mid-portion of the spindle to its original length.

If during this shortening resistance is met, arresting the shortening of the muscle, the stretch reflex will increase the extrafusal fibre activity. As the intrafusal muscle fibres continue to contract at the original rate, stretching of the sensory region of the spindle will occur. The discharge of the spindle afferents will then increase, leading to a reflex excitatory input of the α-motoneurones and a more powerful muscle contraction overcoming the new loading. In this way, the stretch reflex can act to regulate the ongoing contraction and generate an initial, rapid response to errors in the planned movement. This response can be powerful and damaging. Meeting an unexpected obstruction to a step that stretches the calf muscles whilst the ankle is being extended can lead to such a brisk response that the Achilles tendon may be torn from the heel.

The stretch reflex is part of a complex control system and during movement corrective changes are also made by central structures such as the cerebellum and the motor cortex (see p. 231).

Central pattern generation

Subjects with transected spinal cords have provided evidence for the presence of independent **central pattern generators** (CPGs) located within the spinal cord. These CPGs generate basic elements of locomotor movements even in the absence of any descending, supraspinal control. It appears that there is a CPG for each of the limb girdles, though their activities are coordinated. Their output produces the alternating patterns of extension and flexion that form the basis of walking. Sensory feedback and descending commands serve to modify these basic patterns to meet needs of the current situation.

These central pattern generators can be shown to be present in neonates. If a week-old baby is held with its feet just touching a moving walkway it will make recognizable stepping movements. These become less obvious as the higher centres of the brain develop their spinal connections.

Summary

Spinal reflexes

- Muscle receptors form the sensory component of the segmental spinal reflexes.
- Long-loop reflexes involve the motor cortex in control of the hands.
- Spinal reflexes are important in the maintenance of posture and the control of ongoing muscle contraction.
- Pattern generators of basic locomotor movements exist in the spinal cord.

Supraspinal control of movement

Introduction

The spinal cord, independently of the brain, is capable of mediating a range of reflex actions whose purpose is to provide rapid regulation of ongoing postural and locomotor activities. Through central pattern generators, the spinal cord may also be capable of maintaining basic patterns of motor output for rhythmic movements. The main centres for the control of motor behaviour, however, lie in the brain. The motor commands are transmitted to the spinal cord via the **descending motor pathways**. The neurones of these and other motor pathways are confined to the CNS and are referred to as **upper motoneurones**. Some of these upper motoneurones make direct connection with the α- and γ-motoneurones (the **lower motoneurones**) and so can directly evoke muscle contractions. Other upper motoneurones connect with interneurones in the spinal cord and so influence the lower motoneurones by a less direct route, via the reflex pathways (see Clinical Example: Upper and lower motoneurone lesions).

Generation of an accurate, voluntary movement necessitates the development of a 'motor plan' which depends initially on the processing of a large amount of sensory information; for example, internal information such as the current position of the limbs, their ongoing movements and the degree of contraction of the different muscles, in both the limbs and trunk of the body; and external information such as the position of the target in relation to the body and the presence of any obstacles. This information, combined with previous experience, is used to produce the motor plan which encodes the movement in terms of the timing and amplitude of the muscle contractions.

Recordings of electrical activity in the brain show that the motor areas of the cerebral cortex become active up to 1 second before the onset of the voluntary movement. These motor areas are central to the generation of the motor plan and they form part of two looped pathways: one with the basal ganglia, the other with

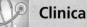

Clinical Example

Upper and lower motoneurone lesions

Hughlings Jackson defined disorders of the motor systems as producing two possible effects: negative signs represent the loss of some motor function while positive signs (release phenomena) represent the appearance of an abnormal motor behaviour previously held under inhibitory control.

The lower motoneurones are those that have their cell bodies in the spinal cord or brainstem and which innervate the skeletal muscles. Lower motoneurone lesions leave the muscles denervated, giving rise to a flaccid paralysis in which the muscles can no longer be made to contract (except by direct electrical stimulation) and undergo progressive atrophy; there is, of course, no resting muscle tone.

The term upper motoneurone is applied to all neurones wholly within the CNS motor pathways, and therefore upper motoneurone lesions have a variety of effects. One of the most common such lesions is defined by neurologists as pyramidal tract syndrome and is frequently caused by bleeding into the internal capsule – a stroke. The characteristic signs are contralateral spasticity with major impairment of fine voluntary movements and a positive Babinski sign; if the outer border of the sole of the foot is stroked, the great toe goes upward (extends). Spasticity may be defined as being a state of

exaggerated stretch reflexes (hyperreflexia) with increased muscle tone (hypertonia) which acts to resist passive movement of the limb, these effects being most pronounced in the antigravity muscles. Spasticity is therefore clearly distinct from rigidity where there is greatly increased muscle tone to both flexion and extension, usually without hyperactive stretch reflexes (cf. parkinsonism).

Pyramidal tract syndrome, however, is a complex disorder since it represents the lesion of a number of pathways including the cortical projections at the brainstem motor nuclei, so all the motor outputs are affected. Lesions of the pyramidal tract in the medulla or spinal cord are much more limited in effect. There is a marked reduction in manual skill and a modest hypotonia, but voluntary movement can still be made and there may be some recovery of motor skill with time. This reflects the ability of the CNS to utilize the rubrospinal tract to control the distal limb muscles.

Spinal cord lesions result in the most profound deficits, with complete paralysis occurring below the site of a cord transection. In man, spinal cord transection is followed by a period of spinal shock when all spinal reflexes are lost and there is no muscle tone. After a time, the reflexes gradually recover and increase in amplitude reaching a hyperreflexic state, particularly of the flexion reflexes.

the cerebellum. These pathways, operating in parallel, develop different aspects of the motor plan and then the motor commands, which are output via the descending motor pathways (which also operate in parallel to some extent) to the spinal cord. During its execution, the movement is continuously monitored and modified, again by parallel pathways, at the levels of the spinal cord, the cerebellum and the cerebral cortex.

Descending motor pathways

The descending motor pathways, by tradition, have been divided into the **pyramidal tracts**, which originate from the cerebral cortex, and the **extrapyramidal tracts**, the descending paths of which originate in the brainstem. An alternative classification is based on the anatomical locations of the pathways (Table 3.7.1).

Pathways of cortical origin

These motor pathways originate in several distinct areas of the cerebral cortex and descend to terminate in the brainstem at the spinal cord. Recent evidence suggests that in man 60% of the descending fibres originate in the **precentral gyrus**, a region called the **motor cortex** (Figs 3.7.1A and 3.7.3). The remaining fibres come from the adjoining **premotor cortex** and **supplementary motor area** and from the **postcentral gyrus** (the sensory cortex).

From the cortex, the fibres descend through the internal capsule (a region of clinical importance because of its frequent involvement in strokes) to the brainstem. Within the brainstem, one group of fibres, constituting the **corticobulbar tract**, terminates on groups of cranial nerve motor nuclei controlling eye and facial movements (Fig. 3.7.1B).

The major component of the descending fibres constitutes the **corticospinal tract** (Fig. 3.7.1A). These fibres descend directly from the cortex to the grey matter of the spinal cord. As the corticospinal tract passes through the brainstem, collateral branches make connections with the neurones of the **red nucleus** and the **reticular formation**, both of which also project to the spinal cord (reticulospinal and rubrospinal pathways of Table 3.7.1). Within the brainstem the corticospinal fibres divide into two groups. 85% of the fibres cross (**decussate**) the midline of the medulla and descend in the

---

Table 3.7.1 Descending (motor) spinal pathways

	Anatomical location in cord	Major functions
Pathways of cortical origin		
Corticospinal		
Crossed pyramidal	Lateral	Voluntary movements of the body
Direct pyramidal	Anterior	
Pathways of brainstem origin		
Vestibulospinal	Ventromedial	Posture and balance
Tectospinal	Ventromedial	Motor component of visual and audio reflexes
Reticulospinal	Ventromedial	Muscle tone, autonomic system, regulation of sensory end-organs, e.g. muscle spindles
Rubrobulbar	Dorsolateral	Project to medulla
Rubrospinal	Dorsolateral	Extrapyramidal control of flexor muscles

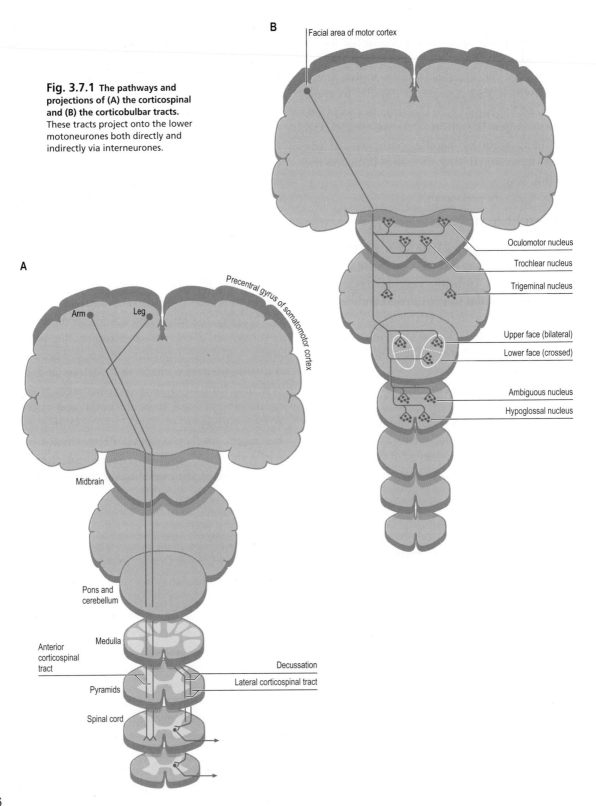

Fig. 3.7.1 The pathways and projections of (A) the corticospinal and (B) the corticobulbar tracts. These tracts project onto the lower motoneurones both directly and indirectly via interneurones.

B | Facial area of motor cortex

Oculomotor nucleus

Trochlear nucleus

Trigeminal nucleus

Upper face (bilateral)

Lower face (crossed)

Ambiguous nucleus

Hypoglossal nucleus

A

Arm

Leg

Precentral gyrus of somatomotor cortex

Midbrain

Pons and cerebellum

Anterior corticospinal tract

Medulla

Decussation

Lateral corticospinal tract

Pyramids

Spinal cord

contralateral spinal cord as the **lateral cortico-spinal tract**. The other 15% of fibres remain ipsilateral, constituting the **anterior cortico-spinal tract**. The anterior tract extends downwards only as far as the upper thoracic cord and projects bilaterally onto the motoneurones and interneurones within the medial portion of the spinal cord. These motoneurones predominantly innervate the muscles of the upper trunk and the neck.

The lateral corticospinal tract fibres subdivide according to their origin within the cortex. The fibres from the sensory regions of the cerebral cortex terminate predominantly in the dorsal horn on interneurones which, in turn, may act to facilitate or inhibit the segmental reflexes by their actions on the incoming sensory activity. Many fibres from the precentral motor areas terminate directly on the α- and γ-motoneurones and constitute the means by which the cerebral cortex can directly evoke muscle contraction. Note that the projection to α- and γ-motoneurones is in keeping with the model of α–γ coactivation for maintaining stretch reflex sensitivity during movement (see p. 217). The lateral corticospinal tract fibres only project contralaterally and predominantly to the lower motoneurones innervating the distal muscles of the limbs, especially of the hand, though there are projections to the more proximal muscles as well. Some fibres of the corticospinal tract from the motor cortical areas terminate on interneurones rather than directly on motoneurones. Whilst all the fibres of the tract are excitatory, where they terminate on interneurones their overall action may be facilitatory or inhibitory depending on the nature of the interneurones.

Functions of the corticospinal tract

The lateral corticospinal tract has a specific role in the control of skilled, voluntary movements as revealed by the distinctive deficits resulting from its transection (see Clinical Example: Upper and lower motoneurone lesions). The monosynaptic connection between the motor areas of the cortex and the α-motoneurones enables the cerebral cortex to exert direct control over the contraction of the distal limb muscles, for example for fine manipulation of the hand. In man the tract shows the greatest degree of development of any primate. This is reflected in the number of fibres constituting the tract, with a greater density of projections onto the lower motoneurones of the distal muscles and with the projections to more proximal muscles, found in man, absent in other primates.

Pathways originating in the brainstem

The tracts of brainstem origin project to the spinal cord where they synapse onto interneurones. There are four main tracts which can be divided into two anatomical groups: the **ventromedial** and the **dorsolateral** pathways (Table 3.7.1).

The ventromedial pathways comprise the **vestibulospinal**, the **tectospinal** and the **reticulospinal** tracts. All these tracts terminate mainly within the motor pools of the axial and proximal limb muscles. The vestibulospinal tract receives major inputs from the vestibular system (see p. 332) and is involved in the reflex control of balance; as such, its main projection is onto the motor pools of extensor muscles. The tectospinal tract is involved in the coordination of eye–body movements, while the reticulospinal tract is particularly concerned with regulating the excitability of extensor muscle reflexes.

The dorsolateral pathways comprise the **rubrobulbar** and the **rubrospinal** tracts which represent an evolutionarily older form of the corticobulbar and lateral corticospinal tracts in that they act as the motoneurone pools of the distal limb muscles. The neurones of the red nucleus receive a major input from the cerebral cortex and are particularly concerned with reflex control of flexor muscles.

The brainstem

The brainstem is important in movement control as a major site of sensorimotor integration, forming the bridge between different higher centres and the spinal cord (see Fig. 3.1.4, p. 144). Two aspects of motor control that are mediated within the brainstem are the control of eye movements (p. 144) and the postural reflexes.

Postural reflexes

A number of reflexes are involved in postural adjustments related to movements of the head and neck, which depend particularly on sensory information from the visual system, the vestibular system and the muscle spindles of the neck. The postural reflexes dependent on vestibular and muscle spindle information are involved in the maintenance of head–body position in space and the relative position of the body with respect to the head.

The semicircular canals of the vestibular system (p. 332) provide information about angular rotation of the head, while the otolith organs signal linear accelerations (horizontal and vertical) and, thereby, the position of the head relative to gravity. Rotational acceleration of the head and body to the right leads to extension of the antigravity muscles on the left and relaxation of those on the right so that the body leans to the right, the response being mediated by the semicircular canal input to the vestibulospinal tract. This leaning of the body into the direction of the acceleration acts to maintain balance. Similar responses are seen during linear acceleration, mediated by the otolith organs (Fig. 3.7.2).

The neck muscles contain dense populations of muscle spindles and these provide an input to the postural reflexes. If the head of a quadruped is tilted upwards on the body, thereby extending the neck, the **tonic neck reflex** causes the forelimbs to extend and the hind limbs to flex, restoring the head–body axis. (*Note:* Extension of the neck is one of the common tricks used when training a dog to sit. If the neck is flexed, the hind limbs extend and the forelimbs relax.) In adult humans, this reflex is not evident but it may be demonstrated in babies.

These postural reflexes therefore serve to maintain the head–body axis in a straight line and to tilt that axis to counter movement that would otherwise lead to falling over.

The visual system also has a powerful input to the postural mechanisms in terms of the information about head position and movement.

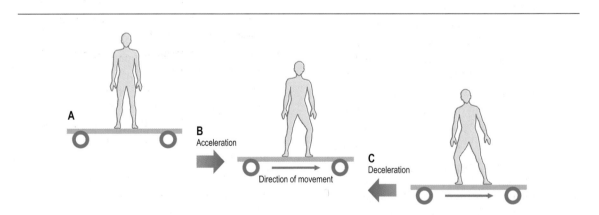

Fig. 3.7.2 Postural reflexes. The subject is standing on a trolley. **A.** With the trolley stationary, the subject stands upright. **B.** As the trolley starts to move, the subject is accelerated and the semicircular canals and vestibulospinal pathway mediate a postural reflex causing the subject to lean into the direction of the acceleration. **C.** During slowing, the subject again leans into the negative acceleration.

An example of this effect is that if one is in an open space, looking straight up at the sky, the effect of clouds passing overhead is to generate an illusion of movement, and the attempts to compensate for this can lead to falling over. This illusion occurs despite the conflicting evidence from the vestibular system that the head is stationary. Maintained conflict between the visual and vestibular systems is a cause of motion sickness.

Some of the most powerful information that helps to maintain posture and an upright stance comes from pressure receptors on the skin. When standing, receptors monitoring the distribution of weight over the soles of the feet are a major factor. In the disease tabes dorsalis, a late stage of syphilis, ascending spinal tracts conveying this information are destroyed. If the sufferer closes his eyes, he falls over in spite of an intact vestibular system. Racing car drivers are said to drive 'by the seat of their pants'. This is not far from the truth.

Movement control by the cerebral cortex

The cerebral cortex has a fundamental role in the control of voluntary movement, this control being exerted directly by means of the corticospinal and corticobulbar pathways (p. 146) and indirectly by means of inputs to the brainstem pathways. The motor output from the cerebral cortex represents the integration of many different inputs from other cortical regions, from subcortical motor areas such as the basal ganglia and the cerebellum and from ascending inputs from the spinal cord.

There are three main motor areas of the cerebral cortex (Fig. 3.7.3A):

- the motor cortex (also called M1 or area 4 of Brodmann's map), which occupies the precentral gyrus
- the premotor cortex (area 6)
- the supplementary motor area (M2, areas 6 and 8).

Summary

Motor pathways

- Neurones of motor pathways in the CNS are called upper motoneurones.
- Motor areas of the cerebral cortex, central to the generation of movement, form looped pathways with the basal ganglia and cerebellum, which output via descending motor pathways.
- The descending motor pathways, called the pyramidal and extrapyramidal tracts, are alternatively called the lateral and medial systems.
- The origin of the motor pathways is 60% from the motor cortex on the precentral gyrus, the remainder from the premotor cortex, supplementary motor area and postcentral gyrus.

- Of the corticospinal tract, 85% decussates in the medulla.
- Many fibres from the motor cortex terminate directly on α- and γ-motoneurones, directly invoking muscle contraction.
- The lateral corticospinal tract controls skilled voluntary movement.
- Motor tracts originating in the brainstem can be divided into the ventromedial (the vestibulospinal, tectospinal and reticulospinal) and dorsolateral (the rubrobulbar and rubrospinal) tracts.
- Motor control is in part modulated in the brainstem by postural reflexes from the neck and vestibular apparatus and the visual system.

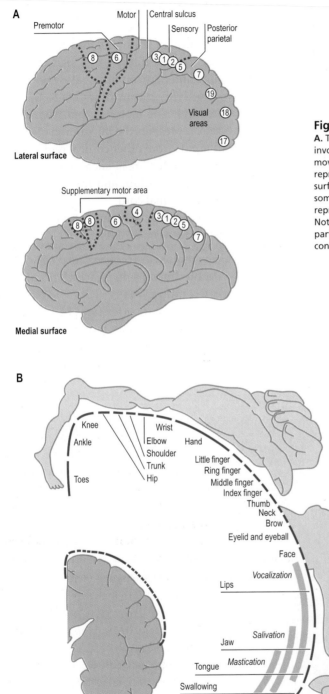

A

Premotor

Motor | Central sulcus

Sensory | Posterior parietal

⑧ ⑥ ③①②⑤ ⑦

⑲

Visual areas ⑱

⑰

Lateral surface

Supplementary motor area

⑧⑧ ⑥ ④ ③①②⑤ ⑦

Medial surface

**Fig. 3.7.3 Movement and the cortex.
A.** The areas of the cerebral cortex involved in the control of voluntary movements, the motor cortex. **B.** The representation of the body areas on the surface of the cortex is in the form of a somatotopic map which can be represented as a 'motor homunculus'. Note that large areas are present for parts of the body capable of fine motor control.

B

Knee | Wrist

Ankle | Elbow Hand

Shoulder | Little finger

Trunk | Ring finger

Toes | Hip | Middle finger

Index finger

Thumb

Neck

Brow

Eyelid and eyeball

Face

Vocalization

Lips

Salivation

Jaw

Tongue *Mastication*

Swallowing

Vertical section

Two other cortical areas which have intimate association with these areas are the **primary somatosensory cortex** (postcentral gyrus, areas 1, 2 and 3) and the **posterior parietal cortex** (areas 5 and 7). These two regions are involved in the processing of sensory information and the posterior parietal cortex is particularly important in the programming of motor plans.

Motor cortex

The motor cortex is the main region of origin of the corticospinal and corticobulbar tracts which make direct, monosynaptic connections with the α- and γ-motoneurones as well as influencing them indirectly by their connections with spinal interneurones. Excitation of the motor cortex therefore evokes muscle contraction directly and alters the strength of the stretch and other spinal reflexes to facilitate the movement. Further, indirect effects are evoked by means of the motor cortical connections with the brainstem pathways, particularly the rubrospinal tract.

The motor cortex is organized **somatotopically** such that electrical stimulation of specific zones of the cortex causes the contraction of muscles in specific regions of the body (Fig. 3.7.3B). The lateral corticospinal tract is especially important for the activation of the distal limb muscles, and the corticobulbar tract for the muscles associated with the face, eyes and vocalization. This is reflected in the large area of representation of the cortex given over to these regions. Lesions of the cortex or of the corticospinal tract therefore remove fine control of the hand muscles, but other pathways from the brainstem can still control the proximal muscles, and some crude control of the hand can be achieved via the rubrospinal tract.

Recordings made from single cells of the motor cortex of primates during learnt, skilled movements show that some of the neurones giving rise to the pyramidal tract start to discharge 20–50 ms before the start of the movement; this time lag corresponds with the calculated conduction delays of a monosynaptic pathway. Different populations of neurones discharge according to the direction of the movement (e.g. flexion or extension), representing the recruitment of agonist or antagonist muscles. The rate of firing of the neurones encodes the force to be generated by the muscles rather than the size of the movement, with some neurones signalling the rate of development of the force whilst others code for the steady-state level.

Single-cell recordings have also demonstrated that the activity of the neurones is dependent on the type of movement being performed. Neurones in the corticobulbar tract are active during a skilled, biting task but are silent when chewing food. Similarly, neurones of the corticospinal tract are activated during precision grip–release manoeuvres by the fingers but not during crude force grips. This illustrates very clearly the role of the pyramidal tracts in the direct control of fine movements and the presence of indirect, parallel pathways via the brainstem so that the CNS can activate the same muscles by different routes according to the task being performed.

The motor cortex receives inputs from sensory receptors in muscle (muscle spindles, tendon organs), joints and skin which are transmitted via the somatosensory cortex or directly via the thalamus. The sensory receptive fields of the cortical neurones are closely related to their field of motor control so that the sensory consequences of the muscle contraction are fed back to the motor cortex.

This pathway may also be the anatomical basis of the **long-latency stretch reflex**. The human stretch reflex comprises two separate components. The classical, monosynaptic, short-latency reflex is elicited by the tendon tap (p. 218). But if a long-lasting, relatively slow stretch is applied there is a longer-latency reflex which precedes any voluntary response to the stretch (Fig. 3.7.4). This long-latency

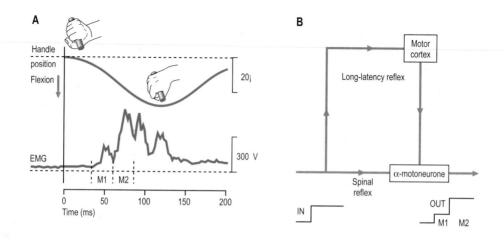

Fig. 3.7.4 Short and long latency responses of a wrist extensor muscle to an imposed flexion. A. The upper trace shows the movement of a handle being held upright by the subject, the downward deflection is the imposed movement which flexes the wrist. The EMG of the extensor muscle is shown on the lower trace; the first element of the response (M1), starting about 30 ms after the onset of the flexion, is a monosynaptic reflex; the second element (M2), starting at about 60 ms, is the long-latency reflex which includes the motor cortex. The last response is voluntary. **B.** The pathways involved in the short- and long-latency responses.

reflex is particularly prominent in the hand muscles (which also have the largest cortical representation). Current evidence suggests that the long-latency reflex is mediated by the motor cortex, at least for the hand muscles, thereby allowing for controlled adjustment of the reflex according to the ongoing activity. Similarly, it appears that the cutaneous inputs can generate reflex activity; for example, during precision gripping of a delicate object between the index finger and the thumb, 'micro-slip' of the object stimulates the cutaneous receptors and leads to reflex tightening of the grip.

Supplementary motor area

In order to produce complex movements, there must be a motor plan that specifies the sequence and extent of the muscle contractions needed to execute the movement itself and to effect the necessary postural adjustments associated with the movement; for example, compensating for a change in the position of the centre of gravity.

The output of the motor cortex activates specific muscles but does not of itself produce complex motor behaviour. This appears to be the role of the supplementary motor area and the premotor cortex (Fig. 3.7.3A).

The supplementary motor area receives inputs from the basal ganglia and the cerebellum (via the ventrolateral nucleus of the thalamus) and from the posterior parietal cortex. It also has outputs going to both the basal ganglia and the cerebellum as well as to the motor cortex and brainstem and a minor component direct to the spinal cord via the corticospinal tract. The input–output loops with the basal ganglia and the cerebellum indicate a role in movement programming.

Electrical stimulation of the supplementary motor area often produces complex, bilateral movements, and measurements of cortical blood flow reveal that the area is active during movements involving extensive coordination, particularly of both hands, but not during simple flexion/extension movements of single joints. Furthermore, the area is active during mental rehearsal of a movement in the absence of any actual movement. Lesions of the supplementary motor area result, for example, in the inability to orient the hand correctly when reaching for a target or to coordinate the hands during bi-manual tasks.

Recordings from single cells show that some neurones become active up to 1 second before the onset of a voluntarily initiated movement, indicating the role in planning and preparation for the movement. Note that this activity occurs significantly earlier in the movement genera-tion than the activity in the motor cortex. There is also evidence that the supplementary motor area is particularly involved in movements that are dependent on **internal cues**, such as proprio-ceptive feedback from the muscle spindles, etc., rather than visually guided movements.

Premotor cortex

The premotor cortex receives its main inputs from the posterior parietal cortex, the cerebellum (via the ventrolateral thalamus) and the supple-mentary motor area. The main outputs project to the motor cortex, the brainstem and the spinal cord via the ventral corticospinal tract.

As with the supplementary motor area, the premotor cortex shows neural activity begin-ning well before movement onset. The pre-motor cortex appears to be involved in postural preparation for the coming movement, as indi-cated by its input to the anterior corticospinal tract. It also has a role in the motor processing of visual information: subjects with a damaged premotor cortex are unable to learn movements dependent on visual information, whereas internally cued movements dependent on inter-nal, proprioceptive information can still be performed.

Posterior parietal cortex

The posterior parietal cortex lies posterior to the somatic sensory cortex (Fig. 3.7.3A). The inputs to the posterior parietal cortex come from the other sensory regions of the cerebral cortex, carrying visual, auditory, cutaneous, proprioceptive, etc., information as well as inputs from the motor areas. This region there-fore appears to be the part of the brain where the sensorimotor information is brought together to generate the conscious map of the body, of the body's position in space and its relationship to other objects in space.

Lesions of the posterior parietal cortex lead to varied symptoms such as the inability to direct attention to sensory stimuli or the condi-tion of hemi-neglect where the patient ignores, and even denies the existence of, one side of the body. Whilst appearing very different, both these symptoms reflect a defect in the normal ability of the brain to create a correct represen-tation of the body and of its relationship with the outside world. In terms of motor function, damage to the posterior parietal cortex does not actually prevent movement but leads to failure of movement planning because of the inability to relate the position of objects in space to that of the body.

Basal ganglia

The basal ganglia have become infamous as the origin of the motor disorders that characterize **Parkinson's disease**, but because they have no direct motor outputs to the spinal cord, their role in movement control has been hard to study and much of it has been inferred from observations of basal ganglia disorders.

The basal ganglia are a group of nuclei lying deep in each cerebral hemisphere and com-prising the **caudate nucleus** and the **putamen** (which together are termed the **neostriatum**), the **globus pallidus**, the **substantia nigra** and the **subthalamic nucleus** (Fig. 3.7.5). The main input to the basal ganglia comes from the cerebral cortex (particularly the supplementary motor area, p. 225) which projects to the neo-striatum. Within the ganglia there are several loops of connections and the main output is via the thalamus back to the supplementary

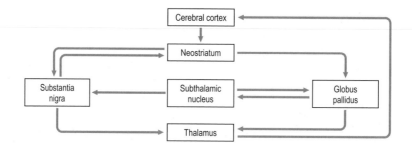

Fig. 3.7.5 The major connections of the basal ganglia. The main flow of information is in a loop from the cerebral cortex (mainly the supplementary motor area) through the ganglia to the thalamus and then back to the cortex. Within the ganglia there are loops processing the information.

motor area of the cerebral cortex. This organization in terms of sets of loops within the main loop from and to the cerebral cortex indicates a role in information processing and programming. Associated with this, many neurones in the basal ganglia are active several hundred milliseconds prior to the onset of the movement.

Disorders affecting the basal ganglia are characterized by either an excess of movement (hyperkinesia) as in **Huntington's chorea** or a slowness (bradykinesia) or lack (akinesia) of movement as occurs in Parkinson's disease. Parkinson's disease is caused by degeneration of the dopaminergic neurones in the substantia nigra that project to the neostriatum. The net effect is a reduced excitatory output from the thalamus back to the cerebral cortex. Affected patients show characteristic symptoms of tremor at rest, rigidity and bradykinesia (see Clinical Example: Parkinson's disease).

Patients with **parkinsonism** show reduced levels of activity in the supplementary motor area before movement, which is associated with reduced and more slowly-developing muscle contractions, though the muscle sequencing is still correct. As a result, movements are slowed in execution and delayed in onset. Complex motor sequences progressively deteriorate

during execution until they may fail completely. On the basis of this it is proposed that the basal ganglia are involved in processing internal, proprioceptive information (cf. the supplementary motor area, see p. 225) as the basis for setting the amplitude and timing of the next movement. Movements performed using visual cues are significantly less affected than those using internal cues; for example, the patient who has great difficulty in walking can do so much more easily if lines are drawn on the floor where the feet are to be placed.

Huntington's chorea shows the opposite symptoms in that patients display uncontrolled movements of the limbs. This disorder is associated with degeneration of neurones within the striatum and results in excess excitation of the thalamocortical pathway.

The cerebellum

The cerebellum has three main functions:

- regulation of ongoing movements
- programming of motor sequences
- regulation of vestibular reflexes.

Implicit within these functions is the importance of motor learning, which is carried out by the cerebellum.

Clinical Example

Parkinson's disease

Parkinson's disease (paralysis agitans) is one of the best known of the diseases affecting motor function. It is a neurodegenerative disorder with highly characteristic symptoms which were first documented by James Parkinson in 1817 as 'involuntary tremulous motion, with lessened muscular power in parts not in action and even when supported with a propensity to bend the trunk forwards, and to pass from a walking to a running pace: the sense and intellects being uninjured'. With the exception of the last phrase, this description remains largely accurate.

The most common form of Parkinson's disease, which affects about 1 in 1000 of the population, is idiopathic (that is, it arises spontaneously and without apparent cause) and usually appears after the age of 50. Parkinson's disease is characterized by pronounced tremor at rest and rigidity of the muscles, both of which are positive signs, and by bradykinesia (slowness of movement, particularly in its initiation), which is a negative sign.

In the 1950s it was found that dopamine constitutes almost 50% of the catecholamine in the brain and that 80% of it is located within the basal ganglia. Post-mortem studies of the brains of people who had suffered parkinsonism revealed that there was a substantial reduction in the levels of dopamine. Subsequent studies revealed the characteristic loss of the dopaminergic neurones from the substantia nigra (other regions are also affected, including the nucleus coeruleus) which project onto the striatum of the basal ganglia (the nigrostriatal pathway). It is proposed that the loss of this inhibitory input to the striatum results in excessive inhibitory output from the basal ganglia to the thalamus, affecting the motor functions.

Current treatment centres around the administration of L-dopa (3,4-dihydroxy-phenylalanine, or its analogues) which is an amino acid precursor of dopamine and which can cross the blood–brain barrier. This treatment serves to reduce the symptoms of Parkinson's disease but does not affect its progression. Recently, studies have been carried out into the effect of implanting fetal cells into the basal ganglia. These fetal cells appear, in some cases, to be maintained and to be capable of synthesizing dopamine, though the initial promise of such studies remains unfulfilled. Another approach to the investigation of the disease has come to light as a result of the discovery of the action of the substance MPTP, which can be a contaminant of heroin. This has enabled the development of models of parkinsonism and thereby greatly enhanced our ability to investigate the disease.

Disorders of the motor system, due to experimental or accidental lesion or due to disease, have played and continue to play a key role in our understanding of the functions and integration of the different structures and pathways within the nervous system.

Cellular organization of the cerebellum

The cerebellar surface is deeply infolded, giving a substantial surface area for the cerebellar cortex. The cortex surrounds a white matter core in which are embedded the deep cerebellar nuclei. The cortex contains five different cell types: the **Golgi**, **basket** and **stellate cells**, which are all inhibitory interneurones; the **granule cells**, which are excitatory and the **Purkinje cells** which are the output cells (Fig. 3.7.6).

Afferent fibres to the cerebellar cortex come via the brainstem and make excitatory connections with the deep cerebellar nuclei before entering the cortex itself. There are two types of afferent fibre called **mossy fibres** and **climbing fibres**. The mossy fibres are the axons of neurones within the brainstem, which receive inputs from a wide range of sources, including ascending sensory pathways from the spinal cord and descending motor pathways. The climbing fibres all originate from the inferior olivary nucleus in the medulla, which, in turn, receives inputs from the red nucleus, cerebral cortex and spinal cord.

Each climbing fibre synapses directly with up to 10 Purkinje cells, making numerous connections with the soma and dendritic tree. Each Purkinje cell, though, only receives an input from one climbing fibre. By contrast, the mossy fibre input shows extensive divergence. Each mossy fibre synapses with many granule cells. The granule cells give rise to axons which intersect with the dendritic trees of the Purkinje cells. The dendritic trees are very extensive, lying in a flat plane perpendicular to the course of the parallel fibres; thus each Purkinje cell receives inputs from about 200 000 parallel fibres and each fibre in turn synapses with several thousand Purkinje cells. The connections made by the inhibitory interneurones have the effect of focusing this Purkinje cell excitation both temporally and spatially (Fig. 3.7.6), the latter being related to the body maps projected onto the cerebellar cortex.

The granule cells fire at relatively high rates (up to 100 impulses/s) in response to the mossy fibre input, this discharge being directly related to ongoing motor activity and/or sensory stimulation. In response to this input the Purkinje cells discharge at a lower rate. The climbing fibres discharge at much lower rates (<1 impulse/s) but each action potential causes the Purkinje cell to fire a '**complex spike**'. These complex spikes significantly alter the response of the Purkinje cells to the ongoing parallel fibre input and are believed to form the basis of the learning mechanism in the cerebellar cortex.

The discharge from the Purkinje cells represents the only output from the cerebellar cortex and is inhibitory in effect. The axons of the Purkinje cells mainly project onto the deep cerebellar nuclei, though some project directly onto the vestibular nuclei in the medulla. The effect of this inhibition is to modulate the activity of the nuclei that is generated by the excitatory inputs from the mossy and climbing fibres.

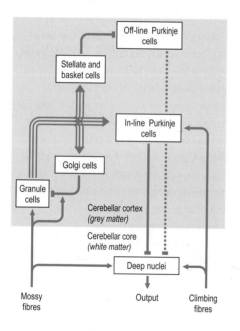

Fig. 3.7.6 The cellular organization of the cerebellum.
The mossy and climbing fibres make excitatory contacts with the deep nuclei. The climbing fibres then excite the Purkinje cells directly while the mossy fibres excite them indirectly via the parallel fibres of the granule cells. The branches of the parallel fibres excite the stellate and basket cells which inhibit 'off-line' Purkinje cells on either side of the active Purkinje cells. This produces a clear distinction between the excited and inactive groups of neurones, sharpening the somatotopic map of the body on the cerebellar surface. The Purkinje cell axons pass to deep nuclei and inhibit their activity. The feedback from Golgi cells focuses the activity in line by inhibiting the granule cells.

Cerebellar functions

The cerebellum can be divided into three functional regions: the **vestibulocerebellum** (archicerebellum), the **spinocerebellum** (palaeocerebellum) and the **cerebrocerebellum** (neocerebellum) (Fig. 3.7.7).

Vestibulocerebellum

The main input–output connections of the vestibulocerebellum are with the vestibular nuclei of the medulla, and it is chiefly involved in the regulation of balance, via the vestibulospinal tract to the motoneurone pools of the axial muscles, and the control of eye movements.

Lesions of the vestibulocerebellum lead to disturbances of balance with the patient displaying **ataxia**: the gait is unsteady, characterized by rolling, with the feet widespread, the so-called 'drunken sailor' gait. Eye movements are also disturbed, often with a maintained, coarse **nystagmus** (pronounced oscillation of the eyes).

Lesions of the vestibulocerebellum also clearly illustrate the role of the cerebellum in learning. Normally the vestibulo-ocular reflex (p. 243) results in the eyes moving in the opposite direction to rotation of the head. If prisms are worn so as to reverse the visual field, a normal subject learns to reverse the vestibulo-ocular reflex to compensate. Patients with vestibulocerebellar lesions, however, are unable to adapt to the new input and the original reflex is maintained, even though it is now inappropriate.

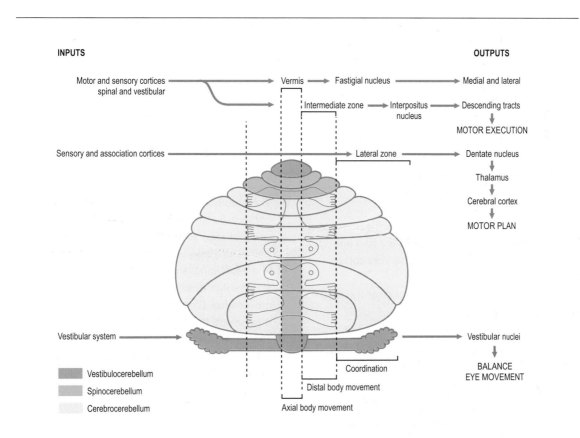

Fig. 3.7.7 **The anatomical localization of the main functions of the cerebellum** (shown with the lobes unfolded, somewhat in the fashion of a hedgehog uncurled).

Spinocerebellum

The spinocerebellum receives a wide range of sensory input from the spinal cord as well as from the motor areas of the cerebral cortex. The functional role is twofold, to regulate the execution of ongoing movements and to control muscle tone.

The regulation of movements is probably achieved by comparison of the descending motor commands with the ascending sensory feedback which signals the results of the ongoing movement. The spinocerebellar output to the motor cortex and particularly to the medial and lateral brainstem motor pathways enables correction for deviations from the required movement. This control is manifest in the regulation of the sequence of agonist/antagonist muscle activation during movements. A characteristic feature of lesions of the spinocerebellum is 'past-pointing'. During ballistic movements such as pointing at different targets, the sequence of muscle contractions is disturbed so that the pointing movements become irregular and frequently overshoot the target. Such disturbed coordination and inaccuracy of movement is termed **dysmetria**. Patients with spinocerebellar lesions also show pronounced tremor at the end of movements and a general decrease in muscle tone.

Cerebrocerebellum

The cerebrocerebellum has major reciprocal connections with the cerebral cortex, particularly the premotor cortex (p. 233) and is involved in the planning and initiation of movement. Lesions within this region lead to delays in the initiation of movement, particularly those dependent on visual cues, and a profound disturbance of the coordination and sequence of muscle contractions. There may also be dysmetria and slowing and slurring of speech (**dysphonia**). Note that, unlike the majority of the motor areas, the cerebellar input–output operations remain **ipsilateral** and therefore a unilateral lesion will result in an ipsilateral deficit.

⚹ Summary

The motor cortex

- The motor cortex is divided into the premotor cortex and supplementary motor area and associated with the primary sensory cortex and posterior parietal cortex.
- The motor cortex evokes muscle contraction directly and alters the strength of spinal reflexes.
- The motor cortex is organized somatopically into a 'homunculus'.
- The motor cortex receives inputs from receptors in muscles, joints and skin via the somatosensory cortex or directly from the thalamus.

- The supplementary motor area and premotor cortex are activated up to 1 second before the complex manual activity in which they are particularly involved begins.
- The basal ganglia process proprioceptive information to set amplitude and timing of movements. Disorders lead to Parkinson's disease and Huntington's chorea.
- The cerebellum regulates ongoing movement, programmes motor sequences and regulates vestibular reflexes as a result of prior motor learning.

Clinical Example

Epilepsy

An epileptic seizure is a convulsion or altered state caused by paroxysmal discharges from cerebral neurones usually seen on electroencephalogram (EEG) recordings as a mixture of transient spikes or sharp waves with slow frequencies. Epilepsy is the name for the disease state where there is a continuing probability that seizures will occur.

Epilepsy is a common clinical condition that can have its onset at any age. Up to 3% of the population suffer two or more seizures during their lives.

During an epileptic seizure large numbers of neurones are activated, there is a loss of the inhibitory connections between the cortical neurones and high degrees of synchronization of cortical activity result in the formation of EEG spikes. This gives the characteristic high-voltage spike and wave pattern seen on the EEG in epilepsy.

When this abnormal electrical activity is isolated to one part of the cortex the resulting seizure is manifest as a specific pattern of symptoms and signs. These seizures are called *focal* or *partial seizures*. Generally the patient is conscious during a partial seizure.

If the abnormal discharge spreads to both hemispheres, the resulting seizure is classified as a *partial seizure with secondary generalization*.

Seizures involving loss of consciousness or amnesia are termed *generalized seizures* and these in turn can be subdivided into *tonic–clonic (grand mal)* or *absence (petit mal) seizures*.

All types of epilepsy have similar characteristics. They all involve transient changes in consciousness, movement, behaviour or perception. They also all have characteristic changes in the EEG which occur during seizures.

Humans have a seizure threshold which is defined as the point above which seizure activity occurs and this varies from person to person. Seizures may be triggered by light, sound or chemicals. In rarer cases seizure activity is triggered by psychological factors such as fear or anxiety; these are by definition psychogenic seizures.

Types of epilepsy

Generalized seizures (consciousness is impaired)

Tonic–clonic seizures (grand mal). There is often a prodromal phase (nausea, headache, etc.) followed by a tonic phase. During the tonic phase the body becomes rigid, the tongue may be bitten, and the patient may fall to the ground, call out, and be incontinent of urine or faeces. There is also loss of consciousness. The tonic phase may last for a minute or more.

The clonic phase follows immediately and is the convulsive phase of the seizure. The muscles of the body contract rhythmically, lasting from several seconds to minutes. Following the clonic phase the patient enters the postictal period, which may last several hours; during this phase the patient may be drowsy, disoriented or even in a comatose state.

Absence seizures (petit mal). This type of seizure occurs almost exclusively in children; only 10% of sufferers experience this type of seizure in adulthood. By definition absence seizures are accompanied by 3 Hz spike and wave patterns on the EEG.

Most attacks last less than a minute; typically the child will become very still, pale and will stare. This may be followed by a few jerks, lip-smacking or blinking and the child will usually be unaware that the seizure has occurred.

Clinical Example *(Continued)*

Partial seizures

Focal seizures (consciousness generally unimpaired). Focal seizures are typically the result of discharge from a focal group of neurones. The clinical features of the ensuing seizure usually give an indication of the anatomical site of the epileptic discharge.

Focal seizures can be motor, sensory or autonomic. Motor seizures (or jacksonian seizures) often begin at one point and spread. For example, a motor seizure may begin as twitching in the muscles of the thumb. Then, as the seizure progresses, the twitching spreads to the arm and eventually will involve the whole of the contralateral side of the body from the epileptic focus in the brain. This spread of epileptic activity is called the march of the seizure and can be recorded on the surface of the cortex.

Focal seizures may also be sensory, affecting perceptions such as vision, hearing, taste, balance and smell.

Complex partial seizures (consciousness generally impaired). Complex partial seizures are usually focused in the temporal or frontal lobes of the brain. In temporal lobe epilepsy there is often a prodromal sense of fear associated with gastrointestinal disturbance. There are often bizarre olfactory experiences and short-lived hallucinatory experiences are common. This form of epilepsy is also often accompanied by feelings of unreality or detachment.

Precipitating factors in epilepsy

Genetic predisposition. Family history is very important when diagnosing epilepsy. Approximately one-third of patients with epilepsy have a first-degree relative with a history of seizures.

Birth injury. Brain injury at birth, particularly that associated with haemorrhage, is associated with epilepsy. Extreme prematurity and anoxia at birth can also result in subsequent epilepsy. Pyrexia in children under 5 years often causes generalized seizures (febrile convulsion) but these do not tend to lead to epilepsy in later life. Children and adults with learning disabilities have much higher rates of epilepsy, which may in part be related to birth trauma.

Head injury. Trauma to the head is often associated with epilepsy. It may be an early complication of the injury or may develop many years later.

Intracranial disease. Mass lesions and infarcts can both act as epileptic foci, leading to either partial or secondary generalized seizures. The onset of seizures in an adult should be thoroughly investigated because in almost 3% of cases of adult-onset epilepsy an occult mass lesion will be discovered.

In encephalitis and meningitis, seizures are often the first indication of the underlying disease process.

Drugs and alcohol. Some antipsychotic, antidepressant and stimulant (e.g. amphetamine and caffeine) drugs can provoke seizures and are thought to lower the seizure threshold. Anticonvulsant drugs and benzodiazepines increase the seizure threshold; however, rapid withdrawal of these drugs can result in rebound epileptic activity.

Chronic alcohol abuse is a common cause of epileptic seizures, which commonly occur during withdrawal from alcohol.

Seizures also occur in cases of drug toxicity following overdose, e.g. lithium carbonate has a narrow therapeutic range and can cause seizures in overdose.

Clinical Example *(Continued)*

Degenerative brain disease. Epilepsy can occur in most types of dementing illness but is common in both Alzheimer's disease and multi-infarct dementia. Epilepsy is also common in demyelinating diseases such a multiple sclerosis.

Metabolic imbalance. Epilepsy can be a feature of the following metabolic abnormalities:

- uraemia
- liver failure
- hypokalaemia
- hyponatraemia
- hypoglycaemia
- hypocalcaemia
- hypoxia.

Diagnosis

Diagnosis is usually established by informant history of the seizure, clinical examination and EEG. CT scanning is routine in adult-onset epilepsy.

Treatment

Anticonvulsant medication is indicated in repeated seizures. Different drugs are prescribed for the different seizure types.

Status epilepticus

Status epilepticus is the situation where there is either an extended seizure or several seizures follow each other without recovery of consciousness. This is a medical emergency with a mortality of about 15%. Treatment is usually in the form of immediate administration of rectal diazepam solution or as bolus i.v. diazepam followed by i.v. infusion of diazepam.

Prognosis

Following diagnosis of epilepsy up to 40% of patients will remain fit-free for 5 years. Poorer prognosis is associated with combinations of generalized seizures with other seizure types.

The production of a voluntary movement

We can now bring together the major elements of the motor system that have been described to form an overview of their interactions during the planning and execution of a voluntary movement. For the sake of making it comprehensible, much of the detail will be omitted.

Figure 3.7.8 shows a diagram of the main components of the motor system. The voluntary movement begins with an idea in the association areas of the cerebral cortex. This idea embodies the objective of the movement, e.g. 'I want to pick up that pencil.' For this action to be performed, the brain must first evaluate the sensory information, particularly the visual information about the position of the pencil in relation to the body and the proprioceptive feedback regarding the present position of the limbs and the body. This main visual processing is carried out in the posterior parietal cortex, while the proprioceptive information is relayed to the spinocerebellum and via the thalamus to the somatosensory and motor areas of the cerebral cortex and to the posterior parietal cortex.

The posterior parietal cortex communicates with the supplementary motor area and the premotor cortex where movement planning takes place. About 1 second before the onset of the movement the supplementary motor area becomes active and, via the basal ganglia loop,

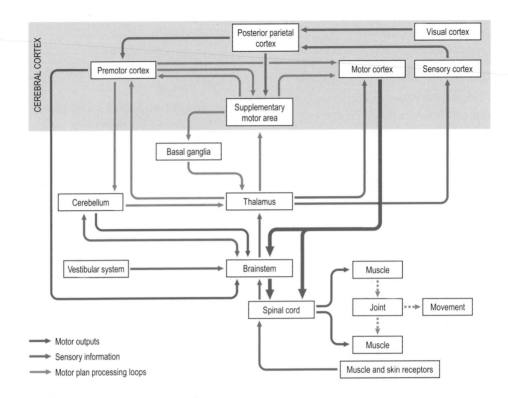

Fig. 3.7.8 Summary of the motor system. The major pathways of the system are shown, including the descending motor output pathways, the ascending sensory pathways and the looped pathways.

the internal cues for the movement initiation and sequence are established along with the amplitude setting for the components of the movement. The coordination of bilateral operations is also set up. At the same time, the premotor cortex–cerebrocerebellum loop becomes active for the development of the coordination and timing of agonist/antagonist muscle activities based on interpretation of the visual information.

The supplementary motor area and the premotor cortex output their command sequences to the motor cortex. The premotor cortex, via the anterior corticospinal tract and connections to the brainstem ventromedial pathways, initiates the postural adjustments required to enable the reaching process. The motor cortex, via the lateral corticospinal and, indirectly, the

corticorubrospinal tracts, sets in train the activation of the prime mover muscles, the muscles that will actually generate the reach–grasp movement. This process of activation both directly excites the appropriate α-motoneurones and, via the γ-motoneurones and spinal interneurones, alters the sensitivities of the spinal reflexes to optimize the movement performance.

During the course of the movement, there is continuous proprioceptive feedback from the muscles and joints, which leads to adjustment of the ongoing movement via the spinal reflex arcs, which directly modulate α-motoneurone activity via the spinocerebellum (which alters the outputs of the brainstem pathways) and via the motor cortex itself. There is also visual feedback, which alters the motor output at the cortical and cerebellar levels.

The process of ongoing supplementary motor area and premotor cortical activity and output of motor commands, modulated at the different levels by the sensory feedback, continues throughout the execution of the movement.

The existence of a coherent plan has been demonstrated by the use of magnetic stimulation of the motor cortex during the preparation for a timed motor task. The effect of a single pulse of stimulation is to delay the onset of the movement without altering the sequence or amplitude of muscle activations. The plan is therefore prepared and stored and executed in sequence, so delaying the onset does not affect the motor output.

 Summary

Voluntary movement

- The idea of movement begins in the association areas.
- Sensory, particularly visual, information relating to the postulated movement is analysed in the posterior parietal cortex.
- The posterior parietal cortex activates the supplementary motor area and premotor cortex to plan the movement about 1 s before muscle contraction begins.
- At the same time, the basal ganglia loop and the cerebrocerebellum loop are inputting amplitude settings and coordination respectively to the plan.
- The supplementary motor area and premotor cortex then command the motor cortex, while at the same time the premotor cortex initiates the postural adjustments required.
- The motor cortex via the lateral corticospinal and corticorubrospinal tracts activate α- and γ-motoneurones to bring about movement directly and by altering spinal reflexes.

Control of eye movements

The eyes are moved by three pairs of antagonistic muscles innervated by the oculomotor (III), trochlear (IV) and abducens (VI) cranial nerves. The motoneurones of these nerves have their cell bodies in the brainstem and are interconnected via neurones of the medial longitudinal fasciculus. There are two direct inputs to the motor nuclei of the eye muscles: from the vestibular nuclei and from the gaze centres. There are two gaze centres, one located in the pons (the horizontal gaze centre) and one in the midbrain (the vertical gaze centre). There are also several indirect inputs from the superior colliculus and the frontal and occipital lobes of the cerebral cortex.

Eye movements are predominantly associated with rotation of the eyeball to fix a target on the fovea and then to maintain that fixation despite movements of the target or of the head. **Saccades** are the rapid, ballistic movements that flick the eye from one target to another. The motoneurones can discharge at very high rates (up to 600 impulses/s) for brief periods, giving a very rapid onset of contraction. Because the eyeball has very low inertia (compared with moving a skeletal joint) and the vitreous humor acts to critically damp its movement, a fast contraction can accelerate it to high velocity very quickly, but this movement can be precisely controlled. Rapid execution of the movement is important in minimizing blurring of vision while the movement is in progress.

Once the target is fixed on the fovea, it is maintained there by two types of eye movement. Movement of the target elicits a **smooth pursuit** response; as the target moves off the fixation point on the fovea, the eyeball is rotated to restore and then maintain fixation. Conversely, if the target is stationary and the head is rotated, the eyes will be rotated in the skull in the opposite direction but at the same speed as the head is moving so that the target remains fixed on the fovea. This **vestibulo-ocular reflex** is mediated by the sensory input from the semicircular canals of the vestibular system (p. 332).

243

When the target is moving relatively slowly, smooth pursuit movements enable tracking of the target within the range of rotation of the eyes. For larger angles of rotation, the movement of the eyes may be combined with rotation of the head and, if necessary, of the whole body to maintain tracking; the eye–body movements being mediated by the tectospinal tract (p. 227). If a large target is moving rapidly or if the tracking angle is limited, then the form of the movements changes. Initially the eye will track an object by smooth pursuit until approaching the limit of rotation; at this point a saccade is performed in the opposite direction, a new target point is fixated and another pursuit movement is performed. The alternation between smooth pursuits and reverse saccades is termed **optokinetic** movements. Such movements can easily be observed, for example, in someone watching out of the window of a fast moving train.

During steady fixation on a target, the eyes do not actually remain stationary but make continuous, involuntary small movements which take the form of slow drifts of less than 1 degree followed by microsaccades. These movements are so small that one is not aware of them but they are essential for continuous vision, since images that are perfectly stabilized on the retina, such as those due to the retinal blood vessels, become invisible. As an extension of the drift–microsaccade pattern of movement, when one is fixating on a target such as a face, the eyes are again continuously moving but the movement takes the form of scanning, with concentration on the key features such as the eyes, nose and mouth (see Ch. 4.1).

Summary

Eye movements

- Three pairs of antagonistic muscles are innervated by motoneurones with cell bodies in the brainstem.
- The motor nuclei of eye muscles receive inputs directly from the vestibular nuclei and the vertical and horizontal gaze centres.
- The vestibulo-ocular reflex keeps the eyes fixed on a stationary target when the head is rotated.

Sensory mechanisms

Introduction

Sensory information is essential to our ability to respond to the external environment or to the internal state of the body. For the most part, external sensation is experienced consciously, as well as being used at subconscious levels. Much of the sensory information regarding the internal state of the body, however, does not reach the level of conscious awareness.

There are two main divisions of the nervous system concerned with sensation:

- The general sensory system. This includes:
  - somatic sensation – the mechanical, chemical and thermal stimulation of the body and the face
  - visceral sensation relating to the internal organs.
- The special senses. These include vision, hearing, taste and smell and balance, which is mediated by the vestibular system.

The sensory systems contain a wide variety of receptors which respond to these different stimuli by means of a change in membrane potential, a process which is called **transduction**. Detection of an appropriate stimulus is then signalled by action potentials in the afferent axons.

The stimulus

The stimulus has features which are important for its interpretation by the sensory system: modality, quality, intensity, duration and location.

The modality of the stimulus refers to its general nature. Thus, the classical five senses of sight, hearing, touch, taste and smell are each sensory modalities, as are other, less obvious sensations such as temperature and internal senses such as thirst, breathlessness and so on. Each modality can usually be divided into submodalities or qualities. For example, the qualities of taste are sweet, sour, salty or bitter (Fig. 3.8.1) and the qualities of vision are the colours red, green and blue.

Detection of a specific modality of sensation depends on the interaction between the stimulus and a specific type of receptor. Under normal circumstances each type of receptor is sensitive to a specific stimulus. Thus, the receptors in the retina of the eye are sensitive to light, whilst the hair cells of the cochlea are sensitive to sound waves. The stimulus to which a receptor is specifically sensitive is termed the **adequate stimulus**.

Transduction

The arrival of an appropriate stimulus at a receptor is signalled in terms of a change in the **receptor potential**. This receptor potential is then encoded as a train of action potentials depending on its intensity and duration. The processes involved in the development of the receptor potential in response to a stimulus are referred to as sensory transduction.

In most receptors, transduction involves the opening of cation-selective channels and depolarization of the receptor membrane. The simplest such process occurs in mechanoreceptors, where stretching of the membrane leads to opening of stretch-activated channels (Fig. 3.8.2). Chemoreceptors are dependent on receptor–ligand binding, when a molecule of the chemical stimulant binds with the receptor in the cell membrane. This may lead to channel opening directly or indirectly via a second messenger system. The mechanism in a photoreceptor is the opposite of these two mechanisms in that the channels are open in the dark. Arrival of a photon of light leads, via a second messenger system (p. 65), to channel closure and effective hyperpolarization of the receptor cell.

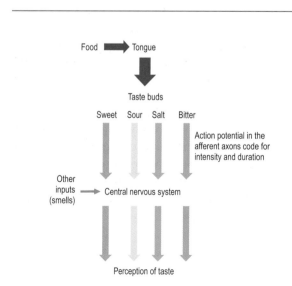

Fig. 3.8.1 The modality of taste. The stimulus (flavoured solutions) stimulates receptors on the tongue. Different receptors respond selectively to sweetness, sourness, salt and bitterness. The receptor discharge signals the intensity and duration of the stimulus as a train of action potentials.
Within the CNS these signals are integrated with other sensory information, olfactory and tactile (from the buccal cavity) to produce the perception of food.

In all receptor systems the final stage of the transduction process, the generation of an action potential, takes place in the peripheral terminals of the primary afferent axon itself.

In some receptors the depolarizing receptor potential is produced in the terminal of the primary afferent fibre and acts to move its membrane potential towards the threshold for action potential generation (Fig. 3.8.3) and action potentials are initiated, usually at the first node of Ranvier.

In other systems a mechanical transduction takes place before this final stage. Then the receptor consists of two elements, the primary afferent fibre and cells of non-neural origin such as the Merkel disks in the skin or hair cells in the cochlea. The receptor potential is produced in these sensory receptors, and their depolarization leads to release of an excitatory neurotransmitter which, in turn, depolarizes the terminals of the primary afferent axon. This latter depolarization, referred to as a **generator potential**, is then encoded as a train of action potentials within the neurone.

Adaptation

An important property of all sensory receptors is that their receptor potential progressively decreases in amplitude in response to a sustained stimulus – adaptation. Receptors vary in their rates of adaptation and therefore signal different temporal features of the stimulus. Some, such as the Pacinian corpuscle, which is a subcutaneous receptor, adapt very rapidly, responding with a brief burst of impulses at the start and end of a maintained stimulus (see Fig. 3.8.4). The duration of the stimulus is therefore signalled by 'on' and 'off' responses. Such receptors are particularly sensitive to the rate of change of the stimulus and also capable of responding to high-frequency stimulation, such as vibration, with a single impulse to each stimulus.

Slowing adapting receptors, such as the Merkel receptor or the muscle spindle will maintain a discharge throughout the duration of the stimulus but the rate of discharge decreases (often exponentially) as the stimulus persists. The rate of discharge is dependent predominantly on the intensity of the stimulus rather than its rate of change.

The mechanism of adaptation may be due to changes in the excitability of the receptor membrane, such as time-dependent inactivation of cation-selective channels or activation of K^+ channels, often as a result of increasing internal Ca^{2+} concentrations. Adaptation may also depend

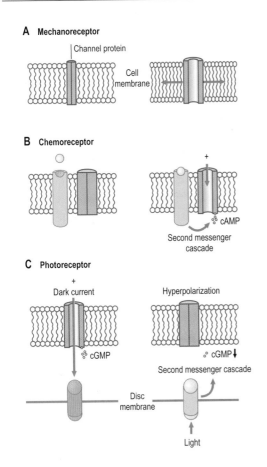

Fig. 3.8.2 Receptor transduction mechanisms. A. Stretching of a membrane opens an ion channel directly. **B.** An agonist acting on a chemoreceptor may open a channel directly or produce a second messenger that then interacts with an ion channel to open it. **C.** In the case of the photoreceptors of the rods and cones of the eye, photons reduce the concentration of cGMP at membrane channels. This allows the channel to close. The 'dark current' is thus switched off hyperpolarizing the membrane (see p. 39).

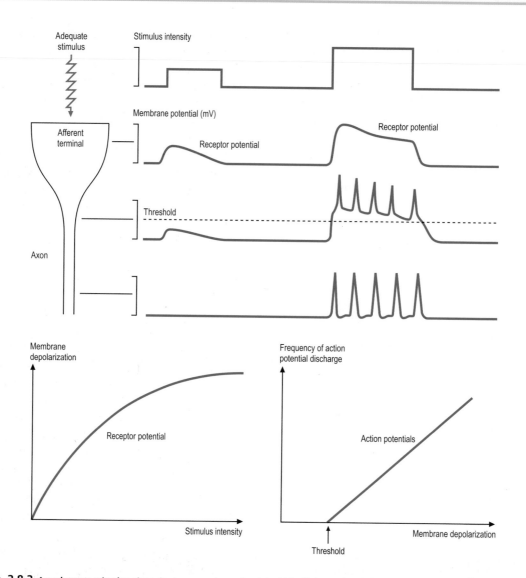

Fig. 3.8.3 An adequate stimulus gives rise to a receptor potential which, if above threshold, excites action potentials in the axon. The receptor potential increases with the intensity of the stimulus but saturates at high intensities. The rate of action potential discharge is related to the extent to which the receptor potential exceeds the threshold.

on the properties of the non-neural structures associated with the receptor, particularly for mechanoreceptors. In the Pacinian corpuscle the nerve ending is surrounded by concentric layers of connective tissue like the skin of an onion. When the corpuscle is mechanically deformed, the deformation is transferred to the sensory ending via the layers of the capsule. These layers, however, slide relative to each other so that the maintained deformation of the outermost layer is no longer reflected by deformation of the inner layers and so the ending stops discharging; the receptor is rapidly adapting. If the capsule is removed and the stimulus is applied directly to the nerve terminal, the response becomes that of a slowly adapting receptor.

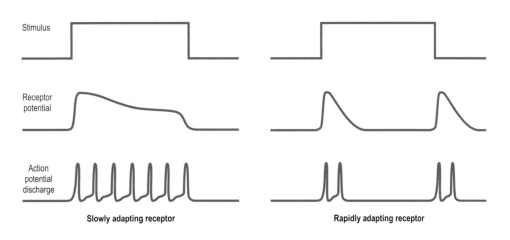

Slowly adapting receptor   Rapidly adapting receptor

Fig. 3.8.4 **Receptors adapt to stimuli.** They do this at different rates. In the case of a slowly adapting receptor the response to a continuous stimulus is maintained but declines. In the case of rapidly adapting receptors (e.g. Pacinian corpuscles) the response is limited to an off and on signal.

Receptor specificity

Note that a receptor may also respond to other stimuli if they are strong enough. For example, a blow to the eye can make one 'see stars'; the mechanical stimulus has evoked a response from the retina but this is still interpreted by the brain as a visual signal because of the labelled line by which the signal reaches the brain.

Information coding

The intensity of the stimulus is a measure of its strength or amount. For most stimuli there is a minimum intensity below which there is no change in action potential discharge in the afferent axon. This minimum intensity that elicits a response in the afferent axon is called the **threshold**. Smaller stimuli may evoke a change in membrane potential of the receptor itself but this will be insufficient to generate action potentials. Increasing stimulus intensities, above threshold, leads to increases in the frequency of action potential discharge, the relationship often being exponential (Fig. 3.8.3). This sensory threshold, which generates action

potentials in a sensory nerve, should not be confused with the membrane threshold of a neurone, which is the membrane potential at which an action potential is triggered (p. 44).

A stimulus that is above threshold for a single receptor may not, however, give rise to sensory perception. The attention of the CNS has to be 'caught'. Perception of a stimulus may only occur when the action potential discharge is above a certain frequency so that there is temporal summation of the synaptic input to the second neurone in the afferent pathway, or when more than one afferent is discharging and these afferents converge onto the second neurone giving spatial summation.

The duration of the stimulus may be encoded by a similar duration of increased discharge in the case of slowly adapting receptors. Rapidly adapting receptors, conversely, do not respond to maintained stimuli but give a burst of impulses at the onset of the stimulus; the end of the stimulus may also be marked by an 'off' burst of impulses (Fig. 3.8.4). However, the responses of even the slowly adapting receptors are not constant for a maintained stimulus; even they show a steady decline or adaptation to the stimulus (although this decline may be very slow; Fig. 3.8.4). The perceived intensity of a constant, maintained stimulus, similarly has a steady decline.

Central processing of information

Each receptor responds to a specific stimulus and the afferent nerve fibre makes specific connections within the nervous system. This specificity of wiring, referred to as a labelled line, is the basis for the ability of the nervous system to interpret a train of action potentials in one axon, for example, as signalling a change in temperature whilst a similar pattern of firing in another axon indicates touch.

Receptive fields

The location of a stimulus is signalled by the activation of a particular receptor or group of receptors. Which receptors are activated is determined by the receptive fields and the area of the stimulus.

The receptive field of a sensory neurone is the area over which stimulation causes the neurone to discharge. For a cutaneous receptor, the receptive field of the peripheral afferent neurone is a region of skin, whereas for a cone receptor in the eye, the field would be the degrees of arc of the visual field over which light fell on the receptor.

Receptive fields vary markedly in size: human fingertips have about 2300 receptors per square centimetre, which are innervated by 300 afferent axons with each afferent axon innervating up to 20 individual receptors and each receptor being innervated by up to three axons. Thus, even though the receptive field of each afferent axon is very small, there is also considerable overlap of the fields. Moving up the arm, the receptive fields on the forearm are significantly larger, and on the trunk of the body the receptive fields are about 100 times larger than those on the fingertips. Peripheral receptive field size is one of the major factors determining the ability to localize stimuli accurately.

The afferent neurones connect with sensory neurones in the CNS, each of which also has a receptive field. Because there is considerable convergence and divergence of the sensory information at each relay point in the sensory pathways, the receptive fields of the central sensory neurones are often larger than those of the peripheral afferents (Fig. 3.8.5) and there is still a significant overlap between receptive

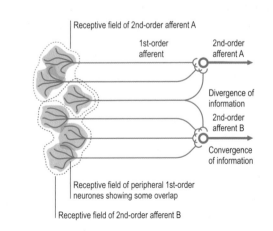

Receptive field of 2nd-order afferent A

1st-order afferent

2nd-order afferent A

Divergence of information

2nd-order afferent B

Convergence of information

Receptive field of peripheral 1st-order neurones showing some overlap

Receptive field of 2nd-order afferent B

Fig. 3.8.5 Receptive field organization. The receptive fields of individual peripheral afferent neurones frequently show a degree of overlap. Where these afferents synapse onto the second-order neurones there is both convergence and divergence of activity so that the receptive fields of these neurones are usually larger than that of the first-order afferents but again show overlap. This pattern is repeated at each level of the sensory pathway.

fields. Note, however, that in most cases the central neurones only receive convergent inputs from neurones mediating the same modality of sensation, thereby maintaining the specificity of the labelled line.

The receptive fields of the first-order afferent neurones (those innervating the receptor itself) are excitatory in that stimulation leads to afferent depolarization and the discharge of action potentials (but see visual transduction, p. 302). The receptive fields of more central neurones, however, may have both excitatory and inhibitory regions, the most common being a central excitatory region surrounded by an inhibitory region (Fig. 3.8.6) such that stimulation of the surrounding region results in inhibition of the neurone's activity. These inhibitory effects are very important in the generation of a sharply defined spatial distribution of the activity resulting from a given stimulus.

Lateral inhibition

Inhibitory mechanisms are very important in the ability to localize a stimulus accurately and the ability to discriminate between two stimuli that are very close together, called **two-point discrimination**.

The effect of convergence and divergence in the afferent chain would tend to reduce spatial discrimination as the excitation is spread to more neurones at each step. However, the central neurones also connect with inhibitory interneurones that act to inhibit the adjacent neurones. The neurone that displays the greatest activity will therefore also exert the greatest inhibition on its neighbours and so the representation of the stimulus within the CNS becomes focused and can be localized accurately (Fig. 3.8.7).

When two stimuli are close together, each will activate a group of receptor afferents innervating the area around the stimulus site. In the absence of lateral inhibition, the effect of convergence and divergence would result in the

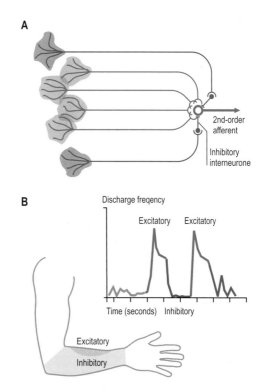

Fig. 3.8.6 Facilitatory and inhibitory receptive fields of central sensory neurones. A. The blue area represents the excitatory receptive field, the area over which stimuli cause excitation of the neurone. Surrounding this is an inhibitory field in which stimuli inhibit the central neurone via an inhibitory interneurone. **B.** The effect of stimulating excitatory and inhibitory fields on discharge frequency in the second-order afferent.

merging of the two stimuli as the zones of excitation showed increasing overlap at each relay stage. However, the effect of the inhibitory interconnections is that each stimulus is spatially defined by a central zone of excited cells, surrounded by a field of inhibition. Therefore the two stimuli are clearly distinguished in terms of two populations of excited cells with a distinct separation between them. Two-point discrimination, like the accuracy of localization, is dependent on receptive field size and for touch is finest on the fingertips where it is about 2 mm compared with 40 mm for the arm.

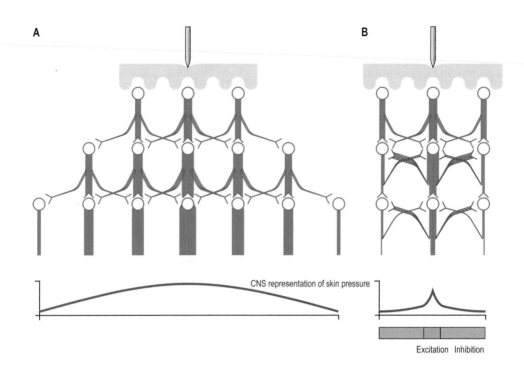

Fig. 3.8.7 **The importance of lateral inhibition. A.** In the absence of lateral inhibition, convergence and divergence at various levels blur the excitation distribution in the CNS. **B.** In the presence of lateral inhibition, the excitation is focused.

Summary

Sensory mechanisms

- Much sensory information about the internal state of the body does not reach conscious awareness.
- Physical energy (light, pressure, heat, etc.) is changed into afferent potentials by the process of transduction.
- Sensory receptors show a high degree of specificity to their adequate stimulus.

- Adaptation is the reduction in frequency of action potentials with time in response to a constant stimulus and ranges from rapid to slow.
- Intensity, type and position of a stimulus are signalled by frequency of action potentials, labelled lines and somatotopic representation of receptive fields respectively.
- Lateral inhibition improves the contrast around a receptive field.

General
sensory system

Introduction

The general sensory system comprises the systems of somatic and visceral sensation. Both these systems are organized hierarchically with receptors providing the input for first-order neurones which project onto second-order neurones in the central nervous system and so on to higher-order neurones (Fig. 3.9.1). At each level of the hierarchy there is convergence and divergence of the projections, leading to processing of the information in terms of its modality, location or intensity (p. 237) or, at the higher levels, in terms of specific characteristics such as shape or texture. Similar processing occurs in the pathways of the special senses.

Sensory pathways

The lowest level of the hierarchy is the first-order afferent neurone. In the periphery these neurones terminate either in a specific receptor structure or as free nerve endings. The first-order neurones may be divided into two groups on the basis of their innervation of either musculoskeletal receptors or cutaneous and visceral receptors. They are then classified according to the sensation they mediate and their axonal diameter (and hence conduction velocity). This classification has been described already in Chapter 3.5 (Table 3.5.1). These neurones respond to the stimulus and conduct

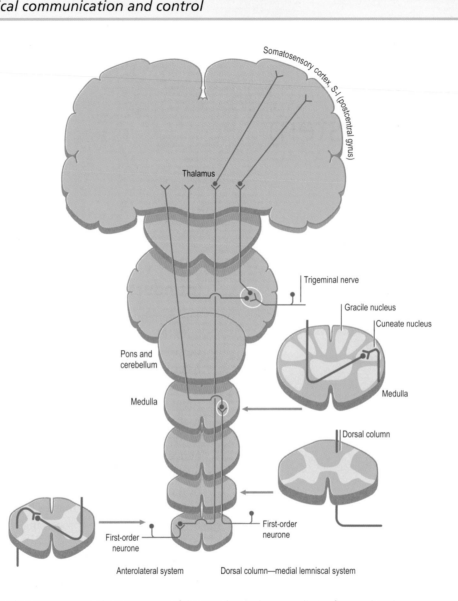

Fig. 3.9.1 **Ascending sensory tracts.** The arrangement of the ascending pathways mediating fine touch and proprioception (dorsal column–medial lemniscal pathway) and crude touch, temperature and pain (anterolateral system). In each case the second-order neurone crosses the midline (decussates) carrying information to the contralateral side of the brain. The level of the first synapse and the decussation is different for the two pathways. The trigeminal nerve, from the face, has some uncrossed fibres.

action potentials to the CNS. The first-order afferents conveying somatic information from the limbs and trunk of the body have their cell bodies in the dorsal-root ganglia of the spinal cord. There are two major pathway systems of conscious sensation from the body: the dorsal column–medial lemniscal system and the anterolateral system (Fig. 3.9.1).

Dorsal column–medial lemniscal system

The dorsal column–medial lemniscal system mainly mediates tactile sensation and proprioception (Table 3.9.1). The first-order afferent neurones have predominantly large-diameter, myelinated axons which course from the

Table 3.9.1 Main ascending pathways

Tract	Termination of afferents			
	Main 1st order	1st order	2nd order	3rd order
Dorsal column–medial lemniscal system	Aβ I, II	Medulla	Thalamus	S-I cortex (primary somatosensory cortex)
Anterolateral system				
Lateral spinothalamic tract	Aδ, C, III, IV	Spinal cord	Thalamus	S-I cortex
Anterior spinothalamic tract	Aδ, C	Spinal cord	Thalamus	S-I cortex
Spinoreticular tract	Aδ, C, III, IV	Spinal cord	Reticular formation of brainstem	Higher-order projections to the thalamus and cortex
Spinomesencephalic tract	Aδ, C, III, V	Spinal cord	Tectum of midbrain	Higher-order projections to the thalamus and cortex
Dorsal spinocerebellar tract	I, II	Spinal cord	Cerebellum	Higher-order projections to the thalamus and cortex
Ventral spinocerebellar tract	I, II	Spinal cord	Cerebellum	Higher-order projections to the thalamus and cortex
Cuneocerebellar tract	I, II	Spinal cord	Cerebellum	Higher-order projections to the thalamus and cortex

periphery to the spinal cord and ascend in the dorsal columns of the cord to terminate in the dorsal column nuclei in the ipsilateral medulla (Fig. 3.9.1). Within the cord the axons are topographically arranged, those from the distal parts of the lower leg running most medially while those from more proximal regions run more laterally.

The second-order neurones, originating in the dorsal column nuclei, receive convergent inputs from the first-order neurones and from interneurones. As a result, their individual receptive fields are usually larger than those of the first-order afferents and, depending on the interneuronal input, they may have both excitatory and inhibitory zones (see Fig. 3.8.7, p. 252).

In most cases the convergence will be from neurones mediating the same sensory modality (cf. labelled line, p. 250). Some second-order afferents, however, are polymodal in that they receive, and respond to, inputs from more than one type of peripheral receptor. Their firing characteristics such as adaptation rates, however, tend to be the same as those of the first-order afferent.

The second-order neurones cross the midline (decussate) in the medulla and project, as the medial lemniscus, to the ventral posterolateral nucleus of the contralateral thalamus. The third-order neurones project to the **primary somatosensory cortex**, this projection retaining the somatotopic organization of the pathway as a whole. Higher-order neurones make interconnections within the primary somatosensory cortex and with neurones in other regions of the cerebral cortex.

At each level, in this and other pathways, the synaptic connections permit the processing of the information, not only as a result of divergence and convergence of the ascending pathways but also because of inputs from other ascending and descending pathways via interneurones which may be excitatory or inhibitory in effect.

Anterolateral system

The anterolateral system mainly mediates pain and thermal sensation, though there is also a contribution to crude touch sensations (Table 3.9.1). The main pathway is the **lateral spinothalamic** tract (Fig. 3.9.1). The first-order afferents are usually small-diameter myelinated (Aδ) and unmyelinated (C) fibres which run from the periphery to the spinal cord where they terminate, within one or two spinal segments of their entry point, in the **substantia gelatinosa**.

The second-order afferent neurones cross the midline and ascend in the contralateral cord to the ventral posterolateral nucleus as well as to the central lateral nucleus of the thalamus from where the third-order neurones project to the sensory cortex. Two other pathways are also involved in the anterolateral system: the **spino-reticular** and the **spinomesencephalic** tracts. Both these tracts respond to noxious stimuli. The spinoreticular tract terminates in the reticular formation of the brainstem from where neurones project to the thalamus and on to the cerebral cortex. The involvement of the reticular formation indicates that this tract may be involved with direction of attention and arousal related to pain. The spinomesencephalic tract terminates in the tectum of the midbrain (in the superior colliculus) and also has projections to the mesencephalic periaqueductal grey matter, which is important in the descending regulation of pain (p. 272).

The synaptic connections in the pathway enable information processing as in other pathways. Of particular importance is the modulation of pain transmission via descending and other ascending pathways. As with the dorsal column–medial lemniscal system, the second- and third-order neurones may remain specific in terms of their sensory modality or they may be polymodal as a result of convergent inputs. In some cases this leads to a pattern of response that covers a wide range of stimulus intensities, for example from innocuous touching to frankly painful squeezing of the skin. In certain pathological conditions, such neurones with a wide dynamic range may underlie the effect whereby normally innocuous stimuli may produce pain sensations (p. 274).

Cerebellar pathways

Three pathways convey predominantly proprioceptive information to the cerebellum: the dorsal and ventral **spinocerebellar** tracts carry information from the trunk and legs, while the cuneocerebellar pathway relates to the arms and neck.

Spinal lesions

The organizational differences of the ascending pathways give rise to important differences in the effects of spinal injuries. This is best illustrated by a hemisection of the spinal cord, the Brown-Séquard syndrome (Fig. 3.9.2). The dorsal column pathway is ipsilateral in the cord and therefore there will be a loss of touch, etc., on the same side as the injury. Conversely, the anterolateral pathways ascend in the contralateral cord, and therefore pain and temperature sensation will be lost from the side of the body opposite to the injury site.

Sensation from the head and face

Most of the conscious sensation of the face and oral cavity is carried in the trigeminal nerve, the fifth of the cranial nerves (Fig. 3.9.1). The trigeminal nerve innervates the cutaneous receptors of the face, the proprioceptors of the muscles and joints serving the mouth and provides the sensory outflow from the teeth, the oral cavity and the dura mater.

The trigeminal nerve comprises three main branches and three sensory nuclei:

- tactile sensation of the face is mediated in the principal nucleus in the pons
- pain and temperature are mediated in the spinal nucleus in the medulla

- proprioception is mediated in the mesencephalic nucleus in the midbrain.

The second-order afferents decussate and project to the thalamus, and third-order afferents project to the somatosensory cortex. The basic organization is therefore similar to that for the ascending pathways from the spinal cord. The trigeminal nerve is of particular interest in terms of its transmission of the pain involved in toothache and headache.

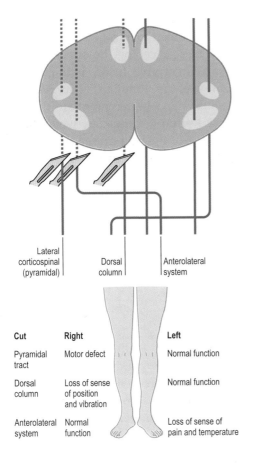

Cut	Right	Left
Pyramidal tract	Motor defect	Normal function
Dorsal column	Loss of sense of position and vibration	Normal function
Anterolateral system	Normal function	Loss of sense of pain and temperature

Fig. 3.9.2 Brown-Séquard syndrome. The effect of cutting across one half of the spinal cord is to interrupt the dorsal column conveying sensory information from that side and the anterolateral pathway conveying sensory information from the opposite side of the body. Motor tracts to the ipsilateral musculature are also cut.

Summary

Sensory tracts

- The sequence of neurones carrying an afferent message is designated in order, from the most peripheral: first-order neurones, second-order neurones, etc.
- Sensation enters the spinal cord via the dorsal roots and ascends in the dorsal column–medial lemniscal system (touch, proprioception) and the anterolateral system (pain, temperature, crude touch).
- Both sensory systems decussate, but at different levels.
- The spinoreticular and spinomesencephalic tracts are involved with the anterolateral system in transmitting noxious stimuli and arousal relating to pain.
- The cerebellum receives information about the trunk and legs from the dorsal and ventral spinocerebellar tracts and from the arms and neck in the cuneocerebellar pathway.
- Sensations from the face and mouth are carried in the trigeminal nerve.

Sensory receptors

The sensory receptors of the somatovisceral system range from highly complex sense organs such as the muscle spindle, through the cutaneous end-organ structures to simple, free nerve endings. Each of the afferent neurones innervating the periphery can be distinguished according to:

- the form of its peripheral terminal
- its sensitivity to particular stimuli
- the diameter of the axon and hence its conduction velocity, and
- the presence or absence of a myelin sheath, which again influences the conduction velocity (Table 3.5.1).

Cutaneous sensory receptors can be subdivided into three groups: **mechanoreceptors**, **thermoreceptors** and **nociceptors**. Sensation from the musculoskeletal and visceral systems is derived predominantly from mechanoreceptors and nociceptors.

Cutaneous receptors

Mechanoreceptors

Most of the mechanoreceptors in the skin take the form of the terminal of a large diameter (Aβ) myelinated axon in association with a non-neural structure. The mechanical properties of these non-neural structures determine, to a great extent, the response properties of the afferent neurone. For example, the afferent axon innervating a Pacinian corpuscle responds preferentially to high-frequency stimuli and adapts rapidly to maintained stimuli. If the membranous corpuscle itself is removed, leaving only the nerve ending, the afferent will respond in a slowly adapting manner. The structure and mechanical properties of the corpuscle act as a filter and determine what components of the stimulus actually pass through to the nerve ending. Conversely, the thermoreceptors and nociceptors (including those responding to noxious mechanical stimuli) are bare (free) nerve endings with small-diameter myelinated (Aδ) or unmyelinated (C) axons.

The mechanoreceptors are sensitive to mechanical stimuli such as stroking or indentation of the skin and they can be subdivided into rapidly adapting and slowly adapting receptors. They also vary according to their distribution in hairy and non-hairy (glabrous) skin and their depth with respect to the skin surface (Fig. 3.9.3A).

The main rapidly adapting mechanoreceptor in hairy skin is the hair follicle receptor, its counterpart in glabrous skin being the Meissner's corpuscle. Both hairy and glabrous skin are supplied with slowly adapting Merkel's receptors (though their organization is slightly different). All these receptors lie superficially and have small receptive fields, permitting good localization of the stimulus (Fig. 3.9.3A).

The subcutaneous receptors are the slowly adapting Ruffini's corpuscles, which respond to stretching of the skin caused by indentation or lateral pressure, particularly in terms of vibration; and the rapidly adapting Pacinian corpuscles, which are particularly sensitive to high-frequency stimulation. Because of their relative depth in the skin these receptors provide poor localization of the stimulus, though they do display a small zone of particularly high sensitivity (Fig. 3.9.3B).

Thermoreceptors

Temperature sense is provided by two classes of thermoreceptors: cold receptors and warm receptors, the cold receptors being more numerous, with the greatest receptive densities occurring on the face. Both receptor types are slowly adapting. Receptor adaptation is very important for the perception of temperature since any change of temperature is perceived relative to the starting temperature. This is clearly illustrated by Weber's three-bowl experiment: three bowls are filled with water, one cold, one lukewarm and one warm. To start, one hand is placed in the cold and the other in the warm

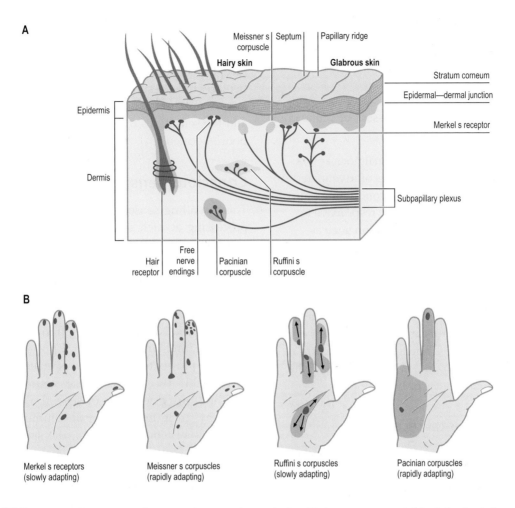

Fig. 3.9.3 Receptor adaptation. A. All receptors (except nociceptors) adapt. Their response to a maintained stimulus declines. The rate of adaptation varies. In the skin the most superficial Merkel's receptors are slowly adapting and have small receptive fields. Deeper Meissner's corpuscles rapidly adapt but also have small receptive fields. The deeper Pacinian corpuscles adapt very rapidly but respond well to vibration, whereas Ruffini's corpuscles adapt slowly. These deeper receptors have wide receptive fields. In hairy skin the hair receptor replaces the Meissner's corpuscle and adapts rapidly. The hair acts as a very localized detector. **B.** The relationship between depth within the skin and size of receptive field in four receptor types. Deep or superficial receptors may be rapidly or slowly adapting as shown. Ruffini's corpuscles are most excited by stretch of the skin in specific directions, as shown by the arrows. The red areas are regions of highest sensitivity.

water for several minutes until the sensations of the two hands have adapted. Both hands are then placed in the lukewarm water which will evoke sensations of warmth from the first hand and cold from the other. Associated with the effects of adaptation is the effect of slow changes in temperature such that continuous adaptation takes place so the receptors do not respond to the temperature change until it has become quite large. This is particularly true of slow cooling and can result in significant heat loss from the body before the subject becomes aware and acts to reverse the change.

The cold receptors are innervated by small-diameter myelinated (Aδ) axons and the warm receptors by unmyelinated (C) axons. As well as their role in conscious temperature sensation, thermoreceptors are also important in the unconscious regulation of body temperature.

Nociceptors

There are two main classes of cutaneous nociceptor:

- The mechanical and thermal nociceptors, which are the free-endings of myelinated Aδ fibres. These are the fast-conducting pain fibres and are particularly responsive to strong mechanical stimulation such as pinching or pricking.
- The polymodal nociceptors, which respond to a range of noxious stimuli, chemical (e.g. chemicals such as potassium released as a result of tissue damage) and thermal. These nociceptors are the free endings of unmyelinated C fibres which are slowly conducting (up to 2 m/s) and mediate the sensations of ache or burning pain.

Musculoskeletal receptors

The musculoskeletal system is richly endowed with mechanoreceptors, which are mainly concerned with providing proprioceptive information about limb position and movement. The main receptors are the muscle spindle, tendon organ and the joint receptors which are described in dètail in Chapter 3.6. This sensory information is of great importance for the motor control system but also reaches consciousness to give a sensation of limb position and a sense of effort and movement (kinaesthesia).

Nociceptors are also present in muscle and joints. Both mechanical, which are innervated by myelinated group III afferents, and polymodal nociceptors, unmyelinated, group IV afferent axons, are present.

Visceral receptors

The viscera are supplied with many specialized receptors such as chemoreceptors, baroreceptors, etc., which are involved in the autonomic regulation of organ function (e.g. respiratory and cardiac regulation). There are very few thermoreceptors or touch receptors. Nociceptors, particularly those responsive to mechanical stimuli, are present though they are sparsely distributed and the sensations they give rise to are usually poorly located.

Conscious sensation

The ascending sensory information undergoes processing at each synaptic relay in the pathway as a result of the convergence and divergence of ascending and descending signals (p. 250). This process progressively modifies the information that eventually reaches the level of conscious perception in the sensory regions of the cortex. Neurones arising from the thalamus (predominantly the ventral posterolateral nucleus) project to the primary somatosensory cortex (S-I) (Fig. 3.9.4). These neurones are the third-order neurones of several ascending pathways including the dorsal column–medial lemniscal system (touch, etc.), the spinothalamic tracts (pain, temperature) and the pathways projecting from the trigeminal nerve (sensory information from the head).

The primary somatosensory cortex lies on the post-central gyrus of the cerebral hemisphere (Fig. 3.9.4) and can be subdivided along the anteroposterior axis (sagittal plane) into four functional areas: Brodmann's areas 1, 2, 3a and 3b. Areas 1 and 3b are dominated by cutaneous inputs, whereas proprioceptive inputs, from muscles and joints, dominate areas 2 and 3a. Perpendicular to this axis (i.e. the coronal plane), the S-I cortex is organized as a distorted map of the body. The ascending pathways retain their somatotopic organization throughout and the area of the cortex occupied by the representation of each body region corresponds to the density of the sensory innervation and the functional importance of that region in sensory terms. Thus, the fingers and the mouth area have large representations compared with the trunk or thighs.

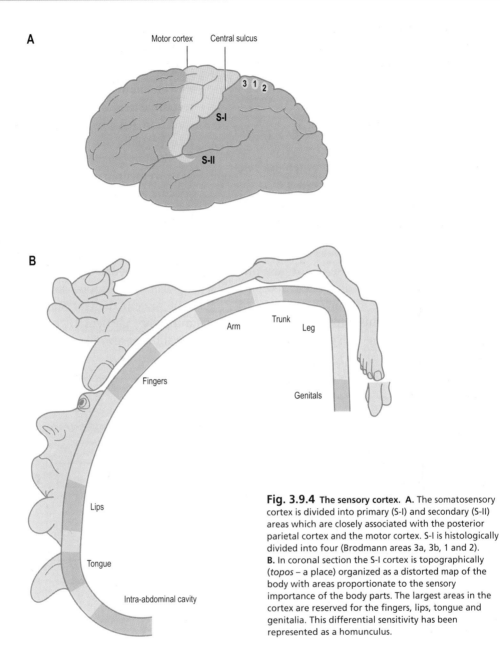

A

Motor cortex   Central sulcus

3 1 2

S-I

S-II

B

Arm   Trunk   Leg

Fingers

Genitals

Lips

Tongue

Intra-abdominal cavity

Fig. 3.9.4 **The sensory cortex. A.** The somatosensory cortex is divided into primary (S-I) and secondary (S-II) areas which are closely associated with the posterior parietal cortex and the motor cortex. S-I is histologically divided into four (Brodmann areas 3a, 3b, 1 and 2). **B.** In coronal section the S-I cortex is topographically (*topos* – a place) organized as a distorted map of the body with areas proportionate to the sensory importance of the body parts. The largest areas in the cortex are reserved for the fingers, lips, tongue and genitalia. This differential sensitivity has been represented as a homunculus.

Within each of these representational areas of the S-I cortex, the neurones are organized in a columnar fashion; that is, all the neurones along a line perpendicular to the cortical surface have similar response properties and similar receptive fields. Thus, within a specific column in area 3b all the neurones might respond to activation of rapidly adapting mechanoreceptors from a fingertip, whereas a neighbouring column might be responsive to slowly adapting mechanoreceptors. Similar columnar organization occurs in other primary sensory areas of the cortex, particularly the visual cortex (Brodmann's area 17, see p. 309) and in output areas such as the motor cortex.

Feature detection

The thalamic inputs to the S-I cortex project mainly to areas 3a and 3b. The receptive fields of the neurones in these regions remain relatively small and the neurones respond to discrete stimuli of the appropriate modality. Areas 3a and 3b, in turn project to areas 2 and 1 (which also receive some thalamic input) and to the secondary somatosensory cortex (S-II). In these regions the response of the neurones becomes more complex and their receptive fields are larger owing to convergence of various input signals. Thus groups of neurones respond specifically to movement across the

surface of the skin. Such movement detectors can be divided into three types:

- motion-sensitive neurones that respond to movement in any direction across the receptive field (Fig. 3.9.5)
- direction-sensitive neurones that respond preferentially to movement in one direction
- orientation-sensitive neurones that respond to movement in either direction along a specific axis.

Furthermore, whereas the neurones of areas 3a and 3b only respond to stimulation within a small receptive field, for example one (or at most two) phalanges of a digit, the neurones in areas 1 and 2 might respond to stimulation of any part of several fingers. Such complex, higher neurones are particularly active during tactile exploration of an object when determining its

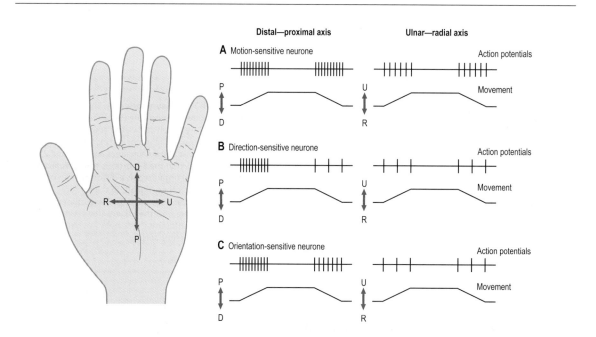

Fig. 3.9.5 Feature extraction. Responses of three types of movement detector neurones in the S-I cortex. The stimulus is stroking the hand. **A.** Motion-sensitive neurones respond while the stimulus is moving in any direction. **B.** Direction-sensitive neurones respond most to stroking in one orientation and direction. **C.** Orientation-specific neurones respond to movement in only one orientation but in both directions.

shape and texture. The combination of this information with the proprioceptive inputs also enables estimation of the object's size and its weight, the latter for example, being derived from the sense of effort related to lifting the object as well as the pressure the object exerts on the skin. The S-I and S-II cortices make projections to the posterior parietal cortex (areas 5 and 7) where this complex sensory information is integrated with information arising from the visual, auditory, olfactory systems, etc., in the generation of a map of the body's relationship with the surrounding space. The sensory cortices also make direct projection onto the motor areas and this is important in the control of ongoing movement, particularly, for tactile exploration.

Summary

Sensory receptors

- Cutaneous sensory receptors are mechanoreceptors, thermoreceptors and nociceptors. Sensory receptors of the musculoskeletal and visceral systems are largely mechanoreceptors and nociceptors. The viscera have baroreceptors and chemoreceptors but few thermoreceptors or nociceptors.

- Non-neural structures frequently modify the properties of receptors (Pacinian corpuscle).
- The primary (S-I) and secondary (S-II) somatosensory cortex lie on the post-central gyrus, are somatotopically organized and arranged in columns of neurones processing the same modality.

Pain

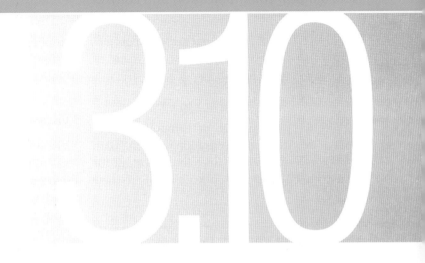

Introduction

Pain is very much a mixed blessing. Its primary purpose is, of course, a protective one. It is clearly of great benefit to withdraw quickly from a stimulus which is causing tissue damage, and individuals with an abnormally high pain threshold as a result of nerve damage, for example, can suffer considerable injury as a result of their reduced perception of pain.

But pain is an experience, not merely a sensation. The perception that pain produces is not only the product of the intensity of the noxious stimulus, but is influenced by a number of factors, many psychological. Military personnel can incur severe battlefield injuries while appearing to feel no pain at the time. Many mothers recall being in very little pain during childbirth, although at the time the pain seemed very severe. On the other hand, the pain experienced during terminal malignant disease can result in a devastating degree of suffering. Furthermore, the debilitation and misery produced by chronic pain can often be reduced by psychological techniques although the severity of the pain, as reported by the patient, remains essentially unchanged.

Classification of pain

English which can express the thoughts of Hamlet and the tragedy of Lear, has no words for the shiver and the headache. The merest schoolgirl, when she falls in love, has Shakespeare and Keats to speak for her; but let a sufferer try to describe a pain in his head to a doctor and language at once runs dry.

Virginia Woolf, 'On Being Ill'

Despite the philosophical and linguistic problems of describing any sensation let alone pain to another person, it is clinically important for patients to be able to describe their pain to their doctor.

Somatic and visceral pain

Pain can be divided into visceral and somatic which can itself be divided into superficial and deep pain (Fig. 3.10.1).

Somatic pain

The pain that is most often felt by the majority of individuals is superficial; in other words it arises from the skin or other superficial structures in the body. This pain characteristically occurs in response to actual or threatened injury to these tissues. The pain is well localized by the individual to the point of injury and is usually focal; in other words the perceived pain is limited to the site of tissue injury. The function of this pain is clearly a protective one, and usually leads to a withdrawal or other

response which limits tissue injury. Deep pain is frequently associated with connective tissue, bones, muscles and joints.

Visceral pain

Visceral pain is the pain that arises from internal organs, and differs in many respects from deep and superficial pain. The stimuli which lead to visceral pain are often very different from those producing superficial pain. Many internal organs such as the liver and kidneys appear to be insensitive to stimuli such as cutting and crushing which are very effective in producing superficial pain in the skin. However, other visceral organs such as the mesentery, gonads and liver capsule are very sensitive to these sort of stimuli. The distension of hollow organs characteristically leads to pain which may be further exacerbated by the contraction of smooth muscle in the wall of the organ. This is the sort of pain that is felt in colic. Often, the degree of distension which produces pain is very much less than that required to produce any degree of tissue damage and so the role of such pain is not clear. Inflammation is another very potent pain-producing stimulus to most internal organs. The pain of appendicitis or an inflamed gall bladder are both examples of pain arising by this mechanism. Internal organs are also very sensitive to ischaemia. The most obvious example of this is the pain of angina due to cardiac ischaemia but many other internal organs such as the gut are painfully sensitive to a lack of oxygen.

Unlike deep and superficial pain, visceral pain is usually diffuse and poorly localized. Typically, the victim feels the pain arising 'from inside' but cannot pinpoint it exactly. The pain is often more widespread than superficial pain. For example, the pain from a gastric ulcer may be felt over a large area across the upper abdomen, despite arising from a very small inflammatory structure. In many cases, the pain arising from an internal organ may be felt in an area distant from the organ itself. Thus, the pain

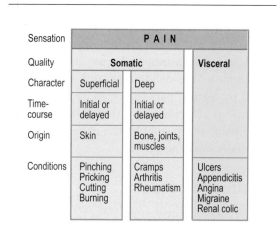

Sensation	PAIN		
Quality	Somatic		Visceral
Character	Superficial	Deep	
Time-course	Initial or delayed	Initial or delayed	
Origin	Skin	Bone, joints, muscles	
Conditions	Pinching Pricking Cutting Burning	Cramps Arthritis Rheumatism	Ulcers Appendicitis Angina Migraine Renal colic

Fig. 3.10.1 A scheme for describing pain.

of a myocardial infarction is often felt not only in the chest, but also in the left arm or the neck. This phenomenon is known as **referred pain**. Table 3.10.1 lists some common sites of pain referral from internal organs. Structures to which the pain of internal organs is referred are usually innervated from the same spinal segment and it is likely that referral results from primary or secondary neurones innervating both the internal organ and the site of referral. In addition to differences in its quality, the pain arising from internal organs differs from that of superficial pain in the degree of systemic upset that it causes. Increased activity of the sympathetic nervous system with visceral pain leads to sweating and circulatory changes, and the pain is often accompanied by malaise, nausea or even vomiting.

Abnormal pain

Pain is usually associated with tissue injury. The pain may have a protective function, and it diminishes and finally disappears as the tissue injury heals. This is the type of pain experienced by everybody from time to time, and is described by many authors as physiological pain. However, pain may not adhere to this time-course and may become chronic and debilitating. Pain may become long term as a result of a long-term stimulus, for example in rheumatoid arthritis. However, as described below, a long-term pain stimulus may lead, over time, to changes in the central activity of the pain pathway, altering the perception the painful stimulus. For example, neuropathic pain is the chronic pain which results from neuronal damage. The pain that this sort of damage produces is characterized by phantom limb pain, the intractable pain that an amputee feels to be coming from his amputated limb, although of course the limb is no longer present. This pain has no obvious physiological role because the initial tissue injury has now ceased. Neuropathic pain is often continuous, but may be intermittent or brought about by innocuous stimulation. For example, trigeminal neuralgia (tic douloureux) may be triggered by very light stimulation of the face of an affected individual.

The pathophysiology behind abnormal and chronic pain syndromes is unclear, but is likely to involve changes in the central and peripheral

Table 3.10.1 Referral of pain from internal organs

Organ	Site of referred pain
Meninges	Back of head, back of neck
Heart	Central chest, arms (usually left), neck, occasionally abdomen
Trachea	Behind sternum
Diaphragm	Shoulder tip
Oesophagus	Behind sternum
Stomach, duodenum	Upper abdomen, epigastrium
Small bowel, pancreas	Around umbilicus
Large bowel, bladder	Lower abdomen above pubic bone

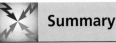

Summary

Classification of pain

- Pain perception is affected by the context in which it is experienced.
- Pain is arbitrarily categorized into somatic – superficial and deep – and visceral pain.
- Visceral pain is sometimes referred to another site.
- Structures to which the pain is referred are innervated by the same spinal segment as the origin of the pain.
- Pain may arise from phantom limbs or be triggered by inappropriately mild stimulation in abnormal conditions.

nervous system. Treatment of chronic pain is often difficult and now forms part of a specialized field, which includes not only primary analgesic therapies, but also cognitive therapies to help the patient cope with a long-term pain which may never be relieved by conventional means.

Pain pathways

Pain is appreciated when what is by definition a painful stimulus causes activation of peripheral pain receptors (nociceptors) resulting in nervous impulses being conducted along a series of neurones, starting with peripheral primary nociceptor afferents and continuing with spinal and supraspinal neurones terminating in higher brain centres (Fig. 3.10.2). It would be very wrong, however, to think of the pain pathway as merely representing a series of neural relays from the periphery to the cerebral cortex. Throughout the length of the pain pathway,

nervous impulses and transmission are modulated by extraneous factors, including inflammatory mediators at the periphery, and local and descending nervous pathways in the spinal cord and above (Fig. 9.3.2).

Peripheral nociceptors

Pain usually results from a noxious stimulus applied to the periphery. A noxious stimulus is one that may result in tissue damage. Nociceptors are the sensory receptors which respond to noxious stimuli and are formed from branched free nerve endings of unmyelinated C fibres and small-diameter myelinated Aδ fibres. They are all high-threshold receptors, which therefore respond to stimuli associated with tissue injury while not usually responding to less noxious stimuli.

Various workers have classified nociceptors on the basis of the type of stimulus to which they most readily respond. Thus, mechanoreceptors

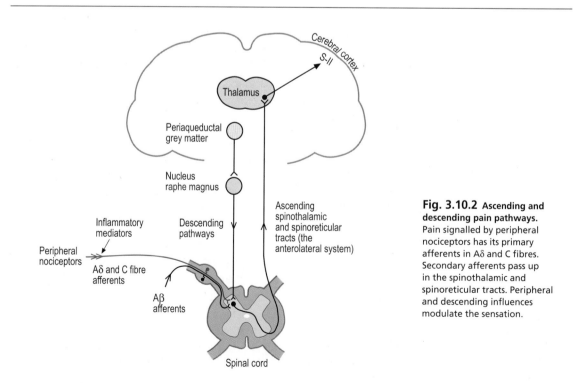

Fig. 3.10.2 Ascending and descending pain pathways. Pain signalled by peripheral nociceptors has its primary afferents in Aδ and C fibres. Secondary afferents pass up in the spinothalamic and spinoreticular tracts. Peripheral and descending influences modulate the sensation.

and thermoreceptors, which respond to excessive tissue distortion and extremes of temperature, have been described together with polymodal nociceptors, which respond to a wide range of noxious stimuli. The concentration of peripheral nociceptors varies between different parts of the body and correlates well with the sensitivity of that part of the body to pain.

Nociceptor primary afferents

There are two types of nociceptor primary afferents: Aδ and C fibres. Aδ fibres are small-diameter (1–5 μm) myelinated afferents with conduction velocities of 3–30 m/s and account for about 20% of nociceptor primary afferents. Aδ fibres arise from thermo- and mechano-receptors as well as from polymodal receptors, and the pain produced by their discharge is characteristically sharp, well localized and is perceived almost immediately the noxious stimulus is applied. C fibres account for about 80% of the nociceptor primary afferents. C fibres are unmyelinated fibres of small diameter (<1 μm) and low conduction velocities, typically less than 2 m/s. C fibres arise from polymodal nociceptors, and the pain that their discharge produces is typically described as dull or aching and cannot be well localized to the body surface. The pain conveyed by C fibres typically begins 1 second or so after noxious stimulation, which is due, at least in part, to the slower conduction velocities of these fibres.

The cell bodies of the primary afferents of this system lie within the dorsal root ganglia of the spinal cord (or within the trigeminal ganglion in the case of afferents arising from parts of the head) and the axons terminate in the dorsal horns (trigeminal nuclei) of the spinal grey matter.

Peripheral nociceptors and inflammation

The reaction of peripheral nociceptors and primary afferents to noxious stimuli is variable and can be altered by a number of different factors, particularly the presence of inflammation.

Inflammation is a characteristic response which tissues make to injury and is directed to removing the source of injury and to promoting tissue healing. The so-called cardinal signs of inflammation are *rubor* (redness), *dolor* (pain), *calor* (heat production), *tumor* (swelling) and are all produced by the action of inflammatory mediators. These mediators are produced in response to tissue injury by many different cells, including vascular endothelial cells, platelets and mast cells, and many of them act on peripheral nociceptors and pain afferents. Amongst these mediators are prostaglandins and leukotrienes.

In response to cell injury, arachidonic acid is liberated from membrane lipids by phospholipases. **Prostaglandins** and **leukotrienes** are produced by the breakdown of arachidonic acid by cyclo-oxygenase and lipoxygenase respectively (Fig. 3.10.3) and decrease the pain threshold by their action on peripheral nerves. However, although they decrease the pain threshold, these substances do not cause pain themselves when administered to experimental subjects. Cyclo-oxygenase is inhibited by non-steroidal anti-inflammatory drugs (NSAIDs) such as ibuprofen, and the decrease in prostaglandin production peripherally is, in part, responsible for their analgesic action.

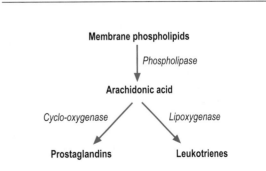

Fig. 3.10.3 The production of prostaglandins and leukotrienes from cell membrane phospholipids.

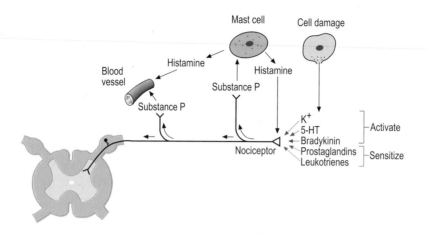

Fig. 3.10.4 **The origins and effects of pain mediators.** Activation of nociceptors is frequently brought about by damage but does not require the nociceptor itself to be damaged. For example, release of chemical mediators by damaged cells leads to the sensitization and activation of nociceptors, which in turn releases substance P by an axon reflex. Substance P then degranulates mast cells to release histamine, which stimulates nociceptors in a feedback loop.

Bradykinin is produced in the plasma from its precursor kininogen by the action of the enzyme kallikrein which is itself produced from prekallikrein. Among its many pro-inflammatory actions, bradykinin stimulates nociceptors, this action being potentiated by the prostaglandins. Other inflammatory mediators thought to sensitize or stimulate peripheral nociceptors include 5-hydroxytryptamine (5-HT), interleukins, hydrogen ions and potassium ions released from damaged cells, and substance P released from nerve endings by axon reflexes from the originally stimulated nociceptor (Fig. 3.10.4).

Although the presence of inflammation tends to result in an increased sensitivity and stimulation of peripheral nociceptors, there is also good evidence that in the presence of inflammation, pain afferents express opioid receptors. Activation of these receptors by endogenous or exogenously administered opioids may result in a degree of analgesia.

Summary

Nociceptors

- Nociceptors are free endings of C fibres (80%) and Aδ nerve fibres (20%).
- Nociceptors are high-threshold receptors.
- Aδ fibres produce sharp well-localized pain, C fibres produce dull aching poorly localized pain.

- Inflammatory mediators, including prostaglandins and leukotrienes, increase the sensitivity to pain.
- Nociceptor axon reflexes release substance P which degranulates mast cells.

The spinal cord and the modulation of the pain pathway

The spinal cord is a very important part of the pain pathway because a good deal of information processing takes place here, particularly in the dorsal horn of grey matter. Synapses here are not merely relays in the pain pathway, but are part of a complex neural system which may lead to an increase or a decrease in the intensity of perceived pain. Aδ and C pain fibres synapse initially in the dorsal horn with secondary neurones which pass into the ipsilateral and contralateral spinothalamic tracts and ascend to the thalamus (Fig. 3.10.2). At the level of the dorsal horn, the pain pathway may be modulated by other sensory afferents at the same spinal level, by neural pathways descending from higher centres in the brain, or by the duration and intensity of long-term painful stimulation.

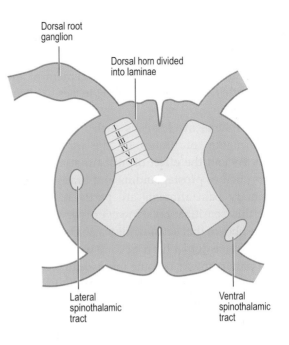

Fig. 3.10.5 **Section of the spinal cord.** The laminae of the dorsal horn of the grey matter are shown together with the ventral and lateral spinothalamic tracts.

Synapses in the dorsal horn

The dorsal horn of the grey matter of the spinal cord is conventionally divided into six numbered layers or laminae, on the basis of light microscope appearance (Fig. 3.10.5). Pain afferents terminate in laminae I and II and Aδ fibres project to deeper laminae. Lamina II is known as the **substantia gelatinosa** because it does not take up stain well and so has a translucent appearance on light microscopy. It is thought that much of the spinal modulation of the pain pathway takes place here.

A number of neurotransmitters have been identified in the dorsal horn, which are thought to be released by primary pain afferents. These include excitatory amino acids such as glutamate and peptides such as neurokinin, calcitonin gene-related peptide (CGRP), vasoactive intestinal peptide (VIP), bombesin, substance P and somatostatin.

The application of neurotransmitters to secondary neurones in the dorsal horn results in the production of excitatory postsynaptic potentials (EPSPs). These add together and, if a large enough membrane potential results, an action potential is produced in the nerve axon. Nerve recordings have suggested that different neurotransmitters may evoke EPSPs of different latency and duration in the same secondary neurone. EPSPs produced by the action of glutamate on amino-3-hydoxy-5-methylisoxazole-4-propionic acid (AMPA) receptors have a short latency and short duration. EPSPs of longer latency and duration are produced by the action of other transmitters such as the neurokinins, CGRP and substance P. Longer-duration EPSPs can also be provoked by glutamate acting on *N*-methyl-D-aspartate (NMDA) receptors. The summation and interaction of these EPSPs may be in part responsible for the phenomenon of central sensitization.

Central sensitization

It has long been recognized that prolonged peripheral tissue injury can lead to **hyperalgesia**,

271

in which an exaggerated response is elicited by painful stimuli, and **allodynia**, in which a normally innocuous stimulus is perceived as painful. In addition, an enlargement of the receptive fields of nociceptor neurones has been described.

Peripheral mechanisms such as mechanical deformation of tissues by the inflammatory process and the effect of inflammatory mediators such as prostaglandins and bradykinin on primary pain afferents are partly responsible for this sensitization. However, nerve studies have shown that sensitization also occurs at the level of the dorsal horn. Secondary neurones in the pain pathway become more excitable.

The interaction of EPSPs is thought to be one mechanism responsible for this sensitization. It has been postulated that chronic stimulation causes summation of EPSPs, which leads to the membrane potential of the secondary neurone being closer to the threshold for firing. This summation is further enhanced by the upregulation of receptors such as those for neurokinin and CGRP, the stimulation of which provokes EPSPs.

Central sensitization may be reduced experimentally by the administration of opioids or antagonists to receptors to NMDA, CGRP and neurokinin. Often the effect is more pronounced if the drug is administered pre-emptively, and there is limited clinical evidence that the pain following surgery is reduced if analgesia such as opioids or local anaesthetics is administered before or during the operation.

Pain inhibition by the activation of Aβ fibres

Aβ fibres are responsible for conveying the sensations of light touch and temperature. It has been known for some time that C-fibre-mediated pain pathways can be inhibited by the activity of Aβ fibres innervating the same spinal segment. This inhibition is thought to be as a result of both presynaptic inhibition of C fibres and postsynaptic inhibition of secondary neurones

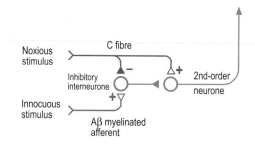

Fig. 3.10.6 A model of the 'gating' of pain. The spontaneously active interneurone acts on the second-order neurone inhibiting it. Activity in the C fibre inhibits the interneurone and excites the second-order neurone to produce the sensation of pain. Activity in the myelinated afferent restores the activity in the inhibitory interneurone.

in the dorsal horn of the spinal cord (Fig. 3.10.6). Furthermore, these electrophysiological data have been supported by behavioural studies in man and animals.

This interruption of the C-fibre-mediated pain pathway by Aβ fibre stimulation forms the **gate control theory** of pain regulation. It is thought that the analgesia that is brought about by rubbing or applying heat or cold to a painful area is as a result of this mechanism. The gate control theory also accounts for the analgesic effect of transcutaneous electrical nerve stimulation (TENS), a method of pain relief that involves applying a small electrical current to the skin, of sufficient intensity to produce a light paraesthesia. It is possible too that part of the analgesic effect of acupuncture may also be explained in this way.

It is thought that inhibitory interneurones are involved in the interruption of the pain pathway produced by Aβ stimulation, although the exact neural mechanisms have yet to be elucidated. It may be that opioids are not involved, as the analgesia produced by TENS is not blocked by naloxone, a selective opioid antagonist.

Descending inhibitory pathways

It has been established that electrical stimulation of selected discrete areas of the brain produces a profound analgesia. Furthermore, it was established that during stimulation of these areas, neurones in the dorsal horn of the spinal cord became less responsive to painful stimuli and that section of the dorsolateral funiculus of the spinal cord abolished the analgesia. These results suggested that descending pathways from the brain were responsible for modulating the pain pathway at the level of the dorsal horn of the spinal cord (Fig. 3.10.2).

Areas of the brain which appear to be involved in the descending pain modulating pathways include the **periaqueductal grey matter** in the midbrain and the area around the nucleus raphe magnus in the medulla.

The periaqueductal grey matter receives neuronal inputs from a variety of sources within the CNS including the thalamus, hypothalamus and cerebral cortex, as well as the spinal cord. It is likely that the periaqueductal grey matter brings about most of its analgesic effect by stimulation of the nucleus raphe magnus and the adjacent medulla, probably via neurones containing glutamate or aspartate.

The most important pain-modulating neurones projecting from the medulla to the dorsal horn are neurones containing 5-hydroxytryptamine (5-HT) and noradrenaline (NA). 5-HT-containing neurones arise mainly from the nucleus raphe magnus, whereas the noradrenergic neurones arise mainly from the adjacent medulla. The analgesic effects of electrical stimulation of the periaqueductal grey matter and the nucleus raphe magnus can be partly abolished by 5-HT and NA antagonists, and analgesia can be produced by 5-HT agonists such as tramadol, the tricyclic antidepressants and α_2 adrenergic agonists such as clonidine. Clonidine has a particularly effective analgesic effect when administered epidurally or into the cerebrospinal fluid around the lumbar spinal cord.

Opioids

For centuries the analgesic properties of opiate agents such as opium, laudanum and morphine,

derived from the seed case of the poppy *Papaver somniferum*, have been known. Endogenous opiate-like substances were first isolated in the 1970s and include leu-enkephalin, met-enkephalin, β-endorphin and the dynorphins. They occur throughout the body and are intimately involved in the modulation of pain, as well as being neurotransmitters outside the pain pathway. Leu-enkephalin and met-enkephalin are both pentapeptides which differ from each other only in the terminal amino acid which is leucine in the case of leu-enkephalin and methionine in the case of met-enkephalin. Both enkephalins are formed from the cleavage of a pro-enkephalin, a larger precursor polypeptide. β-endorphin is a 31-amino-acid polypeptide which contains the amino acid sequence that forms met-enkephalin. It is cleaved from the precursor pro-opiomelanocortin. The dynorphins include dynorphin itself, α-neoendorphin and β-neoendorphin, which are formed from the precursor polypeptide prodynorphin.

The enkephalins are found throughout the nervous system, but of relevance to their role in analgesia is that they are found in the dorsal horns of the spinal cord, the periaqueductal grey matter and the nucleus raphe magnus. The dynorphins are found in the spinal cord and the periaqueductal grey matter, and β-endorphin is found in the hypothalamus.

Opioids act on opioid receptors, classified as μ, δ, κ and ε receptors. Initially, a σ receptor was described, although this receptor is now thought to be a form of NMDA receptor. A proposal that there may be two subclasses of μ receptors, μ_1 and μ_2, has not been supported by the recent cloning of a single μ receptor. The International Union of Pharmacology has recently proposed the renaming of the μ, δ and κ receptors as OP_3, OP_1 and OP_2 receptors respectively, although use of the older terminology is still widespread.

The administration of opioids to the dorsal column results in a decrease in the release of excitatory neurotransmitters by the primary pain afferents and a decreased sensitivity of the secondary neurones. This effect is brought about by the inhibition of calcium ion channels and possibly by the inhibition of adenylyl cyclase, the enzyme which catalyses the formation of cyclic AMP. Administration of opioids to the periaqueductal grey matter results in a very profound analgesia, and much of this analgesic effect is mediated by the descending pain-modulating pathways. Opioids are among the most powerful analgesic drugs available, and their use is widespread despite their numerous side-effects including tolerance, addiction, nausea, vomiting and respiratory depression.

Ascending pain pathways from the spinal cord to the cerebral cortex

Secondary pain neurones ascend in the contralateral spinothalamic and spinoreticular tracts. Within the spinal cord, the spinothalamic and spinoreticular tracts are not separate and only become distinct within the brainstem. Some spinothalamic tract neurones may be activated weakly by tactile stimuli but more powerfully by noxious stimuli, and are called **wide-dynamic range cells**. They mainly signal noxious events but may be activated to produce the sensation of pain under pathological conditions. Other **nociceptive-specific** or **high-threshold cells** are only activated by noxious stimuli (Fig. 3.10.7). The wide-range cells may, under non-pathological conditions, exert something like lateral inhibition (p. 252), reducing overlap, not in terms of receptive fields (lateral inhibition) but in terms of modalities, between pain and touch for example. This effect may be involved in the 'gating' of pain (p. 272).

Fibres in the spinothalamic tract arise from laminae I and V of the dorsal horn and synapse in the ventrobasal thalamic nuclei. These nuclei project fibres within the posterior part of the internal capsule to areas of the cerebral cortex including the somatosensory cortex.

Fibres in the spinoreticular tract, including some medial fibres from the spinothalamic

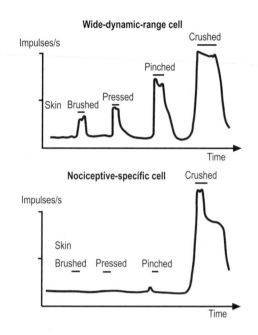

Fig. 3.10.7 Response of two main types of spinothalamic tract cells to increasing intensity of stimulation. The wide-dynamic-range cell receives input from mechanoreceptors and nociceptors, responding to a wide range of stimuli. The nociceptive-specific cell only receives input from first-order nociceptors and only responds to noxious stimuli.

tract, arise from deeper layers in the dorsal horn and project to nuclei in the midbrain reticular formation, the nucleus raphe magnus, the periaqueductal grey matter, the hypothalamus and the medial nuclei of the thalamus. Projections from these areas pass to the many different parts of the brain, including the cortex and the limbic system.

These two distinct pain pathways are believed to subserve different sensory aspects of pain. The pathway including the spinoreticular tract is thought to be involved in feedback control of pain intensity via the descending pathways and it is also thought to be involved in many of the affective and motivational aspects of pain. The spinothalamic–somatosensory cortex pathway is thought, on the other hand, to be involved in the appreciation of the spatial and sensory aspects of pain.

A complex neuronal network

One of the earliest and most interesting descriptions of the modulation of pain comes from the explorer Henry Livingstone, who was mauled by a lion in Africa. Livingstone records that after the first shock and intense pain the sensation became much less appalling. A profoundly religious man, he postulated that this mechanism had been instituted by a benevolent God to reduce the suffering of creatures who were by necessity the prey of other animals.

Pain is a complicated experience and its purely sensory elements are complemented by complex emotional and psychological aspects. The pain pathway itself is a complicated neuronal network and is continuously modulated throughout its length. Pain usually has a clear physiological benefit, yet some individuals suffer over periods of many years with a pathological form of pain that has no obvious purpose. The relief of pain has been one of the aspirations of physicians for centuries, and although our catalogue of analgesic drugs and techniques is larger than it has ever been, there is still much we do not understand about this complicated aspect of human suffering.

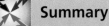

Summary

Ascending and descending pathways

- Much modulation of the pain pathway takes place in the dorsal horn of the spinal cord grey matter.
- The gate control theory postulates that Aβ fibres inhibit the effect of C fibres by inhibiting secondary neurones in the dorsal horn.

- Descending pathways releasing 5-HT and noradrenaline produce analgesia by acting at the dorsal horn.
- Natural and synthetic opioids act at the spinal cord and higher levels.
- Secondary afferents ascend to the thalamus and reticular system before passing to the sensory cortex, particularly the region S-II.

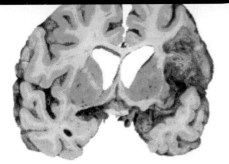

3.11

Stroke

Introduction

In the developed countries, stroke represents the third most common cause of death after coronary heart disease and cancer and is the most common cause of physical disability. Whilst the probability of occurrence of strokes is clearly associated with ageing, with 75% of stroke victims being over 65 years old, strokes may occur at almost any age and are associated with a characteristic set of risk factors. General risk factors include:

• increasing age
• hypertension
• smoking
• increased blood cholesterol levels
• diabetes mellitus.

The following are examples of specific indicators for stroke:

• coronary heart disease (angina pectoris, etc.)
• transient ischaemic attacks
• peripheral vascular disease (thrombosis, etc.).

The term stroke (or cerebrovascular accident) may be defined as a rapidly developing loss of cerebral function which is of vascular origin, being focal or global in extent, and which results in death or symptoms of more than 24 hours' duration. The symptoms of a stroke are due to the death of neurones in the area of the brain affected by the disruption to the blood supply.

The brain represents about 2% of the body mass but

receives about 14% of the resting cardiac output. The blood supply is distributed by means of complex networks of arteries arising from four main arteries: the two internal carotid and the two vertebral arteries (Fig. 3.11.1). The two vertebral arteries link together to form the *basilar artery* which, in turn, is linked with the carotid arteries at the *circle of Willis*. The cerebellum and brainstem receive their blood supply from vessels arising from the vertebral and basilar arteries, while the cerebral arteries arise from the circle of Willis. The territories of the arteries show a degree of overlap so that a particular region of the brain may be supplied by two arteries. Such collateral circulation can be important in limiting the damage caused by disruption to one of the arteries.

The most notable feature of the cerebral circulation is its efficient system of regulation, such that the overall blood flow to the brain can be maintained almost constant irrespective of changes in demand placed on the cardiovascular system by the rest of the body (see Ch. 6.7, Special circulations). The maintenance of a constant blood supply is critically important because the brain, of all the body's organs, is very vulnerable to any disturbance to that supply. A reduction in the blood supply lasting only a few seconds can lead to loss of

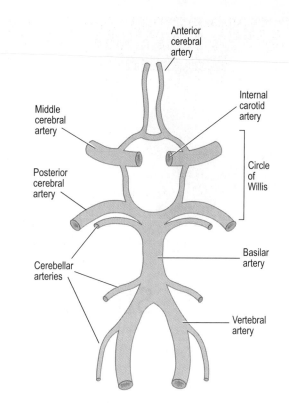

Fig. 3.11.1 The major blood vessels to the brain. The flow in the circle of Willis comes from the basilar artery and the two internal carotid arteries.

vision ('blackout') and fainting, as many people have experienced from getting up too quickly. Interruption of the blood supply for more than 1 or 2 minutes leads to neuronal cell death and irreversible damage to the affected region of the brain. Disruption of the blood supply may arise spontaneously as the result of cerebrovascular disease or it may result from traumatic injury.

Cerebrovascular disease gives rise to two main classes of spontaneous disorder, both of which are included in the term 'stroke'. A stroke may be *ischaemic* in origin, because of occlusion of an artery, or *haemorrhagic*, owing to bleeding.

Ischaemic stroke

Ischaemic stroke represents 80% of stroke cases. There is an insufficiency or total lack of blood supply within the territory of that artery. If the ischaemia is severe or complete, then ischaemic cell death will occur, a process termed *infarction*. The extent of the resulting neurological

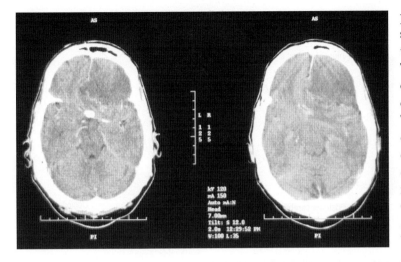

Fig. 3.11.2 CT/MRI scan of infarct. This illustrates the use of computerized tomography to localize an ischaemic infarct which can just be seen in the left frontal region. Compare with the effect of angiography (Fig. BS3.11.1). (Courtesy of Dr Margaret Jones.)

deficit will depend on the size and location of the infarct (Fig. 3.11.2).

The duration of symptoms for more than 24 hours (see above) distinguishes a stroke from a markedly less severe event, the *transient ischaemic attack* (TIA). As its name suggests, the TIA results from brief occlusion of an artery with restoration of the supply before irreversible damage takes place. The symptoms depend on which artery is affected but commonly include monocular loss of vision and contralateral weakness. The symptoms develop rapidly, within a few seconds, and disappear within a matter of minutes or a few hours. Loss of consciousness is very rare and the signs are usually focal; a TIA should therefore be distinguished from *syncope*

(fainting) due to a brief reduction in blood supply to the whole brain, often as a result of sudden systemic hypotension. The occurrence of TIAs may be regarded as a warning sign since they are frequently indicative of underlying cerebrovascular disease.

Most ischaemic strokes and TIAs result from complications arising from *atheroma* (degeneration of the arterial walls). Arterial occlusion in these cases may be due to *thrombosis*, the formation of a clot (thrombus) on the arterial wall, or due to an *embolism*, in which part of a thrombus (or another blocking agent) breaks off from its site of origin and is transported via the bloodstream till it lodges in another vessel. Atheroma is usually widespread, and other

parts of the body may be similarly affected (particularly the coronary circulation). The most common sites of occlusion are the branch points of the arteries (see Fig. 3.11.1). The presence of collateral circulations, such as the circle of Willis, means that occlusion of an artery in the neck may not cause cerebral infarction. Occlusion of the cerebral arteries themselves or of their branches will probably cause cerebral infarction because there is less capacity for collateral supply.

As with a TIA, the symptoms of ischaemic stroke develop rapidly, reaching their maximum extent within a few minutes. Assuming that the patient survives, then there is usually some functional improvement during the first few weeks, though 40% of survivors from a cerebral infarct will still be dependent at 6 months. The specific symptoms resulting from an ischaemic stroke depend on the artery affected, and therefore the territory of the brain that has been affected.

Middle cerebral artery

Infarction in the territory of the middle cerebral artery is the most common of the ischaemic strokes. The middle cerebral artery is the largest of the branches arising from the internal carotid artery (see Fig. 3.11.1) and it supplies the lateral surfaces of the frontal,

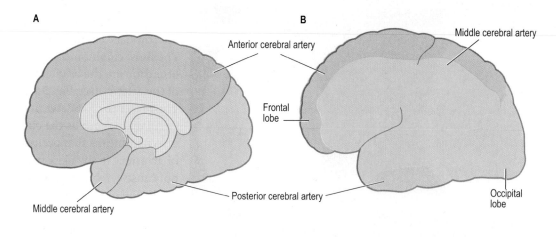

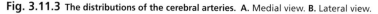

Fig. 3.11.3 The distributions of the cerebral arteries. **A.** Medial view. **B.** Lateral view.

parietal and temporal lobes (Fig. 3.11.3).

Complete occlusion of the middle cerebral artery therefore has profound consequences, including contralateral sensory loss and motor weakness with a positive Babinski sign (Ch. 3.6) indicative of upper motoneurone lesions. There is usually loss of half of the visual field (hemianopia) owing to damage to the tracts connecting the lateral geniculate nucleus to the visual cortex (p. 307).

Depending on which side of the brain is affected, there will also be impairment either of language or of spatial perception. In the majority of individuals, the left hemisphere is dominant for language. Damage to these regions of the cerebral cortex gives rise to *aphasias* which are

disorders of language affecting the generation of speech and its understanding (as distinct from disorders affecting articulation or hearing), often accompanied by difficulties in reading and writing. Complete occlusion of the middle cerebral artery gives rise to global aphasia with inability to read, write, speak or comprehend language. More circumscribed infarcts as a result of occlusion of one of the arterial branches can give rise to characteristic language deficits, and the study of such deficits has been of great value in the investigation of language processes. Damage to the frontal lobe may affect Broca's area (see Fig. 3.11.4), giving rise to Broca's aphasia in which comprehension of language is relatively undisturbed but language production (and writing) is affected with an

inability to construct sentences or speak with any fluency.

Note that because Broca's area is located near the motor cortex and the internal capsule, lesions affecting Broca's area also usually give rise to contralateral weakness (hemiparesis).

Infarcts within the temporal lobe can affect Wernicke's area (Fig. 3.11.4), giving rise to Wernicke's aphasia. Patients displaying Wernicke's aphasia show impairment of comprehension of language, both heard and read. Production of language is fluent but the patient will frequently use the wrong words and cannot convey ideas, so-called 'empty speech'. A number of other aphasias are also recognized and lesions of other areas may also lead to language impairment; for example, right hemisphere

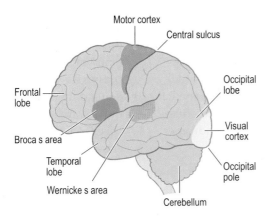

Fig. 3.11.4 **The location of some of the functional areas affected by infarcts in the territories of the middle and posterior cerebral arteries.** Occlusion of the left, middle and posterior cerebral arteries may affect Broca's area or Wernicke's area, giving rise to aphasias (speech defects). Occlusion of the posterior cerebral artery affects the visual cortex.

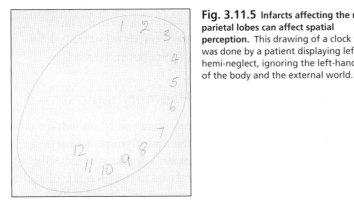

Fig. 3.11.5 **Infarcts affecting the right parietal lobes can affect spatial perception.** This drawing of a clock face was done by a patient displaying left hemi-neglect, ignoring the left-hand side of the body and the external world.

the medial surfaces of the frontal and parietal lobes and the corpus callosum as well as a strip along the upper part of the lateral surface. Occlusion of this artery will therefore affect the regions of the motor and sensory cortices representing the contralateral lower leg (cf. Fig. 3.7.3, p. 230, the motor homunculus) causing motor weakness and sensory loss. The supplementary motor area (p. 229) may also be affected, leading to poor coordination of bilateral movements.

Posterior cerebral artery

The posterior cerebral artery arises from the basilar artery (see Fig. 3.11.1) and supplies the occipital lobe and part of the inferior surface of the temporal lobe (see Fig. 3.11.3). One of the main functional areas affected by occlusion of one posterior cerebral artery is therefore the visual cortex, giving rise to homonymous hemianopia, the loss of half of the visual field on the same side for both eyes. The occipital pole, which is the very posterior tip of the occipital cortex (see Fig. 3.11.4), receives its blood supply from the middle cerebral artery and therefore there is usually sparing of the central vision, which is represented in the occipital pole.

Occlusion of the posterior cerebral artery may also affect the thalamus, giving rise to

lesions may lead to loss of the *affective* component of language so, for example, the patient may speak in a monotone, irrespective of the emotional content of the sentence.

Infarcts within the right cerebral hemisphere, particularly those affecting the parietal lobe may give rise to a variety of bizarre disturbances of spatial perception. For example, in hemi-neglect,

patients may fail to recognize the left-hand side of their bodies and any object within the left visual field, though the visual processing itself is undisturbed (Fig. 3.11.5).

Anterior cerebral artery

The anterior cerebral artery arises from the internal carotid artery and forms part of the circle of Willis (see Figs 3.11.1 and 3.11.3). It mainly supplies

281

contralateral sensory loss, and the subthalamic nucleus, in which case the patient will display chorea-like symptoms (p. 234) contralateral to the affected nucleus.

The interior of the brain is mainly supplied by relatively fine penetrating arteries which arise from the cerebral arteries and the circle of Willis. Occlusion of one of these arteries causes infarction in small brain areas, the infarcts being called *lacunae*. The effect of such lacunae is very circumscribed, ranging from no effect at all to quite major deficits, for example contralateral hemiparesis if the lacuna lies in the internal capsule.

Vertebral and basilar arteries

The brainstem and cerebellum receive their blood supply from arteries arising from the vertebral and basilar arteries, including the paramedian branches of the basilar artery and the cerebellar arteries (see Fig. 3.11.1). Infarctions involving the brainstem usually have profound results because of the large number of ascending and descending tracts, the vital centres (respiratory, cardiovascular, etc.) and the reticular formation which, among other things, is involved in the control of arousal. Many such infarctions will therefore result in coma or death.

The effects of an infarction depend critically on its location but a simple classification is to divide brainstem syndromes into lateral (occlusion of the cerebellar arteries) and medial (occlusion of the paramedian branches). Lateral syndromes may include:

- ipsilateral Horner's syndrome (disruption of the sympathetic nerves leading to drooping of the upper eyelid (ptosis), constriction of the pupil and absence of sweating)
- lesion of the spinothalamic tract with contralateral loss of pain and temperature sensation
- lesion of the trigeminal sensory pathway causing ipsilateral loss of cutaneous sensation
- lesion of the interconnections with the cerebellum giving rise to ipsilateral ataxia (p. 237).
- disruption of the vestibular system with nausea, nystagmus (p. 237) and loss of balance
- lesion of specific cranial nerves, depending on the level of the infarct.

Medial lesions may include:

- lesion of the corticospinal tract with contralateral hemiparesis (p. 146)
- lesion of the dorsal column–medial lemniscal pathway causing contralateral loss of fine touch sensation, etc.; but the spinothalamic tracts are spared so crude touch, pressure, pain and temperature sensation are preserved
- depending on the level of the lesion, there will be specific deficits due to cranial nerve lesions, such as disorders of gaze.

Occlusion of the basilar artery itself can lead to bilateral infarction of the ventral pons, interrupting the corticospinal and corticobulbar tracts on both sides, giving rise to a condition called 'locked-in' syndrome. The patient is quadriplegic and unable to make facial movements other than those of the eyes and eyelids.

Haemorrhagic stroke

Spontaneous haemorrhage is the underlying cause of 20% of strokes and is commonly related to the presence of an aneurysm (a balloon-like swelling that develops on the wall of an artery because of congenital deformation or degenerative vascular disease) or an arteriovenous malformation (AVM) in which there is an abnormal connection (fistula) between an artery and a vein. Hypertension is a major risk factor in haemorrhagic stroke. The most common intracranial haemorrhages are:

- subarachnoid haemorrhage (SAH), bleeding into the subarachnoid space

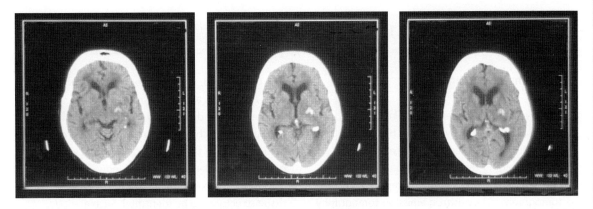

Fig. 3.11.6 CT scan of an intracerebral haemorrhage. The haematoma (white area) is associated with a bleed into the left internal capsule and is surrounded by a region of oedema (dark area). (Courtesy of Dr Margaret Jones.)

- primary intracerebral haemorrhage (PICH), bleeding within the brain
- ventricular haemorrhage, bleeding into the ventricles
- subdural haematoma, bleeding into the subdural space.

Subarachnoid haemorrhages commonly occur as a result of rupture of an aneurysm on the circle of Willis or the base of one of the cerebral arteries. The onset of the haemorrhage may be precipitated by activities that raise the blood pressure, such as heavy exertion or straining. Onset is marked by a sudden, usually severe headache. In severe cases, coma and death may ensue within minutes, particularly if there is brainstem involvement, and 50% of patients die within the first month.

Primary intracerebral haemorrhage (Fig. 3.11.6) is typically associated with hypertension and the symptoms, particularly in less severe cases, may not be distinguishable from infarction due to arterial occlusion.

In severe cases, death results because of herniation of the brain tissue by the volume of blood.

Subdural haematomas may occur spontaneously but are often the result of traumatic injury. The onset of symptoms is often slow and related to compression of the underlying brain tissue giving rise to headaches, episodes of confusion and drowsiness. Early diagnosis is important since evacuation of the fluid can lead to full recovery.

Basic Science 3.11.1

Brain imaging techniques

The investigation of neurological disorders and the study of the living brain have been dramatically enhanced by the development of new imaging techniques. Of particular importance are angiography, computerized tomography (CT), positron emission tomography (PET) and magnetic resonance imaging (MRI).

Angiography

Angiography allows detailed examination of the blood supply to the brain by means of intravascular injection of a radio-opaque material followed by X-ray radiography to record the location of the dye within the vasculature (Fig. BS3.11.1). This can therefore be employed to locate occlusions, aneurysms, etc., in the blood vessels and their territories.

Computerized tomography

Computerized tomography involves projecting a set of narrow X-ray beams from a source on one side of the head, to a detector on the opposite side. The source and detector are rotated progressively and the X-ray transmission is measured at each site. The result is a picture of a section through the brain (Fig. BS3.11.2) which, because of the large number of individual transmission measurements, enables the soft tissue structures to be identified. Such a technique enables localization of an infarct or haemorrhage, or a tumour, etc.

Positron emission tomography

Positron emission tomography (PET) is based on the principle of CT and the production of images that represent levels of activity within the brain. The subject receives a dose of a radioactive isotope, such as ^{11}C or ^{13}N, which is substituted within a molecule such as the analogue of glucose, 2-deoxyglucose. The isotopes emit positrons, which collide with electrons, generating two gamma rays, which travel in opposite directions. The gamma rays are recorded by detectors placed around the head, enabling the localization of the point of

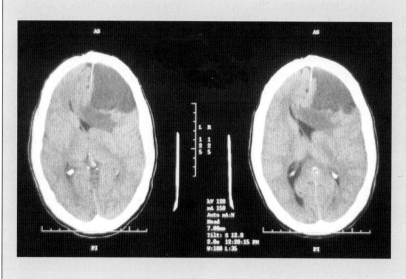

Fig. BS3.11.1 Angiography. Contrast medium injected into the blood supply of the brain shows up this left frontal infarct which is shown without contrast in Figure 3.11.2. (Courtesy of Dr Margaret Jones.)

Basic Science *(Continued)*

emission. Since the glucose analogue will be taken up more by areas that are actively metabolizing, these areas will appear bright on the resultant image of the brain, enabling determination of the dynamic state of activity.

Magnetic resonance imaging

Magnetic resonance imaging is also based on computerized tomography but has the advantage of higher resolution without the use of X-rays or radioactive material. The principle of the technique is based on the phenomenon that when elements with an odd atomic weight, such as hydrogen, are exposed to a strong magnetic field, the nucleus behaves as a magnet and spins within the field. Normally the axis of rotation is parallel with the magnetic field but this can be perturbed by a pulse of radio waves. When the pulse is turned off, the nucleus

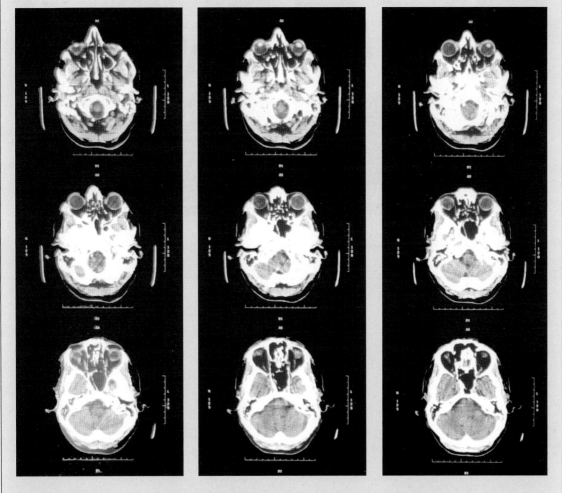

Fig. BS3.11.2 A CT scan provides images of slices of the brain. (Courtesy of Dr Margaret Jones.)

Basic Science *(Continued)*

returns to its original orientation within the magnetic field, releasing energy as radio waves as it does so. The frequency of the radio waves emitted and the rate at which the nucleus returns to its original state (the relaxation time) are characteristic for the nucleus within each specific compound, so, for example, the relaxation time for hydrogen in fat is more rapid than in water. Both these characteristics can be measured and used to produce images that allow contrast between the different tissues (Fig. BS3.11.3).

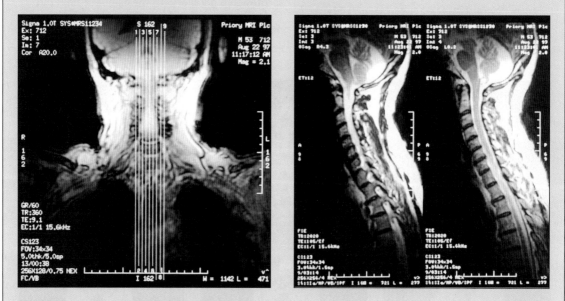

Fig. BS3.11.3 Magnetic resonance imaging. The vertical lines in the large image show where the 'slices' (two of which are shown) in editor Professor Davies's brainstem and cervical spinal cord were imaged.

Further reading

Carpenter R H S 1996 *Neurophysiology*, 3rd edn. Arnold, London.

A first-class read. Concise but comprehensive approach to a difficult subject book comes with interesting PC program of interactive simulations of neural processes.

Fillenz M 1990 *Noradrenergic neurons.* Cambridge University Press, Cambridge.

A monograph covering the development of our understanding of noradrenergic mechanisms.

Goldberg S 2000 *Clinical neuroanatomy made ridiculously simple*, 2nd edn. MedMaster Inc, Miami.

Unique, highly entertaining little book intended for medical students but useful to others. It reduces neuroanatomy to a minimum and includes relevant clinical examples of pathology.

Hammond C (ed) 1996 *Cellular and molecular neurobiology.* Academic Press, London.

A novel problem-based approach to the molecular aspects of neurobiology. Its illustrations demonstrate many of the classical experiments on which our modern knowledge are based and the text encourages students to formulate hypotheses to be tested. .

Shepherd G M 1994 *Neurobiology*, 3rd edn. Oxford University Press Inc, New York.

Aimed primarily at students on neuroscience courses, this book will be of interest to the student of medical sciences wishing to put his basic knowledge into the context of biological levels of organization and comparative biology.

Stjarne L, Misghina M, Stjarne E 1990 *Upstream regulation of the release probability in sympathetic nerve varicosities.* Neuroscience 36: 571–587.

A stimulating review of the contentious aspects of the regulation of the local control of sympathetic nerve varicosities.

Zigmond, M J et al (eds) 1999 *Fundamental Neuroscience (book and CD-ROM).* Academic Press, London.

Superb comprehensive cover of the subject with outstanding illustrations. A first-class reference for those interested in this subject.

Questions

Answer true or false to the following statements:

3.1

Nervous control:

A. Involves electrical and chemical signals.
B. Depends on tightly regulated exocytosis.
C. Is always excitatory.
D. Makes use of voltage-operated and ligand-operated channels.
E. Is more rapid when the nerves involved have a small diameter.

3.2

Sympathetic nerves:

A. Usually have shorter preganglionic fibres than parasympathetic nerves.
B. Leave the spinal cord in the S2,3,4 region.
C. Release adrenaline from their postganglionic nerve terminals.
D. Release acetylcholine from their preganglionic fibres.
E. Have a positive chronotropic effect on the heart.

3.3

Noradrenaline:

A. Is synthesized by hydroxylation of dopamine.
B. Is more potent in activating β-adrenoceptors than α-adrenoceptors.
C. Is degraded by monoamine oxidase within the junctional gap between nerve and target cell.
D. Is released from the adrenal medulla.
E. Release is limited by feedback inhibition.

3.4

Neuromuscular transmission in skeletal muscle:

A. Relies on cholinergic stimulation of nicotinic receptors.
B. Is suppressed in low $[Ca^{2+}]$ solutions.
C. Generates an all-or-nothing endplate potential.
D. Is promoted by inhibitors of acetylcholinesterase.
E. Activates a cationic membrane current through ligand-gated channels.

3.5

Motor units:

A. Consist of a muscle fibre and all the motoneurones which innervate it.
B. In large postural muscles have a low innervation ratio.
C. Contain α-motoneurones with their cell bodies in the ventral horn of the spinal cord.
D. Containing glycolytic muscle fibres tend to be recruited before those containing oxidative muscle fibres.
E. Can contribute to an increased force of contraction by increasing action potential amplitude.

3.6

In the muscle stretch reflex:

A. The receptors are sensitive to changes in muscle tension.
B. The sensitivity of the muscle spindles can be adjusted by changes in γ-motoneurone activity.
C. Reciprocal inhibition relaxes muscles antagonistic to the stretched muscle.
D. The excitatory reflex arc is monosynaptic.
E. The afferent output from primary sensory endings on the muscle spindles adapts more rapidly than that from secondary endings.

3.7

Defects of the cerebellum:

A. Are associated with reduced muscle tone.
B. Cause ataxia.
C. Are classically associated with difficulty in initiating voluntary movement.
D. Cause dysmetria.
E. Involving the right side of the cerebellum will cause symptoms on the left side of the body.

3.8

Sensory pathways:

A. Carrying proprioceptive information ascend ipsilaterally within the spinal cord.
B. Originate as primary sensory neurones whose axons enter the spinal cord via the ventral root.
C. For all sensory modalities pass through the thalamus before they are consciously perceived at the cortical level.
D. Give rise to conscious awareness of touch through neuronal connections with the somatosensory cortex in the precentral gyrus.
E. Involving rapidly adapting receptors are activated strongly by high-frequency stimuli.

3.9

In sensory transduction:

A. The amplitude of the stimulus is coded for by the frequency of the sensory action potentials.
B. The amplitude of the stimulus is coded for by the amplitude of the receptor potential.
C. Stimulation of the receptor always leads to membrane depolarization.
D. Lateral inhibition in primary sensory neurones enhances contrast perception.
E. The perceived sensory modality is entirely dependent on the nature of the stimulus.

3.10

Pain:

A. Pathways contain exclusively myelinated fibres.
B. From viscera may be referred to skin innervated by the same spinal segments.
C. Pathways may be activated directly by prostaglandins.
D. Transmission in the spinal cord can be inhibited when other afferent neurones to the same spinal segment are stimulated.
E. Transmission in the spinal cord can be inhibited by activation of descending pathways from the medulla.

(Answers overleaf →)

Answers

3.1

A. **True.** Electrical action potentials lead to release of chemical neurotransmitters.

B. **True.** This is the basis of transmitter release.

C. **False.** It may be excitatory or inhibitory.

D. **True.** Action potentials depend on voltage-operated channels but transmitters act on ligand-operated channels.

E. **False.** Large axons conduct more rapidly (especially if also myelinated).

3.2

A. **True.** These often terminate in pre- and paravertebral sympathetic ganglia.

B. **False.** They exit the spinal cord between T1 and L2/3.

C. **False.** They release noradrenaline.

D. **True.** This acts on nicotinic receptors on the postganglionic cells.

E. **True.** They increase heart rate, an important β_1-adrenoceptor effect.

3.3

A. **True.**

B. **False.** It is more potent at α-adrenoceptors; adrenaline has similar potencies at both α- and β-receptors.

C. **False.** Monoamine oxidase is located in mitochondria within the nerves.

D. **True.** The adrenal medulla releases adrenaline and noradrenaline in a ratio of approximately 10:1.

E. **True.** This is mediated by α_2-adrenoceptors on the nerve terminal (presynaptic receptors).

3.4

A. **True.**

B. **True.** This inhibits exocytosis of transmitter, which requires Ca^{2+} influx.

C. **False.** The EPP is a graded potential, unlike the action potential.

D. **True.** This slows the breakdown of transmitter within the neuromuscular cleft.

E. **True.** A mixed Na^+/K^+ current flows through the nicotinic receptor/channel when activated by acetylcholine, i.e. the ligand.

3.5

A. **False.** A motor unit is a single motoneurone and all the fibres it controls.

B. **False.** It tends to be high in these muscles, i.e. a lot of fibres are controlled by one motoneurone.

C. **True.**

D. **False.** Slow oxidative motor units are recruited before faster glycolytic ones.

E. **False.** Action potential amplitude is fixed; frequency of firing and number of active motor units can be increased to increase force.

3.6

A. **False.** Muscle spindles are sensitive to changes in muscle length.

B. **True.** These innervate the contractile regions of the spindles.

C. **True.**

D. **True.** This is the simplest possible reflex arc.

E. **True.** The primary endings provide both a dynamic and a static response to stretch; secondary endings mainly show a static response.

3.7

A. **True.**
B. **True.** Unsteadiness reflects loss of cerebellar regulation of posture.
C. **False.** This is more typically a feature of defects of the basal ganglia.
D. **True.** This is due to loss of the motor predictive role of the cerebellum.
E. **False.** The cerebellum causes symptoms ipsilateral to the defect.

3.8

A. **True.** They ascend within the dorsal columns. This information crosses from one side of the CNS to the other at the level of the medulla oblongata.
B. **False.** The sensory roots enter dorsally.
C. **False.** The exception is the olfactory pathway, which connects directly with the olfactory cortex. It also makes connections with the thalamus, however.
D. **False.** The somatosensory cortex is in the postcentral gyrus.
E. **True.** This type of receptor responds best to rapidly changing stimulus strength.

3.9

A. **True.**
B. **True.** This in turn controls action potential frequency.
C. **False.** This is usually true but in some cases, e.g. photoreceptors, the response is hyperpolarization.
D. **True.** This also improves spatial localization of touch, e.g. in two-point discrimination tests.
E. **False.** The perceived sensation depends on the receptor which is activated, e.g. mechanical stimulation of the retina by intense pressure on the eyeball is perceived as light. The principle that stimulation of a given receptor always leads to the same perceived sensation is called 'the labelled line' principle.

3.10

A. **False.** Pain is carried by a mixture of Aδ and unmyelinated C fibres.
B. **True.**
C. **False.** Prostaglandins lower the threshold for receptor activation but do not activate the nociceptors directly.
D. **True.** Inhibition of pain transmission in the spinal cord following activation of Aβ sensory fibres is sometimes referred to as 'pain gating'.
E. **True.**

Special senses and higher functions

4

Introduction

Our sense of the world around us and our position in it is largely made up of information provided by what are known as 'special senses', the senses of sight, sound, balance, taste and smell. The organs of special sense, the eyes, ears and taste-buds, are each superbly sensitive to one specific type of energy and turn it into our sensations. Although, as we will see in this section, the organs of special sense deal with very small parts of our sensory surroundings we perceive a whole (a *Gestalt*) which we recognize as consciousness. Although most people can provide a fairly good working definition of consciousness, closer scrutiny reveals philosophical difficulties with the concept and that of 'mind' which is generally considered the basis of consciousness. Although there are few who would now agree with Aristotle that the heart is the physiological basis of mind there are still philosophers who will argue Descartes' proposition that mind is something immaterial and separate from the brain. Such considerations are beyond the scope of this book. We need only accept that consciousness is a state requiring a series of processes to be going on in the brain.

The concept that the brain is the 'processor' of consciousness is reinforced by the ability to follow the individual pieces of sensory information from the environment to specific regions of the brain. Thus activity from specific photoreceptors in the eye travel through pathways in the brain where highly specific individual characteristics of the optical image on the retina are extracted; characteristics, for example, as basic as whether or not a line is vertical. These characteristics are not sensed as such; we perceive a face as a face even though the lines that make it up may alter considerably. This is why what we sense depends on previous experience and why the process of learning is included in this section on special senses.

Section overview

This section outlines:

- The nature of special senses and specific stimuli
- How visual accommodation is brought about
- The reflex control of eye movements
- The structure and properties of the retina
- Central visual pathways and the visual cortex
- Sound conduction and impedance matching in the ear
- Processing of auditory signals
- The inner ear in detection of movement and rotation
- Taste and odour transduction
- Consciousness in sleep and arousal
- Learning and memory mechanisms.

Vision

4.1

Seeing

As you read this page you have a perception of a single coherent object. If you look around the environment in which you are at present, it is likewise a single coherent space. Your perception of objects and your environment is one created by your nervous system from the constant flow of information from your senses. The degree of agreement between this perception and reality depends on the quality of that information and the ability of your CNS to process it. The importance of the latter is illustrated by the effectiveness of camouflage in nature. A brown leveret set in its form surrounded by green grass is not seen. If its presence is pointed out you see it clearly. The image on the retina of the eye has not changed, only the CNS interpretation.

Seeing is not a passive process. We scan our environment constantly with varying attention. Indeed, if an image is experimentally fixed within our **visual field** it disappears from our perception in a few seconds. Small eye movements prevent this happening in normal life. We do not see the shadow of the retinal blood vessels through which the light has to pass to the **retina** because they are always in a fixed relation to the retina.

In viewing a complex image, our eyes follow the contours of the image, stopping where two contours meet. We also fixate on features we

Basic Science 4.1.1

Spherical lenses

When a beam of light passes from air into a more dense medium like glass or water it is bent towards the perpendicular (Fig. BS4.1.1). This is due to the light being slowed up as it enters the more dense medium and is referred to as refraction.

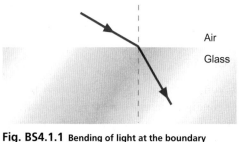

Air

Glass

Fig. BS4.1.1 Bending of light at the boundary between materials of different optical density.

This effect is used in lenses. Spherical lenses have surfaces which are parts of a sphere. They can be convex (positive) where the glass itself is part of a sphere (Fig. BS4.1.2A) or concave (negative) where the glass is hollowed out as if a sphere were pushed into it (Fig. BS4.1.2B). The properties of spherical lenses are very well known and can therefore be accurately used to correct defects of vision.

A lens forms one of two types of image. A *real* image is one that can be focused on a screen or piece of paper and is formed by convex lenses as a result of converging beams of light (Fig. BS4.1.3).

A *virtual* image cannot be focused on a screen because the relevant light rays are diverging, and as an image is a theoretical concept (Fig. BS4.1.4). A virtual image can be converted into a real image by a convex lens system such as the eye, and in fact the rays of light which form our view of the world around us are diverging or at the most parallel from distant objects.

The strength of lenses is described in terms of their *focal length*. Light from very distant objects is travelling in parallel beams; a lens focuses such

A

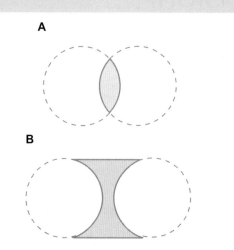

B

Fig. BS4.1.2 Spherical lenses. **A.** Convex. **B.** Concave.

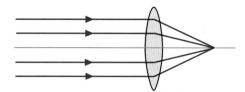

Fig. BS4.1.3 A convex lens converges light rays.

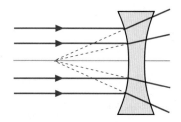

Fig. BS4.1.4 A concave lens diverges light rays.

a beam at its *focal point* which is a point on the optical axis of the lens at a distance of 1 focal length away from the lens. A positive lens has its focal point on the opposite side from the object which forms the image. It has a positive focal length (Fig. BS4.1.5A). A negative lens has its virtual image on the same side as the object producing it. It has a negative focal length (Fig. BS4.1.5B).

Basic Science 4.1.1 *(Continued)*

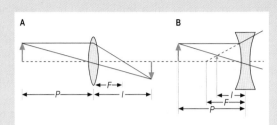

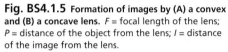

Fig. BS4.1.5 Formation of images by (A) a convex and (B) a concave lens. *F* = focal length of the lens; *P* = distance of the object from the lens; *I* = distance of the image from the lens.

There is a simple relationship between the distance of an object (*P*) and its image (*I*) from a lens and the focal length of the lens (*F*):

$$\frac{1}{F} = \frac{1}{P} + \frac{1}{I}.$$

You can see from this the truth of the statement that when light is coming from a very distant object it forms an image at the focal length, because 1 divided by a very large number = 0 and $1/F = 0 + 1/I$, so $F = I$.

If *F* is measured in metres then $1/F$ is the strength of the lens in dioptres (D).

So a positive lens of focal length 0.1 m has a strength of +10 D. A negative lens of focal length −0.5 m has a strength of −2 D.

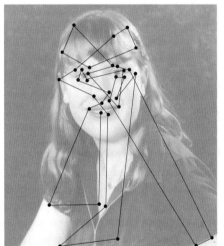

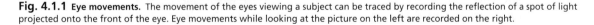

Fig. 4.1.1 Eye movements. The movement of the eyes viewing a subject can be traced by recording the reflection of a spot of light projected onto the front of the eye. Eye movements while looking at the picture on the left are recorded on the right.

consider significant. If the image is of a human face, the eyes and mouth are fixated particularly often (Fig. 4.1.1).

We have some understanding of the collection of information by the visual system but do not have a neurophysiological understanding of its conversion into a perception.

The eye

The important structures of the eye are illustrated by an anterior view and a horizontal section (Fig. 4.1.2).

The intact view of the eye shows the eyelids, the conjunctiva covering the visible **sclera**, and

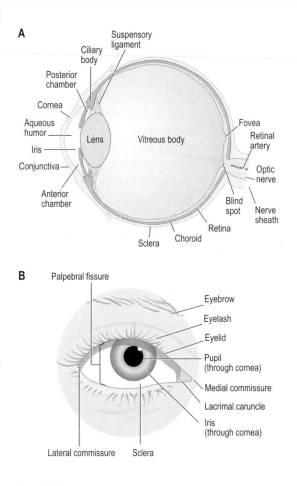

A

Suspensory
ligament

Ciliary
body

Posterior
chamber

Cornea

Aqueous
humor

Iris

Conjunctiva

Anterior
chamber

Lens

Vitreous body

Fovea

Retinal
artery

Optic
nerve

Blind
spot

Nerve
sheath

Retina

Sclera

Choroid

B Palpebral fissure

Eyebrow

Eyelash

Eyelid

Pupil
(through cornea)

Medial commissure

Lacrimal caruncle

Iris
(through cornea)

Lateral commissure   Sclera

Fig. 4.1.2 The eye. A. Horizontal section through the right
eyeball. The anterior and posterior chambers make up the
anterior segment. The vitreous body occupies the posterior
segment. **B.** Surface anatomy of the right eye.

the transparent **cornea** showing the **iris** whose
contraction varies the diameter of the **pupil**.

The visible part of the eye is covered with a
thin fluid layer. This **lacrimal fluid** is produced
by the tear glands situated under the upper
temporal part of the eye socket and is spread
over the exposed surface of the cornea and conjunctiva by continuous involuntary blinking. It
is similar in composition to an ultrafiltrate of
blood plasma. It prevents the exposed living
cells of the cornea and conjunctiva from drying
out, rinses small foreign bodies from the con-
junctival space and has bactericidal properties.

The horizontal section of the eye shows its
internal structure. The sensory apparatus of
the eye is the retina whose acuity, the ability
to separate two close images, is far greater at
the **fovea** than elsewhere. A sharp image of
the environment on the fovea is produced by
refraction of the light by the lens and at the
corneal–air interface. The lens only accounts for
about 25% of this refraction but adjustment of
its power by the action of the **ciliary muscle** is
the basis of **accommodation** when a close object
is studied.

The **anterior segment** (anterior compartment)
of the eye is filled with transparent fluid, the
aqueous humor, which is formed by the **ciliary
bodies**, circulates through the **anterior** and **posterior** chambers, which make up the anterior
segment, and drains into the **canal of Schlemm**.
The formation and removal of the aqueous
humor determines the pressure within the
eyeball.

The **posterior segment** is filled with a transparent, gelatinous, vitreous body. It is a gel of
hyaluronic acid. One important function of the
vitreous body is to damp the movements of
the eye.

The retina is nourished by two vascular networks. The **choroid plexus** supplies the outermost layers nearest to the sclera (the fibrous ball
of the eye). The choroid is also densely pigmented to prevent light scattering in the eye.
Those retinal cells close to the vitreous body are
supplied by branches of the central artery of the
retina, which enters the eye through the papilla
of the optic nerve. These blood vessels are optically between the lens and the retina but are
sparsest in the region of the fovea.

The blink reflex

This is a very important reflex that protects the
eye from damage. It is very robust and is one of
the last to be lost during general anaesthesia.
The afferent side of the reflex arc can be either
the visual system – something seen rapidly
approaching the face will cause a blink – or

tactile stimuli to the cornea or conjunctiva – a small foreign body 'in the eye' will cause blinking. The usefulness of this latter response together with the increased lacrimation that is also caused by dust on the cornea is obvious. However, if a foreign body is sharp, and blinking causes scratching of the surface of the eye, the pain inhibits the blink reflex and the eyelids are shut. This protects the cornea from abrasion, which is slow to heal.

If you ever anaesthetize the cornea for any purpose you must cover and protect the eye until sensation is fully recovered. Should you fail to do this and a bit of grit does get in the eye, the normal continuous involuntary blinking, which spreads lacrimal fluid, will in a short time severely abrade the cornea of that eye.

Accommodation

The adequate stimulus for vision is light falling on the retina. A real inverted image of the object is produced on the retina. The information content of the image is related to the sharpness with which the refractive surfaces focus the image. Accommodation is the adjustment of this focus for objects at differing distances from the eye. At rest in the normal, **emmetropic**, eye distant objects are in focus. This is known as the **far point** of the eye. Maximum accommodation in the young will focus objects a few centimetres from the eye. This is known as the **near point**.

Accommodation to near objects is the result of a fattening of the lens which increases its refractive power. The lens is normally under a radial tension generated by the pressure within the eyeball (the intraocular tension) acting on the lens via the suspensory ligaments. This tension flattens the lens and reduces its refractive power.

When a near object is studied, contraction of the ciliary muscle takes the tension off the suspensory ligament and the lens relaxes, returning to its fatter shape, which increases its refractive power (Fig. 4.1.3). With age, the elasticity of the lens is lost and, so, when unloaded, less accommodation is possible. The near point moves away from the subject. Children have a near point of some 10 cm (an accommodation of 10 D – 1 m/10 cm) and this increases more or less linearly with age. By the age of 50, it has deteriorated to 50 cm (2 D) and by 70 it is at more than 1 m (<1 D). This defect is called

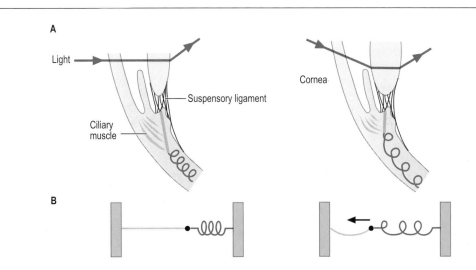

Fig. 4.1.3 Accommodation. A. In accommodation for viewing a near object, the ciliary muscles take up the tension transmitted from the wall of the eye to the lens capsule and allow it to become more spherical and therefore more powerful in refracting light. **B.** An analogy is a rope held in tension between two posts by a spring – pulling on the spring takes the tension off the rope and allows it to sag.

presbyopia and this loss of the ability to increase the refractive power for viewing near objects is compensated for by wearing reading glasses with convex lenses.

Emmetropia is the condition in which the refractive system matches the size of the eyeball. If there is a mismatch between the diameter of the eyeball and the power of the refractive system, a defect is present. If the eyeball is too long for the refractive system only near objects can be focused. This is **myopia**, shortsightedness. The excess of power of the refractive system can be corrected by wearing concave (negative) lenses that produce, at the far point of the myopic eye, a virtual image of the object. The lens is reducing the converging power of the eye's optics (Fig. 4.1.4). If the eyeball is too short for the refractive system, then distant objects can only be focused by accommodation, whose useful range is thus reduced. This is **hypermetropia**, farsightedness. This lack of refractive power can be corrected by wearing convex (positive) lenses that increase the converging power of the eye's optics (Fig. 4.1.4).

In the case of **astigmatism**, the eye's refractive system does not have equal power in all planes. The curvature of the system is greater in one plane than another, and if a sun-burst of lines is viewed, only those in one plane can be focused at any time (Fig 4.1.5). It is as if a cylindrical lens were present in the eye's optics. This defect is corrected by wearing glasses containing an appropriately aligned cylindrical lens whose power equals that of the eye's defect. This equalizes the power of the refractive system in all planes.

Damage to the cornea can produce scarring that results in the refractive system behaving as though it were made up of lenses of many different powers. Any image on the retina is blurred. This defect can be corrected by contact lenses that allow the cornea to interface with tears that fill the space behind the lens, very much reducing the refractive index change at the cornea.

Eye movements and their reflex control

When an object close to the observer is studied, not only must the eye accommodate but eye movement must occur to keep the images in the two eyes on both their foveae. The eyes

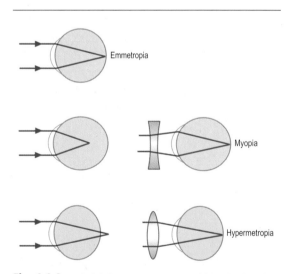

Fig. 4.1.4 Optical defects. In emmetropia (the normal eye) the image is focused on the retina. In myopia, where the eye is too long for the power of its optics, the image is focused in front of the retina; this can be corrected by a concave, diverging, lens. In hypermetropia, where the eye is too short for the power of its optics, the image is focused behind the retina; this can be corrected by a convex, converging, lens.

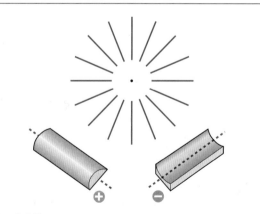

Fig. 4.1.5 Astigmatism. An eye with astigmatism sees lines in one direction on the 'wheel' less clearly than those in other directions. This can be corrected by adding a positive or negative cylindrical lens.

converge. The control of this **convergence** is in part driven by the accommodation needed to keep the object in focus (convergence occurs during accommodation even if one eye is covered) and is due in part to an image comparison by the central visual system.

If the object moves it has to be tracked. An object must be held stationary on the fovea to allow the visual system to extract the maximum information. This process involves not only the control of the movement of the eye in the orbit, and the head on body movements that facilitate tracking, but also many postural reflexes that stabilize the position of the head in space (see pp. 228 and 243). You can easily fixate a fly and track its movement at a distance of 20 m. The control system is complex and involves processing of the visual input at a high level in the CNS. The eye and its extraocular muscles have evolved to allow precise movement control. The extraocular muscles have very small motor units – single motor neurones that do not branch extensively and innervate few muscle fibres, which are themselves small. The force produced can therefore be graded in small increments. The vitreous body of the eye is important as a damper of eye movement. It is a viscous gel. When the eye moves the vitreous body lags behind. The friction between it and the moving eye acts as a damper and creates what is known as a critically damped system. If you have floaters, small opacities in the vitreous body which cast shadows on the retina, you can see this happening if you look at a bright plane surface and move your fixation point. Your floaters will initially lag behind your eye movement and then catch up, usually without overshooting.

If a series of objects move rapidly past an observer or the observer rotates in a stationary environment, such as swivelling on an office chair, eye movement transiently fixes and tracks individual objects and then flicks backwards and fixes a new object. The eye is described as moving in **saccades**. This type of movement is also produced by semicircular canal stimulation (see p. 336).

Movements of the iris

Movement of the iris changes the diameter of the pupil. This will control the amount of light falling on the retina.

Reflex changes in the pupil size also accompany accommodation unrelated to the changes in light intensity. Changing fixation from a distant to a near object causes the pupils to constrict. This is called the near point or convergence response. Objects are usually brought close to the face for detailed examination. Pupillary constriction improves the quality of the image on the retina by restricting light entering the eye to that passing through the more optically perfect centre of the cornea.

The most obvious changes in pupil size occur in response to changes in the brightness of the environment. This allows the visual system to operate efficiently in conditions of rapidly changing illumination; the pupil opens as the illumination falls and constricts as it rises. Light need only be shone into one eye to produce a constriction of both pupils, whose diameter is normally identical. Dissimilar pupil diameters always require medical explanation. When light is shone into only one eye, the response of the pupil of the illuminated eye is called the **direct light response**, that of the other eye the **consensual response**.

The overall sensitivity of the eye to light can be varied over several orders of magnitude. However, adjustment of pupil diameter will only compensate for small changes in illumination. You will be dazzled by car headlights at night and you will initially see little if you walk out of a well-lit room into a starlit night. In both instances your vision will improve with time. You will adapt. The basis of this adaptation is dramatic changes in the sensitivity of the light-sensitive cells of the retina, the **rods** and **cones** (see p. 303).

Summary

Physics of the eye

- Lacrimal fluid and the blink reflex are important protection for the cornea and conjunctiva.
- Aqueous humor formed by the ciliary bodies fills the anterior and posterior chambers and drains into the canal of Schlemm.

- The viscous gel which fills the chamber behind the lens dampens eye movement.
- Accommodation brought about by allowing the lens to bulge is reduced with age.
- Convergence of the eyes on a near object is accompanied by constriction of the pupil.
- The major adaptation to changing levels of light is by changing the sensitivity of the retina.

The retina

The retina is the light-sensitive part of the eye that occupies the position and function of the film in a photographic camera. It is not a uniform structure. The optic nerve with its central artery penetrates the retina and at this point there are no rods or cones; this produces a '**blind spot**'. You can experience your blind spot by fixating (staring fixedly and unblinkingly) on the cross in Figure 4.1.6 with your right eye (left eye closed) at a distance of about 25 cm. Move the book towards or away from you slowly until the spot disappears. If you are good at this sort of visual trick, the pattern behind the dot will appear to fill the gap as a result of the visual system 'extrapolating'.

At another point close to the centre of the retina is the **macula lutea** (yellow spot). In the centre of this is a slight depression, the **fovea centralis**. Here the overlying blood vessels are at a minimum and retinal cones most numerous, making this the region of greatest visual acuity and the point at which we focus an image in the eye.

The rods and cones that make up the photoreceptors of the retina differ from each other in structure, function and neural connections. The activity of cones is dominant in bright light to give us **photopic vision** with its high acuity,

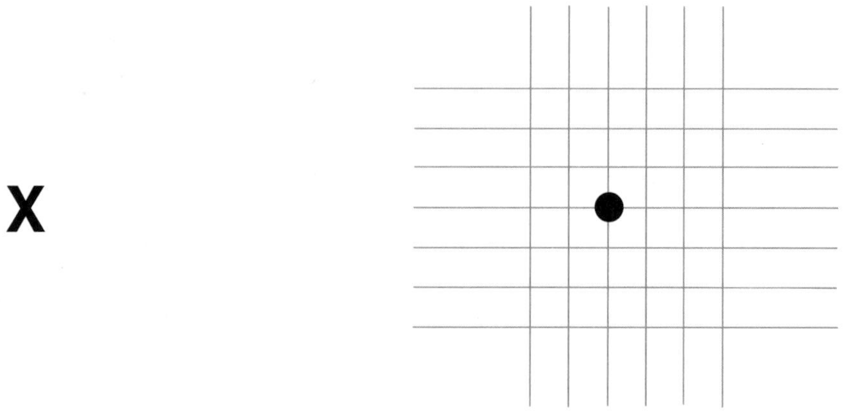

Fig. 4.1.6 The blind spot. Hold the book about 25 cm from your face. Close your left eye and fixate with your right eye on the cross. Slowly move the book towards or away from you and you will find a place where the dot disappears. The grid behind appears to be continuous.

colour and pattern recognition. During low levels of light, **scotopic vision** prevails and 'in the dark all cats are grey' because only the rods are being stimulated and, although very sensitive, they cannot differentiate colours.

The neural elements of the retina are outgrowths of the brain and it is a whimsical thought that when you look into someone's eye with an ophthalmoscope you are looking at part of that person's brain.

Rods and cones

The rods and cones of the visual system have very different functional characteristics. This is in part due to the way they are connected in the nervous system. For example, there are more rods connected to a **ganglion cell** in the rod system than cones to a ganglion cell in the cone system and, while the ratio of photoreceptors to ganglion cells is 1 : 1 in the fovea, there is considerable convergence in other parts of the retina with the overall ratio being about 100 photoreceptors to each ganglion cell. The rods collect light from a greater area to ensure excitation of their ganglion but in doing so sacrifice optical resolution of detail in the image (Fig. 4.1.7). The structure of rods and cones is similar with some differences (Fig. 4.1.8). Both consist

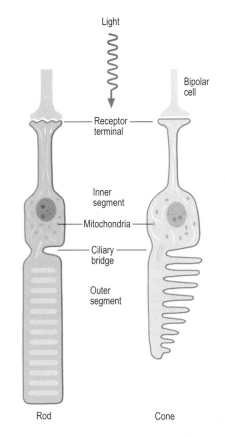

Fig. 4.1.8 Structure of rods and cones. The outer segment of both rods and cones forms 'discs' from the cell membrane. In rods, these are replaced at a regular rate; no similar mechanism exists in cones. This representation is diagrammatic – in actual rods and cones there are about 1000 membrane discs or infoldings per cell.

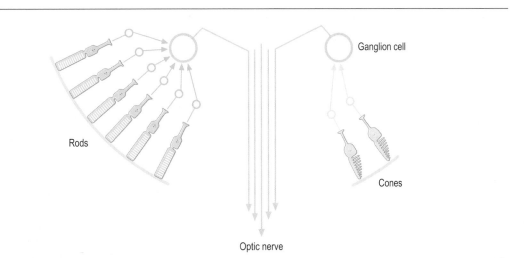

Fig. 4.1.7 Convergence in the retina. A ganglion cell in the rod system receives input from a converging system of rods which cover a larger field in the retina than that served by a ganglion cell in the cone system.

of an inner segment which is continuous with the receptor's terminal; and an outer segment that is connected to the inner by a ciliary bridge.

The outer segment of the receptors contains an elaborate system of about 1000 stacked discs which are formed from the cell membrane and contain the visual photopigments, molecules arranged in such a way as to maximize the chance of them being hit by photons of light. The extensive folding of the membrane also increases the area for light trapping. The rods and cones of the vertebrate eye are a unique type of receptor. In the absence of their specific stimulus (light) their membrane potential is only about −30 mV and a large 'dark current' flows through the cell membrane. In the light, the membrane resistance increases, membrane current falls and the membrane hyperpolarizes to a more negative voltage. This is the opposite of what happens in all other receptors when stimulated (except hair cells in the cochlea of the ear; their membrane potential oscillates either side of zero).

The hyperpolarization is initiated by the absorption of a photon by the **visual pigments** of the rods and cones. The visual pigment **rhodopsin** in rods is made up of two parts, one of which (retinal) is chemically closely related to vitamin A_1. Retinal can exist in two forms and the impact of a photon (particularly of a wavelength of about 500 nm) on the *cis* (bent-tail) form straightens it out into the *trans* form. This is the only point at which light is involved in the whole process of vision. One photon will drive a molecule of rhodopsin into a higher energy state, which decomposes into a colour-less opsin and vitamin A_1, a process known as bleaching of the visual pigment. Rods have one type of visual pigment, rhodopsin; cones are of three subtypes according to which of three visual pigments they contain, pigments which are most sensitive to blue, green or red light.

The process of bleaching rhodopsin is linked by a G-protein to the activation of phosphodi-esterase, which in turn converts the cyclic neuc-leotide cGMP to GMP. Sodium channels in the plasma membrane are maintained open by cGMP so its reduction by light causes the rod or cone to become hyperpolarized. Calcium is involved in this process, probably influencing the rate of receptor adaptation.

In the short term there is a logarithmic rela-tionship between the intensity of illumination (I_1), the previous level of illumination (I_2) and the amplitude of the receptor potential (A):

$$A = k \times -\log \frac{I_1}{I_2} \, \text{mV}.$$

The negative sign means that the change is hyperpolarization.

The electrical activity of the retina can be recorded on the surface of the body as the **elec-troretinogram** detected by electrodes placed about the orbit of the eye. The retina creates a voltage difference such that the cornea is posi-tive. This potential can be used to detect eye movement and also the response of the retina to flashes of light.

Dark adaptation

Vision in bright environments (photopic vision) and in low light conditions (scotopic vision) has several distinctive features.

In the long term the sensitivity of the pho-toreceptors is determined by their previous exposure to light. The bleaching of the visual pigment by light is reversed by metabolism. This process, **dark adaptation**, is not very fast (Fig. 4.1.9).

The time-course of dark adaptation is bipha-sic. An initial rapid change is almost complete by between 5 and 10 minutes. This is followed by a further slower increase in sensitivity over the next half hour. The early component is related to cone adaptation, the later to rod adaptation.

The reason for the biphasic shape of the adaptation curve is that rods and cones adapt at different rates. Rod adaptation reaches a maxi-mum only after 30 minutes, whereas full cone adaptation occurs in less than 10 minutes but is 1000 times less effective than that of the rods.

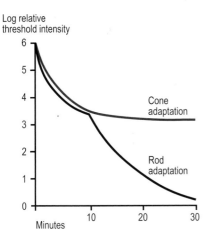

Log relative
threshold intensity

Cone
adaptation

Rod
adaptation

Minutes

Fig. 4.1.9 Dark adaptation. The threshold at which your eyes detect light falls the longer you stay in the dark (you become more sensitive to light). This increase in sensitivity is biphasic because the cones (tested with red light, to which rods are not very sensitive, focused on the fovea, which is mainly cones) adapt more rapidly than rods. The red line is produced with red light; the black line with white light.

The process, in rods, if fully complete, can raise their sensitivity to the theoretical maximum. Fully dark-adapted rods will respond to a single photon.

Since rods have only one pigment and dominate scotopic vision, colour perception is not possible at low light levels. Also, because the fovea has few rods, visual acuity is low in poor light conditions and the sensitivity of the fovea is greatest at its edges. Look at a dim star at night. It may disappear when you fixate it, only to reappear when you look slightly to one side of it. The ability of rods to report flicker is also less than that of cones. The upper limit of temporal resolution, the **flicker fusion frequency**, is lower away from the fovea and during scotopic vision.

Light adaptation is more rapid than dark adaptation, being complete within a minute. Dazzle at night by car headlights is an important problem and occurs during the initial phase of this adaptation, when perception is impaired.

Signal processing in the retina

Seeing is not simply the detection of a visual stimulus on the retina. As one might expect for a part of the brain, the retina carries out a great deal of processing of the signals produced by rods and cones. The next link in the visual pathway, after the rods and cones, is the **bipolar cells** (see Fig. 4.1.10). Some are in contact with rods and the photoreceptors' transmitter, glutamate, causes them to depolarize. Glutamate from *cones* hyperpolarizes most of the bipolar cells they make contact with but in a minority there is depolarization.

Horizontal cells, receiving information from rods and cones over a wide area of the retina, are the basis of lateral inhibition which aids visual discrimination. Horizontal cells and **amacrine cells** respectively modulate the activity of the vertical elements of the retina and provide the only lateral link between the bipolar and ganglion cells, which are the final common pathway out of the retina for visual information that has already been extensively analysed.

It should be remembered that the only part of this system which can produce action potentials for transmission to the visual cortex is the ganglion cells; all other components produce receptor potentials which modulate the rate of production of action potentials.

Like most neural networks the retina is never silent, even when it is not being stimulated. If you remain in the total dark for some time, you will experience the sensation of the darkness lightening so that you are surrounded by a grey fog in which you may even be able to see lighter patches or shapes. These effects are due to spontaneous activity in the nerve cells of the retina.

Again, like other sensory systems, the response of the retina to changed conditions (a stimulus) depends on the original condition to which the system has adapted, and from which the change takes place (an example from another system is the way moderately warm water feels hot to cold hands).

In the case of the retina, *local adaptation* gives rise to **after-images**. If you carry out the experiment in Figure 4.1.11, the parts of the retina exposed to the black circle will have become

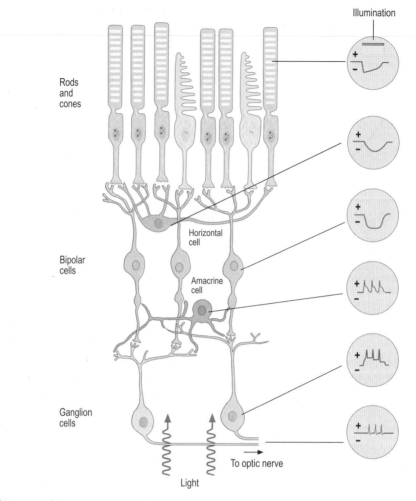

Illumination

Rods
and
cones

Horizontal
cell

Bipolar
cells

Amacrine
cell

Ganglion
cells

To optic nerve

Light

Fig. 4.1.10 **Diagram of the horizontal and vertical elements of the retina and the electrical potentials they produce.** The vertical and horizontal arrangement of cells is the anatomical foundation of many of the neurophysiological characteristics of the retina. The ganglion cells are the only ones to produce action potentials.

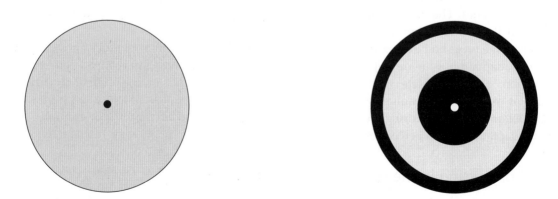

Fig. 4.1.11 **After-images.** Fixate with one eye on the centre of the image on the right for about 30 seconds and then fixate on the centre of the circle on the left. You will see a light centre to the image.

more sensitive than the parts exposed to the light areas. Another good example of this is to look at a bright sky through a window with glazing bars on it. If you then close your eyes an after-image of the bars remains but now as a negative of light images against a dark background.

The chemical processes in the light-sensitive elements of the retina, and the way the neural elements are connected vertically *and* horizontally can explain the visual phenomena we have described and others such as **simultaneous contrast** (see below). These vertical and horizontal connections within the retina give rise to the concept of receptive fields.

Receptive fields

It was suggested more than 100 years ago that vision was made up of two antagonistic systems: one that 'sees' white and the other that 'sees' black. The physiological basis of these two systems was found by the study of what are known as **receptive fields**. The whole visual field is made up of receptive fields which are areas of the retina that send their information to a *single* ganglion cell. The fields of adjacent ganglion cells can overlap considerably owing to the horizontal propagation of information in the retina. Each ganglion cell's activity can be changed by light stimulating even a small region of its receptive field. This receptive field can be subdivided into central and peripheral regions, and illumination of each produces complementary changes in the ganglion cell's activity. The size of the central and peripheral regions is not constant. The centre shrinks in bright illumination.

Some ganglion cells are classed as *on-centre*; their activity is increased by illumination of the centre of their receptive field. Other ganglion cells are *off-centre*; their activity is decreased by illumination of the centre of their receptive field. The antagonistic systems that 'see' white and black are the on-centre neurones and off-centre neurones respectively (Fig. 4.1.12).

Simultaneous contrast

Physiological receptors generally respond to changes rather than absolute levels. In the retina these changes are spatial as well as temporal. The brightness of an object is related to that of the adjacent areas. This leads to edge enhancement and a bright surround to a dark object (Mach's band). Any ganglion cell whose central field just touches an intensity transition will lose the effect of some of its peripheral field, releasing the effect of its centre. If this is an on-centre ganglion cell that is just in a bright field, then it will fire at a higher rate than a neighbouring cell totally within the bright field (Fig. 4.1.13).

Visual pathways

The information from the retinal ganglion cells is carried to the visual areas of the **occipital cortex** via the **lateral geniculate body**. The information from the right half of the visual field travels to the left visual cortex via the left lateral geniculate and the left half via the right lateral geniculate to the right cortex. Fibres from the nasal side of the retina that are stimulated by light from objects in the temporal field of that eye pass along the optic nerve as far as the optic chiasma where they cross over and join fibres from the temporal field of the opposite eye, which have also been stimulated by the same object.

Damage to the visual pathway can be localized because of the characteristic visual field defects produced (see Fig. 4.1.14).

Branches from the retinal ganglion cells also pass from the optic tract to the pretectal region of the midbrain and the superior colliculus where they form the afferent limb of the visual reflexes. Connections with the supraoptic nuclei of the hypothalamus are responsible for various circadian endocrine and other light-driven rhythms.

The lateral geniculate body

The fibres from the retinal ganglion cells synapse in the lateral geniculate body where

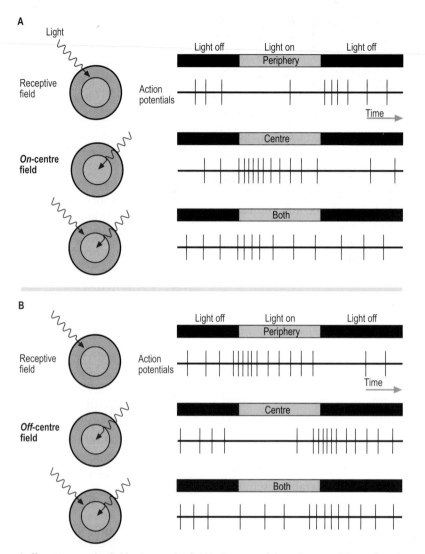

Fig. 4.1.12 On- and off-centre receptive fields. A receptive field is that area of the retina containing rods and cones that serve a single retinal ganglion cell. Ganglion cells are the only parts of the retina that produce action potentials for the optic nerve.
A. On-centre fields increase the rate of action potential discharge when the centre of the field is illuminated. They 'see' white.
B. Off-centre fields decrease the rate of discharge when the centre of the field is illuminated. They 'see' black. In both cases when both the centre and periphery are illuminated, the effect of the centre dominates.

further processing of the visual information is carried out. Information on shape, depth, colour and texture is processed separately from information on movement and changes in light intensity.

The lateral geniculate body consists of six distinct layers arranged rather like the loops of a fingerprint with two large-celled layers and four small-celled layers. It is the large-celled layers that receive input from large retinal ganglion cells and further process movement and flicker information. The small-celled layers receive input from small retinal ganglion cells and further process information about shape, depth, colour and texture (Fig. 4.1.15).

In each layer there is a precise point-to-point representation of the retina. Layers 1, 4 and 6 receive input from the eye on the opposite side

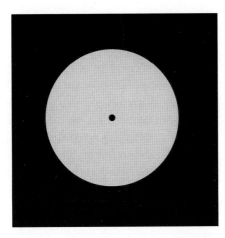

Fig. 4.1.13 **Simultaneous contrast.** The two inner circles are equally uniformly grey but set against different backgrounds the phenomenon of simultaneous contrast causes the outer edge of the left-hand circle to appear lighter and that of the right-hand circle darker than the rest.

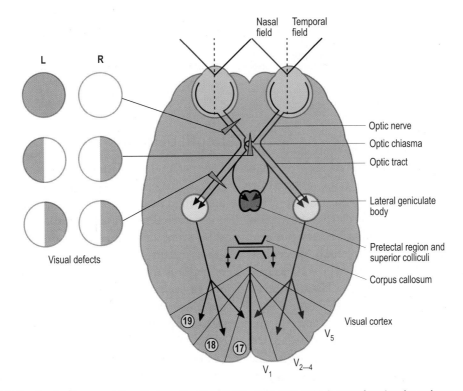

Fig. 4.1.14 **The visual pathway and the effects on the visual fields of the right and left eyes of cutting the pathway at various places.** The visual association areas are labelled with their Brodmann numbers on the left side of the diagram.

and layers 2, 3 and 5 from the eye on the same side. In the different layers these connections are aligned so that information from any single object in the environment is represented in the individual layers so as to form a locus perpendicular to the plane of the layers at that point.

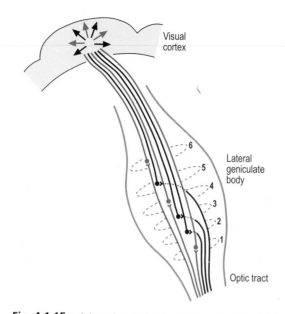

Fig. 4.1.15 Left lateral geniculate body. Fibres from the right eye, shown in red, synapse in layers 1, 4 and 6. Both in the geniculate bodies and on the visual cortex, fibres are arranged in the same order as in the retina (topographical representation) with the retinal fovea being represented by a disproportionately large area for its size.

The visual cortex

The output of the lateral geniculate body connects to the **primary visual cortex** (V_1) in a point-to-point manner. The **visual association areas** (V_2, V_3, V_{3A}, V_4 and V_5) surrounding the primary visual cortex receive information largely from the primary visual cortex but also have some input from the lateral geniculate body. ($V_1 = 17$, V_2–$V_4 = 18$, $V_5 = 19$ in the Brodmann system (see Fig. 4.1.14), another example of too many names for the same thing.)

The result of the further processing of the information within the cortex is that individual cells become more selective in their response. Some cells respond to bars or edges with a particular orientation in the visual field. Others, particularly in the visual association areas, require even more complex stimuli.

The cells of different areas tend to share common general requirements for activation. Cells within V_5 generally respond to motion without selection of colour. V_4 cells discriminate on the basis of colour and form. V_3 and V_{3A} discriminate form but not colour.

Areas V_1 and V_2 are necessary for the conscious awareness of a visual stimulus. People with lesions of area V_1 are blinded. Though they have no awareness of visual stimuli, if asked to guess the nature of a visual stimulus they distinguish between colour and direction of motion more reliably than random guessing. This is called **blind-sight**.

Central visual processing

Before we become aware of our environment, the incoming information is extensively processed to produce a construct of what has been seen. The image constructed is based not only on the retinal images but also upon previous experience and expectation. We all know how difficult it is to spot errors in typescript. Spelling errors often go unnoticed. However, once your attention is drawn to the error it sticks out like the proverbial sore thumb.

Depth perception

The perception of depth is possible because each eye receives an image of the world that has horizontal disparity relative to the other. You do not perceive two images but construct a solid object from them. This allows us to create **stereograms**, pictures with depth, by presenting a pair of pictures that differ slightly in point of view, one to each eye. In the 19th century this was a popular entertainment achieved by means of a stereoscope, or by the use of red/green printing and a pair of filters.

Recently, single image stereograms have been produced. These have been very popular as Magic Eye pictures. The system is based upon the observation by Julesz that camouflaged objects that could not be identified in either photograph of a stereogram pair became obvious when both images were viewed in a stereoscope. Adding depth information allows the brain to extract more information from a scene.

Colour perception

Colour is so important in our lives it is little wonder that its nature has been the subject of scientific investigation from even before Sir Isaac Newton demonstrated the spectrum of colours that make up white light.

We have seen that the on-centre and off-centre neural systems provide us with the sense of black and white, and between these two extremes the human eye can distinguish about 40 steps in what is known as the **grey** or **achromatic scale**. Added to this sensation is that of colour, that property of light that is independent of its brightness. This property of colour has three qualities:

- **hue** – which depends on the pure frequency of the light and is close to what is popularly known as colour
- **saturation** – which is determined by the ratio of black or white to colour present (brown is red with black added, pink is red with white added)
- **lightness** or **intensity** – which is determined by *what* is added to the colour in terms of the achromatic component that makes up the saturation (from black through the greys to white).

It has long been known that three colours of light, red, green and blue, can be used to match any known colour and these three colours with their peak wavelengths of 700 nm, 550 nm and 450 nm approximately match the peak absorbencies of the three visual pigments found in the three types of cones; pigments called **erythrolabe**, **chlorolabe** and **cyanolabe** respectively.

The peak sensitivity for photopic (bright light, colour, cone) vision is about 560 nm while that of scotopic (twilight, black and white, rod) vision is about 500 nm, which explains why as twilight falls red flowers appear almost black while blue flowers seem to glow (the Purkinje shift).

The commercial importance of exact colour matching has resulted in its intense study. The existence of three independent monochromatic mechanisms that contribute to the hue of a colour mean that a colour can be duplicated exactly by the correct combination of the three primary monochromes (red, blue and green). This fact is completely described by the 'colour matching equation':

$$a[C_1] + b[C_2] + c[C_3] = C_x$$

where $=$ means 'matches' and a, b and c are the intensities of the three monochromatic primary colours.

This formula may suggest the process of vector addition and, in fact, this is what happens in commercial devices such as the 'colour triangle' DIN 5033 in which the effect of combining different proportions of red, blue and green are graphically displayed (Fig. 4.1.16).

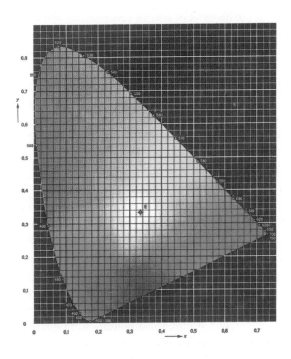

Fig. 4.1.16 The German colour standard DIN 5033. Any colour can be precisely matched from its coordinates between the red–green–blue points. (From Schmidt R F 1987 *Fundamentals of Sensory Physiology*. Springer-Verlag, Heidelberg, with permission.)

Clinical Example

Clinical defects of vision

The sense of vision represents an interaction between our nervous system and a system of physical optics which provides it with the most basic and important special sense which connects us with the outside world. Defects of this system are many and for most of us even the normal processes of ageing bring restrictions to our sight.

The conjunctiva and cornea

The optics of the eye demand that the cornea and its overlying conjunctiva be transparent and optically correct. To this end they are made up of non-keratinizing stratified squamous epithelium. By far the most common defect of the conjunctiva, at least in the western world, is acute bacterial or allergic conjunctivitis where pain and hyperaemia demand medical attention before serious damage to the optics of the eye occurs. Much more serious is *trachoma,* a long-standing chlamydial infection of the cornea where an inflamed mass replaces the superficial layers. This disease is the most common cause of blindness in underdeveloped countries.

Glaucoma

Behind the cornea is the anterior chamber, filled with aqueous humor produced by the ciliary body and removed by the trabecular meshwork and the canal of Schlemm. Pressure of aqueous humor should not exceed 20 mmHg. This is measured in the clinic as the pressure of a stream of air required to indent the cornea. Glaucoma is an increase in intraocular pressure sufficient to cause degeneration of the optic disc and nerve. It is a disorder affecting 4% of people over 40 years of age. The most common cause is obstruction of outflow of aqueous humor.

This obstruction is of two major types, causing respectively primary open-angle glaucoma and closed-angle glaucoma.

Primary open-angle glaucoma

Primary open-angle glaucoma is responsible for 90% of cases of raised intraocular pressure. A chronic slow rise in pressure is attributable to microscopic abnormalities in the canal of Schlemm. Constriction of the pupil with drugs such as pilocarpine relieves pressure on the canal and aids aqueous flow. Surgical treatment can be successful in severe cases. Treatment arrests visual loss but cannot reverse existing damage.

Closed-angle glaucoma

Closed-angle glaucoma is so called because the outflow of aqueous humor is impeded by a change in the angle between the iris and cornea through which the humor leaves the anterior chamber. This acute ophthalmological emergency is usually precipitated by dilatation of the pupil in preparation for fundoscopy in patients with an anatomical predisposition. The rapid increase in intraocular pressure causes severe pain and if not treated by osmotic agents such as mannitol and pupillary constrictors such as pilocarpine can cause complete blindness in days.

The lens

Refraction of light to form focused inverted real images on the retina is the result of the light passing through media of different refractive indexes from air through cornea, anterior chamber, lens and posterior chamber. Most refraction takes place at the air–corneal interface, but this is fixed. Accommodation, which focuses light from different distances by changing the thickness of the lens, is mediated by the parasympathetic branch of the

Clinical Example *(Continued)*

oculomotor nerve. By the age of 60 most of the flexibility of the lens to accommodate has been lost. This phenomenon and the mismatch between the optical and biological lengths of the eye that results in the conditions of myopia (nearsightedness) or hyperopia (farsightedness) are so common as to hardly warrant the description pathological. They are therefore dealt with in the main section of this chapter.

Cataracts

Cataracts are cloudy or opaque areas which develop in the lens. They may be congenital, inherited in an autosomal fashion, due to fetal infection, especially rubella, or associated with chromosomal abnormalities or a variety of traumas to the adult lens. Their incidence increases as the lens enlarges with age. The lens has no blood supply and receives its nutrition from the aqueous humor. It consists of a mass of modified epithelial cells of the ectoderm from which it is derived. In advanced cataracts these cells break down and undergo dissolution, becoming opaque. High levels of glucose in diabetes produce sorbitol which exerts an osmotic effect, damaging the cells. Clinically, cataracts produce halos or spots in the visual field which result in a progressive loss of visual acuity. Current treatment involves removing the lens and replacing it with an artificial one.

The retina

The delicate structure of the retina is susceptible to damage from a variety of sources as well as a spectrum of genetic disorders.

Retinopathy of prematurity

Premature infants frequently suffer from respiratory distress syndrome which requires hyperbaric oxygen. The immature retina responds to increased partial pressure of oxygen with vasospasm and proliferation of retinal vessels into the vitreous humor. Oedema and leakage of blood then leads to retinal detachment and blindness. Careful control of oxygen therapy of the newborn is therefore essential.

Retinitis pigmentosa

Retinal degeneration is the hallmark of a group of inherited degenerative disorders known as retinitis pigmentosa. Beginning in early life at the periphery of the retina, loss of rods, cones and ganglion cells progresses slowly to blindness by the age of 50.

Retinal detachment

Detachment of the neuroepithelial layer of the retina from the pigmented layer may be the result of:

- fluid exudation
- contraction of fibrous tissue formed as a result of haemorrhage
- a hole developing in the retina which allows ingress of liquefied vitreous humor between the layers.

One in 10 persons over 40 years of age have such holes in their retinas. Retinal detachment deprives the neuroepithelial layer of its blood supply and causes degeneration within 4–5 weeks. This manifests itself as sudden loss of part of the field of vision. Untreated, the detachment progresses to involve the whole retina. Laser treatment is effective in arresting the progression of visual loss.

Colour blindness

This rather extreme description is applied to persons who, owing to inherited or acquired

313

Clinical Example *(Continued)*

factors, do not see colours in the way generally agreed. Acquired defects in colour vision can be divided into those affecting the outer retina, which relate to blue vision, and those affecting the inner retina, which affect red–green vision.

Because there are three types of cones carrying three photopigments there can be three types of defect in colour vision. The absence of the red mechanism is called protanopia, absence of the green is deuteranopia, and absence of the blue tritanopia. Some individuals do not suffer from a frank loss of one or more of the colour mechanisms but are less sensitive to one of the primary colours. These people are said to suffer from an anomaly (protanomaly, deuteranomaly, tritanomaly).

The gene for red–green colour blindness is recessive and located on the X chromosome. Because men have only one X chromosome, the presence of this recessive gene inevitably results in red–green colour blindness. Women with their

XX combination of chromosomes can carry the gene but only express it if it is on both chromosomes. About 8% of European men have a red–green defect, whereas only 0.4% of women show this defect. The gene for the blue cone mechanism is autosomal.

Some people lack all three cone mechanisms and are known as achromats.

It has been suggested that diseases of the outer retinal layer produce tritanopia while those of the inner layer and optic nerve produce protan-deuteranopia because the larger number of very fine fibres which serve red and green cones will be more likely to be affected by a disease of the inner layer.

These defects are detected by a number of methods, the best known being Ishihara's Test Charts in which a number, made up of a series of dots of a specific colour, is invisible against a background of dots of other colours unless the mechanism for detecting the number's colour is present (Fig. CE4.1.1).

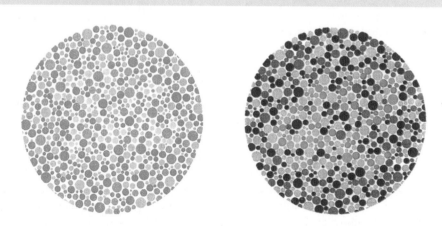

Fig. CE4.1.1 Colour blindness. Ishihara charts are often used to assess colour blindness. Normal individuals can see one number (in this case 74 on the left, and 42 on the right), while colour-blind individuals see a different number or no number at all. For accurate testing of colour deficiency, original test charts should be used, as imitations or reproduced copies might not be reliable and give false positive or false negative results. Ishihara's Tests are published by Kanehara Trading Co. and copyright is owned by the Isshinkai Foundation, Tokyo, which granted permission for these charts to be reproduced here.

Optical illusions

'So you cannot believe your eyes.' Many common illusions of pattern demonstrate how much we add from experience to interpret our visual experience (Fig. 4.1.17).

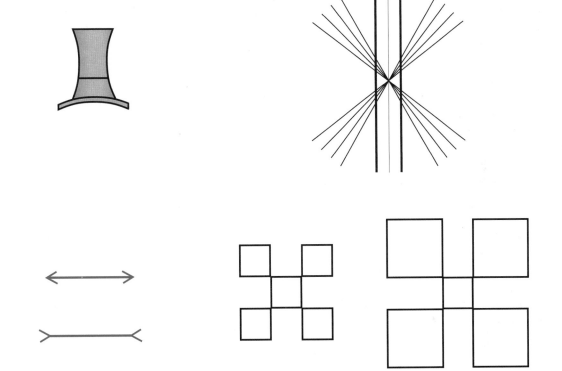

Fig. 4.1.17 Illusions. Physiological mechanisms such as lateral inhibition aid discrimination between stimuli that differ only slightly from each other, by enhancing the difference in neural activity each provokes. This can be used where two lines form an angle to produce illusions. The brim of the hat is the same length as its height. The shafts of double-headed arrow and the forked stick are the same length. The two thick lines are parallel and the two central squares are the same size.

Summary

Visual signal processing

- The photoreceptors of the retina are rods and cones in the ratio of 20:1 with cones concentrated in the fovea.
- The photosensitive substance in the rods is rhodopsin and in the cones rhodopsin-like colour-sensitive pigments.

- The visual cortex (V_1) has association areas (V_2–V_5) which respond to highly specific features (movement, colour, form) of the visual field.
- The perception of three-dimensional space is the result of horizontal disparity between the images formed by our two eyes.

Hearing

4.2

Introduction

The auditory system enables us to detect sound over a very wide range of frequencies and intensities. That ability alone would be notable; however, we are also capable of highly detailed analysis of the sounds in our environment such that we can extract specific pieces of information from the background noise and interpret both the signal content (for example speech) and the direction of its source.

The nature of sound

The sound generated by a violin string, a loudspeaker or someone's vocal cords is transmitted through the air as a series of sinusoidal pressure waves. Figure 4.2.1 shows the effect of a pure tone emitted by a tuning fork; the forwards and backwards oscillations of the prongs alternately compress and rarefy the surrounding air so that the pressure varies sinusoidally. As shown in Figure 4.2.1B, the air molecules oscillate to and fro in the direction of propagation of the wave, leading to a sequence of alternate waves of lower and higher pressure.

The structure of the ear

The ear can be divided into three main sections: the external ear, the middle ear and the inner ear.

Basic Science 4.2.1

The physics of sound

Sound is a series of pressure waves in air. The amplitude of the wave, the extent of movement of the individual molecules, is termed the sound pressure, which we detect as the loudness (intensity) of the sound (see below). The changes in sound pressure are a form of physical energy and the rate of delivery of energy (to the ear in this case) is power. We can compare the sound pressure (p) of the sound we are interested in to a standard sound (p_o), as a ratio, in decibels (dB):

$$\text{Sound pressure level (in dB)} = 2 \times 10 \times \log_{10}\frac{p}{p_o}$$

$$= 20 \times \log_{10}\frac{p}{p_o}.$$

The 'bel', named in honour of Alexander Graham Bell, $\log_{10}(p/p_o)$, is very large, hence we use the smaller unit, the decibel. The decibel system can be used to compare any two signals in the same type of any form of energy (electrical, magnetic, sound, etc.). When comparing sound intensities, including '2' in the equation compares the power of the sounds, which is proportional to the square of the signal amplitude – the log of the square of a number is twice the log of that number. p is the recorded pressure and p_o is the reference pressure which is usually taken as:

$$p_o = 2 \times 10^{-5} \text{ N/m}^2.$$

This corresponds approximately to the average threshold for hearing at the most sensitive range of the auditory system. If the intensity of the sound recorded was $p = p_o$, then this would be 0 dB (Fig. BS4.2.1). A sound pressure 100 times as great would have a loudness of 40 dB.

Fig. BS4.2.1 Range of hearing. A. The range of hearing of a young adult is limited to sound between 20 and 16 000 Hz. The threshold varies with frequency and is lowest at about 3000 Hz. Higher and lower frequencies are less easily detected. Very high levels of sound are painful. **B.** Some landmark frequencies are shown. Note that the predominant frequencies of speech coincide with the greatest sensitivity of the system.

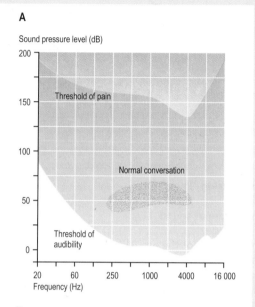

A

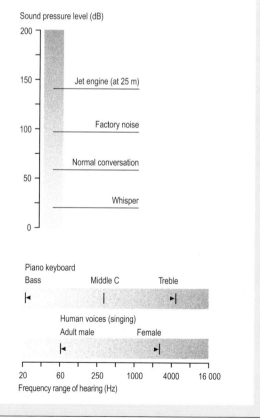

B

Basic Science 4.2.1 (Continued)

Conversational speech is about 65 dB and sound pressures over 100 dB are likely to cause damage to the sensory apparatus. Overall, the ear responds to sound over a range of 120 dB, which represents a millionfold range in sound pressures.

To distinguish this measure of sound from other measures that use dB the notation for sound pressure levels is dB SPL.

The wavelength of a given sound wave is the distance, in metres, between two corresponding points on the cycle (see Fig. 4.2.1) and is inversely correlated with the frequency of the wave, which is the number of full cycles per second. We refer to the frequency of a pure tone as its pitch; for example middle C on a piano has a frequency of 256 Hertz (Hz, cycles per second). The adult human ear is sensitive to frequencies over the range 20 Hz – 16 kHz, though the upper frequencies are lost with ageing. The auditory system, however, is not equally sensitive over the whole of this range; the range of greatest sensitivity is 1000–3000 Hz (Fig. BS4.2.1); therefore sounds of lower or higher frequencies will have to be louder in order to have the same perceived loudness for the subject listening to them.

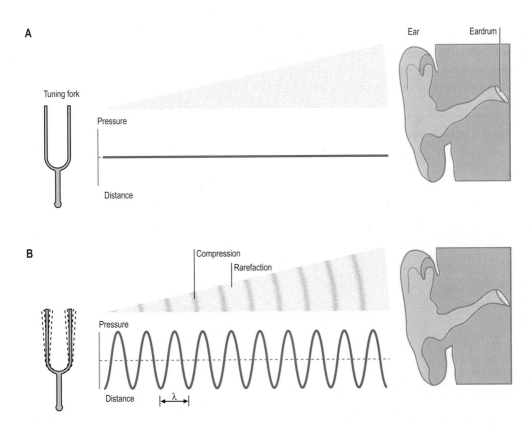

Fig. 4.2.1 The properties of sound. Sound is generated when the tuning fork vibrates producing alternating compression and rarefaction of the surrounding air. Pressure waves spread out like ripples on a pond after a stone is thrown into the water. When these waves reach the eardrum the drum is vibrated by the wave. **A.** The state of the air molecules at an instant in time. **B.** The distribution of the air molecules is described in terms of the local pressures. Sound is described in terms of its volume (amplitude) and pitch (frequency or wavelength). Wavelength and frequency are inversely related: frequency ∝ 1/wavelength.

External ear

The external ear comprises the **pinna** and the **external auditory meatus** (the auditory canal) which leads to the **tympanic membrane** (eardrum) (Fig. 4.2.2). The pinna is important in many vertebrates for transferring sound to the ear canal and for determining the directional sensitivity to sound.

Middle ear

The middle ear is an air-filled cavity which contains three small bones (**ossicles**), the **malleus** (hammer), **incus** (anvil) and **stapes** (stirrup), so called because of their characteristic shapes. These bones form a mechanical linkage between the tympanic membrane and the **oval window**, a membrane-covered opening into the fluid-filled inner ear (Fig. 4.2.3). A second, membrane-covered opening, the round window, also links between the middle and inner ears. Two muscles in the middle ear can act to reduce excessive movement of the ossicles; the **tensor tympani** acts on the malleus and the **stapedius** on the stapes (Fig. 4.2.3).

The mean pressure across the eardrum is normally zero. The middle ear is maintained at atmospheric pressure by means of the eustachian tube which opens to the nasopharynx (Fig. 4.2.2). The eustachian tube is normally closed but opens during swallowing or yawning. Differences in pressure between the middle and outer ears can arise as a result of rapid changes in atmospheric pressure, for example during ascent or descent in an aeroplane. If these pressures are not equalized, this can lead to painful stretching or even rupture of the tympanic membrane. Airlines flying planes with limited pressurization hand out boiled sweets during take off and landing to encourage their passengers to swallow and equalize the pressures across the eardrum.

Inner ear

The inner ear is a cavity lying within the temporal bone which contains the **cochlea** and the **vestibular apparatus** (p. 333). The cochlea is a

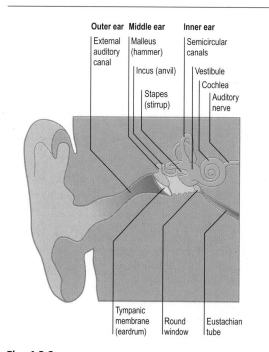

Fig. 4.2.2 The structure of the external ear and middle ear and their relation to the cochlea.

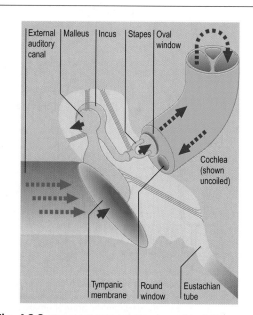

Fig. 4.2.3 The middle ear showing the ossicle chain connecting the tympanic membrane to the oval window.

spiral structure of two and a half turns, formed as a hollow within the temporal bone, the so-called bony labyrinth (Fig. 4.2.2). The cochlea itself may be divided into three fluid-filled compartments, the **scalae** ('stairways'). The **scala tympani** follows the outer contours of the cochlea and ends at the round window (Figs 4.2.3 and 4.2.4). At its other end (the centre of the spiral), the scala tympani is continuous with the inner compartment, the **scala vestibuli**, the region where they join being called the helicotrema ('spiral hole'). The scala vestibuli ends in the vestibule, an expanded region which links with the oval window. Both the scalae tympani and vestibuli are filled with fluid, the

perilymph. These two compartments are separated by a membrane-bound compartment, the scala media or cochlear duct (Figs 4.2.3 and 4.2.4), which is filled with **endolymph**. Within the cochlear duct lies the organ of Corti, which is the sense organ itself. The cochlear duct is bounded by the basilar membrane, along which the organ of Corti lies, and Reissner's membrane, which forms the roof of the duct.

The **organ of Corti** is a complex structure comprising a structural frame (the rods of Corti), various supportive cells and two groups of **hair cells**, the outer hair cells which are in rows of three, and a single row of inner hair cells. The **stereocilia** of both sets of hair cells

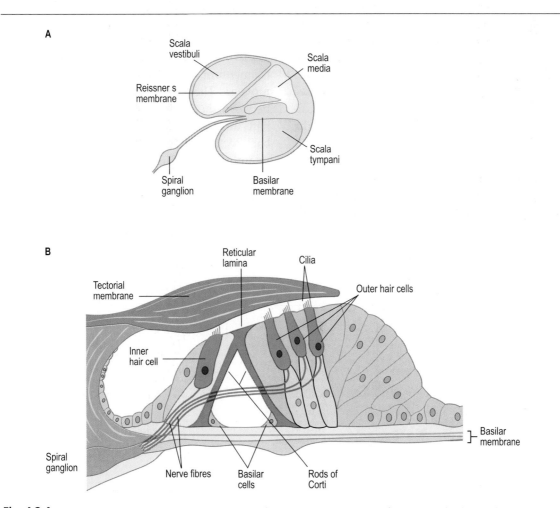

Fig. 4.2.4 The organ of Corti. A. Cross-section of one turn of the cochlea. **B.** The organ of Corti on the basilar membrane contains the receptor (hair) cells.

contact the **tectorial membrane** which forms a roof, overhanging the organ (Fig. 4.2.4). The hair cells are innervated by afferent axons, whose cell bodies lie in the spiral ganglion, and which project to the brainstem as part of the VIIIth cranial nerve, the auditory nerve. The hair cells also receive a motor, efferent, innervation.

Sound conduction

Sound waves entering the auditory canal cause the tympanic membrane to vibrate in phase with the alternating compressions and rarefactions (p. 319) of the sound pressure. The movement of the tympanic membrane directly acts on the malleus so that it and the incus and stapes, in turn, oscillate in response to the sound (Fig. 4.2.3). The base of the stapes connects with the oval window so that movements of the ossicles cause the oval window to move in and out. The tympanic membrane and ossicles provide a mechanism for transferring the sound wave in air into movements of the fluid within the cochlea. If the sound waves were conducted directly from the air to the perilymph, most of the energy would be lost by reflection at the air–fluid interface.

The lever action of the ossicles and the mechanical advantage provided by the ratio between the large surface area of the tympanic membrane and the small area of the oval window serve as an **impedance-matching** device so that there is minimal loss in the conduction pathway. The tensor tympani and stapedius muscles act on the ossicles to reduce the amplitude of the movement in response to very loud sounds, varying the sensitivity of the ear.

Impedance matching

The role of the ossicles as an impedance-matching system between the air and the perilymph is illustrated by considering what happens if two suspended steel spheres collide and the collision is elastic.

Consider what happens if one sphere is very much bigger than the other. If the smaller is in motion and collides with the larger (Fig. 4.2.5A), it will rebound retaining most of its momentum. The larger sphere will scarcely be moved. There is little energy transferred between the spheres. If you bounce an elastic ball on the earth, the ball bounces almost back to the height from which it was released, retaining most of its energy.

If the larger sphere is in motion and collides with the smaller (Fig. 4.2.5B), it will continue along its path carrying the smaller with it. The larger thus retains most of its momentum. The smaller sphere will gain little momentum. There is little energy transferred between the spheres.

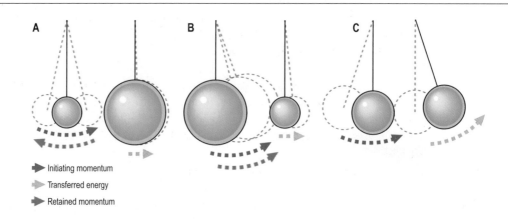

▶ Initiating momentum
▷ Transferred energy
▶ Retained momentum

Fig. 4.2.5 The executive toy. A model of impedance matching. See text for description.

If the two spheres are of equal size (Fig. 4.2.5C), then after the collision the stationary sphere will move off with a velocity and in a direction equal to that of the original moving sphere, which will remain stationary at the point of collision. After the collision, the momentum will have been transferred from one sphere to the other. There is complete energy transfer between the spheres.

By a similar process of impedance matching the energy imparted to the tympanic membrane by the sound waves is transferred to the perilymph. Since the perilymph is effectively incompressible and the organ of Corti is in the rigid petrous bone, the fluid movements due to the oscillation of the oval window occur because of the presence of the round window (Fig. 4.2.3).

Sound transduction

The basilar membrane varies in width and stiffness along its length, such that it is narrow and stiff at the basal end, close to the oval window, and is wide and flexible at the apical end. The movement of the perilymph in the scala vestibuli sets up a travelling wave (Fig. 4.2.6A) along the basilar membrane (similar to the wave form seen when one shakes one end of a long rope). As a result, portions of the membrane respond preferentially to different frequencies. The apical end responds maximally to low frequencies (Fig. 4.2.6B) and the basal end to high frequencies (Fig. 4.2.6C). Overall, the response in the auditory nerve fibres varies according to the origin of each fibre along the length of the cochlea.

As the basilar membrane oscillates, it moves with respect to the tectorial membrane causing the stereocilia to bend and straighten (Fig. 4.2.7). As for the basilar membrane, the stereocilia have different mechanical properties, being short and stiff at the basal end and long and flexible at the apical end. Therefore the hair cells are tuned to respond mechanically to a limited range of frequencies of sound energy.

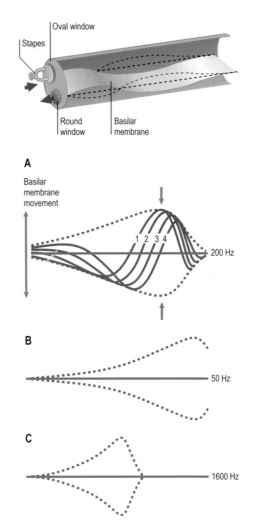

Fig. 4.2.6 Movement of the basilar membrane. Movement of the stapes creates a travelling wave in the basilar membrane. **A.** At successive short intervals in time the displacement of the membrane is shown (1, 2, 3 and 4). The dotted red lines indicate the envelope of these movements, which reach a maximum amplitude (resonate) at the point indicated by the arrows. **B.** At 50 Hz the largest movements are far from the stapes. **C.** At 1600 Hz they are near to the stapes.

There is also evidence of electrical tuning in terms of the time constants of the receptor membranes.

At the point of contact between the basilar membrane and the external wall of the cochlea is a highly vascularized structure, the **stria vascularis** which actively secretes ions into the endolymph, maintaining a potential of about +85 mV between it and the perilymph. This is

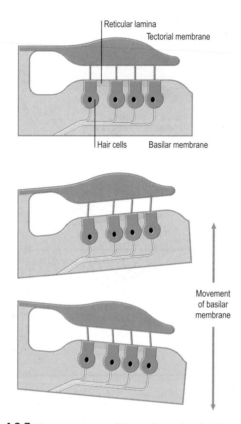

Reticular lamina

Tectorial membrane

Hair cells   Basilar membrane

Movement
of basilar
membrane

**Fig. 4.2.7 The arrangement of the basilar and tectorial
membranes.** This is such that when they move a shearing action
takes place, bending the stereocilia and leading to a receptor
potential in the hair cells.

called the **endocochlear potential**. The resting
potential of the hair cells is –85 mV with respect
to the perilymph; therefore the potential
across the receptor membrane of the hair cells
can be as large as 170 mV, creating very large
electrochemical gradients for several cations.

The transduction process is as follows. The
bending of the stereocilia of the hair cell in one
direction leads to opening of cation channels
and an inward current that depolarizes the hair
cell. When the direction of bending reverses, the
cell hyperpolarizes. Thus the receptor potential
varies with the oscillation of the sound stimulus
but overall there is net depolarization.

If the electrical potential of the perilymph
at the round window is measured, this is found
to oscillate, reproducing faithfully the sound

being heard. This signal is called the cochlear
microphonic. It has zero latency, no threshold
and is thought to be the sum of the receptor
potentials generated by the hair cells.

The hair cell, at its basal end, releases an
excitatory neurotransmitter in response to
depolarization by the receptor potential. This
transmitter depolarizes the terminals of the first-
order afferent neurone, which, if depolarized
sufficiently, generates action potentials.

About 90% of the afferent fibres innervate
the inner hair cells, which appear to be the sites
of sound transduction. The outer hair cells
receive afferent and efferent innervation and
are probably involved in modulating the tuning
sensitivity of the organ of Corti. There are about
3000 inner hair cells and each one is innervated
by about 10 afferent axons, with each axon only
innervating one hair cell.

Since each inner hair cell is tuned to respond
to a specific sound frequency band and each
afferent axon only connects with one hair cell,
recordings from the afferent axons show
sharply defined **tuning curves** (Fig. 4.2.8). This
has the effect that the afferent has a low threshold to stimulation at its characteristic frequency.
The threshold rises rapidly (i.e. the sensitivity
rapidly decreases) for lower or higher frequencies. Note that the response characteristics of
the basilar membrane–inner hair cell arrangement, the cochlea and the first-order afferent
axons arising from it are described as being
tonotopically organized. Place and frequency
response are linked, afferents from the basal
end responding to high frequencies, those from
the apical end responding to low frequencies.
This tonotopic mapping is preserved in the central projections of the auditory nerve.

For low frequencies of sound (~20 Hz) afferent axons show a phase-locked response by discharging one or more action potentials at a
given point in each cycle of the input sound
stimulus (Fig. 4.2.9A). Such a response is
restricted at high frequencies by the maximum
rate of firing possible by the afferent axon. At
intermediate frequencies each afferent retains a

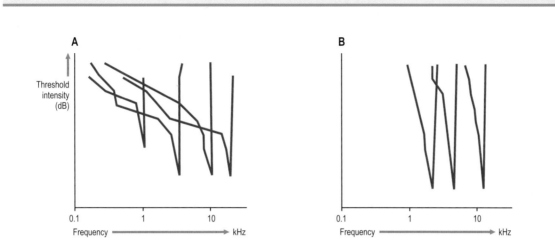

Fig. 4.2.8 Tuning curves for (A) four VIIIth nerve fibres and (B) three neurones in the inferior colliculus. The neurones of the inferior colliculus show a sharper tuning of their bandwidth of sensitivity than those of the VIIIth nerve because of neuronal processing of the input.

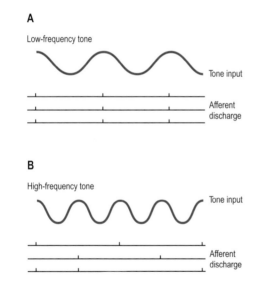

Fig. 4.2.9 Low- and high-frequency discharge. **A.** With low-frequency sound the afferent discharge of the VIIIth nerve fibres is locked to the sound frequency, one action potential for each cycle of the sound wave. **B.** With higher frequencies, some cycles are missed but the discharge still retains a relationship to the cycle phase (phase locking).

phase-locked relationship but responds to every second or third cycle (Fig. 4.2.9B). Since each hair cell is innervated by several afferent fibres, the combined response still signals the stimulus frequency, a process called **volley coding** which has been observed for frequencies up to 8 kHz.

At higher frequencies tonotopic location of the afferent axon signals the frequency of the stimulus. Place coding might also be important in our ability to perceive lower frequencies, but volley coding is also involved.

In either case the intensity of the sound is encoded by the rate of discharge and the number of afferents discharging.

Summary

The auditory process

- The eardrum passes sound vibration to the auditory ossicles, which efficiently pass it to the perilymph by impedance matching.
- The oval window on which the stapes sits is one end of the scala vestibuli of the cochlea. The other end, the helicotrema, leads to the scala tympani which terminates at the oval window.
- Specific regions of the cochlear basilar membrane and specific hair cells are tuned to respond to certain frequencies.
- The very large (170 mV) potential across the hair cell's membrane is modulated by the bending of its cilia.

Processing of auditory signals

Homo sapiens relies upon sound for communication by speech. The extraction of meaning from complex sounds involves much processing by the CNS. In man the auditory cortex is large. Much processing also occurs at subcortical levels.

The afferent neurone of the VIIIth cranial nerve terminates in the **cochlear nucleus** of the pons. From here there are major pathways projecting directly to the **superior olivary nuclei** and the **inferior colliculus,** with further projections from the superior olivary nuclei to the inferior colliculus (Fig. 4.2.10). From the inferior colliculus there are projections to the **medial geniculate nucleus** of the **thalamus** and thence to the **primary auditory cortex** (A_1, Brodmann's areas 41 and 42).

Sound localization

Within the superior olivary nuclei, the incoming signal is processed to identify the localization of the source of the sound. A sound coming from a point to the right-hand side of the head will arrive at the right ear sooner and will be louder in comparison with the signal reaching the left ear, the left ear being partly shielded by the bulk of the head. Furthermore, at any instant, because of the timing differences, the signals arriving at the two ears will be at different points of the sound wave. The two signals therefore show phase differences due to the different distances they have to travel. This means that it is still possible to localize maintained tones on the basis of timing as well as intensity. The neurones of medial superior olivary nuclei receive inputs from both of the cochlear nuclei

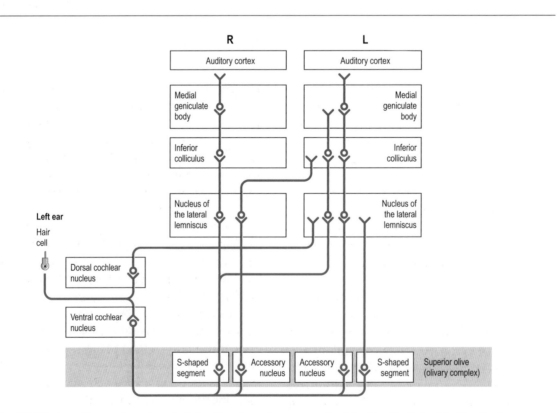

Fig. 4.2.10 The auditory pathway from the hair cells to the auditory cortex. R = right side of brain; L = left side of brain.

and respond to differences in the timing of these inputs, the phase differences. The cells of the lateral olivary nuclei also receive inputs from both right and left auditory nerves. They detect differences in the intensity of the signals from the two ears.

Cortical information processing

The cells of the inferior colliculus receive binaural inputs. The specific convergence of inputs produces a sharpening of the tuning curves for the inferior colliculus cells (Fig. 4.2.8B), thus increasing the ability to discriminate pitch. These cells project to the thalamus and thence to the primary auditory cortex. Within the cortex, a **tonotopic map** is preserved, although the higher the neurone is in the system the more complex the pattern of the sound that is needed to excite it. Within the cortex the process of pattern recognition is completed and cells extract elements of information from a stimulus. The similarity between this function in the auditory and visual cortices can be seen (see p. 310).

Within the auditory cortex the neurones are organized in a **columnar** fashion, partly resembling the ocular dominance columns of the visual cortex (p. 309). These columns reflect binaural processing with an alternating pattern of summation and suppression columns. In summation columns, the neurones respond preferentially to inputs coming from both ears rather than just from one. Conversely, the neurones of the suppression columns respond more strongly to sounds that stimulate one ear rather than both, one ear being dominant in each column. It is likely that the organization of these columns is involved in sound localization.

In addition to the VIIIth nerve afferent pathway from the cells of the organ of Corti up to the primary auditory cortex, there is also a **descending pathway** from the cortex, via the thalamus and inferior colliculus to the cochlear nucleus. From here, efferents project to the outer hair cells and to the first-order afferents. It is possible that these connections are involved in modifying the tuning and specific sensitivity of the organ of Corti and the afferent pathway. This could help direct attention to specific sounds.

Auditory testing and deafness

The auditory system normally operates with sounds over a wide range of frequencies (10 Hz – 20 kHz) and intensities (100 dB). Central neural processing of the input renders the system capable of extracting important signals from sound which includes much background noise. With normal ageing, however, the sensitivity of the system deteriorates and it is also vulnerable to various other defects.

The reduced ability to hear, deafness, is a common problem affecting a large fraction of the older population to a serious extent. Two broad classes of deafness can be identified: **conductive deafness** and **sensorineural deafness**.

Conductive deafness

Conductive deafness involves impairment of the transmission of sound energy from the air to the inner ear. It can result from relatively minor conditions such as an excessive build-up of wax (cerumen) in the external auditory meatus, reducing the conduction of sound to the eardrum. Otitis media, inflammation of the middle ear, reduces conduction through the ossicles of the middle ear. Secretory otitis media (glue ear) is common in children. An accumulation of fluid in the middle ear impedes the movement of both the eardrum and the ossicles. This is often treated by perforating the eardrum and insertion of a 'grommet', to allow drainage of the fluid. Otosclerosis is an hereditary disorder which causes progressive deafness in adult life as a result of excessive growth of the bone in the inner ear causing the stapes to become locked in the oval window. Otosclerosis can usually be treated surgically.

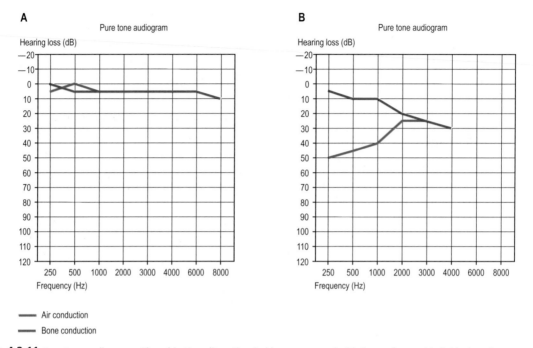

A Pure tone audiogram

B Pure tone audiogram

Air conduction

Bone conduction

Fig. 4.2.11 Pure tone audiograms. The subject's auditory thresholds are compared with those of normal individuals and any deviations are presented graphically. (Audiograms for one ear only are presented.) **A.** Normal individual in which neither the threshold for air-conducted (blue) or bone-conducted (red) sound is raised. **B.** An individual with hearing problems. Bone-conduction thresholds are raised particularly with higher frequency sounds. In addition, air conduction is also impaired, most obviously at lower frequencies. The loss in bone-conducted response is characteristic of the elderly and reflects damage to the cochlear innervation. A simple cause of the air-conducted response might be wax in the ear but damage to the ossicle chain would have the same effect.

Sensorineural deafness

Sensorineural deafness results from damage to the cochlea and hair cell apparatus or the ascending afferent pathways. Cochlear hair cells are easily damaged by repeated exposure to loud sounds. Cochlear lesions result in deafness on that side. Since most of the projections from the cochlear nuclei are bilateral, a unilateral lesion of the cochlear nuclei will affect transmission of signals from both ears.

The ageing processes results in loss of hair cells. The most obvious loss during normal ageing is the inability to hear high frequencies. With age, the upper limit drops from the child's 20 kHz. The auditory threshold rises at all frequencies (Fig. 4.2.11) but is most evident with high frequencies.

Exposure to excessive noise (peak sounds in excess of 120 dB or maintained noise levels over 80–100 dB), even for short periods, leads to damage of the hair cells and reduced sensitivity, particularly at higher frequencies. Continued exposure can lead to a permanent deafness. Exposure to damaging intensities of sound at specific frequencies will damage the hair cells sensitive to those frequencies. Industrial noise and excessively loud music are common causes of cochlear damage. Personal stereo-players often produce sound through their headsets that exceed 100 dB and many young people now have serious hearing defects from their use. The degree of deafness and determination of the frequencies affected can be assessed by audiometry. Each ear of the patient is tested with pure tones over a range of frequencies and intensities. The threshold intensities are plotted against the frequencies and compared with the expected thresholds to give a measure of the hearing deficit.

Tests

Conductive and nerve deafness can be distinguished using Rinne's test. A tuning fork is struck and placed close to the ear; when the patient can no longer hear the sound as the amplitude of the vibration decreases, the stem of the fork is placed against the mastoid process of the temporal bone. If the patient again hears the sound, this implies that conduction through the bone is better than conduction through the air and that there is therefore a conductive deficit.

A unilateral cochlear defect can be sensitively detected by Weber's test. If a vibrating tuning fork is placed on the forehead in the midline, a unilateral cochlear defect will cause the sound to be reported as coming from the opposite side to the defect.

Summary

Processing of signals

- The auditory system is tonotopically organized from the basilar membrane to the auditory cortex.
- Location of a sound source is identified within the superior olivary nuclei from the difference in loudness and phase at each ear.
- Descending nerve pathways modify the specific sensitivity of the organ of Corti.
- The ageing process results in a preferential loss of hair cells sensitive to high frequencies.

The vestibular system

Introduction

The vestibular system is part of the membranous labyrinth of the inner ear and is sensitive to movements of the head and the position of the head in space. The system comprises two interconnected organs, the **semicircular canals** and the **otolith organs**. The semicircular canals respond to angular (rotational) acceleration of the head and the otolith organs respond to linear acceleration. The output from these organs gives rise to the sense of balance. Unlike many of the senses, the sense of balance does not normally form a major input to our consciousness. Disturbance of that sense, however, with the resulting giddiness and nausea, forms all too powerful an input. The vestibular system plays a key role, at the subconscious level, in a range of motor functions including the control of posture, movement coordination and the control of eye movements.

The vestibular system lies within the bony labyrinth of the inner ear and is continuous with the cochlear duct (p. 320). Like the cochlear duct, the membranous labyrinth forming the vestibular apparatus is filled with endolymph. The surrounding spaces, between the bone and the membrane, are filled with perilymph, continuous with the scalae tympani and vestibuli (Fig. 4.3.1 and see p. 321).

Basic Science 4.3.1

Inertia and momentum – Newton's laws

Sir Isaac Newton (1642–1727) formulated three beautifully simple laws which precisely describe the motion of objects (bodies). They can be stated in modern English as follows:

1. Every body continues in its state of rest or uniform motion in a straight line unless acted on by an impressed force.
2. The impressed force produces a rate of change in momentum proportional to the force, which takes place in the direction of a straight line along which the force acts.
3. To every action there is an equal and opposite reaction.

The first law describes how mass has the property of inertia (the tendency to stay still or to continue to move in a straight line unless acted on by a force).

The term 'impressed force' means an external force acting on the body.

Newton's genius was such that he subscribed to the atomic theory of matter, and he probably would not be surprised by the recent proposition that the property of 'mass' or 'inertia' resides with a single type of subatomic particle.

The second law tells us that the more rapidly you change the velocity of an object, that is the more violently you accelerate or stop it, the greater the force required.

The third law tells us that when you push an object with a certain force to accelerate or stop it, the object pushes back at you with an equal force.

These laws apply to liquids as well as solid objects and their importance to the vestibular system, which we are dealing with in this chapter of this book, is that the endolymph in the semicircular canals of the ear has inertia and obeys the laws.

When you rotate your head the endolymph 'remains in its state of rest' for a while (Law 1). When you stop rotating your head the endolymph 'continues in its state of motion' (Law 1).

The more rapidly you accelerate your head into motion the greater this effect will be (Law 2).

To bring the endolymph up to the speed of rotation of the head, the ends of the semicircular canals provide the 'impressed force', and in accordance with Law 3 the endolymph presses back against the ends with 'an equal and opposite reaction' which stimulates the hair cells in the cupula of the canals and provides the sensation of rotation.

The semicircular canals

There are three semicircular canals, which lie in three planes approximately at right-angles to each other; the *anterior* and *posterior* canals lie in two vertical planes, both perpendicular to the horizontal canal. The orientation of the canals within the head is such that the anterior canal on one side lies in the same plane as the posterior canal on the opposite side (Fig. 4.3.1B) and they therefore form functional pairs. The horizontal canals lie in the same plane on each side.

Each of the canals connects at both ends with the **utricle** and, next to the point of joining, one end swells to form the **ampulla** (Figs 4.3.1 and 4.3.2). Within the ampulla there is a thickening of the epithelium to form the **ampullary crest**, which contains a number of receptor cells, the **vestibular hair cells**. From the apical surface of each of the hair cells extend 40–70 **stereocilia** and a single **kinocilium** (Fig. 4.3.2A). The stereocilia are arranged in an ascending order of length with the longest stereocilium next to the kinocilium, the whole series being in line with the plane of the canal. The stereocilia project into the **cupula**, a gelatinous structure that extends from the surface of the ampullary crest to the roof of the ampulla, effectively occluding the canal.

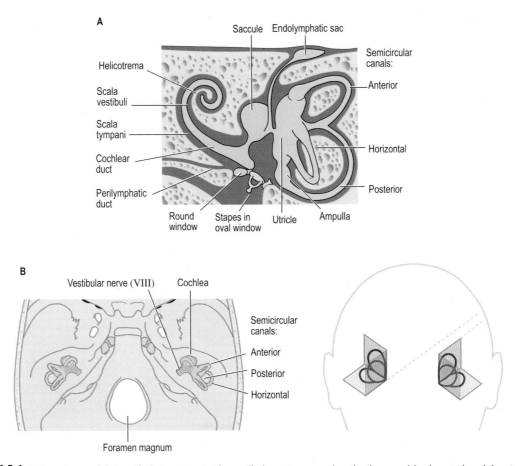

Fig. 4.3.1 **Basic anatomy of the vestibular system.** **A.** The vestibular system comprises the three semicircular canals and the otolith organs (utricle and saccule). Lying within the inner ear it is connected with the cochlear duct. **B.** The semicircular canals are oriented to receive information concerning acceleration in all three planes.

Rotational acceleration of the head moves the labyrinths but the endolymph within has inertia and its acceleration therefore lags behind (Fig. 4.3.2B). As a result, the endolymph exerts a force on the cupula causing it and the hairs to be bent in the reverse direction to the movement. The displacement of the cupula is maximal at the centre of the ampullary crest; therefore the hair cells at the centre are most sensitive to acceleration. Increasing acceleration stimulates progressively more cells towards the periphery of the crest.

The process of transduction is effected by the bending of the bundle of hairs by displacement of the cupula. The stereocilia of all the hair cells

of each ampulla are oriented the same way. Bending of the hair bundle towards the kinocilium opens cation channels leading to depolarization of the hair cell. At rest, about 10% of the transduction channels are open and these are closed by bending of the bundle away from the kinocilium, thereby hyperpolarizing the hair cell.

The hair cells are innervated by the terminals of the first-order afferent neurone. At rest, because some transduction channels are open, there is a steady release of neurotransmitter from the hair cell and therefore the afferent neurone discharges action potentials at about 100 impulses/second. Rotational acceleration of the

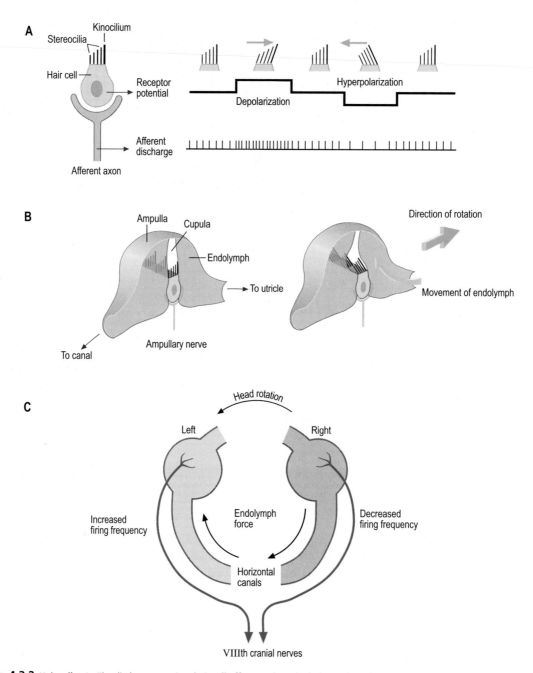

Fig. 4.3.2 **Hair cells.** **A.** The discharge rate in a hair cell afferent when the hairs are bent in opposite directions. **B.** How rotation of the head displaces endolymph to bend hairs – in either direction. **C.** How head rotation increases firing frequency in canals on one side and reduces it on the other.

head is therefore signalled by an increase or a decrease in the rate of firing of the afferents depending on the direction of movement (Fig. 4.3.2C).

As shown in Figure 4.3.1, the semicircular canals can be viewed as being paired on the two sides of the head. The signals in the two VIIIth cranial nerves arriving at the brainstem in response to acceleration will therefore be acceleration of discharge from one side and deceleration from the other, reflecting the opposed orientations of the hair cells on the two sides of the head.

Otolith organs

There are two otolith organs, the **utricle** and the **saccule** (Fig. 4.3.1). As in the ampullae of the semicircular canals, the utricle and saccule show thickening of the epithelium to form the **macula** which contains the hair cells (Fig. 4.3.3). The macula is covered by the **otolithic membrane**, a gelatinous substance which contains numerous crystals of calcium carbonate, the otoliths. The stereocilia and kinocilia of the hair cells project into the otolithic membrane so that movement of the membrane, as a result of linear acceleration of the head, will produce bending of the hairs.

The macula of the utricle lies in the horizontal plane while that of the saccule is oriented vertically. The hair cells are not arranged in an ordered manner in relation to the kinocilia as they are in the semicircular canals. As a result, the otolith organs in combination are sensitive to linear acceleration in any plane. This will relate both to actual movement of the head and to the acceleration due to gravity, the latter providing information regarding the position of the head in space.

Central pathways

The first-order afferents are carried in the VIIIth cranial nerve and have their cell bodies in the **vestibular ganglion**, which lies close to the auditory meatus, and projects from there to the **vestibular nuclei** of the medulla. There are four distinct sets of nuclei, the **lateral**, **medial**, **superior** and **inferior** vestibular nuclei. These in turn project to the **cerebellum** (p. 234), the oculomotor nuclei where they mediate the **vestibular reflex** (p. 228), the spinal cord (particularly as the **vestibulospinal tract** is concerned with postural adjustments) (p. 228) and also to the **reticular formation**.

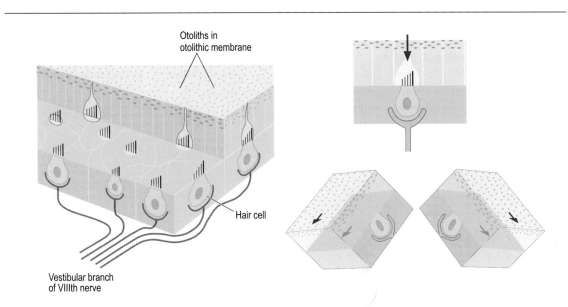

Otoliths in otolithic membrane

Hair cell

Vestibular branch of VIIIth nerve

Fig. 4.3.3 **Structure of the macula of the utricle.** The hairs extend from the hair cells into the gelatinous otolithic membrane. Unlike in the ampulla, the hair cells are not all oriented in the same direction; therefore the movement of the otolithic membrane will depolarize some and hyperpolarize other hair cells.

Disturbances to the vestibular system

Disturbances to the vestibular system can be extremely distressing, resulting in vertigo (a sensation of giddiness and an inability to maintain balance) and nausea. A common experience of such problems occurs during rotation on a roundabout. Initially the semicircular canals signal the acceleration but as the rotation proceeds at constant speed, the endolymph no longer exerts a force on the cupula so the vestibular system no longer signals rotation. When the roundabout stops therefore, particularly if it stops quickly, there is an apparent acceleration in the reverse direction due to the momentum of the endolymph. This lasts for several seconds so that there is an illusion of movement when the body is actually stationary; as a result it is difficult to stand upright and there may be a feeling of nausea. This type of sensation is also related to motion sickness on a ship, for example. Here, if one is inside the ship, the visual system does not detect the movement, which is signalled by the vestibular system, and the conflicting inputs lead to nausea.

Ménière's disease (see Clinical Example) is an example of a vestibular disease. It results from overproduction of endolymph, which disturbs both vestibular and auditory function. It is characterized by attacks of severe vertigo with nausea and often tinnitus (ringing in the ears). Testing of the vestibular system may be carried out by measuring **nystagmograms**. This depends on the intimate relationship between the vestibular system and oculomotor reflexes. If the endolymph of one vestibular system is moved by blowing warm air into the ear canal, it will set up currents within the fluid of the semicircular canals as would rotation of the head. Since one set of canals is affected but not the other, the input to the brainstem is asymmetric. Measurements of the size and frequency of the eye movements when in the dark are indicative of the input from the vestibular system.

Summary

Balance

- Unlike many senses, the sense of balance signalled by the vestibular system is rarely conscious.
- The semicircular canals of the inner ear signal rotation of the head; the utricle and saccule signal linear acceleration.
- The four vestibular nuclei receive acceleration sensation and project to the oculomotor nuclei, cerebellum and spinal cord, coordinating balance and posture.
- Conflicting information from the visual and vestibular systems can lead to vertigo and nausea.

Clinical Example

Ménière's disease

Ménière's disease is an uncommon condition of the inner ear, producing both auditory and vestibular symptoms. It therefore probably involves both the cochlea and the labyrinth. The cause is not known and infection, allergy and vascular conditions have all been suggested. The patient is usually a middle-aged man with a history of unilateral deafness (less than 25% of cases are bilateral). He presents with a history of unilateral deafness, tinnitus (ringing in the ears), vertigo, vomiting and ataxia lasting several hours. The patient describes a sensation of fullness of the ear and the attack is often accompanied by nystagmus. Attacks recur over months and years and the vertigo ceases when deafness is complete. The progress of the disease may be so slow that this never occurs.

Pathology is the result of a build-up of endolymph with a resulting increase in pressure which eventually destroys the cochlear hair cells and results in deafness.

Treatment with drugs is difficult. Phenothiazines are dopamine antagonists which block dopamine receptors in the chemoreceptive trigger zone of the vomiting centre. They, like antihistamines, are useful in treating many types of vertigo and nausea, although Ménière's disease tends to be resistant. Interestingly, betahistine, a histamine analogue, may give some relief, apparently by reducing endolymphatic pressure. If the condition is particularly distressing, it may be necessary to surgically destroy the affected labyrinth, usually using ultrasound. This of course results in total deafness on the treated side.

Taste and smell

Introduction

Taste and smell are chemical senses that provide information regarding the external world. Although they are mediated by separate receptor mechanisms, during eating the two senses operate in concert. The full appreciation of good food depends on both its taste and smell; when the nose is blocked, the appreciation of food is diminished.

Although in humans these senses are less obviously important than in many other animals, they still enable a remarkable degree of discrimination, as demonstrated by professional wine tasters who claim to distinguish over 100 different components of taste and smell when identifying wines.

Taste and particularly smell also have unique features. They send information to areas of the brain that affect emotional states and trigger memories and associations with great potency. Odour is used as a signalling mechanism especially with powerful emotions such as fear or sexual arousal.

Taste

Taste is a major element in food selection and has an important protective role. It is sensitive. Quinine can be detected in concentrations less than 1×10^{-3} g/litre.

The sense of taste (**gustation**) is mediated by specialized receptor cells, clustered together to form **taste buds**, which are mainly found in the epithelia of the tongue and also on the palate, pharynx, epiglottis and upper oesophagus. On the tongue, the taste buds are grouped in **papillae**, of which there are three types (Fig. 4.4.1B):

- **Fungiform papillae** are mushroom-like and are located on the anterior two-thirds of the tongue.
- **Foliate papillae** are folded to form leaf-like structures on the posterior edge of the tongue.
- **Circumvallate papillae** are large, round structures encircled by a groove, located on the posterior part of the tongue.

The fungiform papillae lie on the region of the tongue innervated by the VIIth cranial nerve (the **chorda tympani** branch of the facial nerve), while the posterior part of the tongue is innervated by the **glossopharyngeal nerve** (IXth cranial nerve) (Fig. 4.4.1A). There may be several thousand taste buds in each papilla.

Each taste bud contains between 50 and 150 gustatory receptor cells along with basal cells and supporting cells (Fig. 4.4.2). There is a continuous turnover of the receptor cells, which are replaced by differentiation of the associated cells. The taste buds are embedded in the epithelium and are exposed to the surface by a small opening called the **taste pore**. The apical surfaces of the gustatory receptor cells give rise to microvilli that extend through the pore and make contact with the fluids in the mouth. These microvilli are the only parts of the receptor cell that are exposed to the external medium and it is on this surface that sensory transduction is initiated.

Taste transduction

The qualities of taste are classified in four main groupings: sweet, salty, sour and bitter. The receptor cells mediating these qualities are located in different regions of the tongue (Fig. 4.4.1C) with sweet receptors at the tip, salty and sour along the lateral margins and bitter at the

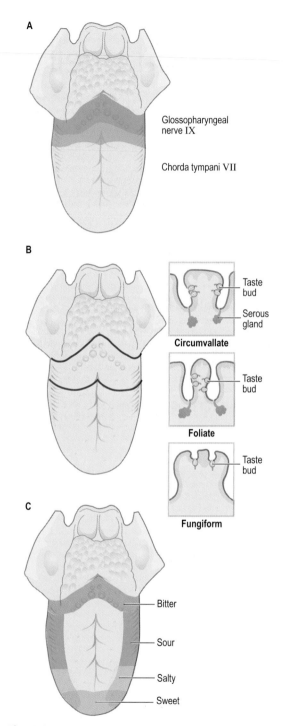

Fig. 4.4.1 The innervation and distribution of papillae and taste qualities on the tongue surface. A. The innervation of the posterior third of the tongue is by the glossopharyngeal (IX) cranial nerve. The anterior two-thirds are innervated by the corda tympani (VII). **B.** The three types of papillae and their distribution on the surface of the tongue. **C.** The regions where each of the four qualities of taste predominate.

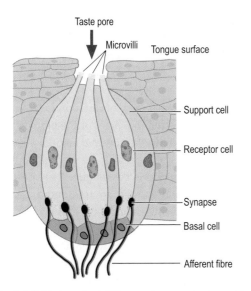

Fig. 4.4.2 The taste bud. This comprises receptor, supporting and basal cells. The afferent axon branches to innervate several receptor cells, contact being in the form of chemical synapses. The microvilli of the receptor cells project into the taste pore where they are exposed to the fluids in the mouth.

back. These qualities differ in the transduction process involved, salty and sour being directly mediated whereas sweet and bitter involve second messenger systems.

Saltiness. This has the simplest of the transduction mechanisms since it does not require any specific membrane receptors; rather there are passive Na$^+$ channels on the microvilli through which Na$^+$ enters the receptor cell, depolarizing it (Fig. 4.4.3). It is likely that the Na$^+$ within the cell is then pumped out via an Na$^+$/K$^+$ ATPase on the basolateral membrane.

Sourness. This quality is evoked by acids, the intensity of the taste being dependent on the H$^+$ concentration. The hydrogen ions act to block the K$^+$ channels which are present on the apical membrane. Na$^+$ and Ca^{2+} channels on the basolateral membrane are not exposed to the H$^+$ and are unaffected. The blockade of the K$^+$ channels and movement of K$^+$ out of the cell therefore leads to depolarization of the receptor cell.

Sweetness. Sweet taste is dependent on the binding of sugars to specific membrane receptors (Fig. 4.4.3) leading to an elevation in the concentration of the second messenger cAMP. Cyclic AMP has been shown to reduce the K$^+$ conductance, probably by blocking K$^+$ channels on the basolateral membrane, and thereby producing depolarization.

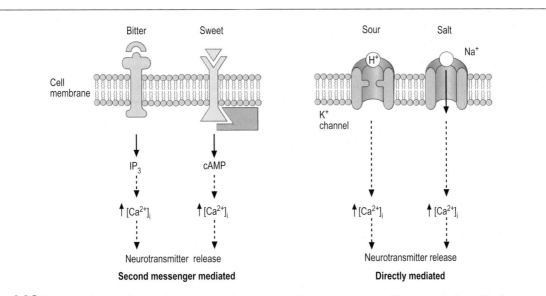

Fig. 4.4.3 Taste transduction. Bitter and sweet are mediated by second messenger systems while sour and salt are directly mediated; sour by closing a K$^+$ channel and salt by direct influx of Na$^+$ through an Na$^+$ channel. All the mechanisms result in an increase in intracellular Ca^{2+} concentration leading to neurotransmitter release.

Bitterness. Bitterness is evoked by a range of chemical compounds which bind to specific membrane receptors. As for sweetness, bitterness depends on a second messenger system probably involving inositol trisphosphate (IP_3) which leads to an increase in the intracellular Ca^{2+} concentration by release from intracellular calcium stores.

Each receptor cell is innervated by a branch of an afferent neurone. Each neurone innervates several taste buds and several receptor cells within each bud. The result is to increase the sensitivity of the system at the cost of localization. The specific chemical stimuli produce a depolarization of the receptor cell and, in consequence, an influx of Ca^{2+} through voltage-dependent Ca^{2+} channels on the basolateral membrane. The increase in intracellular Ca^{2+} concentration triggers the release of neurotransmitter to depolarize the first-order afferent neurone.

Central connections

The first-order gustatory afferents form part of one of the **cranial nerves** (VII, IX and X) projecting to the medulla. Here they form a columnar grouping, the **gustatory nucleus**. The second-order afferents project to the **thalamus** and thence to the **cerebral cortex**. At each level the gustatory fibres are separated from other sensory modalities and are unusual in that they remain ipsilateral. Within the cerebral cortex, the central coding for the interpretation of taste depends on the different levels of activity within the whole population of neurones. There is comparison of the activities of different groups of afferents which have preferred primary stimuli.

Olfaction

The olfactory system can sensitively detect and discriminate many odours. The subdivision into qualities is less satisfactory but there are considered to be seven primary qualities of smell: peppermint, musk, floral, ethereal, pungent, putrid and camphoraceous.

Summary

Taste

- Taste and smell send information to phylogenetically old areas of the brain associated with memory and emotion.
- The groups of taste buds are segregated to specific regions on the tongue.
- Saltiness and sourness are transduced directly; sweetness and bitterness involve second messengers.
- In sensing a taste, activity in neurones of all four qualities, i.e. the whole population of taste neurones, is compared.

Specific odours may be detected at concentrations of less than a few parts per billion. The foul-smelling methyl mercaptan can be detected at a concentration of 5×10^{11} molecules/litre of air, 1 molecule of mercaptan per 50 000 molecules of air.

The sense of smell is mediated by sensory receptors located in the olfactory mucosa, a small, specialized region of epithelium (about 5 cm² in total area) lying deep within the nasal cavity (Fig. 4.4.4). The receptors are bipolar neurones with a short peripheral process that expands into an **olfactory knob**. The surface of the olfactory knob gives rise to cilia that extend into the mucous layer and serve as the site of sensory transduction. The receptor cells are associated with basal and supporting cells in the epithelium which generate the new receptor cells as turnover takes place.

Odour transduction

The act of sniffing directs the incoming air onto the olfactory mucosa. Odorants entering the nasal cavity are absorbed into the mucous layer overlying the receptors. They may then diffuse through the layer till they contact the cilia.

A

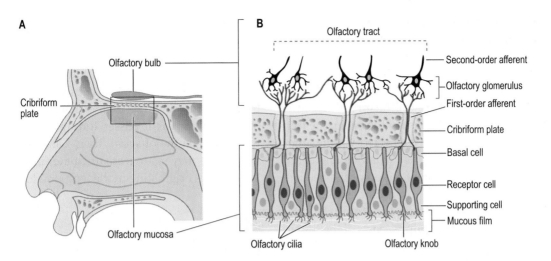

Olfactory bulb

Cribriform plate

Olfactory mucosa

B

Olfactory tract

Second-order afferent

Olfactory glomerulus

First-order afferent

Cribriform plate

Basal cell

Receptor cell

Supporting cell

Mucous film

Olfactory cilia

Olfactory knob

Fig. 4.4.4 **The olfactory mucosa. A.** The anatomical location of the olfactory mucosa and its relation to the olfactory bulb. **B.** The cellular organization of the pathway to the olfactory bulb where the first synaptic relays are found in the olfactory glomeruli.

Within the mucus they may become attached to an **olfactory binding protein** which is thought to act as a carrier.

The odorants binding with receptors on the surface of the cilia lead to the activation of second messenger systems. The most common second messenger is cAMP which causes the opening of an Na$^+$ channel, the inward current then depolarizing the receptor. The evidence suggests that there are a large number of receptors with different specificities though it is unclear how finely tuned these receptors are, whether they will respond to a single odorant or to a few but with differing degrees of response so that the combined responses of a number of such receptors would encode the specific odorant. Within the olfactory mucosa the receptors are grouped according to their primary qualities.

An obvious feature of the olfactory transduction process is that it exhibits adaptation to a high degree. The survival value of detecting new odours in the environment is obvious. The extent of adaptation possible is clear from the common observation that after being in any place for a few minutes it ceases to have a pronounced smell.

Central connections

The central processes of the bipolar receptor neurones are unmyelinated axons that are aggregated into bundles in the olfactory nerve (the first cranial nerve). The olfactory nerve passes through the sieve-like cribriform plate into the cranium. The first synaptic relay of the olfactory nerve is the ipsilateral **olfactory bulb** in the telencephalon. The transmitter in this synapse is probably carnosine. This pathway is unique among the sensory systems in that there is a direct projection to the evolutionarily old parts of the cerebral cortex before projecting onto the thalamus and then radiating to other areas of the cerebral cortex. This probably reflects the early phylogenetic development of the olfactory system compared with the other senses.

Within the olfactory bulb are specialized regions called **glomeruli** where the synaptic connections take place (Fig. 4.4.4B). There are two types of second-order neurones, the **mitral cells**, which are large with extensive dendritic fields, and smaller, **tufted cells**. There are also numerous **granule cells** which are inhibitory interneurones and which are involved in the processing of the incoming information.

343

It appears that there is some degree of functional mapping within the glomeruli, since the activity of cells within specific glomeruli increases in response to specific odorants.

The second-order afferents from the olfactory bulb project, as the **olfactory tract**, to a number of sites at the base of the brain; the two olfactory bulbs are also connected via the anterior commissure. Via the thalamus there are inputs to the orbitofrontal region of the neocortex, which is probably concerned with odour discrimination. There are also inputs to the amygdala and hippocampus, parts of the limbic system (p. 353) which are involved in the effective response to odours.

The sense of smell is important in feeding, in a social context (identifying outsiders) and in sexual behaviour. In the latter context, odour information that is not consciously appreciated influences both the physiological and the emotional sexual response. These scent cues are called pheromones.

Disturbances of taste and smell

The perceptual sensitivity of both taste and smell may be reduced by minor infections, such as head colds, that reduce the access to the olfactory mucosa giving rise to **hypo-osmia**. **Anosmia**, the inability to smell, and the inability to taste may be specific for certain stimuli which may, for example, be genetically determined. Complete anosmia may be caused after head injury by the severing of the filaments of the olfactory nerve as it passes through the cribriform plate on the olfactory tract. Olfactory hallucinations may result from **uncinate fits**, which are seizures originating in the temporal lobe.

Summary

Olfaction

- The olfactory mucosa is only about 5 cm² and lies deep within the nasal cavity.
- Cilia on the olfactory knob of smell receptors bind with odorants to activate second messenger systems.
- There are many more qualities of odour than the four qualities of taste.
- There is functional mapping of specific odours to specific regions within the olfactory tract.

Higher functions

Introduction – consciousness

The integrative processes of the central nervous system that are described as its higher functions are not simply the processing of sensory inputs or controlling motor activity, irrespective of how technically sophisticated or complicated that processing may be. Integrative activity involves the integration of sensation with memory and learned activity into consciousness and the selection of a behavioural pattern in response to that consciousness. The level of consciousness of an organism and the 'menu' of options of behaviour available to it depend on its level of evolution, and this gives us a clue to the physical basis and determinants of consciousness. Even among mammals, differences in the structure of the brain, as we compare one species to another, give us clues to the physical origin of our human consciousness.

Areas of the cerebral cortex of mammals can be identified as the termination of sensory pathways and origins of motor systems. They are called the sensory and motor cortex respectively (Fig. 4.5.1).

There are, however, regions of cortex which do not fall into either of these categories and appear to be involved with the association of one part of the brain with another. They are therefore called the **association cortex**. The vast increase in the association cortex in human beings is responsible for the relative increase in the size of our brains and the folding of the

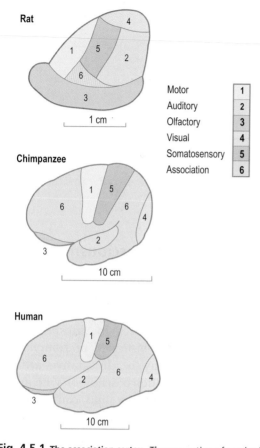

Rat

Motor	1
Auditory	2
Olfactory	3
Visual	4
Somatosensory	5
Association	6

Chimpanzee

Human

Fig. 4.5.1 The association cortex. The proportion of cerebral cortex occupied by areas in three mammalian species. The difference in the number of neurones involved can be gauged from the differences in the overall size of the brains and the fact that the neurones in all three are the same size.

cortex which give the brain its wrinkled appearance. These facts suggest two things:

- The association cortex is the physical basis of our human consciousness.
- Other animals, because they too possess this structure, to a greater or lesser degree, share our consciousness.

The neural systems of communication and control we have described so far, made up as they are from neural elements and systems of increasing complexity as we approach the higher regions of the brain, are only outposts of the physical basis of what must be one of the greatest physiological and philosophical

puzzles: What is consciousness? We have already, in Figure 3.2.1 (p. 150), superficially characterized consciousness as an observer of our sensory environment and director of our motor response.

Although the definition of consciousness is a daunting task, we can begin by defining the boundary conditions necessary for it to exist, and some of the higher functions that make up the state of consciousness.

The electroencephalogram

As consciousness must clearly be the result of specific electrical activity of the brain, we need methods of studying that activity if we wish to study consciousness.

When you consider how small the voltage changes involved in the activity of a single neurone are (less than 0.01 V), it is surprising that you can record brain activity on the surface of the skull. Such a recording can be made between two points on the skull or between a single skull electrode and a so-called indifferent electrode attached to the body. The ability to record this activity at such a distance from the tiny neurones of the brain immediately and correctly suggests that it must result from the synchronous activity of a great number of those neurones. Such a recording is called an **electroencephalogram** (EEG).

Just like the electrocardiogram, the electroencephalogram has become a routine diagnostic and experimental tool in which the position of the electrodes and description of the signals recorded has been standardized (Fig. 4.5.2, Table 4.5.1), allowing comparisons between recordings.

The form of the EEG is highly dependent on the level of consciousness (Table 4.5.2). When the subject is relaxed with eyes closed, waves with a slow rhythm (about 10 Hz) appear at the same time at many recording sites. These are called **alpha waves** and because this activity occurs simultaneously at several sites the recording is called a **synchronized EEG**.

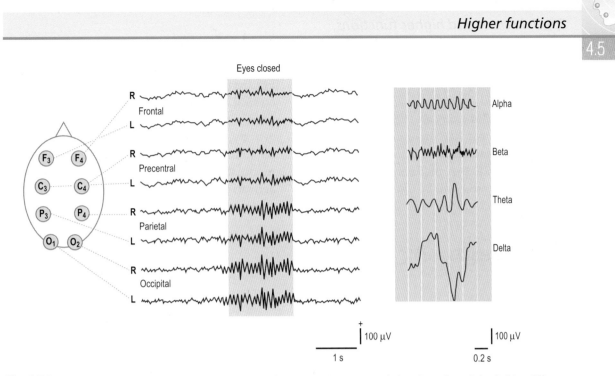

Fig. 4.5.2 The electroencephalogram. The electrical activity of the cerebral cortex recorded on the surface of the skull has different amplitudes and rhythms depending on the recording site and mental activity. When a relaxed subject closes the eyes the activity 'synchronizes' into alpha waves. As the subject slips deeper into sleep, the waves become deeper and slower until rapid eye movement sleep intervenes.

Mental activity, or sensory stimulation such as opening the eyes, suppresses the synchronized alpha waves in a process known as 'alpha blocking'. The EEG becomes irregular, with the recordings from the various sites being widely different in amplitude and frequency. The EEG has become 'desynchronized'. In place of the alpha waves smaller higher-frequency **beta waves** (about 20 Hz) dominate the picture.

On the other hand, if the subject falls asleep, larger slower **theta waves** (about 6 Hz) and **delta waves** (about 3 Hz) appear. In children these slower waves are seen even when awake.

It is clear that the EEG arises from the neurones of the cerebral cortex. Direct recordings from these neurones and the frequencies of the EEG waves demonstrate that the EEG is the result of slow changes in the membrane

Table 4.5.1 Frequency bands that constitute recognizable EEG waves

Wave	Frequency
Delta	0.5–3.5 Hz
Theta	4–7.5 Hz
Alpha	8–12 Hz
Beta	13–30 Hz

Table 4.5.2 EEG patterns in different behavioural states

Behavioural state	EEG wave pattern
Excited	Highly variable, low voltage, mainly beta activity
Alert (eyes open)	Mainly beta activity, low voltage
Relaxed	Alpha bursts (usually when eyes closed)
Drowsy	Low alpha activity, slow waves, mainly theta and delta activity
Sleep	No alpha activity, sleep spindles and slow waves

potentials of cortical neurones (excitatory and inhibitory postsynaptic potentials) and are not due to the traffic of action potentials.

Each electrode in an EEG samples the synchronized activity of more than 1 000 000 cortical neurones below its site of attachment to the skull, and the more synchronized the activity the greater will be the amplitude of the EEG. This activity is not synchronized to produce the alpha rhythm by the cortex itself but by the thalamus controlling the rhythm of cortical activity. Cells in the thalamic nuclei are known to generate a spontaneous 'pacemaker' activity at a frequency of about 3 Hz. The thalamus in turn has its rhythmic activity modulated by inputs mainly from the **reticular activating system**, which is important in influencing our cycle of sleeping and waking.

Clinical Example

Implications of the EEG

The electroencephalogram (EEG) was first described in 1929 by the psychiatrist Hans Berger. He discovered that the electrical activity of the human brain could be measured through the skull. Since this time the EEG has become a valuable investigative and diagnostic tool used widely in both psychiatry and neurology.

Despite its widespread use, the physiological basis of the EEG is not entirely understood and the interpretation of EEGs is a highly skilled and difficult task.

The EEG measures the voltage difference between electrodes attached to the scalp. This voltage is related to the electrical activity of the underlying neurones of the cerebral cortex; the tiny electrical signals are amplified and recorded. Intracellular recordings from individual neurones may measure several millivolts, whereas the EEG recorded on the skull may measure between 10 and 100 microvolts.

The EEG wave characteristics recorded depend on several factors including physical factors such as the degree of folding of the underlying gyri of the cerebral cortex and the degree of bone thickness (and therefore electrical resistance) of the skull. The type of wave form recorded on the EEG also depends on the amount of synchronization of the underlying neurones; the greater the degree of synchronization the greater the voltage recorded and therefore the greater the amplitude of the EEG wave.

High degrees of synchronization of cortical activity result in EEG spikes. These are defined as waves lasting 70 milliseconds or less. EEG spikes are seen in disease states such as epilepsy, which is often diagnosed using electroencephalography in addition to a clinical history of convulsions.

The physiology of what happens at the cellular level to produce an ECG is still unclear but it is known that the pyramidal cells in the cortex have afferent inhibitory and excitatory connections which result in the conduction of changes in the neuronal action potential as axon spikes. Axon spikes are conducted to the postsynaptic membranes causing electrical changes, and it is assumed that the summation of these can be recorded on the scalp as the EEG.

The normal EEG

In the normal individual the amplitude and frequency of the EEG are dependent on behavioural state (see Table 4.5.2) and age. The EEG of an infant under 1 year typically has a dominant slow occipital rhythm with generalized slow-wave delta and theta activity. This is a very different picture from that of a normal adult where there is usually dominant alpha activity over the posterior quadrant of the skull. Slow-wave delta and theta activity is normal in the very young and in adults during sleep.

Clinical Example *(Continued)*

The abnormal EEG

Certain EEG patterns are indicative of distinct clinical disorders. The following are descriptions of a small sample of clinically important disorders that display characteristic EEG abnormalities:

- *Petit mal epilepsy* classically has a 3 Hz spike and wave pattern.
- *Grand mal epilepsy* is identified by large 8–12 Hz spikes in groups during tonic–clonic seizures.
- *Migraine* can be difficult to distinguish from cerebrovascular disease, especially if the presentation is with acute hemiplegia. The EEG in these migraine sufferers shows localized slow wave activity. Generally in migraine the EEG changes are non-specific.
- *Creutzfeldt–Jakob disease* is a neurodegenerative disorder caused by prion disease which presents clinically with dementia and myoclonic jerks (often elicited by startle). The EEG contains periodic repetitive discharges, typically at a rate of 1–2/second, occurring bilaterally. This feature, while not always present early in the illness, is strongly suggestive of the diagnosis.
- *Huntington's chorea* shows a generalized flattening of the EEG trace that is thought to be due to loss of basal ganglia cells.
- *Alzheimer's dementia* is characterized by reduced alpha activity on EEG.
- *Delirium* usually shows slow alpha activity and increased delta activity on EEG.
- *Herpes simplex encephalitis* is characterized by discharges occurring every 1–3 seconds with slow-wave activity prominent in the temporal areas. These abnormalities on the EEG typically occur within the first 2 weeks of illness.

Psychiatric disorders unfortunately do not show EEGs of unvarying character that could be used diagnostically. There are, however, a few useful associations:

- *schizophrenia* – no characteristic pattern is found uniformly, although many non-specific patterns have been reported
- *depression* – the normal characteristic, of a latent period of about 1 hour before an REM sleep EEG pattern occurs, is disturbed, with REM pattern occurring sometimes in a matter of minutes after falling asleep
- *dementias* – the associations in Huntington's chorea and Alzheimer's disease are described above.

As might be expected, drugs can alter EEGs:

- *hypnotics and sedatives* – increase beta wave activity
- *tricyclic antidepressants* – increase theta and delta waves and reduce alpha waves
- *alcohol* – increases theta waves.

Clinical significance

The EEG is a useful diagnostic test but it should be noted that corroborative clinical features are required. EEG is particularly helpful in that it can suggest the possibility of abnormality in the function of the brain despite normal structure (e.g. a normal CT scan in a patient with severe epilepsy).

In addition to its role in the diagnosis of disease states, EEG has proved to be a useful tool in the study of the physiology of sleep and sleep disorders.

It should be noted that despite widespread use in medicine, EEG has its limitations. Up to 30% of patients with epilepsy have a normal EEG between fits, while up to 15% of normal individuals show abnormalities in their EEG. Therefore all EEG results need to be interpreted in the context of the overall clinical picture.

Summary

The electroencephalogram (EEG)

- Development of human consciousness is closely related to dominance of the association cortex in the human brain.
- The electroencephalogram records activity in the cerebral cortex synchronized by the thalamus.
- Patterns of EEG depend on the level of arousal and are used diagnostically.
- Drugs affect the pattern of the EEG.

Sleep and arousal

Every day we each experience changes in consciousness that are beyond the explanation of neural science, we wake up and go to sleep. We have detailed descriptions of what happens to us during sleep and the devastating effects of being deprived of it but its actual physiological function still eludes us.

It is most people's experience that they perform best at some specific time during the day. They say they are 'morning people' or 'evening people' (very few claim to be 'afternoon people'). These differences in performance and perception are the result of *circadian rhythms* (see Ch. 1.5) and one of these rhythms is linked with the desire to sleep.

While depth of sleep can be simply gauged by the strength of stimulus required to wake the sleeper the EEG provides a more objective analysis of types of sleep.

Sleep is not a uniform state; when we first drop off to sleep we can be easily wakened but as time passes we sink deeper into sleep. As sleep deepens, the EEG becomes slower until deep sleep brings with it a trace composed almost entirely of large slow delta waves. The visible physical correlates of this deep sleep are the slow breathing, low heart rate and profound muscular relaxation we see in the contented sleeper.

A night's sleep is not uniform, however; about every 90 minutes our sleep lightens, respiration and heart rate speed up, and muscle tone briefly returns. Then follows a period during which there is profound relaxation of the skeletal muscles *except for salvoes of rapid eye movements*; these periods are called **rapid eye movement (REM) sleep** and last about 15 minutes (Fig. 4.5.3).

During REM sleep, the EEG is similar to that of someone who has just fallen into shallow sleep, but paradoxically the subject is very difficult to awaken, as if he or she is in deep sleep. For this reason REM sleep is sometimes called *paradoxical sleep*.

The profound skeletal muscle relaxation which accompanies REM sleep has a dangerous aspect to it. The tone of the muscles of the pharynx normally holds the pharynx open during respiration. When this tone is removed in REM sleep, the negative pressure of inspiration in the airways can cause the pharynx to collapse, blocking the airway and preventing breathing, in what is known as *obstructive sleep apnoea*.

One of the dangers with obstructive sleep apnoea is that it causes the sufferer to wake just for a few seconds and, as this occurs during REM sleep, the subject is deprived of REM sleep, an essential component of normal sleep. Sufferers of sleep apnoea find themselves suffering the symptoms of sleep deprivation and dropping off to sleep during the day. If they are driving or operating machinery when that happens the results can be fatal.

Subjects who are woken during a period of REM sleep, frequently report that they were dreaming. This and other evidence strongly suggests that dreams take place largely during REM sleep. If subjects are deliberately deprived of REM sleep they undergo mood changes (for the worse), and go through brief REM phases even with their eyes open. It is not clear whether the detrimental effects of sleep deprivation come from the lack of REM sleep or the

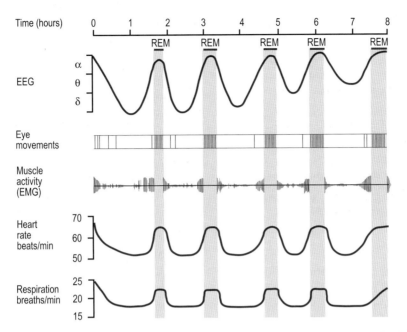

Fig. 4.5.3 Sleep cycles. A night's sleep is cyclical, depth being gauged by the EEG, getting shallower as the night progresses. During rapid eye movement (REM) sleep, skeletal muscle tone diminishes and respiratory and heart rate increase.

lack of dreams. After a period of REM sleep deprivation, subjects spend a larger percentage of their total sleep than normal in REM sleep. You cannot, however, go straight to REM sleep; you must first have a period of non-REM sleep, however brief.

It would be very reasonable to consider sleep as a period of necessary 'rest' for the brain. It has been suggested that there is an accumulation, or depletion, of chemicals which must be corrected at regular intervals. No such accumulation or depletion has been measured and it is clear from the EEG that sleep is a different but no less active state of the brain. In this and other ways, sleep differs from coma, another state of absence of consciousness but which depends on suppressed brain activity.

Without making the perhaps unwarranted assumption that wakefulness is the natural state, we can at least discover what arouses consciousness from sleep. In the brainstem are found specific sensory pathways and

non-specific projections. Destruction of this area of the brainstem or its projections to the cerebrum results in coma. Electrical stimulation of this **ascending reticular activating system** arouses a subject from sleep. General anaesthetics and stimulants such as amphetamines act in this area. Two nuclei, the **locus coeruleus** and the **raphe nucleus**, are central to the sleep–wake–sleep cycle. These nuclei, either directly or via giant reticular neurones which have enormous fields of activity throughout the brain, have dendrites which end close to all the cells of the cortex. The raphe nucleus secretes serotonin (5-hydroxytryptamine), which appears to be essential for the induction of non-REM sleep which precedes REM sleep. REM sleep is then induced by noradrenaline secreted by the locus coeruleus (Fig. 4.5.4).

A clue to the need for sleep comes from the fact that infants and young children spend a much greater fraction of their day asleep than adults, and a greater fraction of an infant's sleep

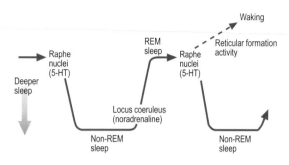

Fig. 4.5.4 **Sleep–wakefulness.** The rhythm between REM and non-REM sleep is established by release of serotonin (5-HT) and noradrenaline in the brainstem. Activity in the ascending reticular activating system promotes wakefulness.

is spent in REM. The total duration of sleep and the fraction devoted to REM sleep decreases in an almost linear fashion throughout life, and it may be that REM sleep is important for the maturation of the brain of young individuals.

Summary

Sleep and arousal

- Sleep can be categorized as non-REM and REM (rapid eye movement).
- Circadian rhythms divide sleep into approximately 90-minute periods of non-REM sleep separated by 15-minute intervals of REM sleep.
- During REM sleep, the subject has the appearance of being in a very shallow sleep except for profound skeletal muscle relaxation.
- Dreams take place during REM sleep.
- Cycling between REM and non-REM sleep involves the locus coeruleus and raphe nucleus, while the level of arousal depends on the ascending reticular activating system.

Learning and memory

Learning and memory are probably the most evolutionarily advantageous developments in neurophysiology. The acquisition of information, **learning**, and its storage in **memory** enable an organism to repeat success and avoid failure by utilizing its past experience.

In our own experience we remember very little of our past; about 1% of our experience is stored long term and a great deal of that is forgotten. This process is important to prevent us being overwhelmed by information, and it seems that the amount already stored and the information acquired after a fact has been added to our memory determine the likelihood of the fact being retained.

Although we are only beginning to understand the neuronal mechanisms of memory, models of how memory works have been about for some time. It is generally accepted that there are several levels of memory (Fig. 4.5.5).

It is generalizations and concepts that are stored in memory and the details are filled in while it is being retrieved.

Information from the environment is first received by modality-specific sensory stores. Visual **sensory memory** is known as **iconic memory** and material stored here begins to decay in less than 1 second. Auditory, **echoic memory**, shows significant decay if not reinforced in 5 seconds. Human ability to verbalize both abstract and concrete ideas is a great adjunct to memory and it appears that verbalization of the unit of memory, the so-called **engram**, takes place before it is passed on to **short-term memory** where it has a life of seconds unless it is supported by practice, that is attentive repetition. This is the stage of the telephone number just read from the 'phone-book being repeated while you go to the telephone. Practice appears to be reinforcing an engram resonating in a neural network (Fig. 4.5.6); it also helps the transfer of information to the large permanent **secondary memory**.

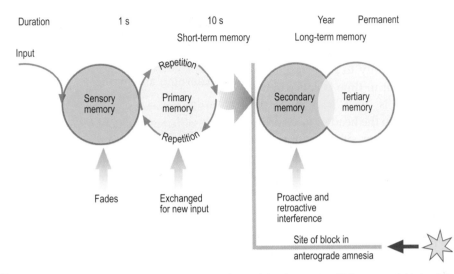

Fig. 4.5.5 Types of memory. Only a part of the memory stored at each level passes to a higher, more stable level. Repetition helps, but does not guarantee transfer from primary to secondary memory. Anterograde amnesia prevents storage of memory after the event (for example, a blow) which produces it.

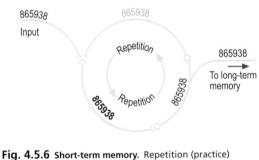

Fig. 4.5.6 Short-term memory. Repetition (practice) reinforces an engram resonating in a neural network in short-term memory and helps its transition to secondary memory. The loop-like appearance of this model should not suggest that memory is like magnetic tape or disk.

Figure 4.5.6 is dangerous if it suggests to you that your memory is like a magnetic tape or computer disk which picks up information until the input stops or the disk is full. That this is not so is clearly demonstrated by the fact that it is easier to remember a short sequence of letters or numbers than a long one. It is in secondary memory, where storage takes place from minutes to years. Here the erosion of the stored material by material already stored, proactive inhibition, or things learned later, retroactive inhibition, takes place. Material in secondary memory that is used regularly, like

your name, or how to write, passes into **tertiary memory** and is never forgotten unless trauma or disease intervene.

The location of memory

Models of the type shown in Figure 4.5.5 do not tell us much about the physical basis of memory. Our information about the location of that part of the brain involved in the processing of information to form memory comes from some fairly disastrous operations carried out in America to relieve certain types of epilepsy. The tips of the **temporal lobes** of the cerebral hemispheres were removed and the unfortunate patient found that while his epilepsy was not relieved he now could not remember for more than 10 minutes anything that happened after the operation although his memory of before the operation was unimpaired. It is probable that this disability resulted from damage to the **limbic system**, which lies within the temporal cortex itself. This is supported by the observation that alcoholics frequently show degenerative changes of the limbic system and suffer from a type of anterograde amnesia known as the Korsakoff syndrome.

This phenomenon is clearly an interference with the processing of new information and it seems that **long-term memory** is more diffusely or robustly stored. Inability to retrieve memories from before a point in time is called retrograde amnesia and is well known to be associated with blows to the head or electroconvulsive therapy. Even after such treatments it appears to be *access* to secondary memory rather than the memory itself that is damaged because, with recovery, the forgotten period gets shorter.

While these findings tell us of the gross locations of structures associated with memory, they do not tell us what the essential changes in synaptic transmission must be to establish memories. The idea that information is first stored as a dynamic engram of resonating activity has already been described in our consideration of short-term memory. Long-term memory requires a structural engram to be established, and of all the possible ways this might occur long-term potentiation is the current favourite.

Long-term potentiation

It is a seductive theory that long-term engrams are 'written' as circuits in the brain, these circuits being pathways of reduced resistance through the synaptic network. Support for this theory comes from the phenomenon of **long-term potentiation** (LTP).

LTP is the enhancement of synaptic transmission in certain brain synapses (particularly in the hippocampus) which follows a brief conditioning burst of presynaptic stimulation. Subsequently, transmission is easier at that synapse for days or weeks. A low resistance path has been 'etched' in the brain.

LTP involves the excitatory amino acid (EAA) synapse specifically stimulated by *N*-methyl-D-aspartate (NMDA). Conditioning these cell membrane receptors makes transmission easier by both presynaptic and postsynaptic mechanisms, the former involving enhanced release of transmitter.

Summary

Learning and memory

• There are several levels of memory with different durations of retention and mechanisms of storage.
• The step from short- to long-term memory is the point most vulnerable to disruption. Here anterograde amnesia exerts its effect.
• The limbic system is profoundly involved in the process of memory.
• Long-term potentiation enhancing synaptic transmission along neural pathways provides a potential physical explanation for long-term memory.

Lateral dominance

A striking anatomical characteristic of the central nervous system is its **bilateral symmetry** as defined by the longitudinal fissure of the brain and the anterior fissure and median septum of the spinal cord. We have not made much of the crossing over of visual information at the **optic chiasma** nor the **decussation** of sensory and motor pathways (Fig. 4.5.7) nor the massive connections between the right and left sides of the brain which make up the **corpus callosum**. In fact the anatomy of the central nervous system might lead us to believe that there is a right and left half acting together and in parallel. This concept of neat symmetry is disturbed by the overwhelming tendency of most individuals to be right- or left-handed and by a group of patients known as 'split brain' individuals.

In an attempt to restrict the spread of devastating epileptic episodes from one side of the brain to the other a number of patients have had the corpus callosum, which joins the cerebral cortices of the two sides of the brain, cut. Apart from their original problem, these patients seem to suffer few ill effects from this

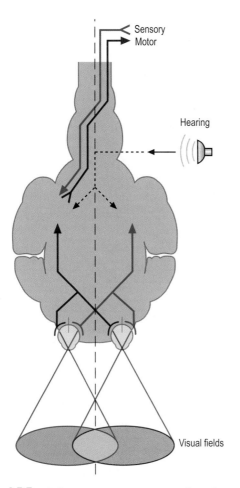

Fig. 4.5.7 Split brain. How sensory, motor and visual systems are segregated to the contralateral cortex of the brain. If the brain is split down the middle, sensation and motor activity is served by the opposite side of the brain. Hearing from each ear goes to both sides.

⚡ Summary

Lateral dominance

- Right and left cerebral hemispheres are mainly connected by the corpus callosum.
- Cutting the corpus callosum demonstrates that the left hemisphere of the brain – connected to the right side of the body – has all the attributes of a complete human brain.
- Experiences going to the right hemisphere cannot be expressed verbally or in writing; this hemisphere is bereft of language.

hemisphere and the subject behaves like a normal individual.

Objects placed in the *left* visual field cannot be named, but the subject can be instructed verbally, or by using writing placed in the *left* field, to correctly select objects. However, even after selecting them the subject cannot name them. He cannot express experiences going to his *right* cerebral hemisphere verbally or in writing.

Thus the left hemisphere of the brain is indistinguishable in its abilities from the whole normal brain. The right hemisphere and its subcortical structures, however, appear to lead an independent life, bereft of language even in normal individuals.

Because our human consciousness is so dependent on our ability to verbalize our experience, it is tempting to suppose that the physical substrate for human consciousness resides in the left side of our brain, even though our right cerebral hemisphere and its subcortical structures show abilities such as musical understanding and spatial awareness which exceed those of the left.

heroic procedure. That is, until we restrict the sensory information presented to the subject to one side of the body.

A normally right-handed subject who has undergone this 'brain splitting' can recognize objects and read words in the *right* side of his visual field, (Fig 4.5.7) and can recognize objects placed in his right hand. This sensory information is being fed to his *left* (dominant) cerebral

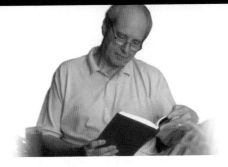

4.6

Ageing and the special senses

Introduction – patterns of ageing

The Concise Oxford Dictionary defines the verb to age as 'to grow old or mature'. In this chapter we look at ageing and the special senses in this light, i.e. including two simultaneous processes – growing old, and maturing. Growing old can be taken to correspond to the negative aspect – deterioration of function. Maturing can be taken to correspond to the positive aspect – increasing ability to respond appropriately to challenges. The human life span, nowadays most commonly 70–80 years, can be viewed as a combination of maturation and deterioration – of build-up and

run-down. Although the two processes coexist, maturation (including both physical growth and increasing skills) dominates in the first two to three decades and deterioration dominates in the last two to three decades of life. Figure 4.6.1 indicates the concept and some components of the processes of maturation and deterioration. Before applying these concepts to the special senses, they will be reviewed briefly in physiological terms.

Maturation

The major growth in body tissues and their assumption of the adult state takes place in the first 15 or so years of life.

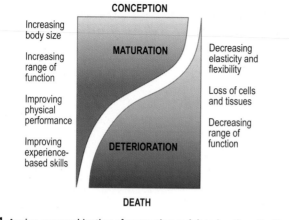

CONCEPTION

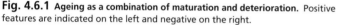

Increasing body size

Increasing range of function

Improving physical performance

Improving experience-based skills

MATURATION

Decreasing elasticity and flexibility

Loss of cells and tissues

Decreasing range of function

DETERIORATION

DEATH

Fig. 4.6.1 **Ageing as a combination of maturation and deterioration.** Positive features are indicated on the left and negative on the right.

Physical performance tends to improve for a further similar period, with increasing muscle strength, particularly in the male, and improved neurological control. After this, function can continue to improve with experience and even centenarians can experience and participate in new activities. Throughout the life span much of this maturation is due to developments in the brain and this is highly relevant in regard to the special senses. Large regions of the brain are concerned with the interpretation of patterns obtained from the eyes and from the ears. These regions are organized during maturation and contribute in turn to our ability to carry out skilled physical activities and make appropriate judgements. There is increasing evidence that quite localized brain regions are involved in critical decisions. Such evidence is provided by modern scanning techniques which can, for example, show increased activity in a specific area when people are matching patterns with different colours. Further evidence comes from patients with small cerebral tumours whose only symptoms may be loss of a specific skill, in one case the skill to identify paintings by specific artists.

Deterioration

As indicated in Figure 4.6.1, this occurs to some extent even in the fetal state and infancy, e.g. loss of elasticity and flexibility with gradual drying out of the body and deterioration chemically in major body components such as collagen and elastin. Increasingly with age the effects of loss of irreplaceable cells and tissues, e.g. brain cells, teeth, cartilage, becomes apparent, leading to a severe decrease in the ability to vary function in old age. This may range from less ability to deal with the fluid loss of intestinal infections to increased vulnerability to excessive heat and cold. This diminishing range of functions is also evident in the special senses.

The causes of the deterioration are the subject of much research, and may include cell self-destruction – apoptosis – and accumulation of toxins, including the currently fashionable oxygen free radicals. In more general terms, some of the major causes of accelerated ageing, or deterioration, are environmental and, to some extent, preventable – cigarette smoke, radiation, including solar radiation, and in the case of hearing overuse in the form of sustained loud noise.

The combined effects of maturation and deterioration of the special senses will now be examined – mainly with respect to vision and hearing.

Vision

Patterns of maturation will be discussed first, followed by problems with maturation and then patterns of deterioration.

Maturation

At the time of birth the human infant is suddenly exposed to a bright and colourful world with which life in the uterus can provide little comparable experience. The infant shows little evidence of appreciating the significance of these new surroundings and only gradually develops the ability to distinguish and respond to various faces and objects. Research in other species suggests that without normal visual stimuli (e.g. with the eyes permanently covered) the visual cortex fails to develop and normal vision is impossible. This is confirmed, as discussed later, in children where a refractive error or squinting can lead to blindness in one eye. Thus it is possible to have a structurally normal eye which is useless to the individual because the related and linked cortical areas of the brain are not available to interpret the visual patterns reaching that eye.

Problems with maturation

Normal maturation includes synthesis in the brain of the patterns obtained from the two eyes into a single three-dimensional picture – normal **binocular vision**. Development of binocular vision can be hindered or totally prevented when problems in the eyes make it difficult or impossible for the infant/child to focus comfortably on objects with the two eyes simultaneously. In general such problems lead to squinting.

Squinting is present when the visual axes of the two eyes do not normally converge on the object being looked at (Fig. 4.6.2). The effect is that the fixing eye receives a clear image of the object on the macula lutea (the most sensitive part of the retina with the best visual acuity) and this clear image is conveyed to the visual cortex. The squinting eye, however, receives a different part of the visual field on its macula and the object seen by the fixing eye is relatively peripheral and indistinct. The visual cortex fails to receive the simultaneous clear pictures from the two eyes which are necessary for development of the connections leading to

binocular vision with its three-dimensional quality and sense of distance. Where two coherent images should be available for blending and interpretation, there are conflicting images. The only solution it seems is for the central visual processes progressively to ignore the less clear and relevant information from the squinting eye. This is what happens with the so-called 'lazy eye'. The images from the 'lazy', i.e. squinting, eye may eventually be completely suppressed and that eye is essentially blind – the individual at this final stage can see nothing when the

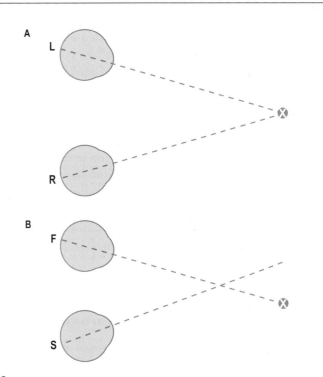

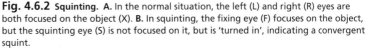

Fig. 4.6.2 Squinting. A. In the normal situation, the left (L) and right (R) eyes are both focused on the object (X). **B.** In squinting, the fixing eye (F) focuses on the object, but the squinting eye (S) is not focused on it, but is 'turned in', indicating a convergent squint.

dominant, fixing, eye is covered. This process occurs in childhood and when complete there is no known way of regaining vision for the squinting eye. To prevent irreversible changes, the fixing eye may be covered intermittently so that the squinting eye retains function while remedial measures are arranged.

Diagnosis and treatment of the condition are necessary to prevent the eye becoming blind. Squinting is often noticed by parents and can be confirmed by expert examination. It is often related to refractive problems in the eyes, commonly *myopia* (short-sight) or *hypermetropia* (long-sight). In myopia, the eye is long relative to the refractive power of the eye, so that the image, particularly at a distance, is formed in front of the retina. In hypermetropia the opposite is the case and the image is formed behind the retina. In both cases blurring results. These refractive errors can be corrected by appropriate spectacles with a concave lens for myopia and a convex lens for hypermetropia.

Correction of refractive errors increases the clarity of objects for both eyes and reduces the burden on the child who may avoid squinting only by excessive activity in the ciliary muscle which controls lens convexity and in the external ocular muscles which determine direction of gaze – the squint in such cases may appear intermittently when the child is tired.

Imbalance of the extraocular muscles is a second major cause of squinting. In this case the resting position of the two eyes may be excessively convergent or divergent. Eye surgery, by moving the site of attachment of one or more of the extraocular muscles, can rotate the visual axis of the eye. Thus, in Figure 4.6.2, the visual axis of the squinting eye (S) would be moved to correspond to that of (R) in the upper diagram. When these corrections are made early in life the squinting can be cured and binocular vision developed. This can be both assessed and assisted by exercises in which the child is presented with separate images to the two eyes and encouraged to blend them, e.g. an image of a bird in one eye and of a cage in the other perceived as a bird in a cage.

Thus improved optical function in the two eyes leads to improved cortical organization in the brain which in turn allows the two eyes to be used optimally for binocular vision.

Deterioration

Macular degeneration

All aspects of the eyes and vision are subject to deterioration. Thus the rods and cones of the retina are gradually lost, leading to a reduced ability to distinguish small items such as the differences between letters at a distance. This ability is carried out mainly in the macula lutea because the closely packed cones there provide the basis for distinguishing tiny objects from one another. Macular degeneration is increasingly common in older people. In severe cases the middle of the visual field becomes a featureless blur, and vision is greatly impaired despite the vast majority of the retinal area functioning normally. Cigarette smoke and solar radiation are two specific causes which accelerate ageing changes in the macula. An extreme example is solar burning due to staring at the sun during an eclipse.

Glaucoma

Glaucoma is another example of deterioration of vision associated with ageing. It causes almost the opposite effect to macular degeneration – tunnel vision, where the visual fields contract to relatively small central discs. The mechanism is increased intraocular pressure due to accumulation of excessive aqueous humor. This fluid is secreted by the ciliary gland in the posterior chamber of the eye, and absorbed in tiny channels which lead to a circular canal at the corneoscleral angle in the anterior chamber. This canal communicates with local veins. In glaucoma the channels become blocked so that absorption is decreased and fluid pressure rises. This rise in pressure can become severe, so that increased pressure is transmitted back through the vitreous body to the retina. The back of the eye then bulges at the optic disc and this 'cupping' can be seen when looking at the back of the eye with an ophthalmoscope. The pressure is severe enough to damage fibres of the optic nerve, which leave the eye here. Random loss of fibres progressively reduces the number of rods and cones that can send signals to the visual cortex. Since the macular region has by far the highest concentration of sensory cells (all cones) it retains reasonable vision when peripheral vision has been lost.

Diagnosis of glaucoma is made by measuring ocular pressure using a delicate instrument (tonometer) which presses on the front of the eye and registers the resistance. The aim is to recognize the condition before serious damage has been done and the visual fields have contracted as demonstrated by perimetry. Two methods of treatment are available – reducing secretion of aqueous fluid and improving drainage. *Carbonic anhydrase inhibitors* reduce secretion, suggesting that this active process relies on carbonic anhydrase or a similar enzyme. Drainage can be improved in the short term by drugs which constrict the pupil since this moves the iris towards the centre of the cornea and away from the drainage channels in the corneoscleral angle. Surgical removal of a segment of iris has a similar effect.

Cataract

Cataracts constitute one of the commonest causes of remediable blindness throughout the world and are a good example of deterioration of function (this time of the lens) which is strongly associated with ageing. It may seem strange that the word for opacity of the lens of the eye is the same as for a series of falls on a river. However, the ancients used the same word since in both cases the condition offered an obstruction – in one case to the passage of boats along a river and in the other to the passage of light through the refractive media of the eye. Removal of cataracts provides one of the most dramatic of modern medical treatments. With finely developed skills (relying on excellent vision developed during maturation of the surgeon's eyes!) and using local anaesthetics, the opaque lens can be removed with little disturbance to the patient. In addition, a replacement lens can be inserted. Naturally the removal of the lens greatly reduces the refractive power of the eye leaving an impractically distant near point. Formerly this was corrected by powerful convex lens spectacles, but the inserted lens is much more convenient.

Occasionally results are disappointing. Since the cataract is opaque it is not possible to assess clearly the state of the macula and if this has deteriorated while the cataract was present then vision may remain poor. In contrast, many patients notice not only vastly improved clarity of vision but also the return of vivid colour vision. The reason is that a cataract usually affects mainly central vision. Thus the patient retains peripheral vision, but since this is mediated largely through rods it is strongly monochromatic – likened to a sepia print. Return of cone vision brings full colour vision.

Presbyopia

One feature of visual deterioration is so strongly linked with age that it is called 'the vision of the elderly', i.e. presbyopia – presby, referring to the elderly and opia, referring to vision. This is due to a further aspect of age-related deterioration of the lens. To understand it we need to understand that focusing on nearby objects relies on the ability of the lens to spring into a relatively convex shape.

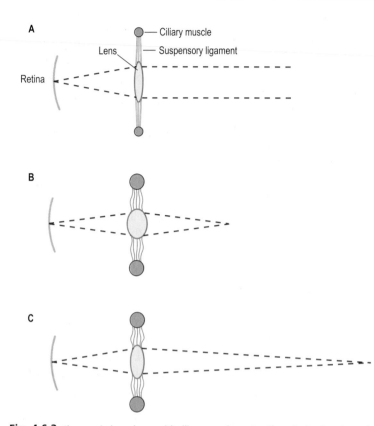

Fig. 4.6.3 Changes in lens shape with ciliary muscle contraction. **A.** A relaxed muscle and a flattened lens focusing an object at infinity on the retina. **B.** A contracted ciliary muscle and a lens which has sprung into a convex shape (exaggerated here), focusing an object at the near point on the retina. **C.** In contrast, when the ciliary muscle contracts and relaxes the suspensory ligaments in the presbyotic eye, the lens shows much less increase in convexity, so the near point has receded much further from the eye.

Figure 4.6.3A shows the eye in the resting state. The ciliary (smooth) muscle is relaxed. Being shaped like a sphincter round the corneoscleral junction, the relaxed state is associated with maximal separation of opposite sides of the muscle, so the suspensory ligaments of the lens pull on its margins and flatten it. The eye is focused on infinity. The middle diagram (Fig. 4.6.3B) shows the opposite state (effects are exaggerated to make the point). Vision is actively 'concentrated' on a nearby object and the ciliary muscle is maximally contracted. The gap in the middle of the 'sphincter' narrows, releasing the pull of the suspensory ligaments on the margin of the lens. The lens of its own 'elasticity' springs into a more convex shape and focuses on the near point.

The bottom diagram (Fig. 4.6.3C) shows the contracted ciliary muscle in the presbyopic eye. Although the suspensory ligaments are relaxed, the lens has much less ability to spring into a convex shape, so the same effort by the ciliary muscle leads to much less convexity and the near point is now much further away. Thus small print which could be read by the eye in the middle diagram is too distant to be read by the one in the bottom diagram. If the print is held closer, there is blurring and again it cannot be read. Eventually the lens becomes hardened, stiffened and virtually rigid so that the near point moves well away from the eye – perhaps to as much as a metre.

These changes occur universally. The result is that while young children have a near point of around 5 cm, the near point is about 10 cm in the late teens and continues to recede to 50 or more centimetres by the age of 50. At this stage the lens has virtually lost its ability to accommodate (change shape with ciliary muscle contraction) and there is little further change. Put technically, the accommodating power of the lens is around 15 dioptres in early childhood, about 10 in the twenties, 5 in the forties and 1 from the mid-fifties. The problem can be dealt with by using a convex lens (magnifying glass or spectacles) which restores the ability to focus on objects near the eye, and makes use of the relatively good retinal function present in most people. Because a small aperture and good light give a sharper picture for optical reasons, the presbyopic eye can read much better in a bright than in a dim light.

Hearing

Again, some aspects of maturation will be considered, followed by patterns of deterioration.

Maturation

While the complexities of three-dimensional vision are linked to skilled movements such as sporting abilities, maturation of hearing is strongly linked with speech. Just as the totally blind cannot compete in sports with the visually normal, so the totally deaf cannot speak normally. The development of hearing patterns and consequently speech takes place largely in early childhood. This early maturation is manifest in a greatly superior ability to acquire language, particularly the nuances of pronunciation, in early childhood compared with adulthood. Thus treatment such as the artificial cochlea must be applied at this stage. With lesser degrees of deafness, as with squints and refractive errors, correction by appropriate hearing aids and the use of lip-reading need to be applied as soon as practical to aid central maturation and the acquisition of optimal speech and related education.

Deterioration

Just as the lens of the eye is the site of the common pattern of deterioration of vision with ageing, so deterioration of hearing is determined largely by deterioration in a specific locality – the part of the cochlea concerned with detecting high frequencies. This is the basis of presbyacusis – 'the hearing of the elderly'.

Presbyacusis

Like presbyopia, this is an almost universal finding. It is quantified in the audiogram, which conventionally plots sound frequency on the x-axis and hearing loss (downwards) on the y-axis. Figure 4.6.4 shows diagrammatically some normal audiograms and the progression of presbyacusis. Normal audiograms can be produced for air conduction (sound transmitted through external and middle ear) and for bone conduction (sound transmitted through bone to the inner ear). The normal line for both passes through zero, because *zero hearing loss equals average normal hearing* by both methods, even though bone conduction is less efficient than air conduction.

In the early stages of presbyacusis hearing loss is mainly evident at the higher frequencies and this is increasingly so in severe presbyacusis, where hearing for low frequencies is only

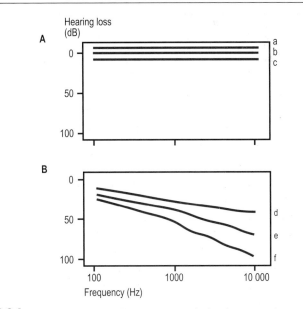

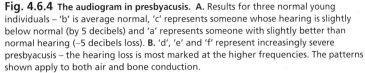

Fig. 4.6.4 The audiogram in presbyacusis. A. Results for three normal young individuals – 'b' is average normal, 'c' represents someone whose hearing is slightly below normal (by 5 decibels) and 'a' represents someone with slightly better than normal hearing (–5 decibels loss). **B.** 'd', 'e' and 'f' represent increasingly severe presbyacusis – the hearing loss is most marked at the higher frequencies. The patterns shown apply to both air and bone conduction.

moderately affected, whereas hearing for the high frequencies is virtually abolished. What is the reason for the difference? It can be explained by the fact that high frequencies are perceived in the initial part of the organ of hearing near the oval window, whereas low frequencies are perceived further up and along greater lengths of the cochlea. As people age and as presbyacusis progresses, it is this early part of the cochlea that deteriorates most. This is not surprising as it is the most delicate part of the cochlea and is subject to very high-frequency shaking. It is of interest that the deafness produced by working for long periods at very high noise levels (85 decibels and over) shows quite similar patterns and in many respects is an accelerated form of presbyacusis.

What is the effect of this pattern? High-pitched sounds like whistles and birdsong become undetectable. Even more significantly, the condition has a serious effect on perceiving speech. Intelligibility of speech depends heavily on consonants, which are of relatively high frequency. Their frequency is around 2000–3000 Hz and they may be indistinguishable to those with moderate to severe presbyacusis, leading the hearer to make guesses, which may seem amusing to others but can be frustrating and humiliating to the older person. Clear enunciation is the best way of communicating. Sound amplification may be of little help or may make matters worse by reaching unpleasant levels of noise without improvement in clarity. More sophisticated hearing aids may eventually give better assistance but prevention of the condition by reducing general ambient noise levels would seem a more logical approach.

A further factor plays a major role in the difficulties of the elderly in understanding speech, particularly when rapid. This is a loss of efficiency in central (brain) processing, including slowing of the processes. Not uncommonly an elderly person will have worked out what has been said just as the words are being repeated. Time to 'digest' the message, rather than a repeat at a higher level of decibels may be what is needed.

Other senses

Other senses show parallel deterioration with time owing to loss of the fine structures mediating the senses. The organs of balance, adjoining the cochlea, work in a very similar way by means of hair cells and, with ageing, their function too is blunted. Since they make a vital contribution to maintenance of posture, their loss contributes significantly to unsteadiness and falls in the elderly. Balance is maintained by a combination of proprioception, including the organs of balance, and vision, so elderly people with loss of the sense of balance are much more likely to fall in a dark or dimly lit environment. A possible compensation is that travel sickness which is due to excessive stimulation of the organs of balance (nausea is derived from the word for a boat, hence nautical) declines with loss of function in the vestibular system.

Another sense that declines in the elderly is chemo-reception in the nasal and palatal mucosa. Receptors here give rise to both the sense of smell and the finer aspects of taste other than the simple salt, sweet, sour, bitter, pain (curries!) sensations in the tongue. Food tends to lose its flavour and the loss of smell may sometimes remove a warning of danger, for example from toxic gas.

Further reading

Gregory R L 1997 *Eye and brain: the psychology of seeing*, 5th edn. Oxford University Press, Oxford.

Intended for students of the psychology of visual perception this book is of considerable general interest being accessible to the lay reader. The phenomenon of visual illusion is its major and entertaining theme which is well illustrated.

Malzack R, Wall P D 1996 *The challenge of pain*, 2nd edn. Penguin Books, London.

A popular explanation of this topic by the workers who propounded the 'gate theory' of the processing of pain and at a stroke provoked a revolution in this subject.

Nicholls J 2001 *From neuron to brain*, 4th edn. Sinauer Associates Incorporated, Sunderland, Massachusetts.

That this book has remained in press for 25 years to reach its 4th edition should say enough. Brought right up to date, this edition is appealing to students of the subject and those without specialized background in biology.

Pickles J O 1988 *An introduction to the physiology of hearing*. Academic Press, London.

Although 13 years old now this book still gives the student a clear and concise presentation of how the auditory system processes sound. Cochlea mechanics and function and hair cell transduction are particularly well covered.

Robinson, J O 1999 *The psychology of visual illusions*. Dover Publications, New York.

This is an unabridged replication of the book originally published by Hutchinson & Co in 1972. It includes an excellent collection of visual illusions.

Sacks O 1986 *The man who mistook his wife for a hat*. Picador, London.

Funny and yet serious, this book gives a wonderful insight into brain function by describing its malfunctions in a truly skilful narration.

Questions

Answer true or false to the following statements:

4.1

During accommodation for near vision:

A. The ciliary muscle contracts.
B. The sympathetic nerves to the eye are activated.
C. The pupil constricts.
D. Images from distant objects are focused behind the retina.
E. The focusing power of the lens is increased.

4.2

With regard to photoreceptors:

A. Cones are responsible for scotopic vision.
B. Incident light causes an increase in intracellular cyclic GMP levels.
C. Foveal receptors link to ganglion cells in a 1:1 ratio.
D. Light converts the *cis*-retinal to the *trans*-retinal form.
E. Rods have a much lower stimulus threshold than cones.

4.3

With regards to visual defects:

A. Damage to the macular region of the retina is likely to impair visual acuity.
B. Hypermetropia can be corrected using a convex lens.
C. The blind spot is caused by absence of photoreceptors from the optic disc region.
D. Loss of vision in the left visual field of both eyes may be caused by damage at the optic chiasma.
E. Damage to the right optic tract affects signals from the left retinal field of each eye.

4.4

In the ear:

A. The ossicles link the tympanic membrane to the oval window.
B. The cochlea contains receptors for both sound and balance.
C. All the sensory receptors affect activity in the VIIIth cranial nerve.
D. The hearing threshold changes with sound frequency.
E. The hearing threshold for air conduction is normally lower than that for bone conduction.

4.5

During sound transduction:

A. Vibration of the basilar membrane causes bending of the hair cell cilia.
B. Hair cell depolarization causes release of excitatory neurotransmitter.
C. The frequency of sound is coded both by phase locking of the afferent signal and by the position of the maximally activated hair cells.
D. High-frequency sounds cause maximum vibration of the basilar membrane at the apical end of the cochlea.
E. Sound amplitude is coded by the frequency of the sensory action potentials.

4.6

In the vestibular system:

A. The semicircular canals respond to rotational acceleration more than to constant rotation.
B. The cupula is distorted by the inertia of the perilymph during angular acceleration.
C. The utricle is more sensitive to vertical acceleration than is the saccule.
D. There are central connections to four vestibular nuclei in the pons.
E. Signals from the vestibular nuclei project to the oculomotor nuclei.

4.7

Taste:

A. For saltiness is mainly located at the back of the tongue.
B. For sourness (acid) is transduced by direct blockade of apical K^+ channels on the receptor cells.
C. For bitterness is transduced through a second messenger system.
D. From the anterior of the tongue is transmitted via the chorda tympani.
E. Sensations are projected centrally to the contralateral cortex.

4.8

The EEG:

A. Reflects the generation of excitatory and inhibitory potentials in a large number of neurones.
B. Typically consists of high-frequency (approximately 20 Hz), low-amplitude beta waves during sleep.
C. Consists mainly of large-amplitude, low-frequency delta waves during REM sleep.
D. Has an amplitude of approximately 1 V.
E. Demonstrates alpha waves during relaxed consciousness.

4.9

The left cerebral hemisphere:

A. Receives most modalities of sensory information from the right side of the body.
B. Contains the main areas for the understanding and production of speech in most individuals.
C. Is the dominant cerebral hemisphere in most individuals.
D. Is connected to the right by the corpus callosum.
E. Is usually larger than the right.

4.10

Learning and memory:

A. May be interfered with by previously learned material.
B. May be interfered with by subsequently learned material.
C. Are promoted by rehearsal.
D. Involve temporal lobe components of the limbic system.
E. Are believed to be related to long-term potentiation of synaptic transmission.

(*Answers overleaf* →)

Answers

4.1

A. **True.** This allows the suspensory ligaments to relax, so the natural elasticity of the lens pulls it into a more spherical shape.

B. **False.** Contraction of the ciliary muscle is stimulated by parasympathetic nerves.

C. **True.** Pupils constrict to light and to accommodation; this is another parasympathetically mediated reflex.

D. **False.** Light from distant objects will be over-refracted, i.e. focused in front of the retina.

E. **True.** This is because of its increased convexity.

4.2

A. **False.** They provide photopic vision; rods are scotopic.

B. **False.** Levels of cGMP fall during light stimulation.

C. **True.** This is one of the reasons why the foveal cones produce vision with high levels of spatial resolution.

D. **True.** This is the first step in phototransduction.

E. **True.** Rods provide high-sensitivity, low-resolution, monochromatic vision, i.e. scotopic vision.

4.3

A. **True.** This is the region of high acuity in the eye, with the fovea at its centre.

B. **True.** The optical system is too weak for the length of the eyeball, so images from near objects tend to be focused behind the retina. A convex lens adds additional focusing power.

C. **True.** The optic disc is the area of the retina where the optic nerve leaves the eye.

D. **False.** Damage at this point classically causes bitemporal visual loss, i.e. loss of the right visual field in the right eye and of the left visual field in the left eye.

E. **False.** Unilateral damage to an optic tract inhibits transmission from the ipsilateral retinal field in both eyes. This causes defects in the contralateral visual fields because images are laterally and vertically inverted on the retina.

4.4

A. **True.** This transmits sound vibrations from the auditory canal to the perilymph in the cochlea.

B. **False.** The cochlea transduces sound only; the vestibular apparatus is in a separate, though connected, part of the inner ear.

C. **True.** The vestibulocochlear nerve.

D. **True.** The threshold is high for high- and low-frequency sounds, and low, i.e. sensitivity is maximum, for frequencies of about 2000–3000 Hz.

E. **True.** Air conduction is more efficient than bone conduction except in cases of conductive hearing loss.

4.5

A. **True.** This is the basis of the generation of the hair cell receptor potential.

B. **True.** This activates the afferent sensory neurones in the cochlear portion of the VIIIth nerve.

C. **True.** Phase locking is important up to about 8 kHz. Tonotopic coding is important above this, and may play a role at lower frequencies too.

D. **False.** The basilar membrane resonates to high-frequency sounds close to the oval window, and to low-frequency sounds near the apex.

E. **True.** Increased sound amplitude leads to increased receptor potential amplitude in the hair cells. They release more neurotransmitter and a higher frequency of sensory neurone action potentials results.

4.6

A. **True.** The deflection of the cupula is maximal when rotation is changing, when the fluid in the canal is moving at a different velocity from that of the canal itself.

B. **False.** The fluid inside the canal is endolymph, not perilymph.

C. **False.** The horizontal orientation of the macula in the utricle makes it relatively insensitive to vertical acceleration. The macula in the saccule is vertical.

D. **False.** The vestibular nuclei are in the medulla oblongata.

E. **True.** These projections link eye movements to the position and movements of the head. This can cause nystagmus of the eyes following rapid rotation or in vestibular disorders.

4.7

A. **False.** Saltiness is mainly near the tip; bitterness is at the back.

B. **True.** The H^+ ions block these channels, depolarizing the receptors.

C. **True.** The process is probably IP_3 based.

D. **True.** This is a branch of the VIIth, or facial, cranial nerve.

E. **False.** Unusually, taste is projected ipsilaterally.

4.8

A. **True.** It is the cumulative changes in EPSPs and IPSPs, rather than action potentials themselves, which are detected.

B. **False.** Beta waves are typical of alert wakefulness.

C. **False.** These are characteristic of non-REM or deep sleep; the waves have a higher frequency and smaller amplitude during REM sleep but the patient is harder to arouse; hence this is paradoxical sleep.

D. **False.** The amplitude is less than 1 mV.

E. **True.**

4.9

A. **True.** The exceptions are taste and smell, which are projected ipsilaterally.

B. **True.** These are sometimes referred to as Wernicke's and Broca's areas.

C. **True.**

D. **True.**

E. **False.** The two hemispheres are usually almost identical in size.

4.10

A. **True.** This is called proactive inhibition of memory.

B. **True.** This is called retroactive inhibition of memory.

C. **True.** This is the conscious repetition of information or learned actions.

D. **True.** These regions seem to be involved in storing new memories.

E. **True.** This is believed to be one of the cellular mechanisms which underlie memory, making it easier to activate certain neural pathways in the brain.

The endocrine system

5

5.7 **Applied physiology: Temperature regulation** 477

Introduction

We have established that the nervous and endocrine systems represent two parts of the continuum of control systems that maintain homeostasis in our bodies. The similarities of the two systems will become clear as you read this section. The difference between these systems is basically one of time. The nervous system responds in fractions of a second, whereas the endocrine system, while capable of responding in seconds, is more often associated with control of cellular metabolism over cycles of days, months or even years. The obvious limitation on the speed of action of the endocrine system is that imposed by the circulation. Like the nervous system, the endocrine system depends on chemicals to exert its influence. Unlike the nervous system, which relies on diffusion to carry its chemical agents over very short distances to exert their influence, the endocrine agents (hormones – from the Greek word to set in motion) are carried by the circulation to distant sites before they then diffuse to the cells on which they act. Another important difference is that between the stereotyped and localized response obtained when a nerve is stimulated (a poke in the eye produces a flash of what appears to be light, although light is in no way involved in this dramatic experiment) and the response to a hormone, which may be widespread throughout the body and depends as much on the tissue being stimulated as the nature of the hormone involved. Such considerations should not lead us away from the principle of integration of the nervous and endocrine controls of homeostasis, and that principle is most clearly seen in the hypothalamus of the brain and the pituitary gland where the two systems are linked.

Section overview

This section will:

- Explain the integration of the nervous and endocrine systems

- Describe the nature of a hormone

- Explain the mechanisms of hormone actions

- Relate the hypothalamus to the anterior and posterior pituitary gland

- Differentiate between the mechanisms of production and actions of the anterior and posterior pituitary hormones

- Explain the importance of iodine to thyroid function

- Outline the metabolic importance of the thyroid hormones

- Describe the control of production of thyroid hormones

- Differentiate between the secretions of the two parts of the adrenal gland

- Emphasize the relationship of the adrenal medulla to the sympathetic nervous system

- Compare the actions of adrenal cortical mineralocorticoids, glucocorticoids and androgens

- Outline the hormone control of the gastrointestinal tract and its associated exocrine glands

- Compare the actions of pancreatic hormones on blood glucose levels

- Describe calcium homeostasis.

General principles of endocrinology

Introduction

The endocrine system is the second major extra-cellular communication system in the body and achieves control of its target cells through the synthesis and release of molecules known as hormones. By contrast, the nervous system is characterized by mediating its activity through nerves that directly innervate the cells being controlled, releasing regulatory molecules known as neurotransmitters to achieve the desired effect (Fig. 5.1.1). Both systems enable the body to respond to a wide range of internal and external stimuli by eliciting appropriate responses that ensure that the physiological functioning of the body is as effective as can be achieved in the prevailing circumstances. While it is possible to cite examples to the contrary for each system, in general the actions of the nervous system are associated with rapid, time-limited responses such as muscle movement, and hormones tend to be thought of in terms of responses that take longer to establish and that last for longer once elicited.

Hormones are implicated in four main areas of physiological function:

- growth and development
- maintenance of the internal environment (homeostasis)
- regulation of energy metabolism
- reproduction.

A Endocrine system

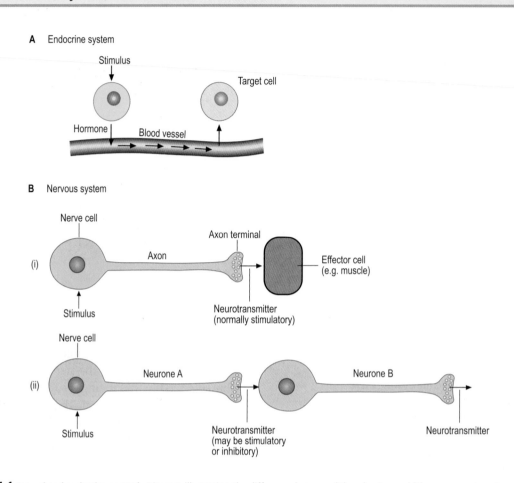

Fig. 5.1.1 Neural and endocrine control. Diagram illustrating the difference between (**A**) endocrine and (**B**) nervous systems in delivery of regulatory secretions to target cells.

Historically, the nervous and endocrine systems were perceived to act entirely separately, but there are many examples where a stimulus will evoke both a nervous and an endocrine response. We now know that there is close integration of the two systems in order to achieve optimum function, and this is the basis of the science of neuroendocrinology. Molecules considered to be hormones in one context are also produced in the nervous system, and nerves are capable of synthesizing and secreting molecules into the blood that act as circulating hormones. Additionally, cells in both systems are capable of secreting directly into the bloodstream, being depolarized and generating electrical potentials.

How do the nervous and endocrine systems interact?

There are many examples of activity in the central nervous system resulting in changes in endocrine activity; these include changes in photoperiod stimulating reproductive activity in seasonal breeders, physical and emotional stress stimulating the pituitary–adrenal axis, and release of TSH following stimulation of hypothalamic temperature-regulating centres by exposure to cold. Integrated neural and endocrine responses are also well documented. The body's response to haemorrhage involves both systems, with the blood loss resulting

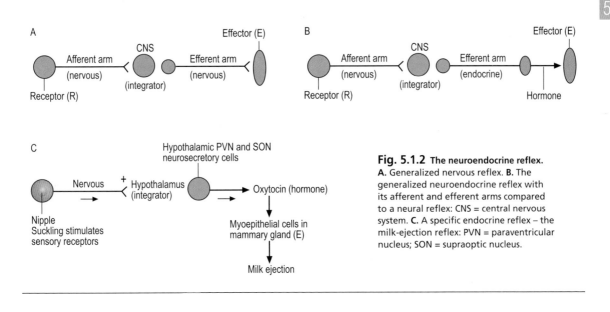

Fig. 5.1.2 **The neuroendocrine reflex.** **A.** Generalized nervous reflex. **B.** The generalized neuroendocrine reflex with its afferent and efferent arms compared to a neural reflex: CNS = central nervous system. **C.** A specific endocrine reflex – the milk-ejection reflex: PVN = paraventricular nucleus; SON = supraoptic nucleus.

in nervous stimulation causing compensatory changes in the cardiovascular system, as well as release of the neurohormone ADH to cause increased water reabsorption by the kidney, and secretion of hormones from the adrenal cortex and medulla.

A further example of neuroendocrine integration is the existence of a number of neuroendocrine reflexes (Fig. 5.1.2). These are similar to purely nervous reflexes except that the efferent arm of the reflex is hormonal rather than nervous. A good example is the milk-ejection reflex (Fig. 5.1.2C). Suckling at the nipple sends nervous stimulation via the spinal cord to the hypothalamic neuroendocrine cells that produce oxytocin. Depolarization of these cells causes release of oxytocin, from the nerve terminals in the posterior pituitary, into the bloodstream for circulation back to the myoepithelium in the mammary glands. Contraction of these cells forces milk from the alveoli into the ducts and out through the nipple to the suckling infant. The reflex is abolished by anaesthesia, thus providing evidence of the involvement of the nervous system in this response.

This is an example of integration of the nervous and endocrine systems in the process of **neurosecretion**. This was first suggested as the

mode of action of the neurones arising in the paraventricular and supraoptic nuclei of the hypothalamus, whose axons pass down the pituitary stalk and into the posterior pituitary. There they terminate in close association with blood capillaries, not in a synaptic connection with other nerve cells as would normally be the case. It was hypothesized that these neurones did not produce classical neurotransmitters at the nerve terminal (Fig. 5.1.3A), but peptide material in the nerve cell body, where the synthetic apparatus for protein synthesis resides (Fig. 5.1.3B). The resulting neuropeptide is then transported down the axon by axonal transport and stored in vesicles at the nerve terminals.

The evidence for this was established by ligating the pituitary stalk, resulting in the accumulation of secretory product proximal to the ligation (Fig. 5.1.4); this accumulation was relatively easy to visualize because the neuropeptide is packaged with an electron-dense carrier molecule, neurophysin. The peptide is released into the blood capillaries by the passage of an action potential down the axon, using the same mechanism as release of classical neurotransmitter, but in this case, the peptide passes into the circulation and acts as a

A

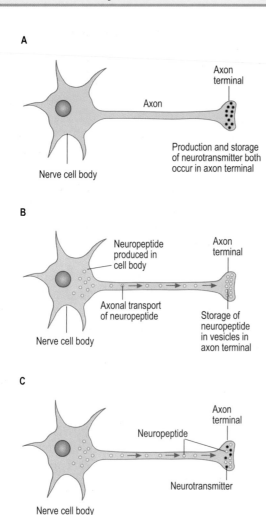

Axon terminal

Axon

Production and storage of neurotransmitter both occur in axon terminal

Nerve cell body

B

Neuropeptide produced in cell body

Axon terminal

Axonal transport of neuropeptide

Storage of neuropeptide in vesicles in axon terminal

Nerve cell body

C

Axon terminal

Neuropeptide

Neurotransmitter

Nerve cell body

Fig. 5.1.3 Neurosecretion and neurotransmission: the difference in production of neuropeptides (by neurosecretion) and neurotransmitters. A. Neurotransmitter production: depolarization of the axon terminal causes release of neurotransmitter by exocytosis. **B.** Neurosecretion: depolarization of the axon terminal causes release of neuropeptide by exocytosis. **C.** Depolarization of the axon terminal causes simultaneous release of neuropeptide and neurotransmitter.

A

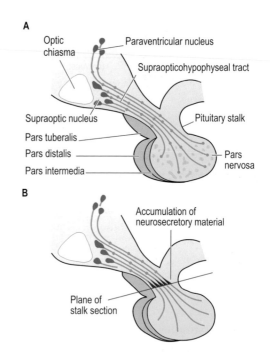

Optic chiasma

Paraventricular nucleus

Supraopticohypophyseal tract

Supraoptic nucleus

Pituitary stalk

Pars tuberalis

Pars distalis

Pars nervosa

Pars intermedia

B

Accumulation of neurosecretory material

Plane of stalk section

Fig. 5.1.4 Axonal transport. The postulated mechanism of axonal transport in the pituitary gland (**A**) was demonstrated by ligating the stalk (**B**) where secretory products accumulated proximal to the ligation.

elucidated further. Research has established that neurosecretions can act in any of three modes:

- **hormone**
- classical **neurotransmitter**
- **neuromodulator.**

Further, the same molecule may act in one mode at one site and in a different mode at another site. It has also been established that some neurones produce a classical neurotransmitter at the nerve terminal, and a neuropeptide in the cell body (coexistence) (Fig. 5.1.3C). An example of this can be found in the salivary glands, where the neurotransmitter acetylcholine is produced at the nerve terminals and the neuropeptide VIP in the soma. The acetylcholine stimulates the activity of the acinar cells

hormone that proved to be ADH. Subsequently, the second posterior pituitary hormone, oxytocin, was identified and its actions described.

Since these first experiments, the overlap in function between the two systems has been

Summary

Nervous and endocrine system interaction

- The nervous and endocrine systems form the two extracellular communication systems of the body.
- The endocrine system exerts its effects on growth, homeostasis, energy metabolism and reproduction via hormones.
- Integration of the nervous and endocrine systems takes place in neuroendocrine reflexes where the afferent arm of the reflex is neural and the efferent arm is hormonal.
- Neurosecretion is the release by nerves into the bloodstream of substances that act as hormones, neurotransmitters or neuromodulators.

in the glands to produce saliva, while the VIP causes local vasodilatation, ensuring a good supply of plasma from which more saliva can be formed.

What is a hormone?

The existence of hormones was firmly established when it was shown that the presence of acid in the small intestine elicited the secretion of alkaline pancreatic juice from a denervated pancreas. The only possible mechanism could be the release of a chemical (which was called secretin) from the small intestine, which then travelled in the blood vessels linking the small intestine and the pancreas. This chemical was called a hormone (from the Greek, to excite to activity; although we now know that some hormones act by inhibition), and the science of endocrinology was established.

Once this discovery had been made, observations that had been recorded over thousands of years but which had not been satisfactorily explained began to make sense. Probably one of the oldest examples is the effect of castration on the human male to produce a eunuch, a male who is no longer reproductively capable. Throughout history, doctors have documented clinical syndromes that we now know to be due to hormone dysfunction, such as cretinism (undersecretion of thyroid hormones in developing infants) and acromegaly (oversecretion of growth hormone in the adult).

As our knowledge of how the endocrine system works increases, potential definitions of a hormone become more complex and need to include a number of elements and exclude those molecules produced in the body that also have a regulatory function but are not hormones, for example the regulation of ventilation by carbon dioxide. The definition of a classical hormone is as follows:

A hormone is a chemical messenger synthesized by specialized cells, often grouped together to form a ductless endocrine gland, and secreted directly into the circulation in response to a specific stimulus. The amount of hormone secreted varies with the strength of the original stimulus, and the blood concentration is always low (picomolar to micromolar). Once in the blood, the hormone circulates to distantly located target cells where it interacts with specific receptors to elicit specific effects involving the regulation of cellular activities.

This traditional definition of a hormone has become blurred by a number of discoveries resulting in the recognition of molecules acting as **autocrines**, **paracrines** or **neurocrines** (Fig. 5.1.5). A hormone is acting in autocrine mode when, in addition to any action it may have elsewhere in the body, it also has an effect in the cell that synthesizes it, or on neighbouring identical cells

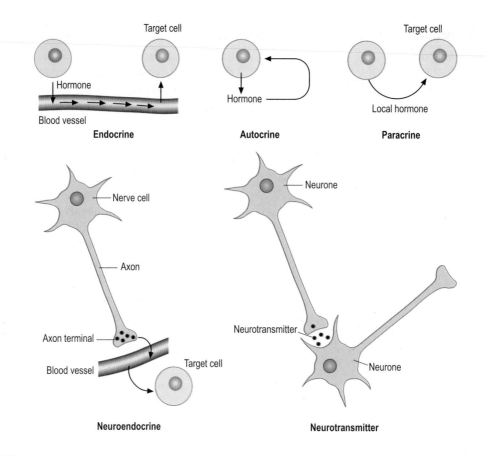

Fig. 5.1.5 Cell-to-cell signalling. The variety of pathways for cell-to-cell signalling by hormones.

(for example, noradrenaline released from nerve endings modulates the release of the same substance from neighbouring nerves). A paracrine substance will diffuse locally within a tissue and exert an effect on neighbouring, but different, cells (for example, the local effect within the testes of testosterone on spermatogenesis). An example of a neurocrine substance is ADH, the hormone that regulates reabsorption of water in the kidney, a peptide molecule produced in nerve cell bodies in the hypothalamus by neurosecretion, and secreted into the general circulation from the nerve terminals in the posterior pituitary.

Hormone families

The recognized endocrine glands are derived from different embryological layers, and this has an effect on the chemical nature of the hormones produced by each gland. Chemically, hormones fall into two categories:

- **peptides** and amino acid derivatives
- **steroid** derivatives of cholesterol (Table 5.1.1).

The chemical nature of a hormone has implications for its transport in blood and its mechanism of action at the target cell. A hormone is

Table 5.1.1 The embryonic layer from which each endocrine gland differentiates, and the chemical nature of the hormone(s) produced by each gland

Embryonic layer	Endocrine gland	Chemical nature of hormone	Hormones*
Ectoderm	Adrenal medulla	Amine derivative	Adrenaline
	Posterior pituitary	Peptide	ADH/vasopressin (8), oxytocin (8)
	Anterior pituitary	Protein	FSH, LH, prolactin, GH, TSH, ACTH
Mesoderm	Adrenal cortex	Sterol derivative	Glucocorticoids (cortisol) Mineralocorticoids (aldosterone)
	Testis (male gonad)	Sterol derivative	Testosterone
	Ovary (female gonad)	Sterol derivative	Oestrogens, progesterone
Endoderm	Thyroid	Amine derivative Peptide	T_3, T_4 (thyroxine) Calcitonin (32)
	Parathyroid	Peptide	Parathyroid hormone (84)
	Islets of Langerhans (endocrine pancreas)	Peptide	Insulin (21), glucagon (29)

* Number of parenthesis = number of amino acids in the peptide chain

considered to be a protein if it consists of more than 75 amino acids; hormones containing fewer amino acids than this are polypeptides. The smallest polypeptide hormone is TRH, thryotrophin-releasing hormone, a tripeptide secreted by the hypothalamus. Any protein or polypeptide hormone that also contains a carbohydrate residue may be called a glycoprotein. Hormones classified as amino acid derivatives include thyroid hormones, catecholamines secreted by the adrenal medulla, and melatonin from the pineal gland.

Steroid hormones that have an intact steroid nucleus, the cyclopentanoperhydrophenanthrene nucleus, include the hormones of the adrenal cortex and gonads. Specificity of action of these hormones is conveyed by the nature of the side-chains and groups attached to the nucleus (Fig. 5.1.6). The steroid hormones in which the B ring of the nucleus has been split are the metabolites of vitamin D_3.

What is the endocrine system?

Classically, the endocrine system comprises a series of ductless glands whose locations in the body are shown in Figure 5.1.7. Each of these endocrine glands is discussed in detail in subsequent chapters, and their most important actions are only briefly previewed here.

Hypothalamus

The hypothalamus produces a range of release and release-inhibiting hormones controlling the synthesis and secretion of anterior pituitary hormones. They are:

- growth hormone-releasing hormone (GRH) and somatostatin (SS), controlling growth hormone (GH)
- corticotrophin-releasing hormone (CRH), controlling adrenocorticotrophic hormone (ACTH)

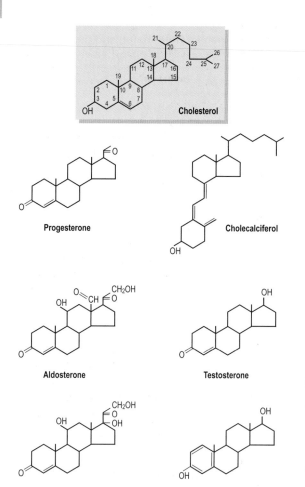

Fig. 5.1.6 **The cholesterol basis of steroid hormones.** The relationship between the cyclopentanoperhydrophenanthrene steroid nucleus and biologically active steroid hormone molecules.

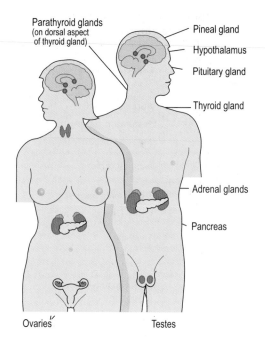

Fig. 5.1.7 Location in the body of the classical endocrine glands.

Anterior pituitary (adenohypophysis)

- Growth hormone influences the growth of almost all cells and tissues including the skeleton, and plays an important role in glucose homeostasis.
- Adrenocorticotrophic hormone controls the activity of the glucocorticoid-producing zona fasciculata layer in the adrenal cortex, and has a permissive role in the activity of the mineralocorticoid-producing zona glomerulosa.
- Thyroid-stimulating hormone stimulates the thyroid gland to produce thyroid hormones.
- Follicle-stimulating hormone stimulates follicle growth in the female ovary and sperm production in the male testis.
- Luteinizing hormone is necessary for ovulation in the female, and also stimulates the production of oestrogen and progesterone by the ovaries and testosterone by the testes.

- thyrotrophin-releasing hormone (TRH), controlling thyroid-stimulating hormone (TSH)
- prolactin-inhibiting hormone (PIH – dopamine), controlling prolactin (PRL)
- gonadotrophin-releasing hormone (GnRH), controlling the gonadotrophins, luteinizing hormone (LH) and follicle-stimulating hormone (FSH).

Posterior pituitary (neurohypophysis)

- Antidiuretic hormone (ADH or vasopressin) is responsible for causing water reabsorption by the kidney, thus maintaining water homeostasis, and at high levels will cause vasoconstriction.
- Oxytocin causes enhanced contraction of uterine smooth muscle during parturition, and milk ejection from the breast in the lactating female.

Thyroid gland

- Thyroxine (T_4) and tri-iodothyronine (T_3) cause an increase in the metabolic activity of almost all cells in the body.
- Calcitonin causes a lowering of blood calcium levels.

Parathyroid gland

Parathyroid hormone controls plasma calcium homeostasis in conjunction with vitamin D and calcitonin.

Adrenal cortex

- Aldosterone, the principal mineralocorticoid, causes sodium retention and potassium excretion by the distal nephron.
- Cortisol, the principal glucocorticoid, has important functions in relation to carbohydrate, fat and protein metabolism, and is also a vital component in the body's defence against stress.

Islets of Langerhans (endocrine pancreas)

- Insulin stimulates the movement of glucose into many tissues in the body, principally muscle and liver.
- Glucagon stimulates the release of glucose from body glycogen stores, mainly in the liver.

Ovaries

- Oestrogens stimulate the development and maintenance of the female sex organs and secondary sexual characters, and are required for the operation of the reproductive cycle.
- Progesterone causes the tissues previously primed by oestrogen activity to become secretory.

Testes

Testosterone stimulates the growth and maintenance of the male sex organs and secondary sexual characters, and is vital for spermatogenesis.

Other hormones

In addition to the hormones produced by these endocrine glands, other hormones to be remembered are vitamin D, whose precursors are in the diet or are manufactured in the skin, and the various growth factors (sometimes referred to as somatomedins) made in the liver.

Biosynthesis and storage
Peptides and amino acid derivatives

Peptide hormones are synthesized using the same biochemical processes as other proteins. The starting point is the transcription within the cell nucleus of a hormone gene causing the formation of a specific messenger RNA (mRNA) and transfer RNA (tRNA). The mature mRNA is transported from the cell nucleus to the cytoplasm, where it becomes bound to ribosomes that are themselves attached to the rough endoplasmic reticulum. The tRNA molecules also pass into the cytoplasm where they become attached to specific amino acids. Once combined with amino acids, the tRNA links to the mRNA on the ribosomes in a predefined sequence, gradually adding more amino acids to the growing peptide chain. This is the translation stage of the process, when the amino acid

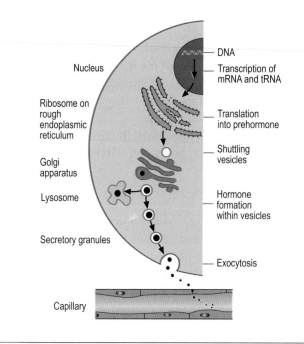

Nucleus

Ribosome on
rough
endoplasmic
reticulum

Golgi
apparatus

Lysosome

Secretory granules

Capillary

DNA

Transcription of
mRNA and tRNA

Translation
into prehormone

Shuttling
vesicles

Hormone
formation
within vesicles

Exocytosis

Fig. 5.1.8 Biosynthesis of protein and peptide hormones. Transcripted mRNA and tRNA from the nucleus are translated into prehormones at the ribosomes. These are transported in shuttling vesicles to the Golgi apparatus, where they mature into hormones. The Golgi apparatus forms secretory granules, which are released to the extracellular space by exocytosis. Some granules are hydrolysed by lysosomes (crinophagy).

sequence coded in the mRNA is converted to the formation of an actual peptide chain (Fig. 5.1.8).

Synthesis of the peptide chain always starts at the amino-terminal and ends at the carboxy-terminal. Normally, a molecule longer than the biologically active form of the hormone is formed; this is called a **prehormone**. In some instances an even longer molecule, or **pre-prohormone**, is formed. The prehormone contains a signal peptide, which is removed by peptidases present in the reticular cisternae through which the newly formed peptide travels before being transferred to the Golgi apparatus. During this journey, any further modifications take place. Once inside the Golgi apparatus, the hormone is packaged into membrane-bound vesicles, the secretory granules. If the hormone is in the form of a prohormone, it may be packaged together with the inactive form of a specific catalytic enzyme. The secretory granules travel from the Golgi apparatus to beneath the cell membrane prior to release, often aided by the presence of microfilaments and microtubules. Cleavage of the prohormone to the active form of the hormone normally takes place as part of

the secretion process (an exception to this is angiotensin I, which is converted to the active angiotensin II once in the circulation).

Storage of peptide hormones within the body is minimal, the exception being thyroid hormone, which is stored in precursor form sufficient for up to 3 months' requirements. Secretion of peptide hormone usually requires a stimulus, which may itself be hormonal. The hormone molecules leave the cell by a process of exocytosis into the bloodstream.

Steroids

Steroid hormones, by contrast, are not stored in cells in a biologically active form, but are synthesized from intracellular precursors as required (Fig. 5.1.9). Cells that produce steroid hormones contain fat droplets made up mainly of cholesterol esters. When the stimulus for hormone formation is received, the cholesterol esters are hydrolysed to cholesterol, which is then transferred into the mitochondria. In the mitochondria, cholesterol is converted to pregnenolone, the first stage in the formation of any

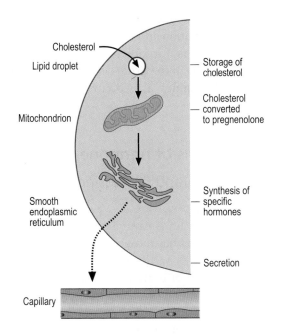

Fig. 5.1.9 **Biosynthesis of steroid hormones.** Cholesterol is stored as esters in lipid droplets. It may be immediately synthesized into hormones by specific hormones within the cytoplasm or move to the mitochondria where it is converted into pregnenolone. Pregnenolone is then transported to the smooth endoplasmic reticulum where it is converted to steroid hormones. Steroid hormones are released from the cell by diffusion and transported in the blood bound to plasma proteins.

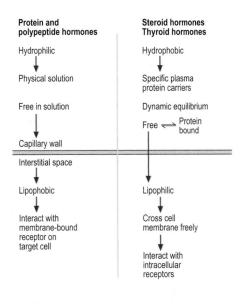

Fig. 5.1.10 Transport of hormones in the blood.

steroid hormone, which in turn is transferred from the mitochondria to the smooth endoplasmic reticulum. The steroid hormone or hormones synthesized within any particular cell are dictated by the enzyme profile of that cell, and steroid hormone deficiencies are often linked to the lack of specific synthetic enzymes. Because of the lipophilic characteristics of the steroid hormones, they probably diffuse across the cell membrane and into the blood as they are synthesized.

Transport of hormones in blood

The chemical nature of a hormone dictates the optimum method by which it is transported (Fig. 5.1.10). Protein and peptide hormones are hydrophilic, which means that they are water-soluble and largely circulate in the blood in physical solution. Any hormone in solution is free to leave the capillaries and enter the extracellular tissue space for interaction with target cells. Conversely, thyroid and steroid hormones are hydrophobic and require specific transport plasma proteins to act as carriers in plasma. There is also a degree of transport of these hormones using the low-affinity, high-capacity binding sites on **albumin molecules**. Hormone carried by protein is referred to as 'bound' hormone, and is in dynamic equilibrium with unbound (or 'free') hormone in the plasma. It is only the free hormone that can easily escape from the capillaries into the tissue spaces, and thence to interact with target cells. As the amount of free hormone decreases, it is replaced by release of bound hormone from the carrier protein, thus restoring the bound : free ratio for that hormone in the plasma. The degree to which a hormone is bound is reflected in the biological **half-life** of the hormone; the greater the binding, the longer the half-life.

Summary

Hormones and the endocrine system

- Hormones are chemical messengers that act as autocrines, paracrines or endocrines.
- Chemically, hormones are peptides and amino acid derivatives or steroids derived from cholesterol.
- Hormones are secretions of the ductless glands that make up the endocrine system, vitamin D formed in the skin, and somatomedins made by the liver.
- Peptide hormones are synthesized by the same biochemical processes as other proteins and are stored intracellularly in small amounts (except thyroid hormone, which is stored as several months' supply).
- Steroid hormones are not stored but synthesized and released as required.
- Protein and peptide hormones (hydrophilic) are carried in solution in the plasma.
- Thyroid and steroid hormones (hydrophobic) are carried bound to specific plasma binding proteins.

Hormone metabolism and excretion

Hormones cannot be allowed to accumulate in the body since this will lead to prolongation of their effect. Following action on the target cells, the hormone is normally inactivated by the action of degrading enzymes, and the resulting metabolites are then excreted. The two main sites of inactivation and excretion are the liver and kidney. For hormones inactivated in the liver, the metabolites may be excreted via the bile and faeces, or pass into the blood for excretion via the kidney. The kidney is the site of both inactivation and excretion for some hormones, whereas for others, excretion of the intact hormone in the urine occurs. Inactivation of some hormones also occurs in the target tissue.

Mechanisms of hormone action

Recognition and processing by target cells

Before any hormone can interact with a target cell, it needs to be 'recognized' by a receptor specific to that particular hormone. This is how specificity of hormone action is achieved. Receptors for any given hormone may be found in a variety of different tissues and the receptor, once activated, will give rise to a signal that initiates changes within the target cell. However, the changes observed in each tissue may not be the same. For example, growth hormone will stimulate protein synthesis in muscle cells but the breakdown of fat in adipose cells. One hormone may exhibit multiple actions. Conversely, multiple hormones may exhibit one function in the same tissue, such as the breakdown of liver glycogen (glycogenolysis) by glucagon, growth hormone, glucocorticoids, adrenaline and thyroxine.

The response of any tissue to hormones is not 'all or none' as seen in nerve activation, but depends on a number of factors. As a result, a dose–response curve can usually be plotted for a hormone and, characteristically, these curves are sigmoid in shape (Fig. 5.1.11). Whatever the hormone action, there is usually a basal level of activity prior to hormone exposure. Increasing amounts of hormone will result in an increase in the activity being measured, which provides the steep part of the curve. The response becomes maximal when all the receptors are occupied.

If, when a tissue is exposed to a hormone concentration that should elicit a maximal response, it gives a lower than maximal response, the

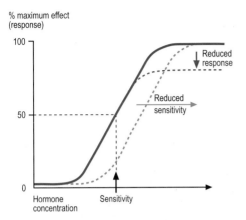

% maximum effect
(response)

Fig. 5.1.11 A hormone dose–response curve. In the dose–response curve of an organ or tissue to a hormone, sensitivity is often expressed as the concentration of hormone that produces half-maximum effect. Changes in responsiveness and sensitivity move the curve as shown.

responsiveness of the tissue is said to be decreased (Fig. 5.1.11). Factors that might cause this are:

- a decrease in the number of functional target cells
- a reduction in receptor numbers
- a fall in intracellular components in the pathway of hormone action
- the presence of a non-competitive antagonist of the hormone.

If it takes a much greater hormone concentration than normal to achieve a maximal response, the **sensitivity** of the tissue is said to be decreased (Fig. 5.1.11). Factors responsible for this include:

- a decrease in receptor number or affinity
- a fall in intracellular components
- an increase in hormone degradation
- the presence of a competitive antagonist.

A tissue may exhibit a combination of both decreased responsiveness and decreased sensitivity.

Changes in the circulating levels of hormone will have an effect on the extent of the change in the physiological parameter being measured, with higher levels of hormone giving a greater response, and lower levels of hormone a lesser response.

The number of receptors available for interaction with the hormone will also have an effect. Receptor populations are described as **labile**, meaning that their number can increase or decrease depending on the prevailing circumstances. The higher the number of receptors, the greater the response of a tissue to any given level of circulating hormone; this increases the sensitivity of the tissue. For example, oestrogen causes an increase in the number of oxytocin receptors in uterine smooth muscle, rendering the muscle more sensitive to circulating oxytocin, with the result that contractility increases without a large increase in the amount of circulating oxytocin. An increase in receptor number is described as **upregulation**, while a decrease is **downregulation**.

Also of importance will be the length of time for which the tissue is exposed to a hormone. Any failure in the degradation mechanism of the hormone will result in its prolonged action. Other factors that may have an effect include length of time between consecutive exposures to the hormone, any changes in intracellular conditions pertaining to the action of the hormone, and effects of antagonist or synergistic hormones acting simultaneously on the tissue.

Target cell receptors

Earlier we described different groups of hormones as being hydrophilic or hydrophobic. By contrast, molecules that are hydrophilic tend to be lipophobic, and vice versa. These characteristics have implications for the way in which hormones interact with the target cell. Protein and peptide hormones are generally lipophobic and therefore unable to pass through the cell membrane. In consequence, the receptors for these hormones are found embedded in the cell membrane, with the hormone-binding site facing outwards. Steroid and thyroid hormones can cross the cell membrane easily, and specific receptors for these hormones are intracellular, usually within the nucleus. Receptor types and mechanisms have been dealt with in Section 1 (p. 63).

Control of the endocrine system

Optimal activity of the endocrine system depends on effective homeostatic control systems. When a target tissue requires more hormone, the gland producing that hormone has to be stimulated to synthesize and secrete it in greater quantity. Equally, when hormone levels need to be attenuated, the gland must be informed and any excess hormone in the body must be degraded in order to avoid prolongation of hormone effects. Normally, endocrine glands are constantly receiving information from a variety of signals; they integrate this information and the amount of hormone secreted is constantly adjusted to meet the body's needs. This is achieved by extrinsic feedback control and a number of different systems operate.

Direct stimulation

This usually involves receipt of a nervous stimulus, when hormones are secreted to bring about an immediate, and often short-term effect. Two examples of this are the release of oxytocin by suckling at the nipple to give milk ejection, and the release from the adrenal medulla of adrenaline in response to sympathetic stimulation.

Direct negative feedback

Here there is direct interaction between the controlling hormone and the controlled metabolite (Fig. 5.1.12). An example of this is the control of plasma calcium levels. When plasma calcium falls it is detected directly by parathyroid cells, and parathyroid hormone (PTH) synthesis and secretion are increased. Conversely, an elevated

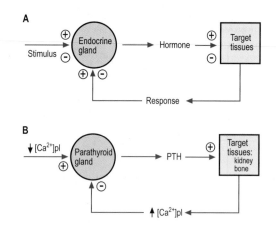

Fig. 5.1.12 **Direct negative feedback.** **A.** General principle. **B.** Example of direct negative feedback using PTH and its effect on plasma calcium.

level of plasma calcium directly inhibits further PTH release.

Indirect negative feedback

Some peripheral endocrine glands (thyroid, adrenal cortex and gonads) are dependent on the regulation provided by hormones released from the anterior pituitary, whose release is in turn dependent on the endocrine activity of the hypothalamus (Fig. 5.1.13). In this situation, the hypothalamic neuroendocrine cells are frequently integrating information from a variety of sources, including the circulating levels of the hormone secreted by the peripheral endocrine gland. For example, in addition to responding to the levels of thyroid hormone in the blood, hypothalamic TRH-producing cells will also be receiving information from the temperature-controlling centres in the hypothalamus. Short-loop feedback may also exist, where the hypothalamic cells respond to the levels of the anterior pituitary hormone whose secretion they regulate. There may even be ultrashort-loop feedback by a hypothalamic hormone on its own secretion.

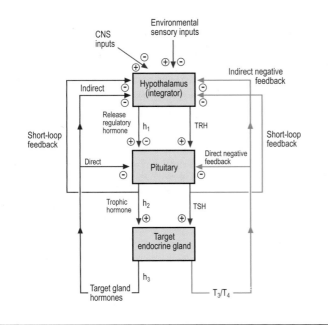

Fig. 5.1.13 Indirect (and direct) negative feedback. The pathway on the left illustrates the general principle. That on the right illustrates the principle as applied to the hypothalamo-pituitary–thyroid axis. The relative importance of the direct negative feedback at the pituitary and indirect negative feedback at the hypothalamus varies with each axis.

Positive feedback

Positive feedback exists when a hormone is able to stimulate its own production. Such situations are rare and the only example that is well documented relates to ovulation and 17β-oestradiol, which achieves positive feedback by stimulating the release of hypothalamic GnRH; this causes the release of pituitary FSH and LH, which in turn stimulates the production of more 17β-oestradiol by the ovary.

Rhythms

Many hormone systems exhibit a characteristic pattern or rhythmicity of release over timecourses varying from minutes to months. Pulsatile or episodic secretion describes the small but regular swings in secretion occurring from every few minutes to every few hours. This is often a background pattern of secretion on which bigger changes in secretion pattern may be superimposed. For example, LH exhibits a constant pulsatile release pattern on which the LH surge responsible for ovulation is superimposed. A second type of rhythm is shown by

hormones such as cortisol, which exhibit a regular daily (circadian) cycle of secretion. A third type of rhythm is the primate female monthly pattern, and finally some hormones even have a seasonal release pattern.

Summary

Mechanisms of hormone action

- One hormone may produce multiple effects and several hormones may produce the same effect.
- A target organ's responsiveness and sensitivity to hormone stimulation may change, frequently as the result of changes in its receptor population.
- Extrinsic feedback control of an endocrine gland may be direct or indirect, positive or negative feedback.
- Many hormone systems generate biological rhythms.

Basic Science 5.1.1

Assessment of endocrine function

Anecdotal evidence gathered over many years led to a good qualitative knowledge of how the classical endocrine glands worked. During the 20th century, the development of techniques that allowed the quantitative measurement of hormones in a range of biological fluids has resulted in a much greater understanding of the endocrine system, and the accurate diagnosis of endocrine disorders. All assay systems need to address four criteria of reliability; these are:

- accuracy
- specificity
- sensitivity
- precision.

   In reality, any assay is usually a compromise among these criteria, depending on the relative importance of each when developing the assay. For example, if the highest priority is precision, it may be necessary to sacrifice a degree of sensitivity.
   How do we define these criteria?

- Accuracy is the closeness with which any measurement approaches its true value, and is usually assessed by running a standard sample of known concentration.
- Precision is the repeatability of any hormone measurement, and plus or minus 10% is an acceptable level of precision in optimal conditions; this is measured by running samples in duplicate or triplicate.
- The specificity of an assay is the determination of a particular chemical entity to the exclusion of all others, and may cause problems where hormones of similar structure may be present in the system.

- The sensitivity of an assay is the smallest single result that can, with some assurance, be distinguished from zero. Any assay system needs to be sensitive enough to detect the hormone at the concentrations at which it is present.

   Assays also need to be practicable in terms of speed, cost and the skill required to perform them.

Assay systems

Initially, biological assays (bioassays) were developed and these were widely used to characterize hormones, using both in vivo and in vitro systems. In general, they tended to lack precision and sensitivity and were often impracticable, being expensive (using many animals) and slow because of the slow time-course of the action being measured. Every hormone has one or more biological end-points that it should be possible to quantify, and this quantification gives a good indication of the level of hormone activity. An example of an in vivo system is testing the potency of androgen in a preparation by measuring its ability to increase seminal vesicle weight in male rats or mice. ADH activity can be measured in an in vitro system by measuring the effect on sodium transport across toad bladder. However, it is not possible to measure the physiological concentrations of a hormone by bioassay.

   In the latter part of the 20th century, binding assays were developed which allow the measurement of minute amounts of hormone in biological fluids, commonly blood and urine. It is important to remember when using binding assays to determine endocrine function that very often a single hormone measurement is not

Basic Science *(Continued)*

sufficient; hormone measurement needs to be combined with a knowledge of how the particular hormone axis functions to ensure that hormone measurements are made at an appropriate time. For example, it may be necessary to allow for normal diurnal variations in secretion, as shown by cortisol, or for surges in hormone secretion such as in growth hormone following the onset of deep sleep.

In the 1960s, Berson and Yalow developed the radioimmunoassay (RIA) for the measurement of insulin, and Ekins the competitive protein-binding assay for the measurement of thyroxine, in both cases for clinical use. Subsequently, the technology was quickly embraced by both clinicians and researchers and allowed very rapid progress in all areas of endocrine research. Binding assays depend on the ability to label the hormone, normally using a radioactive tag. Both assay types also require the availability

of a high-affinity binding protein for the hormone. In the case of RIA, this is a specific antibody generated in a different species for use in the assay, and the method has been extended to allow for the measurement of small protein and non-protein molecules (such as steroids) by coupling the molecule to be measured to a larger antigenic protein molecule so that specific antibodies can be generated. In the competitive binding assay, a naturally occurring binding protein is harvested. A variation on these systems is the use of the hormone receptors to bind to the hormone, giving us the receptor assay.

Both assay systems require calibration by running samples of known hormone concentration (standards) to provide a standard curve against which unknown samples can be read. The particular conditions required for each assay will differ but the basic principles apply (Fig. BS5.1.1). A fixed amount of antibody (Ab)

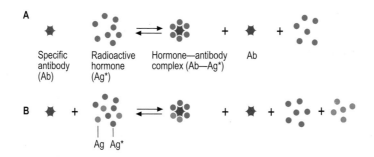

Fig. BS5.1.1 General principle of radioimmunoassay (RIA). A. Specific antibodies (Ab) bind with radioactive hormone (Ag*) to form hormone–antibody complexes (Ab–Ag*). **B.** When unlabelled hormone (Ag) is also introduced into the system, less radioactive hormone binds to the antibody. The assumption is that competition for binding sites on the antibody is in direct proportion to the relative proportions of labelled and unlabelled hormone in the system.

Basic Science *(Continued)*

and radioactively labelled hormone (Ag*) are incubated with either standard or unknown hormone (Ag) samples. At the end of the incubation, antibody-bound moieties (AbAg* and AbAg) and free moieties (Ab, Ag and Ag*) will be present in the system.

The next stage is the separation of the bound and free moieties, and various methods are commonly used, such as the use of a second antibody to remove the bound molecules, or dextran-coated charcoal to absorb the free hormone. The radioactivity in either the bound or free fraction is then counted; values from the standard samples are used to plot a standard curve against which the hormone content in the unknown samples (a and b) can be read (Fig. BS5.1.2).

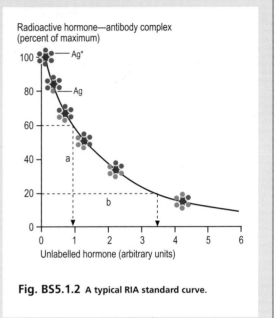

Fig. BS5.1.2 **A typical RIA standard curve.**

The hypothalamus–pituitary gland relationship

5.2

Introduction

The hypothalamus and pituitary together form the site of structural and functional integration between the nervous and endocrine systems, and the study of the relationship between them is termed *neuroendocrinology*. It had been long recognized that the hypothalamus is the region of the brain responsible for controlling many aspects of the autonomic nervous system and body temperature. Its endocrine function was established conclusively in the 1950s. The endocrine function of the hypothalamus is controlled directly by inputs from the higher centres of the brain and other regions of the hypothalamus, indirectly by inputs from the peripheral nervous system, and by blood-borne signals. In response to all these signals, the hypothalamus synthesizes and secretes by a process of *neurosecretion* a range of release hormones, some stimulatory and others inhibitory, which regulate the activity of hormone-secreting cells in the anterior pituitary (**adenohypophysis, pars distalis**), and the two hormones stored and released from the posterior pituitary (**neurohypophysis, pars nervosa**).

The existence of the pituitary gland (synonym: hypophysis from the Greek: *hypo*, under and *physis*, growth) has been known for over 2000 years, with its position and appearance (Fig. 5.2.1) leading Aristotle to describe the infundibulum (Latin for funnel) as draining one of the four cardinal humours, the phlegm

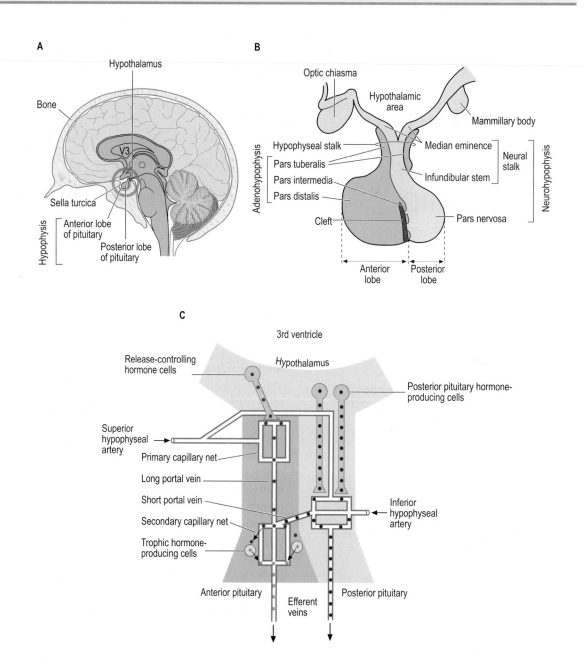

A

Hypothalamus

Bone

V3

Sella turcica

Hypophysis

Anterior lobe
of pituitary

Posterior lobe
of pituitary

B

Optic chiasma

Hypothalamic
area

Mammillary body

Adenohypophysis

Hypophyseal stalk

Pars tuberalis

Pars intermedia

Pars distalis

Median eminence

Infundibular stem

Neural
stalk

Neurohypophysis

Cleft

Pars nervosa

Anterior
lobe

Posterior
lobe

C

3rd ventricle

Release-controlling
hormone cells

Hypothalamus

Posterior pituitary hormone-
producing cells

Superior
hypophyseal
artery

Primary capillary net

Long portal vein

Short portal vein

Secondary capillary net

Trophic hormone-
producing cells

Inferior
hypophyseal
artery

Anterior pituitary

Efferent
veins

Posterior pituitary

Fig. 5.2.1 Anatomical relationship between the brain and the pituitary gland. A. Mid-sagittal section of the brain. The pituitary gland (hypophysis) lies within the sella turcica of the sphenoid bone. It abuts the optic chiasma and hypothalamus (neural tissue of the lower part of the third cerebral vesicle, V3. **B.** The hypothalamo-pituitary area. Anterior and posterior lobes of the pituitary gland are separated by a cleft (space) and linked with the base of the brain by the pituitary stalk. The hypothalamus extends between the optic chiasma and the mammillary bodies. At the median eminence, it makes contact with the pituitary tissue. **C.** Schematic representation of the anatomical and functional relationship between the hypothalamus and the pituitary regions. Arrows indicate the direction of blood flow and movement of hormone molecules. There is direct arterial support to the pars nervosa, but indirect supply via the pituitary pool to the pars distalis (non-neural in origin). The exchange of hypothalamic neurohormones and of pars distalis trophic hormones between the interstitial space and blood occurs at capillary plexi.

(Latin: *pituita*), from the brain, some of it escaping as nasal mucus. Early in the 19th century, it was observed that the pituitary developed by fusion of neural and glandular tissues to form the neuro- and adenohypophyses.

Later, the different functions of the structures comprising this *hypothalamo-hypophyseal complex* began to be recognized, and acromegaly (a disease in adults, involving soft tissue and skeletal enlargements of the hands, feet and head) was linked to the presence of pituitary tumours. In 1895, the physiologists Oliver and Schäfer reported that pituitary extracts contained 'vasopressor activity', which raised blood pressure. Such observations focused attention on the detailed effects, chemistry and sources of active substances present in pituitary extracts, the effects of partial or complete pituitary removal (hypophysectomy) in treating patients, and the extent to which normal pituitary function required that the pituitary be attached to the hypothalamus by its stalk.

Research on the hypothalamo-hypophyseal complex during the 1930s suggested the existence of a vascular link carrying blood from the hypothalamus to the anterior pituitary (the hypothalamo-hypophyseal–portal vessels), culminating in the 1950s in work describing conclusively the process of neurosecretion and the details of the hypothalamo-adenohypophyseal neurovascular link. In consequence, the hypothalamus became recognized as a site of neuroendocrine integration and as an endocrine tissue in its own right.

The hypothalamus secretes two neurohormones into the systemic circulation via the neurohypophysis:

- vasopressin (more commonly and correctly known as **antidiuretic hormone (ADH)**, because of its principal physiological role of controlling water metabolism)
- **oxytocin** (involved in the regulation of parturition and the control of milk ejection).

The hypothalamus also secretes a range of release-controlling hormones into a portal circulation to the adenohypophysis to control the secretion of pituitary trophic hormones, which regulate:

- growth and development (**growth hormone (GH)**)
- milk secretion (**prolactin (PRL)**)
- secretion of other hormones:
  - **thyroid-stimulating hormone** (TSH) controlling the thyroid gland
  - **adrenocorticotrophic hormone** (ACTH) controlling the adrenal glands
  - **luteinizing hormone** (LH), **follicle-stimulating hormone** (FSH) and prolactin controlling the reproductive glands.

Prior to clarification of the endocrine role of the hypothalamus, the pituitary had frequently been referred to as the 'conductor of the endocrine orchestra'. Now that we know so much more about its functionality, it could be argued that this 'conductor' role should be ascribed to the endocrine hypothalamus.

The hypothalamo-hypophyseal complex

Development

The functional links within the hypothalamo-hypophyseal complex are more easily appreciated by first considering its development. Around week 6 in the human embryo, adjacent regions of the mouth epithelium (buccal ectoderm) and the floor of the brain third ventricle (neural ectoderm) bulge towards each other. The non-neural buccal upgrowth (Rathke's pouch) then becomes detached from its origin and invaginates and surrounds the neuroectodermal downgrowth (infundibulum) (Fig. 5.2.2A,B). Rathke's pouch develops into the non-neural anterior lobe of the pituitary, lying in juxtaposition with the posterior neural lobe. By week 10, the compound pituitary gland has developed from this structure, lying within a cavity (the *sella turcica*, or *pituitary fossa*) of the developing sphenoid bone and already

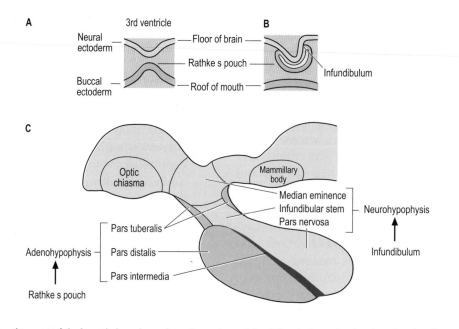

Fig. 5.2.2 **Development of the hypothalamo-hypophyseal complex: origin of the pituitary gland regions forming the adenohypophysis and neurohypophysis. A.** Formation of Rathke's pouch by upgrowth of the mouth (buccal) non-neural ectoderm, accompanied by downgrowth of neural ectoderm. **B.** Rathke's pouch apposed to the developing infundibulum. **C.** Compound pituitary gland. In the adenohypophysis (non-neural origin) the pars distalis secretes pituitary trophic hormones, the pars intermedia is vestigial in human adults, and the pars tuberalis is poorly understood. The neurohypophysis (essentially an extension of the hypothalamus) secretes hypothalamic release-stimulating hormones in the median eminence and conveys nonapeptide neurohormones via the infundibular stem for release at the pars nervosa.

containing its major hormone-secreting cell types. In the human adult, the weight of the pituitary gland ranges from 0.5 g in the male to 1.0 g in the pregnant female, with the adenohypophysis comprising some 75%.

In the mature pituitary (Fig. 5.2.2C), the neurohypophysis consists of three neuroectodermal tissues: the hypothalamic median eminence, the infundibular system (pituitary stalk) and the *pars nervosa* (infundibular process). The adenohypophysis comprises three buccal ectodermic tissues: the *pars tuberalis* and *pars distalis* and the *pars intermedia*, which is vestigial in the human adult.

Structure

Hypothalamic areas

The hypothalamus occupies only about 2% of brain volume. It regulates and integrates a wide range of homeostatic processes including food intake and energy balance, fluid balance, body temperature, cardiovascular function, reproduction, alertness and emotional behaviour. These functions depend upon its close interconnection with the limbic system, the brainstem autonomic centres and the pituitary gland.

The hypothalamus lies at the base of the diencephalon (see Fig. 5.2.1A). The medial portion is rich in nerve cell bodies that are grouped bilaterally to form pairs of hypothalamic nuclei (Fig. 5.2.3), while the lateral portions contain nerve fibre tracts and relatively few such nuclei. The hypothalamo-pituitary link begins with two nerve fibre tracts of unmyelinated neurones that carry the hypothalamic peptide neurohormones from the hypothalamus down their axons towards the pituitary – the hypothalamic tuberoinfundibular tract and the hypothalamic neurohypophyseal tract.

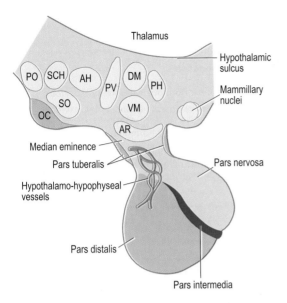

Fig. 5.2.3 The hypothalamic nuclei. AH = anterior hypothalamic; AR = arcuate; DM = dorsomedial; OC = optic chiasma; PH = posterior hypothalamic; PO = preoptic; PV = paraventricular; SCH = suprachiasmatic; SO = supraoptic; VM = ventromedial.

The hypothalamic tuberoinfundibular tract. This tract transports the release-controlling hormones to the median eminence and infundibular stem, a highly vascularized region that drains into the hypothalamo-hypophyseal portal vessels, which are essential to the regulation of anterior pituitary lobe function. The neurones in this tract are parvicellular neurones with relatively small cell bodies, containing dense-cored vesicles of 80–120 nm diameter within the terminals. These neurones mainly populate the hypophysiotrophic areas of the hypothalamus and are responsible for synthesizing and secreting the hypothalamic release and inhibiting hormones.

The hypothalamic neurohypophyseal tract. This carries ADH and oxytocin to the posterior pituitary lobe. The neurones in this tract are magnocellular neurones with large cell bodies, and are the site of production of the hormones secreted from the posterior pituitary. They are characterized by marked axonal swellings

and terminals containing secretory granules of 120–200 nm diameter.

Studies on the effects of removal of the posterior pituitary lobe provided some of the first evidence for its functional link with specific nuclei in the hypothalamus: there was selective degeneration of the magnocellular neurones whose cell bodies are confined to the **supraoptic nucleus** (SON) and the **paraventricular nucleus** (PVN). Histochemical labelling techniques have shown that the paraventricular nucleus also contains parvicellular neurones that project to the median eminence, the brainstem and the spinal cord. Thus, the paraventricular nucleus provides integrated autonomic nervous and endocrine activity in the homeostatic processes listed above. Table 5.2.1 summarizes the distribution of the two types of neurone among the hypothalamic nuclei that are involved in pituitary function.

The blood vessels of the hypothalamo-hypophyseal complex are shown in Figure 5.2.4. The paired inferior and superior hypophyseal arteries are branches of the internal carotid arteries. They serve networks of fenestrated capillaries and sinusoids (see below). In turn, these converge upon short veins that lead to the internal jugular veins via the nearby cavernous sinuses.

Hypophyseal areas

Nomenclature

Anatomical divisions. The detailed structure of the pituitary gland is quite complicated. Histologists and embryologists would divide it up as shown in Table 5.2.2.

Functional divisions. Most physiologists, however, would robustly use the following synonyms:

- anterior lobe = adenohypophysis = pars distalis = pars anterior
- posterior lobe = neurohypophysis = pars nervosa.

The stalk is of little functional consequence in man.

Table 5.2.1 Distribution and characteristics of hypothalamic neurones involved in pituitary gland function

Nerve fibre tract	Neurone type	Hypothalamic nucleus	Neurosecretion
Neurohypophyseal	Magnocellular	Supraoptic	Antidiuretic hormone (vasopressin), oxytocin
		Paraventricular	Antidiuretic hormone (vasopressin), oxytocin
Tuberoinfundibular	Parvicellular	Paraventricular	Release-controlling hormones
		Preoptic (medial)	Release-controlling hormones
		Periventricular	Release-controlling hormones
		Arcuate	Release-controlling hormones

Table 5.2.2 Anatomical divisions of the pituitary gland

	Adenohypophysis (from buccal cavity)		Neurohypophysis (from hypothalamus)		
Anterior lobe {	Pars distalis +		Median eminence		
	Pars tuberalis	+	Infundibular stem	=	Infundibulum (stalk)
	Pars intermedia	+	Pars nervosa	=	Posterior lobe

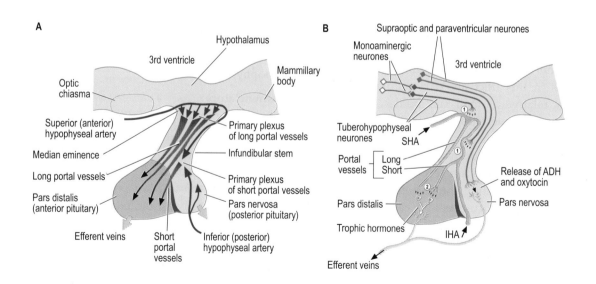

Fig. 5.2.4 The vasculature and functional interrelationships of the hypothalamo-hypophyseal complex. Hypophysiotrophic hormones enter the primary portal capillaries at ① and leave these vessels to influence the adenohypophyseal cells at ②. IHA = inferior hypophyseal artery; SHA = superior hypophyseal artery.

Posterior lobe (neurohypophysis). The posterior lobe is functionally an extension of the hypothalamus. The axons of the magnocellular neurones run from the supraoptic nucleus and paraventricular nucleus down the neurohypophyseal tract. This passes through the internal zone of the median eminence (Figs 5.2.4B) and terminates in the pars nervosa. Here, action potentials cause the release by exocytosis from the axon terminals of ADH and oxytocin, which diffuse into blood within fenestrated sinusoidal capillaries of the inferior hypophyseal arteries.

Anterior lobe (adenohypophysis). The anterior lobe is very sparsely innervated.

It receives almost all its arterial blood supply indirectly via the external zone of the median eminence (Figs 5.2.4A and 5.2.5) and the upper infundibular stem. The superior hypophyseal arteries form the primary capillary plexus of a **hypothalamo-hypophyseal portal system** that distributes hypothalamic release-controlling hormones through long portal veins. These large, parallel vessels terminate at secondary sinusoidal capillary beds in the pars distalis.

In addition to this main route of communication between the hypothalamus and pars distalis, the primary capillaries of a plexus formed by the inferior hypophyseal arteries converge in the lower infundibular stem to form a group of short portal vessels that convey release-controlling hormones to the secondary beds in the pars distalis. The short portal vessels may also function as a vascular link between the posterior and anterior pituitary lobes. The portal system provides a neurovascular link conveying hypothalamic neurohormones in high concentration to their target cells, the **trophs**, in the pars distalis.

The functions of the adenohypophyseal pars intermedia and pars tuberalis in humans are poorly understood. The pars intermedia, though prominent in the developing fetus and enlarged in pregnant women, is normally small in adults (Fig. 5.2.2). Its two known secretions are α-**melanocyte-stimulating hormone** (α-MSH) and **corticotrophin-like intermediate-lobe peptide** (CLIP), both peptides in the proopiomelanocortin (POMC) family. It is well developed in animals such as amphibians that alter skin pigmentation in conformity with their surroundings; if these animals are placed on a dark background, α-MSH secretion increases, causing the skin to darken by stimulating the dispersal of a tyrosine-derived pigment called

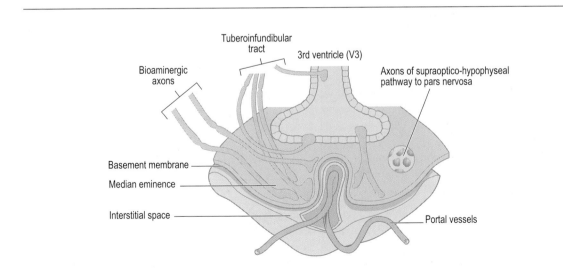

Fig. 5.2.5 The detailed structure of the median eminence.

melanin within melanocytes. Administration of α-MSH to dark-skinned humans can intensify epidermal pigmentation, but since it is normally absent in adults, it is presumed not to be involved in sun tanning. However, in pregnant women a characteristic darkening of the skin at certain sites may be caused by fetal and/or maternal α-MSH production. Surgical disconnection of the pars intermedia from the hypothalamus in several species results in hypertrophy of the pars intermedia and increased α-MSH production. Thus, normal control of secretion may involve tonic inhibition, either through the (dopaminergic) innervation of the pars intermedia or through the hypothalamo-pituitary vascular link.

The pars tuberalis is a marked glandular sheath that surrounds the pituitary stalk (Fig. 5.2.2), but its function is even less clear than that of the pars intermedia.

Summary

Hypothalamo-hypophyseal structure

- The hypothalamo-hypophyseal complex is a major interface between the nervous and endocrine systems.
- The hypophysis (pituitary gland) is a compound, bilobed endocrine structure consisting of:
  - a posterior lobe (neurohypophysis), essentially an extension of the hypothalamus, derived from neural ectoderm
  - an anterior lobe (adenohypophysis), derived from non-neural ectoderm.
- The hypothalamus controls secretions of the pituitary via a portal blood vessel system (anteriorly) and a nerve tract (posteriorly).

Hypothalamus–posterior pituitary function

Antidiuretic hormone and oxytocin are each secreted by separate types of magnocellular neurone with cell bodies in both the supraoptic nucleus and paraventricular nucleus. In addition to either ADH or oxytocin, these neurones contain neurotransmitters and other neuropeptides, such as corticotrophin release-stimulating hormone and the opioid peptides (see below). The existence and functional significance of such co-localization of neuromodulators is controversial. The following outline of ADH and oxytocin physiology is expanded in Chapters 8.4–8.6 and 10.3.

Synthesis and transport of ADH and oxytocin

ADH and oxytocin are cyclic nonapeptides, the disulphide bonds linking cystine residues at positions 1 and 6 being essential for hormone activity (Fig. 5.2.6). Their synthesis accords with the principles already described in Chapter 5.1.

Within the endoplasmic reticulum of the neuronal cell body, a polypeptide pre-prohormone is converted to a prohormone by removal of its

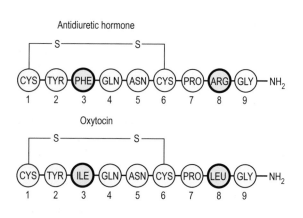
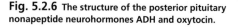

Fig. 5.2.6 The structure of the posterior pituitary nonapeptide neurohormones ADH and oxytocin.

signal peptide. The resulting secretory granules are transferred for transport down the axon to the terminal in the neurohypophysis. As they move along the axon at a rapid rate (8 mm/h), there is cleavage of the prohormone within secretory granules. Each hormone cleavage of the secretory granule yields the active hormone together with a cleavage product, once regarded as a carrier protein, either ADH-associated neurophysin (nicotine-stimulated neurophysin; neurophysin II) or oxytocin-associated neurophysin (oestrogen-stimulated neurophysin; neurophysin I). In mature secretory granules, cleavage of precursor is complete.

Passage of an action potential down the axon causes release, by exocytosis, of both the hormones and cleavage products from the axon terminals. The cleavage products have no known function. Because the circulating active hormones remain unbound, they are subject to rapid degradation in the liver and kidneys (plasma half-life approximately 2 min), principally by enzymic reduction of the disulphide bonds and cleavage of the peptide chains.

ADH – action and effects

Two main effects, the antidiuretic effect and the vasopressor effect, are mediated by specific ADH receptor subtypes (V_1, V_2) located on the surface membranes of its target cells.

Antidiuretic effect

This consists of enhanced back-diffusion of water from urine within the kidney collecting ducts, resulting in raised urine osmolality and in decreased urine volume. This stimulation of water reabsorption is mediated by V_2 receptors on the serosal surface of the target kidney epithelial cells and a resultant increase in the intracellular level of the second messenger cAMP. cAMP acts indirectly to increase the water permeability of the epithelial cell luminal surface membrane through the activation of channels allowing the transcellular flow of water into the high tissue fluid osmolarity of the renal medulla. V_2 receptors are stimulated by lower concentrations of ADH than are required to stimulate the smooth muscle V_1 receptors that mediate the vasopressor effect (see below).

Deficient ADH secretion results in the daily excretion of large volumes of hypotonic urine, as in the disease diabetes insipidus. Additional effects of ADH of less certain physiological significance include stimulation of glucose production by liver cells through increased rates of glycogenolysis and gluconeogenesis, stimulation or facilitation of ACTH secretion by the adenohypophysis, and enhancement of learning and of memory consolidation.

Immunocytochemistry has also shown that ADH may be produced in the periphery. This is evident in the ectopic secretion of abnormally high levels of the peptide by lung tumour and other tissues in the context of the syndrome of abnormal ADH secretion (SIADH), despite the absence of the normal osmotic or volume stimuli (see below).

Vasopressor effect

ADH is a potent vasoconstrictor. It stimulates V_1 receptors, causing arteriolar smooth muscle cells to contract. This involves a rise in the intracellular levels of the second messenger IP_3 and of Ca^{2+}. Venous constriction by the same mechanism removes blood from the periphery, increasing venous return and central venous pressure. Thus, the net immediate effect of ADH is to raise the blood pressure and lower the heart rate. ADH and its analogues have been used pharmacologically to assist haemostasis in severe cases of blood loss, and ADH may contribute to raising vascular tone when secreted in response to haemorrhage.

Control of secretion of ADH

ADH is one of several peptides involved in the control of water and sodium balance. Its secretion is principally determined through two pathways: one mediated by osmoreceptors, the other by volume/baroreceptors.

Osmoreceptor-mediated control

A very small change (1%) in normal plasma [Na⁺] is sensed by hypothalamic **osmoreceptor neurones**, altering plasma ADH levels. Osmoreceptor neurones have been located in the anterolateral hypothalamus. The osmoreceptors lie outside the supraoptic nucleus and paraventricular nucleus and have cholinergic input to the ADH-secreting magnocellular neurones. Below a plasma osmolality of approximately 280 mOsm/kg water, osmoreceptors are quiescent and plasma ADH remains at its resting level of 1 pmol/l (Fig. 5.2.7). In the narrow range 280–290 mOsm/kg water (i.e. a 3–4% increase upon resting osmolality), osmoreceptors

are stimulated progressively and the plasma ADH rises to a level (5 pmol/l) that stimulates antidiuresis maximally. Separate central osmoreceptors with a higher response threshold (approximately 295 mOsm/kg water) are involved in triggering the sensation of thirst and the desire to drink.

Volume/baroreceptor-mediated control

A large change (>10%) in effective circulating blood volume sensed by circulatory stretch receptors affects plasma ADH levels. Stretch receptor systems in the low- and high-pressure compartments of the circulation monitor effective circulating blood volume. Decreased effective circulating volume, for example after haemorrhage, causes:

- decreased activation of volume receptors in the large intrathoracic veins and the cardiac atria, thus reducing the firing rate in afferent vagal nerve fibres
- decreased activation of baroreceptors in the aortic arch and carotid sinus, thus reducing afferent glossopharyngeal nerve fibre activity.

The primary synapses of these afferents lie in the brainstem. ADH secretion increases exponentially in response to reduction in effective circulating volume beyond 10% of normal (Fig. 5.2.8). It is thought that this response is mediated by noradrenergic neurones that project from the brainstem to the hypothalamic supraoptic nucleus and paraventricular nucleus. In common with the osmoreceptor-mediated responses to plasma hyperosmolality, thirst is stimulated less readily than ADH secretion in the context of the volume/baroreceptor response to hypovolaemia (Fig. 5.2.9).

Interactions between the pathways

There is interaction between volume/baroreceptor-mediated and osmoreceptor-mediated ADH secretion. With severe hypovolaemia,

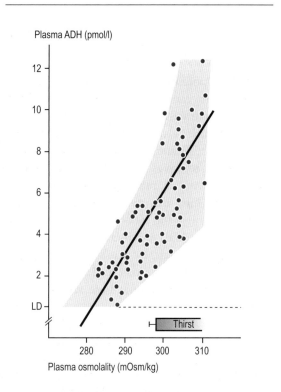

Fig. 5.2.7 Plasma ADH as a function of plasma osmolality and plasma sodium concentration.

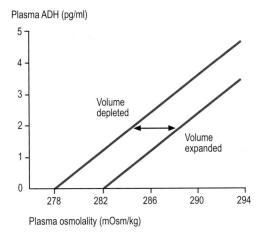

Fig. 5.2.8 Effect of alteration in circulating blood volume on the relationship between plasma ADH concentration and plasma osmolality.

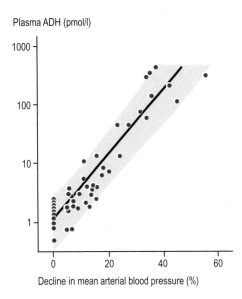

Fig. 5.2.9 Effect of decreasing blood pressure on the plasma ADH concentration.

ADH secretion is stimulated even if there is concurrent plasma hypo-osmolality (and hyponatraemia) sufficient otherwise to suppress it. Thus, volume/baroreceptor control can override osmoreceptor control, and it is notable that even small changes in blood volume can modify the relationship between plasma osmolality and ADH secretion (as reflected in plasma ADH) (Fig. 5.2.8).

Other factors affecting ADH secretion

Several secondary factors affect ADH secretion, usually transiently. Nausea is a potent stimulus to secretion. Intestinal traction during abdominal surgery can elicit ADH secretion and so account for postoperative antidiuresis. Swallowing suppresses release: the oropharyngeal–neuroendocrine reflex triggered by drinking includes a feed-forward component that offsets the effect of ingested and absorbed water to dilute body solutes, but does not override the osmoreceptor control based upon direct monitoring of ECF osmolality.

Among the other neuropeptides within the neurohypophysis, the morphine-related opioid peptides can inhibit ADH release. The antidiuretic and vasopressor effects of ADH are the respective osmoreceptor- and volume/baroreceptor-mediated homeostatic responses appropriate to the signals that cause ADH secretion. These feedback loops are summarized in Figure 5.2.10; and the mechanisms are discussed further in Chapter 8.2 in the context of the integrated control of water and sodium balance.

The effects of abnormal production of ADH

When a deficiency of ADH secretion occurs, patients produce excessive amounts of hypotonic urine (up to 20 litres per day) and exhibit increased thirst. The condition is described as *diabetes insipidus*, and usually results from damage to the cells producing the hormone, or from the growth of a tumour. Total deficiency of ADH is treated by hormone replacement, given

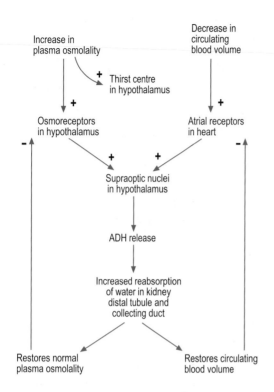

Fig. 5.2.10 Summary of the pathways involved in control of ADH secretion.

as a nasal spray with absorption of the hormone occurring across the nasal mucosa, whereas partial deficiency is treated by drugs that potentiate the action of ADH in the kidney. Very rarely, *nephrogenic diabetes insipidus* may occur because of the kidney failing to respond to ADH. In the rare situations where there is overproduction of ADH, the urine becomes excessively hypertonic through increased reabsorption of water, and the increased water load in the body may cause water intoxication. Treatment includes restricting fluid intake and/or administration of an antagonist to ADH action in the kidney.

Oxytocin – action and effects

The principal effects of oxytocin occur in the context of reproduction (see Ch. 10.3).

Summary

Hypothalamo-hypophyseal function

- Hypothalamic neurosecretory cells synthesize and release:
    - two nonapeptides (ADH, oxytocin) into systemic blood at the pars nervosa region of the neurohypophysis
    - several release-controlling hormones (peptides, amines) into the pituitary portal circulation for delivery in high concentration to specific target cells (trophs) nearby in the pars distalis of the adenohypophysis.
- ADH secretion is stimulated by raised plasma osmolality and by decreased effective circulating blood volume; ADH corrects these deviations through antidiuretic and vasopressor mechanisms respectively.
- Trophic hormones (specific cases shown in brackets) may:
    - stimulate secretion of peripheral hormones by endocrine peripheral target cells of:
        a. the classical peripheral endocrine glands: adrenal cortex (ACTH); thyroid follicles (TSH); gonads (the gonadotrophins FSH and LH)
        b. the liver (GH)
    - regulate the activity of non-endocrine peripheral target cells (GH, PRL).
- Hormone secretion within each hypothalamoadenohypophyseal–endocrine peripheral target cell axis is determined by:
    - primary drive derived in the hypothalamus
    - secondary modulation by:
        a. feedback (usually negative) effects of the circulating levels of the hormones themselves
        b. interoceptive signals (other circulating products; neural afferents)
        c. exteroceptive signals (environmental change).

Hypothalamus–anterior pituitary function

The hypothalamo-adenohypophyseal neuro-vascular link was defined through description of the portal vessels (Fig. 5.2.4) and of the direction of blood flow within them, and by observing the effects of cutting through the pituitary stalk and of transplanting the pituitary gland to a remote site (see Fig. 5.2.12). The nomenclature of the trophic hormones and release-controlling hormones is confusing because of the use of a range of synonyms and abbreviations; these full names and their variants are summarized in Table 5.2.3.

Surgical removal of the adenohypophysis (as in hypophysectomy – removal of the whole pituitary gland) has more profound effects than removal of the neurohypophysis. Hypophysectomy causes atrophy of certain peripheral endocrine glands, namely the adrenals, thyroid and gonads, disturbance of the metabolism of many tissues, and the cessation of body growth. Specific effects of hypophysectomy are reversed by administering pituitary extracts containing selected trophic hormones, or extracts of peripheral endocrine glands. Removal of the neural lobe alone has much less serious consequences, because neurosecretion is not confined to the posterior lobe of the pituitary and the hypothalamic nuclei continue to secrete ADH and oxytocin.

The six currently established trophic hormones are produced by five granule-containing cell types (**trophs**) within the pars distalis. Their effects on non-endocrine peripheral target cells are explained by a combination of:

- direct actions (notably of GH and PRL) on some non-endocrine peripheral target cells
- indirect actions (notably of ACTH, TSH, FSH, LH, and GH) through stimulating secretion of appropriate peripheral endocrine gland hormones, which in turn act on non-endocrine peripheral target cells.

These relationships are depicted schematically in Figure 5.2.11.

The trophic hormones can be put into three families based on their structures – structural similarity within families causes overlaps in biological effect and cross-reactivity in assays.

- **The ACTH-related or pro-opiomelanocortin family** consists of ACTH (adrenocorticotrophic hormone) and other similar peptides.
- **The glycoprotein family** consists of TSH (thyroid-stimulating hormone), and FSH (follicle-stimulating hormone) and LH (luteinizing hormone); FSH and LH are synthesized together as gonadotrophins within gonadotrophs.
- **The somatomammotrophin family** consists of growth hormone and PRL (prolactin).

Each trophic hormone also shows structural variation between species, GH being notably species specific. Thus, GH extracted from animal pituitaries was found to be inactive in patients with GH deficiency; but the production of a suitable GH by genetic engineering techniques has enabled this problem to be overcome. Some of the trophic hormones are also synthesized at extrapituitary sites, notably in the brain.

Hypothalamic release-controlling hormones (releasing hormones)

The existence of releasing hormones was inferred from experimental evidence for hypothalamic control of trophic hormone secretion (Fig. 5.2.12). Thus, transplantation of the adenohypophysis from the sella turcica to an ectopic site (where it became vascularized and remained viable) resulted in permanently reduced secretion of all trophic hormones except PRL, permanently increased secretion of PRL, and permanent impairment of the ability to alter trophic hormone secretion by hypothalamic stimulation (e.g. electrically, through implanted

Table 5.2.3 Nomenclature and targets of hypothalamic release-controlling hormones and anterior pituitary trophic hormones

Hypothalamic release-controlling hormones			Anterior pituitary trophic hormones		
Hormone and (synonym)	**Common abbreviations**	**Target cells in the anterior pituitary (staining property)**	**Hormone and (synonym)**	**Common abbreviations**	**Target tissue**
Corticotrophin-releasing hormone	CRH	Corticotrophs (basophils)	Adrenocorticotrophic hormone (corticotrophin)	ACTH	Adrenal cortex, mainly zona fasciculata
Thyrotrophin-releasing hormone	TRH	Thyrotrophs (basophils)	Thyroid-stimulating hormone (thyrotrophin)	TSH	Thyroid
Gonadotrophin-releasing hormone	GnRH	Gonadotrophs (basophils)	Follicle-stimulating hormone	FSH	Ovary/testis
			Luteinizing hormone	LH	Ovarian follicle Leydig cells in testis
Growth hormone-releasing hormone (somatoliberin)	GHRH	Somatotrophs (acidophils)	Growth hormone (somatotrophin)	GH (STH)	Multiple targets
Growth hormone-inhibiting hormone (somatostatin)	GHIH	Somatotrophs (acidophils)			
Prolactin-releasing hormone	PRH	Lactotrophs (acidophils)	Prolactin	PRL	Breast tissue and testis
Prolactin release-inhibiting hormone	PIH	Lactotrophs (acidophils)			

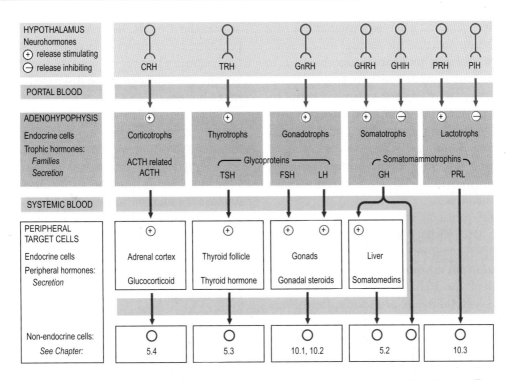

Fig. 5.2.11 Summary of the set of hypothalamo-adenohypophyseal–peripheral target cell (H-A–peripheral target cell) axes.
Hypothalamic release-controlling hormones (releasing hormones) pass via pituitary portal fenestrated vessels to the adenohypophysis where they control the secretion of trophic hormones by trophs bearing specific releasing-hormone receptors. In turn, trophic hormones are delivered via the systemic circulation to their endocrine and non-endocrine target cells. The endocrine peripheral target cells respond by secreting peripheral hormones into the systemic blood, through which they reach their target cells. The details of each H-A–peripheral target cell axis are discussed in the chapters indicated. The full names of the hormones are given in Table 5.2.3.

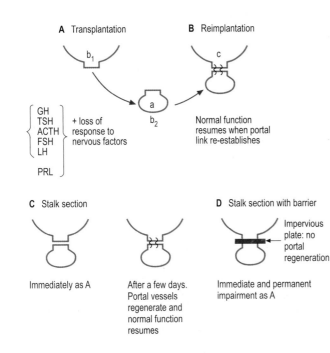

Fig. 5.2.12 The effects of hypophysectomy on trophic hormone release. A. The intact pituitary (a) is separated from the hypothalamus (b₁) and implanted at a distant (ectopic) site (b₂). **B.** Later, it is reimplanted in its anatomical position (c). **C.** In separate experiments, its stalk is cut and there is an immediate effect equivalent to transplantation. Normal function results after re-establishment of vascular connections. **D.** Following section of the pituitary stalk, an impenetrable barrier is placed in the cut to prevent revascularization.

electrodes) (Fig. 5.2.12A). Reimplantation of a viable transplant into the vacant sella turcica, where it became revascularized, resulted in restoration of normal function (Fig. 5.2.12B). The reason why a transplanted pituitary exhibits impaired function, even after vascularization, is that the concentration of release-controlling hormones in the systemic circulation is too low to support normal pituitary function, even following electrical hypothalamic stimulation.

Simple transection of the pituitary stalk (leaving the pituitary gland in situ) resulted in initial changes in secretion of trophic hormones resembling those after transplantation. Subsequent revascularization of the gland within days brought about a resumption of normal trophic hormone secretion (Fig. 5.2.12C). Insertion of a barrier across the pituitary stalk immediately after simple stalk transection (to prevent revascularization) resulted in permanent changes in trophic hormone secretion, resembling the transplantation effect (Fig. 5.2.12D).

Around 1950, Harris and co-workers concluded from such findings that secretion of pituitary trophic hormones is controlled by hypothalamic release-stimulating 'factors'. In order to act, the release-controlling 'factors' must be delivered directly through the pituitary stalk portal vessels to their target cells in the adenohypophysis. PRL secretion is similarly controlled by a hypothalamic factor; it is, however, a release *inhibiting* factor. Seven factors have now been identified. Five of them have activity that stimulates release (commonly termed 'releasing hormones') and two inhibit it ('inhibiting hormones'). The relationship between the hypothalamus, adenohypophysis and peripheral target cells is termed the hypothalamo-adenohypophyseal–peripheral target cell (H-A–peripheral target cell) axis. In Table 5.2.3 and Figure 5.2.11, the established releasing hormones (six peptides and one catecholamine), their appropriate trophic hormones and peripheral target cells are grouped together. With the exception of growth hormone, the trophic hormones of the anterior pituitary are considered later in this section in the context of their peripheral target glands and actions; growth hormone is discussed in further detail below.

Other hypothalamic peptides include members of the pro-opiomelanocortin family, first identified in pituitary corticotrophs (see above), and peptides first discovered in the gut (see Ch. 5.6), but at present their functions are unclear. Similarly, some releasing hormones have additional hypothalamo-pituitary actions and/or extrahypothalamic sites of synthesis that are of uncertain significance.

Primary drive

The initiating signal or primary drive for secretion of pituitary trophic hormones consists of input from the CNS. This signal triggers regularly repeated, episodic (pulsatile) bursts of hypothalamic releasing-hormone secretion, which in turn controls trophic hormone secretion. The pulsatile nature of the stimulus leads to fluctuating levels of controlled pituitary hormones in the peripheral circulation. This must be remembered when assessing endocrine adequacy by measuring peripheral blood hormone levels.

A surgically isolated hypothalamo-pituitary unit continues to control the peripheral target endocrine glands. This episodic secretion is an inherent property of hypothalamic neurones within the suprachiasmatic nucleus (Fig. 5.2.3). The physiological importance of this mechanism has become evident through attempts to stimulate it, for instance in treating abnormalities of gonadotrophin secretion. Thus, in treating some forms of infertility, administration of pulsatile gonadotrophin-releasing hormone to simulate the physiological secretory pattern (about 1 pulse per hour) succeeds in stimulating gonadotrophin secretion, whereas a higher frequency or continuous (tonic) administration does not. Furthermore, abnormally high gonadotrophin secretion in precocious puberty can be lowered by the continuous gonadotrophin-releasing hormone regime. These effects are interpreted in terms of target cell (gonadotroph) responsiveness to the hormone, continuous gonadotrophin-releasing hormone producing receptor desensitization and down-regulation.

Secondary modulation

Hormonal feedback

Partial or complete removal of individual peripheral endocrine glands increases the secretion of specific trophic hormones. This is prevented by administration of the peripheral endocrine gland's hormone(s). Conversely, trophic hormone secretion is suppressed when exogenous peripheral endocrine gland hormone(s) are administered. Similar changes in the secretion of specific trophic hormones occur if there is hypo- or hypersecretion of specific peripheral endocrine gland hormone(s). This occurs because the hypothalamo-pituitary–endocrine axes form negative-feedback control systems. Increases (or decreases) in target peripheral endocrine gland hormone levels cause decreases (or increases) in trophic hormone secretion. The exception to this is the transient positive-feedback effect of oestrogen on LH secretion that precedes egg release from the ovary. In general, the so-called 'long-loop' feedback effect of peripheral endocrine gland hormones (Fig. 5.2.13) involves either a direct action of circulating hormones on pars distalis trophic cells (trophs), modulating their responsiveness to releasing hormone, or an indirect action modulating releasing-hormone secretion by the hypothalamus.

Manipulation of this feedback relationship is the basis for many tests of endocrine function. Additional hormonal negative-feedback control mechanisms also exist. 'Short-loop' feedback by the trophic hormones suppresses their own release through modulation of releasing-hormone secretion at the hypothalamus

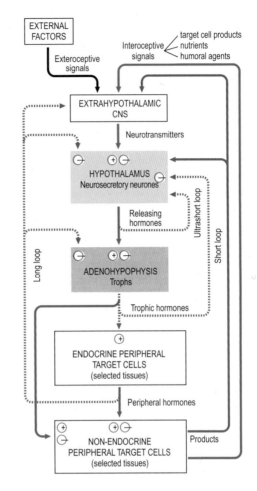

Fig. 5.2.13 Feedback loops in a typical hypothalamo-adenohypophyseal–peripheral target cell (H-A–peripheral target cell) axis. The H-A–endocrine peripheral target cell elements (shaded area) may be any of those designated in Figure 5.2.11. They operate in a closed-loop feedback mode to maintain relatively steady plasma levels of the hormones concerned, subject to modifications of the hypothalamic drive by inputs from outside the body (exteroceptive signals). Long-loop and short-loop negative feedbacks involve respectively the peripheral hormones and the trophic hormones.

(Fig. 5.2.13). 'Ultrashort-loop' feedback by the releasing hormone acts on its own secretion, directly (cf. feedback control of noradrenaline release by sympathetic nerves, p. 165) or indirectly through interneurones.

407

Other modulatory inputs

These hormonal feedback control systems can be modified by neural afferent activity from peripheral receptors, circulating products (secretions, metabolites) monitored by the hypothalamus and extrahypothalamic CNS, and by exteroceptive signals from the outside world that converge on the hypothalamus. These signals include temperature, photoperiod, pheromones (scent signals) and stress (both physical and psychological). The interplay of influences on trophic hormone secretion is illustrated by GH, which circulates unbound in plasma with a half-life of 20–50 minutes. Throughout life, GH influences protein, carbohydrate and fat metabolism through direct and indirect actions on multiple peripheral target cell types.

Growth hormone (GH) actions

Direct actions

Direct actions of GH are important in the provision of circulating metabolic fuels to tissues under conditions of fasting, physical exercise and other stresses (Fig. 5.2.14). They involve production of substrates by:

- stimulation of free fatty acid (FFA) release from stored triacylglycerol (TAG) in white fat cells
- stimulation of glucose release from glycogen in liver cells
- inhibition of glucose uptake by muscle cells.

Together, these supply glucose for obligatory glucose-utilizing cells (notably nerve) and alternative fuels for non-obligatory glucose-utilizing cells (notably muscle) (see Ch. 5.6).

Indirect actions

The indirect actions of GH are important in tissue growth and repair, and development of the skeleton. During skeletal development, GH stimulates sulphation of cartilage by stimulating the liver to synthesize and secrete an active mediator, sulphation factor (somatomedin C; insulin-like growth factor 1; IGF1). Once formed, the cartilaginous template becomes mineralized to form bone. Bone remodelling continues throughout life; a process influenced by a number of hormones. A group of peptide growth factors, including insulin-like growth factors, transforming growth factors, fibroblast- and platelet-derived growth factors, which are secreted by most tissues in response to raised plasma GH concentration, reach their peripheral target cells through endocrine (from liver), paracrine and autocrine routes, and stimulate amino acid uptake and protein synthesis.

Growth hormone (GH) secretion

Primary drive

The primary drive is the intermittent, pulsatile secretion of stimulatory and inhibitory releasing hormones (respectively growth hormone-releasing hormone (GHRH, **somatoliberin**) and growth hormone-inhibiting hormone (GHIH, **somatostatin**)) by neurones in the median eminence. In part, this involves input from the hypothalamic ventromedial nucleus (VMN) (Fig. 5.2.3). An important outcome is the underlying circadian rhythm of secretion, which causes the plasma GH concentration to peak at the onset of deep sleep (sleep stages 3 and 4). This accounts for about 70% of daily GH secretion and may underlie a daily cycle of tissue repair.

Secondary modulation

Secondary modulation is provided through long-loop negative feedback by circulating **somatomedin** at pars distalis somatotrophs, by inhibiting the action of GHRH to stimulate GH secretion, and at hypothalamic neurosecretory neurones, by stimulating GHIH secretion. In addition, there appears to be hypothalamic monitoring (in part by the VMH) of the altered circulating levels of substrates (amino acids, glucose, free fatty acids) that result from the actions of GH and somatomedin (among other regulatory factors) on non-endocrine peripheral target cells. Knowledge of these modulators has been applied in clinical tests of pituitary function involving the ability of administered glucose to inhibit GH secretion and of administered arginine to stim-

ulate it. Finally, there is evidence for short-loop negative feedback by GH through stimulation of hypothalamic somatomedin production, and for ultrashort feedback by GHRH stimulation of GHIH secretion. At present, their importance relative to the above modulators is unclear and, for simplicity, they are omitted from Figure 5.2.14.

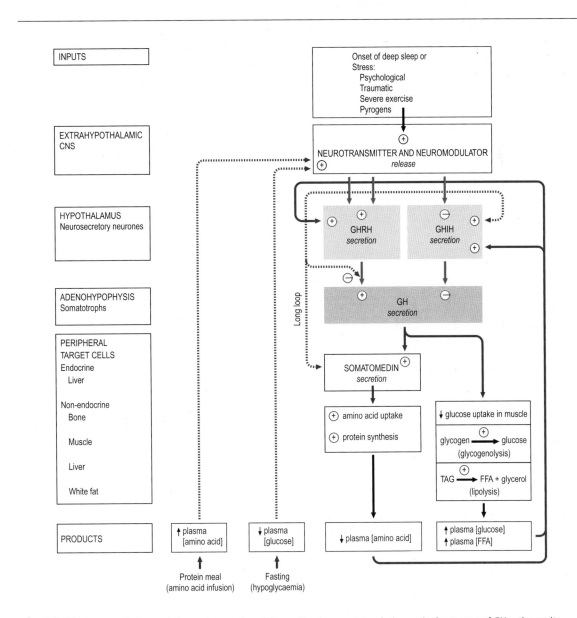

Fig. 5.2.14 The control of growth hormone secretion. GH secretion by somatotrophs is seen in the context of GH action on its peripheral targets and of other inputs (onset of deep sleep; stress). The primary drive by hypothalamic GHRH and GHIH is modulated by the circulating levels of somatomedin and of substrates produced through the actions of GH on liver and most other tissues (important examples are shown). TAG = triacylglycerol; FFA = free fatty acid.

Summary

Hypothalamo-adenohypophyseal function

- Hypothalamic oxytocin stimulates the contraction of specific types of smooth muscle cells during specific reproductive phases, namely:
  - myometrial cells (in the uterus) in childbirth and for haemostasis at the placental site after delivery
  - mammary alveolar myoepithelial cells (in the breasts) promoting milk ejection
  - reproductive tract smooth muscle during sexual arousal and orgasm in both sexes.
- In addition to being produced in the paraventricular nucleus, oxytocin is synthesized in the extrahypothalamic CNS and peripherally.
- Secondary effects of oxytocin resemble those of ADH on vascular and kidney mechanisms.
- The two hormones have shared peptide sequences. Thus, oxytocin can interact with ADH receptors.
- Distinct oxytocin and ADH receptors exist in different vascular beds.
- Oxytocin is relatively more effective in stimulating contraction of human umbilical arteries and veins, while aortic smooth muscle is extremely sensitive to ADH but unresponsive to oxytocin.

Clinical Example

Clinical disorders of the anterior pituitary

It is rare for a single anterior pituitary hormone to be over- or undersecreted; it is more common for a number of hormones to be affected. The most common cause of oversecretion is the development of a benign tumour, or adenoma, and the patient may first present with symptoms due to the enlargement of the pituitary, such as persistent headaches or visual problems caused by increased pressure from the enlarging pituitary, rather than the peripheral effects of hormone overproduction. Radiology and computerized tomography will identify whether a tumour is present. The hormones most commonly subject to oversecretion are growth hormone, prolactin and ACTH; it is quite rare for TSH and the gonadotrophins to be produced in excess. Some tumours may not result in excess hormone production at all and in these cases medical treatment is not usually an option; surgery, radiotherapy and subsequent hormone replacement therapy are normally required.

Growth hormone oversecretion

The manifestations of excessive growth hormone secretion depend on whether it occurs pre- or post-puberty. Before puberty, there is excessive skeletal growth resulting in giantism and, if untreated, the individual can grow up to 7 feet tall. The excess growth is particularly noticeable in the length of the limb bones, and the hands and feet. In adulthood, these individuals are prone to cardiovascular problems due to the increased distance from the feet to the heart.

It is more common for oversecretion to occur after puberty when the epiphyses in the long bones

Clinical Example *(Continued)*

have fused and no further increase in the length of the long bones is possible. Increased bone growth is then confined to pre-existing cartilaginous areas such as hands, feet, parts of the skull, shoulder blades and chest. This condition is known as acromegaly. There may also be thickening of soft tissue such as the tongue. These changes to the extremities may occur so slowly that the patient is unaware of them, and the patient frequently visits the doctor with associated problems such as those described earlier, or diabetic symptoms due to the increased insulin resistance caused by the excessive growth hormone levels. Treatment will depend on the age of the patient, the size of the tumour and the extent of the symptoms present. Wherever possible, treatment will be conservative through the prescription of antagonists such as bromocriptine, but in extreme cases, surgery may be necessary.

Adrenocorticotrophin oversecretion – Cushing's disease

When a pituitary tumour is restricted to excessive ACTH production it is often too small to be detected radiologically, but can be diagnosed by hormone assay. The treatment of choice will be surgical removal of the adenoma. Excess ACTH results in increased glucocorticoid secretion and if the patient is treated by removal of the adrenal glands, rather than removal of the source of excess ACTH, this has the effect of removing negative feedback by the glucocorticoids on ACTH production, which will increase still further.

When this occurs, the patient frequently develops increased skin pigmentation through the ability of excessive ACTH to stimulate melanocyte activity.

Prolactin

Excessive prolactin secretion (prolactinaemia) is more common in females, who often present with changes in sexual functioning. This may simply be loss of libido or changes in the menstrual cycle; in men, impotence may result. In both cases, the peripheral effects are thought to be due to prolactin inhibiting the effect of the gonadotrophins, particularly on sex hormone synthesis by the gonads. Treatment is normally by administration of bromocriptine, which inhibits prolactin secretion and causes the tumour to shrink.

Hypopituitarism

Reduced pituitary function may arise for a variety of reasons. Trauma is a possible cause of hypofunction. This might be due to damage to the pituitary stalk, or direct damage to the pituitary gland itself by tumour, haemorrhage or thrombosis. Once hyposecretion occurs, it will become manifest through reduced hormone activity of the various target endocrine glands. Deficiency of growth hormone or prolactin appears to have little effect in the adult, although growth hormone deficiency before puberty will result in dwarfism. Deficiency in the other pituitary hormones will require permanent hormone replacement therapy in the form of cortisol, thyroxine and gonadotrophins.

Thyroid hormones

Introduction

The thyroid gland is a bilobed organ situated just below the larynx in front of the trachea. It is unique among endocrine organs in that it maintains a large extracellular store of precursors and the two hormones it synthesizes, **thyroxine** (T_4) and the more potent **tri-iodothyronine** (T_3). The gland's location renders any abnormal enlargement, termed a goitre, readily visible (Fig. 5.3.1 and Table 5.3.1). Goitres may be non-toxic, resulting in low or normal rates of thyroid hormone output, or toxic, resulting in abnormally high rates of output.

Around 500 BC in China, successful reduction of goitre was achieved by feeding patients dried seaweed and sea-sponge, now known to be a rich source of iodide (I^-). In the 1930s, a clear relationship between dietary I^- deficiency and non-toxic goitre was established, when it was shown that the high incidence of endemic goitre among inland populations could be prevented by as little as 2 g of potassium iodide taken twice yearly. Alternatively, iodide can be added to dietary components such as bread and salt. This observation is explained by the fact that the gland hypertrophy in iodide-deficiency goitre results from the raised secretion of an anterior pituitary trophic hormone (thyroid-stimulating hormone – TSH), and that TSH secretion is normally subject to negative feedback regulation by the thyroid hormone.

413

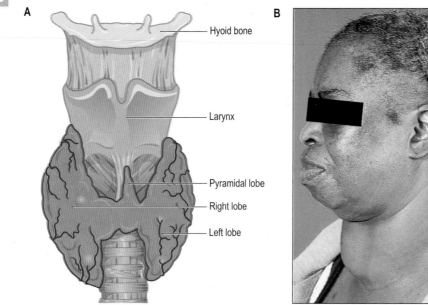

A

— Hyoid bone

— Larynx

— Pyramidal lobe

— Right lobe

— Left lobe

B

Fig. 5.3.1 The thyroid gland. **A.** Gross structure of the human thyroid gland. **B.** A woman with endemic goitre due to dietary iodide deficiency. (From Forbes CD, Jackson WF 1997 Colour Atlas and Text of Clinical Medicine, 2nd edn. Mosby, London. Courtesy of Dr WF Jackson.)

Table 5.3.1	The major causes of goitre
Type	**Causes**
Non-toxic	Dietary I⁻ deficiency
	Dietary goitrogen action
	Hashimoto's thyroiditis (autoimmune disease)
	Thyroid neoplasm
	Genetic defects:
	Hormone synthesis
	Target cell receptors
Toxic	Graves' disease
	Hashimoto's thyroiditis (hyperthyroid phase)
	Thyroid neoplasm
	TSH-secreting pituitary gland tumour

Thyroid hormones have widespread effects in the body. In the developing individual, they are essential for development and growth, particularly of nervous and skeletal systems. Throughout life, they are required as regulators of metabolic rate (O_2 consumption and heat production) in most adult tissues, the exceptions including brain. Their effects involve modulation of the actions of other physiological ligands, including hormones and neurotransmitters.

The thyroid gland

Development

The gland begins development in the 4-week-old human embryo as an out-pocketing of the endoderm near the tongue buds in the pharyngeal region of the gut. The tissue extends caudally to associate with pharyngeal pouch derivatives (parathyroid glands) and to incorporate neural crest cells (parafollicular C cells) from the ultimobranchial bodies. The thyroid tissue is attached to its point of origin by the thyroglossal duct, which normally atrophies by week 7. The gland can respond at the onset of pituitary TSH secretion around week 22. In common with thyroid tissue, salivary and gastric glands can concentrate I⁻ into their secretions. The endocrine thyroid is thought to have evolved from a similar exocrine structure, perhaps one resembling the mucus-secreting endostyle of the larval lamprey, a primitive eel-like fish.

Structure and histology

In adults, the gland weighs 10–20 g and consists of two large lateral lobes connected by a narrow isthmus, from which a smaller pyramidal lobe may project as a remnant of the thyroglossal duct (Fig. 5.3.1A). In women, the gland usually enlarges in the second half of the menstrual cycle, in pregnancy and in lactation. Relative to its weight, the thyroid receives an enormous blood supply (estimated range 4–6 ml/min per gram of tissue). The rich lymphatic system may also have a role in delivery of hormone to the circulation. The sympathetic postganglionic nerve fibres from the middle and superior cervical ganglia, and the parasympathetic vagal preganglionic fibres may regulate blood flow rather than secretory cell activity.

Thyroid hormone-secreting cells are arranged within many thousands of functional units termed thyroid follicles (Fig. 5.3.2). In each follicle, epithelial cells surround a lumen filled with a colloid consisting of the iodinated glycoprotein **thyroglobulin** (TG), the precursor of the hormones T_3 and T_4. This colloid is sufficient for about 100 days of hormone secretion. The size of an individual follicle (20–900 µm), the height of its epithelial cells (squamous/cuboidal/columnar), and the extent of their uptake of colloid from the lumen are all directly related to the level of stimulation of the gland by TSH (Fig. 5.3.3).

Parafollicular C cells, responsible for the secretion of thyrocalcitonin, a calcium-regulating hormone, lie adjacent to follicular epithelial cells within the follicular basement membrane (Fig. 5.3.2) and constitute around 10% of the gland's cell mass. Fenestrated capillaries and a connective fibre network surround the follicles. The interfollicular mast cells may mediate increased blood flow through their release of 5-HT and histamine in response to TSH and to sympathetic stimulation.

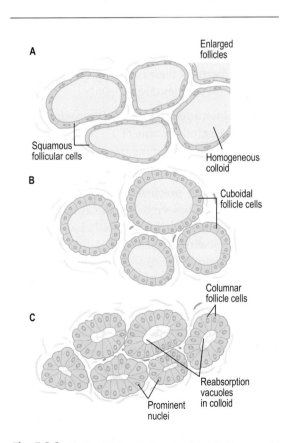

Fig. 5.3.3 Effect of TSH on the thyroid gland. A. Hypothyroid follicles. **B.** Euthyroid (normal) follicles. **C.** Stimulated hyperplastic follicles.

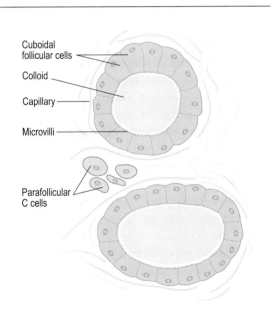

Fig. 5.3.2 Normal thyroid gland follicle. Calcitonin-producing parafollicular C cells are also shown.

Summary

The thyroid gland

- The thyroid gland consists of follicles containing colloid, which stores the thyroid hormones, thyroxine and tri-iodothyronine.
- Parafollicular 'C' cells secrete calcitonin involved in Ca^{2+} regulation.

- Four parathyroid glands, whose secretion has opposite effects to calcitonin, are found behind the thyroid gland in the neck.
- The thyroid gland has a large blood supply and the potent I^--trapping ability necessary to form thyroid hormones.

Thyroid hormones

Biosynthesis, storage and release

Thyroid follicles synthesize the high molecular weight (660 kD) TG, within which specific tyrosine residues are iodinated to yield mono- and di-iodotyrosine moieties (**MIT, DIT**). The proximity of these iodinated tyrosines within the TG molecule permits their coupling to form three main iodothyronines (Fig. 5.3.4):

- 3,5,3',5'-tetra-iodothyronine (thyroxine, T_4)
- 3,5,3'-tri-iodothyronine (T_3)
- 3,3',5'-tri-iodothyronine (reverse $T_3 - rT_3$).

The newly formed (nascent) iodinated TG is thus a hormone precursor, in this case a pre-prohormone. It is secreted at the apical plasma membranes of the follicular epithelial cells and stored extracellularly within the follicular colloid compartment. Subsequently, endocytotic reuptake and proteolytic cleavage of the TG are performed by the epithelial cells, with resultant daily release of T_4 (approximately 130 nmol), T_3 (approximately 7.5 nmol) and rT_3 via their basal membranes into the blood circulation. T_4, the major secretory product, is considered to be a circulating prohormone, the precursor of the more potent, active hormone T_3. Relatively little T_3 or rT_3 is secreted by the thyroid gland, most being formed by enzymic 5'- or 5-deiodination of T_4 in liver and kidneys, and in target cells (Fig. 5.3.4).

Several component processes are stimulated acutely in the follicular epithelial cells by TSH through cAMP.

Eight distinct stages have been described in the TSH-stimulated sequence of synthesis, storage and release of T_3 and T_4 (Fig. 5.3.5).

The first step is the uptake of precursors at the epithelial cell basal membrane. I^- crosses the membrane against an electrochemical gradient by means of an Na^+/K^+-ATPase-linked I^- pump ('trap'), which is specific, saturable and energy-dependent. The active I^- transport can be inhibited by competing anions such as pertechnetate ($^{99m}TcO_4^{-}$), a short-lived radioactive ion, which is used to image the gland radiographically, and perchlorate (ClO_4^{-}) and thiocyanate (SCN^-), competitive inhibitors that have been used in diagnostic tests and in treatment of hyperthyroidism. Normally, the thyroid-to-plasma free iodide concentration ratio [T/P] is about 25. Stimulation by TSH can raise this 10-fold. The uptake of glucose and amino acids, including tyrosine, involve mechanisms similar to those in cells generally, and both are stimulated by TSH.

Next, synthesis of TG precursor occurs within the epithelial cells. The mature glycoprotein is composed of two apparently identical precursor subunits, which are synthesized on polyribosomes, glycosylated during transfer to the Golgi apparatus and delivered in small vesicles to the apical plasma membrane, where release into the colloid occurs by exocytosis.

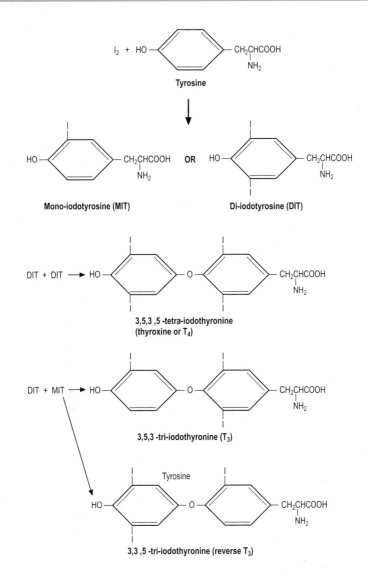

Fig. 5.3.4 Pathway of thyroid hormone synthesis.

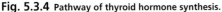

During this transfer, the TG is transformed into the mature dimer and iodinated.

The iodide that has been concentrated in the follicular cells is oxidized at the apical membrane to form active iodine.

Once formed, the iodine is used in the fourth stage of the sequence, iodination of tyrosine residues in TG at the apical membrane. Active iodine is transferred to an acceptor tyrosine followed by coupling of iodotyrosines at the apical membrane. Drugs containing a thionamide (N–C–SH) grouping, such as propylthiouracil (PTU), thiourea and methyl mercaptoimidazole (methimazole, MMI), are potent inhibitors of hormone synthesis that act upon stages 3–5 in the sequence with progressively increasing sensitivity. They are used in the treatment of hyperthyroidism.

The sixth stage is the extracellular storage of mature TG in the colloid. The luminal colloid

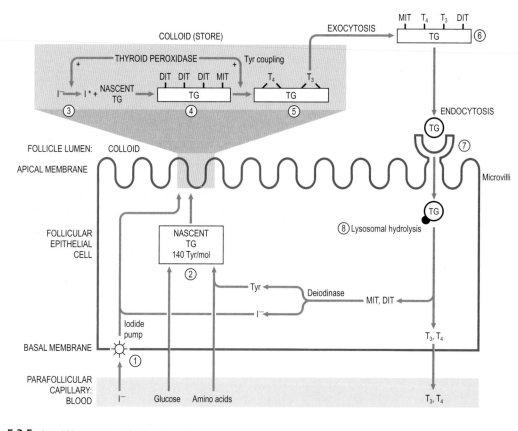

Fig. 5.3.5 Thyroid hormone synthesis and secretion.

store accounts for about 30% of the mass of a normal thyroid gland, and about 90% of the total body iodine.

Endocytotic reuptake of colloid at the apical membrane occurs during the seventh stage in the sequence. Pseudopodia and cytoplasmic microfilaments and microtubules at the apices of active epithelial cells engulf colloid droplets and translocate them basally in the cytoplasm to coalesce with lysosomes moving apically.

Finally, there is release of iodinated residues from TG and subsequent secretion of hormones. Lysosomal proteases digest the iodinated TG with resultant release of MIT, DIT, T_3 and T_4 into the cytoplasm. Normally, little or no TG escapes the gland. MIT and DIT are deiodinated within the cytoplasm by the enzyme deiodinase, providing for recovery and recycling of I⁻ for

further T_3 and T_4 synthesis. Thus, little or no MIT and DIT are secreted normally, but patients genetically deficient in thyroid deiodinase suffer symptoms of I⁻ deficiency and excrete MIT and DIT in their urine. T_4 and T_3 are released via the basal plasma membrane into the bloodstream in a molar ratio of about 17:1, probably by diffusion down their concentration gradients.

Transport in blood

The iodothyronines have the following normal plasma concentration ranges: T_3, 0.9–2.8 nmol/l, and T_4, 50–150 nmol/l. Each consists of two fractions, a small free (unbound) fraction and a larger fraction bound to plasma proteins (Table 5.3.2). The free fraction accounts for only 0.3% of total T_3 and 0.03% of total T_4, and it is

Table 5.3.2	Approximate normal values for thyroid hormones in the blood		
	Total	Percentage free	Absolute concentration free
T_4	100 nmol/l (80 µg/l)	0.03	30 pmol/l (24 ng/l)
T_3	1.8 nmol/l (1.2 µg/l)	0.3	5 pmol/l (0.4 µg/l)

only this free hormone that can diffuse from the blood to act on target cells or be degraded. The vast majority of the thyroid hormones are carried in the plasma bound to a number of plasma proteins. This provides a metabolically inert extrathyroidal reserve that buffers short-term fluctuations. These macromolecular complexes escape renal glomerular filtration, so that very little hormone is excreted in urine.

Three thyroid hormone binding proteins have been identified (Table 5.3.3), all synthesized in the liver.

- **Thyronine-binding globulin** (TBG; formerly termed thyroxine-BG) normally carries about 75% of both total T_3 and T_4.
- **Albumin** binds significant quantities of T_3 and T_4, some 25% of T_3 and 10% of T_4. Although it is present at a much higher concentration than TBG, it has a relatively low affinity for binding with thyroid hormones.
- **Thyroxine-binding pre-albumin** (TBPA) carries T_4 preferentially. Although its concentration is more than 16 times that of TBG, its binding affinity for T_4 is weak and it

carries only 15% of the total T_4 and, normally, no significant T_3.

Thus, TBG is the major T_3 and T_4 binding protein. Since there is one iodothyronine-binding site per TBG molecule, its binding capacity is equal to its plasma level (260 nmol/l). Its 10-fold lower affinity for T_3 accounts for the higher proportion of free T_3 than free T_4 in plasma. Changes in its concentration can affect total T_3 and T_4 levels significantly. For instance, the elevated plasma oestrogen level in normal pregnancy (and in women taking certain oral contraceptives) enhances TBG glycosylation, the resultant more negatively charged molecule is less readily taken up by the liver for clearance, and plasma TBG, T_3 and T_4 levels become raised.

Metabolism and excretion

The carriage of T_3 and T_4 by plasma proteins results in their unusually long half-lives in plasma (T_3, 1 day; T_4, 6–7 days). The metabolism of the unbound molecules (Fig. 5.3.4) involves progressive enzymic mono-deiodination, largely but not exclusively in liver and kidneys. T_4 is thereby converted to active T_3 and inactive rT_3, then to the more rapidly cleared, apparently inactive metabolites di- and mono-iodothyronine (T_2 and T_1) and thyronine (T_0). Oxidative deamination of T_3 and T_4 also occurs in liver and kidneys. Conjugation takes place in liver and kidneys for excretion. A minor fraction in bile is cleaved by intestinal bacteria to yield T_4 and T_3, which are reabsorbed in a so-called 'enterohepatic cycle'.

Table 5.3.3	Thyroid hormone binding proteins			
	Concentration (µmol/l)	Binding affinity	Actual binding T_4 (%)	Actual binding T_3 (%)
TBG	0.3	Very high	75	75
Albumin	640	Very low	10	25
TBPA	5.0	Low	15	0

TBG = thyronine-binding globulin; TBPA = thyroxine-binding pre-albumin

Extrathyroidal deiodination of T_4 and T_3

In normal young adult humans, daily turnover of the active hormone T_3 is found to be around 50 nmol; and since around 7.5 nmol is secreted by the thyroid gland, some 85% of production must be extrathyroidal by the deiodination of T_4.

Since 80% of secreted T_4 is deiodinated and 85% of active hormone (T_3) production is included in this, there is great interest in the regulation of the deiodinases and in their potential for determining thyroid status in normality and disease. Three types (I–III) of microsomal deiodinase with distinct physiological roles have been proposed in relation to their tissue locations, substrate preferences and sites of action (Table 5.3.4).

Most tissues can deiodinate T_4, but some have been studied more intensively than others.

- In liver, kidney and (probably) skeletal muscle the type I enzyme is quantitatively important in the peripheral production of circulating T_3 and in clearance of rT_3. Thus, in short-term fasting and in moderately severe illness, the plasma $[T_3]$ falls, while $[rT_3]$ rises and $[T_4]$ is unaffected. This is attributed to a reduction in the activity of the type I enzyme resulting from lowered NADPH-dependent generation of a cytosolic SH-containing cofactor.

- In CNS and brown fat tissue, the type II enzyme is thought to mediate 5′ deiodination of T_4 within target cells, thereby providing the local T_3 levels critical respectively for normal development of the CNS and for response to cold stress in the young perinatally. In pituitary gland, the intracellular generation of T_3 by this enzyme is required for growth hormone (GH) production and for feedback control in the hypothalamo-pituitary–thyroid axis (see below).

- The type III deiodinase may protect the CNS and, in the case of the placenta, the fetus from excess T_3 by converting T_4 to rT_3 and T_3 to T_2, and it may be the major enzyme for rT_3 production.

Table 5.3.4 The three types of iodothyronine deiodinase

Tissue location	Type I	Type II	Type III
Liver	+		
Kidney	+		
Thyroid gland	+		
Skeletal muscle	+		
CNS	+	+	+
Pituitary gland	+	+	
Brown fat tissue		+	
Placenta		+	+
Skin			+

Summary

Thyroid hormones

- Iodine combines with tyrosine attached to thyroglobulin in the thyroid follicles to begin hormone formation.
- Thyroxine (T_4) is formed in greater quantities than tri-iodothyronine (T_3) but is less active. The duration of action of T_4 is longer than that of T_3, so its overall effect is about the same as that of T_3.
- The hormones can be stored in the follicular colloid for several months.
- Most free T_3 is generated in extrathyroidal sites from T_4.
- The hormones are transported in the blood bound to thyronine-binding globulin, thyroxine-binding pre-albumin and albumin.
- On entering target cells, thyroid hormones again bind to proteins and are then slowly released.

Physiological effects of thyroid hormones

At some stage, almost all cells require adequate exposure to thyroid hormone for normal function. Selected examples will be considered here in order to illustrate general principles. Although the underlying mechanism of action involves the regulation of gene transcription through nuclear T_3 receptors (see p. 386), different aspects of cell function are affected in each case.

Development and growth

Differentiation and maturation of tissues in the fetus, newborn and child are dependent upon adequate thyroid hormone production. Uncorrected deficiency results in cretinism. In the brain perinatally there is an absolute requirement for thyroid hormone for nerve myelination and axon branching, the latter possibly involving stimulation of nerve growth factor (NGF) synthesis. If not corrected at this critical stage, thyroid insufficiency results in permanent mental retardation. Neonates are now routinely screened to check their thyroid status, with thyroid hormone replacement therapy being administered when appropriate.

Skeletal growth in infancy and childhood is diminished in the absence of thyroid hormone and restored by hormone therapy within a less critical time-frame. The hormone acts indirectly at the anterior pituitary gland to stimulate synthesis and to facilitate secretion of GH, and at bone to facilitate GH (or somatomedin) action. In contrast, skeletal maturation (fusion of growth plates) is stimulated directly by T_3.

Metabolic rate

Administration of thyroid hormone raises the resting (basal) metabolic rate (BMR). It stimulates oxygen consumption and heat production (thermo- or calorigenesis) in whole animals and in most tissues studied in isolation. Brain, anterior pituitary, spleen, testis and uterus do not exhibit calorigenesis in these experiments. In the whole organism, there are associated increases in other processes. Oxygen delivery to the tissues is enhanced by increased ventilation, cardiac output and red cell mass. Thyroid hormone increases the intestinal absorption of glucose and mobilization of glycogen, fat and protein, thus providing metabolic fuels. The increased cardiac output and fuel mobilization may involve raised sensitivity to noradrenaline and adrenaline, since thyroid hormone increases the number of β-adrenergic receptors and the efficiency of their coupling to adenylyl cyclase in several of the tissues. Thus, β-adrenergic antagonists (e.g. propranolol) can be useful in the treatment of thyrotoxicosis. The cellular mechanisms underlying increased oxygen consumption and thermogenesis remain controversial.

Hypo-, hyper- and euthyroid states

Thyroid hormone deficiency and excess are respectively termed hypo- and hyperthyroidism. Their causes include malfunction of the thyroid gland itself (primary) and malfunction of the hypothalamo-pituitary axis (secondary). The incidence of autoimmune thyroid disease is similar to that of diabetes mellitus. The signs and symptoms of disease reflect the widespread actions of the hormone, including its enabling of other ligands (Table 5.3.5). Caution is necessary in interpretation of values given for plasma hormone levels. For instance, high or low total plasma levels of T_3 and/or T_4 do not imply respectively hyper- or hypothyroid status. Such levels may be due to altered plasma protein hormone binding. For instance, oestrogen raises binding capacity by raising the TBG level, whereas aspirin lowers the binding affinity of TBG and displaces hormone from it. Such alterations may occur in normality. Because of the feedback control of the free hormone level, functional thyroid status remains normal despite altered plasma protein binding and the subjects are in the normal, or euthyroid, state.

Table 5.3.5 Signs and symptoms of hypo- and hyperthyroidism

Parameter	Hypothyroid	Hyperthyroid
Plasma free [T$_3$ and/or T$_4$]	Low/absent	High
Growth	Deficient	—
Goitre	Present/absent	Present
Thermogenesis/metabolism		
BMR	Lowered	Raised
Body core temperature	Lowered	Raised
Sweating rate	Lowered	Raised
Thermal discomfort	Cold intolerant	Heat intolerant
Protein metabolism	Decreased synthesis	Increased catabolism
Lipid metabolism	High plasma [cholesterol]	Low plasma [cholesterol]
Intestinal absorption	Glucose lowered	Glucose raised
Appetite	Lowered	Raised
Body weight	Gain	Loss
CNS/behavioural effect	Cretinism (perinatal)	—
	Slow mentation/lethargic	Rapid mentation/restless
CVS (resting)		
Heart rate	Lowered	Raised
Cardiac output	Lowered	Raised
Arterial pressure	Lowered	Raised

Hyperthyroidism

The commonest form of hyperthyroidism is Graves' disease (Fig. 5.3.6). Typical presentation is a patient showing heat intolerance, excess sweating, palpitations, skeletal muscle wasting and weight loss, increased appetite, diarrhoea, and nervous irritability. Other signs may include a large goitre, exophthalmos (protruding eyeballs, owing to infiltration of orbital tissues with lymphocytes, mucopolysaccharides and oedema fluid), and myxoedema (puffy, oedematous skin) at certain sites. The causes of exophthalmos and myxoedema are poorly understood. Plasma total [T$_3$] is raised but TSH is not. These patients have present in their blood a substance capable of independently stimulating thyroid gland function; it was at one time called long-acting thyroid stimulator (LATS) because of the delayed onset and long time-course of its action. The active agent is now known to be an autoantibody, thyroid-stimulating immunoglobulin or antibody (TSI or TSAb). It binds to TSH receptors and stimulates cAMP production. The resultant increase in thyroid hormone output inhibits thyrotroph TSH secretion, but not TSI production.

Successful treatment initially requires making the patient euthyroid in order to effect some recovery before taking any measures to prevent disease recurrence. This may involve anti-I$^-$ thyroid agents, surgery, radioiodine, β-adrenergic blockers, and iodine, which paradoxically inhibits hormone release. Gland tissue may then

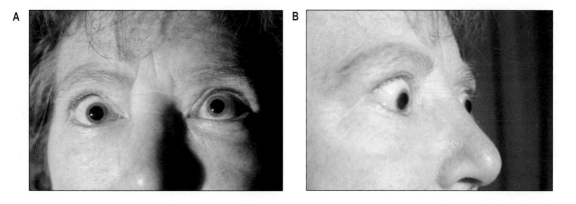

Fig. 5.3.6 Graves' disease. The thyroid gland is diffusely enlarged to form a goitre. The exophthalmosis (proptosis) is due to retro-orbital inflammation, swelling and oedema, which is present in 70% of these patients but is not related to the severity of the disease. (Courtesy of Professor C D Forbes.)

be removed surgically or inactivated by exposure to an iodine radioisotope, with monitoring of thyroid status and appropriate subsequent T_4 replacement therapy. β-adrenergic blockers may be used to control only some of the features of hyperthyroidism, such as palpitations.

Hypothyroidism

Hashimoto's thyroiditis, the commonest form of primary hypothyroidism, is another example of autoimmune disease, and affects approximately 1% of the adult population. Symptoms tend to be the opposite of those characteristic of Graves' disease (see above), additional symptoms including dry, flaky skin and hair loss (alopecia). Goitre is almost always present. Serum free T_4 is decreased, accompanied by elevated TSH because of the reduced T_4 negative feedback. Treatment is by hormone replacement, using a single daily dose of T_4 because its longer half-life provides a more stable level of circulating thyroid hormone over 24 hours. Thyroxine replacement is usually introduced gradually, elevating the dose every 4 weeks

until the euthyroid state is achieved. Over-replacement with thyroxine can initiate cardiovascular problems, and possibly a reduction in bone density resulting in osteoporosis.

The hypothalamo-anterior pituitary–thyroid gland axis

This feedback control system maintains the circulating level of the free prohormone T_4 (Fig. 5.3.7), operating on the general principle described elsewhere (see Ch. 5.2). The tonic, pulsatile release of hypothalamic thyrotrophin-releasing hormone (TRH) into the pituitary portal vessels provides the primary drive for TSH release from pituitary thyrotrophs through an IP_3- and DAG-mediated pathway. In certain animals and in human infants (but not adults) acute exposure to cold raises plasma [TSH] by stimulating TRH release. The lowering of TSH secretion in response to other stresses may be mediated by hypothalamic somatostatin or dopamine, or by glucocorticoids. Most importantly, TSH secretion is modulated normally through feedback inhibition by plasma free [T_4]

Summary

Physiological effects

- The two major effects of thyroid hormones are to increase overall metabolic rate and to stimulate growth in children.
- The mechanism of thyroid hormone action is to stimulate DNA transcription, which increases protein synthesis, enzyme production, size and number of mitochondria and cell membrane transport.
- Hypothyroidism may be *primary* – a defect in the supply of iodine or the functioning of the gland; or *secondary* – a deficiency of TSH (see below).
- Hypothyroidism causes reduced metabolic rate, heart rate, gut motility and mental function.
- Cretinism is irreversible mental retardation resulting from congenital hypothyroidism.
- Hyperthyroidism (thyrotoxicosis) usually results from abnormal autoantibodies overstimulating TSH receptors on the thyroid gland, or a tumour that secretes thyroid hormone.
- Hyperthyroidism elevates metabolic rate and heart rate, and provokes insomnia and anxiety.

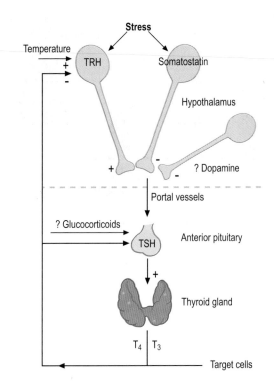

Fig. 5.3.7 Possible factors regulating thyrotrophin (TSH) secretion. TRH = thyrotrophin-releasing hormone.

rather than plasma [T_3], since plasma [TSH] is more closely correlated (inversely) with free [T_4] than with free [T_3].

By modifying DNA transcription within thyrotrophs, T_3 reduces the number of TRH receptors, thus lowering cell sensitivity to TRH. In contrast, at the hypothalamus T_3 suppresses TRH synthesis. Although TSH is the main regulator of thyroid function, its action may be subject to local modulation. Notably, the ability of follicular cells to respond to TSH relates inversely to [I^-]. Thus, in preparing certain hyperthyroid patients for surgery, large iodine doses can be used to reduce gland function and size.

Summary

The hypothalamo-hypophyseal–thyroid axis

- Control of thyroid function is by thyrotrophin (thyroid-stimulating hormone – TSH) from the anterior pituitary gland. TSH stimulates all stages of thyroid hormone synthesis.
- Thyrotrophin release is primarily regulated by negative feedback of thyroid hormones onto the anterior pituitary.

- Higher centres exert an effect on thyrotrophin release by modulating hypothalamic neurosecretion of thyrotrophin-releasing hormone (TRH) into the hypothalamo-hypophyseal portal blood vessels.
- Somatostatin from the hypothalamus has a minor inhibitory effect on TSH release.

The adrenal gland

Introduction

The adrenal glands are paired and comprise
two distinct tissues, an inner **medulla** and an
outer **cortex**, each with different secretions.
They are situated on the upper poles of the kidneys. In 1855, the physician Addison proposed
that a group of symptoms including progressive fatigue, hypotension and increased pigmentation of the skin (later termed Addison's
disease) could be caused by degeneration of the
adrenals. Shortly after, the physiologist Brown-
Séquard showed that bilateral removal of the
adrenals was fatal. The different functions of
the medulla and cortex were not understood
until the end of that century. The physiologists
Oliver and Schäfer (1895) reported the blood
pressure-raising effect of medullary chromaffin
tissue extracts. The catecholamine adrenaline
(also called epinephrine) was then isolated and
synthesized. By 1930, steroid-containing cortical tissue extracts were found to be effective in
the treatment of Addison's disease. The major
active adrenal cortical steroids were identified
and synthesized in the next 20 years.

They were classified, on the basis of their function, into two groups:

- the **mineralocorticoids** (typified by aldosterone in humans), named for their effects on electrolyte balance
- the **glucocorticoids** (typified by cortisol), named for their effect of increasing the concentration of glucose in blood and the storage of glycogen in liver.

Later, a third group, the masculinizing adrenal **androgens**, was identified. The glucocorticoids were found to have a broad spectrum of effects including the suppression of inflammation and of immune system function.

The compound adrenal gland: medulla and cortex

Development

Adrenal medullary and cortical tissues form from separate embryonic tissues:

- medullary **chromaffin cells** from the neural crest (neuroectoderm)
- cortical cells from the mesothelium lining the body cavity (coelomic mesoderm).

They become closely juxtaposed to form the adrenal glands. The adrenal medulla develops with the peripheral sympathetic nervous system. Adrenal medullary cells arise from the neural crest cells that also form nerve fibres. The chromaffin cells synthesize noradrenaline until just before birth; then adrenaline becomes the major adrenal medullary hormone. This change accompanies the stimulation of glucocorticoid secretion from the cortex by pituitary adrenocorticotrophic hormone (ACTH).

The adult cortex begins to form distinct zones at this time and replaces the regressing fetal cortex during the first year postnatally. Isolated groups of ectopic cortical or medullary cells (crests) occur frequently in the fetus, and in fetal life most catecholamine is secreted by such extramedullary chromaffin cells. They

regress postnatally, but can remain as tumours called phaeochromocytomas.

Zonation, vasculature and innervation of the adrenal gland

Cortical arteries and medullary arteries in the capsule serve separate circulations that drain into a common central adrenal vein. The cortex consists of steroid-producing cells that secrete the corticosteroid hormones. The medulla consists of chromaffin cells, of which:

- those exposed to corticomedullary portal blood secrete adrenaline
- those exposed to medullary arterial (systemic) blood alone secrete noradrenaline.

There are some isolated chromaffin cells in the cortex.

Catecholamine secretion is determined by preganglionic neuronal activity, each neurone serving many chromaffin cells. Corticosteroid secretion is determined by factors circulating in the blood.

The combined weight of the adrenals in adults is 8–10 g, of which 80–90% is cortex, made up of three histologically distinct zones:

- the outer zona glomerulosa
- the zona fasciculata
- the inner zona reticularis (Fig. 5.4.1).

The cortex surrounds the central medulla and the whole gland is enclosed by a capsule.

Blood from a rich subcapsular primary arteriolar plexus flows via corticomedullary portal vessels into a secondary sinusoidal plexus at the junction of the zona reticularis and medulla. Some small arteries directly form a separate medullary plexus. Both sets of vessels drain into a central adrenal vein.

In each gland, sympathetic preganglionic neurones innervate medullary chromaffin cells. The few chromaffin cells that are scattered within the cortex may have a local hormonal (paracrine) function.

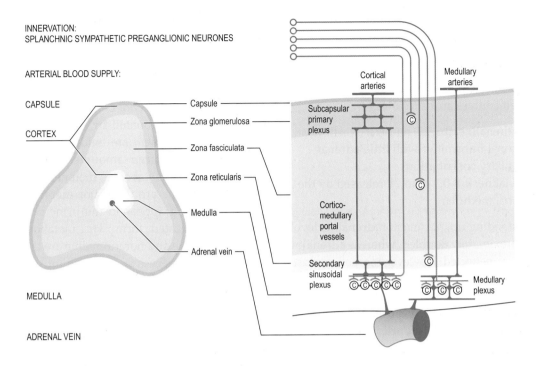

Fig. 5.4.1 The adrenal gland. C = chromaffin cell.

Summary

Adrenal structure

- The adrenal glands are compound endocrine glands, comprising an inner neuroectodermal medulla and an outer mesodermal cortex.
- The medulla consists of chromaffin cells, which secrete the catecholamines noradrenaline and adrenaline when stimulated by splanchnic preganglionic sympathetic neurones.
- The cortex comprises the *zona glomerulosa*, which secretes mineralocorticoids; the *zona fasciculata*, which secretes glucocorticoids; and the *zona reticularis*, which secretes glucocorticoids and adrenal androgens.

Adrenal medullary hormones: noradrenaline, adrenaline and met-enkephalin

Synthesis, storage, release, metabolism and excretion

Medullary catecholamine secretion comprises noradrenaline and adrenaline in a molar ratio of $1:4$. Noradrenaline is secreted by medullary tissue perfused directly by systemic blood via the medullary arteries. Adrenaline is secreted by the cells lying adjacent to fenestrated vessels that carry portal blood containing cortisol from the cortex. High local **cortisol** levels induce (stimulate) the cytosolic enzyme phenylethanolamine-*N*-methyl transferase (PNMT), which is necessary for adrenaline synthesis. These cells also contain the protein pre-pro-enkephalin, and are the source of the circulating opioid peptide met-enkephalin (see Ch. 3.10). The effects of release of noradrenaline and adrenaline are shown in Figure 5.4.2. Plasma levels of catecholamines are often measured as an indicator of sympathetic activity. In resting, conscious, supine subjects the normal catecholamine plasma levels and their sources are as follows:

- noradrenaline: 0.6–2.0 nmol/l, overflow of neuronal transmitter with little adrenal medullary contribution
- adrenaline: 0.1–0.3 nmol/l, released by the adrenal medulla.

On standing up, plasma noradrenaline levels are approximately doubled, whereas adrenaline levels are unaffected. However, marked increases in plasma adrenaline levels are provoked by stressor stimuli including moderate to severe hypoglycaemia, heavy exercise and surgery. Circulating adrenaline is functionally important, whereas only rarely does plasma noradrenaline exceed the threshold for production of systemic effects.

Catecholamines have a short half-life in the circulation measured in minutes. They are methylated by catechol-*O*-methyl transferase (COMT) and deaminated by monoamine oxidase (MAO), which are widely distributed and present in large amounts in the liver. The methylated metabolites metanephrine and normetanephrine are the major metabolites of the amines and appear in the urine both free and in conjugated form. The metabolites of both adrenaline and noradrenaline are taken up into aminergic nerves and smooth muscle. This is the mechanism by which the effects of neuronally released noradrenaline are terminated and which allows its reuse by sympathetic nerves.

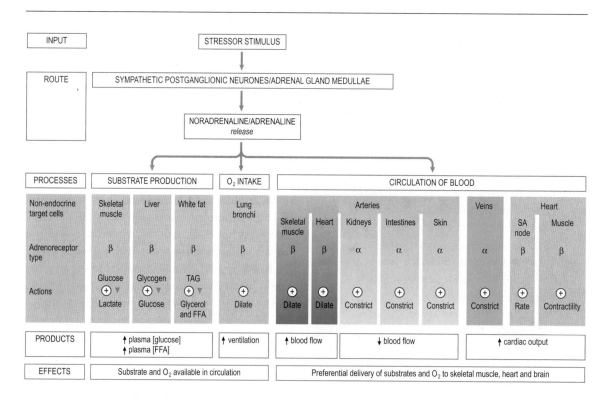

Fig. 5.4.2 The release of adrenaline and noradrenaline from the adrenal medulla and their subsequent actions.
TAG = triacylglycerol; FFA = free fatty acids.

Physiological effects and mechanisms of action

In 1929, the physiologist Cannon portrayed the sympatho-adrenal system as an emergency mechanism activated in situations of 'fight or flight'. This response dramatically illustrates the system's effects but in an exaggerated form. The most important role of the system is as a homeostatic mechanism. Except in extreme stress, the system functions normally, even if the adrenal medullae are removed. Release of catecholamines from nerves produces only localized responses. Adrenal catecholamines affect all tissues via the circulation and reinforce the actions of the neurotransmitter noradrenaline in response to stressors. There is evidence that the two catecholamines can be released independently from the medulla (see below and Ch. 3.2).

The fight or flight reaction

During the fight or flight reaction catecholamines acting on α- and β-adrenoceptors facilitate increased substrate and oxygen delivery to active tissues. There is rapid mobilization of glycogen and triacylglycerol (TAG) from stores. Oxygen uptake and supply to active tissues is ensured at the expense of that of less essential tissues. Blood is preferentially supplied to brain, heart and skeletal muscle. Catecholamines increase metabolic rate and arousal. These effects require sufficient tissue levels of thyroid hormone and cortisol, and involve alteration of the secretion of other hormones including insulin.

Patients with phaeochromocytomas (rare tumours of chromaffin cells) can suffer uncontrolled, intermittent or sustained hypersecretion of the catecholamines. Their problems include hypertension, increased metabolic rate and hyperglycaemia.

Control of adrenomedullary hormone secretion

It must be emphasized that the activity of the autonomic system is always circumscribed and directed. The fight or flight reaction should not be seen as typical. The medulla is innervated and controlled by the central autonomic nervous system via preganglionic sympathetic fibres in the splanchnic nerves (see Ch. 3.2). Each neurone innervates many chromaffin cells and releases **acetylcholine** to act on nicotinic receptors of the ganglionic type.

Summary

Functions of the adrenal medulla

- The adrenal medulla secretes the catecholamines noradrenaline and adrenaline; it is the main source of adrenaline in the body.
- The effect of catecholamines is to stimulate substrate mobilization and oxygen uptake and cause the redistribution of blood flow.

- The adrenal medulla is not essential to life except under conditions of extreme stress, when adrenal catecholamines reinforce the actions of the noradrenaline released from sympathetic nerve endings.

Adrenal cortical hormones: mineralocorticoids, glucocorticoids and adrenal androgens

Biosynthesis, storage and release of adrenal steroid hormones

Steroid-producing cells of the adrenal cortex have abundant smooth endoplasmic reticulum (SER) and large mitochondria. The cells obtain **cholesterol** mainly from circulating plasma low-density lipoprotein cholesterol (LDL-cholesterol) made by the liver. It is taken up by endocytosis, attached to membrane LDL receptors, and stored as lipid droplets. Individual cortico-steroids are produced by different cells according to their enzyme complement (Fig. 5.4.3). Absence of an enzyme critical for the synthesis

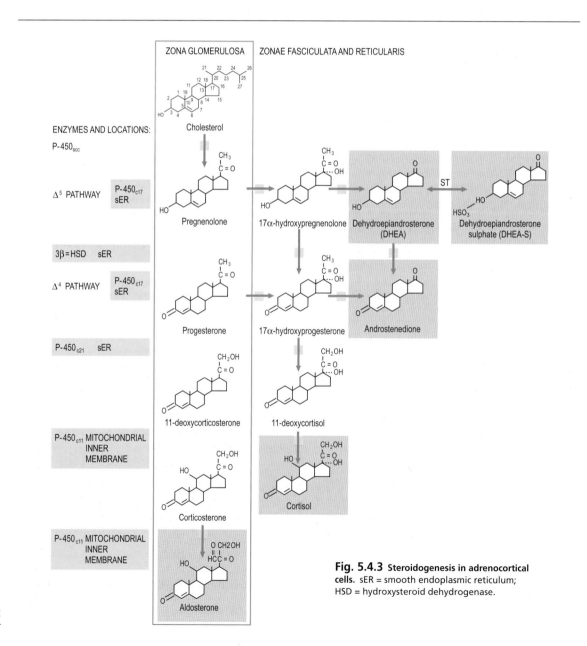

Fig. 5.4.3 Steroidogenesis in adrenocortical cells. sER = smooth endoplasmic reticulum; HSD = hydroxysteroid dehydrogenase.

of any corticosteroid results in a deficiency of that hormone, accompanied by characteristic clinical manifestations of that deficiency. **Aldosterone** synthesis is by the zona glomerulosa, with a cortisol and weak androgen output by both zona fasciculata (mainly cortisol) and zona reticularis (mainly androgen).

Corticosteroids are lipophilic and thus diffuse rapidly into the circulation. There is little storage. Thus, stimulation of secretion is by the turning on of synthesis. The mechanisms underlying functional zonation in the cortex are not well understood. Subcapsular cells can differentiate into all three zonal cell types. However, cells isolated from each zone can produce similar secretions in tissue culture. It may be that, in vivo, the synthesized steroids and by-products (notably lipid peroxidation metabolites) flowing from outer to inner cortex, in passing, control the synthetic enzymes.

Transport of adrenal steroids in the blood

The plasma concentrations of the major adrenocorticosteroids in normal humans are summarized in Table 5.4.1. The normal ranges are very wide. Single measurements must be interpreted with care. Like thyroid hormones, corticosteroids are carried in the plasma bound to plasma proteins. The nature and extent of plasma protein binding of individual steroid hormones differ (Table 5.4.2). Three major binding proteins are involved, all being produced by the liver.

- **Corticosteroid-binding globulin** (CBG; transcortin) is a glycosylated alpha-2-globulin with a low capacity but high affinity for cortisol. It has, relative to cortisol (1), lower affinities for aldosterone (0.03) and dehydroepiandrosterone/dehydroepiandrosterone-sulphate (DHEA/DHEA-S) (0.001). Binding of all these steroids is to a common site; thus, increases in total cortisol level cause displacement of aldosterone into the free fraction and increase its destruction by the liver.

Table 5.4.1 Carriage of adrenocortical hormones in blood

	Total plasma concentration (nmol/l)	Percentage bound
Cortisol		
08:00	Up to 700	Approx. 95%
24:00	Less than 140	(half-life 50–90 min)
Aldosterone		
Supine	0.02–0.15	Approx. 60%
Ambulant	0.3–0.55	(half-life 15–25 min)

Table 5.4.2 Plasma protein binding of corticosteroids

	Cortisol (%)	Aldosterone (%)
Corticosteroid-binding protein (CBG)	90	20
Albumin	6	40

- **Albumin** has lower binding affinity but is present in 800 times greater amounts than CBG.
- **Sex hormone-binding globulin** (SHBG) is a glycosylated molecule with high affinity for androgens and oestrogens.

Changes in total plasma cortisol levels occur because of altered CBG production. As with the thyroid hormones and thyronine-binding globulin (TBG; see p. 419), only the free hormone is available to react with its receptors and suppress pituitary adrenocorticotrophic hormone secretion. However, CBG (and SHBG) is an allosteric protein with a cell surface membrane-binding site as well as a steroid-binding site. The globulin–steroid complex is capable of internalization. Thus, bound hormone is also effective in peripheral tissues.

Metabolism and excretion of adrenal steroids

In the liver, steroids are inactivated by enzymes causing their reduction, oxidation and hydroxylation. Their excretion by the kidney is also promoted by conjugation with glucuronic acid or sulphate to yield water-soluble derivatives that, once filtered by the glomerulus, remain in the renal tubular fluid to be excreted in urine. These inactivation mechanisms have a very large capacity. (This is exploited during the use of the short-acting steroid general anaesthetics, e.g. althesin.) The binding of corticosteroids reduces their availability for metabolism. Their half-lives in plasma relate directly to the extent of their plasma protein binding (Table 5.4.2). The low level of binding and short half-life of aldosterone are functionally important.

The major glucocorticoid, cortisol, has an 11-keto analogue **cortisone**. Cortisone was the first glucocorticoid agent to be isolated and used therapeutically. Cortisone itself is inactive. Its effectiveness depends upon conversion, in liver, to **cortisol** by the reversible cytosolic enzyme 11-hydroxysteroid dehydrogenase (11-HSD).

The weak androgens DHEA, DHEA-S and androstenedione include the most abundant products of the adrenal cortex. **Testosterone** and **oestrogens** are derived from DHEA and androstenedione in tissues such as muscle and fat. In women, this source of testosterone is essential for the development of libido and growth of pubic and axillary hair, and the non-ovarian source of oestrogens may be important postmenopausally (see Clinical Example, p. 889).

Physiological effects and mechanisms of action of adrenal hormones

Progressive destruction of the adrenal cortex (for example by tuberculosis) leads to Addison's disease, which if untreated by administration of glucocorticoids is fatal. This is due to a number of factors:

- Loss of body fluids from extra- and intracellular compartments results in poor blood circulation and tissue hypoxia.
- The reduced ability to mobilize stored glucose, fatty acids and amino acids for energy provision and synthesis of essential proteins, coupled with loss of appetite, causes considerable weight loss.
- The inability to respond satisfactorily to a wide variety of potentially harmful events, termed stressors, results in crises triggered by normally trivial infections. This is the most common cause of death of patients with Addison's disease.

The underlying mechanisms that are disrupted reflect the widespread effects and essential nature of the mineralocorticoids and glucocorticoids. The adrenal androgens are dispensable.

The effects of mineralocorticoids

The lack of aldosterone results in circulatory shock through decreased plasma volume. Aldosterone contributes to electrolyte (Na^+ and K^+) and water homeostasis, and hence to maintenance of cardiac output by acting on several target tissues. The main site of action is in cells of the late distal convoluted tubules and collecting ducts in the kidneys (see p. 743). The late segment of the distal tubule has two important functions: reabsorption of Na^+ from the tubular fluid in exchange for K^+ and secretion of H^+ into the tubular fluid in exchange for K^+. Administration of aldosterone, after a delay of 0.5–1 hours, stimulates Na^+ reabsorption and K^+ excretion by the kidney. It acts on intracellular mineralocorticoid (glucocorticoid type I) receptors in the distal tubule to induce synthesis of three proteins that together exchange tubular Na^+ for interstitial fluid K^+ (Fig. 5.4.4).

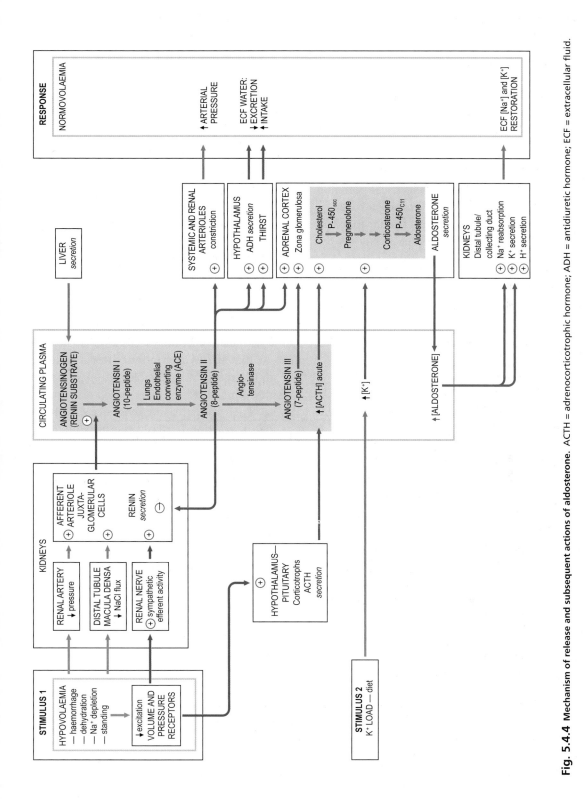

Fig. 5.4.4 Mechanism of release and subsequent actions of aldosterone. ACTH = adrenocorticotrophic hormone; ADH = antidiuretic hormone; ECF = extracellular fluid.

These are:

- luminal (apical) plasma membrane Na$^+$ channels
- mitochondrial ATP-generating enzymes
- serosal (basolateral) plasma membrane sodium pumps (Na$^+$/K$^+$ ATPase).

The resulting Na$^+$ reabsorption creates an electrochemical gradient across the luminal membrane down which K$^+$ diffuses into the lumen, and a transepithelial electrical potential difference down which Cl$^-$ moves, between the cells (paracellularly), from tubular to extracellular fluid (ECF). Aldosterone promotes the synthesis of an H$^+$ ATPase that excretes H$^+$ across the luminal membrane of the distal tubular cells.

Aldosterone also controls the synthesis of the sodium pump in several other cell types, notably muscle fibres. In the presence of aldosterone, simultaneous administration of glucose and insulin lowers plasma K$^+$ concentration by stimulating K$^+$ uptake into muscle. As glucose moves into the cells K$^+$ goes with it. This is useful therapeutically as an immediate treatment for K$^+$ intoxication.

Simple aldosterone deficiency has a number of effects. It would lead to hypotension resulting from the depletion of plasma volume that follows loss of ECF Na$^+$ and water in urine, tissue hypoxia and metabolic acidosis resulting from inadequate tissue perfusion. A raised plasma K$^+$ concentration (hyperkalaemia) is also observed. This results from a decreased K$^+$ uptake from the ECF into muscle, loss of K$^+$ from the ICF by cell surface membrane K$^+$–H$^+$ exchange, and decreased K$^+$ secretion into urine, all of which lead to hyperkalaemia and a lowering of the resting membrane potential of excitable (e.g. cardiac) cells.

Adrenocortical deficiency can be treated by administration of mineralocorticoids, such as the synthetic steroid fludrocortisone. The effects of simple aldosterone deficiency are mitigated by cortisol, which has mineralocorticoid potency but only around 1/500 that of aldosterone.

The effects of glucocorticoids

The glucocorticoid cortisol has multiple effects (see Table 5.4.3). The hormone is essential for optimal functioning of virtually all tissues. The physiological response to many challenges requires that the tissues have previously had adequate exposure to cortisol. Glucocorticoids permit the synthesis of proteins by their target cells. These proteins include regulatory agents, enzymes, receptors and other components of cellular receptor–effector systems. This action is called the **permissive action** of glucocorticoids.

Inhibition of ACTH and CRH release by the hypothalamo-pituitary unit. Glucocorticoids inhibit the release of corticotrophin and its releasing hormone, thus forming a negative-feedback system controlling their own release. Administration of exogenous glucocorticoids inhibits corticotrophin secretion to such an extent that if this is continued for any length of time (days), irreversible adrenal atrophy results, which leads to a decreased resistance to stress. There is increasing evidence for physiological interaction between the inflammatory/immune system and the hypothalamo-pituitary–adrenal cortex axis.

The effect of glucocorticoids on intermediary metabolism. Glucocorticoids influence intermediary metabolism profoundly. Their effect is to raise the plasma glucose concentration. This involves several target cell types upon which they have numerous effects (Fig. 5.4.5). The response of target cells to several other stimuli are modified, notably an increased responsiveness to catabolic hormones and to sympathetic stimulation, and a decreased sensitivity to the hormone insulin, leading to lower glucose uptake from plasma by non-obligatory glucose-utilizing cells. In certain cells, glucocorticoids inhibit glucose uptake directly.

The classical effects of the glucocorticoid cortisol to raise plasma glucose concentration and liver glycogen content are shown in Figure 5.4.5. They centre on the mobilization of gluconeogenic intermediates (amino acids, glycerol) from

Table 5.4.3 Peripheral effects of glucocorticoids (cortisol) in man

	Effect
Intermediary metabolism	Glycogenesis, particularly in liver. Also in heart and skeletal muscle
	Gluconeogenesis in liver. Substrate provided in part by cortisol-induced protein catabolism, especially in skeletal muscle
	Lipolysis in adipose tissue, releasing fatty acids to serve as alternative energy substrate (excess results in redistribution of fat stores)
	Anti-insulin effect blocks uptake of glucose into peripheral cells
	Acid secretion increased in stomach – tendency to ulceration
Immunological function and inflammation	Depressed immune and inflammatory responses increase susceptibility to infection
	Involution of lymphatic and thymic tissue
Musculoskeletal system and connective tissue (excess secretion)	Protein catabolism leads to muscle atrophy, weakness and fatigue
	Connective tissue – inhibition of fibroblasts and synthesis of ground substance
	Prolonged exposure – thin skin that bruises easily and osteoporotic bones
Fluid and electrolyte balance	Sodium retention and redistribution of body fluids. Hypertension may develop
Central nervous system	Necessary for normal CNS function
	Behavioural changes and disruption of sleep patterns described in patients with excess/deficiency
Developmental	Lung – stimulates formation of type II pneumocytes, which secrete surfactant
	Adrenal medulla – stimulates differentiation of neural crest cells into chromaffin cells

protein and TAG stores, and the enhancement of gluconeogenesis and glycogenesis through induction of several enzymes. For simplicity, the effects of unopposed cortisol action are indicated in the diagram: the effects of the counter-regulatory hormone insulin are considered elsewhere.

An insufficiency of cortisol (e.g. Addison's disease) has multiple effects. The rate of glycogenesis, glycogenolysis and gluconeogenesis in liver are all reduced. Proteolysis occurs in muscle, lymphoid and connective tissue, and there is lipolysis in white fat tissue. There is thus insufficient glycogen reserve together with

impaired ability to produce glucose and fatty acids in response to stressors such as fasting and exercise. This, together with the unrestrained action of insulin, leads to an increased tendency to hypoglycaemia and a sluggish recovery from it. This is particularly damaging to neurones, which are obligatory users of glucose. The glucocorticoids have therefore been described as the hormones of starvation.

Cardiovascular and renal function of glucocorticoids. The proper functioning of the cardiovascular and renal systems is cortisol dependent. The effects of cortisol deficiency include hypotension and impaired ability to

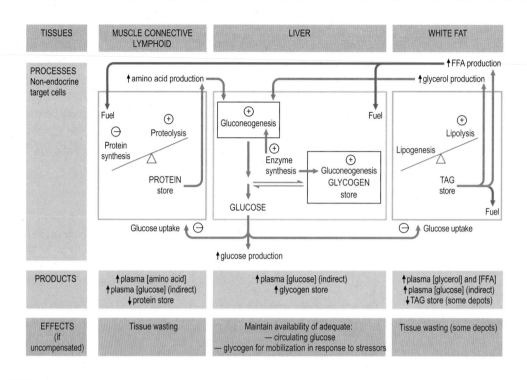

Fig. 5.4.5 Main effects of glucocorticoids on intermediary metabolism. TAG = triacylglycerol; FFA = free fatty acids.

excrete a water load. Reduced sensitivity of myocardium and arteriolar smooth muscle to catecholamines results in poor myocardial performance and loss of vasomotor control. This effect is aggravated by an increase in vascular endothelial permeability. When coupled with aldosterone deficiency (see above), these would hinder vascular compensation for hypovolaemia.

Cortisol deficiency often leads to water intoxication, which occurs for several reasons:

- hypothalamic secretion of antidiuretic hormone (ADH) is disinhibited
- the kidney's sensitivity to ADH is increased
- there is reduced glomerular filtration rate
- Na⁺ loss occurs because of aldosterone deficiency; aldosterone secretion is itself dependent on cortisol.

Modification of inflammatory and immune responses by glucocorticoids. Adrenalectomy

or the administration of the glucocorticoid receptor antagonist RU486 (mifepristone) results in exaggerated responses to infection or even in spontaneous inflammation. Glucocorticoids normally restrain the complex inflammatory and immune responses to tissue injury and infection. Administered in large (pharmacological) doses, they are used to suppress autoimmune disease and allergies and to prevent the rejection of transplanted tissue.

In inflammation, glucocorticoids restrain the activities of mast cells, epithelial cells, and fibroblasts and inhibit the migration of leucocytes (see Table 5.4.3). These effects involve high-affinity glucocorticoid receptors and induction of specific inhibitory proteins and their receptors. One such protein is **vasocortin**, which also inhibits histamine release. Another is **lipocortin-1**. Lipocortin-1 is located at several sites including the epidermis and epithelium. It is a protein with receptors on monocytes and neutrophils (but not lymphocytes) that inhibits the production of the eicosanoids and platelet-activating factor. This in turn limits chemotaxis and other pro-inflammatory functions of leucocytes.

Other effects of glucocorticoids. Glucocorticoids affect development and growth. In the nervous system, cortisol deficiency causes increased sensitivity to auditory, gustatory and olfactory stimuli, while cortisol excess can cause neurone damage (see below).

The expanding catalogue of glucocorticoid effects makes it difficult, but ever more important, to recognize a pattern to these effects. It is suggested that the effects can be remembered more readily by regarding glucocorticoids as *preventive agents*. Thus, in the normal adult subject, cortisol:

- prevents undersupply of *nutrients* to tissues by maintaining both production of fuels and blood flow; it is the hormone of starvation
- prevents excessive *fluid* retention by promoting water excretion
- prevents inappropriate activation of the *inflammatory* and *immune* reactions.

Control of aldosterone secretion

ACTH and aldosterone secretion

The control of aldosterone secretion is not directly mediated by ACTH from the pituitary. The normal role of ACTH is to maintain the responsiveness of the zona glomerulosa to other controlling factors. However, when ACTH secretion by corticotrophs is stimulated through the hypothalamo-pituitary axis (see below) by stressors such as haemorrhage the large rise in plasma ACTH concentration stimulates not only cortisol secretion but also that of aldosterone.

Major stimuli for aldosterone secretion

Aldosterone secretion by the zona glomerulosa controls the circulating blood volume and fluid balance (see pp. 602 and 755), maintaining ECF volume and preventing K^+ accumulation in the ECF. The major stimuli for its secretion are:

- decreased kidney perfusion operating through the renin–angiotensin system
- increased plasma K^+ concentration operating directly on aldosterone synthesis in the zona glomerulosa.

The interplay of factors affecting its release is summarized in Figure 5.4.4.

Juxtaglomerular apparatus of the nephron and the renin–angiotensin system. Renin is a proteolytic enzyme secreted into blood by the juxtaglomerular apparatus of the kidney (see p. 754). Renin is secreted by juxtaglomerular cells in response to several stimuli. These include:

- increased renal sympathetic efferent nerve activity
- decreased afferent arteriolar pressure
- decreased glomerular filtration leading to reduced NaCl flux in the nearby macula densa.

The substrate of renin is angiotensinogen, which is converted in a series of steps into angiotensin II and III.

Effects of angiotensin II. In zona glomerulosa cells both angiotensin II and III stimulate aldosterone synthesis and secretion through the IP_3/DAG second messenger system. In addition, angiotensin II, as its name implies, potently stimulates systemic and renal arteriolar vasoconstriction. In the presence of cortisol, it promotes NaCl and water reabsorption by the renal proximal tubules. In the hypothalamus, it stimulates ADH secretion and thirst. Collectively these effects restore blood volume after blood loss.

Plasma K^+ and aldosterone secretion. Rising plasma K^+ concentration is a potent and important stimulus for aldosterone secretion. Raised extracellular K^+ concentration depolarizes the zona glomerulosa cells, opening voltage-gated Ca^{2+} channels and thus causing Ca^{2+} influx. This leads to activation of steroidogenesis.

Glucocorticoid interactions with salt and water balance

Cortisol has some limited mineralocorticoid effect. This is important in aldosterone deficiency (see above) or during chronic cortisol hypersecretion, as in Cushing's syndrome. More importantly, cortisol modulates angiotensinogen synthesis in the liver and atrial natriuretic peptide (ANP) synthesis in the heart. When ANP secretion rises in response to hypervolaemia, it inhibits aldosterone secretion by zona glomerulosa cells. By dilating renal afferent and efferent arterioles, ANP also mediates the glucocorticoid-induced increase in GFR (see above).

Control of cortisol secretion

The hypothalamo-pituitary–adrenal cortex axis

In normal subjects there is a basal circadian rhythm in the plasma concentration of total cortisol that is related to the sleep–wakefulness cycle (see Ch. 1.5). The concentration is at a maximum a few hours before awakening and falls to a minimum around the onset of sleep (Fig. 5.4.6). Blood sampling has shown that the rhythm results from bursts of hormone secretion. Each burst produces a sharp rise in

plasma cortisol concentration followed by a slow decline determined by the long half-life of cortisol in plasma (1–1.5 h). The increased frequency of bursts during sleep causes plasma cortisol to rise. The periodic pattern of secretion implies that the time and conditions of sampling must be defined closely when assessing glucocorticoid status clinically. Single time measurements are not interpretable.

There is a pulsatile release into hypophyseal portal blood of the 41-amino acid peptide **corticotrophin-releasing hormone** (CRH) by parvicellular neurones of the hypothalamic paraventricular nucleus. The suprachiasmatic nuclei determine the circadian pattern of secretion related to the dark–light (photoperiod) and sleep–wakefulness cycles. CRH, acting via cAMP, rapidly stimulates ACTH release by corticotrophs. Stimulation of ACTH synthesis occurs more slowly, within hours. CRH and ADH release have a similar pattern and may interact at the corticotroph.

At adrenal cortical cells, the ACTH has multiple effects, mediated by cAMP, all resulting in stimulation of steroidogenesis. First, there is acute (within minutes) activation of cholesterol ester hydrolase and of the side-chain cleavage enzyme P-450$_{scc}$ (see Fig. 5.4.3), which is rate limiting. This is followed by chronic (within hours or days) increases in the synthesis of LDL receptors and enzymes required for cholesterol uptake and processing. Finally, it stimulates the production of a local growth factor (insulin-like growth factor 2, IGF-2) that maintains adrenal gland mass.

The secretion of glucocorticoids is controlled by two negative-feedback loops:

- Long-loop negative feedback by cortisol on to the corticotroph, hypothalamus and limbic cortex inhibits both secretion and synthesis of corticotrophin-releasing hormone, ADH and ACTH.
- Short-loop negative feedback by ACTH inhibits its own secretion by inhibiting CRH release.

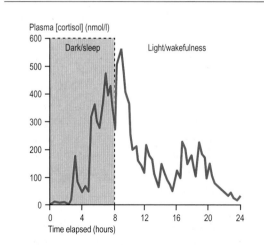

Fig. 5.4.6 Circadian pattern of secretion of cortisol.

Pituitary corticotrophs respond within seconds to the rate of rise in plasma cortisol concentration. This response may involve a cell membrane-stabilizing effect of the hormone. They also have slowly responding glucocorticoid type II receptors of low affinity. Feedback via the hippocampus in the limbic cortex involves high-affinity type I as well as type II glucocorticoid receptors. The feedback control interacts with stressors such as fear and anxiety, trauma, infection and hypoglycaemia at the hypothalamic level. These pathways are summarized in Figure 5.4.7.

Control of adrenal androgen secretion

Adrenal androgen secretion is stimulated by ACTH and largely parallels that of cortisol. Androgen output increases at puberty (termed the **adrenarche**, see p. 888) and decreases with ageing.

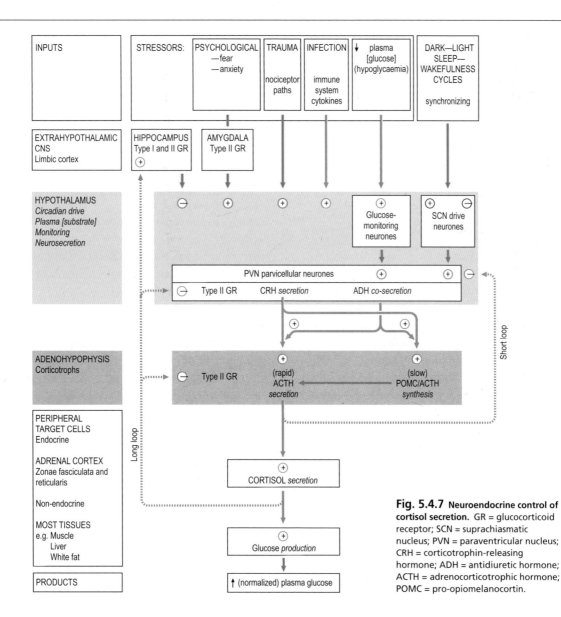

Fig. 5.4.7 Neuroendocrine control of cortisol secretion. GR = glucocorticoid receptor; SCN = suprachiasmatic nucleus; PVN = paraventricular nucleus; CRH = corticotrophin-releasing hormone; ADH = antidiuretic hormone; ACTH = adrenocorticotrophic hormone; POMC = pro-opiomelanocortin.

Clinical Example

Hypo- and hyperfunction of the adrenal cortex

The appearance of an individual can provide important clues about underlying disease. For instance, in Cushing's syndrome, characteristic truncal obesity, thin limbs, 'moon' face, plethora and skin stretch marks (striae) result from overaction of the adrenal cortex. In Addison's disease, equimolar hypersecretion of ACTH and α-MSH is caused by lack of cortisol feedback inhibition at the hypothalamo-corticotroph level. A characteristic skin hyperpigmentation results from stimulation of melanin synthesis by the α-MSH.

Hypofunction – adrenal insufficiency

Adrenal insufficiency may be primary, secondary or tertiary.

Primary adrenal insufficiency – Addison's disease

This is due to destruction of the adrenal cortex. ACTH is elevated because of loss of negative feedback control by cortisol.

Symptoms and signs. Patients consistently present with symptoms of weakness, tiredness, fatigue and anorexia, commonly associated with gastrointestinal symptoms of nausea, vomiting, constipation and abdominal pain. Signs include weight loss, hyperpigmentation (due to elevated ACTH) and hypotension (due to lack of aldosterone).

Secondary adrenal insufficiency – deficient pituitary ACTH

ACTH and cortisol levels are decreased; aldosterone may be low in chronic cases.

Symptoms and signs. Hyperpigmentation is not present (because ACTH levels are not elevated) and hypotension does not occur (because aldosterone secretion is less disrupted). Other signs and symptoms are similar to those of primary adrenal insufficiency, but with decreased incidence of gastrointestinal problems.

Tertiary adrenal insufficiency – deficiency of secretion of CRH or other ACTH secretagogues

ACTH and cortisol levels are depleted; aldosterone levels may be low in chronic cases. The symptoms and signs are the same as those of secondary adrenal insufficiency (see above).

Hyperfunction

Hypercortisolism – Cushing's syndrome

Cushing's syndrome may be either ACTH dependent (Cushing's disease) or ACTH independent when the adrenal cortex secretes excess cortisol because of tumour, dysplasia or hyperplasia.

In Cushing's disease, ACTH levels are elevated but not necessarily anterior pituitary in origin. ACTH can be secreted by ectopic (non-pituitary) tumours. ACTH may also be secreted in response to elevated CRH secretion, which can be hypothalamic or ectopic in origin.

Symptoms and signs. Clinical presentation is variable, but the most common manifestations are centripetal obesity, weakness and proximal myopathy, facial plethora, hirsutism, glucose intolerance, hypertension and psychological changes.

Adrenal glands and the response to stressors: a general model

A stressor is anything that tends to disrupt homeostasis. Stressor stimuli are recognized at many levels from the cerebral cortex to the brainstem, and defensive reflexes activate the sympathetic nervous system and adrenal glands. The paraventricular nuclei of the hypothalamus are important in integrating these outflows. Figure 5.4.8 shows a general model for the coordination of the immediate response to stressors.

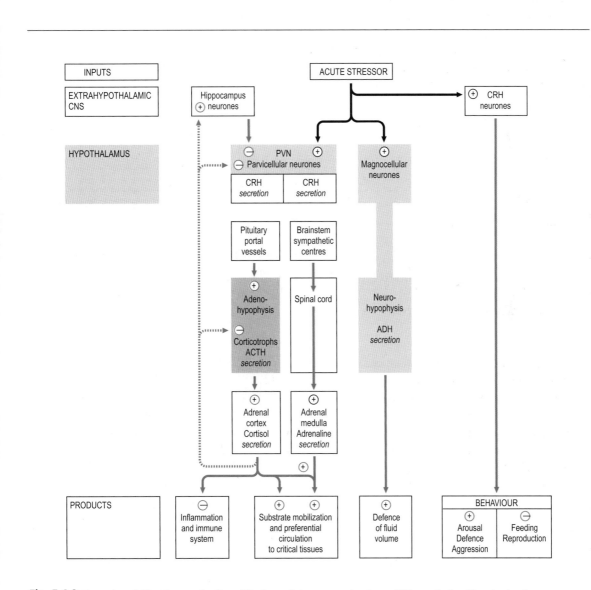

Fig. 5.4.8 General model for the coordination of the immediate response to stress. CRH = corticotrophin-releasing hormone; PVN = paraventricular nucleus; ADH = antidiuretic hormone.

Stressors cause release of corticotrophin-releasing hormone from paraventricular nuclei parvicellular neurones, which stimulates ACTH (and thus cortisol) secretion and sympathetic activation (see above). Corticotrophin-releasing hormone has a wide range of behavioural effects leading to increased arousal, defence and aggression. If high levels are maintained, feeding is reduced, and amenorrhoea occurs in women, while men become sterile. Corticotrophin-releasing hormone inhibits not only its own release but also that of other hypothalamic releasing hormones, including gonadotrophin-releasing hormone, and the catecholamine dopamine, which inhibits prolactin secretion.

To maintain homeostasis, cortisol acts, with adrenaline, on many tissues. The circulation to vital organs (brain, heart, lungs, selected skeletal muscles) is maintained at the expense of the supply to others (kidneys, digestive system, reproductive system). Catabolic pathways are activated to provide energy; and anabolic pathways inhibited (fuel storage, tissue repair and growth). Chronic stress leads to sustained cortisol secretion and hypertrophy of the adrenal cortex.

Summary

Functions of the adrenal cortex

- The adrenal cortex secretes three types of steroid hormones: mineralocorticoids (by the zona glomerulosa); glucocorticoids (mainly by the zona fasciculata); and adrenal androgens (mainly by the zona reticularis).
- Aldosterone, a mineralocorticoid, prevents excessive loss of extracellular fluid Na^+ (with water) or accumulation of K^+.
- Aldosterone secretion is stimulated by angiotensin II and III generated in response to hypovolaemia, and by increased plasma $[K^+]$.
- Cortisol, a glucocorticoid, exerts a 'permissive' action, which determines the responsiveness of most tissues to many other stimuli.
- The classical glucocorticoid effect is to raise plasma glucose concentration.
- Cortisol actions on cardiovascular and renal functions prevent excessive water retention.
- Cortisol prevents inappropriate inflammatory and immune responses.
- Cortisol secretion is stimulated by corticotrophin (ACTH), determined by corticotrophin-releasing hormone (CRH).
- Cortisol secretion follows a circadian basal rhythm, and is increased by many stressor stimuli.
- There is coordinated activation of adrenaline and cortisol secretion in response to acute stress.

Clinical Example

Response to life-threatening physical stress

Severe physical stress produces a very marked neuroendocrine response, which is essential for survival. Following severe injury such as in a road traffic accident, severe burns or scalding, or during and after major surgery, a patient in an intensive care unit is literally 'fighting for his or her life'. In this situation, the body must carry out many functions in order to survive. The heart beats more rapidly and strongly than usual to maintain the circulation in the face of an inadequate blood volume. The liver processes toxins released from damaged tissues, and other chemical processes such as blood coagulation and those involved in the release and actions of cytokines in damaged areas add to the activity. All this additional activity requires the use of additional energy, so the metabolic rate of the body is increased, and this increase must be maintained for days or weeks during recovery.

Although the sympatho-adrenal system and many hormones such as vasopressin, aldosterone and thyroxine are involved, one hormone stands out above all others – the adrenal cortical hormone, cortisol. Evidence for this is that in the absence of this hormone, patients suffering severe physical stress are much more likely to die, whereas replacement of the hormone in such patients largely reverses this effect on survival. The particular problem with deficiency of cortisol is circulatory collapse (a progressive and fatal fall in arterial blood pressure that cannot be reversed by treatment other than cortisol replacement), so a vital role of cortisol is to maintain an adequate circulation. The details of how it does this are still unclear.

How does the body produce the cortisol response? How does the brain of an unconscious patient 'know' to send out signals via the hypothalamus and pituitary? The input seems to be via pain receptors throughout the body. In someone with widespread tissue damage, the products of the damaged cells (e.g. prostaglandins, potassium ions, substance P) stimulate large numbers of pain endings, and impulses pass via the spinothalamic tracts to the hypothalamus. Even in the unconscious patient (where the cerebral cortex is not functioning adequately), the hypothalamus and nearby areas can receive information from the nearby thalamus and send signals to the pituitary via hypothalamic-releasing hormones and the pituitary portal circulation. This leads to release of adrenocorticotrophic hormone and other hormones from the pituitary and, hence, stimulation of the adrenal cortex to release cortisol. Evidence for this has been found in that the blood cortisol level is raised following injury, and the degree of elevation is related to the severity of the injury.

The daily cortisol rise and fall (circadian rhythm) is replaced by a surge to much higher levels for the time during which the patient is 'fighting to survive'. As a result of sustained high cortisol levels, body tissues are broken down (catabolism) to provide the energy needed for the life-saving processes that maintain the circulation and permit survival. When the crisis has passed, the cortisol level declines to the normal levels where healing and return of function occur (anabolism) during convalescence. These processes have been likened to the tide going out (ebb) and later returning (flow) – the body's reserves and, indeed, body mass ebb away during the acute, catabolic phase, and are restored (flow back) during the convalescent anabolic phase.

Clinical Example *(Continued)*

There are two fundamental reasons why patients sometimes cannot mount this response:

- the cortisol signal may be deficient
- the necessary body substrate on which the signal acts may be inadequate.

One cause of a deficient signal is bilateral disease of the adrenal cortex so that cortisol cannot be released. However, a much commoner cause is depression of the cortisol response because of long-term glucocorticoid therapy for inflammatory conditions such as rheumatoid arthritis. In these patients, the constant negative feedback to the pituitary causes depression of the cells that produce adrenocorticotrophic hormone. Secondly, the cells that produce cortisol are also depressed. Such patients are encouraged to carry a note indicating their therapy so that cortisol supplements can be given should they be admitted to hospital unconscious with severe injuries.

Lack of the necessary substrate of body reserves is present in the seriously malnourished patient with poor energy stores and depleted body protein as indicated by a low plasma albumin level. Such a patient tends to have a poor hormonal response, but even if given cortisol, still has a high risk of dying, owing to inability to produce energy for the responses necessary for survival.

Endocrine function of the gastrointestinal tract and pancreas

5.5

Introduction

The gastrointestinal tract (gut), together with two of its associated exocrine glands, the liver and pancreas, secretes a number of peptide hormones. The cells secreting these do not form discrete glands, as in most endocrine glands. Rather, the hormone-secreting cells of the gut, liver and pancreas are dispersed throughout these organs. The hormones secreted by the liver hepatocytes, the insulin-like growth factors (IGFs), are considered in Chapter 5.2, while the gut hormones are considered in Section 9 as well as in this chapter.

Gut hormones are principally involved with regulation of secretion and motility in the stomach and intestine and secretion in the exocrine pancreas. Pancreatic hormones are mainly responsible for controlling blood glucose levels as part of the body's overall regulation of energy metabolism. Additionally, a trophic action has been described for some of them, as being essential for the initial development and continued structural maintenance of different parts of the gut. Collectively, the cells secreting all these hormones are known as the **gastro-enteropancreatic endocrine system**, with around 30 hormones or hormone-like peptides having been identified to date.

Embryologically, the cells in this gut endocrine system are thought to be endodermal in origin, derived from a common precursor stem

447

cell from which cells in the nervous system are also derived; these cells are known as **APUD** (amine precursor uptake and decarboxylation) cells. Consequently, many of the peptides secreted by the gut and pancreas have also been isolated from cells in the nervous system, a further example of the intimate relationship existing between these two systems.

Hormones of the gastrointestinal tract

The peptides secreted by the gastroentero-pancreatic endocrine system are known collectively as the **gut regulatory peptides**: some have been ascribed full hormonal status (Table 5.5.1); some are still considered to be putative

Table 5.5.1 Gut hormones

Hormone	Origin	Factors causing release	Site of action	Primary effects
Secretin	Duodenum/jejunum	pH <4.5 in duodenum	Pancreatic acini	Bicarbonate-rich pancreatic secretion
Gastrin	G cells, stomach antrum Duodenum/jejunum	Peptide and pH <3 in pyloric antrum and duodenum	Stomach parietal cells	Acid secretion
Cholecystokinin – CCK (pancreozymin)	Duodenum/jejunum	Amino acids, fatty acids, low pH in duodenum	Pancreatic acini	Enzyme-rich pancreatic secretion
			Gall bladder	Gall bladder contraction
Glucose-dependent insulinotrophic peptide	Proximal small intestine	Carbohydrate and fat in duodenum	Pancreas (islets of Langerhans)	Insulin secretion
Motilin	Duodenum/jejunum	Not known	Stomach, upper small intestine	Increased smooth muscle contractions
Enteroglucagon	Lower small intestine and colon	Food in stomach	All GI tract	Mucosal growth
Neurotensin	Lower small intestine	Food in stomach	Stomach	Inhibits gastric acid secretion and gut motility
Vasoactive intestinal polypeptide (VIP)	Neurone cells in gut and pancreas	Not known	Stomach	Inhibits acid secretion
			Liver	Glucose release
			Pancreas	Insulin release and secretion of bicarbonate-rich juice

hormones; and others are thought to be acting in a neurotransmitter/neuromodulation role. Those with full hormone status include secretin, cholecystokinin (CCK), gastrin, glucose-dependent insulinotrophic peptide (GIP), motilin and enteroglucagon. Gut peptides that have also been isolated in the central and peripheral nervous systems include gastrin, somatostatin, CCK, vasoactive intestinal peptide (VIP), insulin, neurotensin, substance P, bombesins and enkephalin. Whether they act in endocrine, neurotransmitter or neuromodulation mode is not clear. Structurally, the gut hormones appear to be organized into two homologous families; the first contains gastrin and CCK, while the second includes secretin, VIP, GIP and glucagon.

Secretin

In 1902, Bayliss and Starling established that the presence of acid in the duodenum causes the secretion of bicarbonate-rich pancreatic juice from the exocrine acini and ducts of the denervated pancreas, demonstrating that a humoral agent must be responsible. Thus, the existence of hormonal control was established experimentally, and they named this hormone **secretin**. However, it was a further 60 years before the 27-amino acid chain molecule could be isolated and synthesized. Secretin is released from duodenal mucosa when the luminal pH falls below 4.5; bile has also been shown capable of stimulating secretin release, and the action of secretin in the pancreas is potentiated by gastrin and CCK.

Gastrin

Gastrin was described in 1905 when it was demonstrated that distension and the presence of secretagogues, especially small peptides and amino acids, in the denervated stomach resulted in gastric acid secretion. Vagal activity during the cephalic phase of gastric secretion also stimulates gastrin release. The existence of gastrin remained controversial for some 30 years because of the separate discovery of histamine, a paracrine that also stimulates gastric acid secretion. The separate existence of gastrin was finally established in 1938, and it was chemically isolated and synthesized in 1964. Gastrin is synthesized in **G cells** in the antral gastric mucosa and is found in the plasma in two forms, G34 and G17, with 34 and 17 amino acids respectively and the biological activity residing in the four identical C-terminal amino acids in each molecule. In addition to its primary effect on acid secretion, gastrin also influences gastric peristalsis and potentiates the action of secretin. Its homologous structure to CCK results in weak CCK-like activity, and its ability to stimulate enzyme synthesis and secretion by the pancreas is thought to be of physiological significance. Gastrin secretion is inhibited when the pH of gastric contents falls below 2.5.

Cholecystokinin

Cholecystokinin (CCK) was first described in 1928 with regard to its ability to stimulate contraction of the gall bladder. In 1943 a hormone was described which was called **pancreozymin** (PZ), primarily because it was responsible for stimulating the synthesis and secretion of digestive enzymes by the pancreatic acinar cells. Subsequently, in 1964, it was established that CCK and PZ were the same molecule, synthesized by mucosal cells scattered throughout the duodenum and jejunum. CCK exists in multiple forms, but biological activity resides in the C-terminal octapeptide, CCK-8, which is therefore the smallest form with biological activity. The main stimulants for CCK release are thought to be the presence of amino acids and fatty acids in the duodenum.

In addition to gall bladder contraction and pancreatic enzyme secretion, CCK has been shown capable of potentiating pancreatic juice secretion, inhibiting gastric emptying, stimulating pancreatic endocrine secretion, inducing satiety ('fullness'), and exhibiting a trophic function in the pancreas.

Glucose-dependent insulinotrophic peptide (GIP or gastric inhibitory peptide)

The action first attributed to this molecule was that of slowing gastric emptying and inhibiting gastric acid secretion, hence its original name of **gastric inhibitory peptide** (GIP). This hormone, secreted by cells in the mucosa of the upper small intestine in response to the presence of carbohydrate and fat in the duodenum, stimulates the release of insulin. It is now accepted that this is the physiological role of GIP, which has been renamed **glucose-dependent insulinotrophic peptide** (GIP). The action of GIP may explain why an oral dose of glucose is metabolized faster than an intravenous dose of similar proportions. GIP's effects in the stomach are weak in comparison, and it is thought to be one of a number of negative-feedback factors that regulate secretion and motility in the stomach.

Motilin

Another peptide secreted by endocrine cells in the mucosa of the duodenum and jejunum, **motilin**, mainly influences motility in the stomach and upper small intestine by increasing contractions. It is present in the blood even in the fasting state, and it is not entirely clear what causes its secretion. A specific role has yet to be described for motilin, and it is thought to generally stimulate gastric and intestinal motility to prevent stasis of luminal contents.

Enteroglucagon

Although similar in structure to pancreatic glucagon, **enteroglucagon** has very different actions. Unlike the gut hormones already discussed, enteroglucagon is secreted by cells dispersed throughout the intestine, with release occurring rapidly following a meal and being maintained for several hours. Its role is thought to be mainly a **trophic** one in maintaining the integrity of the intestinal mucosa by stimulating the growth of new cells. This theory is supported by the fact that starvation leads to atrophy of the intestinal mucosa, a situation associated with depleted levels of enteroglucagon.

Neurotensin

Although **neurotensin** was first described in brain tissue, its largest concentrations by far are located in the intestinal mucosa. Its main actions appear to be inhibition of gastric acid secretion and gastric emptying. It is a 14-amino acid peptide synthesized by endocrine cells in the mucosa of the ileum and secreted into the blood following a meal – the larger the meal the greater the secretion of neurotensin. While a specific role has not been described, neurotensin is thought to help 'pace' the rate at which chyme is allowed to enter the small intestine, helping to optimize the digestive and absorptive processes.

Vasoactive intestinal peptide (VIP)

VIP is found mainly in neurones in the muscle layers of the gut, and although intestinal actions can be elicited by pharmacological amounts of VIP, it has yet to be established what its physiological role might be. VIP has been shown capable of inhibiting gastric acid secretion and stimulating the release of insulin and pancreatic juice from the pancreas and of glucose from the liver. All these are actions primarily associated with hormones with amino acid sequences similar to those of VIP – GIP, secretin and glucagon. No specific stimulus for its release has been identified.

![Summary icon] **Summary**

GIT hormones

- Hormone-secreting cells are dispersed throughout the gastrointestinal tract and its associated exocrine glands, the liver and pancreas.
- Gut hormones are principally involved with the regulation of secretion and motility, while the pancreatic hormones insulin and glucagon are mainly responsible for controlling blood glucose levels.
- Gut hormones (or gut regulatory peptides) are derived from a common precursor stem cell, from which cells in the nervous system are also derived – endodermal APUD (amine precursor uptake and decarboxylation) cells.
- Gut hormones appear to be organized into two structurally homologous families; one includes gastrin and CCK, the other secretin, VIP, GIP and glucagon.

Pancreatic hormones

The pancreas is a mixed gland, 98% of which is exocrine tissue responsible for secretion of digestive enzymes and alkaline pancreatic juice. The remaining 1–2% of the pancreas comprises between 2 and 18×10^5 islets of Langerhans, small islands of endocrine tissue with the principal function of secreting insulin and glucagon, hormones involved in the regulation of blood glucose concentration. The islets also secrete the peptides somatostatin and pancreatic polypeptide. Embryologically, the pancreas arises from endodermal outgrowths from the fetal foregut. The origin of islet cells can be traced to the ductal epithelium. Islet cells are well vascularized and receive autonomic innervation.

Four cell types have been identified in the islets. The α- (A) cells comprise up to 30% of the islets and secrete **glucagon**, up to 80% are **insulin**-secreting β- (B) cells, with the remaining cell population consisting of δ- (D) cells secreting **somatostatin** together with F cells scattered throughout the islets and exocrine pancreas and secreting **pancreatic polypeptide** (PP). All of the cell types contain granules that release their hormones into the capillaries, and hence the general circulation, by exocytosis.

Insulin

Synthesis and release

Insulin was first described by Banting and Best in 1922, thus providing the potential to develop life-saving therapy for individuals suffering from *diabetes mellitus*. Synthesized initially as a large precursor pre-proinsulin molecule, insulin is a polypeptide molecule consisting of a 21-amino acid α-chain joined to a 30-amino acid β-chain. It has been estimated that β-cell granules represent a store of approximately 10 times the normal daily requirement of insulin. Synthesis and storage processes are independently regulated, with the release of insulin from the granules being calcium dependent. Both basal and stimulated release have been demonstrated, with basal release occurring when blood glucose concentration is less than 5 mmol/l.

Insulin release is regulated mainly by blood glucose levels, with a rise in glucose stimulating both synthesis and secretion of the hormone, and a fall suppressing it (Fig: 5.5.1). Glucose is thought to stimulate the entry of calcium ions into the β-cells, thus triggering a calcium-dependent exocytosis mechanism involving microtubules. In the circulation, insulin has a half-life of 5–10 minutes and most is degraded by the liver and kidneys by enzymic disruption. In muscle and fat, the insulin appears to be broken down by proteolytic enzymes.

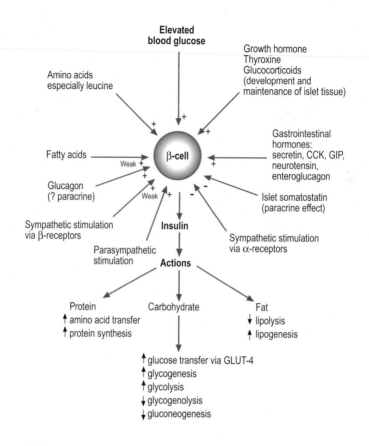

Elevated
blood glucose

Growth hormone
Thyroxine
Glucocorticoids
(development and
maintenance of islet tissue)

Amino acids
especially leucine

Gastrointestinal
hormones:
secretin, CCK, GIP,
neurotensin,
enteroglucagon

Fatty acids

β-cell

Weak +

Glucagon
(? paracrine)

Weak +

Islet somatostatin
(paracrine effect)

Sympathetic stimulation
via β-receptors

Insulin

Parasympathetic
stimulation

Sympathetic stimulation
via α-receptors

Actions

Protein
↑ amino acid transfer
↑ protein synthesis

Carbohydrate

Fat
↓ lipolysis
↑ lipogenesis

↑ glucose transfer via GLUT-4
↑ glycogenesis
↑ glycolysis
↓ glycogenolysis
↓ gluconeogenesis

Fig. 5.5.1 **Factors affecting insulin secretion and an outline of the actions of insulin.** GLUT-4 = glucose transport protein-4.

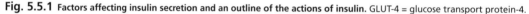

A number of other stimuli have been shown capable of causing insulin secretion by β-cells, but all seem dependent on the presence of glucose in the blood for them to be effective. Amino acids, especially leucine, are thought to have a physiological role in stimulating insulin secretion, and, while free fatty acids, volatile fatty acids and ketone bodies have been shown to exert a weak stimulatory effect, their physiological significance is questioned.

Several hormones are known to influence islet function. Growth hormone, thyroxine and glucocorticoids have been shown to be necessary for the normal development of islets, and they are also thought to exert a trophic maintenance influence in the adult. Several gut hormones stimulate insulin release, either directly or by potentiating the effects of glucose; these include GIP, secretin, CCK, neurotensin and enteroglucagon. Glucagon is capable of increasing the rate of insulin secretion, and somatostatin of decreasing it, although the physiological significance of these actions is not fully understood. It is also likely that glucagon and somatostatin act in paracrine mode, influencing β-cells directly by diffusing throughout islet tissue.

Autonomic nerve terminals synapse with β-cells and the dominant effect of sympathetic stimulation is the inhibition of insulin release via α-receptor activation. Activation of β-receptors causes a mild stimulation of release, and parasympathetic stimulation also causes enhanced insulin secretion.

Actions

The action immediately associated with insulin is its ability to *lower blood glucose*. Although the main one, it is only one of several actions of insulin in relation to its overall involvement in the regulation of energy metabolism. Blood glucose concentration is maintained within a range of 4–8 mmol/l by the complex interaction of a number of hormones. All cells use glucose as an energy substrate; some are independent of insulin (liver, CNS, RBCs, kidney), while others depend on it for the transport of glucose into the cell (principally skeletal and cardiac muscle and adipose tissue). When insulin is absent, this second group of tissues switches to using free fatty acids as energy substrate, resulting in an accumulation of keto- and other acids, which in turn cause a metabolic acidosis to develop (see p. 777). If untreated and the pH falls below 7, this can result in acidotic coma and death (Fig. 5.5.2).

Insulin is the hormone primarily responsible for preventing the persistence of raised levels of glucose in the blood; this is called its **hypo-glycaemic effect**. It achieves this by stimulating a facilitated diffusion process in the target cell membranes that utilizes the insulin-sensitive glucose transporter GLUT-4. Other membrane effects are the transport of amino acids into liver and muscle by stimulating an active transport mechanism, inhibition of lipolysis in adipose tissue, and stimulation of potassium uptake by cells.

Significant intracellular effects of insulin include the stimulation of glycogenesis in liver through the production of glycogen synthetase, inhibition of glycogenolysis and depression of gluconeogenesis. Other intracellular actions

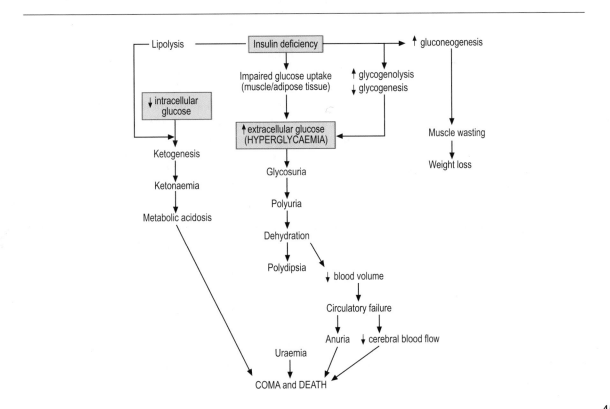

Fig. 5.5.2 Consequences of persistent insulin deficiency.

include stimulation of protein synthesis in peripheral cells and lipogenesis in liver and adipose tissue. The action of insulin in target cells is via the stimulation of a cyclic AMP-independent protein kinase.

Insulin deficiency

Insulin deficiency manifests itself as the clinical syndrome *diabetes mellitus*, first described over 2000 years ago. The name is derived from two major symptoms associated with the syndrome, *diabetes* referring to the characteristic polyuria (increased frequency and volume of urination) and polydipsia (increased thirst), and *mellitus* describing the sweet smell of the urine that results from the presence of glucose (Fig. 5.5.2).

Normally, all glucose present in the kidney glomerular filtrate is reabsorbed in the proximal tubule. When the level of glucose in the filtrate exceeds the concentration beyond which it cannot be further reabsorbed (approximately 11 mmol/l), glucose is lost in the urine (glycosuria). This glucose takes water with it by osmotic action, causing the polyuria, and induces body dehydration, which leads to thirst and polydipsia.

We now know that diabetes is a group of disorders based on a variety of genetic and environmental, including lifestyle, factors. It is characterized by persistent hyperglycaemia with glucose levels in excess of 11 mmol/l, which if untreated results in grave consequences for the individual (Fig. 5.5.3). In a normal individual, following an oral dose of 75 g of glucose, blood glucose levels should return to normal within 2 hours. In patients where the blood glucose level remains above 10 mmol/l after 2 hours, diabetes can be diagnosed. This glucose meal is called a glucose tolerance test.

Secondary diabetes can occur as a result of disruptions that cause hyperglycaemia in other endocrine disorders, for example the elevated secretion of cortisol (Cushing's syndrome), growth hormone (acromegaly), catecholamine (phaeochromocytoma) or glucagon

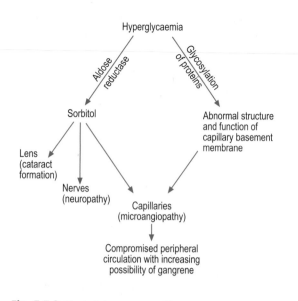

Fig. 5.5.3 Physical changes caused by persistent hyperglycaemia. Glycosylation of proteins causes swelling of the basement membrane, and sorbitol produced by abnormally high levels of glucose exerts a damaging osmotic effect on nerves and the lens of the eye.

(glucagonoma). However, it is possible that these disorders may require a simultaneous inability of the pancreas to secrete insulin before a true diabetes mellitus is established.

Primary diabetes mellitus falls into two types:

- **type I**, which is insulin dependent (IDDM)
- **type II**, which is not insulin dependent (NIDDM).

Type I diabetes accounts for up to 30% of all cases, usually starts in childhood, and is due to near-total or total failure of the pancreas to secrete insulin owing to autoimmune destruction of the β-cells. Patients with type I diabetes are dependent on daily injection of insulin to reduce their blood glucose levels.

The more common type II diabetes occurs in adults. Onset is usually after the age of 40, and the condition is often described as late-onset, or maturity-onset diabetes. Typically, insulin secretion is severely depressed rather than completely absent. The condition is often familial, and is most common in obese individuals. Depending on severity, the condition may be controlled by diet, stimulation of insulin production by prescribing sulphonylurea-based drugs such as tolbutamide, regulation of glucose metabolism by non-insulin drugs (biguanides), inhibition of starch absorption from the gut using α-glucosidase inhibitors, or insulin injection. Obesity has been linked to insulin insensitivity, and weight loss is sometimes all that is required to restore this sensitivity.

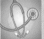 **Clinical Example**

Modern insulin treatment of diabetes mellitus

For some years after the introduction of insulin, many patients were maintained on a single daily injection, which was gradually released into the circulation over the subsequent 24 hours. This produced a dramatic improvement in the outlook of patients with diabetes, but longer-term problems tended to arise because the pattern of insulin release from a single injection is quite different from the normal pattern of insulin release. Current treatment aims to come as close as possible to this normal pattern.

The normal pattern of insulin release is closely related to food intake, because insulin is essentially the hormone that causes intracellular storage of nutrients after their absorption from the intestine. Thus, most of the daily insulin secretion takes place in the 3–4 hours after each meal. More insulin is secreted after a large meal than after a small meal or snack. Relatively little is secreted once a meal has been absorbed and during the night. Inevitably, a single daily injection of insulin leads to a fairly steady level throughout the day and this cuts across the normal pattern of rise and fall. Therefore, once the food has been absorbed and little insulin is required, the artificial level is too high, and *hypoglycaemia* may develop. On the other hand, during the absorption of meals the insulin level will be too low, leading to considerable loss of nutrients because their reabsorption threshold in the renal tubules is exceeded. Loss of glucose in the urine is the main consequence, and is referred to as *glycosuria*.

Even in the early days of insulin treatment, some patients with a scientific background discovered that giving themselves two or three injections of insulin a day, with each main meal, led to better control and well-being. The dose was dictated by the presence or absence of sugar in the urine – a test available for many years before the current convenient blood-testing equipment. Patients found that they felt best if most urine samples showed a modest content of glucose. This meant that the peak glucose levels were somewhat above the level at which glucose spilt into the urine (renal threshold for glucose). This may seem a disadvantage, since the blood level was probably then above the normal maximal level. However, it meant that the minimal glucose levels were much less likely to fall to levels risking the dangers of serious hypoglycaemia. This careful attention to maintaining levels of insulin and glucose as close as possible to physiological values seemed to reduce the long-term complications of diabetes mellitus as well as improving immediate well-being.

Modern treatment aims to come even closer to the physiological situation in two ways. Firstly, insulin is administered in a pattern very close to

Clinical Example *(Continued)*

the normal and, secondly, regular blood testing gives improved feedback on the primary variable of blood glucose rather than the secondary variable of glucose in the urine. The aim is to have a low background level of insulin throughout the 24 hours, such as occurs naturally, together with a booster of insulin with each meal. This booster is related closely to the nutrient content and hence to the amount of insulin that would normally be secreted during the absorption of the meal. One method of achieving this is to have a pen-type of insulin injector that contains a computer; the content of the meal is 'dialled in' and the device calculates and delivers the appropriate amount of insulin. Thus, insulin is seen as part of the food menu – the hormone that allows the various components of the meal to be stored in cells.

One factor that can still present problems is the reduction of insulin required when the patient takes a substantial amount of physical exercise. Strenuous exercise produces body changes, hormonal and cellular, which greatly aid the uptake of glucose into cells. This means that a patient who has taken the normal insulin dose a few hours previously is at serious risk of hypoglycaemia. With experience, sports participants anticipate this and reduce their insulin prior to severe exercise; otherwise, they may need to take glucose or other food supplements during and after the exercise. Thus, even the best replacement treatment lacks the flexibility to deal with unexpected and irregular patterns of food intake and physical exercise. Pancreatic islet cell transplants, if and when they become generally practicable, may overcome these problems.

Insulin excess

The consequence of an excess of insulin is **hypoglycaemia** and it occurs rarely in non-diabetics, and usually as a result of neoplasia (insulinoma). More commonly, it occurs as a side-effect in insulin-dependent diabetics who may exhibit the effects of insulin excess for a number of reasons. Following an injection of insulin, the patient may leave too long a delay before eating, or may eat too little food, or the patient may have exercised excessively causing a rapid reduction in blood glucose levels. In these situations hypoglycaemia results, with blood glucose levels falling below 2 mmol/l.

The brain and peripheral nervous system are largely dependent on glucose as an energy substrate, and in hypoglycaemia the central nervous systems fails to function normally, with all the symptoms of hypoglycaemia being manifestations of this CNS failure. Initially the patient becomes confused, and may appear lethargic and tired. There may be signs of increased sympathetic activity such as sweating, anxiety and tachycardia. Vision may become blurred and the patient may have difficulty in speaking. If untreated, the patient may collapse and have convulsions, leading to coma and, possibly, to respiratory paralysis and death.

Treatment in the early stages of a hypoglycaemic attack is by oral administration of glucose, such as glucose tablets or a sugary drink, and the patient normally recovers within minutes. Hospitalization may be necessary for the unconscious patient, and diabetics often keep an injection of glucagon in the refrigerator in case unconsciousness occurs at home.

Glucagon, which needs to be administered intramuscularly, will stimulate release of glucose from liver glycogen (see below).

Glucagon

Synthesis and release

As with insulin, glucagon is formed initially as a large precursor pre-glucagon molecule, which is modified within the Golgi apparatus of the α-cells, first to proglucagon, then to the single-chain, 29-amino acid glucagon molecule, which is stored in granules prior to release by exocytosis. It has a plasma half-life of 5–6 minutes, and appears to be degraded mainly in liver and kidney. Hypoglycaemia, a fall in blood glucose levels, is the main stimulus for glucagon release, and amino acids such as arginine and alanine have also been shown to stimulate secretion (Fig. 5.5.4). Other hormonal effects on glucagon secretion are stimulation by CCK, and inhibition by insulin and pancreatic somatostatin. Stimulation of both branches of the autonomic nervous system results in increased glucagon secretion.

Actions

Glucagon's primary role is the *elevation* of blood glucose, and it achieves this through a number of actions (Fig. 5.5.4). In liver, glucagon stimulates glycogenolysis and gluconeogenesis, and inhibits glycogenesis, all of which have a direct

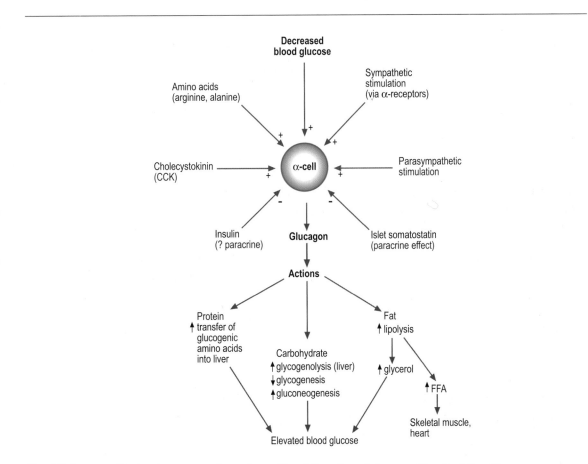

Fig. 5.5.4 Factors affecting glucagon secretion and an outline of the actions of glucagon. FFA = free fatty acids.

and positive effect on blood glucose. There is some evidence to suggest that glucagon stimulates the uptake of glucogenic amino acids into liver, thus helping to provide substrate for gluconeogenesis. In adipose tissue, glucagon stimulates lipolysis. The glycerol released into the blood can be used by the liver in the gluconeogenic pathway, and the fatty acids by some tissues, such as cardiac and skeletal muscle, as an alternative energy substrate to glucose, thus preserving the glucose for those tissues that are dependent on it as their sole source of energy substrate.

Somatostatin

Somatostatin was first described in the hypothalamus where its release inhibits the secretion of growth hormone by the anterior pituitary. It is a single-chain, 14-amino acid molecule synthesized in the pancreas by islet δ-cells and stored in granules prior to release. It is also synthesized in the central nervous system, and in other gastrointestinal sites including stomach, pancreas, large and small intestine, and salivary glands. Stimuli that cause secretion of pancreatic somatostatin include elevated blood glucose, amino acids (arginine and leucine), secretin and CCK.

Wherever it is secreted, somatostatin appears to have a general *inhibitory action*. Within the islets it is thought to act in paracrine mode, diffusing to the α- and β-cells and inhibiting the release of glucagon and insulin. Inhibitory actions described at other sites are probably due to somatostatin secreted in that location, rather than to somatostatin that has circulated there from the pancreas.

Pancreatic polypeptide (PP)

Pancreatic polypeptide is synthesized in F cells scattered through both islet and exocrine pancreatic tissue. It is secreted in response to parasympathetic and hormonal (mainly CCK) stimulation of the F cells. Protein digestion products in the intestine and acute hypoglycaemia have also been shown to stimulate secretion. Its main actions appear to be the inhibition of gall bladder contraction and of pancreatic enzyme secretion, although the physiological significance of these actions remains unclear.

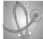 **Clinical Example**

Hypoglycaemia

Widespread use of insulin therapy for patients with diabetes mellitus has made episodes of seriously low circulating glucose (hypoglycaemia) a major hazard. As with many bodily functions, the blood glucose level can vary to some extent without problems. It can approximately double before glucose is lost in the urine. In the other direction, it can fall somewhat without problems, but at around half the fasting level, the symptoms and signs of hypoglycaemia begin to appear. As the level falls further, the patient lapses into coma, and death may result.

The brain is the main organ affected, for three reasons:

- it normally relies almost entirely on glucose for its metabolism
- brain cells, especially in the cerebral cortex, have a very high metabolic rate and lose their function when their metabolism is depressed

Clinical Example *(Continued)*

- the brain does not have significant energy stores – unlike, for example, striated muscle, which has considerable stores of glycogen and lipid.

The effect on the patient of depressed brain function in hypoglycaemia follows a common pattern that can be produced by anything which interferes with brain metabolism – including lack of oxygen, severe changes in hydrogen ion concentration, hypo- and hyperthermia and various drugs and toxins, including excessive alcohol.

The loss of brain function progresses from the highest level of cortical function towards the lower centres around the brainstem. Early loss of cortical function impairs *critical discriminatory function*. One well-known physician revealed his early signs of hypoglycaemia by abruptly becoming quite unreasonable at committee meetings. Often patients show subtle changes in personality that are, however, obvious to those who know them well. If the condition develops while the patient is driving a car, impaired judgement could lead to an accident, as with alcohol.

As the condition progresses, the resemblance to alcoholic intoxication is maintained, with slurring of speech and unsteadiness of gait, as lower parts of the cerebrum are affected. As the brainstem alerting centres are depressed, the patient loses consciousness. Finally, again as with alcohol, hypoxia, etc., the vital centres controlling breathing and the circulation may be affected and death can result.

In addition to these direct effects of hypoglycaemia, the body produces quite dramatic compensatory responses, which can abort mild attacks and draw attention to the condition at a relatively early stage.

Compensatory responses include activation of the autonomic nervous system and secretion of hormones that tend to raise the level of blood glucose. The sympathetic system is particularly helpful in mobilizing glucose from glycogen stored in the liver (a beta-adrenoceptor response). Other features of the sympathetic component of autonomic activation include a hyperdynamic circulation (rapid heart rate with a strong bounding pulse), tremor and sweating, all of which can act as danger signals to patients and observers.

The parasympathetic system, through the vagus, increases activity in the gut, giving the sensation of hunger, and facilitating absorption of food that is taken as a result. Less dramatically, hormones such as glucagon, growth hormone and cortisol help to prevent a dangerous drop in the blood sugar level.

Families and friends are particularly important in recognizing early hypoglycaemia, since the patient's awareness of what is happening may be blunted. Sometimes this makes patients resist the necessary treatment, which is to take rapidly absorbable food immediately by mouth (unless the patient is unconsciousness, when intravenous injection of glucose is needed). Because of the increased gut activity mentioned earlier, any glucose-containing carbohydrate is transported rapidly to the intestine and absorbed within minutes.

Finally, several situations can be mentioned where hypoglycaemia is either particularly likely or particularly dangerous.

- Physical exercise utilizes large amounts of glucose and increases its uptake into the exercising muscle. This considerably lowers the insulin requirements of the patient. Many diabetics successfully participate in strenuous and prolonged exercise, but they are aware that they usually have to reduce their insulin intake considerably beforehand to avoid episodes of hypoglycaemia.

- During the perioperative period when patients are under general anaesthesia it is particularly important for patients on insulin (and some on oral hypoglycaemic agents) to receive a continuous intravenous infusion of glucose.

A solution of 5% glucose contains many times the normal plasma concentration of glucose and prevents hypoglycaemia.

- Nocturnal hypoglycaemia is a hazard, particularly for the diabetic patient living alone. Care is needed to avoid blood levels of insulin that could cause profound hypoglycaemia and death when the patient is asleep and unable to respond to warning signs.

Endocrine control of energy metabolism

All cells require energy to function, and the fuel most commonly utilized is glucose. Indeed, the nervous system is almost solely dependent on glucose as an energy substrate. It is unable to synthesize it; neither does it store significant amounts of glycogen. So, while other tissues can switch to alternative energy sources, blood glucose levels need to be maintained in order to ensure a constant supply of energy for the nervous system. Prolonged severe hypoglycaemia is fatal, owing to brain and nervous system dysfunction.

Conversely, persistent hyperglycaemia results in the body losing valuable glucose in the urine; this glucose carries water with it by its osmotic action and the patient produces excessive amounts of urine (polyuria), with the consequent dehydration causing excessive thirst (polydipsia) in an attempt to replace the lost water. Long-term hyperglycaemia produces deleterious changes in the circulation, eyes, kidneys and nervous system accompanied by symptoms that are distressing for the patient (Fig. 5.5.3). Regulation of blood glucose

levels is therefore essential for the optimal functioning of the body, which inevitably involves the regulation of alternative energy substrates, and this total energy metabolism is regulated by hormones. The system is complicated because of the many variables that need to be considered.

The body uses three different fuels (carbohydrate, fat and protein), and metabolism of these substrates is regulated by six hormones working in a number of tissues in situations that provide ever-changing demands on the regulatory mechanisms.

Following digestion and absorption, the way in which the body treats its energy sources varies with the nutritional state of the individual. In times of 'food plenty' the body stores as much of the excess energy as it can, with glucose being converted to glycogen, mainly in liver and skeletal muscle, and fat being stored as adipose tissue. The body cannot store excess protein, which is broken down in the liver and excreted via the kidney. Normally, the body's carbohydrate stores, in the form of glycogen in liver and skeletal muscle, constitute less than 1% of the total energy stores, with adipose tissue contributing 80% and muscle protein 20%.

Conversely, when the body is short of a ready supply of energy substrate, such as during fasting, starvation and exercise, and in response to cold stress, glycogen is converted back to glucose, adipose tissue is mobilized to provide an alternative energy substrate to glucose for cells other than in the brain and nervous system, and amino acids are converted in the liver to glucose by the process of gluconeogenesis.

All of these metabolic pathways are regulated by six hormones – insulin, glucagon, growth hormone, cortisol, adrenaline and thyroid hormones (Fig. 5.5.5). Insulin is essentially the 'hormone of plenty', stimulating the transport of glucose into skeletal muscle and adipose tissue for storage, increasing lipogenesis in adipose tissue, and stimulating amino acid uptake and protein synthesis in many cell types (Fig. 5.5.1). Growth hormone supports insulin in promoting amino acid uptake and protein synthesis. Insulin inhibits lipolysis in adipose tissue, gluconeogenesis in liver, and protein catabolism to release amino acids for gluconeogenesis.

When availability of energy substrate, essentially glucose, is decreased, several hormones act to reverse the situation (Fig. 5.5.5). These hormones bring this reversal about in three main ways:

- release of glucose from glycogen stores (glycogenolysis)
- mobilization of free fatty acids (FFA) from adipose tissue to provide an alternative energy substrate to glucose (lypolysis)
- manufacture by the liver of new glucose from amino acids and other substrates (gluconeogenesis).

When glucose levels fall below 3.3 mmol/l, insulin secretion stops and the body is in a state of hypoglycaemia. In the absence of circulating insulin, the glucose remaining in the blood cannot enter those cells that require the presence of insulin for glucose transfer, thus preserving the glucose for brain and nerve cells, which are dependent on it as their energy source but do not depend on insulin for glucose uptake.

The falling blood glucose levels directly stimulate the secretion of glucagon from the α-cells in the pancreatic islets; this circulates to the liver where it stimulates glycogenolysis, releasing glucose into the circulation. Adrenaline, released from the adrenal medulla in response to severe hypoglycaemia, has a similar effect but acts principally on muscle glycogen. Both hormones act via stimulation of a cyclic AMP-dependent protein kinase. Other hormones capable of stimulating glycogenolysis include glucocorticoids, growth hormone and thyroid hormones.

Hypoglycaemia stimulates growth hormone secretion from the anterior pituitary, which acts to preserve blood glucose levels in two ways:

- In muscle, it exerts an anti-insulin effect, decreasing the uptake of glucose into muscle cells; this is sometimes described as exerting a brake on the peripheral utilization of glucose. Glucocorticoids exert a similar effect.
- In adipose tissue, growth hormone stimulates lipolysis, and the free fatty acids released into the circulation are taken up by non-nervous cells, principally cardiac and skeletal muscle, which can switch to using FFA as an alternative energy substrate to glucose. Glucagon and adrenaline also stimulate lipolysis in adipose tissue.

The body's third line of defence against hypoglycaemia is gluconeogenesis, the formation in the liver of glucose from amino acids. The hormones mainly responsible for this process are the glucocorticoids, secreted by the adrenal cortex in response to hypoglycaemia and acting in two sites. They stimulate the breakdown of protein, mainly in skeletal muscle, thus increasing the level of circulating amino

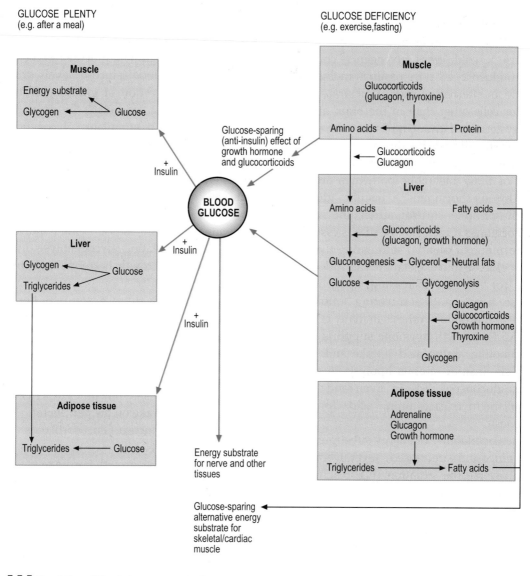

GLUCOSE PLENTY
(e.g. after a meal)

GLUCOSE DEFICIENCY
(e.g. exercise, fasting)

Fig. 5.5.5 Regulation of blood glucose concentration.

acids, which are taken up by the liver in the presence of both glucocorticoids and glucagon. In liver, glucocorticoids stimulate the formation of transaminase enzymes, which act in a metabolic pathway promoting the conversion of amino acids to carbohydrate.

Hypoglycaemia has also been shown to act on the feeding centre in the hypothalamus, inducing a feeling of hunger. If food is available, feeding will occur and this will also serve to restore blood glucose levels and the body's depleted energy stores.

Summary

Feast and famine

- The pancreatic hormones insulin and glucagon are secreted from islets of endocrine cells dispersed throughout the exocrine pancreas – the islets of Langerhans.
- Maintenance of blood glucose levels within closely controlled limits is achieved through the regulatory actions of a number of hormones.
- Insulin is the single hormone responsible for reducing elevated blood glucose levels (hyperglycaemia) by stimulating glucose uptake into a number of tissues, mainly skeletal muscle, and by stimulating metabolic pathways that result in increasing the body's energy stores – glycogenesis, lipogenesis and protein synthesis.
- Decreased blood glucose levels cause the release of a number of hormones (glucagon, adrenaline, growth hormone, glucocorticoids and thyroid hormones) that elevate blood sugar using a number of mechanisms – glycogenolysis, lypolysis, gluconeogenesis.

Calcium homeostasis

5.6

Introduction

Plasma calcium levels are maintained within very narrow limits in order to support the many physiological functions in which calcium is involved.

- Calcium ions play an essential role in the regulation of membrane permeability, and hence influence neuromuscular excitability.
- They participate in the release of neurotransmitters, and are a vital component in the excitation–contraction process in muscle cells.
- They are also involved in many intracellular metabolic pathways where they act as coenzymes and regulators, and in both endocrine and exocrine cells they are often implicated in excitation–secretion pathways.
- Blood coagulation is dependent on normal levels of calcium, as are bone and tooth formation and milk production.

More than 99% of total body calcium is contained in bone and, although it provides the principal store of calcium, most is incorporated into a complex crystal structure called **hydroxyapatite**, which means that it cannot be released quickly when required. The remaining 1% of the calcium in bone can be readily exchanged, being in the form of calcium phosphate salts that are in equilibrium with plasma calcium and hence provide a convenient buffer to sudden

Table 5.6.1 Distribution of calcium in blood plasma

	Concentration (mmol/l)	Percentage of total
Diffusible		
Ionic Ca^{2+}*	1.2	50%
Combined with citrate/phosphate	0.2	9%
Non-diffusible		
Combined with plasma protein	1.0	41%
Total	2.4	

* Regulated by PTH, vitamin D$_3$ and calcitonin

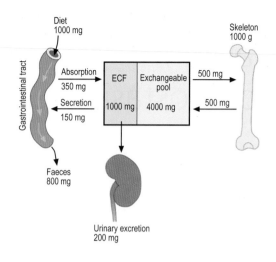

Fig. 5.6.1 Calcium exchange. This figure represents calcium exchanges in an adult human in calcium balance. ECF = extracellular fluid.

changes in calcium levels. Normally, plasma calcium is maintained at 2.3–2.6 mmol/l and is present in three forms (Table 5.6.1): 50% ionized, 41% protein bound and 9% combined with citrate and other acids. The bound and ionized components are in equilibrium with each other and represent the labile fraction of plasma calcium, which is regulated by hormones.

In addition to the daily loss of calcium from the body in nails, dead cells and hair, there is also a daily flux of calcium across the gastrointestinal and kidney epithelia. The net result is a daily loss of some 1000 mg of calcium, which needs to be replaced in the diet (Fig. 5.6.1). Regulation of plasma calcium depends on three hormones:

- **parathyroid hormone** (PTH) from parathyroid glands
- **1,25-dihydroxycholecalciferol** (the active form of vitamin D$_3$)
- **calcitonin** from C cells in the thyroid gland.

Calcitonin acts to decrease plasma calcium, whereas the other two act to raise it. The effects of all three hormones occur at the three sites of main calcium flux: bone, gastrointestinal tract, and kidney.

Hypocalcaemia (a fall in plasma calcium levels) is potentially more dangerous, and more likely to occur, than hypercalcaemia. Hypocalcaemia, if sustained, can cause changes to the endplate region of the nerve–muscle junction, resulting in muscle spasm (tetany), and possibly respiratory death due to spasm of the larynx and diaphragm.

Hormonal regulation of plasma calcium

Parathyroid hormone (PTH)

There are four parathyroid glands attached to the posterior surface of the thyroid gland. For many years it was thought that the thyroid gland secreted PTH, because problems of calcium homeostasis frequently occurred following thyroid surgery – in reality, surgeons were removing the parathyroid glands in ignorance (Fig. 5.6.2).

The parathyroids receive an arterial blood supply, which becomes a capillary plexus. Two cells types are found in the glands:

- **chief cells**, producing PTH
- **oxyphilic cells**, whose function is not yet clear.

Parathyroid hormone is a single-chain, 84-amino acid polypeptide. It is produced as a larger precursor molecule of 115 amino acids, which undergoes cleavage to yield a second precursor of 90 amino acids and a final cleavage within the Golgi apparatus to produce PTH,

which is then packaged into secretory granules. PTH is released in direct response to a lowering of plasma calcium, and it acts to restore plasma calcium concentration (Fig. 5.6.3). Release is biphasic, with an immediate release of PTH from the secretory granules followed by a delayed release of newly synthesized hormone. PTH simultaneously decreases plasma phosphate concentration.

A reciprocal relationship exists between plasma calcium and phosphate, such that a decrease in one results in an elevation of the other, and vice versa. This is frequently due to the dual action of the calcium-regulating hormones. PTH raises plasma calcium concentration by acting at all three sites of calcium flux: kidney, gastrointestinal tract and bone.

Kidney

Normally more than 95% of the filtered calcium load is reabsorbed via a number of active and passive transport mechanisms. Paradoxically, PTH has been shown to inhibit reabsorption of calcium in the proximal tubule while stimulating reabsorption in the distal nephron, with the overall effect of increased reabsorption, thus raising plasma calcium concentration. PTH also inhibits reabsorption of phosphate in the proximal tubule, resulting in its increased excretion.

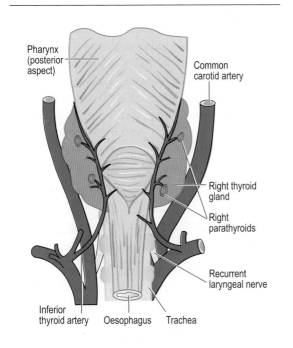

Fig. 5.6.2 Parathyroid glands. The four parathyroid glands are attached to the posterior surface of the thyroid gland.

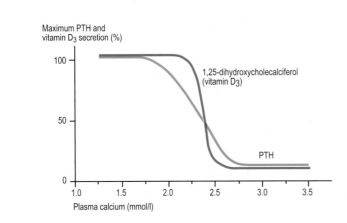

Fig. 5.6.3 Control of plasma calcium. The relationship between plasma calcium concentration and (a) PTH and (b) 1,25-dihydroxycholecalciferol (vitamin D_3).

Gastrointestinal tract

Any direct effect of PTH in the gastrointestinal tract has yet to be identified. However, PTH does influence the gastrointestinal tract indirectly. PTH stimulates manufacture in the kidney of an enzyme, 1α-hydroxylase, which converts circulating 25-hydroxy-vitamin D_3 (25-hydroxycholecalciferol) to the biologically active 1,25-dihydroxy-vitamin D_3 (1,25-dihydroxycholecalciferol), which raises plasma calcium concentration by stimulating calcium absorption from the upper small intestine. Hence, the action of PTH in the GI tract is indirect, by stimulating production of active vitamin D_3.

Bone

99% of the body's calcium is in bone, and 99% of this calcium is contained in a complex mineralized matrix of hydroxyapatite crystals from which calcium ions cannot readily be removed. However, a small proportion of bone is constantly **remodelled** throughout life, which is why bones are able to heal following a fracture. This remodelling is a dynamic equilibrium in which bone resorption roughly equals accretion (bone formation). PTH is able to influence the buffering capability provided by the calcium phosphate salts present in this readily exchangeable bone. It does this by acting in two stages on the bone cells.

Bone contains three cell types: osteoblasts, osteocytes, and osteoclasts.

- **Osteoblasts** cause bone deposition by laying down new bone matrix.
- Once surrounded by new bone, osteoblasts become **osteocytes** with the capability of reabsorbing bone matrix (osteolysis).
- **Osteoclasts** produce proteolytic enzymes that are responsible for bone resorption (and hence calcium reabsorption).

The first stage of PTH action is to stimulate osteolysis by surface osteocytes; the second is to stimulate the reabsorption of calcium from completely mineralized bone by stimulating both the activity of existing and the formation of new osteoclasts. PTH also causes a transient reduction in the activity of osteoblasts. The net effect is a withdrawal of calcium from bone and an elevation of plasma calcium concentration.

Mechanism of action

PTH is a polypeptide molecule and therefore binds to specific membrane-bound receptors at target cells. In kidney and bone this results in the activation of a G protein with subsequent activation of adenylyl cyclase and generation of intracellular cAMP, which in turn stimulates intracellular pathways resulting in the changes in cellular activity associated with PTH stimulation.

Summary

Parathyroid hormone (PTH)

- PTH, a polypeptide produced by chief cells of the parathyroid gland, is released in response to lowered levels of plasma calcium and acts to restore plasma calcium concentration.
- Release is biphasic: an immediate release from the secretory granules is followed by delayed release of newly synthesized hormone. PTH simultaneously decreases plasma phosphate concentration.
- PTH acts on kidney, gastrointestinal tract and bone.
- In the kidney, PTH stimulates reabsorption of calcium, inhibits reabsorption of phosphate and stimulates production of the enzyme, 1α-hydroxylase, which converts 25-hydroxy-vitamin D_3 to active vitamin D_3.
- In the GIT, it acts indirectly by stimulating production of active vitamin D_3.
- In bone, it acts in two stages to stimulate, first, osteolysis and then reabsorption of calcium.

Vitamin D₃ and its metabolites

Vitamin D_3 is not a classical hormone in the sense that it is not secreted by a recognized endocrine gland. Two sources are available to the body. Vitamin D_3 (**cholecalciferol**) is either:

- present in the diet and absorbed in the small intestine, or
- synthesized in the skin from 7-dehydrocholesterol in the presence of **ultraviolet** (UV) **light** (Fig. 5.6.4).

Some populations are more dependent than others on a dietary source of the vitamin. An increased level of skin pigmentation decreases the rate at which UV light can stimulate vitamin D_3 synthesis, and this can be a particular problem when dark-skinned people move to environments where the amount of UV light is decreased. Also at risk are white populations whose exposure to UV light is diminished. The situation in both cases can be balanced by taking a dietary supplement such as cod liver oil, which is a rich source of vitamin D_3.

Vitamin D_3 is biologically inactive and must be converted to the active metabolite 1,25-dihydroxy-vitamin D_3 (Fig. 5.6.4). Circulating vitamin D_3 is exposed to a 25-hydroxylase present in the liver, resulting in the conversion to 25-hydroxycholecalciferol (25-hydroxy-vitamin D_3), which in turn is converted to the active metabolite 1,25-dihydroxy-vitamin D_3 when exposed in the kidney to the converting enzyme 1α-hydroxylase, whose production is stimulated by PTH.

Metabolites of vitamin D_3 are similar to steroid hormones in structure, and so are transported in the blood bound to plasma proteins. 1,25-dihydroxy-vitamin D_3 (1,25-$(OH)_2$-D_3) is the metabolite considered to be the active hormone and it acts in a similar way to other steroid hormones. An intranuclear receptor–hormone complex stimulates mRNA transcription, which causes the formation of proteins involved in the various calcium transport mechanisms associated with the hormone at its known sites of action. The hormone acts in conjunction with PTH to raise plasma calcium levels and acts directly on the gastrointestinal tract, bone and kidney.

Gastrointestinal tract

1,25-$(OH)_2$-D_3 stimulates movement of calcium and phosphate into epithelial cells of the small intestine against a concentration gradient. It achieves this by stimulating the synthesis of a carrier protein for calcium. The presence of this protein in intestinal cells can be correlated with the presence or absence of the hormone.

Bone

The principal role of 1,25-$(OH)_2$-D_3 is to increase calcification of the matrix and hence stimulate bone formation. At least part of this effect is a consequence of the raised plasma calcium following the action of 1,25-$(OH)_2$-D_3 in the gastrointestinal tract. In bone, the hormone also stimulates both the activity and proliferation of

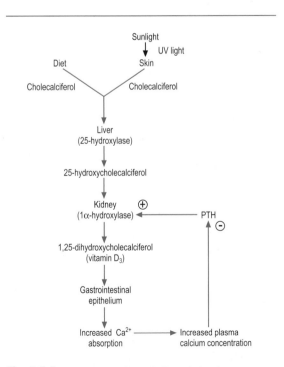

Fig. 5.6.4 The sources and metabolism of vitamin D_3.

469

osteoblasts. This stimulation of bone formation is particularly important during development of the skeleton. Deficiency results in excess osteoid formation in the osteoblastic cavity, meaning that less bone is laid down, and the resulting structure is weak. When this occurs during development, lack of hydroxyapatite, which gives bone its compressional strength, results in the long bones being unable to support the weight of the individual and the bones bow, resulting in a situation known as rickets. This disease is common in children who receive a poor diet and lack exposure to UV (sun) light, thus compromising the two normal sources of vitamin D_3.

At high concentrations, vitamin D_3 causes bone resorption, and normal levels of vitamin D_3 are necessary for the optimal effects of PTH on bone resorption in normal remodelling.

Kidney

Evidence suggests that $1,25\text{-}(OH)_2\text{-}D_3$ stimulates both calcium reabsorption from the distal nephron, and calcium and phosphate reabsorption from proximal tubules. In addition, it inhibits the action of 1α-hydroxylase, providing a negative-feedback effect that limits its own overproduction.

Calcitonin

Calcitonin (sometimes called **thyrocalcitonin**) was originally thought to be produced by the parathyroid glands. It is now known to be secreted by parafollicular C cells distributed throughout the thyroid gland. C cells are derived from cells that have their embryonic origins in the neural crest, and similar calcitonin-producing cells exist elsewhere in the nervous system, further illustrating the relationship that exists between the endocrine and nervous systems. In the nervous system, the molecule produced is **calcitonin gene-related peptide** (CGRP), a vasodilator and cardiac inotropic agent.

Calcitonin is a 32-amino acid polypeptide that is initially synthesized as a larger precursor molecule. It is secreted in response to an elevation in ionized plasma calcium above 2.5 mmol/l. As with PTH, the concentration of calcium in the plasma has been established as directly causing calcitonin release; however, whereas PTH secretion is stimulated by a *fall* in plasma calcium, calcitonin secretion is stimulated by a *rise*. While this is considered to be the primary stimulus for release, in some species such as rodents and pigs, gastrointestinal hormones have been shown to stimulate calcitonin

---

Summary

Vitamin D_3 and its metabolites

- Vitamin D_3 is not secreted by a recognized endocrine gland, but is either obtained from the diet or synthesized in the skin from 7-dehydrocholesterol in the presence of UV light.
- It is biologically inactive and must be converted by two hydroxylation reactions (the first in liver, the second in kidney) to the active metabolite 1,25-dihydroxy-vitamin D_3.

- Metabolites of vitamin D_3 are transported in the blood bound to plasma proteins.
- 1,25-dihydroxy-vitamin D_3 acts in conjunction with PTH to raise plasma calcium levels; it stimulates absorption of calcium and phosphorus in the small intestine, turnover in bone, and reabsorption of calcium and phosphate in the kidney.

secretion, suggesting that calcitonin may be involved in the regulation of postprandial hypercalcaemia.

Physiologically, calcitonin is probably of less importance than PTH and $1,25\text{-}(OH)_2\text{-}D_3$. Calcitonin has minor effects, the reverse of those of PTH, on calcium handling by the kidney and bone. However, calcitonin does not act simply as a direct antagonist to PTH; separate mechanisms may be utilized to elicit the opposite effect to that produced by PTH. Binding of calcitonin to specific membrane-bound receptors in target cells is thought to stimulate a cAMP-mediated second messenger pathway.

Bone

Following release of calcitonin, an immediate inhibition of osteolysis by osteocytes and inhibition of bone resorption by osteoclasts is observed, thus preventing bone resorption.

Kidney

Calcitonin causes increased urinary excretion of both calcium and phosphate, as well as sodium and chloride. Calcitonin receptors have been identified in the loop of Henle and distal convoluted tubule.

The interactions of PTH, vitamin D_3 and calcitonin in controlling ionized plasma calcium are summarized in Figure 5.6.5.

Summary

Calcitonin

- Calcitonin is a polypeptide secreted by parafollicular C cells of the thyroid gland in response to elevated plasma calcium.
- It has minor effects on calcium handling by kidney and bone, which are the reverse of those of PTH – it inhibits osteolysis and bone reabsorption, and stimulates urinary excretion of calcium and phosphate.

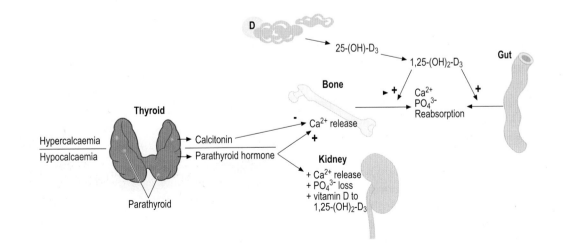

Fig. 5.6.5 Calcium homeostasis. The actions of parathyroid hormone, calcitonin, vitamin D and its products 25-hydroxycholecalciferol (25-(OH)-D_3) and 1,25-dihydroxycholecalciferol (1,25-(OH)$_2$-D_3) on calcium homeostasis.

Disorders of calcium homeostasis

Hyper- or hypocalcaemia, as diagnosed by measurement of total plasma calcium, are not necessarily caused by abnormalities in parathyroid function or vitamin D_3 action; abnormal levels of plasma proteins, for example, will affect total calcium levels. However, there are a number of clinical states that result from abnormalities in the plasma levels of the calcium-regulating hormones. These disorders can be directly linked to elevated or decreased plasma levels of PTH or vitamin D_3.

Hyperparathyroidism

Primary hyperparathyroidism occurs as a result of excessive PTH secretion, often from parathyroid adenoma, and in a significant number of patients is associated with other endocrine tumours. However, secondary and tertiary hyperparathyroidism are also possible, and so a confirmed diagnosis is vital before treating the patient. The elevated secretion of PTH causes hypercalcaemia because of increased bone resorption, which can result in spontaneous pathological fractures, and increased intestinal absorption of calcium via PTH-stimulated activation of vitamin D_3.

Persistent hypercalcaemia and PTH excess cause renal complications, which may finally result in renal failure. Gastric acid secretion is stimulated, causing dyspepsia and possibly ulcer formation. Hypercalcaemia causes generalized tiredness and lethargy, together with muscle weakness owing to proximal myopathy. The elevated calcium levels can cause cardiac arrhythmias, and even heart block in severe cases.

Once primary hyperparathyroidism has been diagnosed, treatment is normally surgical removal of the adenomas, hyperplastic tissue or carcinoma. Postoperative hypocalcaemia is offset by pretreatment with vitamin D analogues. If this hypocalcaemia persists, it may be necessary to give intravenous calcium gluconate.

Secondary hyperparathyroidism occurs when a clinical situation results in hypocalcaemia that in turn stimulates hyperactivity of the parathyroid gland. Examples of such clinical situations are vitamin D deficiency and chronic renal failure. The secondary hyperparathyroidism disappears once the primary cause of the hypocalcaemia has been treated.

Tertiary hyperparathyroidism occurs when adenomas or hyperplasia result from prolonged secondary hyperparathyroidism, and surgical removal of the parathyroids may become necessary in extreme cases.

Hypoparathyroidism

Hypoparathyroidism results in PTH deficiency accompanied by hypocalcaemia. The condition may arise as a result of an autoimmune disorder, but is more likely to follow accidental surgical removal of parathyroid tissue during thyroid surgery. Mild hypocalcaemia is often asymptomatic, but once serum calcium falls below 1.8 mmol/l, symptoms associated with increased neuromuscular excitability are usually observed. To test for hypocalcaemia, the two signs most commonly induced are facial twitch (Chvostek's sign) by percussion of the facial nerve, or carpal spasm (Trousseau's sign, Fig. 5.6.6) by ischaemia of the arm. If the

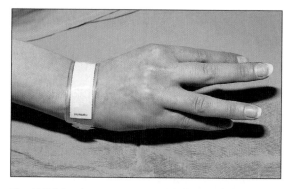

Fig. 5.6.6 Position of the hand in hypocalcaemic tetany (Trousseau's sign). (From Munro JF, Campbell IW eds 2000 *Macleod's Clinical Examination*, 10th edn. Churchill Livingstone, Edinburgh.)

hypocalcaemia is untreated, and remains progressive, there is a risk of tetany (muscle spasms) developing, which in extreme cases can prove fatal if respiratory muscles become involved.

Immediate treatment of the hypocalcaemia is by intravenous administration of calcium gluconate, followed by long-term treatment with vitamin D analogues to promote calcium absorption across the intestinal tract.

Disorders of bone

Bone disorders can result from vitamin D deficiency. Biologically active metabolites are essential for the normal mineralization of bone. When vitamin D is deficient, the total bone matrix is normal but calcification is deficient, resulting in bone weakness. In children, this manifests as **rickets**, when the weight-bearing bones bend under the weight of the growing child, and in adults as **osteomalacia**, when the weakened bones are liable to pathological fracture.

Vitamin D deficiency can arise for a number of reasons. Normal levels of vitamin D are achieved through a combination of manufacture in the skin under the influence of UV (sun) light and dietary intake. Vitamin D analogue treatment can restore plasma levels, as well as reversing the other causes of rickets and osteomalacia.

Osteoporosis (see Clinical Example box) differs from osteomalacia in that there is overall loss of bone mass including matrix. The results are similar in that there is bone pain and biomechanical bone weakness, often accompanied by pathological fractures. The condition is a particular problem in postmenopausal women owing to the fall in oestrogen levels. It may also occur secondary to Cushing's syndrome, hyperthyroidism and male hypogonadism. Once established, loss in bone density is almost impossible to reverse; premenopausal prevention is the best course of action, but this is dependent on young women responding to health education programmes. Once the menopause has started, evidence indicates that prolonged use of hormone replacement therapy (HRT) will prevent further postmenopausal loss in bone density; unfortunately many women do not like to take HRT, and those that do tend to stop once the classic menopausal symptoms, especially hot flushes and night sweats, have ceased.

Paget's disease (osteitis deformans) is not related to hormonal imbalance, and its cause is not known. It is a softening deformity of bone seen in old age, frequently accompanied by fractures. There is often bone thickening, which may trap nerves, resulting in severe bone pain. Treatment involves administration of both analgesics and drugs that reduce bone turnover.

Summary

Calcium homeostasis

- Calcium is essential for the normal functioning of numerous physiological pathways, e.g. bone and tooth formation, neuromuscular excitability, blood clotting, enzyme pathways.
- Plasma calcium levels are tightly controlled, and calcium balance depends on dietary intake, intestinal absorption and renal excretion.
- Plasma ionized calcium levels are regulated by three hormones: PTH, 1,25-dihydroxy-vitamin D_3 and calcitonin.
- Hormone hyper- and hyposecretion result in well-documented clinical disorders.

Clinical Example

Osteoporosis

This term literally means 'porous bones'. Compared with normal sturdy bones, the bones are sponge-like, insubstantial and brittle. This condition is usually diagnosed from the X-ray appearance when the bones appear less substantial and, particularly, less dense than normal. As with a number of medical terms, the same word is used for a clinical state, a pathophysiological concept and a radiological appearance.

The *clinical state* consists of features such as pain, deformities and fractures caused by relatively slight force on a bone weakened by disease (pathological fractures). Normally, a young person's femur will only fracture when subjected to severe force as in a road traffic accident. However, the osteoporotic femur of an elderly person may fracture spontaneously because of the normal stresses of weight bearing. The *pathophysiological concept* is of a bone that has gradually wasted, particularly through the loss of its collagen fibres, so that the calcium salts are not adequately reinforced. The *radiological appearance* is of bones that cast relatively thin pale shadows. How do we put these concepts together?

A good place to start is with the dictionary definition of osteoporosis (Dorland's): 'abnormal rarefaction of bone, seen most commonly in the elderly'. This draws attention to the effect of age. In fact, the bones of normal people grow and become denser and stronger during childhood and into early adulthood. Genetic, hormonal, nutritional and activity factors play a part in the ultimate strength in early adulthood, and thereafter bone strength gradually declines. Male bones in general are much stronger than female bones – so much so that one of the ways the sex of skeletal remains found by

archeologists is determined is by the size and ruggedness of the long bones, with generally a clear gap between the male and female femur in terms of bulk. This is likely to be related to the increased strength of male muscles, because the pull of muscles and the stresses of gravity combine to develop strength in such bones. Having started smaller, female bones tend to decline in strength more rapidly than male bones, particularly after the menopause. Thus, in octagenarians and nonagenarians the problems of osteoporosis are largely, though not entirely, confined to females. Collapse of vertebrae with curvature of the spine (kyphosis) and loss of height are one manifestation. A more drastic effect is fracture of the femur, referred to above. This may lead to serious illness and death in some cases, but modern techniques of repair with a metal plate or other prosthesis can often avoid this and lead to quite rapid recovery.

The above description refers to the common form of osteoporosis, related to age. The condition can also occur in younger people when the fibrous collagen matrix (which acts like the steel reinforcing in reinforced concrete) is attacked by certain hormonal disturbances. One of these is *excessive glucocorticoid activity*, which can be due to adrenal tumours, but is more often due to therapeutic administration of the glucocorticoids (e.g. prednisone) for conditions such as rheumatoid arthritis, asthma and polymyalgia, and to patients with organ transplants to prevent rejection. Excessive thyroid activity can also lead to a catabolic state in which the protein collagen fibres of bone are broken down.

To prevent osteoporosis as far as possible, children, particularly females, are encouraged to ensure an adequate calcium intake mainly in the form of milk and to exercise adequately to build

Clinical Example *(Continued)*

up strong bones. Adequate calcium and exercise should be continued throughout life – not to prevent loss of bone mass (which seems at present inevitable), but to minimize the rate of loss. Postmenopausal hormone replacement can help to reduce the rate of bone loss, and calcium supplements may help in situations where the condition is marked (assessed by bone scanning) or where glucocorticoid therapy increases the risk of osteoporosis.

Finally, *osteomalacia* can be mentioned. It literally means softening of the bones and it can produce similar effects to osteoporosis. Strictly speaking it is a pathophysiological condition due to inadequate calcium salts in bone (compare inadequate collagen in osteoporosis). This may be due to lack of calcium in the diet or to lack of activated vitamin D (dihydroxycholecalciferol), which is needed for adequate absorption of calcium. In children, because the bones are indeed particularly soft, deformities may be marked (rickets) with severe curvature of spine and leg bones. In adults, the effects are more like those of osteoporosis.

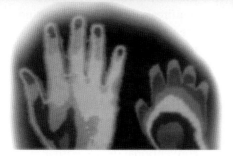

Applied physiology

Temperature regulation

Introduction

Mammals and birds gain considerable advantage from maintaining a high, constant body temperature, which allows them to maintain a full range of activities over a wide range of environmental conditions. They are said to be **homeotherms**.

Stability of body temperature can only, however, be achieved at the expense of a high rate of metabolism and sophisticated control processes that involve, in some way or another, virtually every physiological system of the body. In this chapter we will consider these processes of thermoregulation, but we must start with a very simple question. What do we mean by the term 'body temperature'?

If we quote a single figure, say 37ºC, this implies that all parts of the body are at the same temperature, which is manifestly not the case. We are all aware that, in most environments, our hands and feet are cooler than the rest of us. The only circumstances in which all parts of a body will be at the same temperature are if it is perfectly 'stirred', so that heat can exchange freely between all parts, and if it is perfectly insulated from the surrounding environment, so that heat cannot be lost or gained through its surface. We are clearly not perfectly insulated, and in most environments tend to lose heat constantly through our surface to cooler surroundings. We are, however, fairly well stirred, because the circulation of blood around the body allows heat to exchange to its various parts. The effect of this exchange is that a large part of the inside of us is all at more or less the same temperature – the 'core' temperature, defined as the temperature of the blood in the main vessels leaving the heart.

Surrounding this core, we have a shell of tissues of variable thickness and thermal insulation, through which heat is normally lost to the environment. The temperature of our body surface will therefore vary enormously, depending on the insulation at different points and the temperature of the surroundings – the 'ambient' temperature (Fig. 5.7.1).

Body temperature is therefore normally considered as the temperature of the core.

Measurement of body temperature

Measuring core temperature requires a device for registering the temperature plus some means of getting it into or close to the core. A variety of devices and approaches can be used. Perhaps the most familiar is the mercury in a glass clinical thermometer. This is a conventional device with a column of mercury expanding up a capillary as temperature increases, but modified so that it retains the value of the maximum temperature to which it has been exposed. In this way, it avoids the problem of the device cooling once it has been removed from the body in order to be read. Clinical thermometers are normally used to record temperature in the mouth or the axilla. Neither is a particularly good reflection of the core temperature. The mouth is generally half a degree or so cooler, and subject to variations associated with breathing and the consumption of hot or cold liquids. The temperature at the axilla is that of the body surface, and whilst it will give a general indication of core temperature, it does not accurately reflect small changes that may be significant.

Continuous recording of temperature is normally undertaken with electronic devices connected to thermistor probes. Thermistors are semiconductors whose

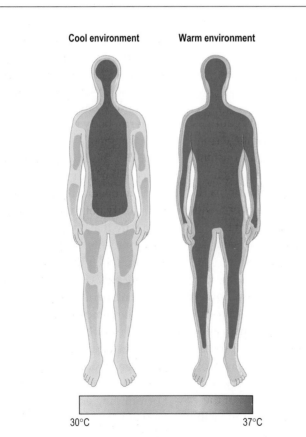

Cool environment **Warm environment**

30°C   37°C

Fig. 5.7.1 Thermal image. The naked body shows a warm core in the cool environment. This core spreads towards the skin and down the limbs in a warm environment.

electrical resistance changes with temperature; the electronics measure these changes in resistance. Thermistor probes may be inserted into a variety of orifices. Most commonly, they are used to measure rectal temperature, which is an accurate reflection of core temperature. They may also, with modification to allow for heat loss via the external auditory meatus, be used to monitor the temperature of the tympanic membrane of the ear, which is a very accurate reflection of the temperature of the blood supply to the brain.

Surface temperature is more difficult to measure. Thermistors may be attached to various sites over the body, or a thermal imaging device may be used to detect infrared radiation from the body surface, the properties of which are determined by the temperature of the surface.

Generally speaking, however, the core temperature is the more important.

What is the normal range of core body temperature?

In normal adults at rest, core temperature varies from about 36ºC to about 37.5ºC. Higher temperatures can be attained in a normal individual during exercise.

Core temperatures outside the range of 36–38ºC are associated with significant functional changes. Increases in temperature are known as **hyperthermia**, and decreases as **hypothermia**. Both can be dangerous.

We are familiar with the effects of small rises in core temperature, such as occur in a febrile illness. Above 38ºC, we become aware of central nervous changes. Concentration is impaired and, as temperature rises further, thoughts and actions may become disorganized, leading eventually to delirium. Temperatures up to 40ºC are tolerable, with only temporary loss of function. Rises in temperature above 41ºC can lead to permanent brain damage. Few people can survive temperatures above 43ºC. As temperature rises, there may also be changes associated with the body's efforts at thermoregulation. Changes in the cardiovascular system and the activity of sweat glands can cause damaging or even fatal circulatory collapse or dehydration.

The effects of falls in body temperature are more insidious. Just as with rises, the initial effects are on the central nervous system. There is a progressive slowing of mental activity. Old folk in particular may become unaware of the fact that they are cold and disinclined to do anything about it, so allowing hypothermia to develop further. As body temperature falls, so does the pace of general metabolism and less heat is generated in the body. Once body temperature reaches about 32ºC, metabolism alone cannot generate enough heat to return body temperature to normal; without external heating the subject will die. Lower body temperature, down to 26 or 27ºC, can, however, be tolerated, provided subjects are rewarmed carefully. On occasion, subjects are deliberately cooled for surgery to prolong the time that vital organs can survive with reduced or absent blood flow.

To maintain optimum function, however, our core body temperature must be maintained within a 2ºC range. This is achieved despite a very wide range of environmental conditions. Humans live in ambient temperatures from −35ºC to about +45ºC. We also have a highly variable rate of internal heat production, which can change 20-fold from rest to hard exercise. The mechanisms of thermoregulation therefore face a substantial challenge. They must maintain body temperature within a 2ºC range in environments whose temperatures can vary over a range of 80ºC, and as metabolic heat production varies by up to 20-fold. How do they do it?

The thermal balance of the body

The temperature of any body is determined by the balance

between heat in and heat out. If these heat flows are the same, then temperature will not change. If heat in exceeds heat out, then body temperature will increase at a rate dependent upon the size of the body – its thermal capacity. If heat out exceeds heat in, then the body temperature will fall, again at a rate dependent on thermal capacity. The thermal capacity of an adult is large; that is to say we can soak up a lot of heat with a relatively small temperature change, so body temperature tends to change only slowly. The thermal capacity of babies is, however, much smaller, making their body temperatures more labile.

The physiological mechanisms of thermo-regulation act to produce a balance between heat gain and loss, so that body temperature remains stable (Fig. 5.7.2). To achieve this, they modulate the normal ways in which the body gains and loses heat, so it is with these that we should start.

Mechanisms of heat gain and heat loss

Heat is gained from metabolic activity and from any part of the environment that is hotter than the body. Consider first metabolic activity. There is a minimum level of metabolic activity necessary to support life, even in an individual who is asleep and starved. This is the **basal metabolic rate** (BMR). The BMR is related to body surface area and is generally about 200 kJ/m² per hour, which for an average individual of surface area 1.8 m² corresponds to about 100 J/s, or 100 W. Even sitting quietly will increase the figure by 50% or so. Exercise may increase it considerably, producing heat outputs for brief periods of heavy exercise of up to 2 kW.

You will perhaps now understand why 100 people active on a disco dance floor can generate enough heat to require substantial air conditioning if the room temperature is not to rise unacceptably.

Heat is gained from the environment via the body surface. Heat exchange between our body surface and our surroundings can, however, occur in either direction, depending on the temperature gradient. Normally, in temperate climates, most of the environment is cooler than we are, and so there is net heat loss rather than gain.

Heat exchanges with the environment by conduction, convection and radiation. In addition, heat can be lost by evaporation of water from the body surface, a mechanism of heat loss with the advantage that it still operates when the environment is hotter than we are.

Heat loss by conduction is generally small. This is because we are usually surrounded by air, which conducts heat rather poorly. We tend to warm up a thin layer of air around our bodies, which then acts as a thermal blanket to limit further heat loss. Clothes accentuate this by retaining the air. Generally speaking, it is not the fabric of the clothes we wear that keeps heat in, but the air trapped between and within the fabric layers.

Conductive heat loss can, however, be considerable under some circumstances. An obvious example is if a subject is immersed in water, which conducts heat well. Lying on cold ground with inadequate insulation

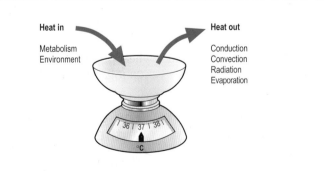

Heat in
Metabolism
Environment

Heat out
Conduction
Convection
Radiation
Evaporation

36 | 37 | 38
°C

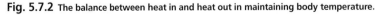
Fig. 5.7.2 The balance between heat in and heat out in maintaining body temperature.

underneath the body can produce rapid cooling. There can also be problems if the warm air layer normally trapped close to the body surface is constantly removed. This happens if subjects are exposed to cold winds, which strip away our natural warm air blanket and produce 'wind chill' (Fig. 5.7.3). The effective temperature of an environment can be very much lowered if there is a strong wind.

Heat loss by convection is a similar process. The warm air blanket around us tends to rise, as it is less dense than the surrounding air, and this streams off the top of the body. More air must be warmed to replace it. Clothes tend to minimize this effect, particularly if they fit tightly around the neck. That is why removing a tie is such an effective way of cooling if we get a little overheated. Some groups utilize convection effects to increase cooling by wearing loose clothes, which maximize the upward flow of air over the body in a sort of 'chimney' effect to assist in cooling, particularly by the evaporation of sweat.

In normal situations, however, neither conduction nor convection contributes significantly to our heat loss. Most loss occurs by radiation. Heat exchanges between surfaces by radiation at a rate that depends upon the temperature difference between them. Radiative heat loss therefore occurs from the outermost surface of the body (i.e. outside of clothes) at different rates to different parts of the environment.

Writing this chapter on a winter's day sitting next to a window, I will be losing most heat to the cool surface of the glass, and relatively little to the rest of the room, which is warmed by the circulation of hot air from the fire.

At rest, in a temperate environment, about 65% of heat loss from the body occurs by radiation, about 10% by conduction, about 5% by convection, and the remainder by evaporation of water (Fig. 5.7.4).

Cooling by evaporation of water involves the change of state of the water from liquid to vapour, which requires energy – the latent heat of evaporation. Some body water must be lost continuously, particularly from the respiratory tract as the air we breathe is humidified. This is associated with heat loss. Some water also evaporates continuously from the body surface, the so-called 'insensible loss'. Overall, respiratory water loss and insensible loss through the skin correspond to a cooling of about 30 W. We never gain heat by condensation of water.

Evaporative heat loss can, of course, be spectacularly

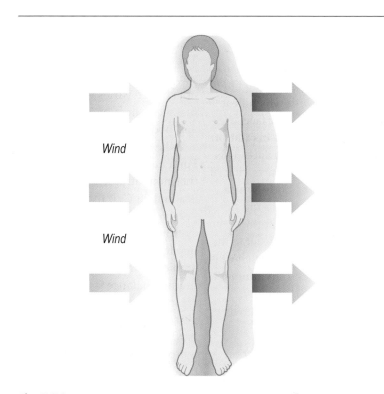

Wind

Wind

Fig. 5.7.3 How air movement enhances cooling.

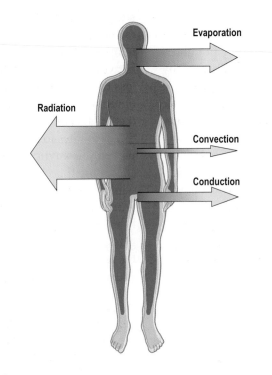

Fig. 5.7.4 Mechanisms of heat loss to the environment.

increased by the secretion of water onto the body surface – sweating. It is, as we shall see, an essential process of thermoregulation.

Factors determining the balance between heat gain and heat loss

Overall, the tendency for body temperature to change is determined by the balance between heat in, coming mainly from metabolism but sometimes from parts of the environment, and heat out to the environment, lost at a rate that depends upon the *surface* temperature of the body.

The relationship between the core temperature and surface temperature is determined by the difficulty with which heat can transfer to the surface, that is to say the **thermal insulation** between core and surface. This insulation has two parts, that of the tissues of the body, which affects heat transfer to the skin surface, and that of clothing, which affects heat transfer to the outer surface, from which heat is actually lost to the environment.

Three factors, therefore, determine the balance between heat gain and loss:

- metabolic heat production
- the effective temperature of the environment, averaged

across its different parts, know as the ambient temperature

- the insulation separating the body core from the outer surface.

If two of these factors are fixed, it is always possible to specify a value for the third that corresponds to an exact balance between heat loss and heat gain and therefore no tendency for body temperature to change.

In practice, we calculate, for specified values of metabolic heat production and insulation, the ambient temperature at which the body is in thermal balance with the environment. This is known as the **thermoneutral** temperature. It is important to understand that there is no single thermoneutral temperature. The ambient temperature at which body temperature will not change varies with metabolic heat production and body insulation.

Take some examples. For a naked adult at rest, the thermoneutral temperature is about 28ºC. If that same person puts on normal indoor clothing, then the extra insulation requires a lower ambient temperature before thermal balance is achieved, typically about 21ºC. If the person then starts to exercise hard, an even lower temperature is required, maybe down to 8–10ºC depending on the level of exercise. If the person is heavily insulated, say, wearing clothing suitable for the Arctic, then the thermoneutral temperature may be well below freezing, and if exercising it may be so low as to be unachievable. This can be a real problem for people who have to undertake physical work in cold climates. They may suffer heat stroke, because the clothes they need to wear to keep them warm at rest may not permit the loss of sufficient heat during exercise.

For any given combination of metabolic activity and insulation, however, there is one environmental (ambient) temperature where thermoregulation is not necessary. If the ambient temperature is above this thermoneutral value, then body temperature will tend to rise. If it is below it, body temperature will fall. This is when mechanisms of thermoregulation must operate. In essence, these mechanisms act to change heat loss or gain in order to make the existing ambient temperature thermoneutral, by 'active cooling' or 'active warming'.

Mechanisms of active cooling

There are many ways in which heat loss from the body may be facilitated. It is rarely possible to reduce heat input from metabolism to aid thermoregulation, though heat gain from the environment may be modified behaviourally.

Both active cooling and warming mechanisms tend to operate as a progressive hierarchy, starting with simple behavioural modifications when little change is required, but ranging up to major physiological changes in extreme situations.

The commonest, and simplest mechanism of active cooling is often forgotten. When we feel hot, we remove clothing. This reduces insulation and allows our outermost surface temperature to rise, so facilitating heat loss to cooler parts of the environment (mainly by radiation). Another important behavioural change is to get out of the way of environmental heat sources (e.g. direct sun).

Eventually, however, limits of propriety are reached and physiological mechanisms become more prominent. The effective thermal insulation between the core and the skin surface is determined by the amount of blood flowing through the most superficial blood vessels in the skin. Here, flow is mainly through arteriovenous anastomoses, and is regulated by sympathetic control of smooth muscle sphincters on their arteriolar side. If sympathetic activity is reduced, more blood flows peripherally, the skin temperature rises, and more heat can be lost.

Often, these changes are insufficient, especially in warm environments, and we therefore activate our principal mechanism of active cooling – the secretion of water on to our body surface in the form of **sweat**.

Sweat glands are modified sebaceous glands. They are spread over the entire body surface, though they are concentrated more in some areas. There are two types:

- **apocrine** sweat glands, found in the axilla and groin and on the feet, where secretions contain protein and other inorganic substances in addition to water and electrolytes
- **eccrine** glands, covering the rest of the body, which secrete principally water and electrolytes.

The eccrine glands are by far the most important in thermoregulation.

Eccrine sweat glands consist of a blind-ending acinus draining into a long, coiled duct that opens on the skin surface. The glands are innervated by the sympathetic nervous system, though the principal neurotransmitter released is not noradrenaline. It is acetylcholine.

When stimulated by acetylcholine, the acinar cells produce a primary secretion of water and electrolytes, which is

483

roughly isotonic with plasma. As the primary secretion passes along the ducts, sodium and chloride are reabsorbed, but not water, leaving a hypotonic solution to be secreted onto the skin. The more sweat is produced, the less opportunity there is for reabsorption of sodium in the ducts, and so the more sodium the final product contains. The concentration of sodium in sweat can range from about 10–60 mmol/l. This means that individuals sweating at a high rate lose much more salt per litre of sweat that those sweating at low rates – a matter of great practical importance.

The maximum rate of sweating varies between individuals, but can be up to 2 litres per hour. Over the first few weeks of exposure to a tropical environment, the number of sweat glands in the skin of Caucasians increases dramatically, and the threshold for the onset of sweating becomes lower, so these 'acclimatized' individuals are more effective at active cooling.

The effects of prolonged sweating on water and salt balance can be very severe. The power of mechanisms of thermoregulation is such that they will drive an individual to death by dehydration and salt depletion in vain attempts to control body temperature.

Mechanisms of active warming

Heat loss from the body may be limited in several ways, but in the case of active warming, there is also the option of increasing metabolism to generate extra heat, a process known as **thermogenesis**.

Again, however, the initial reaction to an environment slightly below thermoneutral is to change behaviour – put on more clothes or move to a warmer situation. Just as with active cooling, it is also possible to modify the insulation between core and skin by, in this case, increasing thermal insulation via a reduction in blood flow to the most superficial vessels. This is achieved by changes in sympathetic activity.

Once the environmental temperature is significantly below thermoneutral, at what is known as the 'critical temperature', active warming involves increases in metabolism brought about by a variety of mechanisms. Acute exposure to the cold leads to **shivering**, which is an exaggeration of the normal tremor in skeletal muscles. This generates plenty of heat, but is very inefficient and would lead rapidly to exhaustion if continued for any length of time. After a few hours, therefore, it is supplanted by **non-shivering thermogenesis** – an increase in metabolic activity in a number of tissues. There are two main components of non-shivering thermogenesis:

- A general increase in metabolism is brought about by increased secretion of thyroid hormones. The hypothalamus produces extra thyrotrophin-releasing hormone, stimulating the pituitary gland to secrete extra thyrotrophin (thyroid-stimulating hormone, TSH), which promotes extra secretion from the thyroid gland.

- In young infants in particular, but also to some degree in adults, the increase in thyroid activity is supplemented by an increase in the metabolism of a specialized form of adipose tissue – **brown adipose tissue**. This is found in various sites, most notably between the shoulder blades, and is a tissue whose cells contain unusual mitochondria in which the consumption of normal substrate has been uncoupled from the production of ATP, so heat is produced instead. The activity of brown adipose tissue is under the control of the sympathetic nervous system.

So long as adequate substrates are available, mechanisms of thermogenesis can maintain body temperature for long periods under harsh conditions. To achieve this, however, individuals must eat a great deal more than usual. It is not uncommon for people working in the Arctic to require two and a half times as much food as those doing a similar job in a temperate climate.

Control of active cooling and active warming

If body temperature is to be maintained, then a wide range of physiological mechanisms must be activated appropriately. This requires sophisticated control. Many of the mechanisms of active cooling and warming involve the autonomic nervous system, and as autonomic function declines with age, thermoregulation inevitably becomes less effective, which is one reason why old folk are particularly prone to hypothermia in winter. As endocrine mechanisms are also involved, an obvious potential site for control is the hypothalamus, and it does appear that this is the principal structure controlling thermoregulation.

Keeping variables constant requires feedback control. The essential elements of a negative-feedback control mechanism are a sensor to monitor the controlled

variable, a comparator to compare the actual value with a 'set point' and effector mechanisms to correct any error detected. We have already described the effector mechanisms, which operate in a complex hierarchy. So, where is the sensor?

As the brain is the part of us most susceptible to changes in body temperature, then it is an obvious place to look for thermoreceptors sensitive to the temperature of the blood passing through it. Neurones with these properties have been found in the hypothalamus. There are several different types.

In all types, the firing rate of the neurone varies with local temperature. In some, firing rate increases steadily as temperature falls below some threshold; in others, it increases steadily as temperature rises above some threshold. Yet others show more complex responses. Overall, however, there is a population of neurones whose firing patterns will give a very clear indication of the temperature of the blood flowing through the hypothalamus.

The action of these neurones can be seen if the hypothalamus is cooled or warmed with no change in general core temperature. If the hypothalamus is cooled, then it will activate all the mechanisms of active warming,

even though the temperature of the rest of the body is still normal. Similarly, if the hypothalamus is warmed independently of the rest of the body, then mechanisms of active cooling will be activated.

In principle, therefore, we can see how body temperature might be controlled. If it becomes too high or too low, this will be detected by appropriate populations of cells in the hypothalamus, which will then, by its connections to the autonomic nervous system and the endocrine system, activate warming or cooling mechanisms in order to bring temperature back to normal.

One problem with this system is the considerable thermal capacity of the body. Temperature changes very slowly, even when the imbalance between heat input and output is considerable. This imposes a substantial delay in the negative-feedback loop, which, as you will have read in Section 1, can have dramatic effects, including large amplitude oscillation in the controlled variable – in this case body temperature.

These oscillations would be harmful. The control system needs to avoid them by, in effect, 'anticipating' the need for active warming and cooling before deep body temperature has actually changed, and taking action to prevent the change. There are mechanisms that allow this to occur. Information from temperature receptors on the skin is fed to the hypothalamus, and modifies the responsiveness of the hypothalamic thermoreceptors. In effect, if the skin is cooled, the central thermoreceptors regard the current body temperature as too low and instigate active warming before core temperature has actually changed.

The end result is very precise control of body temperature. Except in extreme exercise and during illness, deep body temperature does not leave the range 36–37.5°C. Even within this range, variations are not random, because the hypothalamic control mechanisms are affected by a number of influences that, in effect, alter the setting of the body's 'thermostat'.

Controlled changes in body temperature

The setting of the hypothalamic thermostat is affected by a number of factors. One of the most obvious is time of day. Deep body temperature falls to a minimum of about 36.2°C in the early hours of the morning, and reaches its maximum value of around 37.4°C late in the afternoon.

In women, body temperature varies with stage of menstrual cycle. In the luteal phase, when progesterone levels are high, core temperature is about 0.5°C higher than during the follicular phase.

The most dramatic changes in body temperature are seen during illness. A variety of substances, some of external origin, others produced by the body's own immune reactions, act upon the hypothalamic mechanisms to elevate body temperature set point. These **pyrogens** produce **fever**. Fever is not an uncontrolled rise in temperature. As the pyrogens act, mechanisms of active warming are invoked as though body temperature had fallen. The subject feels cold, vasoconstricts peripherally and begins to shiver. As a result, temperature rises. Mild fever is probably beneficial, as it enhances the body's defences against invading organisms. As the action of the pyrogens subsides, and the set point returns to normal, then mechanisms of active cooling are invoked to bring the body temperature down.

In many infections there are alternate waves of active warming and active cooling until the infection subsides.

Some drugs, such as paracetamol and aspirin, counteract the effect of pyrogens upon the hypothalamus, and so limit the extent of fevers.

Further reading

Fuller P, Shulkes A (guest eds) 1994 *The gut as an endocrine organ*. In: Baillière's Clinical Endocrinology and Metabolism series, Baillière Tindall, London

Given that the discipline of endocrinology began with the study of the gut, most textbooks of endocrinology give the system scant coverage. This interesting little book redresses the balance with topics ranging from the evolution of the gastrointestinal endocrine system to the influence of gut hormones on growth and malignancy.

Griffin J E, Ojeda S R (eds) 2000 *Textbook of endocrine physiology*, 4th edn. Oxford University Press Inc, New York.

Intended for medical students studying physiology, this book deals nicely with clinical knowledge in terms of basic science to explain pathology. Particularly interesting are the new sections on obesity and appetite and the interactions of the immune and endocrine systems.

Laycock, J F, Wise P H 1996 *Essential endocrinology*, 3rd edn. Oxford University Press, Oxford.

In discussing clinical and diagnostic principles, the author reinforces basic endocrinology.

Sapolsky R M 1992 Neuroendocrinology of the stress-response. In: Becker J B, Breedlove S M, Crews D (eds) *Behavioral endocrinology*. MIT Press, Cambridge, Mass, pp 287–324

This is part of a larger volume on behavioral endocrinology and provides a fascinating description of the useful protective neuroendocrinological mechanisms that have evolved to protect organisms during crises. These are compared with the responses to long-term stress, using examples from primates and human social situations.

Wilson J D, Foster D W, Kronenburg H M, Larsen P R (eds) 1998 *Williams textbook of endocrinology*, 9th edn. W B Saunders, Philadelphia

An authoritative text which links basic science with clinical observations and practice.

Questions

Answer true or false to the following
statements:

5.1

Endocrine control:
A. Always depends on depolarization to
   trigger the release of a messenger.
B. Is integrated with neural control at the level
   of the hypothalamus.
C. Is often dependent on protein hormones.
D. Relies on endocytosis of messenger
   molecules.
E. Depends on secretion by ducted glands.

5.2

Hormone transport by plasma proteins:
A. Is a characteristic of lipophilic hormones.
B. Is important for hormones that act on
   extracellular receptors.
C. Reduces the hormone's half-life in the
   circulation.
D. Limits fluctuations in hormone activity.
E. Is important in the case of parathyroid
   hormone.

5.3

The posterior pituitary:
A. Develops from Rathke's pouch.
B. Is an important site of peptide hormone
   synthesis.
C. Releases antidiuretic hormone in response
   to hypertonic plasma.
D. Releases oxytocin in response to mechanical
   stimulation of the breast nipple.
E. Releases vasopressin in response to
   hypovolaemia.

5.4

The anterior pituitary:
A. Is controlled by hypothalamic hormones.
B. Controls the function of several peripheral
   endocrine glands.
C. Secretes hormones manufactured in the
   hypothalamus.
D. Secretes growth hormone during periods of
   psychological stress.
E. Becomes enlarged during pregnancy.

5.5

Thyroid hormones:
A. Are lipophilic.
B. Are manufactured from iodinated tyramine
   molecules.
C. Are present in the blood mainly in the
   T_4 form.
D. Are converted from T_4 to active T_3 by
   microsomal deiodinases in peripheral
   tissues.
E. Are required for normal perinatal brain
   development.

5.6

Aldosterone:
A. Has a longer half-life than the adrenal
   glucocorticoids.
B. Is secreted in response to an increase in
   plasma $[K^+]$.
C. Promotes renal absorption of Na^+ and H_2O.
D. Deficiency may cause a metabolic alkalosis.
E. Deficiency is likely to cause a large increase
   in [ACTH].

5.7

Glucocorticoids:

A. Inhibit hypothalamic CRH production leading to short-loop negative feedback.
B. Are anabolic steroids.
C. Promote gluconeogenesis in the liver.
D. Demonstrate a diurnal rhythm with maximal plasma concentrations before waking.
E. Can lead to fluid retention and hypertension when present in excess.

5.8

With regard to gastrointestinal hormones:

A. Secretin is stimulated by acid in the duodenum.
B. Cholecystokinin stimulates enzyme secretion from the endocrine pancreas.
C. Gastric acid secretion is stimulated by neurotensin.
D. Gastrin secretion is partly stimulated by vagal activity.
E. Enteroglucagon promotes intestinal motility.

5.9

Hypoglycaemia:

A. May result from an insulin-secreting tumour.
B. Increases the secretion of adrenal catecholamines.
C. Dramatically reduces energy release in cardiac muscle.
D. Can be treated with oral glucagon.
E. Occurs most commonly in diabetic patients.

5.10

Parathyroid hormone (PTH):

A. Is released in response to low plasma [Ca^{2+}].
B. Promotes reabsorption of phosphate in the kidney.
C. Stimulates osteoblastic activity.
D. Is under direct negative-feedback control.
E. Is released from parafollicular cells in the thyroid.

(Answers overleaf →)

Answers

5.1

A. False. Depolarization is a feature of neurosecretion but it is not required in many endocrine cells.

B. True. Integration is via the hypothalamo-hypophyseal complex.

C. True. Protein and smaller peptide hormones are common.

D. False. Hormones are released by exocytosis.

E. False. Endocrine glands are ductless.

5.2

A. True.

B. False. Lipophilic hormones cross the plasma membrane to act intracellularly.

C. False. Half-life of the hormone is increased.

D. True. The protein-bound hormone buffers change in free hormone levels and activity depends on free hormone.

E. False. It is important for thyroid and steroid hormones.

5.3

A. False. This is the origin of the anterior pituitary.

B. False. The peptide hormones released from modified axons in the posterior pituitary are manufactured in hypothalamic cell bodies.

C. True.

D. True.

E. True. ADH and vasopressin are the same substance.

5.4

A. True.

B. True. Particularly thyroid, adrenal cortex and gonads.

C. False.

D. True. Growth hormone is one of the 'stress' hormones.

E. True.

5.5

A. True.

B. False. Tyrosine is the amino acid precursor.

C. True.

D. True. T_3 is the biologically active form.

E. True. Perinatal deficit can cause mental retardation.

5.6

A. False. It has a shorter half-life.

B. True. Aldosterone is the main regulator of $[K^+]$.

C. True. It does this by its action on the distal portion of the distal convoluted tubule.

D. False. Deficiency causes metabolic acidosis by reducing H^+ secretion in the kidney.

E. False. The main negative feedback on ACTH secretion is by glucocorticoids; some ACTH is required for aldosterone production but it is not the physiological regulator.

5.7

A. False. This is an example of long-loop negative feedback.

B. False. They are catabolic.

C. True.

D. True.

E. True. Glucocorticoids also have mild mineralocorticoid effects.

5.8

A. **True.** It stimulates alkaline pancreatic secretion in response.
B. **False.** Enzyme is secreted from the exocrine pancreas.
C. **False.** Neurotensin inhibits gastric secretion and emptying.
D. **True.**
E. **False.** It stimulates mucosal growth.

5.9

A. **True.**
B. **True.**
C. **False.** Cardiac muscle can use free fatty acids for energy.
D. **False.** Glucagon is an appropriate treatment but must be injected; like other peptides it cannot be absorbed intact from the gastrointestinal tract.
E. **True.** It occurs when the amount of injected insulin exceeds the carbohydrate load, e.g. because of a delayed or inadequate meal. Hypoglycaemia is not a feature of untreated diabetes mellitus.

5.10

A. **True.**
B. **False.** It promotes renal phosphate excretion.
C. **False.** It stimulates osteocytic and osteoclastic activity.
D. **True.** Increasing $[Ca^{2+}]$ suppresses PTH secretion.
E. **False.** These cells secrete calcitonin, a hormone that lowers $[Ca^{2+}]$.

The cardiovascular system

6

493

Introduction

The functions of the cardiovascular system can be expressed in a single word: transport. It is most immediately concerned with the transport of oxygen to all the tissues of the body and with the transport of carbon dioxide, the 'waste' product of oxidative metabolism, away from the tissues. In this respect it works closely with the respiratory system because this is the route through which O_2 is taken into and CO_2 is lost from the body. It is also concerned with the transport of nutrients from the sites where they are absorbed or synthesised, usually the digestive system or liver respectively, to the tissue cells where they are used. Equally importantly, it transports waste products and toxins away to sites where they can be lost from the body or detoxified, generally the kidney or liver. The cardiovascular system also plays an essential role in the transport of hormones from endocrine organs where they are produced, to the target cells where they act. And, perhaps less obviously, it plays a crucial role in the transport of excess heat from actively metabolising cells to the surface of the body where it can be dissipated to the environment by conduction, convection, radiation and evaporation. Finally, it is important in the transport of protective cells and substances to sites of tissue damage or infection, so allowing a defensive response and repair to be initiated.

The transport medium is, of course, the blood, which is pushed through a system of tubes, the blood vessels, by a pump, the heart (see Fig. 6.1.1, p. 498). In fact, the cardiovascular system is more accurately considered as two sets of blood vessels with a double pump. The right side of the heart pumps blood to the lungs through the **pulmonary circulation** and, from here, blood returns to the left side of the heart from where it is pumped to all other tissues of the body through the **systemic circulation**. Blood is pumped out of the heart into vessels known as **arteries**. It returns to the heart in vessels known as **veins**. The blood that travels in the pulmonary arteries to the lungs has a relatively low O_2 concentration, whereas that which returns from the lungs to the heart in the pulmonary veins is well oxygenated. By contrast, the blood that travels in the systemic arteries towards the body tissues is well oxygenated and that which returns in the systemic veins has relatively low O_2 concentrations. Thus, it can be clearly seen that any particular blood vessel is called an artery or a vein, not on the basis of the oxygen concentration of the blood flowing through it, but on the direction of that blood flow relative to the heart.

The heart itself comprises four chambers: the relatively thin-walled left and right atria into which blood drains from the veins, and the thicker-walled left and right ventricles that pump blood into the arteries. In the pulmonary or systemic circulation, the blood vessels can be subdivided on the basis of their histology and the functional roles they play. The major arterial vessels into which blood is pumped by the ventricles are known as **elastic arteries**. They branch to form **muscular arteries**, which branch repeatedly, eventually forming **arterioles** – arterial vessels of < 50 μm in internal diameter. The arterioles themselves branch several times, eventually forming **capillaries**, the smallest blood vessels in the body through which most of the exchange of nutrients, waste products, hormones, etc. takes place between the blood and the fluid around the tissue cells, the **interstitial fluid**. Capillaries converge, gradually forming the smallest venous vessels, the **collecting venules**, which in turn converge to form small, medium and then large veins that drain into the heart. The functioning of each part of the cardiovascular system, the heart and each type of blood vessel, is affected by the behaviour of and events that occur in the parts that come before and after it in the circuit. It is therefore very much easier to gain a full understanding of the cardiovascular system if you have an overview of how it works as a whole and of the terminology that is used to describe its essential features and functioning, before you try to gain a more detailed understanding of any particular aspect of the system. This is what Chapter 6.1 provides.

Section overview

This section outlines:

- Physical laws that govern flow of liquids, the summing of resistances to flow and the relationship of pressure in a vessel to tension in its walls
- The special nature of the cardiac action potential
- The origin of rhythmic cardiac pacemaker activity
- Spread of electrical activity through the heart
- The origin of the phases of the ECG
- Interaction of the cardiac dipole with the position of recording leads
- Myocyte structure and properties
- Pressure and volume changes in a cardiac cycle

- Heart sounds
- Measurement of cardiac output
- Autonomic nerve effects on the heart
- Starling's Law of the Heart in terms of preload and afterload
- Arterial structure related to function
- Factors regulating arteriolar diameter
- Functions of capillaries
- Structure of venous vessels related to their functions
- Overall control of the cardiovascular system during specific situations.

Essential terminology and concepts

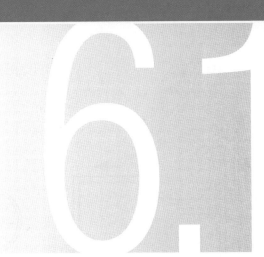

The heart

The **heart** is an intermittent pump: the cardiac muscle that forms it contracts and then relaxes, this cycle being repeated throughout life. The left and right sides of the heart contract and relax more or less synchronously. Each period of contraction is known as **systole**. Each period of relaxation is known as **diastole**. The number of times the heart contracts or beats per minute is known as the **heart rate** or pulse rate. At rest, the heart rate of a normal individual averages 70 beats/min (range ~65–75 beats/min).

Each time the heart contracts, it ejects a volume of blood into the pulmonary and systemic circulations (Fig. 6.1.1). The volume of blood ejected by each ventricle is known as the **stroke volume**. Normally, the stroke volume of the left ventricle is equal to that of the right ventricle. Transient imbalances may occur over a few heartbeats – any longer and the individual will die because blood is accumulating in, or being lost from, the systemic or pulmonary circulation. At rest, the stroke volume of a normal heart is ~70 ml, i.e. each ventricle ejects approximately 70 ml each time it contracts.

The total volume that each ventricle ejects per minute is known as the **cardiac output**. It is the product of heart rate and stroke volume, i.e.:

$$CO = HR \times SV$$

where CO is cardiac output, HR is heart rate, and SV is stroke volume.

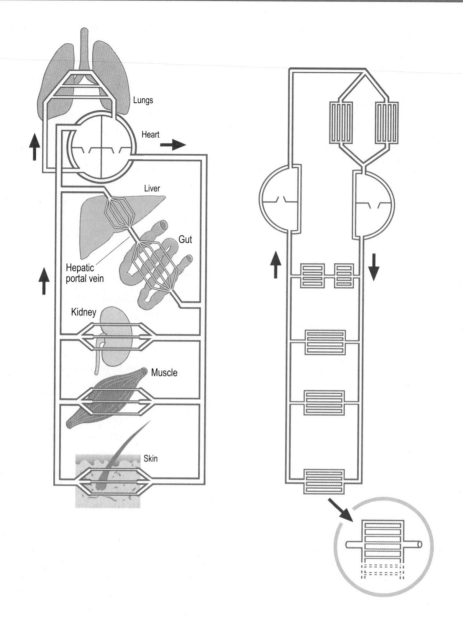

Fig. 6.1.1 The circulation, showing examples of serial and parallel connections of blood vessels. Not all examples are shown. For example, there is serial connection of capillaries in the kidney. The serial connection of the two sides of the heart is shown on the right together with an inset illustrating how the vasculature of organs consists of millions of capillaries in parallel.

From the values given above it can be seen that at rest, the average cardiac output of a healthy human adult is:

70 beats/min × 70 ml = 4900 ml/min.

Or, for ease of remembering, cardiac output at rest is ~5 l/min. As is discussed in later chapters, cardiac output is changed when the activity of the individual deviates from the normal resting state. For example, cardiac output may fall during sleep, whereas it increases in response to exercise.

The amount of blood that returns to the heart per minute is often known as **venous return**. Normally, the venous return to the left atrium is equal to the venous return to the right atrium and, for each side of the heart, the venous return is equal to the cardiac output. There may be transient imbalances over a few beats as is the case for left and right stroke volumes. However, in the steady state the amount of blood leaving the left side of the heart, passing through the systemic circulation and returning to the right side of the heart per unit time, must equal the amount of blood leaving the right side of the heart passing through the pulmonary circulation and returning to the left side of the heart. Inequality results in certain death. The mechanisms that allow the steady state to be achieved even when cardiac output is raised above or below the resting value are discussed in Chapter 6.2.

Pressure and resistance

Since the heart pumps blood, a fluid, into a closed system of blood vessels whose walls tend to resist being stretched, the blood exerts a pressure against the walls. The pressure that a fluid exerts against the walls of its container is known as **hydrostatic pressure**. Because the heart pumps intermittently and because there are valves at the origins of the pulmonary artery and aorta, the pulmonary and aortic valves respectively, that are open only during part of the systole, the hydrostatic pressure in these two arteries waxes and wanes in phase with systole and diastole. For each artery:

- the maximum pressure during systole when blood is being ejected through its valve is known as the **systolic pressure** for its circulation
- the minimum pressure that is reached at the end of diastole and immediately before the valve opens again is known as the **diastolic pressure** for its circulation.

You should note that the systolic pressure in the aorta and pulmonary artery is normally equal to, and occurs virtually simultaneously with, the systolic pressure in the left and right ventricles respectively, because each ventricle and its respective artery is in continuity through the open valve. However, the diastolic pressure reached in the aorta and pulmonary artery is considerably higher than the diastolic pressure in the respective ventricle: the valves close part way through diastole and from then until the next systole there is no continuity between the ventricle and artery and the pressures deviate. Students should note that when the terms systolic and diastolic pressure are used *without* qualification, they refer to systolic and diastolic pressure in the arterial vessels, not the pressures in the ventricles.

A further source of confusion is that when the terms are used without qualification, they refer to the pressures measured in the aorta rather than in the pulmonary artery. This may be particularly confusing because the pressures reached in the aorta are substantially higher than in the pulmonary artery. Given that the left and right cardiac outputs are equal, as is described above, this major disparity arises because the resistance of the systemic circulation is considerably higher than that of the pulmonary circulation. In fact, the absolute hydrostatic pressure present in the aorta or pulmonary artery at any moment of time depends on the volume of blood pushing against the artery wall. This, in turn, is directly related to the volume of blood that is pumped into it per unit time (cardiac output) and on the difficulty the blood has in flowing out of the artery at the other end into the vessels downstream. This last variable is known as **vascular resistance**.

- The resistance of all blood vessels downstream of the aorta is known as **total peripheral resistance** (TPR).
- The equivalent for the pulmonary artery is the **pulmonary vascular resistance** (PVR).

499

Total peripheral resistance is approximately seven times greater than pulmonary vascular resistance.

Put briefly, the reason PVR is so much lower than TPR is that the pulmonary blood vessels are shorter and have larger diameters than the corresponding systemic blood vessels. The consequence of the disparity between the resistances is that the left ventricle has thicker, more muscular walls than the right ventricle. The causal relationship between the thickness of the ventricular wall and the resistance of the circulation that it pumps blood through can be seen in respiratory disease when PVR increases: there is an associated increase in the thickness of the right ventricular wall.

The average pressure present in the aorta over systole and diastole is known as **(systemic) mean arterial blood pressure** (MABP). The equivalent value for the pulmonary artery is **pulmonary mean arterial blood pressure** (pulmonary MABP): it is conventional to state when referring to pulmonary pressure, whereas 'systemic' is assumed. These relationships between pressure, flow and resistance can be expressed mathematically:

Systemic MABP = CO × TPR

Pulmonary MABP = CO × PVR.

These formulae are analogous to Ohm's law for electrical circuits:

$V = i \times R$

where V is voltage, i is current and R is resistance.

These formulae are crucially important for both types of circulation or circuit, for the mean pressure or voltage tells you the energy that is available to push blood or electrons through the blood vessels or wires. When you are considering the cardiovascular system, you may of course rearrange the formula if you wish to calculate CO or TPR from the other two variables. However, from a conceptual point of view, it is important that you do not rearrange the formula, for the pressure in the aorta or

pulmonary artery is dependent on cardiac output and the resistance of the relevant circulation. Neither cardiac output, nor vascular resistance is dependent on the other two variables.

Because TPR is approximately seven times greater than PVR, systemic MABP is approximately seven times greater than pulmonary MABP. The average systemic MABP for a normal individual at rest is 90 mmHg, whereas average pulmonary MABP is 12–13 mmHg. It might be argued that we should move with the times and express arterial pressure in the SI units of kilopascals (kPa). However, the great majority of clinicians and scientists have resisted the trend and still use the traditional units of mmHg, at least in part, because measuring devices are calibrated against a column of mercury. (In my laboratory I have a U-tube full of mercury for measuring high pressure in mmHg and a U-tube full of water to measure low pressure in mmH$_2$O. To move with the times, where can I get a U-tube full of pascals, your author wonders weakly.)

Systemic MABP can increase or decrease when the activity of the individual deviates from the resting state. This can occur because of a change in cardiac output or total peripheral resistance or both. Concomitantly, either systolic or diastolic pressure, or both, may change. Although MABP can change dramatically from the resting value, for example during stress or exercise, there is a control system known as the **baroreceptor reflex** that is organized in such a way as to counteract changes in MABP and to restore it to the resting value. These issues are dealt with in more detail in Chapters 6.4 and 6.6. By contrast, pulmonary MABP is not only lower than MABP, but it changes very little with different levels of activity in the normal individual.

Pressure profiles in systemic and pulmonary circulations

During its passage through the blood vessels, the blood loses energy, which means the pressure falls (Fig. 6.1.2). Most of this loss of energy and therefore pressure is caused by the resistance to the flow of blood offered by the blood vessel walls: energy is lost by the frictional drag between the flowing blood and the vessel wall (see below). The amount of energy lost is substantial, as shown by the difference in pressure between blood in the arteries (90–120 mmHg) and in the large veins where they drain into the right and left atria, normally only 1–2 mmHg. The pressure in the major veins of the systemic circulation where they converge into the right atrium is known as **central venous pressure**. The value of central venous pressure is clinically very important. For example, it is generally raised in heart failure and indicates that the heart is congested or overfilled because the ventricular muscle is not contracting forcefully enough to eject all the blood that is being presented to it.

Because the same amount of blood flows per minute through each type of blood vessel, the shape of the pressure gradient from the beginning to the end of the systemic and pulmonary circulations indicates the relative resistances of the different types of blood vessel: a greater pressure drop means a greater vascular resistance (Fig. 6.1.2). Thus, for the systemic circulation, it can be seen that very little pressure is lost as the blood flows through the elastic and muscular arteries (see below), whereas a great deal of pressure is lost in flowing through the arterioles. The arterioles are in fact, the most important site of resistance in the whole of the systemic circulation, not only because they have the greatest resistance under resting conditions

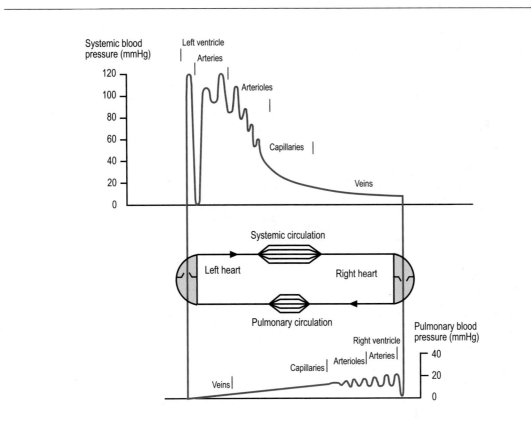

Fig. 6.1.2 Blood pressure. As the same total blood flow occurs in all parts of the systemic and pulmonary circulations, the pressures measured there reflect the resistance to flow. Pressure in the right and left ventricles falls to near zero just before filling begins.

and therefore make the largest contribution to TPR, but because they are the major site of *changes* in vascular resistance (see below). There is a further, significant loss of pressure as blood flows through the capillaries, but very little pressure is lost when blood flows through the whole of the venous section. Rather, all the venous vessels can be regarded as low-pressure, low-resistance or 'capacitance' vessels (see below).

The shape of the pressure gradient in the pulmonary circulation is far less dramatic. There is a gradual loss of pressure as blood flows through the small arteries, arterioles and capillaries and a further, smaller loss of pressure in the venous vessels. There are no high-resistance vessels to correspond with the systemic arterioles. Rather, the whole of the pulmonary circulation can be regarded as a low-pressure, low-resistance circuit.

Relationship between wall structure and function

Elastic arteries

As their name suggests, **elastic arteries** contain a great deal of elastin, which is mainly found in the tunica media (Fig. 6.1.3). Elastin has the property that although elastic, it tends to resist being stretched. Energy is required to stretch it and some of this energy is 'stored' by the elastin. This is important from a functional point of view, because this stored energy is released again when the force that was stretching it is removed. To put it another way, elastin has the property of recoil, just like the rubber sling in a catapult. The energy is 'stored' by the elastin during systole and is given back to the blood during diastole when it helps to propel the blood on its way through the circulation.

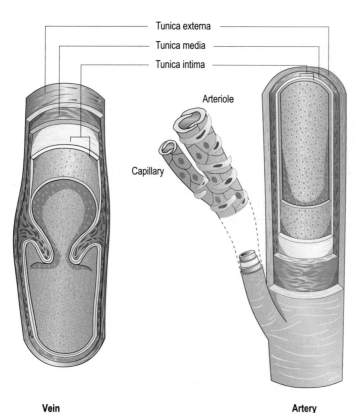

Tunica externa
Tunica media
Tunica intima

Arteriole

Capillary

Fig. 6.1.3 **Structure of blood vessels.** Note the thinner elastic and smooth muscle layer (tunica media) in the vein. The tunica externa is sometimes called the adventitia.

Vein
(showing valve)

Artery

The other important feature of elastic arteries is that they have a thick layer of collagen, which is mainly found in the tunica media and tunica externa. Collagen is a tough material that is highly resistant to stretch. Thus, the elastic arteries are rather like a bicycle tyre comprising an inflatable inner tube that has some intrinsic resistance to being stretched and a non-expandable outer casing that puts a practical limit on the extent to which the inner tube can be filled. These features are discussed further in Chapter 6.4 where you will see that these structural properties allow elastic arteries to convert an intermittent flow of blood from the heart into a continuous flow in the vessels downstream.

Muscular arteries

Although the elastic arteries have smooth muscle, this is not as obvious as it is in the **muscular arteries**, in which the elastin and collagen is reduced and less well organized. As in all blood vessels that have it, the smooth muscle is arranged circularly around the vessel lumen. This smooth muscle layer gradually decreases in thickness as the muscular arteries branch to form smaller arteries and then arterioles, so that the smallest arterioles of all, the terminal arterioles and precapillary arterioles, have only single smooth muscle cells wrapped around the lumen and no collagen or elastin.

Under normal resting conditions, this smooth muscle is partly contracted, which is described as a resting tone. Because the smooth muscle is arranged circularly, further contraction causes the internal diameter of the blood vessel to be reduced. This process is known as **vasoconstriction**. The opposite process, relaxation of the smooth muscle, resulting in an increase in internal diameter, is known as **vasodilatation** (referred to as vasodilation in the US). Although there is the potential for the resting tone to be increased or decreased in the muscular arteries, this potential is generally not used, except in the smaller muscular arteries

within the tissues. Thus, the larger muscular arteries can be regarded as conduit vessels whose most important function is simply to carry blood to the major organs and tissues.

Arterioles

Functionally, the small muscular arteries can be grouped together with the arterioles in that they are resistance vessels. They simply make a smaller contribution to TPR at rest and to changes in vascular resistance than do the arterioles. The many factors that regulate the smooth muscle and therefore the resistance of these vessels are dealt with in Chapter 6.4.

Capillaries

All blood vessels and the heart have a lining of endothelial cells. The endothelial layer has important functions that are discussed in Chapter 6.4. In the capillaries, the endothelial cells are the main constituent of the wall, which has no smooth muscle, collagen or elastin. This means that they are ideally suited to be exchange vessels because there is only the thickness of one endothelial cell between the blood and the interstitial fluid. Since the capillaries have no smooth muscle in their walls, their diameters cannot be actively changed: they cannot constrict or dilate and therefore their resistance cannot be actively regulated. The capillaries branch to form a network and then converge again.

Collecting venules and veins

When capillaries acquire a single layer of smooth muscle, they become known as collecting venules. As more and more of these vessels converge to form small, medium and large **veins** the smooth muscle layer increases in thickness and they gain collagen and a small amount of elastin. However, all venous vessels have thinner walls than their arterial counterparts. Further, in a supine individual, with all parts of the body more or less at the same horizontal level as the heart, the venous vessels are elliptical in cross-section and the collagen is folded, or pleated, around the vessel lumen. This contrasts with the arterial vessels, which are circular in cross-section and with their collagen more or less unfolded. This means that venous vessels can be filled with, or can accommodate, a larger volume of blood with very little change in the pressure exerted by the blood against the vessel wall – the collagen gradually becomes unfolded. The venous vessels are therefore very distensible or **compliant**. Although it is the introduction of an extra volume of blood into the vessel that increases the pressure by stretching the wall, it is usual to represent compliance as Change in volume/ Change in pressure (see p. 659).

$$\text{Compliance} = \frac{\Delta V}{\Delta P}$$

This property of high compliance allows the venous vessels to act as **capacitance vessels** or reservoirs. Additional blood can be held within them under certain conditions and this blood can be 'mobilized' or returned to the right side of the heart, so becoming available to increase cardiac output. Thus, the venous vessels can be said to prime the pump. The conditions that allow the venous reservoirs to fill with more blood and the factors that contract the venous smooth muscle or collapse the veins so that blood is mobilized are dealt with in Chapter 6.5. The larger veins, particularly those of the legs, have **valves** (Fig. 6.1.3); these ensure that when the veins are constricted or collapsed, blood moves in one direction only, towards the heart.

Although venous vessels are very compliant until the collagen becomes unfolded and the lumen circular, once this level of distension is reached their compliance then becomes low (Fig. 6.1.4). The collagen resists stretch, and any further increase in volume produces a large change in pressure. This is essentially what happens in the veins that drain into the heart

in heart failure. The ventricle, atrium and large veins are overfilled with blood because the ventricle is not ejecting blood effectively and therefore the venous pressure is high.

Pulmonary blood vessels

Pulmonary blood vessels are categorized as arterial or venous vessels on the basis of the direction of the blood flowing through them, but from a histological and functional point of view the pulmonary vessels, whether arterial or venous, are comparable to the veins of the systemic circulation. They are thin-walled, have little smooth muscle, and are very compliant. Indeed, the pulmonary circulation is an important blood reservoir.

Tension in blood vessel walls

The pressure that is exerted outwards against the vessel wall (force/unit surface area) is opposed by the tension that is generated in the vessel wall (force/unit cross-sectional area of

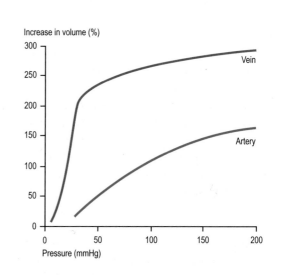

Fig. 6.1.4 Pressure–volume relationships in arteries and veins.

the wall). The relationship between lumen pressure and wall tension in hollow organs is described by the law of Laplace, which was originally put forward by Laplace to describe the balance of forces in a soap bubble. For a tube like a blood vessel (Fig. 6.1.5), consider a unit length of the tube of radius (r) sealed at either end by circular pistons producing a pressure (P). The total pressure on the pistons is πr^2 (the area of a circle) × 2 (there are two pistons) × P (the pressure produced). The total pressure exerted against the wall is thus $2\pi r^2 P$. More correctly, you should consider the transmural pressure rather than the lumen pressure, i.e. the pressure exerted from the inside of the vessel against the wall, minus the pressure exerted from the outside of the vessel against the wall. Although outside pressure is usually near zero it may be raised, for example in skeletal or cardiac muscle when that muscle contracts. The pressure is opposed by the total circumferential tension in the wall ($2\pi rwT$) where $2\pi r$ is the circumference, T is the tension and w is the wall thickness. The tension is the sum of the passive tension exerted by elastin, smooth muscle and,

to some extent collagen when it is being stretched and the active tension generated by smooth muscle when it contracts.

$$2\pi r^2 P = 2\pi rwT.$$

Thus:

$$P = \frac{wT}{r} \quad \text{or} \quad T = \frac{Pr}{w}.$$

The structural constituents of the blood vessel wall must be of sufficient thickness and strength to exert the tension that is required to oppose the lumen pressure. Not surprisingly, the wall composition of each type of blood vessel in the cardiovascular system is appropriate to the range of pressures that are normally found in that vessel. For example, the aorta has a high lumen pressure and a large radius, but the tension that the constituents of the wall have to develop is reduced because the wall is thick. If the wall thickness is reduced, as it is in an **aneurysm**, the tension that the remaining wall constituents must generate for the wall to remain stable is increased and the vessel is liable to burst if lumen pressure increases. On the other hand, capillaries can have thin walls and be stable because both their radius and lumen pressure are low.

Resistances in series and in parallel

The pulmonary and systemic circulations are in series with one another (see Fig. 6.1.1): any given red blood cell passes first through one circulation and then through the other. Similarly, the different sections of the vascular tree are in series with one another: a red blood cell passes first through the aorta, then the muscular arteries, arterioles and so on. The total resistance through blood vessels that are in series with one another is the sum of all the individual resistances (Fig. 6.1.6):

$$R_{\text{total}} = R_1 + R_2 + R_3 + \dots$$

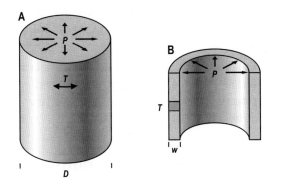

Fig. 6.1.5 Wall tension. A. Laplace's law relating internal pressure (P), diameter (D), and wall tension (T) in an infinitely thin structure (e.g. a bubble). **B.** Modification by Frank to derive tension (T) per unit wall cross-sectional area in a wall of thickness w.

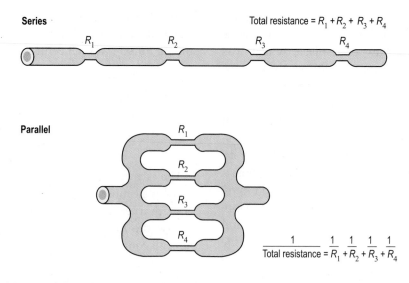

Series

$$\text{Total resistance} = R_1 + R_2 + R_3 + R_4$$

R_1 R_2 R_3 R_4

Parallel

R_1
R_2
R_3
R_4

$$\frac{1}{\text{Total resistance}} = \frac{1}{R_1} + \frac{1}{R_2} + \frac{1}{R_3} + \frac{1}{R_4}$$

Fig. 6.1.6 Vessels in series and parallel. The total resistance of the same resistances connected in the two ways is very different. If each of the resistances in the figure had a value of 2, in series the total resistance would be 8; in parallel it would be $1/2$.

On the other hand, the various organs supplied by the systemic circulation are generally in parallel with one another, and, within each organ and tissue, blood vessels at the same level of the vascular tree, e.g. the capillaries, are in parallel with one another. When resistances are in parallel (Fig. 6.1.6), the reciprocal of the total resistance is equal to the sum of the reciprocals of the individual resistances:

$$1/R_{total} = 1/R_1 + 1/R_2 + 1/R_3 + \ldots$$

A major exception to this general rule for the arrangement of blood vessels in organs is the liver, which receives the majority of its blood supply from blood vessels that drain the capillary bed of the digestive system. There are also exceptions in the pituitary gland and within the kidney where there are two capillary networks in series with one another. This type of circulation is called a **portal circulation**.

When resistances are in parallel, there are several important consequences:

- the total resistance is clearly much smaller than it would be if the same resistances were in series

- if a further parallel resistance is added to the circulation, the total resistance is reduced
- even a large increase in one of the individual resistances produces a relatively small increase in the total resistance.

For portal circulations, the consequences of the resistances being in series are:

- the second capillary network is perfused at a lower pressure because pressure has already been lost in going through the first capillary network
- the blood supplied to the second circulation has already had some oxygen removed from it by the tissue of the first capillary network.

Distribution of cardiac output

For the right ventricle, 100% of its output is ejected into the pulmonary circulation. For the left ventricle, its output is distributed to the various tissues and organs of the body in proportion to their vascular resistances (Fig. 6.1.7). Tissues that have a low vascular resistance

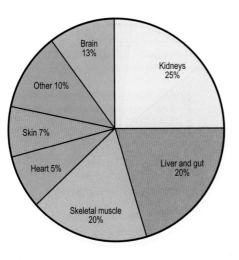

Fig. 6.1.7 Distribution of cardiac output. The distribution of the output of the left ventricle at rest is shown. This distribution changes profoundly during specific activities such as exercise. The whole of the output of the right ventricle goes to the pulmonary circulation.

Flow, velocity and cross-sectional area

Blood flow is a measure of the volume of blood that travels past a fixed point per unit time. **Blood velocity** is a measure of speed or velocity and has the units of distance travelled per unit time.

First, consider a single blood vessel with a narrow region along its length. If a given volume of blood flows into and out of that vessel per unit time, it follows, logically, that the velocity must be higher in the narrow region than it is on either side. In fact, the velocity (v) is directly proportional to the flow (F) and indirectly proportional to the cross-sectional area of the blood vessel (πr^2). Thus:

$$v = \frac{F}{\pi r^2} \, .$$

This means that velocity is higher in a region of a blood vessel that is narrowed by thrombus, or by a partially inflated sphygmomanometer cuff.

Now consider what happens as blood flows from the aorta towards the capillary beds. As the blood vessels branch from one another, so the total cross-sectional area across all the vessels that are in parallel with one another gradually increases. The blood flow in the aorta is the left cardiac output and this same volume of blood per unit time passes through all the arteries, all the arterioles and all the capillaries that are in parallel with one another. Thus, it follows that the velocity falls progressively from the aorta to the capillaries (Fig. 6.1.8). In fact, the velocity falls precipitously by two orders of magnitude (from ~30 to ~0.08 cm/s) from the aorta to the capillaries, because the cross-sectional area increases so dramatically. This means that the velocity of blood in the capillaries is so low that there is normally plenty of time for exchange between the blood and the interstitial fluid.

As the blood passes from the capillaries to the venous vessels and back to the heart, so the blood vessels converge and the total

receive a high proportion, whereas tissues that have a high vascular resistance receive a low proportion. At rest, the vascular resistance of any given organ is determined by the structural characteristics of the blood vessels that supply it, mainly the diameter, length and pattern of branching, and also by the tone of the vascular smooth muscle. The proportions of blood that are distributed to the different organs can be changed by changing the vascular resistances of the organs relative to one another. Because the arterioles are the major site of resistance in the systemic circulation and because their resistances can be changed over a wide range, changes in arteriolar resistance are the most important mechanism for changing the distribution of cardiac output. For example, during exercise, the arterioles in skeletal muscle dilate, while the arteries of the digestive system constrict. Their vascular resistances fall and rise respectively and a higher proportion of cardiac output goes to muscle at the expense of the digestive system.

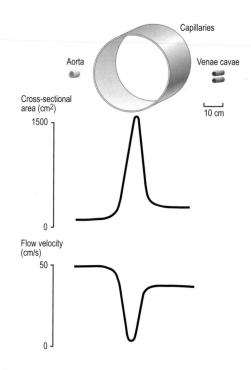

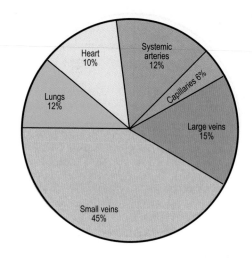

Fig. 6.1.9 **Distribution of blood volume.** The distribution at rest is shown; it varies greatly with changes in activity.

Fig. 6.1.8 **The relationship between total cross-sectional area and flow velocity in the circulation.** Changes in radius of blood vessels has a profound effect on cross-sectional area and therefore velocity because area changes as the square of the radius. In addition, the number of capillaries (in parallel with each other) is vastly greater than the number of any other type of vessel.

cross-sectional area across the branches that are in parallel with one another, decreases. Thus, there is a corresponding increase in the velocity such that velocity in the venae cavae rises to about half that in the aorta (because the cross-sectional area of the venae cavae is about twice that of the aorta).

Distribution of blood volume

The total blood volume is about 5 litres in an adult man, slightly less in the average woman. Approximately 10% of the total is in the heart and the rest is distributed amongst the different types of blood vessels according to their length

and cross-sectional area (Fig. 6.1.9). The greatest proportion (~60%) is in the venous vessels of the systemic circulation in line with their role as a blood reservoir (see above). The arterial vessels of the systemic circulation together contain about 12%, the capillaries contain about 6%, and the whole of the pulmonary circulation contains 12% of the total blood volume.

Blood flow

The blood flow (F, volume/unit time) that passes through a given blood vessel depends directly upon the hydrostatic pressure difference between the two ends of the blood vessel (P) and indirectly upon the resistance that is offered to the movement of blood (R):

$$F = \frac{\Delta P}{R} .$$

Similarly, blood flow through a tissue depends upon the hydrostatic pressure difference across the tissue (pressure in the supplying artery minus pressure in the draining vein) and the vascular resistance of the tissue.

Resistance is determined by the frictional drag between the blood and the blood vessel wall and the friction between the different constituents of the blood. Thus resistance (R) is directly proportional to the length (L) of the blood vessel or blood vessels and is inversely proportional to the fourth power of the radius (r^4) of the blood vessel or blood vessels. The resistance is greater the longer the length and the smaller the radius. The friction between the different constituents of blood is described as its viscosity (η) (see p. 510). When molecules of a fluid slide easily over one another, the viscosity is low; when they do not, the viscosity is high – treacle has a higher viscosity than water. The resistance to blood flow is greater the higher the viscosity.

The French physician Poiseuille, who had trained in mathematics and physics, set himself the task of determining the relationships between the factors that determine the flow of blood in blood vessels, and performed experiments on the movement of water in glass capillary tubes. In 1846, his meticulous experiments enabled him to publish a paper showing that:

$$R \propto \frac{\eta L}{r^4} \ .$$

Subsequently, this relationship was proven mathematically and a constancy factor was incorporated to give:

$$R = \frac{8\eta L}{\pi r^4} \ .$$

Because flow is inversely proportional to resistance (see above):

$$F = \frac{\Delta P \pi r^4}{8\eta L} \ .$$

This relationship is known as **Poiseuille's formula**, in recognition of his work. However, because the relationship was established and verified on the basis of a simple fluid flowing along a rigid glass tube, we need to consider how well these criteria apply to the flow of blood in blood vessels. Put briefly, blood is not a simple fluid, it has cellular constituents, and blood vessels are not rigid glass tubes.

Laminar flow

A simple homogeneous fluid can exhibit **laminar** or streamlined flow. When the fluid in a tube is made to move from a stationary position by the application of a pressure gradient, the molecules of the fluid slide past one another so that the ones in the centre of the tube have the highest velocity and the ones near the outside of the tube have the lowest velocity. The molecules become arranged into a series of extremely thin concentric tubes and the velocity profile across the longitudinal axis of the tube has a parabolic shape (Fig. 6.1.10). Although blood is not a homogeneous fluid, the blood flow in the majority of blood vessels with diameters of greater than 0.5 mm approximates to laminar. The red blood cells align themselves in concentric layers so that the ones in the centre of the vessel have the highest velocity, and the velocity profile is parabolic. Laminar flow is highly efficient in terms of the energy (pressure gradient) required to sustain it.

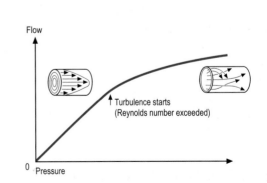

Fig. 6.1.10 The change from laminar to turbulent flow. Many factors determine the onset of turbulence. The dimensionless ratio between fluid velocity, density, tube diameter and fluid viscosity is called Reynolds number, and when this exceeds 2000 in steady flow in a rigid straight uniform tube, turbulence begins.

Turbulent flow

Blood flow can change from laminar to **turbulent**. Eddies of fluid and particles move not only parallel to, but in whirls in all sorts of directions relative to the longitudinal axis of the vessel (Fig. 6.1.10). Turbulence flattens the velocity profile and effectively increases the resistance to flow. A larger pressure gradient is required to produce a given blood flow when the flow is turbulent than when it is laminar. Whether or not turbulence occurs in a simple smooth tube is determined by several factors that can be combined into a formula:

$$Re = \frac{\rho d v}{\eta}.$$

where Re is Reynolds number, d is the diameter of the vessel, v is the velocity of the fluid, ρ is the density of the fluid, and η is the viscosity.

Turbulence generally occurs if Re is > 2000. This means that turbulence is most likely to occur in large blood vessels where the velocity is high. In fact, turbulence usually occurs transiently in the aorta and pulmonary artery during systole. It can occur in other large arteries when the velocity is high, for example in exercise or pregnancy when cardiac output is raised. It can also occur in a region of a blood vessel that has been narrowed by a thrombus, or partially inflated sphygmomanometer cuff, because here the velocity will be high (see above). Turbulence may also occur in smaller blood vessels when blood viscosity is reduced by severe anaemia (see below).

Turbulent blood flow is noisy, whereas laminar flow is silent. Thus, sites of turbulence can be detected by using a stethoscope.

Blood flow in small blood vessels

Clearly, red blood cells cannot be arranged in a laminar fashion in small blood vessels where the size of the cells is large in proportion to the diameter of the blood vessel: in the smallest vessels red blood cells have to move in single

file. This has the effect of flattening the velocity profile across the blood vessel and might be expected to increase the resistance to blood flow, as described above for turbulence. However, this is not the case because the apparent viscosity of blood decreases in small blood vessels and has a counteracting effect (see below).

Viscosity

The viscosity of whole blood is largely determined by the red blood cells. The viscosity of plasma is slightly greater than water and the higher the concentration of red blood cells, the greater the viscosity. The concentration of red blood cells is expressed as a proportion (**haematocrit**) or percentage (packed cell volume) of whole blood and is measured by centrifuging a small sample of blood in a glass capillary tube for a standard period of time at a standard speed. The haematocrit is between 0.4 and 0.5 in a normal adult man and between 0.35 and 0.45 in a normal, premenopausal woman. When viscosity is measured in the laboratory in a standard glass tube (viscometer) of 1 mm diameter, haematocrit has a strong influence on viscosity over the normal range of haematocrit values and the relationship becomes even steeper at higher haematocrit values (Fig. 6.1.11).

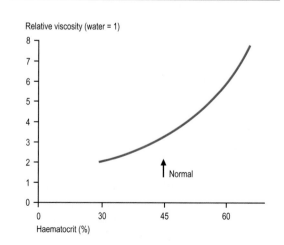

Fig. 6.1.11 Haematocrit related to viscosity.

High haematocrits of 0.6–0.7 occur, for example, in polycythaemia and at high altitude. The viscosity measured in this way would then increase by at least twofold and the resistance to blood flow would be expected to increase by the same proportion.

However, for any given haematocrit, the apparent viscosity varies with the diameter of the tube in which the viscosity is measured (the Fahraeus–Lindqvist effect). The apparent viscosity decreases progressively when the tube diameter decreases below 200 µm (Fig. 6.1.12). Several factors contribute to this phenomenon. The red cells tend to accumulate towards the centre of the tube (**axial streaming**) where they move at a higher velocity, whereas the plasma is largely confined to the margins of the tube where it moves at low velocity. Further, in smaller tubes, this plasma layer or 'sleeve' occupies a larger proportion of the total cross-sectional area of the tube. Thus the plasma has a greater influence on the viscosity and the apparent viscosity tends towards the viscosity of plasma. The apparent viscosity decreases until tube diameter falls below 3 µm and then it increases to infinity (Fig. 6.1.12) because at this point the red blood cells cannot be deformed sufficiently to allow them to pass through the lumen.

This effect of tube diameter is extremely important in the cardiovascular system because so many blood vessels within a tissue have a diameter of < 200 µm. This means that when the effect of haematocrit upon viscosity is measured in a living tissue, the relationship is not what might be expected if viscosity were measured in a standard viscometer tube. The effect viscosity has on resistance is smaller at any given haematocrit than might have been expected and the effect that an *increase* in haematocrit has on resistance to blood flow is much smaller in absolute terms than might have been expected.

The viscosity of blood is also affected by the velocity of the blood flow. At high velocities, axial streaming is more pronounced and apparent viscosity is reduced, but at low velocities, red blood cells tend to aggregate into clumps known as **rouleaux** (sing. rouleau), rather like stacks of coins, and the apparent viscosity is increased. Blood velocity can fall sufficiently for rouleaux to form even in large blood vessels in heart failure or shock when blood pressure is low, and they can also form in small blood vessels downstream of an occlusion when the blood flow is sluggish. Once formed, rouleaux decrease the velocity even further, so creating a positive feedback.

A similar phenomenon occurs at low temperatures such as may be experienced in cold hands and feet and when surgery is done under hypothermic conditions. The viscosity of blood, like that of treacle, increases when temperature falls. This increases the resistance to blood flow (by 2% for a 1ºC fall in temperature), which tends to reduce the velocity and so raise the viscosity further and encourage rouleaux formation.

Length of blood vessels

Length is an important determinant of resistance, whether it is the whole circulation that is being considered, or the resistance of a particular blood vessel. The resistance of the systemic

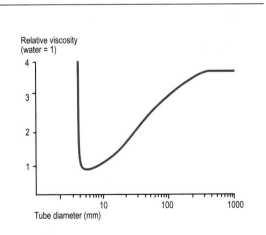

Fig. 6.1.12 The Fahraeus–Lindqvist effect. The measured viscosity of blood flowing in narrow tubes depends on the diameter of the tube.

circulation is greater than that of the pulmonary circulation, partly because the former is a longer circulation. However, in contrast to the other factors discussed above, the length of blood vessels is fixed. The smooth muscle is arranged circularly around the vessel walls and so changes in vessel length cannot be used as a means of changing vascular resistance.

Radius of blood vessels

Poiseuille's formula assumes that the tube through which fluid flows is rigid, not distended by internal pressure, and states that because resistance and therefore flow are related to the fourth power of the radius, a very small change in radius produces a large change in flow.

Some blood vessels, including the venous vessels and all pulmonary vessels, are very distensible, or compliant (see above), and therefore by definition they are not rigid. Increases in driving pressure increase lumen pressure causing distension, increasing vessel radius and reducing vascular resistance, so that blood flow increases disproportionately with increases in ΔP. Systemic arteries and arterioles also show passive distension, particularly at high luminal pressures. The *passive* elastic properties of arteries, and the effects of a reduction in their elasticity with age is shown in Figure 6.1.13, together with the way in which veins change their cross-section more by collapse at low pressures. However, under certain conditions, some arterioles, notably those in brain and kidney, show so-called **myogenic responses** when lumen pressure changes. The smooth muscle actively contracts when lumen pressure rises and relaxes when lumen pressure falls, so that blood flow can remain constant over a range of lumen pressures, usually ~60–160 mmHg (see Fig. 6.4.5, p. 578). Above and below these pressures, the arterioles behave passively, but it is observed that living vascular beds close completely before the pressure in them falls to zero (Fig. 6.1.14). The **critical closing pressure** is determined by wall tension, which in turn is influenced by sympathetically controlled vasomotor tone.

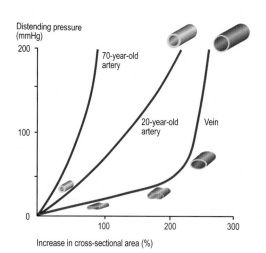

Fig. 6.1.13 Elastic properties of arteries and veins. Changes in diameter of arteries with distending pressure largely depend on the elastic properties of their walls, and hence their age. Veins change their cross-sectional area by collapse more than distension and are therefore less affected in this respect by ageing.

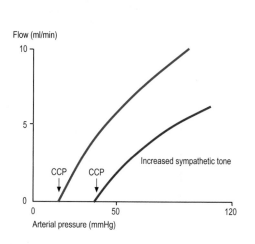
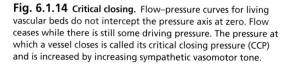

Fig. 6.1.14 Critical closing. Flow–pressure curves for living vascular beds do not intercept the pressure axis at zero. Flow ceases while there is still some driving pressure. The pressure at which a vessel closes is called its critical closing pressure (CCP) and is increased by increasing sympathetic vasomotor tone.

Clearly, any of these deviations from the assumption of vessel rigidity mean the relationship that would be measured between ΔP and blood flow in an individual vessel or tissue at constant length and blood viscosity, would differ from that predicted from Poiseuille's formula. Nevertheless, it is important to note that if ΔP, length and viscosity are kept constant then the blood flow through an individual arteriole is directly related to the fourth power of the radius, as predicted by Poiseuille's formula. This formula was not derived for non-laminar flows or fluids like blood, which are made up of a liquid and solid (cellular) part (see above).

Nevertheless, although Poiseuille's formula cannot be applied accurately to the circulation in vivo to allow us to calculate any one variable from the other four variables that make it up, it is surprisingly useful in indicating in a semi-quantitative way the relationships between the variables. In particular, we can say that under most physiological conditions:

- the most important functions that determine blood flow are the pressure gradient across the vessel tissue and the vascular resistance
- the most important contributor to vascular resistance is blood vessel radius, not only because flow is related to the fourth power of the radius, but because vessel radius is the one variable that can be changed very readily from moment to moment.

We can also go one stage further and say that because arterioles are the major resistance blood vessels, changes in their radius make the most important contributions to changes in vascular resistance.

The heart

6.2

6

The heart is largely made up of muscle. Like all muscles, its contraction is initiated by electrical activity. The repetitive and special nature of this electrical activity reflects the special nature of the activity of the heart.

A heart taken from a living body will continue to beat for some time, showing that the origin of the heartbeat is within the heart itself. The heartbeat is triggered by a wave of depolarization that normally originates from a pacemaker, the sinoatrial node (SA node). This part of the chapter focuses on the electrical activity of both individual cardiac muscle cells and the intact heart.

Cardiac muscle – a functional syncytium

The atrial and ventricular walls are composed of cardiac muscle cells, **myocytes**. The normal pumping action of the heart is dependent upon the synchronized contraction of individual cardiac muscle cells. Cardiac muscle is striated like skeletal muscle, but unlike skeletal muscle it is not dependent upon an external nerve supply for activation. This makes a heart transplant possible. The heart generates its own rhythm. The nerves to the heart speed up or slow down this rhythm. The synchronized contraction of cardiac muscle cells occurs because adjacent cardiac muscle cells are linked to each other at their ends by specialized gap junctions (or nexi). The gap junction is an area where the membranes of adjacent cardiac muscle cells fuse with each other, and bridging channels form pathways of low electrical resistance between the cells. These allow electrical activity to spread rapidly from cell to cell. The term **functional syncytium** is often applied to cardiac muscle to describe how individual cardiac muscle cells are linked such that they function as a single unit, though structurally it is composed of individual cells.

Electrical activity in cardiac muscle cells

Resting membrane potential

The resting membrane potential of cardiac muscle cells is in the range −60 to −90 mV (Fig. 6.2.1). The mechanism producing the negative internal potential of cardiac muscle cells is that common to all cells in the body and is dependent upon high internal and low external concentrations of potassium ions and a low permeability to sodium ions (see Ch. 1.3). The resting membrane potential of cardiac muscle

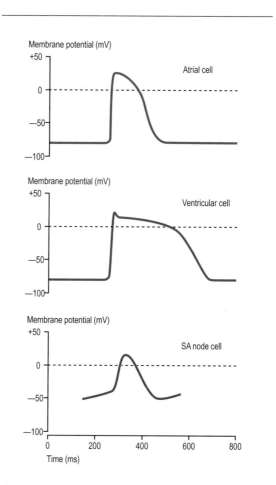

Fig. 6.2.1 Action potentials from cells in the SA node, atrial muscle and ventricular muscle. The different time-courses of these action potentials depend on the different rates of activation and inactivation of membrane channels. The absolute value of the membrane potential of the SA node cell and its rate of depolarization are the result of its 'leaky' membrane.

cells is therefore close to the potassium equilibrium potential (E_{K^+}). The resting membrane potential of the vast majority of cardiac muscle cells remains constant at about 80 mV until the cell is excited by an action potential from a neighbouring cell (Fig. 6.2.1). Cells of the SA node, and some cells of the conducting system, have an unstable resting membrane potential known as a pacemaker potential (see below) which imposes the rhythm of the heart on the majority of typical (non-pacemaker) cardiac muscle cells: their membrane potential does not fall below −60 to −70 mV.

Action potentials in typical (non-pacemaker) cardiac muscle cells

The action potential in contractile (non-pacemaker) cardiac muscle cell has a long duration, from 200 ms in atrial cells to over 400 ms in ventricular cells (Fig. 6.2.1). The cardiac action potential has three distinct components:

- depolarization
- the plateau phase
- repolarization.

Changes in membrane potential during the action potential are caused by changes in membrane permeability to Na$^+$, Ca^{2+} and K$^+$. Although there is movement of ions in and out of the cell during the action potential, and substantial changes in the membrane potential, the actual change in the concentrations of ions that takes place is minuscule, as in other excitable cells.

Depolarization

An action potential in one cardiac muscle cell is normally triggered by an action potential in a neighbouring cell. Current flows from the active to the inactive cell through the gap junctions, causing the membrane of the inactive cell to depolarize. Depolarization in atrial and ventricular muscle cells increases the membrane permeability to sodium ions by opening voltage-sensitive **fast sodium channels** in the membrane. Sodium ions enter the cell passively

down their concentration and electrochemical gradients (Fig. 6.2.2). This is the fast inward sodium current i_{Na}. The positive charge carried by the sodium ions depolarizes the membrane still further and pushes it towards the sodium equilibrium potential (E_{Na^+} of +70 mV, never reached because of the effect of other ions). Depolarization of ventricular cells is extremely rapid and is usually complete within 2 ms. Cells of the SA node and atrioventricular node lack fast sodium channels in their membranes (see below).

Two processes terminate depolarization:

1. the fast sodium channels close after only a few milliseconds
2. a set of voltage-sensitive potassium channels opens, allowing potassium ions to leave the cell down their concentration gradient (Fig. 6.2.2: phase 1).

These two factors cause the membrane potential to start to become more negative, but repolarization is interrupted by the plateau phase of the action potential.

Plateau phase

The plateau phase is a feature unique to the cardiac action potential. It is caused by a second inward current, the **calcium current** i_{Ca}. Depolarization caused by the inward sodium current increases the membrane permeability to calcium ions by opening a set of calcium-selective ion channels, the L-type calcium channels. These allow calcium ions to enter the cell down their concentration gradient (Fig. 6.2.2: phase 2). They remain open for 150–400 ms and determine the length of the plateau phase. Membrane potential during the plateau is relatively constant because the inward flow of calcium ions is balanced by an almost equal and opposite flow of potassium ions out of the cell.

Repolarization

The plateau phase is terminated by closure of the calcium channels and an increase in the

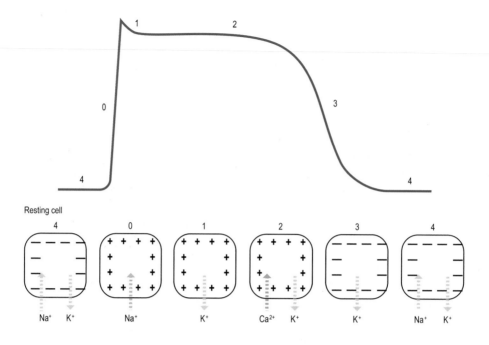

Fig. 6.2.2 **The principal ionic movements during the different phases of the action potential in a cardiac muscle cell.** The important difference between these ionic movements and those that produce the action potential in nerves and striated muscle is the involvement of Ca^{2+}.

outward potassium current. This net outward movement of positive charge returns the membrane to its resting potential (Fig. 6.2.2: phase 3).

Pacemaker activity of the sinoatrial node

Heart rate is determined by the rate at which cells in the **sinoatrial node** generate cardiac action potentials. The sinoatrial node is located in the posterior wall of the right atrium close to the junction with the superior vena cava (Fig. 6.2.3) and consists of a group of specialized small cardiac muscle cells, or myocytes, with few myofilaments.

Pacemaker potentials

Between action potentials, the membrane potential of SA node cells shows a slow depolarization, termed a **pacemaker potential** (Fig. 6.2.4).

When the membrane potential reaches threshold (about −40 mV) the next action potential is generated. Three ionic currents are believed to contribute to the pacemaker potential. Two currents bring positively charged ions into the cell and cause depolarization. The most important of these appears to be an inward current, the so-called 'funny' current (i_f) carried by sodium ions through specific sodium channels opened by repolarization of the membrane. Another inward current, i_{si}, carried mainly by calcium ions through T-type calcium channels makes a contribution during the final phase of the pacemaker potential. These currents are opposed initially by an outward potassium current i_K, which would tend to hyperpolarize the membrane, but as this decays with time, the membrane depolarizes towards threshold under the influence of the Na^+ and Ca^{2+} currents (Fig. 6.2.4).

The rate at which SA node cells generate action potentials is dependent on the rate

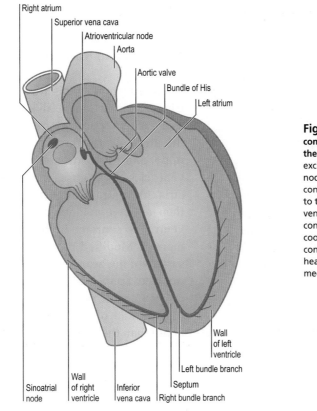

Right atrium

Superior vena cava

Atrioventricular node

Aorta

Aortic valve

Bundle of His

Left atrium

Fig. 6.2.3 The conducting system of the heart. By slowing excitation at the AV node and rapidly conducting excitation to the whole of the ventricles, the conducting system coordinates the contraction of the heart, making it mechanically efficient.

Sinoatrial node

Wall of right ventricle

Inferior vena cava

Right bundle branch

Septum

Left bundle branch

Wall of left ventricle

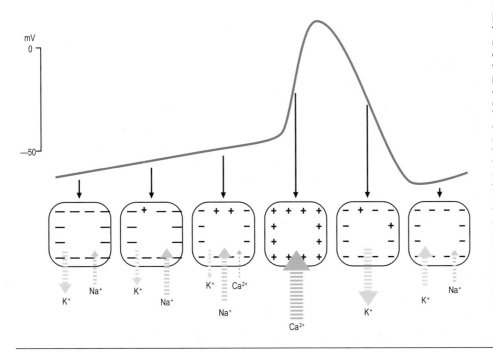

Fig. 6.2.4 The principal ionic movements contributing to the pacemaker potential and the action potential in an SA node cell. The 'leaky' nature of the membrane allows the potential to drift up to threshold where an action potential is triggered. The 'leakiness' and therefore rate of depolarization can be changed by hormones and neurotransmitters and is the mechanism by which the heart rate is controlled.

mV
0

−50

K^+ Na^+

K^+ Na^+

K^+ Ca^{2+} Na^+

Ca^{2+}

K^+

K^+ Na^+

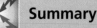

Summary

Cardiac muscle electrical activity

- Cardiac cells can be divided on an electrical basis into pacemaker, conducting system and contractile.
- The cardiac muscle action potential has a very long plateau because of a sustained inward Ca^{2+} current.
- The membrane potential of pacemaker cells rhythmically depolarizes to threshold and triggers an action potential because they have a 'leaky' membrane.

of depolarization of the pacemaker potential and in the absence of any influences from the autonomic nervous system, it is about 2 per second (100–120 beats/min). Cells at the centre of the SA node have the most rapidly changing pacemaker potentials and therefore the fastest rate of action potential generation. Cells from the peripheral regions of the SA node have less rapidly changing pacemaker potentials, but greater numbers of myofilaments. Thus there is a gradual transition in myocyte properties from the central SA nodal cells to the atrial muscle cells proper. A resting heart rate of about 70 beats per minute is dependent upon the 'braking' action the vagus nerve has on the rhythm of the central cells of the SA node (see p. 544).

The spread of excitation through the heart

Cardiac muscle cells are linked by low-resistance pathways associated with the gap junctions of the intercalated discs (see Fig. 6.2.12, p. 534). These enable an action potential in one cell to depolarize and generate action potentials within adjacent cells, which in turn activate

further cells. The combined effect of these individual cardiac action potentials is that a wave of excitation spreads outwards from the centre of the SA node to reach every cardiac muscle cell in the heart.

The function of this wave of excitation is to trigger contraction in all cardiac muscle cells. The excitation spreads relatively rapidly over the atria, slowly through the **atrioventricular node**, and then extremely rapidly through the ventricles. This causes the muscle cells in both atria to contract almost simultaneously, and then about one-tenth of a second later both ventricles contract in the same synchronous manner. Modified myocytes of the conduction system of the heart (Fig. 6.2.3) channel and control the spread of excitation by conducting cardiac action potentials either more rapidly (e.g. bundle of His) or more slowly (e.g. AV node) than the mass of cardiac muscle.

Atrial excitation

Within the atria the wave of excitation spreads from cell to cell at a speed of about 0.3 m/s. Four specialized bundles conduct more rapidly, at about 1.0 m/s, because they contain large Purkinje-like cells (see below). These bundles ensure that both atria contract as a whole. They also conduct the cardiac action potential to the atrioventricular (AV) node. Depolarization of the atria is normally complete within 0.1 s.

Delay at the atrioventricular node

At the AV node, the wave of depolarization passes from the atria to the bundle of His and through it to the ventricles. At all other points, the atria are separated and **insulated** from the ventricles by the ring of connective tissue that contains the valves of the heart. The function of the AV node is to delay the wave of excitation by about 0.1 s before it spreads to the ventricles. The length of the delay depends on the electrical state of the node (the prepotential) at the moment the wave of excitation arrives.

The node is located in the posterior portion of the atrial septum. It is formed by small modified myocytes with diameters of just 2–3 μm. Small cells conduct action potentials more slowly than large cells, and in the AV node the wave of excitation travels at only 0.05 m/s. The delay imposed by the AV node causes the ventricles to depolarize and contract 0.1–0.2 s after the atria. This delay provides time for atrial contraction to be complete and so augment ventricular filling. The length of the delay, determined by the slope of the prepotential, is regulated by sympathetic and vagal activity.

The cells of the AV node connect directly with the Purkinje fibres of the bundle of His.

The bundle of His and rapid ventricular excitation

The wave of excitation passes from the AV node to the ventricular muscle through the **bundle of His** and its branches (Fig. 6.2.3). This is formed from large myocytes, termed **Purkinje fibres**. The bundle of His divides into two major branches, the right and left bundle branches. The right bundle branch passes down the right side of the septum past the apex to supply the right ventricle. The thicker left bundle branch splits into the anterior and posterior fascicles, which course down the left side of the septum to supply the left ventricle.

The Purkinje fibres in these bundles, which are up to 80 μm in diameter and conduct action potentials very rapidly at up to 5 m/s, fan out over the surfaces of both ventricles. The wave of excitation therefore spreads very rapidly from the AV node to the main mass of ventricular muscle, where it is conducted more slowly at about 0.3–0.5 m/s. The first part of the ventricular wall to be depolarized is at the apex (the tip of the heart) and the last is those portions next to the atrioventricular groove. In the ventricular wall the excitation spreads from the epicardial to the endocardial surface, whilst in the interventricular septum it travels from left to right. The spread of the cardiac action potential through the ventricle is very rapid. Depolarization of the bundle of His and the Purkinje fibres is complete within 0.03 s and the last ventricular muscle depolarizes only 0.03 s later. The entire process lasts just 0.06 s.

Alternative pacemakers

The term **sinus rhythm** is used to indicate that the cardiac rhythm is being generated by the SA node. However, the SA node is not the only potential source of pacemaker activity within the heart. Both AV nodal cells and Purkinje fibres exhibit pacemaker potentials, but because the cells of the SA node generate action potentials at a faster rate, they generate cardiac rhythm and determine the heart rate. The heart is 'driven' by the fastest rate available at any time. The intrinsic rate of the AV node cells is about 40–50/min; that of Purkinje fibres is even slower, about 30–40/min. The existence of these alternative pacemakers only becomes apparent during pathological conditions. These alternative pacemakers exhibit electrical instability, which produces rhythms slower than the SA node because their cell membranes are less 'leaky' than those of the SA node (Fig. 6.2.4).

Myocardial cells, other than nodal and conducting tissues, do not normally show spontaneous activity, though occasionally a part of the atrium or ventricle may generate a spontaneous action potential out of phase with the normal sinus rhythm. The term **ectopic focus** describes the site from which it originates and the resulting heartbeat is an extra systole or premature contraction. **Fibrillation** occurs when a number of ectopic foci discharge out of phase with each other. Then some parts of the myocardium contract at the same time as others are relaxing, and coordinated contraction of the myocardium is lost. In ventricular fibrillation the ventricle looks as one would imagine a bag of writhing worms. The normal pumping action of the heart ceases and unless emergency treatment is given immediately, ventricular fibrillation is usually fatal.

Summary

Electrical excitation

- The cardiac rhythm is generated within the heart by cells of the SA node.
- The wave of excitation spreads across the atria from the SA to the AV node, where it is delayed, before conducting to the ventricles via the bundle of His.
- The Purkinje fibres of the ventricular conducting system ensure almost

synchronous depolarization of the ventricular muscle.
- The order of ventricular depolarization is septum (left to right), apex, and then base (endocardial surface first).
- Ventricular repolarization occurs in the opposite direction to depolarization because myocytes at the ventricular base have shorter action potentials than those at the apex.

Basic Science 6.2.1

Voltages, vectors and potential energy

Many investigations in physiology involve measuring voltages. Voltages are differences in electrical energy.

As with many other measurements, the way in which you make the measurement determines the result you get. This is particularly true in cases of electrophysiological measurement such as the electrocardiogram (ECG).

A voltage (*V*) is a measure of electrical potential energy, and potential energy is a measure of the potential to do work. If a battery registers no voltage between its terminals, then it can do no work.

Many forms of potential energy exist – a stone at the top of a hill may roll down, using up its potential energy in producing movement; the higher the hill, the greater the potential energy. Height of such a hill is shown on a map as contours, and so contour lines connect points of equal potential energy.

To exploit the potential energy of the stone in this way it must be free to move, and the stone

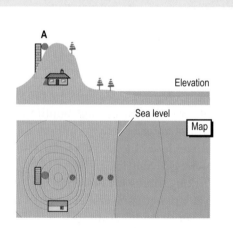

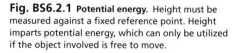

Fig. BS6.2.1 Potential energy. Height must be measured against a fixed reference point. Height imparts potential energy, which can only be utilized if the object involved is free to move.

at A in Figure BS6.2.1, prevented from moving by a wall, is 'insulated' from using its potential energy, just as electrical potential can be insulated, as we will see in a moment.

Basic Science *(Continued)*

Just as the height of a hill is measured against some agreed height (usually sea level), so voltages are frequently measured against an agreed potential (frequently but not invariably the earth). However, voltage, like height, can be measured between any two points, the only absolute requirement being that there must be *two* points to compare. The electrical difference between two points is called the potential difference and is measured in volts.

Measurement of potential difference between the two terminals of a battery requires attaching one lead of a voltmeter to one terminal and the other lead to the other terminal to make a complete circuit so that a tiny current can run through the meter, using up the potential energy to move the meter needle. The greater the potential difference (voltage), the greater is the movement of the needle. If only one lead is attached, there is no circuit and the two terminals are insulated from each other by the air gap. Like the stone on the hill behind the wall, the potential energy, although present, is blocked and cannot be measured. In electrophysiology, voltages are frequently measured against an 'indifferent electrode', which is generally a metal plate attached to the subject's body.

Just as contours round a hill mark points of equal height, so you could mark out points of equal potential round the terminal of a battery if it were surrounded by a conducting medium to carry the current.

If the ends of the two leads of a voltmeter were placed anywhere on the same 'contour' in Figure BS6.2.2, the meter would register 0 volts (O in the figure); with the leads between the two terminals it would register maximum volts (Max in the figure); and at other places an intermediate voltage would be recorded (V in the figure). In this situation, the magnitude of

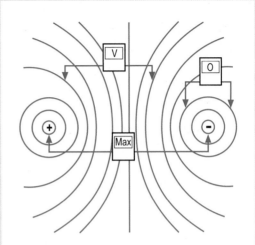

Fig. BS6.2.2 Electrical potential energy.
A charged battery has potential energy. Lines of equal potential can be drawn around its terminals. This potential energy can only be used if the terminals are not insulated from each other and when measured at different points has different values.

the voltage depends on the position at which you measure it, although the voltage of the battery is always the same. In all cases, to be able to make a measurement, you must measure between two points and there must be a complete circuit between the points and through the measuring instrument.

Phenomena that have different magnitudes depending on the direction in which you measure them are called vectors, and the electrical activity of the heart carried to the surface of the body by the conducting tissue fluid is an example of this and is called the ECG. The voltage measured in the ECG changes from second to second; in this case, however, it is not the leads that are moving to produce this effect but a wave of electrical depolarization moving over the heart.

The ECG

The **electrocardiogram** (ECG) is a record of the heart's electrical activity recorded from the surface of the body (Fig. 6.2.5). It is essentially the sum of all the cardiac action potentials of the individual myocytes. Depolarization and repolarization of any excitable tissue entail current flow through the cell membrane and the surrounding extracellular fluid (see Ch. 1.2). Body fluids are good conductors and so mass depolarization of cardiac muscle can be detected at the body surface (Fig. 6.2.6). The size of the signal at the body surface is proportional to the mass of tissue activated and, thus, that from the ventricles of the heart, which is relatively large, is approximately 1 mV. To record an ECG, it is important that the subject be relaxed, to prevent any electrical activity from contracting skeletal muscle obscuring that from the heart.

The ECG can provide a variety of clinical information about the heart, including heart rate and the source of the pacemaker. Various irregularities of the heart produce characteristic changes in the ECG.

The P, QRS and T waves

The ECG shows three main components during the cardiac cycle (Fig. 6.2.5). The first small upward deflection is the P wave. Then the QRS complex occurs. This is usually composed of three separate deflections, but all are not always present. If the first deflection is downward, then it is a Q wave, whilst any upward deflection is an R wave. Any deflection below the baseline following an R wave is an S wave. The last deflection is usually upward and is the T wave. In healthy individuals, a further upward deflection is sometimes present, the U wave.

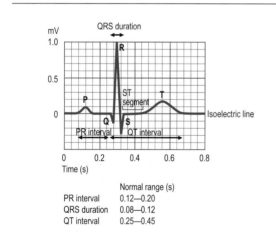

	Normal range (s)
PR interval	0.12—0.20
QRS duration	0.08—0.12
QT interval	0.25—0.45

Fig. 6.2.5 The waves of the ECG. The letters P, QRS and T have no significance in themselves, they are simply the letters chosen by Einthoven to label the various waves of the ECG when he first recorded it in its present form at the turn of the 19th century. ECG machines all run at a standard rate and use paper with standard squares. Each large square is equivalent to 0.2 s and each small square represents 0.04 s. So in this example the PR interval (from the start of P to the start of QRS) = 0.18 s, and the QT interval (from the start of QRS to the end of T) = 0.42 s.

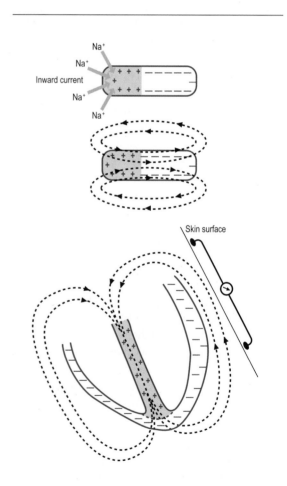

Fig. 6.2.6 Current flow around cardiac tissue. When cardiac cell membranes become permeable during excitation, Na$^+$ currents flow in down the potential difference, which can be detected on the surface of the body.

The P wave is caused by **depolarization** of the atria as the wave of excitation sweeps over them, the QRS complex by **ventricular depolarization** and the T wave by **ventricular repolarization**. The U wave is believed to be caused by slow repolarization of the papillary muscles (see p. 517). Atrial repolarization does produce a small signal but this occurs at the moment of ventricular depolarization and is normally obscured by the QRS complex. The ECG waves and their origin are described in more detail below, but it is important to realize that the ECG is a record of cardiac *action potentials* not contractile activity.

The relationship between the ECG and its source, the cardiac action potential in individual atrial and ventricular myocytes, is illustrated in Figure 6.2.7. It is important to recognize that the waves of the ECG only reflect the rate of depolarization and repolarization of cardiac muscle, and the direction that these events are moving in relation to the recording electrodes. They give little indication of the absolute magnitude of the membrane potential at any time. There is normally no signal in the ECG trace associated with the plateau phase of the cardiac action potential. The flat baseline between moments of depolarization and repolarization is referred to as the **isoelectric line**. This flat line might give the impression that all is electrically quiet within the heart. That is not necessarily so. All it means is that nothing is *changing*. For example, during the brief interval when the atria have depolarized and the action potential is being held up at the AV node before passing into the bundle of His, there is a considerable potential difference between the atria and the ventricles, but *it is not changing*. This is represented on the ECG as the isoelectric PR interval.

The flat isoelectric lines on the ECG that occur when potentials are not changing are the result of the design of the electronic circuits used to record the ECG. The electrical activity is said to be **AC coupled** to the recorder. AC recording is used to record changing

voltages because it ignores any unchanging (DC) voltages present that might interfere with the recording.

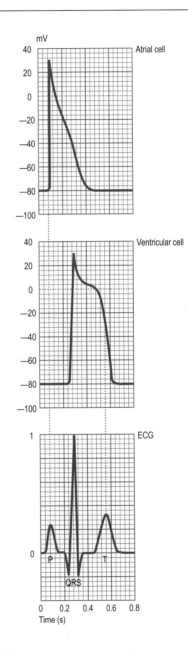

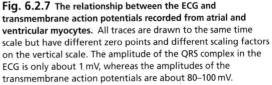

Fig. 6.2.7 The relationship between the ECG and transmembrane action potentials recorded from atrial and ventricular myocytes. All traces are drawn to the same time scale but have different zero points and different scaling factors on the vertical scale. The amplitude of the QRS complex in the ECG is only about 1 mV, whereas the amplitudes of the transmembrane action potentials are about 80–100 mV.

Amplitude and timing

The form of the ECG shown in Figure 6.2.5 is typical of that obtained when the recording is made between electrodes placed on the right arm and left leg (lead II; two electrodes make up one lead, see below). The maximum amplitude of the QRS complex measured from the peak of the R wave to the lowest point of the S wave is approximately 1.0 mV. The amplitude of the P wave is between 0.1–0.3 mV, whilst that of the T wave is from 0.2–0.3 mV.

The normal **PR interval** (so called even though it is measured from the beginning of the P wave to the *beginning* of the QRS complex; see Fig. 6.2.5) is 0.12–0.2 s, with the shorter intervals occurring at higher heart rates. During the PR interval, the cardiac action potential spreads over the **atria** and is delayed at the AV node. A PR interval of more than 0.2 s represents an excessive delay at the AV node, known as **heart block**.

The QRS complex normally lasts from 0.08–0.12 s; a QRS complex lasting more than 0.12 s is suggestive of a type of defect in the ventricular conducting system such that the wave of excitation is conducted by the muscle itself rather than via the more rapidly conducting Purkinje fibres. The ECG is normally isoelectric during the ST segment, i.e. at the same level as the section between the T wave and the next P wave. A **depression** of the ST segment below the baseline occurs if there is myocardial ischaemia – insufficient blood flow to the ventricular muscle. Ischaemia may also cause inversion of the T wave, as there is a pathological reversal of the potential difference between the damaged region and the rest of the heart.

Clinical Example

Heart block

Heart block is a condition in which the spread of depolarization through the AV node or bundle of His is abnormally slow. Normally, the interval between depolarization of the SA node and ventricular depolarization, i.e. the PR interval, is not greater than 0.2 s. About half of this (0.1 s) represents the delay at the AV node. In the simplest form of heart block shown in Figure CE6.2.1A, the PR interval is greater than 0.2 s but each P wave is followed by a QRS complex. This is first-degree block.

If the wave of depolarization sometimes fails to reach the ventricles, then the ventricles do not depolarize during those cardiac cycles. This can be recognized by the absence of a QRS complex and its subsequent T wave between two P waves. Patients can be aware of this and report that 'my heart missed a beat'. This is second-degree block (Fig. CE6.2.1B).

In third-degree (complete) heart block (Fig. CE6.2.1C), depolarization generated by the SA node fails to reach the ventricles. In this situation an alternative pacemaker within the Purkinje fibres of the ventricle generates cardiac action potentials at a rate of about 35 per minute.

There is no relationship between the P waves (arrowed) and the QRS complexes. The QRS complexes have an abnormal shape because ventricular depolarization spreads from the new pacemaker and not from the AV node.

The causes of heart block are various:

- ischaemia of the AV node resulting from coronary artery disease
- compression of the AV node or bundle of His by scar tissue
- electrolyte disturbances
- inflammation of the AV node in diphtheria or rheumatic fever

Clinical Example (Continued)

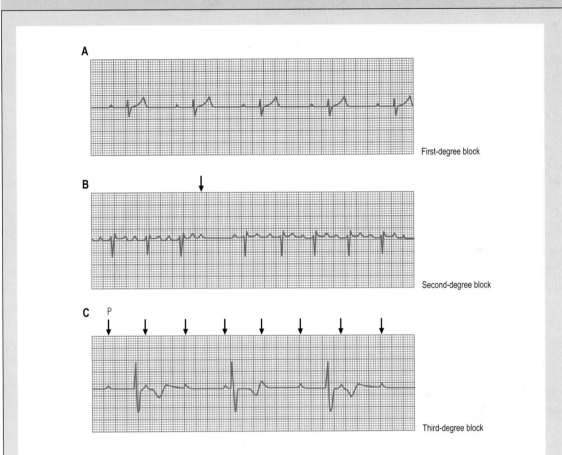

A

First-degree block

B

Second-degree block

C P

Third-degree block

Fig. CE6.2.1 Heart block. ECG traces showing: **A.** first-degree block; **B.** second-degree block; **C.** third-degree block. The P wave of missed beats is arrowed.

- myocardial infarction
- high levels of vagal efferent nerve activity.

Artificial pacemakers are frequently used to treat patients with heart block. Some modern pacemakers are so sophisticated that they detect heart rate and can be used in patients with an intermittent block, they 'step in' with a pulse only when needed.

Understanding the ECG

The concept of a **dipole** (two poles) is essential to the understanding of the changes in voltage that are the ECG. At any instant in the ventricle, there is a resting region that carries positive (+) charges on its surface and a depolarized region with negative (−) charges. These two 'clouds' of charges can be simplified into one positive and one negative charge – like the positive and negative poles of a battery. The voltage of this 'battery' has magnitude and direction (the way it is placed in the body). Things that have magnitude and direction are called **vectors** and their *apparent* magnitude depends on the direction from which you look at them. If you look at the end of a pencil, it looks quite short; turn it through 90° and it looks long (see Basic Science 6.2.1).

To complicate matters even further, in the heart, this dipole, made up of a positive and negative pole, is moving as depolarization spreads over the ventricles with each cycle. The dipole rotates once in an *anticlockwise* direction with each cardiac cycle.

With such a rotating object, the apparent size grows and shrinks with each rotation. Hold your pencil in front of your eyes and rotate it in a horizontal plane, it appears to get longer and shorter. The apparent size at a particular moment depends on the position of the observer. In the case of the ECG, the 'observer' is the electrode. An ECG of sorts can be recorded by placing electrodes at any point on the body surface, and the naming of the position of the leads for recording an ECG have no more significance than the fact that they are convenient and have been agreed by convention.

Thus the apparent magnitude of this **cardiac dipole**, measured on the surface of the body, will depend on the position of the electrodes used to measure it. Vectors (e.g. our dipole) are frequently represented by an arrow, whose length represents magnitude and whose orientation represents direction. The total amount of electrical activity in the ventricles changes as more or less muscle tissue is depolarized and, importantly for the picture seen on the ECG, as the dipole rotates its apparent size changes, depending on the direction from which it is 'viewed'.

Consider two sets of leads measuring the voltage of the cardiac dipole, which rotates in an anticlockwise direction through the cardiac cycle (Fig. 6.2.8). At any instant in a cardiac cycle, each pair is looking at the same electrical activity but because they have different 'points of view', what each records will be different,

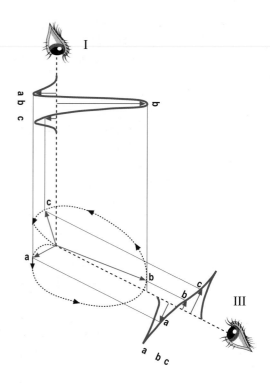

Fig. 6.2.8 The cardiac dipole. The electrical excitation of the ventricles can be considered as a dipole, which being a vector can be represented by an arrow whose length represents magnitude and orientation direction. The cardiac dipole voltage waxes and wanes as the ventricles become activated and then relax. The dipole also rotates in an anticlockwise direction as excitation passes over and through the ventricles. Because of this, the dipole appears to have a magnitude (voltage) that depends on the direction from which it is measured, and at any instant will appear different in different ECG leads.

The cardiac dipole completes one revolution with each ventricular cycle. The shape traced out in the diagram because of this and the growing and shrinking of the dipole voltage appear to many students to be the shape of the heart. This is purely coincidental; this shape is not an anatomical representation.

and the overall shape of the apparent electrical activity will be different (Fig. 6.2.8).

An ECG recording system is so arranged that when a wave of depolarization moves towards the recording electrode it produces an upward deflection of the trace and when it moves away it produces a downward deflection. Similarly, a wave of repolarization moving toward an electrode produces a downward deflection, whereas moving away it produces an upward deflection.

The size of deflection recorded depends on the mass of tissue depolarizing at that time, but also on the direction of movement of that depolarization.

In practice, by convention in electrocardiography, this means that an upward deflection of the trace indicates that the positive (+) pole of a potential difference is directed towards the left arm or leg.

Why are both the QRS complex and the T wave *upward* deflections in the ECG trace in Figure 6.2.5 when the first signal is caused by *depolarization* and the second by *repolarization*? The explanation is relatively simple: myocytes at the base of the ventricle nearest the atria have shorter action potentials than those at the apex, and also, at any level in the ventricles, myocytes in the epicardium have shorter APs than those in the endocardium. The result is that the base of the ventricle is the last portion to depolarize and the first to repolarize and the endocardium depolarizes before the epicardium (Fig. 6.2.9); therefore the wave of repolarization spreads through the ventricle in the opposite direction to depolarization.

In clinical practice, a standard set of electrode positions is employed and the ECG machine compares the electrical potential between these electrodes in different sets known as leads.

The limb leads

The standard bipolar (two electrode) leads record the potential difference between a pair of electrodes attached to the limbs in the following combinations:

- lead I – right arm and left arm
- lead II – right arm and left leg
- lead III – left arm and left leg

the second electrode position in each case being the recording electrode.

The same electrode positions on the limbs are used to form the **augmented unipolar (single) limb leads** (aVL, aVR and aVF). These leads reflect more clearly the activity of that

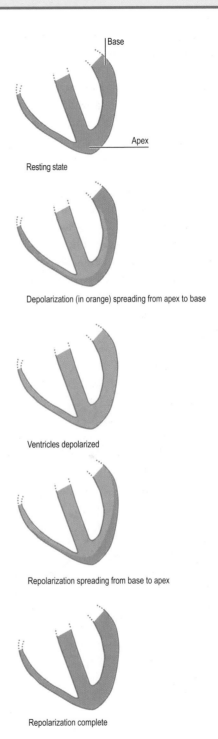

Fig. 6.2.9 The heart and thorax viewed from the front indicating the direction from which each of the limb leads 'looks' at the heart and the normal ECG in each of these leads. The arrow indicates the cardiac axis – the average direction of spread of depolarization in this vertical plane.

part of the heart facing the electrode. Thus, the lead attached to the right arm (aVR) is most affected by the cavity of the ventricles. The potential measured by each of these single leads is usually more amplified than that measured by the standard limb leads, and potentials are compared not to each other but to an electrical zero (since voltage has to be measured between two points) taken as the sum of the voltage at all three electrodes.

The standard limb leads 'look' at the heart in a vertical plane that passes through the head and sides of the body (Fig. 6.2.10A). They all examine the same events, depolarization and repolarization of the myocardium, but from different points of view.

The cardiac axis

Depolarization first arrives in the ventricles, via the bundle of His in the septum, and shortly after on the endocardial surface of the remainder of the ventricle. This results in the cardiac dipole of most people being oriented from about the 11 to the 5 o'clock position as shown by the arrow in Figure 6.2.10A. This wave of depolarization is moving towards lead II where it produces a predominantly upward QRS complex, on the trace, and away from aVR where it produces a downward QRS complex. The wave of atrial depolarization moves in a similar direction from the SA to the AV node, and hence the P wave is also upward in lead II.

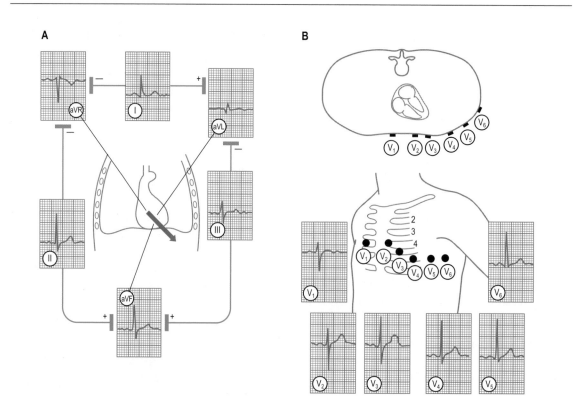

Fig. 6.2.10 The ECG recorded by limb and chest leads. A. The heart and thorax viewed from the front, showing the cardiac axis of depolarization as a broad arrow. The direction from which this is viewed by each unipolar augmented (a) limb lead results in the traces shown. The independent (reference) electrode for each 'a' lead is constructed by joining the other two leads to the negative terminal of the ECG machine through a 5000-ohm resistor. The polarity of the connection of standard bipolar leads I, II, and III to the ECG machine is shown. **B.** The positions of the chest lead, V_1–V_6, the directions from which they 'look' at the heart and the normal ECG in each of the chest leads.

The chest leads

The standard 12-lead clinical ECG comprises the six limb leads described above and six unipolar chest or **V leads**, numbered V_1 to V_6. The electrode positions for the V leads are arranged around the chest such that they 'look' at the heart in a horizontal plane (Fig. 6.2.10B). In V_1 the QRS complex is downward, whilst in V_6 it is upward. The two factors determining the shape of the QRS complex in the chest leads are:

1. The wave of depolarization in the ventricular septum, which, preceding depolarization of the ventricular wall, spreads from left to right.
2. The left ventricular wall is normally much thicker than the right and thus the signal recorded is mainly determined by the left ventricular wall.

The wave of depolarization spreading from left to right across the septum (Fig. 6.2.11A) is directed towards V_1 and thus produces an upward deflection (R wave), and away from V_6 where it produces a downward deflection (Q wave). The wave of depolarization then spreads through the ventricular wall moving both to the left and to the right, but because the left ventricular wall has a much larger muscle mass than the right ventricle, its signal more than outweighs that from the right. The net

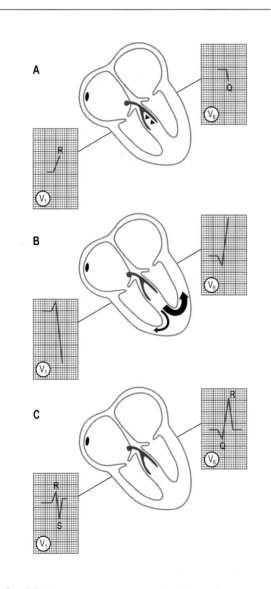

Fig. 6.2.11 Diagrammatic explanation of the different shapes of the QRS complex in the chest leads.

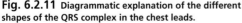

Summary

The ECG

- The ECG is a signal of the heart's electrical activity recorded from the surface of the body.
- Atrial depolarization causes the P wave.
- Ventricular depolarization causes the QRS complex.
- Ventricular repolarization causes the T wave.
- The six limb leads (I, II, III, aVR, aVL and aVF) 'look' at the heart in a vertical plane that passes through the sides of the body.
- The six chest or V leads (V_1–V_6) look at the heart in a horizontal plane.
- A wave of depolarization spreading towards a lead causes an upward deflection in the ECG.

wave of depolarization is thus to the left towards V_6, where it produces an upward deflection, and away from V_1, producing a downward deflection (Fig. 6.2.11B). When the whole of the myocardium is depolarized, the ECG returns to the baseline (Fig. 6.2.11C).

Clinical Example

Cardiac treadmill testing

When patients have difficulties with exercise, it is logical to test them during exercise as well as at rest. The cardiac treadmill is an example of such a test and is widely carried out for people with chest pain suggestive of myocardial ischaemia (inadequate circulation to the beating heart so that painful products of metabolism accumulate). It can also help in the evaluation of abnormal heart rhythms (experienced by patients as abnormal heart movements – palpitations) and heart failure. However, there are certain conditions where such a test would be unjustifiably dangerous and such conditions must be carefully excluded before the test is undertaken. Examples are severe hypertension (systolic pressure above 200 mmHg, diastolic above 100 mmHg) where the load on the heart would be excessive, and severe narrowing of the aortic valve at the outlet of the heart, or severe heart failure at rest where the ability of the heart to increase its output would be seriously impaired.

In preparation for the test, the patient has adhesive electrodes placed on the front of the chest to record, more or less, the usual 12-lead electrocardiogram. The arms and legs have to be kept free for movement, although a blood pressure cuff is placed on one arm to record blood pressure during the test. As the test progresses, the speed and inclination of the treadmill are increased, very gradually for a relatively frail patient and more quickly for someone without serious exercise limitation.

The electrocardiogram is recorded continuously and the blood pressure measured at intervals.

Information from the electrocardiogram is analysed automatically to display the situation of its ST segment. This segment is recorded during the plateau phase of the ventricular myocardium when there is little change in voltage across the membranes of the cardiac cells. The segment is normally isoelectric – it shows zero voltage and follows the same horizontal line as the segment between the P wave and the QRS complex, and, for a longer time, between the T wave and the next P wave. If the segment is slightly above (+1 mm) or slightly below (–1 mm) the isoelectric line, this is within normal limits. However, if the segment drops markedly below the line, this constitutes *ST depression* and is strong evidence that the myocardium is suffering at that moment from ischaemia. A value of –3 mm is taken as the threshold for definite ischaemia. Usually, a number of the leads recorded close to the myocardium (V_1–V_6) will show similar values. When a patient, at the same time, experiences the typical chest pain of cardiac ischaemia, the diagnosis is further reinforced. The importance of this finding is that the patient should then be investigated further, e.g. by visualizing the lumen of the coronary arteries radiologically, and, as necessary, have a procedure to reopen or bypass seriously narrowed vessels.

A further significant finding during the treadmill test is an abnormal rhythm, which may account for symptoms of palpitations and faintness during exercise.

Clinical Example *(Continued)*

The blood pressure measurements help to alert the observers to a serious rise in pressure, but, more importantly from a diagnostic point of view, they may reveal an abnormally low pressure, indicating cardiac failure. During dynamic exercise, such as on a treadmill, the normal heart must increase the force of its ejection of blood, and thus the systolic pressure rises. In a fit individual exercising strenuously, a systolic pressure of 200 mmHg would not be unusual. However, if the systolic pressure fails to rise, and particularly if it falls during exercise, this is strong evidence of cardiac weakness.

A striking feature of the test is that the most dramatic changes may occur in the *recovery period*, after the patient has stopped exercising.

The metabolic 'debts' of the exercise period continue to place a strong demand on the heart, and signs of ischaemia, abnormal rhythms and low blood pressure may appear and persist for a considerable time. This recovery effect is not unknown in normal athletes who have a big debt to repay after a maximal effort and may, in some cases, suffer a degree of post-exercise hypotension. In fact, the test is not without risk for the cardiac patient, but when the information is vital for management decisions, the risk must be taken. On the other hand, if someone has chest pain leading to anxieties about the heart, then the ability to exercise up to a high level without any abnormalities being detected is strongly reassuring.

The pumping heart

Structure of myocytes

Cardiac muscle cells (myocytes) are branching cylinders approximately 30–100 μm long and 10–20 μm in diameter. Each cell has a single central nucleus and is joined to neighbouring cells at its ends rather than its sides. There are many similarities between a myocyte and a skeletal muscle fibre but equally there are a number of crucial differences (see Table 2.1.1, p. 86). The regular arrangement of actin and myosin filaments into sarcomeres bounded by Z-lines gives the myocyte a striated appearance (Fig. 6.2.12). Neighbouring cells are separated at their ends by **intercalated disks**. The gap junction is a specialized region of the intercalated disk where the sarcolemmas (cell membranes) appear to fuse. It provides a pathway of low electrical resistance between adjacent cells. Abundant mitochondria, glycogen granules and lipid bodies within myocytes, together with a high capillary density outside the cells, reflect the myocytes' insatiable demand for energy.

A comparison of the properties of cardiac, smooth and skeletal muscle is made in Table 2.1.1 of the section on muscle (p. 86).

Excitation–contraction coupling

Two tubular systems in the myocyte provide a link between the electrical activity of the membrane and the shortening of the cell during contraction. **Transverse tubules** or T-tubules are formed by the sarcolemma where it invaginates the cell in the form of blind-ended tubes (similar to the hole you would produce if you pushed your finger into a piece of dough). The contents of the T-tubule are therefore in direct contact with extracellular fluid. Their function

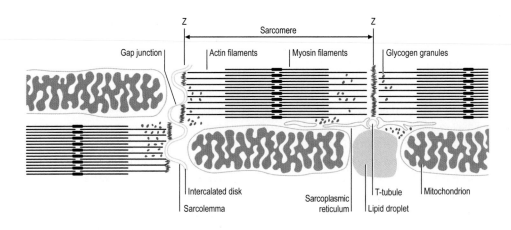

Fig. 6.2.12 The ultrastructure of cardiac muscle. Adjacent cells are joined at their ends by an intercalated disk featuring a gap junction. Much of the cell is occupied by mitochondria. Note the T-tubule at the Z-line and the associated sarcoplasmic reticulum.

is to convey the action potential (that we will see later is the trigger to contraction) to the innermost portions of the cell. There is normally one T-tubule per sarcomere located at the Z-line (Fig. 6.2.12). T-tubules are prominent in ventricular myocytes but poorly developed or absent in atrial muscle, probably because atrial myocytes are thinner than ventricular myocytes.

T-tubules are closely associated with a second tubular system, the **sarcoplasmic reticulum**. This is a closed system of branching tubes within the cell, which courses between the sarcomeres. Close contact with the T-tubules is marked by a flattening of the sarcoplasmic reticulum into sacs termed sarcoplasmic cisternae, though the contents of the two systems cannot mix. The function of the sarcoplasmic reticulum is to act as an internal store for calcium ions, which are an essential part of the excitation–contraction process.

Calcium – the key to contraction

Calcium ions are the key to contraction as they provide the essential link between depolarization of the cell membrane by the action potential spreading over its surface, and sarcomere shortening. The concentration of calcium ions

in a resting myocyte is about $0.1\,\text{pmol/l}$ ($< 10^{-7}\,\text{mol/l}$) but when the cell is depolarized by the action potential this can rise to between $1\text{–}10\,\mu\text{mol/l}$ ($> 10^{-6}\,\text{mol/l}$). The spread of depolarization along the sarcolemma and down the T-tubules initiates the inward calcium current and calcium ions enter the cell down both their concentration and electrical gradients. The calcium entering the cell during the action potential is sufficient to produce only a very small increase in the internal calcium concentration but it acts as a trigger to cause a release of more calcium from the sarcoplasmic reticulum, a calcium-induced calcium release. There may also be a depolarization-induced calcium release from the sarcoplasmic reticulum (Fig. 6.2.13). The importance of extracellular calcium in the contraction of cardiac muscle can be seen if calcium ions are removed from the extracellular fluid; contractile force declines to zero over a number of beats as the internal calcium stores are gradually depleted.

Contractile machinery

The mechanics of contraction in a myocyte are essentially the same as in a skeletal muscle fibre. Calcium binds to the troponin component

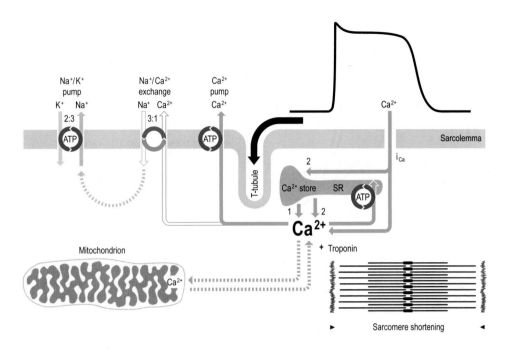

Fig. 6.2.13 Calcium movements during excitation–contraction coupling in cardiac muscle. The action potential triggers a rise in intracellular calcium through the inward calcium current i_{Ca} and both a depolarization-induced (1) and a calcium-induced (2) calcium release from sarcoplasmic reticulum (SR). The degree of sarcomere shortening is proportional to the intracellular concentration. Relaxation results from a lowering of intracellular calcium as it is pumped back into the SR or extruded through the sarcolemma, either by the Na+/Ca2+ exchange pump or to a lesser extent by the calcium pump.

of the tropomyosin complex on the actin filament. This alters the position of the tropomyosin such that it no longer blocks the myosin-binding site on the actin molecule. Crossbridges form and generate force causing the actin filaments to 'slide' between the myosin filaments when the sarcomere shortens (see Ch. 2.2).

The extent to which crossbridges form and generate force depends on the level of the intracellular calcium concentration during the plateau phase of the action potential. Contraction begins to occur at a concentration of approximately 1 µmol/l but the contractile apparatus is only fully activated at about 10 µmol/l. Factors that raise the intracellular calcium concentration increase the force generated, whilst those that lower intracellular calcium decrease the force (see Ch. 2.2).

Relaxation of cardiac muscle occurs during repolarization and is caused by a fall in intracellular calcium. Several factors are involved (Fig. 6.2.13). First, calcium entry into the cell stops as the inward calcium current ceases and release of calcium by the sarcoplasmic reticulum stops. Secondly, calcium is actively removed from the cytoplasm of the cell. An ATP-dependent **calcium pump** returns calcium to the sarcoplasmic reticulum against its concentration gradient in readiness for the next contraction. Calcium is also extruded from the cell by an Na+/Ca2+ exchange pump. The energy to move each calcium ion out of the cell is provided by the entry of three sodium ions. The sodium ions are in turn removed from the cell by the Na+/K+ pump. Some calcium is removed from the cell by a sarcolemmal Ca2+ pump. Mitochondria also serve as internal

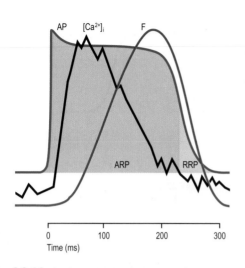

Fig. 6.2.14 The time-course and sequence of events in excitation–contraction coupling. AP, the action potential; $[Ca^{2+}]_i$, the intracellular calcium concentration as indicated by light emission from the calcium-sensitive photoprotein aequorin; F, the force generated. The refractory period (shaded area) lasts almost as long as the mechanical response: ARP absolute refractory period; RRP relative refractory period.

Summary

Myocytes

- Myocytes have low-resistance gap junctions connecting them electrically.
- T-tubules conduct the cardiac action potential deep into the myocytes, where it releases Ca^{2+} from the cisternae of the sarcoplasmic reticulum.
- Influx of Ca^{2+} during the action potential triggers Ca^{2+} release from the cisternae.
- The twitch of a myocyte is about the same duration as the cardiac action potential. Therefore cardiac muscle cannot make a tetanic contraction.

calcium stores but the kinetics of uptake and release are believed to be too slow to be of importance in excitation–contraction coupling.

Twitch contraction

The contraction of cardiac muscle reaches a peak at the end of the plateau phase of the action potential and lasts only fractionally longer than the action potential (Fig. 6.2.14). Cardiac muscle can produce a series of twitches, but it cannot produce a tetanic (or fused) contraction (see p. 100) because of its long refractory period. Once an action potential has been initiated in a muscle cell, it is not possible to initiate another until at least halfway through repolarization, i.e. the membrane is absolutely **refractory**. The relative refractory period lasts until repolarization is complete. It is possible, experimentally, to stimulate cardiac muscle during the relative refractory period. The action potential then produced is atypical and the

ensuing contraction greatly reduced. This type of situation only arises in pathological situations (see ectopic foci, p. 521). Tetanic contraction of cardiac muscle would of course be incompatible with the pumping action of the heart and would result in death.

Mechanical events of the cardiac cycle

Systole and diastole

Effective pumping of the heart is achieved through the contraction of atrial and ventricular muscle coordinated by the controlled spread of electrical activity from the SA node. Remember that the heart is in fact two pumps side by side and that during the cardiac cycle, events on one side of the heart are being carried out at the same time on the other side. The main difference is the greater pressure developed in the left heart. The phase of the cardiac cycle during which contraction occurs is referred to as systole and the phase of relaxation is termed diastole. In this chapter, these terms refer to

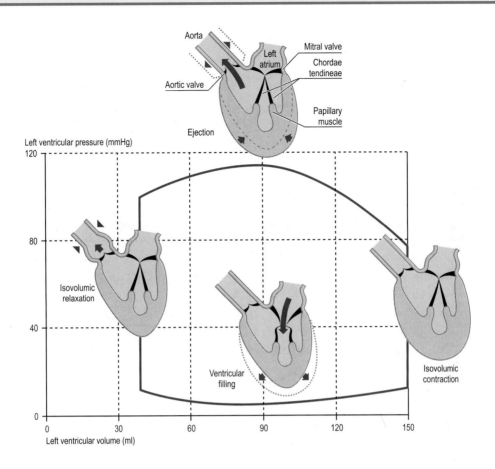

Fig. 6.2.15 The pressure–volume loop of a cardiac cycle. This figure plots the changes in left ventricular pressure and volume during a single cardiac cycle (follow it in an anticlockwise direction). The four sides of the loop represent the four phases of the cycle.

ventricular events, though of course there is also atrial systole and atrial diastole.

Each cardiac cycle can be broken down into four phases:

1. ventricular filling
2. isovolumic ventricular contraction
3. ejection
4. isovolumic ventricular relaxation.

Ventricular filling

The pulmonary and **aortic valves** (semilunar valves) are closed. The **tricuspid** and **mitral valves** (atrioventricular (AV) valves), which separate the atria from the ventricles, are open

(Fig. 6.2.15) because atrial pressure is greater than ventricular pressure. Blood flows from the venae cavae to fill the right atrium and right ventricle and from the pulmonary veins to fill the left atrium and left ventricle. Initially, the ventricles fill very rapidly following opening of the AV valves at the end of the previous cycle (Fig. 6.2.16). When heart rate is 75 beats/min (0.8 s between beats) diastole lasts almost 0.5 s.

Atrial depolarization, signalled by the P wave, triggers atrial contraction late in ventricular diastole. At resting heart rates, most of ventricular filling has already occurred and the contribution of the atria might seem superfluous. However, at higher heart rates when the duration

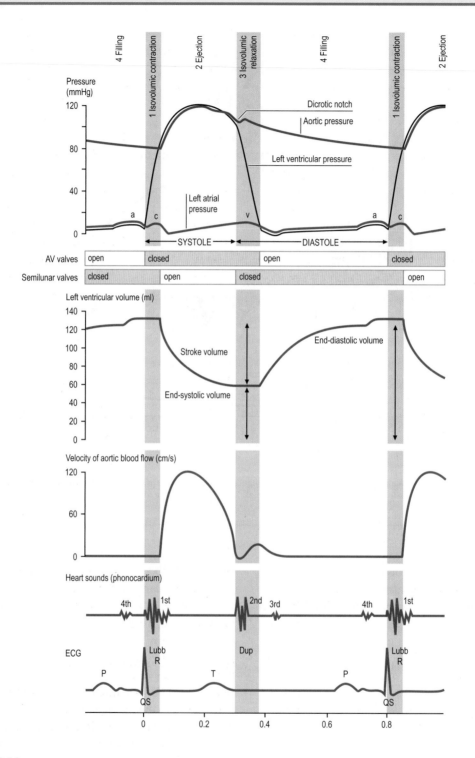

Fig. 6.2.16 The cardiac cycle and associated events.

of diastole is greatly reduced, atrial systole is believed to make an important contribution to ventricular filling. Although the atria lack inlet valves there is little regurgitation of blood into the venae cavae and pulmonary veins during atrial systole owing to the **momentum** of the blood flowing through the atria.

During diastole the volume of blood in the left ventricle of an adult increases from an end-systolic volume (ESV) about 60 ml to an end-diastolic volume (EDV) of approximately 130 ml. The maximum size of the heart during ventricular filling is limited by the **pericardium**. This fibrous sac completely encloses the heart and normally contains a small amount of fluid that acts as a lubricant.

Isovolumic ventricular contraction

Contraction of the ventricles is triggered by ventricular depolarization. Ventricular pressure begins to rise immediately, and the AV valves close as ventricular pressures exceed those in the atria. All four heart valves are now closed (Fig. 6.2.16), making the ventricles closed chambers. Fluids are not compressible and so the volume of the ventricles remains constant as pressure continues to rise, hence the term iso- (same) volumic contraction. The AV valves bulge back into the atria, creating the c wave on the atrial pressure trace, though this bulging is opposed by contraction of the papillary muscles. **Chordae tendineae** of the AV valves are attached to the papillary muscles. They act like guy ropes of a tent; when the papillary muscles contract, the chordae tendineae are pulled down, helping to prevent eversion of the valves. The isovolumic phase lasts about 0.05 s and ends when left and right ventricular pressures exceed pressures in the aorta and pulmonary artery respectively.

Ejection

The aortic and pulmonary valves open when pressure in the ventricles exceeds pressure in the aorta and pulmonary artery. This is usually around 80 mmHg for the aorta and 10 mmHg for the pulmonary artery. With the opening of the aortic valve, cardiac muscle can now shorten and blood flows rapidly into the aorta as ventricular pressure continues to rise towards a peak of 120 mmHg; peak right ventricular pressure is about 25 mmHg. The volume of the ventricle falls rapidly at first and then more slowly after the peak pressure is reached.

Before the peak systolic pressure is achieved, ventricular pressure exceeds aortic pressure. Towards the end of the ejection period, aortic pressure actually exceeds ventricular pressure because aortic wall tension rises as it reacts to being stretched by the blood leaving the ventricle. The momentum of the blood leaving the ventricle is initially sufficient to prevent any back flow but as the ventricle repolarizes and begins to relax, ventricular pressure falls more sharply, there is a slight reflux and the aortic valve closes.

The ejection phase lasts for about 0.25 s and during this time the volume of blood ejected from the left ventricle, referred to as the stroke volume, is about 70–90 ml.

These events are paralleled by events in the right ventricle.

The volume of blood at the end of systole, the end-systolic volume (ESV) is about 60 ml. The proportion of blood ejected from the ventricle in each beat is referred to as the **ejection fraction** and is a clinically useful index of cardiac performance. It is normally about 0.7 but can fall to 0.25 in a diseased heart.

Isovolumic ventricular relaxation

There is a fixed volume of blood in the ventricles once the aortic and pulmonary artery valves have closed; the ventricular muscle relaxes and ventricular pressure falls but the ventricle cannot fill, so the ventricular fibres cannot lengthen. The AV valves open about 0.08 s after the closure of the aortic and pulmonary valves when ventricular pressure falls below atrial pressure. The ventricular muscle continues to relax and can now lengthen as the ventricles again begin to fill with blood from the atria.

Atrial pressure and the jugular pulse

The pressure in the atria shows three peaks or waves during each cardiac cycle (Fig. 6.2.16):

- The **a wave** is produced by atrial systole.
- It is followed almost immediately by the **c wave**, caused by bulging of the AV valves into the atria at the start of ventricular systole.
- The third wave, the **v wave**, is produced by atrial filling and is terminated by opening of the AV valve.

These same three pressure waves can also be seen in the jugular veins of a recumbent subject because there are no valves between the jugular veins and the right atrium. Therefore, inspection of the jugular pulse can provide clinically useful information, e.g. in heart failure there is an elevation of right atrial pressure leading to a distension of the jugular veins.

Heart sounds

Two distinct heart sounds can normally be heard during each cardiac cycle. The first sound, 'lubb', is followed by a shorter sound, 'dup', and then by a pause before the sounds are repeated during the next cycle. The sounds are created by vibrations set up by the closure of the heart valves.

Closure of the AV valves at the start of ventricular systole generates the first sound (Fig. 6.2.16). This is best heard at the position of the apex beat in the fifth rib interspace. The second sound is generated when the semilunar valves close and is best heard in the third left interspace close to the sternum. If one of a pair of valves closes slightly ahead of the other, then a split sound with two components is heard. Delayed closure of the pulmonary valve, particularly during inspiration, creates a split second heart sound and is quite common in normal

healthy young people. Two more sounds may just be heard. A third sound occurs in the early phase of ventricular filling and a fourth sound coincides with atrial systole.

Turbulent blood flow resulting from a narrowed (stenosed) or leaky (incompetent) heart valve creates extra heart sounds, described as murmurs.

Cardiac output

The cardiac output is that volume of blood ejected by **one ventricle** in 1 minute. In an average resting adult male, this is about 5 l/min and, at a resting heart rate of 60–70 beats/min, this would be generated by a **stroke volume** of 70–80 ml/min. A change in cardiac output occurs even when a person moves from a lying to a standing position (down from 5 to 4 l/min) but the biggest changes occur during exercise. In an untrained individual it can increase to over 20 l/min and in a trained athlete to over 30 l/min. The various mechanisms that affect the performance of the heart and cause these changes in cardiac output are described below.

Measurement of cardiac output

Adolph Fick never measured cardiac output but he did describe the principle by which it can be measured, and that is why it is now known as the Fick principle. It states that the amount of a substance taken up from or secreted into the blood by an organ per unit time is equal to the difference between the arterial and venous concentrations of that substance multiplied by the blood flow through that organ. If the body is considered as a single organ, then cardiac output of the left ventricle can be calculated by measuring the oxygen consumption of the body together with the concentrations of oxygen in the blood entering and leaving the systemic circulation.

Oxygen consumption = (Arterial O_2 concentration – Venous O_2 concentration) × Cardiac output.

Oxygen consumption can be calculated from the oxygen content of a known volume of expired air collected over a given time. The oxygen content of arterial blood can be determined from an arterial blood sample. A sample of mixed venous blood must be taken from a catheter with its tip in the pulmonary artery because only here is the blood from various parts of the body sufficiently well mixed for the oxygen concentration to be uniform.

Typical values are:

- oxygen consumption = 250 ml/min
- arterial O_2 concentration = 195 ml/l
- mixed venous O_2 concentration = 145 ml/l.

Cardiac output = 250 ml/min ÷ (195 − 145)
= 250 ÷ 50 = 5 l/min.

The major limitations to this method are that it is slow, very invasive and that cardiac output can only be measured in the steady state.

Dilution methods enable cardiac output to be measured more rapidly over a period of about 20 s. A known quantity of a marker (dye or cold saline) is rapidly added to one point in the circulation, usually the right side of the heart via a systemic vein. Blood samples are taken from a point further on in the systemic circulation via a systemic artery. Cardiac output can be calculated from the mean concentration of the marker substance in these samples and the time it takes for the marker to pass the sampling point. Such techniques are still invasive and do not enable a beat-to-beat measurement of cardiac output.

Cardiac output can now be measured by a method based on the Doppler effect. Pulses of ultrasound are directed at the blood flowing down the long axis of the ascending aorta and reflected back to the probe by red cells in the blood (Fig. 6.2.17). The ejection of blood into the aorta during systole produces aortic flow and the velocity of the red cells increases the frequency of the sound returning to the probe by the Doppler effect. The change in the frequency of the ultrasound signal indicates the velocity of

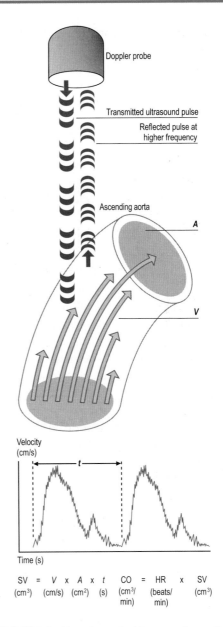

$$SV = V \times A \times t \qquad CO = HR \times SV$$
$$(cm^3) \ (cm/s) \ (cm^2) \ (s) \qquad (cm^3/\ \ (beats/\ \ (cm^3)$$
$$min) \qquad min)$$

Fig. 6.2.17 Pulsed Doppler method for measuring cardiac output. The Doppler probe, positioned at the suprasternal notch, measures the velocity of blood in the ascending aorta. Stroke volume (SV) is calculated from the mean velocity (*V*), the cross-sectional area (*A*) and the duration of the cardiac cycle (*t*). Cardiac output (CO) is the product of stroke volume and heart rate (HR).

blood in the aorta and, if the cross-sectional area of the aorta is measured by echocardiography, stroke volume and cardiac output may be calculated. The obvious advantages of this technique are that it is completely non-invasive and that it can follow beat-to-beat changes in output. However, it is not absolutely accurate because coronary blood flow is excluded and errors in measuring the diameter of the aorta can be large.

Summary

Mechanical events

- The cardiac cycle of systole and diastole can be further divided into four phases: ventricular filling, isovolumic contraction, ejection, isovolumic relaxation.
- The right and left heart contract synchronously.
- The heart sounds, *lubb–dup*, are the sounds of the closing of the AV and semilunar aortic valves respectively.
- Cardiac output is the volume of blood ejected from the left ventricle (and therefore the right ventricle) per minute.
- The Fick principle can be used to measure cardiac output.

Regulation of cardiac output

Controlling the pump

Like all physiological processes, the output of blood from the heart of an organism (cardiac output) is regulated. This endows the organism with the evolutionary advantage of economy of energy under a variety of conditions.

The ways in which the heart is regulated vary from species to species, and we will concentrate on the human condition. The heart as a pump has a number of characteristics in common with mechanical pumps, and several terms in common are used to describe them. The heart can be described as a reciprocating pump; that is, it goes through the same cycle of filling followed by emptying over and over again. It is also classed as a **demand pump**; it does not determine its own output but has it determined for it by demands of external factors.

The output of any reciprocating pump is quantitatively defined by the product of the volume ejected in each cycle (the stroke volume) and the number of cycles completed each second (rate). The rate at which the heart beats is a straightforward concept; stroke volume is slightly more complicated and is illustrated by Figure 6.2.18. The stroke volume of a ventricle of the heart is the difference between the

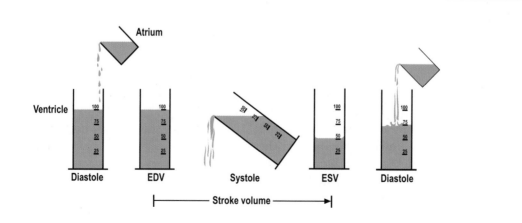

Fig. 6.2.18 Stroke volume. This is the volume ejected from a ventricle in one contraction. It is the difference between end-diastolic volume (EDV) and end-systolic volume (ESV) both of which can be changed.

volume it contains at the end of diastole (EDV) and the volume it contains at the end of systole (ESV). Both these volumes can vary between quite wide limits because the ventricles do not empty completely and can expand to a considerable degree.

Figure 6.2.19 illustrates diagrammatically some of the factors that determine EDV and ESV for the left ventricle. The output of the right ventricle is of course governed by the same principles, and this section will emphasize the important fact that the mechanisms that govern rate, EDV and ESV ensure that, except for very brief intervals, cardiac output (CO) is the same for both sides of the heart since:

CO = Heart rate × (EDV – ESV).

Apart from the venous and arterial pressures illustrated in Figure 6.2.19, which influence cardiac output, there are other factors, neural, humoral and thermal, that affect the functioning of the heart.

Autonomic nerve supply to the heart

The heart is not supplied by voluntary motor nerves but is profoundly influenced in both rate and force of contraction by the autonomic nervous system. Changes in rate (**chronotropic**) and force (**inotropic**) can be either increases or decreases. Increases from the normal rate (50–100 beats/min for adults) are known as **tachycardia**, whereas decreases in rate are **bradycardia**.

Preganglionic neurones of the parasympathetic supply to the heart originate in the nucleus ambiguus and dorsal nucleus of the vagus and run in the vagus nerve. These neurones synapse on the heart itself, and postganglionic fibres are restricted to the atria, particularly in the vicinity of the SA and AV nodes, with none in the ventricles. The effect of an increase in the activity the vagus on the AV node and SA node is to decrease the heart rate and the rate of conduction of the action potential at the AV node.

Sympathetic postganglionic fibres, on the other hand, originate in the paravertebral sympathetic ganglia from T1 to T5 and innervate all parts of the heart, including nodes, conducting system and ventricles. The effect of increase in sympathetic activity is to increase heart rate, shorten delay at the AV node and increase force of ventricular contraction.

The sympathetic and parasympathetic nervous systems exert diametrically opposite effects on the heart. Blocking both systems at the same time shows that the parasympathetic

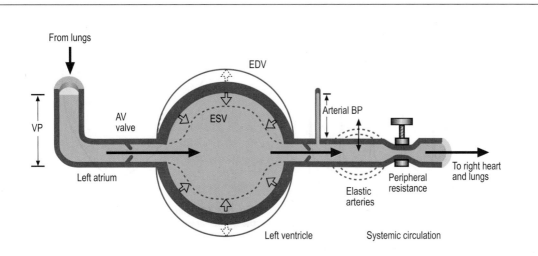

Fig. 6.2.19 A model of the left heart. This illustrates factors that influence EDV and ESV and hence stroke volume. Venous pressure (VP), which determines EDV, is known as central venous pressure (CVP) in the right side of the heart.

'**vagal brake**' normally dominates at rest because, during such a block, heart rate increases to about 100 beats/minute.

Parasympathetic effects

The neurotransmitter of the parasympathetic system is **acetylcholine** (ACh). In the heart, this acts upon M_1 muscarinic receptors, which via a chain of second messengers *inhibits* the formation of cyclic adenosine monophosphate (cAMP). cAMP activates channels that allow Na^+ and Ca^{2+} to leak into the cells (Fig. 6.2.2, p. 518). Reducing this leak reduces the rate of depolarization and the membrane potential takes longer to reach the threshold for triggering an action potential (Fig. 6.2.20).

A decrease in force of atrial contraction results because of reduction in Ca^{2+} current and inhibition of conduction at the AV node. A similar effect of vagal ACh is the opening of specific K^+ channels in the pacemaker (SA node) membrane. Potassium flows out of the cells and they become more hyperpolarized between action potentials. Being hyperpolarized, the membrane potential has 'further to go' to reach the threshold and depolarizes at a slower rate. This parasympathetic activity results in slowing of the rate of triggering of the SA node.

The increase of heart rate that takes place with each inspiration of breathing (sinus arrhythmia) and, more dramatically, the bradycardia of

fainting are due respectively to reduction and augmentation of vagal slowing of the heart.

Sympathetic and catecholamine effects

As might be expected from their antagonistic effects on other systems in the body, the parasympathetic system's slowing of the heart is mirrored by the sympathetic system, which speeds it up.

However, in line with its more extensive innervation of the heart, the sympathetic system, releasing **noradrenaline**, has more wide-ranging inotropic as well as chronotropic effects (Fig. 6.2.21).

These effects are similar to those produced by **adrenaline**, another catecholamine, secreted by the adrenal glands. The receptors responsible for the diverse actions of catecholamines on the heart are exclusively β_1 adrenoceptors, although some α receptors are present, and α receptors have a role in the control of the coronary circulation.

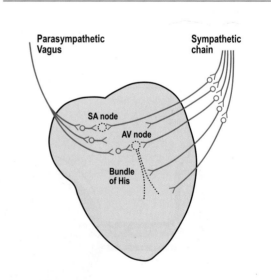

Fig. 6.2.21 Sympathetic and parasympathetic innervation of the heart. Parasympathetic innervation, restricted to the atria, only exerts a negative chronotropic effect, the 'vagal brake', slowing the heart. Sympathetic innervation, and circulating catecholamines exert a positive chronotropic effect on the nodes and bundle of His and, because they reach the ventricles, a positive inotropic effect.

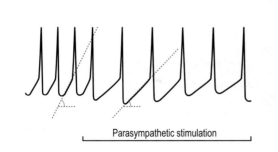

Parasympathetic stimulation

Fig. 6.2.20 Parasympathetic effects on the pacemaker. Acetylcholine secreted by the cardiac branch of the vagus nerve slows the rate of leak of the pacemaker cells, transiently hyperpolarizes them and by both mechanisms slows heart rate.

Whereas acetylcholine decreases the concentration of cAMP in cardiac cells, catecholamines increase it and therefore the inward Na^+ and Ca^{2+} currents. This is the common cause of the different effects of sympathetic stimulation, which include:

- Increase in rate of SA node firing – the inward pacemaker current is increased, and membrane potential therefore reaches the threshold to fire an action potential earlier.
- AV conduction is improved – there is an increased inward Ca^{2+} current and reduced AV node delay.
- Force of ventricular contraction is increased – this is because of increased Ca^{2+} entry and an increase in sensitivity of the contractile mechanism of the ventricular muscle to this extra Ca^{2+}.

The increased vigour of contraction produced by sympathetic stimulation can increase the fraction of end-diastolic volume that is ejected (**ejection fraction**) and the speed of ejection, which in turn shortens systole.

This increased contractility, together with increased filling, is an important contribution to the overall increase in cardiac output in exercise as we will see later.

The price to be paid for this increased activity is a decrease in efficiency and increase in oxygen demand. This reflects a shift in cardiac metabolism from using glucose to using fatty acids. Such an increased demand can be fatal to a heart whose oxygen supply is already compromised by coronary disease.

Reduction in sympathetic activity reduces all of these effects.

Temperature and potassium

Like all chemical reactions, the processes involved in the determination of pacemaker activity are temperature sensitive, increasing heart rate by about 10 beats per minute for every degree Centigrade rise in body temperature. This, in part, explains the tachycardia of fever. More sinister, and much more dangerous, are the changes brought about by changes in the concentration of **potassium** in the blood. These can result from renal failure, acidosis or the use of drugs such as diuretics. Because resting membrane potential depends largely on the difference in potassium concentration across cell membranes, changes in potassium concentration alter the resting potential of cardiac muscle and affect those channels in cardiac cell membranes that are voltage dependent. The overall result of an increase in K^+ concentration (hyperkalaemia) is to reduce the size and duration of action potentials. These puny action potentials are more easily blocked and do not allow sufficient calcium to enter the cells to ensure a vigorous contraction.

Paradoxically, plasma potassium levels may double during exercise, just when vigorous cardiac function is needed, but the heart is protected under these conditions by nerve-released noradrenaline and circulating catecholamines whose levels may increase 20 times to ensure the Ca^{2+} currents that increase contractility.

Summary

The heart as a pump

- CO = Heart rate × (EDV – ESV).
- Parasympathetic fibres innervate the atria; sympathetic fibres innervate the atria and ventricles.

- At rest, the vagal brake on heart rate dominates sympathetic activity.
- Temperature affects rate of depolarization of pacemakers.
- Increasing K^+ concentrations attenuate cardiac action potentials.

Filling and emptying pressures

Figure 6.2.19 represents the left ventricle as a hollow ball of muscle whose contraction ejects blood into the systemic circulation. This may be a gross oversimplification but it clearly identifies the two pressures:

- venous pressure (VP) filling the ventricle
- arterial blood pressure (BP) resisting the emptying of the ventricle

that are the most important hydraulic factors influencing the performance of the heart in terms of the force with which it contracts.

The fact that the force with which a ventricle contracts depends on the volume at which it begins that contraction was demonstrated in amphibian hearts more than 100 years ago. This observation was quickly taken up by Ernest Starling and applied to the *isolated* mammalian heart; that is, a heart taken out of the body, supplied with venous blood at controlled pressure and pumping against controlled resistance. Under these conditions, the heart was found to obey what has become known as **Starling's law of the heart**:

> *The energy of contraction of a cardiac muscle fibre, like that of a skeletal muscle fibre, is proportional to the initial fibre length.*

> Patterson, Piper & Starling (1914)

In other words, the more you stretch a ventricle (up to a commonsense limit of course) by increasing the incoming 'venous' pressure, the more vigorously it will contract.

The actual value of what is a 'commonsense' limit is of considerable clinical importance because it is frequently exceeded in heart disease.

Starling's law is of paramount importance in automatically balancing the outputs of the two sides of the heart. This is a very important task and the way the heart does it deserves our further attention.

Preload, afterload and fibre length

Starling and his colleagues drew attention to the similarity between cardiac and skeletal muscle. What is meant by **preloading** and **afterloading** of a muscle has already been illustrated in Figure 2.2.11 (p. 102).

The difference between functioning cardiac and skeletal muscle is that in the heart, preload is produced not by a weight as in Figure 2.2.11 but by venous pressure (VP) inside the cavity of the ventricle (see Fig. 6.2.19).

Pressure inside the heart or weight on the end of a skeletal muscle produces the same important effect on the skeletal or cardiac muscle fibres; it stretches them. We can therefore modify the experiment in Figure 2.2.11 into that shown in Figure 6.2.22 in which the initial length of a piece of cardiac muscle (represented by the level of the table and determined in real life by the filling pressure of the ventricle) is plotted against the tension it produces when stimulated.

The graph in Figure 6.2.22B shows the isometric tension that the cardiac muscle can produce, i.e. when the muscle cannot lift the *afterload*, which in the case of the intact heart is the arterial blood pressure against which the ventricle is trying to eject blood. This isometric tension is therefore developed in the second of the four phases of the cardiac cycle – isovolumic ventricular contraction – when the aortic and pulmonary valves are closed.

When the pressure in the ventricle exceeds that in the arteries and blood begins to be ejected through the opened valves, we see that the amount of shortening of the fibres depends on the initial length of the muscle as well as the afterload it has to work against. The longer its initial length, the further the muscle can shorten over a range of loads (Fig. 6.2.22C), which is Starling's law.

The explanation for the shape of the curve in Figure 6.2.22B has already been given for skeletal muscle and is illustrated more fully in Figure 2.2.7 (p. 96). The shape relates to the

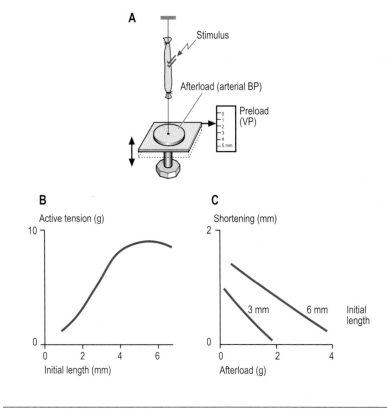

Fig. 6.2.22 **Preload and afterload of cardiac muscle. A.** The strip of cardiac muscle in the diagram is being preloaded (stretched before stimulation) by the level of the table carrying the afterload. The afterload is the weight the muscle has to lift when stimulated. **B.** Graph showing how the active tension that can be produced (afterload) increases as the muscle is increasingly preloaded (stretched) up to a certain limit; then the tension decreases. **C.** Graph showing that the amount the muscle can contract depends on both the afterload it has to lift and its length at the beginning of contraction.

overlap of actin and myosin filaments. When the muscle is below its optimum length, opposing actin filaments overlap each other or even buckle as they reach the end of their range of travel between the myosin filaments. When the muscle is stretched beyond its optimum length, on the other hand, fewer crossbridges are able to form.

In addition, in cardiac muscle, it seems that at moderate rest lengths and tensions all possible crossbridges are not activated by the influx of Ca^{2+} that brings about contraction, and stretching increases the number used. This is called '**length-dependent activation**'.

These effects combine in a heart taken out of the body as in Starling's experiments to give the relationship shown in Figure 6.2.23, if the load against which it is pumping is constant. This is called a **ventricular function curve** or **Starling curve**. In the ascending phase, the heart is said

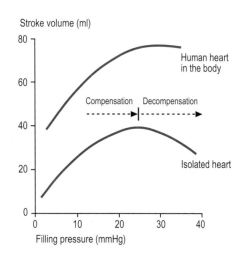

Fig. 6.2.23 **Ventricular function curves.** These are graphical representations of Starling's law that stretching cardiac muscle improves its contractility and therefore the stroke volume of the heart. The human heart in the body behaves in a slightly different way from a heart isolated from the body (which is at a disadvantage and so pumps with a reduced stroke volume), but the principle applies to both.

to **compensate** for increased venous pressure; the descending limb, where the heart is losing efficiency, is **decompensation**. The human heart in the body produces a differently shaped curve (see Fig. 6.2.23) with a long plateau due mainly to the toughness of human myocytes, which become very stiff and resistant to stretch when they reach their optimal extension. It may be that the healthy human heart in situ never reaches the decompensation phase.

Why is Starling's law important?

Reduced to its simplest form, one might restate Starling's law as 'the more blood the heart is presented, the harder/stronger it pumps'. This would lead one to associate this mechanism with the dramatic increase in cardiac output of exercise, but be careful; end-diastolic volume and filling pressure do not change much during exercise. Many additional physiological adaptations are involved in the cardiac response to exercise (see below). Nevertheless, Starling's law has a subtle and vital role – that of **matching** the cardiac outputs of the two ventricles of the heart and contributes to the increase in stroke volume that occurs in exercise.

The heart is clearly two separate pumping systems in series with each other, each pump associated with its own systemic (left side) or pulmonary (right side) circulation.

These circulations might contain 3.5 l and 1.5 l of blood respectively, and cardiac output could be 5.0 l per minute. Suppose that, suddenly, there were just a 1% greater cardiac output of the left heart than of the right heart. The situation would develop as shown in Table 6.2.1. In 30 minutes the pulmonary circulation would be completely empty, if death did not intervene long before that time was reached.

The wonderfully accurate degree of matching that actually occurs is the result of the mechanism described by Starling's law, which, by increasing force of contraction in response to extra stretch, ensures that any additional volume one ventricle receives is immediately passed on and not allowed to build up in either the systemic or pulmonary circulation.

The amazing accuracy of this mechanism can be gauged by imagining that in the example we have used above, the heart was beating 100 times per minute. Stroke volume should therefore be 50 ml. Could you fill beakers with water with an accuracy better than 1 ml at a rate of 100 per minute?

Stroke work

The simplest definition of physical work is the product of a force times the distance it moves its point of application (work = force × distance).

Table 6.2.1 The outcome of mismatching right and left ventricular outputs

Time (min)	Pulmonary circulation		Systemic circulation	
	Volume in circulation (l)	Output (l/min)	Volume in circulation (l)	Output (l/min)
0	1.5	5.05	3.5	5.0
1	1.45	5.05	3.55	5.0
5	1.25	5.05	3.75	5.0
10	1.0	5.05	4.0	5.0
20	0.5	5.05	4.5	5.0

In the case of the pumping heart, external work is the product of arterial blood pressure and the volume of blood ejected (work = pressure × volume ejected). This is external work, and the heart is still doing metabolic work during the isovolumic contraction phase when no blood is being ejected. The **stroke work** of a ventricle is of considerable clinical importance, particularly in a failing heart that may find itself being worked beyond its ability.

Stroke work is best understood by first considering a single stroke of the mechanical pump in Figure 6.2.24. The cylinder is separated from a vertical pipe filled with water by a one-way valve at C. The pressure in the cylinder must exceed the pressure in this pipe before C will open and allow water to be ejected from the cylinder. The relationship between pressure

and volume ejected is the rectangle shown in the figure (a rectangle because the system is rigid and cannot stretch). The work done is the area of the rectangle. For a flexible ventricle that actively changes its tension depending on how much it is stretched and pumps into an elastic system of arteries, the shape is more complicated than in the rigid case, but the principle still applies that the work done is the area inside the lines describing the relationship between pressure and volume.

At 'A' the AV valve opens and the ventricle fills until at 'B' systole begins and increased pressure closes the AV valve. From 'B' to 'C' there is isovolumic contraction until the arterial valves open at 'C'. Ejection takes place until 'D' when isovolumic relaxation takes place until the cycle starts again.

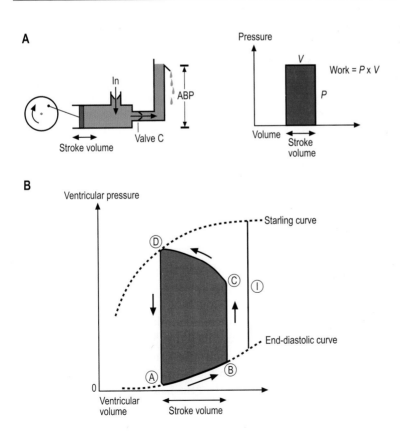

Fig. 6.2.24 Stroke work. The external work of a pump in a single cycle = volume of fluid ejected × pressure against which it is ejected. **A.** The mechanical pump must exceed the pressure (ABP) exerted by the column of water before it can eject its stroke volume and do external work. The work it does in this case is the area of the rectangle = $V \times P$. **B.** The pressure in the ventricle is outlined by the filling pressure (CVP) and the maximum pressure the ventricle can generate at a particular volume (the Starling curve). If arterial pressure is so high that it exceeds this curve, all the ventricle can do is perform an isovolumic contraction (line I), which uses up biological energy but does no useful external work ($V = 0$ in the formula Work = $V \times P$). A normal cardiac cycle is described by the loop ABCD (see text for details) and the work done is the area inside the loop.

Summary

Filling and emptying pressures in the heart

- Preload of the ventricles is provided by venous pressure (VP).
- Afterload is provided by arterial blood pressure.
- 'The energy of contraction of a cardiac muscle fibre, like that of a skeletal muscle fibre, is proportional to the initial fibre length' (Starling's law).
- The mechanism underlying Starling's law is the degree of overlap of muscle filaments.
- Operation of Starling's law matches cardiac output from both sides of the heart.

What determines preload and afterload (CVP and BP)

Preload (CVP)

Preload, the initial stretching of the heart, is the result of a difference in pressure across the wall of the heart. This is a combination of negative pressure outside and positive pressure inside.

Intrathoracic pressure surrounding the heart is usually negative relative to atmospheric pressure. It becomes more negative during inspiration but transiently positive during cough or when lifting heavy weights. This negative intrathoracic pressure exerts an important effect in 'sucking' blood into the chest, while the lowering of the diaphragm increases abdominal pressure and helps to push blood in the abdominal veins into the thorax. This helps to increase venous return to the heart by what is sometimes known as the 'respiratory pump'.

Blood reaches the right heart at **central venous pressure** (CVP) and this pressure is raised slightly by the contraction of the right atrium, which helps filling of the right ventricle.

Blood volume and venous tone (the tension in the walls of the veins) determine pressure in the venous system. The walls of veins are thin and somewhat lacking in smooth muscle when compared to those of arteries, which can give the impression that venous tone is of little physiological consequence. What is forgotten is that the venous system is a low-pressure system and the **sympathetically innervated** smooth muscle, particularly of the skin and splanchnic circulation, is quite adequate to control the volume of the peripheral venous system. Changes in volume of the blood in these veins also alter CVP. As two-thirds of the circulating volume of blood is found in the venous system, this is where changes in blood volume produced by haemorrhage or dehydration exert a major effect.

Gravity and the skeletal muscle pump interact in such a way as to ensure that the venous pooling in the legs, produced by gravity, does not interfere too much with central venous pressure. The pumping action of the muscles of the legs on deep veins within them propels blood toward the heart. The phenomenon of soldiers fainting during long periods of standing at attention demonstrates the importance of this system.

Increased central venous pressure produced by these mechanisms increases the preload and therefore stretching of the ventricles, which helps to increase stroke volume by the mechanisms described by Starling's law. Increased central venous pressure also reduces the flow of blood from the peripheral to central veins, and any inability of the heart to pump the blood it is presented with results in a backing-up of blood in the venous system.

Afterload (BP)

This is the pressure in the arterial system that resists ventricular ejection.

Before the ventricles can begin to eject blood, the pressure inside them must exceed the pressure in the arterial system (point C in Figure 6.2.24). In the extreme case, pressure at point C can be so high that the ventricle cannot reach it and there is no ejection, just isovolumic contraction. In a heart isolated from the body, this situation is approached as arterial blood pressure is progressively raised and the volume ejected gets less and less. However, because less blood is ejected there is more left behind and because venous return continues to 'top up' this volume end-diastolic volume increases. By Starling's law this increases contractility, and stroke volume can increase back to normal provided arterial blood pressure is not too high.

When the heart is in the body, the situation is more complicated; however, Starling's law still operates, as just explained.

Excessively high blood pressure is the consequence of an excessively large cardiac output and/or too high peripheral resistance. Pressure-sensing arterial **baroreceptors** are activated and reflexly reduce sympathetic activity reducing peripheral resistance, cardiac contractility and therefore arterial blood pressure.

Bringing it all together

For convenience of learning, we have artificially divided influences on the performance of the ventricles of the heart into factors that are:

- Physical – CVP and arterial BP, which influence preload and afterload. These effects are described by Starling's law and, graphically, as ventricular function curves.
- Neural and humoral – sympathetic and parasympathetic inputs and circulating hormones, mainly adrenaline, which influence conduction of electrical activity through the heart and contractility.

The most dramatic neural effects on the contractility of myocardium are those of noradrenaline from the sympathetic nervous system (parasympathetic activity, circulating adrenaline and other hormones all have much smaller effects).

Sympathetic activity increases in exercise, stress (particularly haemorrhage) and when you get up from a horizontal or sitting position. This increased activity augments cardiac contractility, so causing a shift in the ventricular function curve (Fig. 6.2.25).

This interaction between neural and physical effects means that there is not one function curve relating CVP to stroke work and cardiac output but an infinite number depending on the level of sympathetic activity.

As with so many physiological systems, the controls of the heart do not act independently, except in those subjects who are unfortunate enough to fall into the hands of physiologists.

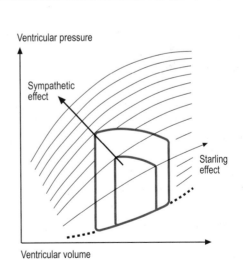

Fig. 6.2.25 Effect of sympathetic activity on ventricular function. Myocardial contractility determines the pressure a ventricle can produce. Contractility can be increased by stretching the ventricle (as described by the appropriate Starling curve) or by moving its operating conditions onto a higher one of the infinite number of these curves that exist. This happens during exercise, mainly as a result of catecholamine stimulation.

The integration of cardiac control is most dramatically seen in the response to vigorous exercise when the heart 'pulls out all the stops' to provide the exercising muscle with blood.

Exercise

Coordination of cardiac and peripheral mechanisms is most clearly seen in exercise.

At light levels of exercise, independence of inotropic and chronotropic mechanisms is seen; increased heart rate accounts for most of the increased output, with stroke volume hardly changing. As the intensity of exercise increases, increases in stroke volume begin to make a contribution. The amount that increased stroke volume can contribute to increase cardiac output largely depends on the resting stroke volume from which the exercise begins, which depends among other things upon posture.

The physical factors that affect CVP and arterial BP during exercise are largely effected by changes in the peripheral circulation. The neural and humoral factors bring about changes in rate and contractility.

Physical:
- The vascular resistance of muscle during dynamic exercise such as jogging or walking is reduced, limiting the rise in arterial blood pressure and therefore afterload.
- Muscle pumps and venoconstriction cause a slight rise in CVP.

Neural and humoral:
- Sympathetic activity to the heart and circulating catecholamines increase up to 20 times, improving contractility so that ejection fraction and stroke volume increase.
- Increased heart rate results from a combination of increased sympathetic and decreased parasympathetic activity.

It is important to remember that unless the cardiac mechanisms to increase cardiac output were coordinated with changes in the circulation, the cardiac changes that tend to increase output would be frustrated. For example, increased cardiac output without peripheral vasodilatation would cause an increase in arterial pressure that might limit the increased output.

Congestive heart failure

A physiological system affected by disease can often tell us a lot about how the system should work normally.

In congestive heart failure we see a heart that is **enlarged**, stretched ('the failing heart is an enlarged heart' is a clinical axiom), and stretching heart muscle generally improves its performance by moving the operating point along a Starling curve.

In congestive heart failure the heart is *congested*, it is over-filled with blood that the heart cannot get rid of. This blood backs up into the veins and increases CVP. This backing-up of blood, particularly in the veins of the neck, is used in the clinical diagnosis of congestive heart failure. The neck veins of the sitting subject, which are normally empty and collapsed, are filled to a level above the heart, which represents the increased CVP in patients with congestive heart failure.

Increased CVP – a good thing?

We have seen that in the normal heart, increasing CVP stretches the ventricles and moves their operating point to the right on the Starling curve (Fig. 6.2.23) and so increases stroke volume. This is 'a good thing' if the heart can compensate and eject the extra blood it is being presented with. However, if the myocardium is weakened in any way, the curve may be depressed, and stretching the heart may move it onto the plateau or even the decompensation part of the curve, 'a bad thing'.

The failing heart is embarrassed by overfilling because:

1. The slope of the Starling curve of failing myocardium is reduced and the myocardium does not respond so vigorously to stretch.

2. The response to adrenaline and noradrenaline is reduced, so the chronotropic response is reduced.
3. Increased diameter of the ventricles (by stretching) reduces the mechanical efficiency of the heart because the tension required to attain a given pressure in the ventricles is greater in an enlarged heart (as described by the Laplace relationship; Fig. 6.2.26).

Distortion produced by overfilling can become so great that it causes the AV valves to leak, further reducing the efficiency of the failing heart.

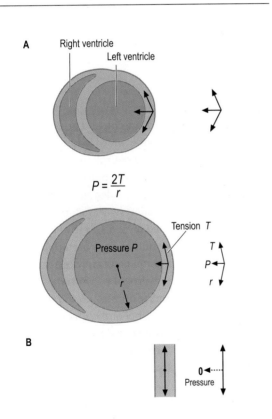

$$P = \frac{2T}{r}$$

A Right ventricle
Left ventricle

B

Tension *T*
Pressure *P*
r

T
P
r

0
Pressure

Fig. 6.2.26 Laplace and the failing heart. To develop the same pressure in a ventricle with a large radius as in a ventricle with a small one requires more tension in the wall, because less of the tension in the 'flatter' large radius is resolved towards the centre. The Laplace relationship ($P = 2T/r$) describes how pressure *P* and wall tension *T* are related in a vessel of radius *r*. If the radius becomes infinitely large (the wall would be flat), any amount of tension would not produce any pressure because 1/infinity = 0.

Congestive heart failure can be due to one or more recognizable conditions:

- high blood pressure may produce chronic overload
- the coronary blood supply may be reduced by artery disease
- myocardial infarction may reduce functional cardiac muscle mass.

In many other cases, however, the cause appears to be biochemical, with the defect being not in the production of energy (in the form of ATP) but in its use, both in the contractile process and, perhaps more importantly, in the transport of calcium, essential in the contraction process, into the sarcoplasmic reticulum.

Treatment of congestive heart failure addresses the three major physiological defects:

1. Cardiac distension is reduced by reducing plasma volume with diuretic drugs.
2. Contractility is improved by cardiac glycosides, although their effect is small (and use restricted nowadays) compared with other therapeutic interventions.
3. Cardiac work is reduced by reducing arterial resistance with vasodilators.

Summary

Bringing it all together

- Preload (CVP) is determined by blood volume, venous tone, gravity, respiratory and muscle pumps.
- Afterload (arterial BP) is determined by cardiac output and total peripheral resistance.
- The ventricular function curve in operation at any time depends on the level of sympathetic activity.
- The fundamental defect in congestive heart failure is the inability to eject the total venous return.

Clinical Example

Cardiomyopathy

In view of the unremitting demands made on it, the need to rapidly alter its output to meet changes in these demands, and its consequent need to rapidly synchronize electrical, physical and biomechanical variables, it is wonderful that the heart does not show more dysfunctional states than it does. Cardiomyopathies are diseases that primarily affect the myocardium. That is, they are not secondary to such cardiovascular disorders as coronary artery disease or valve dysfunction. Most are idiopathic (that is, their cause is unknown), and some are secondary to infection, proliferative disorders or nutritional problems.

Cardiomyopathies are categorized as restrictive, hypertrophic or dilated, terms that describe their pathophysiology.

Restrictive myopathy

This is typified by endomyocardial fibrosis, and usually results from infiltrative diseases of the myocardium, which make the ventricles less compliant and reduces filling. The clinical picture is similar to constrictive pericarditis, with congestive failure as the most common manifestation. There is no specific treatment except cardiac transplantation in severe and suitable cases.

Hypertrophic myopathy

This is best described by its alternative name, *asymmetric septal hypertrophy*. In some people there is a marked inherited tendency to hypertrophy of the ventricles, but particularly of the interventricular septum. This differential growth distorts the architecture of the heart, so beautifully designed to eject blood, and in some severe cases of extreme asymmetry the left ventricular output may be obstructed. Although pathologically powerful in its contraction, the thickened septum is less compliant than normal and diastolic relaxation and ventricular filling are impaired.

Patients present with angina, syncope (typically on exertion) and palpitations. The echocardiogram is diagnostic and treatment consists of treating possible arrhythmias from the disorganized growth of muscle. Surgical resection of the hypertrophic muscle is an option but many patients survive long term on pharmacological treatment.

Dilated myopathy

Sometimes called congestive myopathy, this consists of ventricular dilatation and grossly impaired systolic functions, which lead to heart failure with increased end-diastolic volume and reduced ejection fraction from both ventricles. The symptoms depend on the degree of right or left involvement and reflect heart failure. About half the cases of dilated myopathy are idiopathic; the remainder are a result of viral, bacterial or parasitic infection or autoimmune processes. Heavy consumption of alcohol is involved in a disproportionate number of cases, owing to the direct toxicity of alcohol or it metabolites, the nutritional defects associated with high alcohol intake and the cardiotoxic effects of many additives to alcoholic drinks. The good news is that the myocardial dysfunction can often be reversed if alcohol consumption is reduced or stopped.

The prognosis for other types is not so good and, despite treatment with glycosides, diuretics, corticosteroids and a salt-restricted diet, about 50% die within 2 years of presenting with symptoms.

Blood

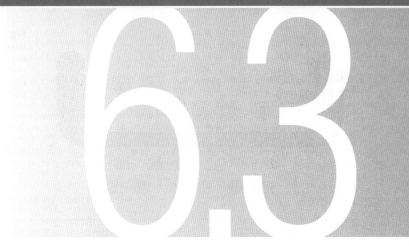

Introduction

Blood is a tissue, as important a tissue of the circulation as is the heart or blood vessels. It is made up of a solid phase of **formed elements** – cells and parts of cells – and a liquid phase – **plasma**. Invertebrates without a circulatory system have no 'blood', only tissue fluid or **lymph** (Latin *lympha* – clear water) surrounding and nourishing their cells. More complicated invertebrates, such as earthworms, have a simple circulation, the blood of which contains respiratory pigment in solution and wandering phagocytic cells. Animals like us with a closed circulatory system maintain a separation between blood and **tissue fluid**, which is formed by the process of filtration through the walls of the blood capillaries. This filtration is brought about by hydrostatic pressure. The filtrate is low in protein compared with blood (in man, tissue fluid has about one-tenth of the protein found in plasma) and is, in part, returned to the venous circulation in blind-ended vessels – the **lymphatics**. Most of the filtered fluid, however, returns to the capillaries by osmosis in a process that circulates the *total plasma volume* out of and back into the blood vessels about *five times a day* (Fig. 6.3.1).

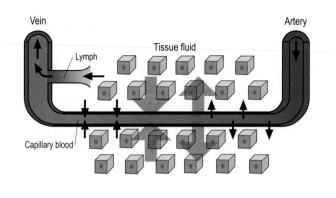

Vein

Artery

Lymph

Tissue fluid

Capillary blood

Fig. 6.3.1 Blood, tissue fluid and lymph. The relationship between blood, tissue fluid surrounding the cells, and lymph in an animal with a closed circulation. Exchange between the capillary blood and tissue fluid is by formation and reabsorption of tissue fluid and by diffusion into and out of the capillary.

The cells of our bodies require their surroundings to be maintained between well-defined limits if they are to function effectively (homeostasis provides this constant internal environment). The evolutionary advantage of a circulation is that it allows specialization of specific organs to control different aspects of our internal environment more efficiently. Specialization of organs brings with it the requirement for a circulation to ensure that the effects of the organs of homeostasis are dispersed throughout the body. This effect on our tissue fluids is only in small part due to the exchange of fluid between the capillaries and the tissue fluids already mentioned. Most of the exchange between blood and cells is the result of diffusion, augmented by facilitated and active mechanisms in the cell walls.

Our blood is a highly evolved tissue. Its importance to survival can be judged by the early stage at which the embryo begins to make its cells. These cells can be divided into red cells, **erythrocytes**, which should really be called **red blood corpuscles (RBCs)** because they do not have a nucleus, and white blood cells, **leukocytes**, and their products, e.g. **antibodies** and **platelets**.

The production of blood cells (haemopoiesis) begins in the embryonic yolk sac at 14 days, with the liver taking over in the second trimester and the bone marrow in the third. These organs mainly make red cells; in the embryo, white cells develop in the mesoderm and then migrate to the circulation.

After birth and for the first 4 years of independent life, the cavities of all bones contain red marrow, which is haemopoietic. Increasing numbers of fat cells appear in the bone cavities to form yellow bone marrow and by 25 years only the skull bones, scapulae, sternum, clavicles, vertebrae, pelvis, sacrum and the proximal ends of the femur and humerus are involved in haemopoiesis. In extrauterine life, white cells develop in the bone marrow with an involvement of the thymus, as we will see later.

Blood fractions

A rough picture of the composition of blood can be obtained simply by adding an anticoagulant to it to prevent clotting and leaving it to stand in a test tube.

The solid components slowly settle under gravity, and after some time the tube contains a layer of RBCs beneath a thinner **buffy coat** made up of white blood cells and platelets (Fig. 6.3.2). This process of settling can be accelerated by centrifuging the blood, and this is frequently done in haematology laboratories to discover the fraction of the total volume of blood occupied by red cells – the **haematocrit**.

After settling, RBCs are packed together at the bottom of the haematocrit tube (with about 5% of the space taken up by plasma between

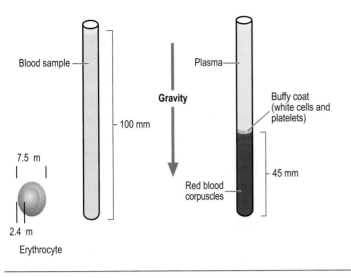

Blood sample

100 mm

7.5 m

2.4 m

Erythrocyte

Gravity

Plasma

Buffy coat
(white cells and
platelets)

Red blood
corpuscles

45 mm

Fig. 6.3.2 The fractions of blood (haematocrit).
If blood treated with an anticoagulant is left to
stand or centrifuged to mimic gravity, the red
corpuscles and white cells separate out. The
percentage of the original volume of blood
then occupied by the corpuscles is called the
haematocrit, in this case 45%. Erythrocytes are
biconcave disks about 7.5 μm in diameter and
2.4 μm thick at their rim.

the corpuscles). The normal haematocrit for men is 40–50%, and for women 35–40%. These figures represent 5.0–5.8×10^{12} and 4.1–5.2×10^{12} corpuscles per litre of whole blood respectively.

The RBC

The normal human erythrocyte is a circular, non-nucleated biconcave disk about 7.5 μm diameter and about 2.4 μm thick. This shape has the advantage over more spherical shapes of presenting a larger area for diffusion. This is particularly important in the case of oxygen, which is carried in the RBC. It enters by diffusion through the cell wall, as does carbon dioxide, whose hydration to carbonic acid (and the reverse reaction) is accelerated by the enzyme carbonic anhydrase carried within the RBC. The size and shape of different erythrocytes is far from constant even in the same individual, and an individual corpuscle changes shape dramatically as it is squeezed through capillaries.

The prime purpose of red corpuscles is to carry and protect haemoglobin, the oxygen carrier of blood (haemoglobin is described in detail on page 680). From this it might be thought that so long as the right amount of haemoglobin (155 g/l for men; 140 g/l for women) is present, it does not matter how it is

carried. This is not so. The size, viability and number of RBCs affect this function and so these factors are often measured in blood.

The number of RBCs per litre of blood (the **red cell count, RCC**) was at one time measured by accurately diluting a sample of blood and counting the number of corpuscles in a section of a tiny trough of known volume, an instrument known as a haemocytometer. This highly skilled technique is now, like so many others, displaced by an electronic device that counts individual corpuscles from a sample of known volume passing though a narrow orifice. Knowing the RCC and the amount of haemoglobin in a litre of blood enables the **mean corpuscular haemoglobin** (**MCH**) to be calculated.

Mean corpuscular volume (MCV), the size of individual corpuscles, is calculated by dividing the haematocrit by the RCC. This is an aid to differential diagnosis of the causes of anaemia when small, microcytic, or large, macrocytic, corpuscles may predominate.

The rate at which the corpuscles settle through the plasma is also of clinical significance and is reported as the **erythrocyte sedimentation rate (ESR)** by haematology laboratories (see Clinical Example: Erythrocyte sedimentation rate, p. 558).

Erythrocyte sedimentation rate (ESR)

Erythrocytes settle out of suspension in plasma during measurement of the haematocrit because they are slightly denser than plasma. The rate at which they settle out is called the erythrocyte sedimentation rate (ESR).

An object falling through a medium less dense than itself will reach a *terminal velocity* when the force of gravity causing it to fall is balanced by viscous drag from its surroundings. For a human being falling through air, a parachutist for example, terminal velocity is about 120 m.p.h. This can be altered by the parachutist changing his effective size by turning in the air and, hopefully, eventually increasing his effective size enormously by opening his parachute.

In the haematology laboratory, ESR is measured as the rate at which the upper surface of the cloud of erythrocytes in a tube of blood containing an anti-clotting agent falls with time. In blood from healthy men, the corpuscles will only have fallen 1–3 mm in an hour; in blood from healthy women, the fall will have been 4–7 mm in the same time. A fall of more than 20 mm is considered pathological.

The most usual cause of an increased ESR is the formation of **rouleaux** of red blood corpuscles. These rouleaux are like stacks of coins and they fall more quickly through the plasma than do the corpuscles that make them up.

Rouleaux formation does not take place to any great extent in normal blood except at low temperature or velocity of flow. It is generally the result of a change in the surface properties of the red corpuscles, which then tend to stick together. This change is brought about by an increased concentration of plasma proteins, the most important of which is fibrinogen, and some immunoglobulins. Increased ESR is therefore a measure of the acute phase response to a challenge that may be immunological, infective, ischaemic, traumatic or malignant.

ESR increases with age.

White blood cells (leukocytes) and platelets

The classification of leukocytes suffers from that common flaw in physiology – too many names for the same thing. But once it is recognized that the major group, granulocytes, is divided into neutrophils, basophils and eosinophils on the basis of their staining with neutral, basic and eosin histological dyes, all should be well (Fig. 6.3.3).

White blood cells make up a large part of the immune system, which protects the body from invasion by material that it recognizes as 'non-self'. This material may be living, parasites, bacteria, viruses (if you can count them as living), or non-living, for example a splinter of wood. The immune system recognizes molecules called **antigens**, which can be *self antigens* which are not normally attacked, or *non-self antigens* to which the immune system's **antibodies** attach themselves, damaging the antigen directly or labelling it for the attention of phagocytes and other defence mechanisms.

The activities of the immune system have become a vast subject, which we will only touch upon here, confining our description of its leukocytes to the following.

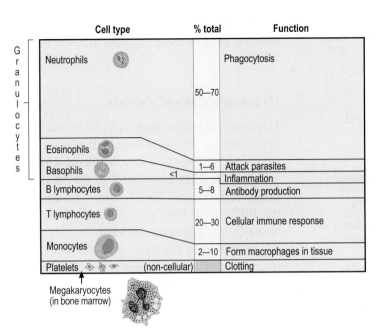

Fig. 6.3.3 Leukocytes. The types and functions of the blood-borne white cells. Numbers vary and are indicative of state of health. Platelets are fragments of megakaryocytes, which are found in bone marrow.

Granulocytes

Neutrophils. 50–70% of all leukocytes are neutrophils. They are phagocytic cells that engulf and digest bacteria and foreign matter.

Eosinophils. 5% of all leukocytes are eosinophils. They are particularly directed against parasites.

Basophils. 1% of all leukocytes are basophils. They release histamine and are involved in inflammation. They play the same role in the blood as mast cells do in the tissue.

Monocytes

1–10% of all leukocytes are monocytes. They can leave the bloodstream to become **macrophages** (big eaters), phagocytosing in the tissues and initiating and controlling specific immune responses. Macrophages play the important role of 'presenting' antigens to B lymphocytes

to 'instruct' the lymphocytes that the antigen is a foreign substance. Some macrophages become permanent residents in the lymph nodes.

Lymphocytes

20–40% of all leukocytes are lymphocytes. These come in two types from common **stem cells** in fetal bone and finish their development either in the bone itself (B lymphocytes) or in the thymus (T lymphocytes). This is why the thymus is large in young animals, while the system is being 'set up', but becomes smaller in later life (Fig. 6.3.4).

B lymphocytes (bone-marrow-formed lymphocytes). The B stands for bursa of Fabricius, which is found in chickens where these cells were first investigated. B lymphocytes act through chemical reactions rather than phagocytosis. They form antibodies that are immunoglobulins (gamma globulins). These act against

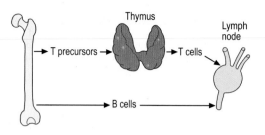

Fig. 6.3.4 B and T lymphocyte formation. Lymphocytes are found in large numbers in lymph nodes, where they proliferate. The original lymphocytes of these colonies originated in stem cells in the bone marrow of the fetus, which underwent differentiation there (B lymphocytes) or in the thymus (T lymphocytes) before being carried to the lymph nodes by the circulation.

substances that the body recognizes as 'non-self' – **non-self antigens**. Antibodies attack non-self antigens in three general ways:

- They **agglutinate** or stick together sites on the antigen. Thus bacteria that are recognized in this way are joined together like criminals on a chain gang.
- They make the offending antigen more obvious to phagocytic macrophages by a process of tagging called **opsonization** (the criminals on the chain gang are made more obvious by their striped suits).
- They activate the plasma **complement system** to attack the offending antigen directly or to respond with more general **inflammation**.

T lymphocytes (thymus-formed lymphocytes). These lymphocytes derive their name from the thymus, from where the various cells that make up the system migrate. Their precursors are found in bone marrow, like B lymphocytes, and they move to the thymus as the first step in their development. They do not secrete blood-borne antibodies like B lymphocytes, but under the complex control of other members of the T lymphocyte 'team', the **killer** and **natural**

killer T lymphocytes attack cells that have been infected by a virus or changed in some way, as in cancer.

Megakaryocytes and platelets

Megakaryocytes are giant cells restricted to the bone marrow. Platelets form within their cytoplasm and are released into the blood when the cell dies. Platelets are colourless spherical, oval or rod-shaped, and about 4 µm diameter. Like the RBCs, they have no nucleus but the presence of Golgi apparatus, extensive endoplasmic reticulum, dense granules, numerous enzymes, microtubules and filaments are all evidence of the platelet's ability to expend considerable energy.

The functions of platelets are:

- haemostasis – the arrest of bleeding (considered later in this section)
- phagocytosis – of viruses, immune system molecules and inert particles
- storage and transport – of 5-hydroxytryptamine (5-HT) and histamine.

Summary

Blood fractions and cells

- Human blood is a liquid tissue made up of formed elements (cells and parts of cells) and plasma.
- The haematocrit, the ratio of the volume of RBCs to the total volume of blood, is approximately 40%.
- RBCs contain the respiratory pigment haemoglobin and have no nucleus.
- White blood cells have specialized roles relating to phagocytosis and immunity.
- Platelets have no nucleus and carry out haemostasis, phagocytosis and carriage of histamine and 5-HT.

Haemopoiesis

The renewal of blood cells lost through ageing or the performance of their normal functions is by a process known as **haemopoiesis**. It results in a fairly steady state in terms of blood cell numbers.

Haemopoiesis in the adult takes place in the bone marrow and involves the development of all types of mature blood cells from pluripotent (having potential to develop into many types) **stem cells** by two processes:

- *differentiation and maturation*, which progressively develops the structure and function of specific cell types
- *proliferation* of a specific type to the numbers required.

Red blood cells complete almost all their development in red bone marrow, only the very last step being completed in the blood. White blood cells start their development in bone marrow but may complete their development there or in the lymph nodes.

The development of red blood corpuscles (**erythropoiesis**, Fig. 6.3.5) differs from that of white cells in that it involves the loss of the nucleus from red bone marrow normoblasts to form reticulocytes (so called because their RNA appears as a network), which enter the bloodstream and circulate as such for 1–2 days before becoming mature erythrocytes.

The production of red blood cells is at a rate that accurately replaces those lost through destruction – mainly in the spleen. Phagocytic cells of the reticuloendothelial system break down haemoglobin, and iron from the haem and amino acids from the globin are recycled. RBCs from the equivalent of 100 ml of whole blood are destroyed each day. The rate of replacement is governed by **erythropoietin** synthesized in the kidneys and is dependent on adequate supplies of iron, vitamin B_{12} and folate (the name of any derivative of folic acid). Erythropoietin production is stimulated by low local levels of O_2. RBCs have an average life span of 120 days.

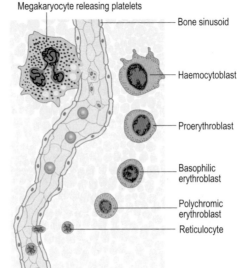

Megakaryocyte releasing platelets

Bone sinusoid

Haemocytoblast

Proerythroblast

Basophilic erythroblast

Polychromic erythroblast

Reticulocyte

Erythrocyte

Fig. 6.3.5 Erythropoiesis. Erythropoiesis takes place in red bone marrow. Haemocytoblasts can form any type of blood cell (they are pluripotent). They form, among other types, CFU-E (colony-forming-unit erythrocyte) cells, which produce large numbers of pro-erythroblasts that are destined to form erythrocytes. Reticulocytes push their way through the endothelium of the sinus to reach the bloodstream.

Functions of blood

This is an appropriate place to reiterate the point already stressed, that blood is of paramount importance in homeostasis. Although it makes little active contribution to homeostasis when compared to the lungs, liver and kidneys for example, it is the medium by which their contributions are brought into close contact with the individual cells. Homeostasis depends largely on the composition of plasma, which is in constant exchange with tissue fluid. Plasma is 90% water, absorbed from the gut. Most of its solid content is protein (8%) with the remaining 2% organic and inorganic substances (Table 6.3.1).

The functions of blood can be considered under the following headings.

Ionic and osmotic balance

Membrane potential and ionic composition of cells depend on the composition of tissue fluid.

Table 6.3.1	The composition of plasma
Constituent	**Proportion/concentration**
Water	92% of total volume
Proteins	7% of total volume
Albumin	31–55 g/l
Globulins	23–34 g/l
Fibrinogen	2–4 g/l
Other solutes	
Bicarbonate	21–27 mmol/l
Calcium	2.1–2.5 mmol/l
Chloride	95–103 mmol/l
Magnesium	0.7–1.3 mmol/l
Phosphate	0.9–1.3 mmol/l
Potassium	4.0–5.0 mmol/l
Sodium	135–142 mmol/l
Sulphate	83–125 μmol/l
Ions (total)	260–280 mmol/l
Cholesterol	3.5–6.5 mmol/l
Glucose	4.5–5.5 mmol/l
Iron	13–32 μmol/l
Urea	2.5–6.7 mmol/l
Uric acid	0.18–0.42 mmol/l

Ions pass rapidly from the blood into tissue fluid and must be in electrical balance in terms of the positive and negative charges present. There are about 300 mmol/l of both inorganic anions and cations in plasma, and for electrical neutrality half the total charge is on anions and half on cations. The **total** osmotic pressure that could be developed by plasma across a perfect semipermeable membrane is 8 atmospheres, 5280 mmHg (800 kPa) (see p. 21). Because the capillary walls are not perfect semipermeable membranes, only the proteins, mainly albumins and globulins, which cannot generally cross the walls, exert any osmotic effect. They create an **oncotic pressure** (osmotic pressure due to plasma proteins) of about 23 mmHg (3.3 kPa).

Nutrition and excretion

Plasma lipids and lipids bound to plasma proteins (lipoproteins), sugars (mainly glucose), amino acids, trace metals and other minor nutrients are delivered to the tissue fluid by the circulating plasma. Hormones controlling function arrive by this route and waste products of metabolism – nitrogenous waste to the kidney, bilirubin to the liver – are carried away.

Blood gases

Carriage of oxygen to and carbon dioxide away from the tissues is greatly augmented by the evolution of carrier systems in the blood, which are considered in Chapter 7.3.

Buffering

We obtain our energy by oxidative metabolism. The word oxygen means 'acid producer' and our homeostasis is under constant threat from production of acid. This acid is first buffered by the blood before being carried to the lungs and kidneys for removal. The mechanism of blood buffering is dealt with in Section 7 (p. 686).

Protection

Perhaps because of its ubiquitous nature, being found in almost all parts of the body, blood has evolved a formidable array of defences for the body.

Non-specific responses such as inflammation, activation of the complement system, and specific responses such as acquired immunity are all protective functions of the blood.

Heat

The enzyme systems of our bodies demand a fairly constant temperature if they are to work efficiently. Blood provides the 'coolant' that carries the excess heat of our metabolism to the 'radiator' of the skin.

Turgor

Fluid formation from the blood provides a large part of the 'tone', or firmness, of skin and other organs. Blood provides the hydraulic pressure to operate the erection of the penis.

Summary

Haemopoiesis and functions of the blood

- Formation of blood cells takes place from stem cells and is called haemopoiesis.
- All except the very last stage of RBC formation (erythropoiesis) take place in bone marrow.
- White cell formation begins in bone marrow and may be completed there or in the lymph nodes.
- Erythropoiesis is controlled by erythropoietin from the kidneys.
- Plasma exerts major homeostatic roles in ionic and osmotic balance, nutrition, buffering and physical support of tissues.

Haemostasis

The unique quality of blood being a liquid tissue brings with it the unique disadvantage that it may leak away. Of course, sophisticated checks are in place, which are aimed at preventing that unfortunate occurrence. The arrest of blood leakage is known as **haemostasis**.

Part, but not all of the mechanism involved is seen if blood in a container is allowed to clot. All materials that produce clotting and all blood cells are bound up in the clot. The clear fluid that remains is called **serum**.

Bleeding time

A skin prick will continue to bleed for a short time if each drop of blood formed is repeatedly wiped away. This is called the **bleeding time** and should be less than 5 minutes. Blood stops flowing, not because of clotting but owing to intense vasoconstriction, or spasm, of the small blood vessels in response to 5-HT released from platelets (see p. 560) and formation of a platelet plug.

Clotting

The mechanisms involved in the bleeding time are inadequate to deal with any but the most trivial haemorrhage. For more serious injury, more substantial interventions are needed. Clotting (coagulation) provides this intervention and clotting can be brought about by an *intrinsic* (plasma-based) pathway or an *extrinsic* (tissue-based) pathway, each of which is made up of many steps involving **clotting factors**, which have been given the Roman numerals I to XIII to identify them.

The intrinsic pathway

This involves factors within the blood and usually begins when vascular damage exposes tissue collagen to circulating platelets. They stick to the injury site and to each other forming a platelet plug. They release adenosine diphosphate (ADP) and thromboxane A_2 (a prostanoid), which increase platelet stickiness and bring about the adhesion of more platelets to the plug. The ADP causes the platelets joining the plug to flatten, send out processes (spicules) and express receptors for fibrin on their surface. This is a positive-feedback situation. All positive-feedback situations must have a mechanism to terminate them or they would run out of control (all circulating blood would clot in this case). In the circulation, prostacyclin, a prostaglandin released by the endothelium of the blood vessel (see p. 580), prevents platelets sticking to undamaged sites.

In the intrinsic pathway, the *Hageman factor* (factor XII) begins a cascade that ends in *prothrombin activator* and results in the conversion of *prothrombin* (factor II) into *thrombin* (Fig. 6.3.6). Thrombin converts soluble *fibrinogen* (factor I) in the plasma into long strands of insoluble *fibrin* by polymerization and ensures that the polymer does not re-dissolve by activating factor XIII (the *stabilizing factor*). Calcium is essential for many of the steps in this intrinsic pathway, and in the extrinsic pathway also (see below).

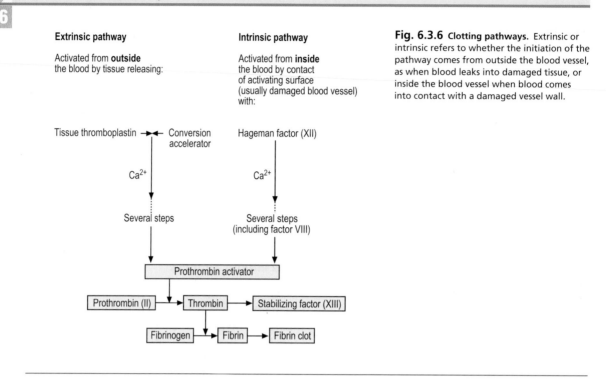

Extrinsic pathway

Activated from **outside**
the blood by tissue releasing:

Intrinsic pathway

Activated from **inside**
the blood by contact
of activating surface
(usually damaged blood vessel)
with:

Fig. 6.3.6 Clotting pathways. Extrinsic or intrinsic refers to whether the initiation of the pathway comes from outside the blood vessel, as when blood leaks into damaged tissue, or inside the blood vessel when blood comes into contact with a damaged vessel wall.

Tissue thromboplastin ▸◂ Conversion accelerator

Hageman factor (XII)

Ca^{2+}

Ca^{2+}

Several steps

Several steps
(including factor VIII)

Prothrombin activator

Prothrombin (II) — Thrombin — Stabilizing factor (XIII)

Fibrinogen ▸◂ Fibrin — Fibrin clot

The extrinsic pathway

This pathway is triggered by tissue damage, which causes the release of tissue *thromboplastin* (factor III). It combines with Ca^{2+} and *conversion accelerator* (factor VII) to form, via a number of steps, *prothrombin activator*, and from here the path is the same as in the intrinsic mechanism (Fig. 6.3.6).

The many steps in the process of clotting serve an important purpose; at each step, a single molecule of enzyme can produce many molecules of the factor that forms the next step. There is multiplication at every step. The disadvantage of a system with many steps is that there are many places at which the process can be disrupted. Defective clotting is known as **haemophilia**. There are several types of this disease, many of which are the result of defects in the genes for clotting factors, the most common of which is an absence of factor VIII (see Clinical Example: Haemophilia, p. 565).

Clot retraction and fibrinolysis

The final stage of haemostasis is retraction that solidifies the clot. The fibrin strands shorten and become denser and stronger. This shortening draws the edges of the wound together and is helped by the actinomyosin-like strands in the platelets, which also contract. Clot retraction begins within minutes of clot formation and is usually complete within an hour.

When the punctured blood vessel has healed or if a clot forms in an inappropriate part of the circulation, it must be removed. Breakdown of blood clots (fibrinolysis) is brought about by *plasmin* (fibrinolysin) a proteolytic enzyme activated during clotting by the Hageman factor (XII) and thrombin. Plasmin splits fibrin and fibrinogen into *fibrin degradation products*. It also digests clotting factors in plasma and so reduces the potential for further coagulation. The most important function of plasmin is the removal of the tiny clots that are continually forming and blocking tiny peripheral vessels, and which would eventually block the entire system if not dissolved.

Summary

Haemostasis

- Spasm of blood vessels is an important mechanism in the prevention of bleeding.
- The fluid left after plasma clots is called serum.

- Clotting can be brought about via an intrinsic (blood) or extrinsic (tissue) system.
- A clot solidifies by retraction and eventually dissolves by fibrinolysis.
- A deficit in the clotting cascade produces the condition haemophilia.

Clinical Example

Haemophilia

The pedigree of the descendants of Queen Victoria provides an excellent example of the sex-linked inheritance of a disease in an inbreeding population.

The Queen carried a defective gene for clotting factor VIII; this is expressed as haemophilia, mainly in males because the defective gene is on the X chromosome. Males have only one X chromosome and a Y chromosome, which only carries a few genes. The defective instruction to synthesize factor VIII is therefore the only one they have. Females have two X chromosomes and rarely inherit a defective gene on both. They therefore have a 'spare' set of genetic instructions on how to synthesize factor VIII,

a 50:50 chance of passing the disease to their sons and a 50:50 chance of passing their carrier status to their daughters.

One of the most famous haemophiliacs in recent times was Alexis, son of Tsar Nicholas of Russia and his wife Alexandra (who was Queen Victoria's grand-daughter), and heir to the throne. The 'mad monk' Grigoriy Rasputin was believed by Alexis' parents to be able to control his bleeding and Rasputin's malign influence over them because of this belief may have hastened the 1917 Russian revolution.

Haemophiliacs are now treated with transfusions of the missing clotting factor and the recent mapping of the human genome offers hope of genetically engineering this defect out of existence.

Immune responses

The immune defences of the body protect against foreign substances and organisms. The defences are generally classified as:

- specific or acquired immunity
- non-specific or innate immunity.

This division of the subject, like many others in physiology, may be counterproductive because these two systems have much in common. For example, the phagocytic cells of the non-specific system must first process antigens and 'present' them to other cells in the system before they can stimulate antibody production in lymphocytes of the specific system.

Specific immunity

We have already discussed those blood cells that form a large part of the specific immune system and observed that the detailed mechanisms of the system are the province of a textbook of immunology. Suffice it to say here that specific antibody-mediated responses protect against bacterial invasion and some viruses by a limited *primary response* to an antigen (Fig. 6.3.7). This is not particularly effective in dealing with the invading antigen because it takes some time to get under way. Its major function is to prepare the system for any further invasion by the same antigen by stimulating the production of **plasma cells,** which secrete antibody to immediately deal with the antigen, and **memory cells** specific to that antigen, which persist after the first exposure is passed. The immune system is made ready by this first exposure to mount a rapid and full-blown response.

Non-specific immunity

This form of immunity does not depend on previous exposure; it is innate against most foreign material and abnormal cells of the host itself (cancer cells for example). The mechanisms involved can be described as:

- inflammation
- the complement system
- natural killer cells.

Inflammation

Inflammation involves:

- increased blood flow
- increased vascular permeability
- phagocyte migration to the tissues.

All of these responses are stimulated by vasodilator substances such as *kinins* (in particular, bradykinin) and histamine from basophils and mast cells, and by prostaglandins.

The complement system

This is particularly directed to defend against bacterial invasion. The system consists of inactive precursors that are activated by proteolytic enzymes in a cascade, which, like other cascade

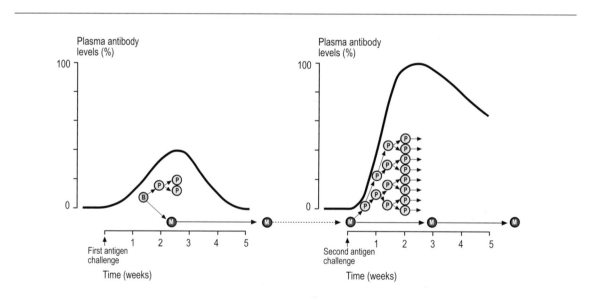

Fig. 6.3.7 Primary and secondary responses of specific immunity. On first exposure, B lymphocytes specific to a particular antigen are relatively slowly activated over a few weeks to proliferate into plasma cells, which produce antibody and memory cells. These provide a reservoir of lymphocytes that respond rapidly and powerfully to subsequent exposure to the same antigen.

systems, multiplies the number of molecules involved at each step. The system can be activated by the specific immune system (the *classical pathway*) or by the non-specific system (the *alternative pathway*). Both pathways end in the production of chemicals known as *complement fragments*, which promote phagocytosis, and a structure known as a *membrane attack complex* (Fig. 6.3.8). This is a ring of complement fragments that inserts itself into the membrane of invading cells, forming a large pore that causes the cell to lyse.

Natural killer cells

These make up less than 10% of blood lymphocytes but are able to identify and destroy cells infected with viruses or tumour cells without previously being exposed to them.

Blood groups

The recognition of an individual's cells as 'self' as opposed to 'non-self', which should be attacked, is brought about by major **histocompatibility antigens** on the surface of almost all cells. These are also known as **human leukocyte antigens (HLA)**.

Red blood corpuscles do not carry this system on their surface. In their case, three major types of antigens are produced by attaching specific oligosaccharides to protein molecules of the corpuscle membrane. The resulting antigen determines whether the blood is group **A**, **B**, or **O**. Group A antigen is obtained when *N*-acetyl galactosamine is attached to the cell membrane, and group B when galactose is attached. Group O carries only a precursor oligosaccharide (H).

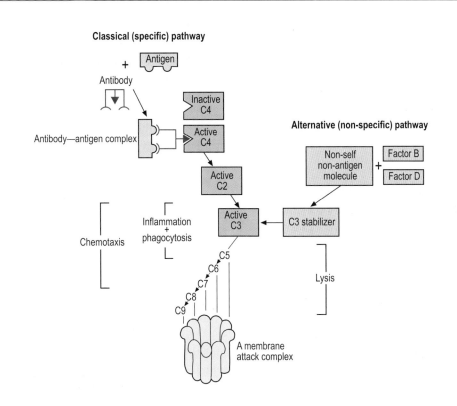

Fig. 6.3.8 The complement cascade. Activation of the cascade can be by the classical specific immune system or by the non-specific production of a C3-stabilizing combination of a non-antigenic but non-self molecule and factors B and D. Like all cascade systems, there is a multiplication of active molecules at each step, and these molecules cause inflammation, phagocytosis, chemotaxis and lysis of cells.

So, of the three blood groups, two can be considered as carrying potent antigens, while the third (O) is blank. You inherit one antigen from each of your parents, so six combinations are available, but since (O) is a blank, there are only four effective groups. In the blood plasma of each individual there is the antibody against the 'non-self' antigen (that is, the one not on the RBC). Thus, group A carries anti-B antibodies and group B carries anti-A antibodies. Group O carries antibodies against both A and B, and group AB has antibodies against neither. There are at least 12 other minor families of blood corpuscle antigens.

When the antigen system on RBCs is activated, the RBCs clump together – **agglutinate**. For this reason these antigens are sometimes known as **agglutinogens**, and the plasma antibodies that attack them **agglutinins**. Large-scale agglutination is a serious problem; the masses of RBCs form thrombi, blocking the circulation and breaking up to release haemoglobin, which damages the kidneys.

This is of considerable importance in transfusing blood, as can be illustrated by two cases of blood transfusion. In each case remember that it is the antibodies in the plasma that do the attacking if there is agglutination; the antigens on the RBCs are passive but offend by being 'non-self'.

- If the RBCs in the donated blood are incompatible with the patient's plasma, they are attacked by the patient's plasma antibodies, agglutinate and lyse, causing things to go terribly wrong. The whole power of the patient's immune system is available to back up the plasma antibodies in their attack.

- On the other hand, if the donated RBCs are compatible but the donated plasma attacks the patients RBCs, it does only a limited amount of damage because the amount of antibody in a litre or two of plasma in a transfusion is small, and

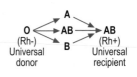

Fig. 6.3.9 The theoretical safe transfusion relationships between blood groups. The rhesus (Rh) antibody status is explained in the text.

the transfused blood cannot call on the body from which it was removed to 'back it up' in its attack.

For this reason it is theoretically possible to transfuse O blood into any recipient and for an AB subject to receive any blood group (Fig. 6.3.9).

In practice, this would be clinically indefensible except in dire emergency and **cross-matching** of the patient's plasma with the cells of the donor blood and the donor's plasma with the patient's cells is carried out.

The RBC antigens that determine blood groups are inherited, and racial differences are quite marked (Table 6.3.2).

The antibodies in plasma are something of a mystery. Antibodies arise as a result of being sensitized by exposure to an antigen. Yet even people who have never had a blood transfusion that would sensitize them have anti-A and/or anti-B antibodies in their plasma (unless they are blood group AB, which cannot by definition have either; see above). Why have these antibodies been formed when there has been no exposure to the antigen usually carried in 'non-self' blood? One theory is that early in our lives intestinal bacteria produce A and B antigens, which may sensitize us.

A second major antigenic factor in blood, the **rhesus factor (Rh)**, can be involved in sensitization.

The rhesus factor

Rhesus antigens (so called because they were discovered from experiments with rhesus monkey blood and not because of any simian traits in those who carry them) are of types C, D or E. Type D vastly predominates and is found on the RBCs of about 85% of Europeans (see Table 6.3.2). Such people are said to be rhesus positive (Rh+).

People without antigen D are rhesus negative (Rh–).

Rhesus-positive people recognize antigen D as 'self' and so do not mount an attack on it. If a rhesus-negative individual is transfused with positive (D-containing) blood, he will mount an immune attack on it, agglutinating it with all the unfortunate consequences already outlined.

A special situation exists where a Rh– mother is carrying a Rh+ baby (who has inherited the antigen D from its father). If some of the baby's RBCs get into the mother's bloodstream at the birth, owing to some rupture of the placenta, she will produce antibodies against antigen D. These antibodies are small immunoglobulins (IgG type) and will cross the placenta during subsequent pregnancies to attack any Rh+ baby in the womb. To prevent this, D-negative mothers are given an injection of anti-D antibodies shortly after the birth. These injected

Table 6.3.2 Racial distribution of blood groups as a percentage of total

Group	[Blood group]				Rh+
	A	B	AB	O	
English	45	8	3	44	83
Scots	34	11	3	52	80
Laplanders	59	16	5	20	98
Nigerians	24	21	3	52	95
Punjabis	21	40	8	31	93
Cantonese	24	26	6	44	99
Japanese	36	23	9	32	100
Native Australians	20	9	1	70	100
Native Americans	16	6	1	77	100
Eskimos	55	5	4	36	100

antibodies destroy any antigen-D in the mother before her immune system can be sensitized by it (Fig. 6.3.10).

This sort of problem does not occur with the A and B antigens on RBCs because the antibodies against these are large immunoglobulins (IgM type) and cannot cross the placenta from mother to baby.

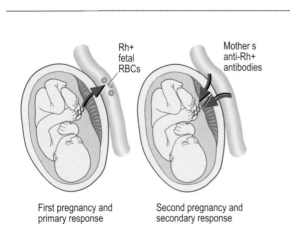

Rh+ fetal RBCs

Mother s anti-Rh+ antibodies

First pregnancy and primary response

Second pregnancy and secondary response

Fig. 6.3.10 Rhesus-negative mother with rhesus-positive baby. The mother may undergo primary sensitization late in pregnancy by the baby's RBCs getting into her bloodstream (usually too late for her immune system to attack the baby). Any subsequent Rh+ baby will be attacked by a powerful secondary reaction from the mother.

Summary

Immunity and blood groups

- Immunity can be specific (acquired) or non-specific (innate).
- Specific immunity depends on memory cells 'remembering' a previous exposure to a specific antigen.
- Non-specific immunity depends on inflammation, the complement system and natural killer cells.

- RBCs carry agglutinogens on their surface, which serve the same function as histocompatibility antigens on other cells.
- The matching plasma antibodies are agglutinins.
- Activation of the agglutinogen/agglutinin system causes agglutination (clumping) of RBCs.
- The main antigen systems on RBCs are the A, B, O system and the rhesus system.

Arterial vessels

Introduction

The general structure of blood vessels has been illustrated in Figure 6.1.3, in which the substantial thickness of the walls of arteries can be seen. These walls are so thick that diffusion of materials from the blood they contain is inadequate to sustain them, and they have their own small blood-vessel network, the **vasa vasorum**.

Structure almost invariably relates to function and the wall structure of arteries relates to their functional classification into **elastic arteries** and **conducting arteries**.

Elastic and conducting arteries

Elastic arteries are those closest to the heart; they have the largest diameter of lumen (1–2 cm) and are few in number. They are the aorta with its major branches and the pulmonary arterial trunk. These blood vessels function as pressure storage (**windkessel**) vessels.

Blood is ejected by the heart in an intermittent fashion (most of each stroke volume in the first third of the ventricular systole) and during diastole there is no flow out of the heart. If our blood vessels were rigid tubes, blood flow through the tissues would therefore stop during diastole and reach a peak during early systole, which is a metabolically and haemodynamically unsatisfactory situation. It is the function of the windkessel vessels to smooth out these pulsations so that flow is more uniform throughout the cardiac cycle. This they do by storing energy in their elastic walls to sustain flow, just like a balloon stores energy as you inflate it and can release that energy to drive out the air it contains when you release the neck. The elastic properties of these arteries are due to the protein elastin in their tunica media. This elastin is many times more easily stretched than rubber. Another protein, collagen, 100 times tougher than elastin, prevents the over-stretching of the artery wall.

Elastic arteries carry out an energy-storing role, and their elastic recoil is used to propel the blood on into the muscular arteries, which are the next stage in the circulation.

Muscular arteries, sometimes called **conduit** or **distributing arteries**, are narrower than elastic arteries (lumen diameter 0.1–1 cm); their tunica media is thicker relative to their diameter and contains more smooth muscle. This smooth muscle can carry out life-saving vaso-constriction, almost completely shutting off the lumen of these arteries if they are damaged. This powerful response can have its disadvantages; surgical trauma, during arterial blood collection for example, has been known to cause such an artery to shut down, cutting off circulation to the tissues it should be supplying.

Blood pressure

This ubiquitous term is usually meant to mean **systemic arterial blood pressure** (ABP) but, of course, the pulmonary circulation contains blood under pressure, although not as great a pressure as in the systemic circulation. It should also be remembered that the pressure in the arterial system is not constant in time, during one cardiac cycle or one lifetime, nor in terms of place in the circulation where it may be measured.

If we return to Figure 6.2.19 (p. 543), we can see all the factors that determine arterial blood pressure. Fortunately for our survival, but unfortunately for our understanding of the

system, these physical and physiological factors change from moment to moment.

Refreshing your memory on a few physical facts about fluids (liquids and gasses) will help the understanding of blood pressure. These physical facts are as follows:

1. Pressure at a point in a fluid is the same in all directions.
2. The deeper one goes in a fluid the greater the pressure (because of gravity).
3. Liquids are incompressible.
4. If no flow is taking place, the pressure at the same horizontal level anywhere in a liquid is the same.
5. If flow can take place, it will be from a region of high to a region of low pressure.
6. Moving fluid has momentum.

These facts are approximations but all we need to know about arterial blood pressure can be explained by using them with reference to Figure 6.2.19 (p. 543). That diagram shows us that the pressure in the large arteries at any instant (which is what we mean by arterial pressure) is determined by:

- the injection of blood into the system by the ventricle
- the elastic properties of the arteries 'upstream' from the outflow (the adjustable clamp in Fig. 6.2.19)
- the degree of resistance to flow offered by that clamp.

We can deal with these three factors in reverse order.

If the clamp were wide open, blood would flow easily from the heart and the 'high' pressure bringing about flow (physical fact 5, above) would not in fact be very high (it is easier to blow through a drainpipe than through a straw).

If the clamp were totally closed and the heart injecting a single pulse of fixed volume into the system, because liquids are incompressible (physical fact 3, above), pressure would depend on the compliance (ease of stretch) of the walls of the arteries (it takes more pressure to put a litre of air into a car tyre than into a child's balloon).

With the clamp partly open, as is the normal situation, pressure depends on the flow into the system from the heart (if you want greater flows through a straw you have to blow harder). If the clamp were totally closed, the *rate of rise* of pressure would depend on the rate of inflow – a rather specialized example of the general condition.

These three factors can be put together in a form we shall meet again in the section on Respiration (p. 663), where we consider airway resistance as equivalent to electrical resistance and restate Ohm's Law in terms of fluid flows as:

$$\text{Resistance} = \frac{\text{Pressure}}{\text{Flow}}.$$

In this case: Resistance is total peripheral resistance; Flow is cardiac output; and Pressure is arterial blood pressure. So:

Arterial blood pressure = Cardiac output × Total peripheral resistance.

Cardiac output has the units of flow (usually litres per second or litres per minute).

If we look at cardiac output at any *instant*, we see that it rises and falls through the cardiac cycle, reaching a peak in the first third of systole and falling to zero during diastole. This explains why pressure in the arteries rises and falls (but never to zero) through a cardiac cycle (Fig. 6.4.1).

The arterial pulse wave is defined in terms of its peak (**systolic pressure**) and its lowest point (**diastolic pressure**). **Pulse pressure** is the difference between these two. The energy stored in a pressurized system like the arteries is represented by the area under the pressure/time trace shown in Figure 6.4.1. The shape of these pressure/time curves is such that about half the area lies below a line one-third of the maximum above diastolic pressure (MP in Fig. 6.4.1). Therefore, average or **mean arterial pressure** is diastolic pressure + $1/3$ pulse pressure.

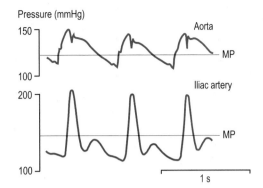

Fig. 6.4.1 Arterial pressure waves. Changes in pressure in the ascending aorta and iliac artery through two cardiac cycles: MP, mean pressure. The shape and height of the wave changes because of the different physical conditions at the two sites. Apparently paradoxically, the peak pressure is greater at the more distal site.

The observant reader will have noticed that the peak pressure in the iliac artery illustrated in Figure 6.4.1 is greater than in the aorta. Also, in Figure 6.1.2 on page 501, peak blood pressure rises in the arteries before falling in the arterioles. This seems to defy physical fact 5 (see above) that blood flows from regions of high to low pressure, but can be explained by the way pressure waves move through the arterial system.

Arterial pressure waves

Two-thirds of left ventricular stroke volume is ejected into the aorta in the first third of systole. This accounts for the initial rapid rise in the aortic pressure wave. The slight reflux of blood, terminated by the closing of the aortic valves, explains the initial falling pressure curve ending in the **dicrotic notch**. Pressure continues to fall during diastole as blood runs out of the elastic arteries through the peripheral resistance.

This sequence of events is very rapid, and the systems involved are not rigid tubes, which results in the pressure waves being more complex than, for example, the pressure developed in a slowly inflated balloon.

The wave of pressure developing in an artery during the cardiac cycle moves much more rapidly than the blood that produces it. That is because blood is incompressible (physical fact 3) and the tubes that contain it are elastic. The interaction of these two facts can be illustrated in the highly artificial situation of Figure 6.4.2. Here the aorta is considered in six segments. The ventricle injects its stroke volume into segment 1. That segment stretches to accommodate one-tenth of the volume. That stretching is not instantaneous and, even when fully stretched, nine-tenths of the volume passes on to the next segment, pushing the blood in that segment forward. Segment 2 does not accommodate the whole of the blood presented to it but instantaneously begins to displace blood from the next segment and so on. The key to the different rates of movement of blood and movement of

pressure in the arteries is that blood is incompressible while arteries are elastic. Taking two extreme cases illustrates the point. If segment 1 were infinitely compliant (easily stretched), it would accommodate all the blood without passing on any pressure to other segments. If segments 1–5 were rigid tubes, pressure would instantly be passed to segment 6.

Another example of elastic and non-elastic systems carrying waves at different speeds can be seen in a children's game played in New Zealand (and probably other countries with a forestry industry). One child listens at the end of a felled tree trunk while another taps the end of the trunk. The listener hears two taps, one almost instantaneously passed down the almost incompressible trunk, and a second, later tap passed through the compressible air.

As you get older, your arteries become less compliant and the pressure pulse travels faster through your arterial system. In young people

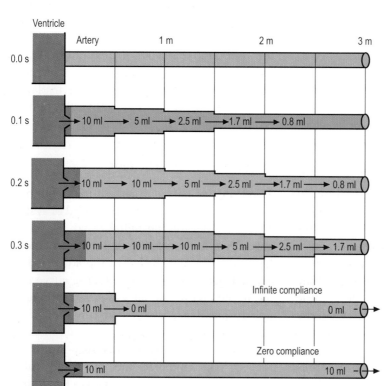

Fig. 6.4.2 The arterial pressure pulse. The model of ventricle and artery shows how a pressure wave is transmitted. The effects of infinite and zero compliance are shown in the lower panels.

the pulse wave travels at about 4 m/s, while the mean velocity of blood flow is 20 times less.

The increase in the pressure wave over the first three generations of arteries is the result of resonance of the elastic arterial wall and the effect of the individual main arteries being tapered so that, although the total cross-sectional area of all arteries increases slightly (owing to their increase in number, but much less than the increase in cross-sectional area that takes place in the arterioles and capillaries), the cross-section of an individual artery gets smaller. This results in a phenomenon similar to that seen in tidal rivers that have wide funnel-like mouths. In these rivers, the rapidly rising Spring tide forms a wave travelling up the river. This wave travels much faster than the sea water entering the river for the reasons given above and is called a *bore*. As the wave moves from the wide river mouth into the narrower reaches of the river upstream, it gets taller because there is less space for the displaced water to occupy. In a similar fashion, the pressure wave in the elastic arteries increases until the viscous properties of blood and the elastic artery wall damp it out.

Summary

Arteries, pressure waves and pulses

- Arteries are elastic (energy storing) or conducting (distributing).
- Blood pressure in the arterial system depends on the rate of injection of blood, elasticity of arteries and the rate of flow out of the arteries through the arterioles.
- The arterial pressure wave is defined by systolic, diastolic, pulse and mean pressures.

These observations are important to our understanding of the structure and functioning of the arterial system but should not obscure the general and important point that large arteries offer relatively little resistance to flow, and that the common clinical procedure of pressure measurement in the brachial artery can be used as an index of pressure in the aorta.

Arterial pressure measurement

The most precise way of measuring arterial blood pressure is by directly connecting a major artery to a transducer via a catheter. This method is of course restricted to intensive care and experimental laboratory situations.

On the other hand, most of us have had our arterial blood pressure measured indirectly by the method invented by Riva-Rocci. This method is invaluable in clinical medicine but you should be aware of the shortcomings of the traditional explanations used to describe it.

A **sphygmomanometer**, consisting of a pressure-measuring device and an inflatable cuff, is used. The cuff is wrapped round the arm above the elbow at the level of the heart, inflated well above arterial pressure and then slowly deflated. The object of this procedure is to squeeze the brachial artery with a known pressure. This objective is, surprisingly, often not achieved when the cuff is too narrow and pressure is not adequately transmitted to the artery, or the cuff is not properly wrapped round the arm.

The auscultatory method

This involves listening for what are known as **Korotkoff sounds**, using a stethoscope placed over the brachial artery in the antecubital fossa of the elbow (Fig. 6.4.3). When the pressure exerted by the cuff is greater than systolic pressure, no blood flows in the artery and no sound is heard. At a pressure slightly below systolic, blood forces its way under the cuff for a short

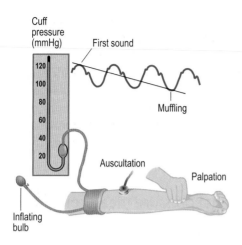

Fig. 6.4.3 Indirect measurement of arterial blood pressure.
The auscultatory and palpatory techniques are shown.

period, just at the beginning of systole when pressure is highest. In the artery under the cuff and when it escapes from under the cuff, the blood flow is turbulent because its velocity is high and produces a sharp **tapping** sound (the first Korotkoff sound). The tapping nature of the turbulent sound is due to there being two distinct states in the artery, open or closed. At this time, the pressure in the cuff and in the artery agree within 10 mmHg in healthy individuals. However, when the wall of the artery is stiffened by arteriosclerosis, it resists closure by the cuff to such a degree that the cuff pressure must be considerably higher than true arterial pressure to close the artery and produce turbulence. Under these circumstances, the pressure measurement is more an index of the arteriosclerosis than a measure of systolic pressure.

As the pressure in the cuff is allowed to fall further, the sound becomes louder and longer, as blood forces its way turbulently under the cuff for a greater part of the duration of systole. Quite suddenly, the sound begins to diminish and changes from a tapping to a muffled character. This muffling is because of the artery still containing turbulent flow but now remaining open for the whole of the cardiac cycle. Since diastolic pressure is the lowest pressure at any time in the cardiac cycle, a cuff pressure higher than diastolic would result in closure, however briefly, of the artery, and the imparting of a tapping characteristic to the sound. The cuff pressure at muffling can therefore be taken as diastolic pressure, although direct measurements indicate that it is a few mmHg above the true value.

A drop in cuff pressure of a further 5 mmHg usually causes the sounds to disappear completely, and it has been suggested that this silence occurs at a cuff pressure more representative of diastolic pressure than the muffling pressure. Silence occurs when blood flow under the cuff changes from turbulent to laminar. Since this change is due to a fall in velocity of blood (which, in both cases, is flowing) and is influenced by factors such as cardiac output and vessel dimensions that have no correlation with diastolic pressure, it would appear that muffling pressure in the cuff would be a better indicator of diastolic pressure than silence. Until recently, this has been the indicator used in the UK. Clinical practice and the British Hypertension Society have now, however, decided that **silence** (sometimes called the fifth Korotkoff sound) gives a better measurement of diastolic pressure, bringing British practice into line with that of the US.

The palpatory method

This involves taking the radial pulse while inflating the cuff (Fig. 6.4.3). The cuff pressure that cuts off the pulse is taken as systolic pressure. Of course, this method cannot measure diastolic pressure, but it provides a wise insurance in patients suspected of hypertension because there is sometimes a silent period within the Korotkoff sounds. It would lead to a serious underestimation of systolic pressure if it were taken to be the lower pressure at which sounds reappeared.

Summary

Arterial pressure measurement

- A sphygmomanometer can be used in the palpatory and auscultatory methods of measuring arterial blood pressure.
- When auscultating an artery, Korotkoff sounds produce tapping at systolic pressure and are muffled then disappear at diastolic pressure.
- Palpation can only measure systolic pressure.

Arterioles – controllers of blood pressure and tissue blood flow

It is common when using a hosepipe to 'pinch' the very tip of the pipe. This reduces flow but increases pressure at the tip to a value closer to that at the tap. The jet therefore goes further – pressure has been 'dammed-up' behind the constriction. If you pinch your hosepipe a few cm back from the tip, however, you get quite the opposite effect. Most of the energy (pressure) is used up in forcing a reduced flow of water through the constriction and the jet emerges at a much lower pressure and flow, trickling out from the end of the pipe. A similar phenomenon occurs in your arterial system. The muscular conducting arteries imperceptibly merge into the terminal arteries and arterioles, which are less than 0.1 mm diameter. It is here that the 'pinch' in the circulation takes place, in terms of both active squeeze on the pipe and its resting diameter. Although individual capillaries are less than half the diameter of arterioles, there are three times as many of them and so the total cross-sectional area of the arterioles is about one-third of that of the capillaries (see Fig. 6.1.8, p. 508). Even 'at rest', this is the narrowest part of the system.

In addition, a most important structural feature of arterioles is the smooth muscle in their walls (it can produce an active pinch of the pipe). Constriction of this smooth muscle reduces arteriolar diameter, and we have established that diameter is the most important determinant of resistance to flow in a tube (see p. 508).

The smooth muscle in the arteriolar walls is richly supplied by sympathetic vasoconstrictor nerve fibres. These control the overall or regional constriction, and therefore resistance, of these vessels, which in turn controls:

- total peripheral resistance
- regional blood flow.

By controlling hydrostatic pressure at the arterial end of capillaries in a region of the body, arterioles also influence capillary exchange.

The vast majority of vascular beds in the body are in parallel with each other (see p. 498). This arrangement means that the flow through individual beds can be varied without disturbing the flow in others, provided ABP is maintained (Fig. 6.4.4).

On the other hand, a large reduction of resistance in one part of the circulation can cause a fall in blood pressure that may deprive others of flow. Thus, very hot weather puts patients with coronary heart disease at risk because dilatation of skin arterioles, to direct blood to the skin to lose heat, reduces ABP and therefore the pressure perfusing the coronary arteries.

The overall resistance of the arterioles determines **total peripheral resistance** and therefore arterial blood pressure (if cardiac output is constant, see p. 600). The arteriolar system must constantly be 'balancing the budget' of ensuring that individual vital organs have sufficient blood flow, while maintaining sufficient total peripheral resistance to provide perfusion pressure for the rest of the body .

Control of arteriolar diameter

Active control of arteriolar diameter is by vascular smooth muscle in the arteriolar walls.

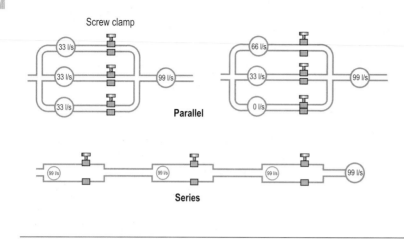

Fig. 6.4.4 Independence of parallel elements. The flow in parallel elements of a circuit can be varied independently. All the elements of a series circuit must carry the same flow.

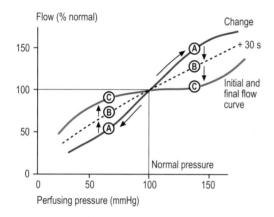

Fig. 6.4.5 Autoregulation. A sudden change from 'normal' perfusion pressure (100 mmHg) of an artery or arteriole produces a change in the rate of blood flow in the direction expected. This then autoregulates back to the 'normal' flow.

The general nature of smooth muscle has been described in Section 2, but vascular smooth muscle has many unique properties. The muscle in arteriolar walls has resting tone; it is partially contracted even under resting conditions. Stretching the arteriole, by increasing the pressure of the blood it contains for example, increases this smooth muscle activity and tone, an intrinsic property of vascular smooth muscle known as **the myogenic response**. This response explains the phenomenon of **pressure**

autoregulation, where a sudden change in perfusion pressure in an artery or arteriole produces a brief change in flow, as would be expected, but this flow very soon returns to near the 'normal' value that existed before the pressure change (Fig. 6.4.5) because of changes in tone in the vessel wall. Note that these changes can be an increase or decrease in tone.

A substantial basal tone must exist in a blood vessel if it is going to be able to respond to conditions that require dilatation. On this basal tone is superimposed *neural, hormonal, endothelial* and *blood-based control*.

Neural control

The autonomic innervation of arteriolar smooth muscle is by:

- sympathetic noradrenergic fibres
- sympathetic cholinergic fibres
- parasympathetic cholinergic fibres.

Sympathetic noradrenergic. This type of *vasoconstrictor* fibre innervates most vascular smooth muscle and contributes to its resting tone. Varicosities on the nerve fibres release predominantly noradrenaline, together with ATP, which recent research suggests acts as a co-transmitter, facilitating the effects of noradrenaline. These transmitters at low concentrations produce a slow sustained increase in muscle tone by **pharmacomechanical coupling**. This phenomenon involves few if any action potentials. Higher concentrations of transmitter (or circulating agonists) provoke an action potential and twitch by the process of **electromechanical coupling**. Thus, increase in sympathetic noradrenergic activity causes vasoconstriction, and decrease causes vasodilatation.

Sympathetic cholinergic. There is some evidence that the sympathetic cholinergic *vasodilator* fibres found in other species supply the arterioles of skeletal muscles of man. This system is in addition to the sympathetic noradrenergic fibres and is only activated during high emotional stress.

NANC fibres. The sympathetic cholinergic fibres serving sweat glands secrete, in addition to acetylcholine, a vasodilatory non-adrenergic non-cholinergic (NANC) transmitter, vasoactive intestinal polypeptide (VIP). VIP is the important transmitter for the sweat gland blood vessels, while acetylcholine is the important transmitter for the acini of the glands.

Parasympathetic cholinergic. These *vasodilator* fibres to blood vessels are restricted to the cerebral and coronary circulations and genital erectile tissue. The neurotransmitter of these fibres is acetylcholine. In the gut, salivary glands and exocrine pancreas, VIP and/or NO may be the parasympathetic transmitter in a situation similar to that seen in the sympathetic VIP fibres that supply the sweat glands (see above).

Hormonal control

As in many other systems, the effects of hormones on the vascular system are long term when compared to the effects of the nervous system. The effects of hormones are also less important than those of nerves in the short term. In the long term, and particularly in control of that most important determinant of blood pressure – blood volume, hormones are very important. Hormonal control includes:

- catecholamines
- antidiuretic hormone (ADH; vasopressin)
- angiotensin–aldosterone system
- atrial natriuretic peptide.

Catecholamines. These exert their effects via **α adrenoceptors** and **$β_2$ adrenoceptors** on the vascular smooth muscle cells. α adrenoceptors cause constriction of arterioles and $β_2$ adrenoceptors cause dilatation. Noradrenaline has a high affinity for α receptors, and adrenaline has about equal affinity for both α and $β_2$ receptors. This explains why both adrenaline and circulating noradrenaline cause vasoconstriction in most tissues, the exceptions being skeletal muscle and liver where $β_2$ receptors predominate and adrenaline causes vasodilatation.

Antidiuretic hormone (ADH). This hormone, produced in the hypothalamus and released from the posterior pituitary gland, is also known as **vasopressin**. However, it is usually, and perhaps more properly, called antidiuretic hormone (ADH) because its major function is to promote reabsorption of water by the kidney (antidiuresis). This is a subtle but very important way of maintaining blood pressure by maintaining plasma volume, and we must never lose sight of the fact that plasma volume is a very important determinant of blood pressure. However, in high concentrations, ADH has a vasoconstrictor (vasopressor) action in all but the coronary and cerebral blood vessels (hence vasopressin as an alternative name). This mechanism helps maintain perfusion of these essential organs when blood pressure falls as a result of haemorrhage. The controls of ADH release are covered in detail in Section 8 (p. 399), but in outline are:

- increases in blood osmolarity – detected by the hypothalamus
- reduction in arterial pressure – detected by baroreceptors

- reductions in blood volume – detected by left atrial stretch receptors
- exercise.

In keeping with its major effect, that on the kidneys, the secretory mechanism for ADH is five times more sensitive to changes in plasma osmolarity than to changes in plasma volume. However, the regulation of blood volume takes priority.

Angiotensin–aldosterone. It is interesting that the initiator of this system of controlling blood pressure is a group of modified vascular smooth muscle cells that make up the juxta-glomerular apparatus in the kidney (see p. 718). In response to sympathetic nerve activity, decreased plasma Na^+, and decreased pressure in the renal arterioles, these cells release the enzyme renin, which by a series of reactions (p. 754) yields angiotensin II. **Angiotensin** II is a potent vasoconstrictor, released when ABP is low. It acts centrally, increasing sympathetic nerve activity, and peripherally it facilitates the release of noradrenaline from sympathetic varicosities. A second, important property of angiotensin II is as one of several stimuli of the adrenal cortex to produce **aldosterone**, which promotes Na^+, and therefore water, reabsorption by the kidneys, so helping to restore blood volume and ABP.

Atrial natriuretic peptide (ANP). Produced by specialized myocytes of the atria in response to distension, this peptide has potent diuretic and natriuretic properties with diametrically opposite effects to the angiotensin–aldosterone system.

Endothelial and blood-based control

Endothelial derived factors. The shear stress caused by blood flowing through blood vessels leads to the formation of an **endothelium-derived relaxing factor** (EDRF). It is now generally recognized that the most important EDRF is nitric oxide (NO). Once formed in the endo-thelium, NO rapidly diffuses into the vascular smooth muscle, which it causes to relax. The endothelium also releases **prostacyclin** (a vaso-dilator) and **endothelin** (a vasoconstrictor). The release of EDRF in vessels 'upstream' to arteri-oles ensures that blood flow is not restricted there, the control of blood flow remaining with the arterioles. As well as the *shear stress* of flow-induced vasodilatation, many agonists (e.g. acetylcholine and bradykinin) can promote the production of NO, although others are not dependent on the endothelium for their action. Entry of extracellular Ca^{2+} into the endothelial cells initiates the chain reaction leading to relaxation shown in Figure 6.4.6. These flow-related effects of EDRF depend on an intact endothelium.

Prostaglandins. Some of this family of vasoac-tive substances generally known as eicosanoids are produced by the endothelium (others are produced by white blood cells). They can be vasoconstrictor (the F series) or vasodilator (the E series and prostacyclin – PGI_2; see above); the vasodilators, generally released from the endothelium in response to chemical agents, also contribute to inflammatory vasodilatation.

Thromboxane (TXA_2). This is mainly produced by blood platelets but can be produced by the endothelium; it constricts arterioles.

Leukotrienes. As their name suggests, these vasoactive substances were first discovered in white blood cells. They are also found in the lung and blood platelets. They are important in causing chemotaxis and leukocyte margination in inflammation. They cause general vaso-dilatation but coronary vasoconstriction.

Platelet-activating factor. This name is mis-leading, since this substance has actions on a wide variety of target cells. It is generated by most types of white blood cell and platelets. As a powerful mediator of inflammation, its effect on arterioles is vasodilatation.

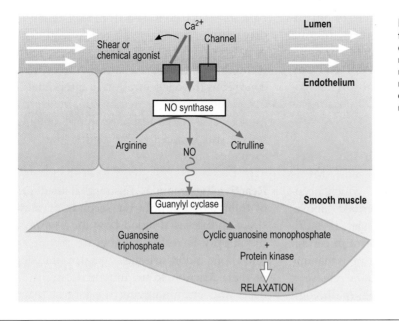

Fig. 6.4.6 Endothelial relaxing factor (NO). Entry of Ca^{2+} into the endothelial cell initiates a chain reaction ending in the second messenger cyclic guanosine monophosphate (cGMP), which causes vascular smooth muscle relaxation.

Histamine. Produced by mast cells and basophils, histamine is stored as granules within their cytoplasm. The process of degranulation releases it under conditions of trauma and allergic reactions, to produce inflammation. Depending on the type of histamine receptor present on the smooth muscle of a blood vessel, it produces vasoconstriction (H_1 receptors – veins) or vasodilatation (H_2 receptors – arterioles). A further important action of histamine is to increase vascular permeability.

Bradykinin. In addition to its role as a regulator of blood flow in the salivary and sweat glands and exocrine pancreas, bradykinin is generated in inflammation. As in the blood-clotting sequence (see Ch. 6.3), bradykinin is formed during inflammation as a result of the action of Hageman factor, activated by contact with a negatively charged surface, interacting with prekallikrein to begin a cascade that ends in bradykinin. It is a potent vasodilator that mediates its effects via NO. It also increases venular permeability.

5-hydroxytryptamine (5-HT). Concentrated by active transport from the plasma into platelets,

5-HT released from activated platelets causes various degrees of constriction of large arteries and veins, dilatation of arterioles, constriction of venules and increased permeability of capillaries.

Metabolic influences

Functional hyperaemia. It is to be expected that the products of metabolism would increase tissue perfusion because part of the purpose of perfusion is to remove those metabolites. Different organs are most sensitive to different metabolites, depending it seems on their metabolic bias, but all show a linear relationship between metabolism and the blood flow that sustains that metabolism. Of course, many organs have a *total* blood flow that far exceeds their metabolic requirements (lungs, kidneys) and these are under separate control. However, the major contributors to vasodilatation are:

- adenosine from ATP breakdown
- CO_2
- hypoxia
- acidosis
- potassium ions.

6

Adenosine. This breakdown product of adenosine triphosphate acts in several ways to bring about relaxation of vascular smooth muscle. These include stimulation of the cAMP pathway (see pp 65 and 66), hyperpolarization of the vascular muscle cells and inhibition of noradrenaline release.

Hypoxia. Hypoxia interferes with the rephosphorylation of AMP to ATP. Instead, AMP is dephosphorylated to adenosine, which accumulates with the results described above. Particularly unfortunately, hypoxia, if sufficiently severe, will cause vasospasm in certain large arteries, most importantly in ischaemic coronary arteries, in part owing to the release of noradrenaline from nerve endings pathologically affected by the lack of oxygen.

Acidosis. Whether from lactic acid or carbon dioxide, acidosis hyperpolarizes vascular smooth muscle and increases release of NO from the endothelium. Both these factors produce dilatation.

Potassium ions. Released from skeletal and cardiac muscle cells during the repolarization phase of action potentials, K^+ may also be released through ATP-sensitive channels under hypoxic conditions. K^+ concentration in interstitial fluid can double from its rest value in exercising muscle, causing hyperpolarization and smooth muscle relaxation by stimulating the Na^+/K^+ exchange pump.

Reactive hyperaemia. Tissues that are deprived of their blood supply for seconds or minutes show an increased blood flow for a while after the supply is restored; they are paying off a 'metabolic debt'. Tissues vary in the degree of their reaction to an impaired supply, with heart and brain showing the largest reaction. Reactive hyperaemia is the result of accumulation of the substances that produce functional hyperaemia, which are listed above, and a myogenic response to the sustained fall in intravascular pressure that occurs during the period of occlusion.

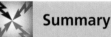

Summary

Arterioles

- Arterioles are the major resistance vessels of the circulation.
- Arterioles control total peripheral resistance and regional blood flow.
- Changes in tension in the abundant smooth muscle in arteriolar walls are responsible for vasomotion, the myogenic response to stretching, and allows pressure autoregulation of blood flow.
- Neural control of arteriolar smooth muscle is mainly by sympathetic noradrenergic nerves but there are also parasympathetic and sympathetic cholinergic fibres to some arterioles.

- Hormonal control of arterioles is by catecholamines, ADH, the angiotensin–aldosterone system and atrial natriuretic peptide.
- Endothelium-derived relaxing factors, including nitric oxide and prostaglandins, have a tonic dilator effect.
- Blood cells and platelets release vasodilators, including histamine, bradykinin, leukotrienes, platelet-activating factor, thromboxane and 5-HT (5-HT constricts large arteries and veins).
- Functional hyperaemia and reactive hyperaemia in tissues are due to arteriolar vasodilatation produced by adenosine, hypoxia, acidosis and K^+ from metabolism.

Clinical Example

Dealing with blocked arteries

Blocked arteries are a major cause of ill health and death. These effects arise when the artery blocked is the sole adequate provider of nutrition and removal of waste products. The result is *tissue ischaemia*, a term referring to inadequate blood flow and its consequences. As the adverse metabolic effects of ischaemia develop (hypoxia, lactic acidosis, lack of nutrients), the patient experiences pain and loss of function in regions such as the arms and legs, and in the heart – where a richly supply of pain fibres can be activated by metabolic changes.

It is possible to experience these effects by putting a blood pressure cuff round your wrist and pumping it up to 30–40 mmHg above your systolic arterial pressure, thereby cutting off all flow to the hand. At first, there will be only slight discomfort from the tightly applied cuff. After some 10–15 minutes, a moderate ache in the hand is likely, and efforts to use the hand muscles make the pain worse. Discomfort is rapidly relieved by removing the cuff.

Removing the cuff leads to a marked flush in the hand – felt as a fullness, as the blood vessels are indeed distended by greatly increased blood flow, and observed as a pink area strictly limited by a line where the proximal margin of the cuff was situated. This increased blood flow is termed *reactive hyperaemia* and illustrates the marked and localized effect of the accumulation of metabolites. It also shows that there are no serious after-effects of the arterial occlusion in the hand.

In general, the peripheries and most tissues can survive considerable periods of ischaemia, unlike the brain, where complete ischaemia leads to unconsciousness in seconds and permanent brain damage in several minutes.

In fact, it is routine in certain operations on the arm or leg to put on a tourniquet to occlude the circulation and provide a *bloodless field* for surgery. The occlusion can safely last for an hour or two. After that, there is an increasing risk of tissue damage and general effects when a flood of 'metabolites' is released into the general circulation.

The crucial point about unblocking arteries is that it can be highly beneficial within a few hours of complete occlusion, but thereafter the chances of complete or even partial recovery steadily decline. The major sites where unblocking arteries is a common and important procedure are the heart and the legs, and these will be considered in turn.

The heart

Unblocking the coronary arteries is needed in two situations. The first is when a moderately narrowed artery can maintain flow at rest but not in exercise – indicated by *angina of effort* (cardiac pain, often in the chest, related to exercise). The second is an acute emergency when a sudden complete blockage, often a *coronary thrombosis*, leads to a *heart attack*, with severe chest pain at rest and a risk of sudden death. A heart attack, or *myocardial infarction*, and its treatment are described on page 616; the treatment of less-sudden narrowing will be considered here.

Narrowing is likely to have been found in an X–ray of the coronary arteries (*coronary angiogram*) undertaken because the patient has angina of effort, with evidence of ischaemia found during a cardiac treadmill test. The narrowing can often be relieved by *angioplasty* (*angio*, a vessel; *plasty*, reconstruction). Here, a cardiac catheter (flexible tube) is passed into the narrowed coronary artery. The catheter is

Clinical Example *(Continued)*

inserted via a major artery such as a femoral, passed up the aorta and into the coronary artery orifice just distal to the aortic valve. The tip of the catheter is passed into the narrowed region, and a balloon surrounding the last few centimetres of the catheter is inflated to a high pressure of several atmospheres to crush the material obstructing the lumen. The dispersed material does not usually cause any harm. Often, a small tube, or *stent*, is inserted to maintain patency of the lumen – it is expanded at the site somewhat like opening an umbrella. Finally, if it is not possible to reopen the vessel in this way (perhaps because a considerable length of artery is severely obstructed) a *coronary artery bypass graft* is made. A segment of the patient's own blood vessels is used. A leg vein can carry out this

function – its wall gradually becomes thickened by smooth muscle (arterialized) – or a nearby internal mammary artery may be used. In both cases, collateral circulations compensate for the vessel removed.

The legs

Problems with inadequate circulation in the legs are also quite often dealt with by a bypass, e.g. of the popliteal artery. Sometimes, a large embolus (dislodged clot) blocks leg arteries and can be removed surgically. As with the heart (see p. 616), if the arterial supply to a leg or legs is suddenly and completely cut off, the tissue can survive for some hours before local tissue death (*gangrene*) develops.

Capillaries and venous vessels

Introduction

In this chapter we deal with the blood vessels where the exchange of materials between blood and tissues takes place, the capillaries, and the somewhat neglected 'Cinderellas' of the circulation, the capacitance or storage vessels, the veins, which have very different functions from the capillaries.

Structure is almost invariably related to function, and this applies to the circulation as much as any other part of the body. Because of the microscopic size of its individual vessels, that part of the circulation made up of arterioles, capillaries and venules is called the **microcirculation**. Do not be deceived by this into thinking that its importance, or physiological activity, is microscopic.

The word capillary means 'hair-like' and these tiny vessels (3–5 μm diameter) have a structure ideally suited to carry out the fundamental purpose of the circulation, the transport of substances to and from the tissues and the exchange of substances within them.

The overall arrangement of the microcirculation depends on the tissue it is serving, but the vessels that make it up have the names and general structures shown in Figure 6.5.1.

The microcirculation can be considered to start with arterioles, which divide into terminal arterioles that have only a single discontinuous smooth muscle layer in their walls. These vessels act as controllers or 'taps'; they regulate flow

585

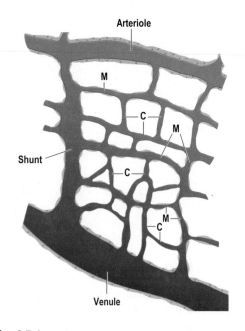

Arteriole

M

C

M

Shunt

C

M
C

Venule

Fig. 6.5.1 **The microcirculation.** A schematic drawing of a microcirculatory bed. The detailed structure and proportions of the vessels depend on the tissue in which it is found. C, small diameter capillaries; M, metarterioles (larger diameter capillaries).

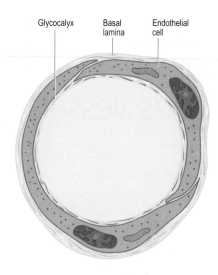

Glycocalyx   Basal   Endothelial
                   lamina   cell

Fig. 6.5.2 **Continuous capillary.** The number of endothelial cells making up the capillary tube may vary between one and three.

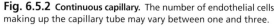

into the capillaries and are themselves regulated by sympathetic nerves (mainly the arterioles) and metabolites (mainly the terminal arterioles). **Arteriovenous anastomoses** form a short cut that bypasses capillaries in the skin of the extremities, in which the microcirculation is involved in temperature control. We will see later that the endothelium of the capillaries themselves exerts a retrograde control of the arterioles supplying them.

The control of flow is so efficient that transit time for blood through a capilliary bed can be varied in individual capillaries from 0.25 s when metabolic rate is high to a few seconds, or even stop, when the tissue supplied is metabolically at rest.

It is in relation to the capillary bed that the greatest variation in the structure of the microcirculation of tissues is seen. These differences are related to the special functions of the tissue being supplied and relate to structure, blood flow and the exchange of substances across the capillary wall.

Capillaries

True capillaries are tubes of approximately 3–4 μm in diameter at the arteriolar end and 5–6 μm at the venular end, and from 0.5–1 mm long. Their wall consists of a single layer of endothelial cells surrounded by a basement membrane.

The tightness of the junctions between the endothelial cells and the presence of 'pores' or 'slits' are used to assign capillaries to one of three categories:

• continuous
• fenestrated
• discontinuous

although these categories merge into each other.

Continuous capillaries

This type of capillary, shown diagrammatically in Figure 6.5.2 and found in skeletal and cardiac muscle, lung, brain, skin and connective tissue, consists of a single layer of flattened endothelial cells. These are lined on the inside by a layer of glycoproteins (the glycocalyx), which act as an important molecular sieve. On the outside, the cells are surrounded by a basement membrane made up largely of collagen, which reinforces the capillary against blood pressure and retards the passage of protein. Pericytes partially surround and support the endothelial cells.

Apart from the extreme thinness of their walls, which aids diffusion, there are other structural arrangements in these capillaries that permit movement of materials into and out of their lumen.

Pores

The sides of the endothelial cells fit against each other like the slabs making up a pavement. The 'fit' between these cells is not perfect and the gaps make up **slit-pores** 10–20 nm wide. This is wide enough to accommodate the largest molecules found in plasma. However, within the slits are found strands that make up **tight junctions** between the cells and form narrow maze-like paths, which molecules passing through the pores must negotiate. These arrangements reduce the effective size of the pores to 4–5 nm (see below). The nature of these paths determines the permeability of this route through the capillary wall, and in the brain these paths are so restricted that they form the **blood–brain barrier**, which is a highly selective filter between the blood and cerebrospinal fluid.

Glycocalyx and basal lamina

The endothelial cells of a continuous capillary are sandwiched between two sleeves of non-cellular material:

- on the inside, lining the capillary, the **glycocalyx**
- on the outside, the **basement membrane** (the basal lamina).

The glycocalyx consists of glycoproteins, which by combining with albumin from the plasma form a molecular sieve (see The effect of pores, p. 590). The basal lamina is a much cruder filter and its major role appears to be strengthening the capillary to withstand blood pressure. It does, however, slow down the passage of proteins.

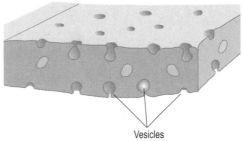

Vesicles

Fig. 6.5.3 Endothelial vesicles. There is little evidence for the exact function of this prominent feature of capillary endothelium.

Vesicles

A unique characteristic of capillary endothelial cells is the presence of many invaginations on the cell surfaces (Fig. 6.5.3). These take up about 25% of the total volume of the cells and, although they do not seem to connect in any way across the cell, they form such a prominent feature that it is tempting to attribute a function to them. Perhaps it is the transport of large molecules, for example proteins.

Fenestrated capillaries

Much more permeable than the continuous capillaries and capable of a high rate of water and solute exchange, these capillaries are found in tissue such as glands, intestinal mucosa and the kidney. They get their name from the fenestrae or circular windows, about 50 nm diameter, in their walls, which may be closed by a thin membrane made up of the inner and outer membrane layers of the cell being closely apposed to form a transcellular route, as in endocrine glands, or be open as in the renal glomerulus (Fig. 6.5.4). The fenestrae account for the increased permeability of this type of capillary over the continuous type.

Discontinuous capillaries

These are the most permeable of all capillaries and are usually found where not just fluid but whole blood cells need to move easily into and

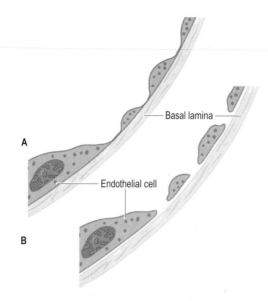

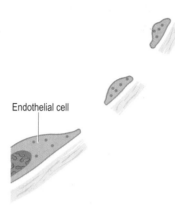

Fig. 6.5.4 **Fenestrated capillaries.** **A.** Endocrine tissue with the fenestrae closed by a membrane. **B.** Renal glomerular capillary with the fenestrae open.

Fig. 6.5.5 **Discontinuous capillaries.** These can have a high endothelium (spleen) or a low endothelium as in the bone marrow or liver.

out of the tissue spaces (bone marrow, liver, spleen). The cells of the endothelium are separated by large discontinuities – gaps of more than 100 nm, and the cells may be of different heights in different tissues (Fig. 6.5.5). This type of capillary frequently forms sinusoids.

Summary

Relationship between capillary structure and function

- The microcirculation starts at the arterioles and ends at the venules.
- Arterioles control flow through the capillaries of the microcirculation.
- Capillaries are a single layer of endothelial cells lined by glycocalyx and surrounded by a basement membrane.
- The glycocalyx and basement membrane are selective filters.
- The endothelial cells of capillaries contain pores, which determine their permeability, and vesicles, which may have a transport function.

- Capillaries can be defined as continuous, fenestrated or discontinuous.
- Continuous capillaries show the most selective movement of substances across their walls, governed by the properties of their cells, pores and tight junctions.
- Fenestrated capillaries have windows in their walls, closed by a thin membrane in some tissues, which accounts for their high permeability.
- Discontinuous capillaries are the most permeable capillaries and frequently form sinusoids.

Basic Science 6.5.1

Membrane reflection, conductance and osmotic pressure

Physicists interested in osmotic pressure of solutions (see Osmotic pressure, p. 21) construct 'perfect' semipermeable membranes out of such esoteric materials as potassium ferrocyanide precipitated into the pores of a ceramic vessel. These 'perfect' membranes produce values of osmotic pressure that are very close to values predicted by applying highly mathematical molecular kinetic theory to the situation. Biological membranes are rather more complicated but more ubiquitous and require at least the following factors to be taken into consideration.

Colloid osmotic pressure

The particles (atoms, molecules, ions) in a gas or liquid are in constant random motion (see Diffusion, p. 27). They bombard the walls of their container. If the gas or liquid is a mixture, the pressure exerted by each of the components of the mixture depends on its concentration, i.e. number of its particles present. In gas mixtures, this pressure is known as the partial pressure (see p. 659). In the case of liquids, dissolving a solute in the liquid reduces the pressure of the solvent because the solute takes over part of the job of exerting pressure. If two solutions of different concentrations of solute are separated by a semipermeable membrane containing pores through which only the solvent can pass, the difference in pressure exerted by solvent on either side drives solvent through and is called the osmotic pressure.

If the solute can pass through the pores, diffusion eventually removes any difference in concentration either side of the membrane and no osmotic pressure exists. Osmotic pressure depends only on the **concentration** of non-diffusible particles involved; their nature has no bearing on the situation. In capillaries, the walls are permeable to almost all dissolved substances except 'colloidal' proteins. These 'colloids' are therefore the major determinant of osmotic pressure in the blood. This pressure is called colloid osmotic pressure (COP) or oncotic pressure (see p. 22).

Although there is a considerable concentration of protein in plasma (approximately 70 g/l), protein exerts a COP of only 25 mmHg because each individual molecule is so massive that the concentration of 70 g/litre is made up of relatively few molecules (0.001 mole/litre). Part of this 25 mmHg pressure is also made up of sodium ions dragged into the plasma by the negative charge on the plasma albumin, which is osmotically the most important plasma protein.

Reflection at a membrane

Development of osmotic pressure depends on non-diffusible particles being in excess on one side of a membrane. 'Non-diffusible' is not an absolute term. It ranges from totally non-diffusible particles, which do not penetrate a semipermeable membrane at all and therefore exert their full theoretical osmotic effect, to particles that are diffusible and therefore exert no osmotic effect.

The reflection coefficient reflects the place of a type of particle on this scale. A reflection coefficient of 1.0 for a substance indicates that the membrane is acting as a perfect semipermeable membrane for that particle, and 0 indicates that the particle passes freely and exerts no osmotic effect.

Hydraulic conductance

Biological membranes such as the walls of capillaries have pores in them that are specific to specific particles (Na+, K+, Cl-, etc.). For each particle, the whole membrane can be considered as a singe tube specific for that particle, which has a specific resistance to flow. The hydraulic conductance for each type of particle is the filtration rate produced by unit pressure difference applied to unit area of membrane.

Transcapillary exchange

Although the true capillaries described above make up the majority of 'exchange vessels' in the circulation, there is not a clear-cut demarcation, and terminal arterioles and small venules take part in exchange to some degree.

The physical processes that bring about exchange between blood and tissue fluid are mainly:

- diffusion
- filtration.
  These processes are influenced by:
- characteristics of the transported molecule (size, shape, lipid solubility)
- characteristics of the capillary membrane (continuous, fenestrated, discontinuous)
- capillary surface area
- hydrostatic and osmotic forces.

Diffusion

Free diffusion is a concept used by physicists to describe molecular movement of solutes through a large volume of solvent. Free diffusion has been briefly described in Basic Science 1.2.5 (p. 26), and its characteristics can be summarized here as:

- Diffusion of a substance through an area (a 'window' in space) takes place from high to low concentration.
- The rate of diffusion is proportional to:
  – the concentration gradient
  – the area (of the 'window') through which diffusion is occurring.
- The rate of diffusion is greater at higher temperatures.
- The rate of diffusion is greater for smaller molecules.

The rate of diffusion across the walls of a capillary is reduced from the ideal state of a dilute solute in a large volume because the **permeability** of the capillary wall depends on its physical and chemical characteristics; its **reflectance** and the **hydraulic conductance** properties of its pores (see Basic Science 6.5.1, p. 589).

Substances that are soluble in fat have the whole of the capillary surface, made up of lipid cell membranes, available for diffusion. This is why volatile anaesthetics and the respiratory gasses oxygen and carbon dioxide move freely between blood and tissues. These substances do not have to rely on movement through pores to move down their concentration gradients.

The effect of pores

Substances that do not readily dissolve in the endothelial cell membrane (e.g. electrolytes, glucose, lactate) pass between blood and tissues at an unexpectedly high rate. This is explained by the presence of pores of different sizes, mainly formed by channels between the cells. These represent less than 1% of the total surface area of the capillary but are of considerable functional significance.

Pores are mainly narrow channels 4–5 nm in diameter with a small minority (1 in 10 000) of large pores, 50–500 nm diameter. These diameters are important in relation to the size of molecule that the pores will admit and should strictly be called **effective diameter** because they have been measured by 'probing' them with molecules of different size rather than measured directly. The permeability of capillaries to these molecules clearly depends on the electrical charge the molecules carry as well as their size and shape. This additional filtering effect is due to the negatively charged glycocalyx layer that covers the entrance and lines the pores. The fibrous glycocalyx molecules trap albumin molecules, which help to form a **molecular sieve**, through which molecules making the transcapillary journey must pass.

Large pores certainly make up a large part of the walls of discontinuous capillaries and probably are involved in the essential passage of plasma protein to the tissues from continuous capillaries. Vesicles in the cell membranes (see above) may also act like large pores, carrying protein molecules in their journey across the capillary wall. Plasma proteins are found in tissue fluid in concentrations up to 50% of that in blood. Their movement, which is passive, is essential for the transport of immunoglobulins and protein-bound substances into the tissue fluid.

The effects of carriers in the membrane

The endothelial cells have specific carriers in their membranes, which allow *facilitated* movement of glucose, amino acids, lactate and pyruvic acid down their concentration gradients.

Filtration (and absorption)

Filtration of fluid across a capillary wall (or through any permeable surface) is a passive process driven by hydrostatic and osmotic pressures. Because the capillary wall is permeable to electrolytes, which therefore distribute fairly

evenly to both sides of it, electrolytes have little osmotic effect. The majority of osmotic pressure is generated by plasma proteins, which produce an **oncotic pressure** (alternatively called a colloid osmotic pressure; see Basic Science 6.5.1).

The other important pressure is hydrostatic pressure. Both osmotic and hydrostatic pressures can force fluid into or out of the capillary (Fig. 6.5.6) and the net flow depends on the balance of:

- hydrostatic forces in and out
- osmotic forces in and out.

Hydrostatic force out. This is produced by arterial blood pressure and falls as you progress along the capillary because it is 'used up' to propel the blood along. This pressure depends on the degree of dilatation of the arteriole serving the capillary and is therefore under sympathetic nervous, metabolic vasodilator and myogenic control. Venous pressure affects the pressure of blood leaving the capillary.

Hydrostatic force in. This is something of a misnomer, which arose from the reasonable expectation that the hydrostatic pressure in the tissue spaces round the capillaries would be positive with respect to atmospheric pressure.

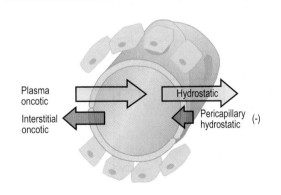

Fig. 6.5.6 Forces of capillary filtration. These pressures are shown as if measured relative to atmospheric pressure. The values of these four pressures change and produce different rates of filtration and reabsorption of fluid.

Pressure in tissue spaces is in fact about 5 mmHg *negative* to atmosphere. This negative pressure is the result of suction of fluid from the tissues by the lymphatic vessels and is about the same for the tissues surrounding the arterial and venous ends of the capillary.

Osmotic force in. Because electrolytes such as sodium chloride can diffuse until they are in equilibrium across the capillary wall, only non-diffusing colloidal protein produces osmotic effects – the colloid osmotic pressure (COP), which varies between 20–30 mmHg. About 75% of this is due to plasma albumin and the Na^+ ions that albumin attracts to itself inside the capillary. This force does not change much as you travel along a capillary because only a small percentage of plasma water and proteins is lost during each transit of the capillaries by blood. The blood is of almost the same composition at the arterial and venous ends of the capillary.

Osmotic force out. The slow movement of proteins out of continuous capillaries and more rapid movement across discontinuous capillaries results in about half the total plasma protein of the body being found in the interstitial space. This movement is accompanied by water, which reduces their concentration but does not alter the substantial total amount. The degree of this dilution determines the colloid osmotic

pressure these proteins exert, which can range from 15–20 mmHg depending on from where in the body the sample of interstitial fluid is taken. Although this osmotic pressure varies from place to place in the body, it is about the same at both ends of the capillary.

The four forces described above result in tissue fluid formation or the reabsorption of tissue fluid into blood vessels. The force that varies most from one end of the capillary to the other, and so controls filtration and absorption, is hydrostatic pressure. But changes in plasma protein concentration are very important and frequently occur, particularly in pathological conditions that produce an excess of tissue fluid – **oedema**.

The great physiologist Ernest Starling combined the effects of these four forces into his 'Theory of tissue fluid formation', which has been refined to the state that it is now accepted that fluid is lost from plasma into tissue spaces at the arterial end of capillaries at a rate of about 8 litres per day. Some is absorbed by venules but of the remainder that passes into the lymphatics almost half is reabsorbed leaving 4 litres per day to be returned to the circulation as lymph (Fig. 6.5.7).

In summary, filtration and absorption are being continuously changed, mainly by changes in arteriolar resistance, but also by changes in plasma protein concentration and venous pressure.

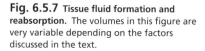

Fig. 6.5.7 Tissue fluid formation and reabsorption. The volumes in this figure are very variable depending on the factors discussed in the text.

Summary

Transcapillary exchange

- Capillaries are the major exchange vessels of the circulation.
- Exchange between blood and tissues and tissues and blood is mainly due to diffusion and filtration.
- Permeability of the capillary wall depends on the chemical properties of its cells and the reflectance and hydraulic conductance of its pores.

- Pores form a molecular sieve; they have an effective diameter that is not necessarily their physical diameter.
- Carrier molecules in the capillary endothelium promote facilitated diffusion.
- Tissue fluid formation is the result of a balance between the sum of hydrostatic forces in and out and osmotic forces in and out.
- A major osmotic force is the oncotic pressure of proteins retained within the capillary.

Clinical Example

Capillaries and burns

Burns to a substantial proportion of the surface of the body constitute a medical emergency where death is threatened, but effective treatment leads to excellent recovery. A major component of the treatment is prompt intravenous infusion of large amounts of fluid. The need for this fluid is related closely to widespread damage to capillaries with perturbation of their normal function.

On admission to the emergency room, an initial priority is to assess the depth and extent of the burns (which may extend into the respiratory tract if hot gas is inhaled). Burns that have destroyed the full thickness of the skin (suggested by anaesthesia of the area resulting from destruction of pain endings in the skin) produce damage to capillaries in the junctional area between destroyed and healthy tissue. This leads to severe loss of fluid from body compartments into the damaged skin. The amount lost is directly proportional to the

surface area of the skin affected by *full-thickness burns*. This area can be estimated from the *'rule of nines'*: each arm contributes 9% of body surface area; each leg $9 \times 2 = 18\%$; front of trunk $9 \times 2 = 18\%$; back of trunk $9 \times 2 = 18\%$; and head 9% (the perineum is allocated 1% to give a total of 100%). Fluid requirements are calculated by a formula related to the percentage of full-thickness burn and the patient's weight. For an extensive burn, several litres of fluid must be given rapidly in the first few hours.

Normally, little fluid is lost from the circulation as the blood passes through capillaries, because the plasma protein gradient across the capillary wall produces a strong osmotic force (*plasma protein oncotic pressure*) which balances the internal hydrostatic pressure driving out water (to which the capillary wall is freely permeable).

When damaged by burns, the capillaries lose their ability to retain protein in the circulation. Thus, in the damaged area, plasma pours out of the circulation. The blood volume falls rapidly and effects on the circulation are similar to

Clinical Example *(Continued)*

haemorrhage (see hypovolaemic shock, p. 635) – arterial pressure tends to fall and compensatory changes are brought about to minimize this effect. As with haemorrhage, there is widespread vasoconstriction, a fall in urinary output, and movement of interstitial fluid into the capillaries in undamaged areas. Although the initial loss is of plasma, interstitial fluid from other sites is also lost, so the net effect is a profound *fall in extracellular fluid volume*. Because the cellular component of blood is conserved, the haematocrit (red cells as a proportion of blood volume) rises steadily and provides an indication of the severity of fluid loss and the effectiveness of replacement.

Just as with haemorrhage, this catastrophic loss of fluid and hence of circulating blood volume threatens death from *peripheral circulatory failure*, and it is for this reason that the extracellular fluid must be replaced promptly. Because sodium and chloride ions are the main constituents of extracellular fluid, the replacing infusions consist largely of normal saline. Such infusions must be maintained until appropriate treatment (including skin grafting) and recovery of the damaged capillaries arrest the abnormal leakage of plasma and interstitial fluid from the burnt area.

Lymphatics

Lymph consists of tissue fluid formed by capillary **ultrafiltration**, which is returned to the circulation by special lymphatic vessels. This system:

- drains the tissues and so prevents accumulations of tissue fluid
- collects digested fat from the intestine and passes it to the plasma
- contains nodes that filter out particles and mount immunological defence reactions.

Tissue lymph vessels are thin-walled like capillaries but blind-ended. Their ability to pump lymph toward the thoracic duct (on the left) and right lymphatic duct, which return lymph to the internal jugular veins, depends on the smooth muscle in the larger lymph vessels, the 'massaging' action of the tissue that surround them; and the presence of valves that ensure a one-way direction of flow. Lymph vessels play an important part in the reabsorption of tissue fluid.

Veins and venules

Venules (3–30 μm diameter) and veins (up to 30 mm diameter) complete the vascular circuit by connecting the capillaries to the heart. These 'Cinderellas' of the circulation have not received as much attention from physiologists as arteries and capillaries, although they are just as important.

These vessels are more similar to each other, with their common structure of thin walls and limited smooth muscle, than are arteries to arterioles.

Blood enters the venules at heart level at a pressure of about 15 mmHg; it enters the heart from the venae cavae at 0–5 mmHg. This small pressure difference is sufficient to return the whole of the cardiac output to the heart, because the resistance to flow of veins is low. Pressure in the venous system is too low to be palpated, but the cyclic changes in pressure in the great veins of the neck can be seen as movements of the skin. These changes in pressure are produced by the cyclic movement of venous blood into the heart.

Because of the low pressure that they contain, venules play an important part in the **reabsorption** of tissue fluid, and changes in pressure and resistance to flow in venules have considerable influence on tissue fluid formation.

There are more venous vessels than arteries and arterioles and they have generally greater diameters, so they offer much less resistance to blood flow. Their number and size results in them having the potential to contain 30 times the volume of blood contained in the arterial system. They thus form the **capacitance vessels** of the circulation. This storage function is neither passive nor simple and is related to their compliance.

Compliance of the venous system

The limited amount of smooth muscle in the walls of venules and veins might suggest that they cannot control their diameters. This would not take into account the fact that they contain blood at low pressure. The smooth muscle in the walls of venules and veins is quite adequate to constrict these vessels against the pressure they contain.

This smooth muscle is innervated by **sympathetic** nerves and the way in which veins are distended by the pressure of blood inside them depends on the activity of these nerves.

In the absence of sympathetic activity, cross-sectional area of a vein shows two distinct phases:

- The first phase (A in Fig. 6.5.8) consists of passive filling with little change in wall tension, something like opening the mouth of a paper bag. This gives the veins a compliance more than 50 times greater than the arterial system.
- The second unstimulated phase (B in Fig. 6.5.8) shows a high resistance to stretch and is due to the collagen in the vessels walls.

When wall smooth muscle is *stimulated*, its compliance curve is a different shape, reminiscent of arterioles, and is displaced to the right,

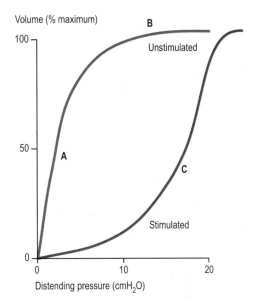

Fig. 6.5.8 Compliance of veins. The compliance of a large vein when the smooth muscle of its wall is relaxed and maximally stimulated is shown. When the stimulated vein reaches 100% volume, its compliance will become as low as phase B of the unstimulated state.

providing a mechanism that, when activated, 'squeezes' blood out of the venous system toward the heart (C in Fig. 6.5.8).

When blood volume is increased, as in a blood transfusion, or decreased, as in haemorrhage, or changed in either direction because of physiological shifts in fluid, the change in volume is distributed among the compartments of the circulation according to their compliances. Therefore changes in blood volume are largely accommodated in the veins.

Venous return

The vessels of the circulation are elastic, with different parts more or less compliant than others. At any moment, this elastic system is filled with a certain volume of blood. There is therefore a 'bottom-line' basic pressure that represents the physical relationship between the system's elasticity and degree of stretch and excludes any biological factors such as reflexes, effects of the pumping heart, and vasomotion. This basic pressure is called the **mean circulatory pressure** and it is on this that the other pressures measured at different points in the circulation and at different times are developed.

The **auxiliary factors** that operate on the veins and assist venous return of blood to the heart are:

- venomotor tone
- venous valves
- the skeletal muscle pump
- the respiratory pump
- suction by the heart.

Venomotor tone

This has been touched upon in relation to venous compliance (above). Neural control of venous smooth muscle is exclusively sympathetic. This neural control is reinforced endocrinologically by circulating catecholamines, which, in physiological concentrations, are less potent than the nervous control. Sympathetic control is important in shifting the distribution of venous blood, as in mobilizing the reservoir of splanchnic blood during haemorrhage and shock. Veins in the skin and superficial tissues respond strongly to sympathetic stimulation, whereas veins of skeletal muscle do not respond at all.

Venous valves

These are thin bicuspid valves, somewhat like two pockets, on opposite sides of the lumen of even the smallest (< 0.1 mm diameter) limb veins. They occur most frequently (every centimetre or so) toward the periphery and not at all in the central abdominal veins.

These valves greatly improve the efficiency of the skeletal muscle pump (see below) because they divide the column of blood in the leg veins into small segments, each at only a small pressure below the one above it. This makes muscle pumping of blood towards the heart easier reduces pressure in the leg veins and helps reduce the likelihood of varicose veins.

In the unpleasant condition of varicose veins, frequently brought on by long periods of standing, the veins of the leg become distended and tortuous, which causes the valves to become incompetent and leads to further distension of the veins in a vicious cycle.

The skeletal muscle pump

Every fluid, gas or liquid, is drawn toward the centre of the earth by gravity. This results, for example, in pressure increasing as you descend below the surface of a swimming pool. By the same mechanism, the pressure in the veins of the foot of a standing man are at a pressure of about 1.8 metres of water (blood) greater than the pressure in the veins in his head. In fact, as the heart, the pump in this pressure system, is below the head in a standing man, the venous pressures in the head are slightly below atmospheric pressure.

The prospect of the heart having to pump blood against a pressure of 1.8 metres of water might be viewed with some alarm unless it is realized that the same force of gravity is also operating on the arterial side of the system. In this respect we are built something like a U-tube (Fig. 6.5.9).

This useful situation is modified, however, by the differences in compliance of the two limbs of the U-tube, and this effect is most clearly seen when a person stands from the horizontal position. Over the first minute after standing, about half a litre of blood accumulates in the more compliant venous limb of the U-tube, flowing in from the high-pressure arterial side and being prevented from flowing back by the valves. This expansion of the venous compartment means that venous return is reduced, which compromises cardiac output and results in the dizziness people sometimes feel on rapidly standing up.

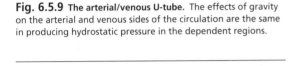

Fig. 6.5.9 The arterial/venous U-tube. The effects of gravity on the arterial and venous sides of the circulation are the same in producing hydrostatic pressure in the dependent regions.

intrathoracic pressure more negative with respect to the atmosphere and compressing abdominal contents. These effects respectively suck and push blood into the thoracic veins. The reverse takes place during expiration.

This stretching of thoracic veins during inspiration helps fill the right ventricle, whose output can alter by 15% during a respiratory cycle because of this effect. The left ventricle, however, has its filling pressure and therefore output reduced slightly during inspiration because of the greater compliance of the pulmonary vessels. This effect is less marked and the left ventricle only alters its output by about 5% between the two phases of the respiratory cycle. The inspiratory and expiratory effects on the left and right sides of the heart are reversed during expiration.

The major veins in the legs are surrounded by skeletal muscle, which squeezes the compartments formed by the valves in a manner similar to someone squeezing a tube of toothpaste. The blood, or toothpaste, is propelled in one direction. During quiet standing, this squeezing by the skeletal muscles is reflexly produced with a rhythm generated by the plantar surfaces of the feet. This results in the slight sway you see in people standing still for some time. During walking and running, of course, the muscle pump is even more active. This mechanism is so important in returning blood from the lower limbs it has been called the 'second heart'.

The respiratory pump

The diaphragm between the thorax and abdomen descends during inspiration, making

Suction by the heart

The ventricles of the heart are thick-walled elastic structures with a clearly defined hollow shape. Just as the heart will return to its 'rest' size when it has been stretched, when it is reduced in size by systolic contraction, it will again return to its rest size. This is the same sort of action you see with the rubber bulb of an eyedropper or when you squeeze a squash ball with a hole in it. In addition, during systole, there is a minor effect due to the ring of tissue bearing the closed atrioventricular valves being pulled down by the contraction of the ventricles. This acts like a plunger in a syringe, drawing blood into the atria.

The factors that affect venous pressure and venous return to the heart are important because they affect not only capillary filtration of fluid (p. 590) but also cardiac filling pressure (p. 546), a major determinant of cardiac function.

Summary

Veins and venules

- Hydrostatic pressure within the venous system is low – between 0–15 mmHg.
- Low hydrostatic pressure promotes reabsorption of fluid into venules.
- The venous system has a very high compliance up to a certain volume; then compliance falls dramatically.
- Venous system compliance is very much reduced by sympathetic stimulation, which mobilizes blood toward the heart.
- As the most compliant part of the circulation, the venous system determines mean circulatory pressure.
- Venous return is assisted by venomotor tone, venous valves, the skeletal muscle pump, the respiratory pump and suction by the heart.
- Venous pressure is a major determinant of cardiac function.

Central control of the cardiovascular system

Introduction

We have established that the business of the circulation is transport; transport involves the flow of a fluid medium, blood. Blood, like any other fluid, flows from regions of high pressure to regions of low pressure. The flow of blood through individual organs and tissues is not constant. It is generally related to the metabolic activity of that organ at that time, and is controlled by a change in the resistance to blood flow through the organ. This **local control** conforms to the economy of effort seen in all systems in the body. Waste of energy is not an evolutionary advantage.

For local controls to operate efficiently, the driving pressure that brings about flow must be sufficient and fairly constant. One of the most important homeostatic mechanisms in our body is the one that maintains **arterial blood pressure** within acceptable limits. These limits are fairly wide: systolic pressure may vary from less than 100 to more than 150 mmHg in a normal day's occupations. However, arterial blood pressure can be compared to the domestic electricity supply, which must have sufficient voltage to drive our machines, but the voltage must not be so high as to damage them.

Arterial blood pressure is determined by the interaction of two variables: **total peripheral resistance** and **cardiac output**.

Arterial blood pressure = Cardiac output ×
Total peripheral resistance.

The only way to alter arterial blood pressure is to alter one or both of these variables, and this is how blood pressure is affected by a series of reflexes. The most important role of these reflexes is to ensure perfusion of the two essential organs, the brain and the coronary circulation of the heart, which are first, and most fatally, damaged by lack of a blood supply.

Changed conditions requiring changes in control of blood pressure may exist for seconds to minutes or months to years. The control mechanisms involved in these different time spans are different. Factors influencing blood pressure may be intrinsic – from within the circulation, or extrinsic – from without.

The mechanism that controls blood pressure is the baroreceptor reflex, and like all reflexes it has afferent and efferent arms joined by a central controller. The efferent arm is the autonomic nervous system and the central controller is, of course, the brain. We will first deal with the afferent 'sensory' mechanisms that sense blood pressure to bring about its baroreceptor-mediated control.

Intrinsic factors

Arterial baroreceptors

These are the most important receptors measuring and ultimately controlling blood pressure on a short-term basis. There is no physiological receptor that measures pressure directly; they all measure the stretch of the walls of the organ in which they are situated. **Arterial baroreceptors** are no exception. They are stretch receptors situated in the adventitia of the **aortic arch** and the **carotid sinuses**, which are situated at the base of the internal carotid arteries either side of the neck. Nerve fibres from the carotid baroreceptors form the sinus nerve, which joins the glossopharyngeal (IXth cranial) nerve and ascends to the nucleus of the tractus solitarius. Fibres from the aortic baroreceptors also reach the tractus solitarius, but in the vagus nerve.

Information about the state of stretch of the arteries containing these arterial baroreceptors is sent to the brain as trains of action potentials. Recordings of these action potentials reveal that the receptors initially respond to stretch by a burst of activity that rapidly adapts (see p. 249) to a new higher level, signalling the new pressure.

When pressure is reduced, the firing rate falls to a subnormal value, which quickly recovers (Fig. 6.6.1).

This transient **dynamic response** is too rapid to be completely accounted for by the viscous properties of the tissue surrounding the receptor, which relaxes after the initial stretch is over. It is probable that K^+ channels are opened by the initial stretch and that this brings about the rapid adaptation. The dynamic response means that the baroreceptors signal the rate of change of pressure and therefore carry out the valuable role of measuring pulse pressure as well as mean arterial pressure. For example, when you stand after lying down for some time, there may be little fall in mean arterial pressure but pulse pressure is reduced because of a reduction in stroke volume; this is corrected by the baroreceptor reflex, which will be described next.

Baroreceptor reflexes

The word 'carotid' comes from the Greek word to stun. Mechanical pressure applied to the baroreceptors of the carotid region will increase their discharge. This increase will reflexly cause:

- an increase in vagal and decrease in sympathetic discharge to the heart, which slows the heart and reduces contractility
- a decrease in sympathetic discharge to splanchnic, renal, skin and skeletal muscle arterioles, which reduces peripheral resistance
- a decrease in sympathetic discharge to venous vessels, which causes venodilatation and decreases central venous pressure.

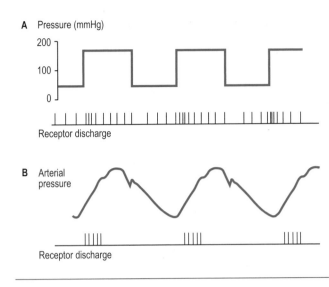

A Pressure (mmHg)

Receptor discharge

B Arterial pressure

Receptor discharge

Fig. 6.6.1 Arterial baroreceptor activity. A. The response of an arterial baroreceptor to stepwise changes in pressure. The dynamic response can be seen early in the increase or decrease of pressure. **B.** The rapid adaptation of many of these receptors means that they only fire during the rising phase of arterial pressure.

These effects cause a fall in blood pressure that, if great enough, will cause a faint, as if stunned. The latency of this reflex is very short, taking effect within one or two beats of the heart.

Falls in blood pressure, resulting from standing rapidly or blood loss, produce the opposite effects to increases in blood pressure:

- a decrease in vagal discharge, and increased sympathetic discharge, speed up heart rate
- increased sympathetic discharge, particularly to the splanchnic, renal, skin and muscle circulations, raises peripheral resistance
- venoconstriction displaces blood from gut and liver veins and increases CVP
- adrenaline, angiotensin and ADH secretion are increased, causing renal retention of extracellular fluid (a mechanism more important in long-term regulation of blood pressure).

A response to increases and decreases in arterial pressure implies that there is an 'ideal' pressure that the system strives to achieve. This is known as the **set point** of the reflex.

The baroreflex set point

The 'ideal' blood pressure that the baroreflex strives to achieve needs to be changed when overall conditions change, and the reflex then 'chases' that pressure. Both the central nervous system (in the brainstem) and the baroreceptors themselves can be involved in this resetting.

During exercise, blood pressure rises. This is useful, as it increases the perfusion of active muscles. It would be counterproductive if the baroreflex struggled to reduce heart rate and dilated non-muscle vascular beds to return pressure to its original value. In fact, the set point, as decided by the brain, is reset at a slightly higher level, although the baroreceptor reflex is working, and the brainstem does not completely restore ABP, reduce cardiac output or produce a general peripheral vasodilatation.

The speed at which the sensitivity of the reflex can be reset is demonstrated by the phenomenon of **sinus arrhythmia**, which is an increase in heart rate with each inspiration and most clearly seen in young people. This is the result of the inspiratory centre in the brainstem reducing the sensitivity of the central connections of the baroreflex to the baroreceptor input. As a result of this inhibition by the inspiratory centre, the cardiovascular centres send out less vagal activity during each inspiration and heart rate rises in phase with inspiration.

These central mechanisms are accompanied by adaptation of the baroreceptors themselves.

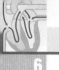

Both these mechanisms result in the baroreflex being most suitable for controlling short-term changes in arterial blood pressure.

Cardiopulmonary reflexes

Low-pressure cardiac receptors

These mechanoreceptors are situated in the atria and venae cavae. Their afferent connections run in the vagus nerves and the reflex effects they produce in response to rapid stretching of the venae cavae and atria are:

- tachycardia, sometimes known as the *Bainbridge reflex*, which is thought to occur only when the receptors are rapidly stretched, as by a sudden infusion of fluid
- decreased sympathetic vasoconstriction to the kidney
- reduced release of ADH by the posterior pituitary, which causes a diuresis.

These receptors clearly play the same role on the low-pressure side of the system as the arterial baroreceptors on the high-pressure side.

Ventricular receptors

Mechanoreceptors in the ventricle wall elicit vasodilatation when stimulated by stretch or powerful ventricular contraction. These receptors were first discovered as a result of injecting the alkaloid veratrine into the heart, which produces the pharmacological rather than physiological hypotensive *Bezold–Jarisch reflex*. The hypotensive reaction to cardiogenic shock may be a similar response to accumulated metabolites stimulating these receptors.

J-receptors

The juxtapulmonary capillary receptors in the lungs may be stimulated during pulmonary congestion produced by severe exercise or high altitude. Their reflex vagal effects are tachycardia and rapid shallow breathing.

Arterial chemoreceptors

Located in the carotid and aortic regions (*and frequently confused with baroreceptors by students*) are tiny highly vascularized organs called chemoreceptors (see p. 692).

The primary function of these **carotid** and **aortic bodies** is to respond to changes in the chemical composition of the blood. They have an enormous blood supply for their size and their specific stimulus is the build-up of metabolites when their supply of oxygen is inadequate for their high metabolic rate. From this we can see that reduction of the amount of oxygen in the blood, or a reduction in blood flow because of a fall in blood pressure, or a combination of the two, will jeopardize their oxygen supply and stimulate these receptors. Their primary response is to stimulate breathing and to produce bradycardia and sympathetic vasoconstriction. Both these effects can only be seen in highly artificial experimental situations because they are normally hidden by the **lung inflation reflex** of mild vasodilatation and marked tachycardia produced by pulmonary stretch receptors in the airways of the lungs (see also sinus arrhythmia, p. 601).

Arterial chemoreceptors are also stimulated by excess CO_2 and H^+ in the blood. Their cardiovascular effects therefore become important during asphyxia (see p. 694) and during severe haemorrhage when pressure has fallen so far that baroreceptors have fallen silent and can therefore make no further contribution to control of blood pressure. Under these circumstances chemoreceptors are strongly stimulated by **stagnant hypoxia** and make a significant contribution to the last-ditch attempt to raise blood pressure to maintain the cerebral and coronary circulation. Arterial chemoreceptors also play a role in the diving reflex (see p. 605). Their effect on breathing is described in the section on Respiration (see p. 691).

Summary

Intrinsic factors affecting ABP

- Arterial blood pressure = Cardiac output × Total peripheral resistance.
- Intrinsic control of blood pressure is control by mechanisms within the circulation.
- Receptors in the reflex control of blood pressure are the arterial baroreceptors.
- Arterial baroreceptor activity increases parasympathetic vagal activity and reduces sympathetic activity.
- The baroreceptor 'set point' is the ideal blood pressure for conditions at that time (rest, exercise, haemorrhage).
- The 'set point' is reset by the brain to suit prevailing conditions.
- Mechanoreceptors with reflex effects are found in the atria and ventricles of the heart.
- Arterial chemoreceptors mainly influence breathing but also produce bradycardia and sympathetic vasoconstriction.

Extrinsic factors

Skeletal muscle receptors

Changes in peripheral resistance, heart rate and contractility during exercise are due in part to:

- Increased activity in motor areas of the brain that bring about muscle contraction stimulating areas of cardiovascular control.
- Reflex activation of receptors in the exercising muscle by mechanical and chemical stimuli. The importance of chemical stimulation, by metabolites, explains why sustained isometric exercise

produces the most powerful effect owing to the high concentrations of metabolites that accumulate.

- The cerebellum, which coordinates muscle movement, contains the fastigial nucleus and vermal cortex, which when stimulated cause renal vasoconstriction as in heavy exercise.

Pain

For reasons other than its subjective nature, pain produces variable effects on the circulation. At low levels, it causes tachycardia and increased arterial pressure (the alerting or defence response, see below). Intense pain may produce bradycardia and hypotension to such a degree as to cause fainting because of circulatory collapse.

Cold

Like the response to pain, the response to cold depends on the intensity. Moderate cold produces vasoconstriction of the skin and piloerection (hair standing on end) via the hypothalamic thermoregulatory areas.

Intense cold will elevate blood pressure by stimulating both cold and pain pathways. The coronary angina sometimes precipitated by intense cold may be due to reflex constriction of the coronary vessels or increased work of the heart pumping against increased arterial pressure.

Ischaemia of the CNS and the Cushing reflex

The CNS and the myocardium are the tissues most easily damaged by the lack of perfusion caused by low arterial blood pressure; these organs are also the most vital for survival. It is little wonder therefore that when arterial pressure falls to 50–60 mmHg, which is sufficient to produce hypotension and ischaemia of the brainstem, there is a powerful general vasoconstriction, the **CNS ischaemic response**, a final effort to maintain perfusion of the brain.

Bleeding inside the rigid cranium that surrounds the brain, or the growth of a tumour, can raise intracranial pressure to a level that, by squeezing the cerebral arteries or forcing the brain down into the foramen magnum (a situation known as 'coning'), also reduces perfusion of the brainstem. The situation provokes a reflex increase in sympathetic tone originating from the brainstem, known as the **Cushing reflex**. This increase in tone elevates blood pressure and may help to maintain CNS perfusion.

The diving reflex

There are many anatomical and physiological observations that demonstrate that we and many other creatures on the earth have a common ancestry. Some of these seem to have little relevance to adult human life, although closer inspection reveals their use under specific conditions. One of these is the diving reflex.

Seals, whales and many other creatures that live by diving for food show profound respiratory and circulatory changes during a dive. These changes include vagal bradycardia, apnoea and intense vasoconstriction of the blood vessels of muscles, kidneys, skin and the splanchnic system. This reflex is activated most strongly by immersion in cold water of the areas of the face served by the trigeminal nerve. It effectively turns the animal's circulation into a heart–brain circuit. This reflex is present in man but to a lesser degree (Fig. 6.6.2). In us, immersing the face in cold water can produce a 20% reduction in heart rate and a 50% reduction in muscle blood flow. In diving animals the

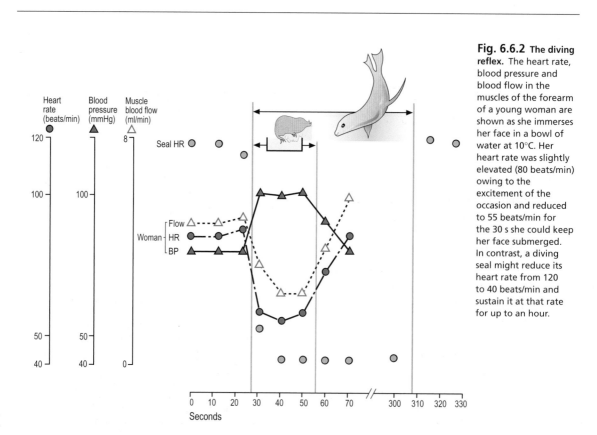

Fig. 6.6.2 The diving reflex. The heart rate, blood pressure and blood flow in the muscles of the forearm of a young woman are shown as she immerses her face in a bowl of water at 10°C. Her heart rate was slightly elevated (80 beats/min) owing to the excitement of the occasion and reduced to 55 beats/min for the 30 s she could keep her face submerged. In contrast, a diving seal might reduce its heart rate from 120 to 40 beats/min and sustain it at that rate for up to an hour.

reflex is powerful enough to allow changes in oxygen and carbon dioxide levels in the blood that would be fatal in man.

The peripheral chemoreceptors (see p. 692) are important in the diving reflex. During breath-holding on the surface (i.e. without the diving reflex) they are stimulated by lack of oxygen and excess carbon dioxide to reflexly produce hyperventilation, bradycardia and vasoconstriction. During the diving reflex, the hyperventilation drive is suppressed but the bradycardia and vasoconstriction remain.

The role of the diving reflex in adult human beings is probably the same as in diving mammals – although clearly rather ineffectual in us. It may also protect against inhalation of noxious liquids and vapours because trigeminal receptors of the nasal passages, pharynx and larynx all produce a response like the diving reflex. During birth, this reflex may inhibit inhalation of contaminated fluid and mucus.

CNS control of the circulation

It was once thought that neural activity controlling the cardiovascular system originated in 'centres' in the brain, but this idea has been superseded by the concept of a flux of activity within and between areas of the central nervous system (Fig. 6.6.3).

The cerebral cortex

The universal experience of emotion, pleasant or otherwise, strong enough to produce cardiovascular effects demonstrates that higher regions of the brain can influence blood pressure.

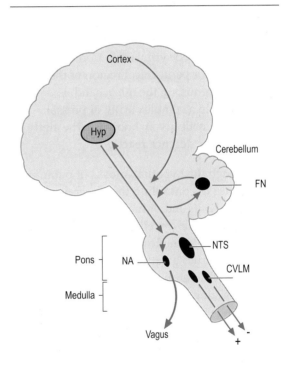

Fig. 6.6.3 Cardiovascular pathways in the brain. The idea of discrete 'centres' in the brain controlling the cardiovascular system has been superseded by the concept of a flux of information between regions such as the caudal ventrolateral medulla (CVLM), fastigial nucleus (FN), hypothalamus (Hyp), nucleus ambiguus (NA) and nucleus tractus solitarius (NTS). This system has efferent connections with the circulation via descending excitatory and inhibitory influences on sympathetic spinal neurones and via the vagus nerve for example. Modified from Levick RJ 1998 *An introduction to cardiovascular physiology*, 3rd edn. Butterworth-Heinemann, Oxford.)

Summary

Extrinsic factors affecting ABP

- Extrinsic control of blood pressure is by mechanisms partially situated outside the circulation.
- Skeletal muscle receptors influence central reflex mechanisms to adjust peripheral resistance, heart rate and contractility during exercise.
- The CNS ischaemic response is a particularly powerful peripheral vasoconstrictor response to maintain CNS perfusion.
- The diving reflex involves vagal bradycardia, apnoea and intense peripheral vasoconstriction in response to immersion of the face.

The hypothalamus and cerebellum

The hypothalamus is so intimately involved in the control of our visceral activities it would be remarkable if it were not involved in control of blood pressure. Various regions within the hypothalamus, if stimulated electrically, have a predominantly pressor or depressor action. As in the case of control of the respiratory system, it is best to ascribe to these areas an increased density of neurones that have the same function, rather than assume there are clear-cut anatomical 'centres' that carry out a specific function (which has been suggested in the past). Nevertheless, there *is* a division of the labour of controlling the cardiovascular system.

* The dorsal anterior part of the hypothalamus produces baroreflex-like effects, suppressing sympathetic activity and activating parasympathetic vagal inhibition of the heart.
* The anterior perifornical region of the hypothalamus, on the other hand, is involved in a complex array of pressor reactions, collectively known as the alerting response or **defence reaction**.

Although the hypothalamus is of paramount importance in controlling the visceral activities of our body, its individual responses are very stereotyped (like a well-trained parrot, which will produce a complicated sentence on cue but cannot construct great literature). The **alerting response** or defence reaction is one such example, consisting of hypertension, tachycardia, dilatation of muscle vessels and splanchnic and renal vasoconstriction. These are the hallmarks of the flight-or-fight reaction but can be elicited under non-threatening situations by electrical stimulation of the **defence area** of the hypothalamus (Fig. 6.6.4) or naturally by pain, sound, touch, etc. The defence area probably receives inputs from the limbic system, which is involved in emotion, because, in human beings at least, these cardiovascular responses can be triggered by emotion alone. The cingulate gyrus is involved in the 'swooning' or 'playing

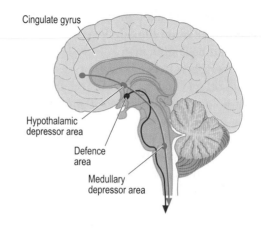

Fig. 6.6.4 The defence and depressor areas. The hypothalamic areas indicated produce the defence and depressor reflexes when electrically stimulated.

possum' seen in some animals in the presence of inescapable danger, and in humans during intense emotion. During its 'swoon' the possum (*Didelphis virginiana*) undergoes a profound hypotension and bradycardia, appearing dead. It is difficult to see the survival value of such a strategy, except being so still as to avoid being seen or avoiding the attentions of predators that do not eat dead prey.

The hypothalamus contains neurones sensitive to blood temperature and others sensitive to osmolality. The former regulate cutaneous vasomotor activity and sweating; the latter ADH release.

The cerebellum is primarily concerned with coordinating muscular movement, and as part of this coordination the increased blood supply to exercising muscle is ensured by redirection of blood away from other tissues such as the kidneys by vasoconstriction.

The brainstem

The pons and medulla, which make up the brainstem, comprise those parts of the CNS that:

* receive afferent information from cardiovascular receptors

- relay this information to specific regions and receive signals from other regions
- output activity to the parasympathetic and sympathetic nerves controlling the heart and blood vessels.

Information from most receptors in the cardiovascular system passes to the *tractus solitarius*. From here, information is relayed to:

- the *nucleus ambiguus*, the origin of the parasympathetic vagus
- the *ventrolateral* medulla, which influences the sympathetic output
- the hypothalamic depressor regions, defence areas, thermoregulatory areas, etc. and the region producing ADH
- the cerebellum.

To summarize and simplify, signals from the cortex, hypothalamus and cerebellum return via the pons (the bridge) to control:

- parasympathetic (vagal) output to the heart
- excitatory output to sympathetic preganglionic neurones in the lateral horn of the spinal cord.

Summary

CNS control

- The cerebral cortex stimulates changes in cardiovascular function associated with emotion and anticipation of exercise.
- The hypothalamus contains areas that produce the defence (alerting) reaction and the diametrically opposite 'swoon'.
- The cerebellum produces muscle vasodilatation as part of its movement coordinating role.
- The brainstem receives information from cardiovascular receptors and higher regions of the brain and outputs to the sympathetic and parasympathetic nerves controlling the cardiovascular system.

Long-term control of blood pressure

The mechanisms described so far control arterial blood pressure on a very short-term basis. Within 2 days of a sustained increase in blood pressure, arterial baroreceptor discharge will have been returned towards normal by adaptation and its effects diminished. A most convincing description of the long-term control of blood pressure has been advanced by the American physiologist Guyton. His description depends on:

- the powerful influence of extracellular fluid volume (including plasma) on arterial blood pressure
- the effect of arterial pressure on renal output or retention of extracellular fluid.

The cardiovascular system behaves somewhat like a beaker in which hydrostatic pressure is determined by the amount of fluid added or lost (Fig. 6.6.5). Although we have stressed the elasticity of arteries, the arterial system is fairly rigid, i.e. it is not very compliant, and any increase in the volume of blood it contains produces a significant change in arterial pressure. Increase in blood volume increases venous return to the heart and increases cardiac output, which increases the amount of blood in the arterial side of the circulation and increases arterial blood pressure.

This is only part of the story. Increased cardiac output causes the tissues of the body in general to be overperfused; they respond by autoregulating their perfusion down toward normal levels (see p. 578). This they do by increasing their resistance, so total peripheral resistance increases as well as cardiac output.

To demonstrate the power of small chronic changes in blood volume to change arterial pressure, Guyton carried out the following calculation.

There is a chronic increase in blood volume of 2%. This increases cardiac filling pressure and

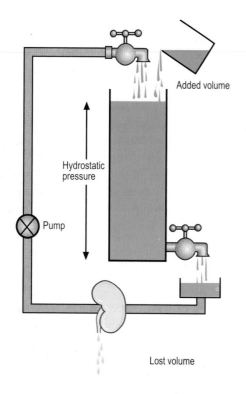

Fig. 6.6.5 **Pressure in a vessel as a balance between input and output.** This simple analogy is a useful but very tenuous one because the mechanisms that determine arterial pressure are more complicated.

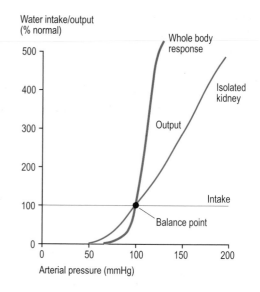

Fig. 6.6.6 **Renal control of arterial blood pressure.** The relationship of arterial blood pressure to urinary output for isolated and intact kidneys is shown. The single point where arterial pressure, renal output and fluid intake are in balance is the point of intersection of the intake and output lines.

therefore cardiac output by 5%. Autoregulation increases total peripheral resistance by 50%.

Cardiac output × Peripheral resistance = Arterial pressure.

Originally: $1 \times 1 = 1$.

Increased volume: $1.05 \times 1.50 = 1.57$.

So a chronic increase of 2% in blood volume could cause a 57% increase in arterial pressure – if the kidneys did not intervene and there were no reflex bradycardia and vasodilatation caused by the baroreflex.

Chronic changes in arterial pressure affect the rate at which the kidney loses water and salt. The relationship in an isolated kidney taken out of the body is a steep one (Fig. 6.6.6) produced by the physical phenomenon of hyperfiltration.

When the biological phenomena of:

- the renin–angiotensin–aldosterone system
- antidiuretic hormone
- atrial natriuretic peptide

are included, the curve becomes even steeper (the *gain* of the control system increases).

The kidney therefore controls the *rate of loss* of fluid from the system.

Plotting a particular *rate of intake* of salt and water (plasma can be considered as a salt solution) on this graph produces a line parallel with the horizontal axis (since water intake is not affected by arterial pressure).

There is only one point where the input and output curves intersect and this determines the arterial blood pressure for those particular intakes and outputs. Any change in the intake of water that would expand or reduce extracellular fluid and produce a change in blood pressure will be vigorously resisted by a change in output by the kidneys.

For this reason, chronic changes in peripheral resistance do not produce chronic changes in blood pressure. The kidneys change blood volume to return pressure to normal.

A remarkable feature of this system is that it can return arterial blood pressure all the way back to normal. To understand why this is remarkable we must go back to Section 1 of this book and control theory. When a variable is disturbed from its normal value, the sensors in a control system note the difference between the new value and the 'set point' the system requires, then switch on the control system that drives the variable towards the set point. When the variable gets *close* to the set point, the sensors cannot tell the difference and switch off the control system, leaving the variable to wander off again until the difference becomes big enough for the sensors to detect it again. There must be a deviation, however small, from the set point before the sensors can activate the control system.

In the case of the kidney's control of blood volume there are no 'sensors' as such. The process is an entirely physical one, hyperfiltration of the plasma, and since there is only one point where arterial pressure, fluid intake and fluid loss balance (Fig. 6.6.6), this physical process will continue at an accelerated or diminished rate until that point is exactly reached.

Guyton explains why a fairly rapid transfusion of half a litre of blood into or out of the system (as in a blood donation) has little effect on blood pressure in a healthy individual as follows. The arterial baroreceptors immediately control cardiac output and peripheral resistance to bring pressure close to the required set point. The kidneys, in the long term, then return blood volume and therefore pressure back to normal. This theory does not receive universal acceptance but is interesting if only because it integrates a separate renal mechanism, other than vasoconstriction, into the long-term control of arterial blood pressure.

Summary

Long-term control

- Arterial baroreceptor discharge returns to 'normal' control value within a few days of a chronic increase in blood pressure. They cannot therefore correct a chronic change.

- The kidneys regulate blood pressure on a long-term basis.
- Plasma volume has a powerful influence on blood pressure.
- The kidneys control plasma volume by retaining or losing water and salt.

Special circulations and conditions

6.7

Introduction: integration of cardiovascular responses

Close inspection of most of the activities of our bodies shows that they involve a number of systems under integrated control. For example, the control of skilled movement involves the learning of a motor program. When the movement is required, the learned program is executed. Fine-tuning of the movement, to compensate for errors caused by unpredictable anomalies in its execution, is brought about by visual and proprioceptive feedback (see Ch. 3.7). An autonomic programme, which can be thought of as providing metabolic 'back-up' in terms of a supply of nutrients and oxygen, has also been learned for each activity. In the case of **vasomotor control** in active tissues, this will attempt to provide just sufficient perfusion to meet the predicted increase in the needs of the active tissue. Any fine-tuning of this part of the program will be in part reflex and in part by local modulation of sympathetic transmission by the local release of metabolites

611

by the active tissue. Other more 'vegetative' activities, such as digesting a meal, also contain a component that involves control of local and overall cardiovascular function.

The control of the perfusion of individual vascular beds illustrates the different ways in which local and central control mechanisms interact.

The coronary circulation

If the heart fails, the circulation fails. An adequate blood supply to cardiac muscle is essential to life. The coronary circulation therefore assumes a very important role in maintaining physiological function in all organs. Total cessation of coronary blood flow for more than a few minutes is lethal. As a result of disease processes, coronary blood flow is frequently compromised and coronary artery disease (ischaemic heart disease) is a major cause of ill health and death in developed countries. Several special factors affect this circulation. For example, ventricular contraction has both direct mechanical effects on the vessel walls themselves and indirect actions through the metabolic products of the cardiac myocytes.

During exercise, cardiac work may increase 5–6-fold. Since coronary oxygen extraction is always very high (70–80% at rest; coronary sinus blood has a very low O_2 content), coronary blood flow must increase **proportionately** with O_2 demand. The mechanisms that control this largely metabolically determined increase in flow are discussed below (p. 614).

Anatomical considerations

The right and left coronary arteries arise at the root of the aorta just beyond the cusps of the aortic valves and supply blood to the whole of the heart (Fig. 6.7.1). The right coronary artery supplies the right ventricle and a part of the posterior wall of the left ventricle, while the left coronary artery, which divides into two major vessels, the left anterior descending and

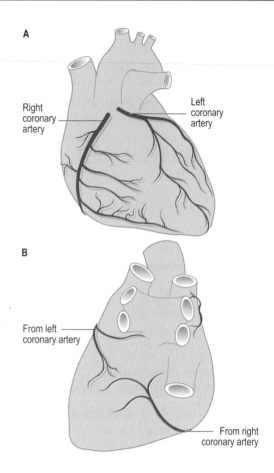

Fig. 6.7.1 The coronary arteries (simplified).

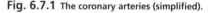

the circumflex arteries, essentially supplies the left ventricle; however, there is some variable overlap.

As the arteries pass across the epicardial surface, small branches penetrate the myocardial substance and end in a rich distribution network of small arterioles and capillaries. From a functional point of view, the potential for these arteries to develop **collateral vessels** becomes important, particularly after their total or partial occlusion (ischaemic heart disease). This potential varies greatly between species and upon the speed of development of the occlusion. With a gradual occlusion, more collaterals become larger, reducing the area of necrosis (cell death) and the potential for cardiac arrest and death. Some studies have demonstrated that in such circumstances coronary blood flow can return almost to pre-control levels within 4–8 weeks.

Collateral vessels are usually small pre-existing arterial vessels, which widen to carry oxygenated blood. There is evidence that following partial coronary artery occlusion, there is also the development of new collateral arteries and an increased growth of myocardial capillaries that may be enhanced by continued low-level exercise. This seems to be related to the development of a lower heart rate (relative bradycardia) associated with a given level of exercise, since it can be observed with paced hearts subjected to chronic bradycardia. The development of new blood vessels may be related to alterations in mechanical stresses or to metabolic sequelae of exercise. Collateral formation can be demonstrated in humans.

After passing through capillaries of the myocardium, most of the venous blood passes back to the right atrium through the coronary sinus, but some 5–7% drains directly into the cardiac chambers.

Capillary density, blood flow and oxygen extraction

The density of the capillary bed surrounding the cardiac muscle cells is high (approx. 3000–4000 per mm³) when compared with skeletal muscle (150–400 per mm³). This reflects the need for delivery of oxygen to cope with the relatively high minimum oxygen consumption of the heart – approximately 20 times greater than resting skeletal muscle.

The high density of capillaries around the cardiac myocytes ensures that there is a large surface area for diffusion and that the diffusion distances between the capillary and the metabolic machinery in the myocytes is short. Both factors facilitate the delivery of oxygen. Under resting conditions, in spite of the high coronary blood flow, the vigorous extraction of oxygen

by the myocardium causes the P_{O_2} in coronary venous blood to fall to approximately 20 mmHg from 100 mmHg in arterial blood, with corresponding falls in oxygen content. There is a high P_{O_2} **gradient** between the blood and the myocytes, as the P_{O_2} in the cardiac muscle cell itself is only 5–6 mmHg. Under exercise conditions, oxygen extraction rises to over 90%, producing a venous P_{O_2} of under 10 mmHg and a cardiac muscle cell P_{O_2} of 1–2 mmHg, despite a very large increase in coronary blood flow. This implies that there is very little left in reserve in terms of O_2 extraction if further demands are made on the heart.

Blood flow during the cardiac cycle

Blood flow through the heart varies considerably throughout the cardiac cycle. The branches of the coronary artery are **compressed** during systole, with the effects being most pronounced in the left ventricle (Fig. 6.7.2).

It can be seen that at the onset of the isovolumic contraction phase, blood flow declines

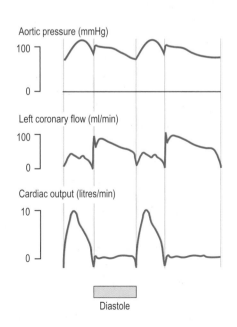

Fig. 6.7.2 Left coronary artery flow.

sharply as myocardial tissue pressure rises to over 120 mmHg, inducing a substantial decrease in transmural pressure across the vessel walls sufficient to cause collapse. When ejection begins, following opening of the aortic valves, aortic pressure begins to rise and flow increases slightly. However, the major increase in flow occurs only after ventricular systole, i.e. during diastole when myocardial tissues pressures have fallen significantly below arterial pressure. There is a transient reversal of flow during early systole. Approximately 80% of flow to the muscle of the left ventricle occurs during diastole. Flow through right ventricular and atrial myocardium is much less affected by contraction, since the intramural pressures, related to the smaller chamber pressures, are much lower.

During tachycardia, the proportion of the cardiac cycle spent in diastole decreases, and therefore the period of restricted flow during each cycle increases. Conversely, when the heart slows (bradycardia), the physical restrictions to flow occupy a smaller proportion of the cycle.

Regional flow in the myocardium of the left ventricle

It is now technically possible to assess tissue pressures and blood flow in the epicardial and subendocardial areas of the myocardium both during a single cardiac cycle and over several cycles.

There are substantial differences in flow across the muscle mass of the left ventricle. Ventricular systole raises **tissue pressure** near the inner endocardium to substantially over 120 mmHg, exceeding aortic pressure. In the subepicardial layers, the pressure rise is less, creating a gradient of pressure across the ventricular wall. Thus, the perfusion of the subendocardial layers of the myocardium is most compromised by this pressure. Inner myocardial layers have a higher capillary density than the outer layers. This partly compensates for the effect of ventricular systole by reducing the diffusion distances between capillary and myocyte. Despite this, under exercise conditions, there is evidence of **anaerobic metabolism** occurring in the inner layers where tissue P_{O_2} is low. The subendocardial layers of muscle are thus most imperilled if the coronary circulation is damaged by disease.

Mechanisms controlling blood flow

As oxygen extraction by cardiac myocytes is high under resting conditions, the only way in which oxygen delivery to the cells can be significantly increased is through an increase in coronary blood flow. In fact, the vasodilatation that occurs during increased work is so great that coronary blood flow is enormously increased in diastole.

Metabolic factors

In normal life there are substantial alterations in cardiac work and oxygen consumption, and a strong linear relationship between oxygen consumption and coronary blood flow over a wide range of workloads (Fig. 6.7.3). Such increases in blood flow could only be achieved by vigorous vasodilatation of resistance vessels. This is **metabolic hyperaemia**. Brief reductions in flow are followed by a vasodilatation whose magnitude and extent are directly related to the period of occlusion (reactive hyperaemia). Important factors that cause this vasodilatation are:

- tissue hypoxia – increasing adenosine production
- increases in $[K^+]$.

Adenosine, which is released in close proximity to the arterioles within the muscle, is particularly important, providing a mechanism that links metabolic usage directly to flow through a negative-feedback loop.

These local vasodilators act directly to relax vascular smooth muscle and also reduce the release of vasoconstrictors by sympathetic nerves. This last is via a presynaptic effect upon

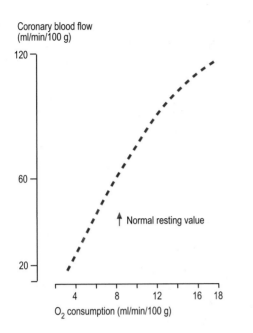

Fig. 6.7.3 **Effect of cardiac metabolic rate (measured as O₂ consumption) on coronary artery blood flow.**

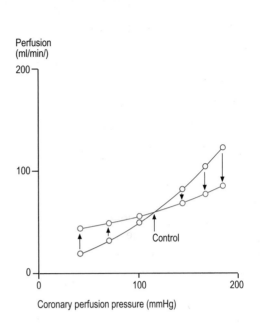

Fig. 6.7.4 **Pressure–flow in the coronary circulation.** Perfusing pressure was rapidly changed from the control value. At first, the pressure–flow relationship was described by the red circles. Autoregulation soon increased or decreased flow back towards the control values.

the quantal content of the transmitter release process (see p. 161) and also via a reflex whose input is from autonomic afferents in the myocardium.

Coronary perfusion pressure and autoregulation

The coronary vascular bed strongly exhibits the phenomenon of **autoregulation** (at least under experimental laboratory conditions). Instead of a positive linear relation between pressure and flow, there is a substantial pressure range (from approx. 60–180 mmHg) over which flow is almost independent of perfusion pressure (Fig. 6.7.4). Essentially, over the auto-regulated zone, resistance (diameter of arterioles) in the vascular bed changes so as to maintain flow constant. The effects are due to myogenic response and active contraction or relaxation of the smooth muscle in vessel walls in response to the actions of metabolites. They illustrate the

power of the feedback loop by which the concentration of vasodilator metabolites at the smooth muscle of blood vessels is held constant, thus matching blood supply to need.

An important role in metabolic vasodilatation has been proposed for **endothelium-derived relaxing factor** (EDRF; nitric oxide) and other agents produced in the endothelial lining of the muscular arteries. In the case of nitric oxide, shear forces produced by the blood flow in the vessel have been shown to trigger its release. High blood flow in a muscular artery would thus dilate it.

Actions of autonomic nerves and neurohumoral agents

The sympathetic innervation of the heart affects the coronary circulation both directly and indirectly.

Direct autonomic vasomotor control. As with all blood vessels, the tone in the wall's smooth muscle, on which vasodilator influences act, is maintained by a steady sympathetic discharge acting via α adrenoceptors. Vasodilator metabolites reduce the release of sympathetic transmitters; therefore when sympathetic activity to the heart and its workload increase, the effect of the sympathetic activity on the coronary vessels is reduced.

Indirect effects of autonomic nerves. Acting via **β adrenoceptors**, the sympathetic innervation of the myocardium increases both the heart's rate and the force of contraction. The consequent increase in metabolism raises, for example, the local concentration of the vasodilator adenosine, helping match blood flow to metabolic needs.

Local perfusion in many tissues is controlled by the interaction of tonic sympathetic discharge with local mediators. In the heart, the power of the local mediators to influence the outcome is very high, as might be expected of this indispensable organ.

Summary

The coronary circulation

- Vasomotor changes are essential parts of motor activities.
- Cardiac oxygen demand per gram of tissue is 20 times greater than that of resting skeletal muscle.
- Oxygen extraction is so high (about 80%) that increased perfusion is the most available response to increased demand (exercise).
- Ventricular wall tension stops coronary flow in the inner part of the left ventricular wall during systole.
- The major factors controlling coronary flow are metabolic (hypoxia and increases in K^+ and adenosine).
- Autonomic effects are important in the response to anticipated exercise.
- Endothelium-derived relaxing factor (nitric oxide) is important in coronary autoregulation and metabolic dilatation.

Clinical Example

Myocardial infarction

This is the usual medical term for what is commonly called a heart attack, coronary thrombosis, or, simply, coronary. The various terms are interconnected, and represent different ways of looking at slightly different things.

Myocardial infarction describes the area of damage in the heart resulting from loss of its blood supply. *Coronary thrombosis* refers to clotting in a coronary artery. This is the usual cause of a myocardial infarction, but the arterial blockage could more rarely be due to a blood clot that travelled from elsewhere – an *embolus*. *Heart attack* refers to a sudden cardiac problem that is often a myocardial infarction due to a coronary thrombosis. However, in some cases the heart attack may lead to an immediate *cardiac arrest*. Cardiac output suddenly stops, because of either asystole or ventricular fibrillation, and the patient literally drops dead, long before permanent damage has been done to the heart. It is difficult to resuscitate someone with *asystole* – complete absence of electrical or mechanical activity in the heart – but *ventricular fibrillation* can often be reversed by *cardiac resuscitation*.

Clinical Example *(Continued)*

In ventricular fibrillation, the ventricles contract feebly around 500 times a minute, and no useful output is produced, just as if the heart had suddenly stopped beating. Provided life is maintained by immediate external cardiac massage and artificial ventilation, the application of a defibrillating electrical current through the chest can cause the heart to resume sinus rhythm. The patient can then be investigated and treated for the myocardial infarction that is likely to be present.

After the interruption of its blood supply, and provided there is no cardiac arrest, the myocardium continues to beat and rapidly accumulates a severely adverse metabolic state. Pain fibres carried with the sympathetic nerves are stimulated. Feeling an intense pain in the centre of the chest, where the heart is known to lie, often gives a feeling of impending death. Severe pain from any source leads to *reflex effects*, including nausea and vomiting, pallor and sweating and autonomic disturbances of heart rate, either slow (bradycardia) or fast (tachycardia). If damage to the heart is extensive, the heart may be unable to maintain an adequate resting cardiac output (*central circulatory failure*). The patient will then be pale, with cold peripheries because of compensatory vasoconstriction, blood pressure falls and urgent treatment is needed. Diuretics reduce circulating blood volume and hence reduce the load on the weakened heart. Occasionally, dramatic mechanical complications develop – the damaged heart wall may *rupture* into the pericardial cavity, which fills up and prevents adequate cardiac filling and hence pumping. Or the interventricular septum may break down, leading to a *ventricular septal defect*.

The fundamental treatment for myocardial infarction is to deal as rapidly as possible with its cause, i.e. unblock the offending coronary artery. Time is of the essence. Fortunately, patients with sudden severe cardiac pain usually seek medical attention promptly. If the artery can be unblocked within an hour or so, there is a good chance that there will be little permanent damage. But if the artery remains blocked for more than 6 hours, the damaged myocardium has probably passed the point of no return. Between these limits, the myocardium may make a fairly good recovery over the next few months, during which the heart is vulnerable and should be protected from avoidable stress, such as non-urgent surgery and anaesthesia.

Treatment consists of giving intravenously a *plasminogen activator*. This is a substance that mimics the normal action of a fibrin clot in the body by converting circulating plasminogen into plasmin, a proteolytic enzyme that effectively digests and breaks down the recent fibrin clot. Unfortunately, this *thrombolytic therapy* can also break down recent thrombus that may be usefully sealing a leaky vessel, especially in an elderly patient. If this leaky vessel is in the brain, bleeding may lead to a *stroke*, illustrating once more that potent beneficial treatment is capable of severe adverse effects.

Similar treatment can sometimes be given for clotting in other sites, including leg vessels. However, since the onset of the clotting is rarely as clear as with a coronary occlusion it is harder to ensure treatment within the short window of opportunity. Sadly, thrombolytic therapy is rarely helpful for patients with strokes. It is difficult to be sure that the problem is due to thrombosis rather than haemorrhage, and there is a risk of bleeding in the infarcted area of brain.

The cerebral circulation

The control of blood flow to the brain and spinal cord is of paramount importance during life and there are special mechanisms that ensure that cerebral blood flow is maintained at the expense of other tissues. In humans, blood flow to the brain is about 750 ml/min (13% cardiac output). The brain does not contain large stores of ATP. There is sufficient present for about 7 seconds of activity, and ATP can only be produced **aerobically** (using O_2). Consciousness is lost if the brain's circulation is arrested for more than a few seconds: longer periods of reduced flow are followed by irreparable damage since, in contrast to most cells, the ability of neurones to maintain their integrity in the presence of a low Po_2 is very limited. Neurotransmission results in a substantial increase in oxygen consumption (see Fig. 6.7.6). Consistent with its local capillary density, blood flow to the grey matter, containing cell bodies and synaptic connections, where most metabolic activity takes place, is much higher than that in white matter, composed largely of axons and fibre tracts.

Whilst considering the control of cerebral blood flow, two important additional areas will also be considered: the formation of cerebrospinal fluid (CSF), and the blood–brain barrier (BBB).

Structural considerations

Blood is delivered to the brain through the internal carotid and vertebral arteries on each side; the latter join to form the basilar artery, which passes along the ventral surface of the brainstem and forms, through connections with the internal carotid artery, the circle of Willis (see Fig. 3.11.1, p. 278). Drainage of venous blood from the brain occurs through the large dural and bony venous sinuses into the jugular veins.

The unique feature of the cerebral circulation is that the brain is wholly contained within the rigid bony cranium. The cranium is full. Space not occupied by the blood vessels and brain tissue is filled with cerebrospinal fluid. Since all of these are incompressible, any change in one must be compensated by an equivalent change in another. Thus, while there can be considerable alterations in local blood flow overall, an increase in arterial blood flow following arteriolar dilatation must coincide with an increase in venous outflow, or a change in CSF space. Under normal circumstances, the volumes of blood and extravascular fluid contained in most tissues vary considerably under different conditions but in the case of the cerebral circulation this is not possible without severe effects, because of the encasing cranium.

Cerebrospinal fluid

The brain is surrounded by cerebrospinal fluid (CSF), which forms a substantial 'cushion' in the space surrounding the brain and spinal cord. This fluid is in direct communication with that in the ventricular system and spinal canal. CSF is derived from blood plasma by filtration, facilitated diffusion and active secretory mechanisms at several sites in the **choroid plexi**. It contains a low level of protein compared with plasma, and different concentrations of certain ions. CSF circulates from the ventricles to the **arachnoid villi**, ultimately draining into the dural sinuses and thence to the blood.

The normal recumbent CSF pressure, measured from a lumbar puncture (Fig. 6.7.5), is 120–180 mmH$_2$O and is well regulated. CSF pressure is normally slightly less than that in the veins of the brain and therefore does not compress them.

Cushing's reflex

An acute increase in CSF pressure can occur for a number of reasons, e.g. by occlusion of drainage. It results in compression of cerebral vessels and cerebral blood flow falls (see above). This provokes Cushing's reflex which is described in the previous chapter. Cushing's reflex occurs *only* under pathophysiological conditions, where it can be an important mechanism for maintaining cerebral function.

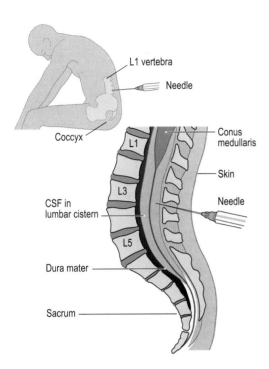

Fig. 6.7.5 Method of lumbar puncture to measure CSF pressure.

Measurement of blood flow

Total cerebral blood flow in a steady state was first measured by Schmidt in 1945 using the gas, nitrous oxide (N_2O) in a modification of the Fick principle (see p. 540).

The development of techniques for counting radiolabelled substances now allows the measurement of total and regional blood flow in the brain using an inert radioactive gas (e.g. xenon-133) or, by using radiolabelled deoxyglucose and positron emission tomography (PET) scanning techniques. In the latter case, the label indicates areas of high metabolic usage, which are generally assumed to be directly associated with local increases in blood flow (see Fig. 6.7.7). Recently, the use of nuclear magnetic resonance (NMR) techniques in conjunction with tomography offers opportunities for dynamic non-invasive assessment in humans (see Basic Science 3.11.1, p. 284).

These computer-based imaging techniques enable local alterations in blood flow evoked by physiological activation of different parts of the brain to be visualized. Localized increases in blood flow (hyperaemia) in different areas of the cerebral cortex associated with voluntary movement of the hand or a mental arithmetic test are illustrated in Figure 6.7.6. Such effects occur rapidly and are short-lived.

Control of cerebral blood flow

The major factors controlling cerebral blood flow are chemical (metabolic) plus local endothelially derived agents such as nitric oxide, which may also come from nerves, and pressure **autoregulation**. As the smooth muscle of cerebral arteries and arterioles has a demonstrable innervation from postganglionic neurones of both sympathetic and parasympathetic systems, it is likely that activity in these nerve fibres provides the background tone upon which the regulatory mechanisms act. Local adjustments to the vascular resistance may be aided by complementary alterations in efferent autonomic activity elsewhere in the body. Changes in baroreceptor and chemoreceptor activity assist in the preservation of adequate cerebral perfusion in face of disturbances to blood gas composition and arterial blood pressure.

Chemical control

The most important factor in controlling cerebral blood flow is the local (interstitial) **carbon dioxide** tension (P_{CO_2}). Small increases in P_{CO_2} cause marked cerebral **vasodilatation**, whereas decreases induce vasoconstriction restricted to the brain circulation (Fig. 6.7.7 shows the effect of hypercapnia on cerebral blood flow). Changes in interstitial P_{CO_2} can be brought about as a result of either changes in local metabolism or changes in arterial Pa_{CO_2}. The changes occur over the physiological range and, for example, a significant cerebral vasoconstriction, which results in dizziness, can be

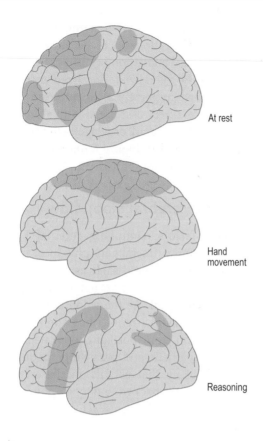

At rest

Hand
movement

Reasoning

Fig. 6.7.6 Cortical blood flow. Hyperaemia of 20% greater than mean in the human cortex during three activities is revealed by the xenon-133 imaging method.

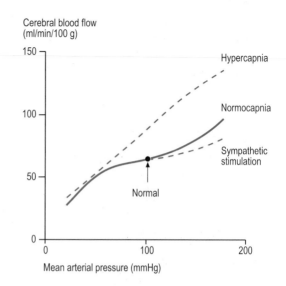

Fig. 6.7.7 Modulation of brain blood flow autoregulation. Brain blood flow autoregulation at normocapnia, the effect of hypercapnia, and the limited effect of sympathetic stimulation, which is only significant at abnormally high arterial pressures.

induced by hyperventilation. Conversely, an increase in Pa_{CO_2} to 45 mmHg doubles cerebral blood flow. Carbon dioxide diffuses to the vascular smooth muscle of the arterioles from the vessel lumen or from the active brain tissue, altering pH in the interstitial space: this is the likely specific stimulus affecting the smooth muscle. Direct intravascular changes in acidity, such as those due to lactic acid in the blood, are ineffective, since the blood–brain barrier prevents the movement of H^+, though diffusion of carbon dioxide occurs.

Changes in arterial Pa_{O_2} can also affect cerebral blood flow. A fall in **oxygen** tension induces vasodilatation; however, oxygen tension has to reach 50–60 mmHg before direct effects on the cerebral vasculature occur. This is why the hyperventilation hypocapnia-induced vasoconstriction described above is not countered by a hypoxic vasodilatation.

Autoregulation

The cerebral circulation strongly exhibits autoregulation; thus, over the physiological range of arterial blood pressure (approx. 60–170 mmHg) any fall in systemic blood pressure is followed by dilatation of the cerebral resistance vessels and maintenance of flow (see Fig. 6.7.7).

At arterial pressures below 60 mmHg, cerebral autoregulation fails as the maximum dilatation that can be achieved by this mechanism has been reached; blood flow then falls steeply. At high arterial blood pressures, where the ability of the autoregulatory mechanism has been exceeded at the other end of its range, cerebral blood flow increases and the increased pressure in small vessels can rupture them in what is known as a **stroke**. Alteration in arterial carbon dioxide tension affects the autoregulatory relationship. Figure 6.7.7 shows the effects of hypercapnia on this relationship.

Effects of autonomic nerves

The vessels of the cerebral vascular bed within the brain tissue itself are innervated by both sympathetic vasoconstrictor fibres and vasodilator fibres from parasympathetic origins. In contrast with virtually every other circulatory bed, reflex effects of these nerves is **minimal** except in conditions of abnormal pressure. The major effect of the sympathetic system is to reduce the range of autoregulation.

Blood–brain barrier (BBB)

The capillaries of the cerebral circulation have a selective permeability, restricting the diffusion of many molecules, including larger ones. Lipid-soluble molecules such as O_2 and CO_2 diffuse freely, but ions like H^+ and larger molecules such as proteins, insulin, and sucrose pass with difficulty. This is important for delivery of certain drugs such as antibiotics, which cannot cross the BBB. This can make treatment of infections of the brain difficult. Pharmaceutical companies are now designing drugs that deliberately either have or do not have the ability to cross the BBB and therefore affect or do not affect the brain.

The barrier is made by a tight investment of capillaries with astrocytes (a type of glial cell), which have 'tight' junctions with endothelial cells. The neuronal environment of the brain is a tightly controlled one in comparison with other parts of the body.

In a few specific areas such as the subfornical organ and area postrema, the blood–brain barrier is absent, and circulating neurohormones and peptides have direct access to the extracellular space surrounding neurones and may modulate their activity.

Summary

The cerebral circulation

- The brain is the most susceptible of all tissue to the effects of lack of perfusion.
- The rigid cranium presents a unique constraint to the cerebral circulation.
- Cerebrospinal fluid is formed by filtration-facilitated diffusion and active transport of the components of plasma.
- Carbon dioxide tension is the most important factor controlling cerebral blood flow.
- Autonomic effects are minimal
- The blood–brain barrier of tight capillary endothelial junctions controls the chemical environment of the brain.

The skin

The perfusion of the skin serves several purposes: the nutrition of the cutaneous tissue, the transfer of heat from the body to the environment and as part of the non-verbal communication mechanisms, like face reddening in anger. The metabolic rate of skin is low and the density of capillaries is not high. However, in 'acral skin', which covers fingers, toes, palms, soles, lips and ears, wide muscular **arteriovenous anastomoses** (AVA) shunts (Fig. 6.7.8) allow high blood flows during heat stress. Like the cutaneous arterioles these shunts are well innervated by sympathetic nerves and flow can be totally arrested if heat has to be conserved or blood loss imperils the circulation. An extensive venous plexus promotes heat loss from the skin when engorged with blood.

Temperature of the surroundings, and body temperature affect skin blood flow in three ways:

- *Direct effect of ambient temperature.* Direct heating seems to reduce the affinity of

A

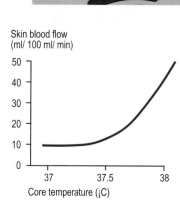

Epidermis

Capillary

A V anastomosis

Arteriole

Venous plexus

B

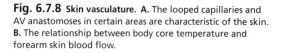

Skin blood flow (ml/ 100 ml/ min)

50
40
30
20
10
0

37   37.5   38

Core temperature (¡C)

Fig. 6.7.8 Skin vasculature. A. The looped capillaries and AV anastomoses in certain areas are characteristic of the skin. **B.** The relationship between body core temperature and forearm skin blood flow.

α_2 adrenoceptors (which are very abundant in skin vessels) for the sympathetic neurotransmitter noradrenaline.

An interesting situation exists in the case of cold vasoconstriction of the hands of some people. After about 10 minutes' exposure to cold, which is sufficient to cause painful vasoconstriction, cold vasodilatation occurs and prevents skin damage. This is the explanation of the reddening of the hands of people who work under cold conditions. This effect is sometimes called 'fish filleter's fingers'.

• *Spinal reflex effect of ambient temperature.* There is a minor effect whereby cold receptors in the skin produce a small reduction in sympathetic vasoconstrictor activity via a spinal reflex.

• *Core temperature effects.* This is the major control mechanism of vasomotor nerves to the skin. Regions that have many AVAs (fingers, toes, palms, face) show vasodilatation when core temperature increases, due to reduction in sympathetic vasoconstrictor discharge to the AVAs, skin arterioles and venous vessels. Regions with few AVAs (limbs, trunk, scalp) contain vasodilator cholinergic sympathetic fibres whose activity is associated with sweating and whose effect is mediated in part by VIP.

The response to heating is graded, with the hands and feet first showing cutaneous dilatation and the limbs and trunk becoming involved at greater heat loads. If overheating is sufficiently extreme, blood flow equivalent to the whole of normal resting cardiac output is diverted to the skin. This requires cardiac output to be increased (which is why hot weather is dangerous to patients with cardiac insufficiency). On the other hand, in very cold conditions, total blood flow to the skin can be reduced to below 100 ml/minute.

Bedsores

The nutrition of the skin does require its perfusion. A reactive hyperaemia is obvious if you observe your own skin after maintained pressure has arrested the skin perfusion for some time. This is presumably due to a myogenic response and the accumulation of metabolites. If pressure is maintained for long periods, then the skin dies and an ulcer is produced. This can easily occur in a deeply unconscious or anaesthetized individual and its prevention by nursing care – 'turning the patient' – is very important.

Splanchnic circulation – the gut

The word *splanchnic* means 'inward parts' – the viscera – and is generally used to refer to the gut. It is sometimes confused with the word *splenic* – relating to the spleen, which of course is only part of it.

The splanchnic circulation is peculiar in its connections, a number of organs of very different structures and functions being connected in **series** and **parallel** (see Fig. 6.1.1, p. 498). In outline, these series/parallel arrangements consist of the elements of the gut and pancreas draining in series to the liver through the portal vein (which carries 70% of liver blood flow) and a parallel arterial supply to the liver from the hepatic artery.

Splanchnic blood flow is considerable, accounting for 20% of cardiac output; 80% of this flows through the intestines and stomach. Intestinal flow is highly variable. After a meal, blood flow per unit weight in regions of the gut can reach levels only exceeded by the brain and kidney.

At a microscopic level, the circulation of the intestine shows another set of parallel blood vessels in the villi, where the arterioles and venules form a countercurrent system that allows high concentrations of Na^+ to exist in the tips of the villi, which aids absorption of water.

Control of blood flow during digestion is very specific, with the supply to the glandular and absorptive layers of the mucosa and submucosa being regulated **independently** of the supply to the musculature, although they both usually increase at the same time during digestion. The mechanisms of control are hormonal (see p. 838) and neural, with the parasympathetic supply increasing flow, probably indirectly by increasing glandular and muscular activity, and a powerful **sympathetic** supply that directly constricts splanchnic vessels. This sympathetic vasoconstriction has considerable significance in the maintenance of arterial and central venous pressure during exercise, haemorrhage or increased body temperature. The power of this mechanism to sustain central venous pressure is due in part to the fact that almost 25% of total blood volume resides in the splanchnic circulation (largely in the veins) and can be mobilized by venoconstriction. As the splanchnic circulation provides 20–30% of the total peripheral resistance, it is very important in the regulation of arterial blood pressure.

Integrated cardiovascular responses

To help understand the physiology of the body, this book has been divided into sections, each one devoted to a particular body system. This is a pure convenience to make understanding easier. No-one would suggest that one system is more important than another, although malfunctions of some have more dramatic effects than others. The body operates as a whole with each part contributing to the maintenance of homeostasis for the whole. The cardiovascular system provides many good examples of this and we can now put together the responses of the parts of the system that combine to respond to some of the changes we meet in day-to-day life.

Standing up from lying down

The average man contains about 5 litres of blood. When he is lying horizontal, gravity distributes this blood more or less in proportion to the amount of tissue present along his length. About 30% can be found in his thorax.

When he stands, there is a delay in the return of blood from the lower limbs to the thorax owing to the effect of gravity and about 500 ml of blood is **retained** in the dependent vessels. This movement is in two phases (Fig. 6.7.9).

On standing, the volume of blood in the thorax is reduced by 25% and central venous pressure is reduced to 1–2 mmHg. This reduces cardiac filling and therefore cardiac output. Pulse pressure falls considerably but mean arterial pressure falls only transiently as baroreceptor reflexes intervene. The vagal brake on the heart is reduced. **Sympathetic outflow**

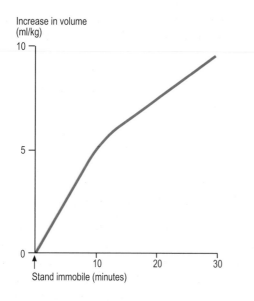

Increase in volume
(ml/kg)

Stand immobile (minutes)

Fig. 6.7.9 Increase in leg volume on standing. The rapid phase is due to a bulk movement of blood. The slow phase is due to transcapillary movement of fluid into the tissue spaces.

increases, increasing heart rate and contractility and constricts splanchnic, skin and skeletal muscle arterioles. This increases peripheral resistance and displaces blood from the splanchnic circulation to compensate for that displaced to the lower body. This downward displacement is resisted by constriction of veins in the legs. Increases in plasma noradrenaline and adrenaline reinforce these reflexes, but hormonal activity plays only a minor role in the rapid response to standing.

During standing, the skeletal muscle pump provided by the leg muscles makes an important contribution to venous return. To stand at all, leg muscles have to be contracted and this limits venous dilatation. The slight swaying movement of standing humans results from proprioceptive reflexes from the plantar surfaces of the feet. These cause rhythmic contractions of the leg muscles, which, by squeezing the underlying veins, counteract the pooling of blood.

Haemorrhage

Any haemorrhage is pathological and so this subject is perhaps more the province of a textbook of pathology, and it is therefore described in more detail in the next chapter (see Hypovolaemic shock, p. 635). However, haemorrhage provides an instructive example of the integrative aspects of cardiovascular control, which can be outlined here. The effects of loss of blood depend, of course, on the volume and rate of loss and the state of the subject before the loss began. 500 ml taken from a healthy individual, the usual amount of a blood donation, causes little change in blood pressure. Rapid loss of 1 litre of blood lowers mean blood pressure and produces the pathological state called **hypovolaemic shock** (see Ch. 6.9). Rapid loss of more than 1500 ml almost inevitably has life-threatening consequences.

Haemorrhage causes an immediate:

- decrease in blood volume
- reduced venous return and cardiac output
- fall in venous and arterial pressure.

If the body can respond effectively to these stresses, it is said to be in a **compensated phase**. If it cannot, the patient is said to have entered the **decompensated phase**.

The compensated phase

Compensation is initiated by baroreflex and volume receptors involves increasing total peripheral resistance by increasing sympathetic outflow. This also produces tachycardia, increased cardiac contractility and venoconstriction; the latter helps to restore cardiac filling pressure. The skin is pale because of sympathetic vasoconstriction and sweating occurs because of the activity of the cholinergic sympathetic fibres to sweat glands. Reduction in capillary pressure because of the increase in sympathetic vasoconstrictor activity and fall in blood pressure brings about an 'internal transfusion' of fluid from interstitial fluid to plasma, particularly in muscle, as the osmotic effects of plasma proteins now dominate transcapillary fluid movement. Hormonal compensation is in the form of angiotensin II and adrenaline, which help to restore arterial blood pressure by peripheral vasoconstriction and venoconstriction. These mechanisms may be sufficiently effective to prevent a significant fall in arterial pressure.

Water and salts are rapidly replaced by satiation of the thirst produced by increased levels of angiotensin II, the most potent thirst-provoking substance known. Increased sympathetic activity reduces renal blood flow and glomerular filtration rate. Salt and water reabsorption by the kidneys is stimulated by increased aldosterone and ADH levels. The formed elements of blood have to be replaced by increased haemopoietic activity and this takes 2–3 weeks.

The decompensated phase

If the loss of blood is too great, or cannot be adequately compensated for so that the stress of loss is sustained for several hours, systems begin to fail and the patient enters the decompensated phase. The first step in decompensation is the failure of sympathetically induced vasoconstriction and tachycardia. Vasodilatation supervenes, producing an irreversible fall in blood pressure, which, as a result of reduced perfusion, causes hypoxic renal failure and finally myocardial hypoperfusion and death.

Exercise and skeletal muscle

Exercise comes in many varieties and intensities. It can be isometric or isotonic, carried out with the subject upright or horizontal, be moderate and aerobic or of an intensity that is anaerobic (see p. 103). Static (isometric) and dynamic (mainly isotonic) exercises have very different effects haemodynamically. These differences mainly result from the sustained pressures generated on muscle blood vessels and intrathoracically and intra-abdominally by static exercise.

The dynamic exercise that most of us are acquainted with presents the body with two major challenges to its circulation:

1. Provide the exercising muscle with sufficient blood flow to sustain its increased metabolism.
2. Meet challenge 1 without compromising circulation to the essential organs.

Resting skeletal muscle takes 20% of our resting cardiac output; during strenuous exercise this can rise to 90%. Although skeletal muscle arterioles are richly innervated by sympathetic vasoconstrictor fibres, blocking their activity only doubles muscle blood flow (maximum activity in these nerves can reduce muscle blood flow to 4% of rest value – virtually zero).

In exercising muscle, the arterioles dilate, so reducing resistance and increasing local flow 20-fold. This is brought about by **metabolic mechanisms**, which overwhelm the increase in sympathetic tone. This functional hyperaemia is accompanied by the recruitment of closed capillaries. In resting muscle, only 20% of its capillaries have flow and many have discontinuous flows. In exercising muscle, all capillaries may have flow, reducing the distance between the blood and mitochondria of the cells. Local blood flow is almost directly related to metabolic rate, and it is thought that release of K^+ ions from muscle cells and increasing interstitial osmolarity are responsible for the arteriolar vasodilatation that helps increase muscle blood flow.

The increased metabolism of exercising muscle cells removes more oxygen than normal from the blood, and so venous blood from exercising muscle is less saturated than normal. This extraction is helped by the presence of **myoglobin** in the muscle fibres (see p. 680), but all these mechanisms are insufficient, even in moderate exercise, to prevent oxygen tension falling to levels where anaerobic metabolism becomes the major source of energy and produces large amounts of lactic acid. This is washed out to be resynthesized by the liver into glycogen or to be used by the heart as a source of energy. Oxygen used in the treatment of this excess lactic acid constitutes the major part of the **oxygen debt** – the increased oxygen uptake seen after exercise ends.

The local increase in blood flow is powerfully modulated by the action of the muscle squeezing the blood vessels (Fig. 6.7.10). This action forms the muscle pump that increases venous return. The increase in capillary pressure and number of perfused capillaries in an exercising muscle results in increased capillary filtration, which is the basis of the commonly observed swelling of muscles immediately after exercise (which body-builders call 'pumping up' your muscles).

Blood flow in exercising muscle can increase by 20 times and, because muscle forms such a large mass, this places large demands on cardiac output. For this to occur without depriving essential organs of blood (challenge 2 above), cardiac output increases and blood is directed away from non-essential organs.

Cardiac output is increased by muscle metabolic and mechanoreceptor reflexes:

- increasing heart rate – by withdrawal of vagal tone and increasing sympathetic activity
- increasing stroke volume by:
  - reducing end-systolic volume by sympathetic activity, and
  - increasing end-diastolic volume by increased venous return
- vasoconstriction in the splanchnic circulation, skin, non-exercising muscle (and in extreme exercise the kidney) by increased sympathetic activity.

Because the pulmonary and systemic circulations are in series, increased blood flow to muscles is matched by an increased flow through the lungs. This is accommodated, as in muscle, by capillary recruitment and distension. In exercise, blood returning to the lungs is less saturated with oxygen and, since arterial blood at rest and during exercise is normally fully saturated, the amount of oxygen picked up and delivered by a given volume of blood during exercise is increased.

If the vasodilatation of exercising large muscles were the only response of the peripheral circulation, blood pressure would fall precipitously as a result of this fall in total peripheral resistance acting as a 'sink' of cardiac output. This would put the vital coronary and cerebral circulations at risk. A general sympathetically mediated **vasoconstriction** in inactive tissues, particularly the renal and splanchnic circulations and non-exercising muscle, protects against this. In severe and prolonged exercise, renal vasoconstriction becomes important. This general vasoconstriction is sufficiently powerful to produce a rise in blood pressure during exercise, which is an important component in ensuring increased perfusion of the active muscles.

The pattern of this perfusion is influenced by the pattern of exercise, isometric or isotonic, which exerts different patterns of pressure on the muscle blood vessels.

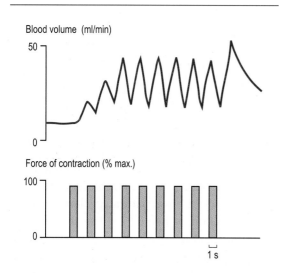

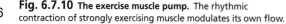

Fig. 6.7.10 The exercise muscle pump. The rhythmic contraction of strongly exercising muscle modulates its own flow.

Summary

Haemorrhage, standing and exercise

- If the compensated phase of a haemorrhage cannot restore the function of circulation, the patient enters the decompensated phase, which may be fatal.
- The neural element of compensation involves increased sympathetic activity, increasing total peripheral resistance and myocardial function.
- The hormonal element of compensation involves adrenaline, angiotensin II and ADH.
- The decompensated phase of haemorrhage begins with vasodilatation and bradycardia, which cause a fall in blood pressure and myocardial hypoperfusion.

- On standing up, gravity reduces central venous pressure and the volume of blood in the thorax.
- The skeletal muscle pump of the legs is activated on standing, to pump blood toward the heart.
- During exercise, the active muscles must be supplied with blood but not at the expense of the vital coronary and cerebral circulations.
- In exercise, cardiac output is increased by increased heart rate and stroke volume.
- General sympathetically mediated vasoconstriction preserves the coronary and cerebral blood supply.

Vasovagal syncope

This is the 'emotional faint' or 'swoon' that one normally comes across in daily life and is slightly different from the fainting that can be produced by standing or by neurogenic shock which causes profound venous pooling. The faint is caused by a sudden reduction in blood pressure, which reduces cerebral perfusion to less than half normal.

Fainting can be induced experimentally by such gruesome procedures as inviting the subject (victim?) who has just undergone venepuncture to drink some of his own blood. There is initially the usual defence response with a rise in blood pressure, tachycardia, muscle vasodilatation, pallor and sweating. The subject then shows all the signs of a massive **vagal discharge** with a profound bradycardia or even total asystole and even more muscle vasodilatation. Sympathetic tone falls and as a result of peripheral vasodilatation coupled with the bradycardia there is a precipitous fall in blood pressure. Interestingly, faints are almost always preceded by a yawn and often by vomiting.

The fainter usually falls to the floor and the horizontal position quickly restores the filling pressure of the heart and normal arterial blood pressure, and consciousness is regained. It is almost universal knowledge these days that forcing a fainter into the upright position is counterproductive; the reasons why are not so universally known.

Cardiac **ventricular receptors** with high thresholds are implicated in fainting and are stimulated by the heart contracting forcefully on a low end-diastolic volume. There is of course an emotional component and these factors are integrated in the lateral hypothalamus.

Cough, micturition and exertion syncope occur more rarely and have the common feature of reduced blood pressure impairing cerebral blood flow.

Sleep

Sleep, or more precisely the lack of it, causes profound changes in human physiology. However, all these changes can be attributed to changes in the functioning of the brain. It seems that although systems of the body can be exhausted, as in our most common experience of muscular exhaustion, these systems do not require the individual to sleep – all they require is rest. Sleep is an **active process** which affects blood flow regionally within the brain and affects sympathetic outflow to the heart and regional vasculature in a clearly patterned way.

During sleep, the systems of the body generally reduce their activity, and resting metabolic rate falls by 10–30%. Sympathetic nervous system activity generally decreases during sleep; the activity of the parasympathetic fibres to the heart may increase. These changes cause blood pressure to fall, typically to values of about 90/50 mmHg. With the fall in metabolic rate comes a reduction in sensitivity to CO_2 and ventilation. This results in a small rise in $PaCO_2$, which, in addition to changes in neural activity causes an increase in cerebral blood flow. As we fall deeper and deeper into sleep, we pass through non-REM into REM sleep (see p. 350). In the initial non-REM phase, the heart rate falls; as we pass into REM sleep there is widespread vasodilatation except in skeletal muscle where there is pronounced vasoconstriction, which contributes to the rise in arterial blood pressure seen in phasic REM sleep.

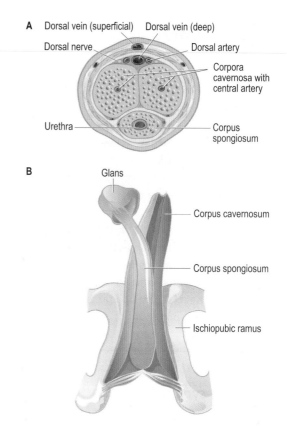

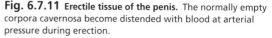

Fig. 6.7.11 Erectile tissue of the penis. The normally empty corpora cavernosa become distended with blood at arterial pressure during erection.

Sexual erection

Erection of the male penis and less obviously the female clitoris is a hydraulic event powered by arterial blood pressure. The erectile tissues of these organs and that around the female introitus consists of cavernous venous sinusoids (Fig. 6.7.11), whose arteriolar supply and venous drainage is controlled by **parasympathetic** fibres in the nervi erigentes of the sacral spinal cord.

During psychic or physical stimulation, parasympathetic activity (and reduction of sympathetic vasoconstriction) in which the transmitter is not acetylcholine but VIP or NO causes arteriolar vasodilatation and constriction of the venous outflow of the penis. This raises the pressure in the cavernous sinusoids and produces erection. Failure of erection is caused by bilateral upper or lower motor nerve lesions as well as by many other physiological and psychological problems.

Ageing

'Maximum achievable heart rate should be 220 minus age in years beats per minute.'

One of the few general 'rules of thumb' in physiological medicine, this rule clearly outlines the fact that cardiovascular performance wanes with age. The overall change that limits the performance of the ageing system is an expression of changes in all parts of the system.

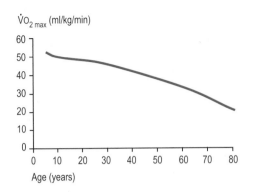

Fig. 6.7.12 How $\dot{V}O_2$ max changes with age. The steady decline in maximum oxygen uptake with age in a population of men.

It is important, however, to look carefully at these changes and distinguish both between their effects on the resting individual and their limitations on exercise and between the effects of normal ageing and the effects of increased incidence of cardiovascular disease which comes with age. This latter distinction is of considerable clinical importance, as there are many similarities between changes resulting from ageing and early coronary heart disease.

The ability of the respiratory and cardiovascular systems to supply the body with oxygen is measured as $\dot{V}O_{2\,max}$.

$\dot{V}O_{2\,max}$ is measured in ml O_2/minute/kg body mass and tends to be highest at about 25 years of age, decreasing by about 1% per year after that, so by the age of 65 it is about 60% of its maximum (Fig. 6.7.12). Sedentary young men have about 33% greater $\dot{V}O_{2\,max}$ than sedentary young women, but they lose this advantage with age.

It is important not to be too pessimistic about the, at first sight, gloomy picture presented by Figure 6.7.12. The healthy cardiovascular system does not restrict the activity of normally ageing individuals; the reduction in $\dot{V}O_{2\,max}$ with age is largely due to a reduction in the requirement for oxygen by all the tissues of the body whose metabolic rate is declining with age. In other words, in health we age as a whole and cannot blame one system more than another for our declining abilities.

One of the most important aspects of ageing of the cardiovascular system is a progressive increase in the ratio of collagen to elastin in the blood vessel walls. This change is general and normal and forms a background to the more patchy atherosclerosis (hardening of the arteries), which may be considered pathological but is almost inevitable. The increase in aortic volume that takes place particularly after 60 years of age is not sufficient to offset the reduction in arterial compliance produced by these effects, and there is an increase in pulse pressure superimposed on a smaller increase in mean arterial pressure. The increased impedance of the arterial system imposes a greater afterload on the left ventricle; this causes an increase in left ventricular chamber size, which, accompanied by a reduction in ventricular compliance, limits end-diastolic volume. All these factors combine to reduce left ventricular stroke volume. Because of the outstanding ability of the healthy cardiovascular system to increase perfusion when required, the limitations imposed by age do not necessarily limit sedentary lifestyles. When the stress of exercise is imposed, the reduced capacity of the cardiovascular system may become apparent.

With increasing age, the dilator capability of vascular smooth muscle, essential as a response to exercise, is decreased. The pulmonary circulation shows an elevated right ventricular end-diastolic pressure during exercise, and the ability to increase ventricular ejection fraction decreases. Stroke volume can still be increased, but the contribution made by decreasing end-systolic volume becomes less important and the ageing heart relies more on an increased end-diastolic volume (the Starling mechanism) during exercise. Increased noradrenaline levels in the elderly fail to stimulate the myocardium as vigorously as in youth, and this is the major cause of the decline in ejection fraction and maximum rate in response to exercise. This is not due to absence of β adrenoceptors but rather to an inability of these receptors to raise levels of **intracellular cAMP** in the myocardium. Orthostatic hypotension (where blood pressure falls more than 20 mmHg on standing from a sitting or recumbent position) is a particular problem for the elderly and is the result of an inadequate heart-rate response owing to this decline in autonomic control.

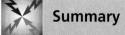

Summary

Syncope, sleep, erection, ageing

- Swoon (vasovagal syncope) results from a massive vagal discharge and reduction in sympathetic tone.
- Peripheral vasodilatation and bradycardia produce a precipitous fall in blood pressure and cerebral perfusion.
- During sleep, there is a decrease in sympathetic tone and a fall in blood pressure.
- Arterial carbon dioxide tension rises in sleep. This and cyclic changes in neural activity increase cerebral blood flow.

- Erection of the sexual organs is a hydraulic event produced by parasympathetic arteriolar vasodilatation.
- The effects of ageing of the healthy cardiovascular system are most apparent during the stress of exercise.
- Reduction in compliance of arteries is a normal part of ageing.
- Orthostatic hypotension in the elderly is largely due to an inadequate heart-rate response.

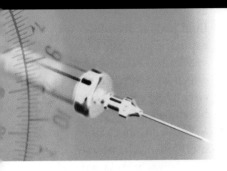

Applied physiology

6.8

Shock

Introduction

Shock is an excellent example of the way more than one system in the body is involved in physiological and pathophysiological situations encountered in real life. Shock involves the response of several systems dealt with in other sections of this book. These include:

- Smooth muscle (p. 109)
- Nervous system: sympathetic nerves (p. 158)
- Endocrine system: adrenocorticotrophic hormone (p. 380); aldosterone (p. 433); anterior pituitary (p. 380); antidiuretic hormone (p. 381)
- Cardiovascular system: cardiac output (p. 543); complement (p. 560); oedema (p. 592); venous return (p. 595)
- Respiratory system: hypoxaemia (p. 692); rapidly adapting receptors (p. 696); ventilation–perfusion mismatch (p. 675).

The term 'shock' is frequently used to refer to 'circulatory shock', which is a wide range of different conditions, including haemorrhagic shock, cardiogenic shock and septic shock. Despite different aetiologies, the feature common to all forms of shock is a *failure of tissue perfusion and oxygenation*. The causes of shock can be reduced to:

- failure of cardiac output (due to cardiogenic failure or mechanical obstruction)
- failure of peripheral circulation (due to hypovolaemia or inappropriate distribution of normovolaemic blood volume).

This failure may be brought about by:

- inadequate circulating blood volume – *hypovolaemic shock*
- an obstruction in the circulation, e.g. pulmonary embolism in *obstructive shock.*
- a failure of the heart because of disease of the cardiac muscle – *cardiogenic shock,* or
- profound vasodilatation of the vascular tree resulting in a reduced perfusion pressure and inappropriate distribution of blood despite an adequate cardiac output – *distributive (normovolaemic) shock* (as in *septic shock* and *anaphylaxis*).

Table 6.8.1 summarizes the different forms of shock. They all share common physiological consequences and, to a large extent, the physiological response to each is similar.

Physiological consequences of shock

In all forms of shock there is a failure of tissue perfusion. In hypovolaemic and cardiogenic shock there is a reduction in cardiac output. In hypovolaemic there is a reduction in circulating volume that results in a reduced venous pressure and ventricular filling, whereas in cardiogenic shock venous pressure is high but there is failure of pumping of the heart. Cardiac failure reduces peripheral perfusion, and this is exacerbated by reflex vasoconstriction.

In septic shock, cardiac output is not initially reduced but the action of bacterial toxins causes widespread peripheral vasodilatation. Since blood pressure is dependent on both cardiac output and peripheral resistance, hypotension and inadequate tissue perfusion result. Later in septic shock, cardiac failure may supervene as a result of the volume of fluid leaking from the capillaries into the tissue spaces and because of the effects of hypoxia and circulating mediators on the heart itself.

In severe shock of whatever mechanism, the pulmonary circulation is impaired and hypoxaemia results because of ventilation–perfusion mismatching (see p. 675). This may be exacerbated if cardiac failure results in pulmonary oedema or if the adult respiratory distress syndrome (shock lung) develops.

As peripheral cells are starved of oxygen and glucose in shock, excess lactic acid is produced by anaerobic metabolism. Following prolonged hypoxia, ATP levels in the cytoplasm start to fall, leading to a failure of ionic pumps in the plasma membrane; sodium, calcium and water leak into the cells and potassium leaks out.

Table 6.8.1	Types of shock			
Hypovolaemic	**Distributive (normovolaemic)**		**Cardiogenic**	**Obstructive**
Haemorrhage	Vagal (faints)		Coronary artery disease	Cardiac tamponade
Burns	Sepsis		Arrhythmias	Pulmonary embolism
Peritonitis	Anaphylaxis		Valve disease	
Vomiting			Cardiomyopathy	
Diarrhoea			Drugs	
Diuresis				

Profound or prolonged shock eventually leads to cell death, although the cells of some organs are more resistant than others. As cell hypoxia and death occur, more vasoactive mediators are liberated into the circulation from disrupted cells and the situation becomes progressively worse.

Responses to shock

The harmful effects of shock are limited by a series of homeostatic physiological responses. These occur as soon as blood pressure and/or cardiac filling begins to decrease. However, not all the responses to the causes of shock are appropriate. For example, in severe infection or trauma, a wide-scale inflammatory response releases 'mediators' that are beneficial against local areas of infection or damage but potentially dangerous systemically.

The responses to shock are a combination of reflexes mediated by the nervous and endocrine systems, whose effects are to:

- conserve fluids and salt
- increase cardiac output, blood pressure and tissue perfusion
- increase plasma levels of glucose and free fatty acids.

The neuroendocrine response is mediated principally by the pituitary gland, the kidney and the

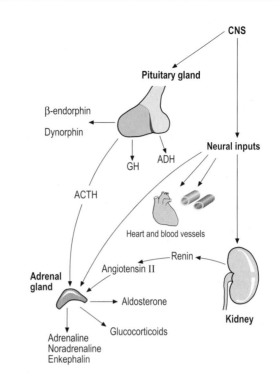

Fig. 6.8.1 The integrated neural and endocrine responses to shock.

adrenal gland as outlined in Figure 6.8.1. The roles of different mediators are summarized in Table 6.8.2.

The neural response

Many neural mechanisms are involved in the response to shock. These include arterial baroreceptors, atrial stretch receptors and chemoreceptors. Shock initially increases activity of the sympathetic nervous system. Sympathetic nerve endings in blood vessels cause a generalized vasoconstriction throughout the circulation, with the notable exceptions of the cerebral and coronary vessels. This vasoconstriction of veins increases central venous pressure filling the heart, and arteriolar constriction increases peripheral vascular resistance and arterial blood pressure. Sympathetic stimulation of the heart increases myocardial contractility and heart rate. All these responses maintain blood pressure and therefore perfusion of organs vital to immediate survival.

The endocrine response

Nervous stimulation of the adrenal medulla stimulates secretion of adrenaline and

633

Table 6.8.2 The neuroendocrine response to shock: a summary of the main elements of the neuroendocrine response to shock together with their physiological effects

Neuroendocrine response	Physiological effect
↑ sympathetic nervous activity	Vaso- and venoconstriction
	Tachycardia and ↑ myocardial contractility
Circulating catecholamines	Vasoconstriction
	Tachycardia and ↑ myocardial contractility
	↑ glucose release from the liver
	↑ glucose uptake peripherally
	↑ plasma free fatty acid concentration
Antidiuretic hormone (ADH)	Salt and water retention in the kidney
	Vasoconstriction
Adrenocorticotrophic hormone (ACTH)	Glucocorticoid release
	Mineralocorticoid release
Glucocorticoids	↑ responsiveness of vascular smooth muscle
	↑ plasma glucose
	↑ plasma free fatty acids
Angiotensin II	Vasoconstriction
	Aldosterone release
Aldosterone	Sodium and water retention

noradrenaline. These circulating catecholamines act on the heart and blood vessels to facilitate the increase in blood pressure. Circulating adrenaline also increases plasma glucose concentrations by opposing the peripheral action of insulin and by promoting the release of glucose from the liver. It also liberates free fatty acids from adipose tissue. These fatty acids are a ready source of energy.

Opioids, particularly enkephalins, are released from the adrenal medulla.

Paradoxically, some of the peripheral actions of opioids may include vasodilatation.

The hormonal response to shock profoundly involves the pituitary gland. ACTH (adrenocorticotrophic hormone) is released from the anterior pituitary, stimulating the adrenal cortex to increase production of steroid hormones, including glucocorticoids and aldosterone. High circulating steroid levels increase the responsiveness of vascular smooth muscle to catecholamines and are also

necessary for catecholamines to exert some of their effects on glucose and free fatty acid metabolism.

In addition, growth hormone from the anterior pituitary affects carbohydrate and fat metabolism in ways similar to catecholamines, increasing plasma glucose and free fatty acid concentrations. Opioids released from the anterior pituitary in response to shock include β-endorphin and dynorphins.

ADH (antidiuretic hormone) from the posterior pituitary acts principally on the renal collecting ducts to conserve water. It is also a vasoconstrictor and stimulates ACTH release from the anterior pituitary.

The kidney is essential in the neuroendocrine response to shock. Initially, the glomerular filtration rate is maintained, although oliguria with concentrated urine develops as a result of the actions of ADH and aldosterone.

In severe shock, constriction of the afferent and efferent arterioles of the glomerulus in the kidney, caused by increased sympathetic activity, reduces the glomerular filtration rate, and acute renal failure can develop. In less severe cases, low arterial pressure leads to increased renin release from the kidney, which in turn leads to an increase in circulating angiotensin II. Angiotensin II is a potent vasoconstrictor and also acts on the adrenal cortex to promote aldosterone release, which causes the kidneys to retain sodium. In severe shock very high plasma ACTH levels increase the production of aldosterone, augmenting its effect.

Severe and prolonged shock of any type generally produces the same physiological consequences. However, different types of shock (see Table 6.8.1) have different pathophysiologies, which result in the different responses outlined below.

Hypovolaemic shock

Hypovolaemic shock is caused by inadequate circulating blood volume.

The commonest cause is acute haemorrhage, following trauma, or gastrointestinal bleeding. Burns result in a considerable loss of fluid of a composition similar to plasma because the waterproof layer of skin has been removed. Inflammation following a burn increases vascular permeability, and in burns victims it is often necessary to replace large volumes of fluid; the volume that is lost is proportional to the surface area of the burn.

Under less acute conditions, dehydration and salt loss may also result in hypovolaemia. Salt and water are lost from the gastrointestinal tract in large volumes in severe diarrhoea, intestinal fistulae and pancreatitis. Water loss alone from the circulating volume is a feature of reduced water intake, diabetes and some renal diseases.

Symptoms

The symptoms and signs of hypovolaemia depend on the circulating volume that has been lost. Other factors include the condition of the individual prior to the volume loss and the rate at which the volume loss occurred. Furthermore, there is considerable variation between individuals with regard to their response to hypovolaemia. Clinically, haemorrhagic shock is divided into four stages corresponding to increasing volume losses (Table 6.8.3).

Treatment

The treatment of hypovolaemic shock is aimed at supporting physiological mechanisms that restore adequate peripheral perfusion and oxygenation. Administering oxygen, arresting the bleeding if this is present, and adequate replacement of circulating volume form the mainstay of treatment. Oxygen administration is important, as the shocked patient is often hypoxaemic because of impaired lung function. In more severely shocked patients, particularly in those whose conscious level is dropping, endotracheal intubation and artificial ventilation of the lungs may be necessary. The physiological responses that have evolved to limit the hypovolaemia are outlined in Figure 6.8.1. Clinical interventions support and supplement these mechanisms.

Initial fluid replacement is usually with 'crystalloid' solutions such as normal saline or 'Hartmann's solution'

Table 6.8.3	Clinical stages of haemorrhagic shock				
Stage	Blood volume lost	Heart rate (beats/min)	Systolic blood pressure (mmHg)	Central venous pressure (mmHg)	Consciousness
I minimal	< 10%	Normal	Normal	Normal	
II mild	10–20%	100–120	Normal	–2 (fall)	
III moderate	20–30%	120–140	100	–5 (fall)	Restless
IV severe	> 40%	> 140	< 80	–8 (fall)	Impaired consciousness

(lactated Ringer's solution). Alternatives include 'colloid' solutions containing particles of relatively high molecular weight, which do not pass across semipermeable membranes and therefore retain water within the circulation more efficiently than crystalloid solutions. They are associated with a small risk of anaphylaxis and the sudden expansion of the circulating volume they produce may occasionally be associated with cardiac failure.

When there has been blood loss, replacement of blood or red cells is indicated, although restoration of the circulating volume is always the primary objective of resuscitation. Research is going on into the use of artificial oxygen-carrying solutions based on either fluorocarbon molecules or haemoglobin polymers. They increase the oxygen-carrying capacity of the circulation while reducing blood viscosity. They remove the risk of infection from donated blood, and their use may be acceptable to religious groups who object to blood transfusion.

When large volumes of blood have been lost, it is also necessary to replace clotting factors and platelets, which do not remain functional in stored whole blood and are removed from red cell preparations. Depletion of these factors leads to a failure of coagulation and exacerbates bleeding.

Distributive (normovolaemic) shock

Septic shock

Septic shock is a severe vascular disturbance in response to infective organisms in the blood (bacteraemia). Many of the responses of the body to this type of shock seem perverse, threatening life. This is because substances released by the foreign organisms distort and disrupt physiological systems and because reactions that would be appropriate in localized infection or necrosis are disastrous when applied systemically.

Toxins from the infective agents release mediators from cells of the immune and vascular systems. These mediators in turn cause a generalized vasodilatation, a leaking of fluid and cells from the vascular system, and depression of the heart. This leads to hypotension. Hypoxia and mediators released by the effects of hypoxia cause capillary damage, which leads to further leakage, reduces local blood flow and causes hypovolaemia. The development of septic shock is outlined in Figure 6.8.2.

Septic shock is always a response to an infective agent, usually Gram-negative bacteria, but other organisms including Gram-positive bacteria, viruses and fungi are also implicated. The roles of

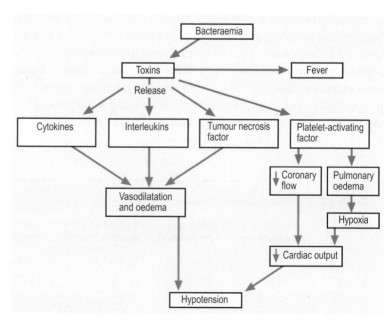

Fig. 6.8.2 Septic shock. The components that contribute to its development.

the mediators in the production of septic shock are described below and are summarized in Table 6.8.4.

Prostaglandins and leukotrienes are released from many different cells, including activated neutrophils, mast cells and platelets. They cause microvascular circulatory changes including either vasodilatation or vasoconstriction, increase vascular permeability leading to oedema, and cause a reduction in circulating volume. Some of them are potent chemotactic agents and can activate leukocytes. Furthermore, they cause pulmonary vasoconstriction and bronchoconstriction, which exacerbates hypoxia.

Cytokines, including leukotrienes, tumour necrosis factor (TNF) and platelet-activating factor (PAF), are released from cells of the immune system as well as from the vascular endothelium in septic shock. They are chemotactic for platelets, neutrophils and other immune cells and promote the adherence of these cells to the endothelium. Adhesion may be followed by the migration of immune cells such as neutrophils and B lymphocytes out of the circulation and into the adjacent tissue. Cytokines also cause vasodilatation or vasoconstriction, increased vascular permeability and decreased myocardial contractility. They often act synergistically, the effect of one cytokine being enhanced by the presence of others.

In septic shock, activation of the complement cascade releases a number of complement fragments including C3a and C5a. These cause vasodilatation, increase vascular leakage and are chemotactic for leukocytes. Other plasma cascades activated include the clotting and fibrinolysis pathways, leading initially to thrombosis of smaller arterioles and capillaries and to the depletion of clotting and fibrinolytic factors in the blood.

Platelets and neutrophils are important cellular mediators of sepsis. Platelets form aggregates in small vessels, blocking blood flow. They release factors that activate other cells and promote

Table 6.8.4 Some mediators in the pathogenesis of septic shock and their actions

Mediator	Actions
Tumour necrosis factor (TNF)	Released by macrophages and endothelial cells. Stimulates the release of other mediators. Toxic to endothelial cells. Chemotactic for leukocytes. Promotes fever
Interleukins	Stimulate the release of other mediators. Attract, activate and promote adhesion of leukocytes. Cause vasodilatation
Platelet-activating factor (PAF)	Stimulates the release of other mediators. Promotes activation and aggregation of platelets. Activates leukocytes. Increases vascular permeability
Prostaglandins (PG), leukotrienes (LTE)	Various actions. Some cause vasodilatation (PGE, PGI), others, vasoconstriction (LTE$_4$)
Coagulation cascade components	Promote platelet activation
Complement cascade components	Promote vasodilatation. Activate leukocytes. Promote release of other mediators
Adhesion molecules	Proteins on cell membranes that promote the adhesion of leukocytes to endothelial cells and the migration of leukocytes through the endothelium
Oxygen free radicals, proteases	Released from neutrophils. Damage vascular endothelium
Nitric oxide (NO)	Released from vascular endothelium. Causes vasodilatation

microvascular changes. Activated neutrophils release oxygen-based free radicals and lysosomal enzymes, which damage the vascular endothelium and other intravascular cells such as erythrocytes. Activated neutrophils bring about vasodilatation in vessels where they are adherent to the endothelial cell membranes. Other cells of the immune system that are thought to play an important role in sepsis include T and B lymphocytes, both activated by interleukins.

The vascular endothelium itself plays an important role in septic shock, releasing a number of factors including cytokines and chemotactic factors. When they express adhesion molecules on their membranes, endothelial cells attract and bind cells of the immune system, which are then activated. The endothelium releases a substance once known as endothelium-derived relaxing factor. This has been identified as nitric oxide, a gaseous compound with a half-life of only a few seconds, which in solution is a very powerful smooth muscle relaxant. Nitric oxide plays a pivotal role in septic shock. In the presence of inflammation, a particular form of nitric oxide synthase, which catalyses the production of nitric oxide, is induced in vascular endothelial cells and in macrophages. Nitric oxide makes a large contribution to

the vasodilatation that occurs in septic shock. Similarly, an induced form of the enzyme cyclo-oxygenase (COX), which produces prostaglandins from arachidonic acid, is expressed in endothelial cells in septic shock, so increasing the production of dilator prostaglandins.

In the early stages of septic shock, much of the hypotension is as a result of generalized vasodilatation. Cardiac output may initially be high and oxygen delivery to the tissues may be normal or even above normal. Tissue hypoxia nevertheless occurs as a result of inadequate perfusion pressures in some organs. Arteriovenous shunting occurs as a result of vasodilatation and damaged and thrombosed capillaries. As fluid leaks from the circulation and as myocardial depression begins to take effect, cardiac output falls, compounding the peripheral circulatory problems.

The pulmonary effects of the mediators of septic shock lead to arterial hypoxaemia as a result of ventilation–perfusion mismatching, right ventricular depression and pulmonary artery hypertension. Septic shock may ultimately lead to frank pulmonary oedema or the acute respiratory distress syndrome.

In severe cases of septic shock, organs such as the kidneys begin to fail, and this exacerbates the situation.

Eventually, the patient reaches a state of 'multiple organ failure' in which a number of different organ systems have failed and require artificial support. It is this group of patients who are most at risk.

Treatment

Treatment of septic shock is aimed at eradicating the underlying infection and supporting the circulation to vital organs.

Antibiotic therapy is started and supportive therapy includes artificial ventilation of the lungs, administration of fluids and the use of vasoactive agents such as adrenaline and noradrenaline. Noradrenaline is a potent vasoconstrictor and most useful in the treatment of hypotension due to vasodilatation.

In severe cases of septic shock, many organ systems require support; for example, it is frequently necessary to provide treatment for renal failure. Many forms of treatment for septic shock have been tried in the past, in particular the use of anti-endotoxin antibodies, but with disappointing results. Steroids have been used to try to reduce the inflammatory response, but with little effect on mortality.

Despite advances in critical care medicine over the past few years, severe sepsis remains one of the leading causes of death in the intensive care unit, and has a mortality that is still around 50%.

Anaphylactic shock

Anaphylaxis is a form of hypersensitivity reaction. It is an exaggerated immunological response to a substance, usually a protein, to which an individual has previously been sensitized.

Initial exposure to the reaction-provoking substance does not result in an anaphylactic reaction but stimulates the production of allergen-specific antibodies from activated B lymphocytes. Amongst these antibodies, those of the IgE class bind to mast cells and basophils. Mast cells are found throughout the body, but are most numerous in the lungs, the gut and the skin. They have a role in fighting infection. It is only following sensitization and the production of antibodies of the IgE class that a true anaphylactic reaction takes place.

If the individual is exposed to the antigen again, a number of the IgE molecules bind to the surface of the mast cell, stimulating degranulation – the release of preformed mediators such as histamine, prostaglandins and leukotrienes.

Histamine released from mast cells (Fig. 6.8.3) and basophils provokes vasodilatation, which results in systemic hypotension. Histamine also increases vascular permeability, leading to oedema and hypovolaemia,

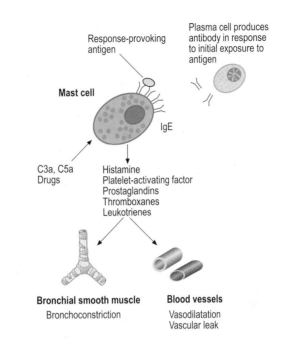

Fig. 6.8.3 **The mast cell.** Its central role in the production of anaphylactic and anaphylactoid reactions.

and so exacerbating systemic hypotension. It also affects the heart, making the myocardium more prone to arrhythmias. All of these effects are mediated by H_1 receptors. Acting via H_2 receptors, histamine increases heart rate and contractility.

In the lungs, histamine is a potent bronchoconstrictor and stimulates pulmonary rapidly adapting ('irritant') receptors that produce reflex bronchoconstriction.

Also important in anaphylactic shock are prostaglandins and leukotrienes. Both are potent bronchoconstrictors and cause inflammation of the bronchial mucosa. Other mediators of anaphylaxis include platelet-activating factor (PAF), which causes vasodilatation increased vascular permeability and hypotension and is chemotactic for immunoactive cells.

Anaphylactoid reactions

In true anaphylactic shock, binding of an antigen to IgE is the first and essential step.

In some cases, a clinically similar condition to anaphylactic shock can take place, which is not mediated by IgE antibodies. This is an anaphylactoid reaction. Many stimuli can provoke such a

639

reaction. Some drugs act directly on mast cells or basophils to cause histamine release. In particular, some muscle-relaxing drugs used in general anaesthesia (e.g. tubocurarine) have this effect. In the majority of individuals, this is of little consequence and may be accompanied by mild skin erythema or occasionally by mild hypotension, but in some individuals a more serious reaction may occur.

Anaphylactoid reactions can also be brought about by elements of the complement cascade activated via either the classical or alternative pathway. The classical pathway requires previous exposure to the antigen. Activation of the alternative pathway does not involve previous exposure. Instead, the first antigen exposure directly activates the cascade. The complement fragments C3a and C5a, whether produced by the classical or alternative pathway, have a direct action on mast cells and basophils, causing degranulation leading to an anaphylactoid reaction.

Clinical presentation

Anaphylactic shock typically follows the intravenous administration of a drug to which the patient has become sensitive. Other causes of anaphylaxis include venomous bites or stings or ingestion of a particular food. The reaction usually occurs within 30 minutes. The patient's skin becomes red and there may be oedema or urticaria. The patient becomes hypotensive and may collapse. In about half the cases of anaphylaxis, bronchoconstriction and airway oedema are prominent features, and ventilation may be impaired as a result. This combined with the cardiovascular reactions leads to hypoxaemia and cyanosis.

Treatment

Initial treatment includes the administration of oxygen, with spasm perhaps necessitating tracheal intubation. Adrenaline may be given to support the failing circulation and counteract the bronchoconstriction. Large volumes of fluid may need to be infused, as plasma volume is frequently reduced as a result of capillary leakiness. Antihistamine drugs and corticosteroids are also administered once the patient's condition has been stabilized.

Vagogenic shock

Vagogenic shock is also known as vagal or neurogenic shock. It is a type of distributive shock in so far as loss of fluid from the vascular system is not the principal cause. The fall in blood pressure in this type of shock is the result of vagal braking effects on the heart coupled with dilatation of the vessels containing the blood and those providing the peripheral resistance, rather than a reduction in the volume of blood.

This dilatation results when sympathetic 'tone' is removed by trauma to the medulla or spinal cord, by interruption of blood, oxygen or glucose supply (as in insulin overdoses), by physical injury or drugs (ganglion blockers), or by parasympathetic stimulation (which inhibits sympathetic activity and slows the heart). Peripheral vasodilatation causes a fall in blood pressure. This constitutes shock.

This type of shock is associated with fainting (syncope). The faint is not the cause of the shock. The fall in blood pressure resulting from the shock causes the faint by reducing blood supply to the brain.

Cardiogenic shock

Cardiogenic shock is caused by impaired myocardial function. The commonest cause is an acute myocardial infarction and coronary artery disease, although almost any form of heart disease may lead to cardiogenic shock.

Failure of the myocardium leads to a reduction in cardiac output. Cardiogenic shock becomes apparent if the cardiac output is less than about 2.5 l/min. As the myocardium fails, the left atrial pressure rises and pulmonary oedema develops. This leads to breathlessness and central cyanosis with widespread crepitations throughout the chest on auscultation. Peripherally, the patient's skin is cool and pale from reduced systemic perfusion resulting from low cardiac output and widespread reflex vasoconstriction in response to low blood pressure.

Hypotension and the neurohumoral response to shock cause a reflex increase in heart rate. This, combined with the increased systemic vascular resistance, leads to an increase in myocardial oxygen requirements. Low perfusion pressure in the coronary arteries and hypoxaemia due to pulmonary oedema mean that the increased demands for oxygen cannot be met and further ischaemia of the myocardium ensues, potentially worsening the degree of shock.

Treatment

Treatment of cardiogenic shock aims to improve oxygenation and support the failing heart. Administration of oxygen is necessary and pulmonary oedema may be relieved by the administration of venodilators such as nitrates. In some patients, endotracheal intubation and artificial ventilation may be required. Ventilating the patient's lungs with positive pressure to the airways can reduce oedema fluid in the alveoli and therefore improve oxygen exchange. Blood pressure is monitored continuously with an intra-arterial cannula, and the central venous pressure is monitored with a cannula in the external jugular or subclavian vein. In more severe cases of cardiogenic shock, a pulmonary artery catheter is sited in order to estimate cardiac output and pulmonary capillary wedge pressure (PCWP), a measure of left atrial filling pressure. Fluid is administered if the PCWP is not high, in order to increase cardiac output. The benefit of fluid administration is monitored by watching its effect on cardiac output. Once a maximum cardiac output has been obtained by this method alone, inotropic drugs such as dobutamine can support the failing heart.

Obstructive shock

Myocardial function can also be impaired by factors that physically interfere with the return of blood to the heart (pulmonary emboli) or physically restrict the pumping action of the heart (cardiac tamponade). In tamponade, fluid exuded inside the tough pericardial sac compresses the heart. The build-up of pressure within the pericardium first prevents filling of the parts of the heart that operate at the lowest pressures – the atria. This obstructs venous return, causes loss of fluid in the form of oedema in the tissues and all the other complications of shock.

Treatment

Despite advances in cardiology and critical care medicine, cardiogenic shock still carries a very high mortality. Treatment is aimed at supporting the failing heart, but for recovery, the myocardium needs to regain some of its lost function, something that it may not be able to achieve, because the failure of the heart as a pump results in reduction in its own coronary flow. This results in further failure as a pump and so on in a vicious downward spiral.

Further reading

Austyn J M, Wood K J 1993 *Principles of cellular and molecular immunology*. Oxford University Press, Oxford.

An interesting approach to the teaching of this subject. The immune system is laid out as a map around which the authors follow the development of an immune reaction. The appendix, which illustrates research techniques may be a little advanced for the average student.

Case R M, Waterhouse J M (ed) 1994 *Human physiology: age stress and the environment*. Oxford University Press, Oxford.

Interesting perspectives on various physiological stresses including their effect on the cardiovascular system.

Hoffbrand A V, Pettit J E 2001 *Essential haematology*, 4th edn. Blackwell Science (UK), Oxford.

A very popular textbook, which has been extensively revised. Well illustrated and laid out.

Jordan D, Marshall J (eds) 1995 *Cardiovascular regulation*. Portland Press for The Physiological Society, London.

A collection of monographs which would bring the student up to date with eight aspects of cardiovascular physiology as understood in 1995.

Levick J R 2000 *An introduction to cardiovascular physiology*, 3rd edn. Arnold, London.

Probably the best book on cardiovascular physiology available to students. If you have to have a book on this subject, this is it.

Noble M, Siva A 2000 *Crash course cardiology*. Mosby, London.

One of an excellent series for use in clinical training but of interest in linking physiology to practice

Roitt, I M 2001 *Essential immunology*, 10th edn. Blackwell Science, Oxford.

Absolutely up to date primer in immunology readable and well illustrated. It has its own web site.

Questions

Answer true or false to the following statements:

6.1

The following would increase net outward capillary filtration in the foot:
A. An increase in interstitial fluid pressure.
B. A decrease in plasma albumin concentration.
C. An increase in capillary permeability.
D. A fall in atmospheric pressure.
E. Arteriolar constriction.

6.2

Systemic veins:
A. Have a lower compliance than systemic arteries.
B. Constrict in response to activation of α adrenoceptors.
C. Are the main resistance element in the circulation.
D. Contain valves that promote venous return during muscle activity.
E. Contain valves that help reduce venous pressure in foot veins during muscle activity.

6.3

Sympathetic nerves:
A. Increase heart rate by acting on α_2 adrenoceptors.
B. Reduce cardiac filling pressure by increasing peripheral resistance.
C. Shift the volume–pressure curve for veins to the right.
D. Promote autotransfusion from the interstitial fluid during hypotension.
E. Are activated by increased baroreceptor activity.

6.4

Regarding parasympathetic nerves:
A. They play an important role in controlling total peripheral resistance (TPR).
B. Their transmitter has a negative chronotropic effect in the heart.
C. Their transmitter has a negative inotropic effect in the heart.
D. They activate muscarinic cholinergic receptors in the heart.
E. They cause arteriolar dilatation in the penis, leading to erection.

6.5

Arterial pressure:
A. Tends to decrease with age because of a fall in cardiac output.
B. Is lower in the pulmonary than the systemic circulation because pulmonary vascular resistance is lower.
C. Is kept constant over weeks to years mainly by the action of the baroreceptors.
D. Increases in the systemic circulation in response to an increase in intracranial pressure.
E. Falls when blood volume is reduced because cardiac filling pressure is reduced.

6.6

Starling's law of the heart:
A. Provides a mechanism that matches the outputs of right and left ventricles.
B. Depends on nervously mediated changes in cardiac contractility.
C. Can be explained using the sliding filament hypothesis of contraction.
D. Provides a mechanism to explain why cardiac output is independent of afterload over a wide range of arterial pressures.
E. Accounts for most of the increase in cardiac output during mild exercise.

(Answers overleaf →)

6.7

Blood flow:

A. To the skin is largely under local metabolic control.

B. To the brain is largely under autonomic nervous control.

C. To the heart is maximal during cardiac systole, when arterial pressure is highest.

D. May be increased locally by endothelial production of nitric oxide (NO).

E. Is inversely proportional to vascular resistance.

6.8

The viscosity of blood:

A. Is increased in anaemia.

B. Is apparently higher in arterioles than in large arteries.

C. Is increased in conditions with high levels of plasma protein.

D. Increases cardiac work.

E. Contributes to vascular resistance.

6.9

During the cardiac cycle:

A. The v wave corresponds with isovolumic ventricular contraction.

B. The first heart sound is caused by closure of the semilunar valves.

C. The ejection fraction is increased by sympathetic stimulation.

D. Atrial systole is responsible for more than half of ventricular filling at a heart rate of 70 beats per minute.

E. The QRS wave of the ECG corresponds in timing with the onset of ventricular contraction.

6.10

In the electrocardiogram (ECG):

A. The P wave is caused by atrial contraction.

B. The signal is recorded using pairs of surface electrodes.

C. The PR interval increases in length in response to parasympathetic stimulation of the heart.

D. The PP interval decreases during inspiration.

E. The T wave is normally positive (upward going) when the wave of ventricular repolarization travels in the same direction as the recording lead.

Answers

6.1

A. **False.** This would oppose filtration.
B. **True.** This would decrease absorption because of the plasma colloid osmotic pressure.
C. **True.**
D. **True.** This decreases the interstitial fluid pressure, making it more negative than normal.
E. **False.** This tends to decrease capillary hydrostatic pressure.

6.2

A. **False.** Veins have a high compliance and so act as capacitance vessels in the circulation.
B. **True.** This is the mechanism underlying sympathetic venoconstriction.
C. **False.** This role is fulfilled by the arterioles.
D. **True.** This is the muscle pump; the valves prevent backflow away from the heart during muscle contraction.
E. **True.** One effect of the muscle pump is to reduce the hydrostatic pressure that would otherwise develop when standing. Varicose veins, in which the valves are incompetent, lead to high venous pressures with oedema and ulcer formation.

6.3

A. **False.** Cardiac adrenoceptors are β_1.
B. **False.** Sympathetic nerves do cause arteriolar constriction, increasing peripheral resistance, but they also promote cardiac filling by causing venoconstriction.
C. **True.** Sympathetically mediated venoconstriction shifts the volume–pressure curve to the right, i.e. the veins have a lower total volume at any given venous pressure.

D. **True.** This is mainly due to the marked arteriolar constriction, which reduces capillary hydrostatic pressure, favouring fluid absorption.
E. **False.** Baroreceptor output inhibits sympathetic activity; reduced baroreceptor output during hypotension leads to increased sympathetic activity.

6.4

A. **False.** TPR is mainly regulated by sympathetic nerves.
B. **True.** Vagal activity slows the heart.
C **False.** The parasympathetic nerves are not distributed to the ventricular muscle.
D **True.**
E. **True.** This leads to vascular engorgement of the penis.

6.5

A. **False.** Systemic pressure tends to increase with age because of decreased arterial elasticity.
B. **True.** The cardiac output is the same on both sides, so the lower pulmonary pressure can only reflect a lower resistance to flow.
C. **False.** Baroreceptors adapt too quickly to provide long-term control of blood pressure. Baroreceptors limit short-term changes over seconds to minutes.
D. **True.** This is the Cushing reaction; increased intracranial pressure compresses cerebral arteries, causing cerebral ischaemia, which directly activates sympathetic vasoconstriction.
E. **True.** Reduced venous return leads to reduced cardiac output by Starling's mechanism, thus reducing arterial pressure.

6.6

A. True. Any mismatch will quickly lead to a change in ventricular volume, causing a compensatory change in stroke volume.
B. False. It is an intrinsic property of the isolated heart.
C. True. The force of contraction increases as the ventricle is stretched because there is less interference between thin myofilaments attached to opposite ends of the sarcomere.
D. True. Any increase in pressure leads to a brief fall in stroke volume that is corrected within a few beats by the resulting increase in ventricular volume.
E. False. This is mainly due to the increase in heart rate caused by increased sympathetic and reduced parasympathetic activity.

6.7

A. False. Cutaneous blood flow usually greatly exceeds metabolic need and is sympathetically regulated to control heat loss from the body.
B. False. Cerebral blood flow is mainly controlled by local metabolic needs, Pa_{CO_2} and myogenic responses.
C. False. Coronary flow is maximal during diastole since ventricular systole compresses the myocardial vessels.
D. True. Nitric oxide causes relaxation of vascular smooth muscle.
E. True. Flow = Pressure gradient/Vascular resistance.

6.8

A. False. The low haematocrit decreases viscosity.
B. False. It is reduced in small diameter vessels – the Fahraeus–Lindqvist effect.

C. True. This is probably because of decreased axial streaming and rouleaux formation.
D. True. It contributes to peripheral resistance.
E. True. Resistance is proportional to viscosity; see page 510.

6.9

A. False. The c wave corresponds with isovolumic ventricular contraction; the v wave corresponds with the period from opening of the semilunar valves to reopening of the atrioventricular valve.
B. False. The first heart sound is caused by closure of the atrioventricular valves.
C. True. The positive inotropic effect.
D. False. Passive filling accounts for about two-thirds of filling at resting heart rates.
E. True. The QRS wave is produced by the spread of ventricular depolarization, which activates contraction.

6.10

A. False. The ECG is an electrical, not a mechanical recording.
B. True.
C. True. The increase in atrioventricular delay reflects slowed conduction at the AV node, which can be caused by increased parasympathetic activity.
D. True. Shortening of the PP interval indicates an increased heart rate during inspiration; this is a feature of normal sinus arrhythmia.
E. False. Spread of repolarization in the same direction as a recording lead gives a downward, or negative, wave. The T wave is normally positive because the wave of repolarization travels in the opposite direction to the main recording leads.

The respiratory system

7

Introduction

The vast majority of the energy necessary to sustain our lives comes from oxidative metabolism; and the vast majority of that metabolism involves the cytochrome-c-oxidase system which produces high-energy adenosine triphosphate by, ultimately, the reduction of oxygen to water. The hydrogen ion (proton) which brings about this final reduction has probably come from a carbohydrate molecule and the 'waste products' of the process are carbon dioxide and water.

In the gaseous phase, therefore, the balance sheet of life simply depends on obtaining oxygen and getting rid of carbon dioxide.

Of course, the atmosphere is our limitless source of oxygen and an inexhaustible sink for carbon dioxide. The process which brings oxygen from the atmosphere to the circulation, which carries it to the cells, and transfers carbon dioxide in the opposite direction is called external respiration (*external* to separate it from the energy-producing chemical processes which go on within the cells, which are called internal respiration and are more the province of biochemists). For the sake of brevity we will omit 'external' when we refer to respiration.

To obtain the amounts of oxygen we need requires an exchange surface which must be moist to dissolve gases, of enormous surface area and extremely thin so as not to impede the transfer. Such a surface is so delicate that evolution has dictated that it must be inside the body, and the study of the mechanisms of bringing fresh air to this, the respiratory surface of our lungs, represents a large part of the physiology of lung mechanics.

Our blood and its circulation, so important to many other systems of our body, are also profoundly modified to effectively carry oxygen and carbon dioxide to and from the tissues.

The respiratory system is unique among the automatic systems of our body in that it is under voluntary control and can be recruited to assist in other functions, communication for example, but when not required for this and other tasks goes about the process of homeostasis without intruding on our consciousness.

Section overview

This section covers:

- Generation of negative intrapleural pressure by lung and chest wall recoil
- The effect of a pneumothorax collapsing the lung
- The liquid lining of the lungs and compliance
- The nature of airways resistance and its distribution in the bronchial tree
- Airway compression during forced expiration
- The work of breathing with different patterns
- The FEV_1
- Anatomical and physiological dead space in ventilation and shunts in perfusion
- The importance of matching ventilation to perfusion
- Haemoglobin as an oxygen carrier
- How the changing properties of haemoglobin while it circulates improve oxygen transport
- How carbon dioxide is carried by the blood
- The role of carbon dioxide in plasma pH regulation
- The sites and sensitivities of respiratory chemoreceptors
- The central respiratory pattern generator.

The mechanics of breathing

Introduction

The movements of the body that make up the outward signs of human respiration are universally recognized as manifestations of life. The primacy of this physiological system in the maintenance of life is demonstrated by the speed with which life is extinguished when respiration is prevented. More insidious interference with respiration – by disease – makes respiratory pathology the third most important cause of premature death and, in the developed world, the most important cause of days lost from work. The ubiquitous nature of respiratory disease can be judged from the reasonable expectation that, whereas most readers of this chapter will pass through life without obvious cardiovascular or renal disease, for example, not one will escape from disease of the respiratory system, if only the common cold.

Overall, human respiration is a circular process (Fig. 7.1.1) with oxygen being taken from the air and carried to the cells of the body by one side of the circuit while carbon dioxide is carried in the opposite direction by the other. We could therefore start a study of this system almost anywhere in the circuit, which fortunately for the student can be broken up into manageable bits, and a study of the mechanical properties of the lungs and chest wall, and the ways these properties affect breathing, is as good a place as any to make such a start.

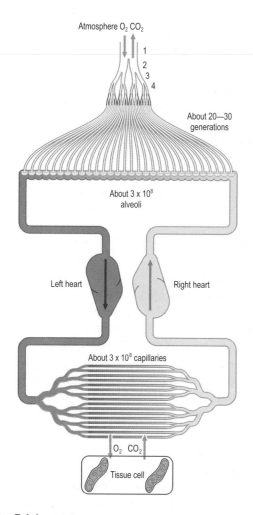

Atmosphere O_2 CO_2

1
2
3
4

About 20—30
generations

About 3×10^8
alveoli

Left heart

Right heart

About 3×10^8 capillaries

O_2 CO_2

Tissue cell

Fig. 7.1.1 A brief overview of respiration. The structure
and function of the respiratory and cardiovascular systems are
designed to facilitate the supply of oxygen to and removal of
carbon dioxide from the tissue cells under all conditions.

Small free-living organisms exchange O_2 and
CO_2 with their environment by simple diffusion. Larger organisms have to develop systems
to permit this exchange over considerable distances. We rely upon the heart to circulate blood
between the active tissues – using O_2 and producing CO_2 – and the lungs where these gases
are exchanged with the atmosphere. At rest, an
adult takes up about 0.3 litres/min of oxygen
and produces a little less carbon dioxide. The
ratio of CO_2 produced to O_2 used is called the
respiratory exchange ratio.

Red blood cells contain haemoglobin, which
binds oxygen at normal atmospheric gas tensions and readily releases it as the tension falls
in the tissues. Haemoglobin is also important in
the carriage of CO_2 as it buffers carbonic acid
formed from CO_2 by hydration. Haemoglobin
increases the ability of blood to transport these
gases by nearly 100 times.

The site of gaseous exchange between the
body and the atmosphere is the alveoli of the
lung. About 3×10^8 of these 0.3 mm diameter
terminal expansions of the smallest airways are
closely associated with the pulmonary capillaries, forming an exchange surface of some 100 m^2.

At rest we breathe approximately 15 breaths,
each of a depth of 0.5 litres, each minute,
about 7 litres/min. This can increase to nearly
100 litres/min during heavy work.

Only that part of the inspired gas that
reaches the alveoli takes part in gas exchange.
The rest remains in the airways, which do not
have gas-exchange surfaces. The volume of this
so-called **dead space** is about 150 ml. During
quiet breathing alveolar ventilation is therefore
about 350 ml per breath. This fresh air mixes, in
the alveoli, with about 3 litres of gas present at
end-expiration (the functional residual capacity; FRC). Increased depth of breathing can be
effected by either increasing inspiration by
about 5 litres to a total lung capacity (TLC) of
nearly 6 litres or by expiring an extra half litre
down to a minimum lung capacity, or residual
volume (RV).

Breathing involves work by the respiratory
muscles. Work is done against the mechanical
resistance of the chest wall, the elasticity of
the lung and against the resistance of the
airways to gas flow. The mechanics of breathing are optimized by neural control of the
pattern of breathing, so that the work of
breathing is minimized at any particular level
of ventilation.

Adaptations of the system occur when either
disease or hostile environment threatens to
impair these processes (see Clinical Example:
Respiratory disease).

Clinical Example

Respiratory disease

Diseases of the respiratory system are extremely common. The airways and alveoli of the lung are exposed to many airborne contaminants; many industrial diseases are related to inhalation of harmful dusts. Droplet infection is a common route for pathogens to invade the body. The upper respiratory tract is attacked by the common cold virus at regular and frequent intervals. Local bacterial or viral infection and consequent inflammation can lead to acute pneumonia or chronic lung disease. Allergic challenges lead to hay fever or asthma, which results when the small airways in the lung are constricted as a response to antigen.

Diseases like asthma which increase the airway resistance are called obstructive diseases. Obstructive disease can also occur if the dead space is increased by expansion of the terminal airways as in emphysema where the airways lack their normal support and collapse during expiration.

Restrictive disease on the other hand, describes the loss of function due to loss of lung expansion. This can be caused by the replacement of the elastic components of the lung structure with collagen.

Disease of the lung can also lead to damage to the pulmonary vascular bed. The resistance to blood flow in this bed is normally low. If disease raises this resistance, the pulmonary artery pressure may rise from its normal level of 25/10 mmHg, with consequential effects on the right ventricle of the heart, which may fail.

Chronic bronchitis and emphysema are the major chronic obstructive airway diseases. They are characterized by the presence of persistent irreversible airway restriction with a chronic cough, producing sputum. There is progressive failure of the respiratory exchange in the lungs with increasing retention of CO_2 and lowered Po_2 of arterial blood.

Chronic bronchitis is associated with damage to the larger airways, with an increase in mucus-secreting cells and a loss of ciliated cells. The mucous membranes are inflamed and thickened. As the disease progresses the smaller airways become affected and become enlarged, while the alveoli become fewer and larger. The fine elastic structure of the lung is destroyed. These later changes are termed emphysema.

The effects of emphysema upon lung function are related to the structural defects outlined above. The chronic nature of the infection and the 'cough and spit' of these patients is a result of increased production of mucus associated with loss of the airway-clearing mechanisms of ciliated epithelia. The hyperinflated 'barrel chest' results from increased airway resistance and the loss of the elastic recoil of the lungs. The patient breathes from a larger functional residual capacity to maintain the small airways open.

It takes effort to breathe. We are going to begin our study of respiration with the way in which this effort brings about breathing and the mechanical properties of the lungs and chest wall which determine how much effort is required. In healthy individuals the work of breathing is small and relates especially to inspiration, but as it may be greatly increased in disease, we need to know the factors that affect it.

Respiratory muscles act to inflate and deflate the lungs through the generation of pressure differences which cause air movement through the airways. The extent of the pressure change required depends on the ease with which the air will flow – the airway resistance. The muscular effort required to generate a given pressure difference depends upon the mechanical properties of the lungs and thorax, and in particular on the ease with which the lungs stretch – the lung compliance. Changes in either variable alter the effort required to breathe.

The lungs and thorax as a mechanical system

The respiratory muscles, the thoracic wall and the muscle sheet separating thorax and abdomen (the diaphragm), operate on the lungs to cause their expansion in volume (inspiration) and, by reducing their effort, allow lung contraction (expiration). The lungs fill the thoracic space and are separated from its walls by two layers of pleura. The potential space between the two layers of pleura is the **pleural space**. Air and blood have access to the lungs via depressions on their mediastinal surface – the hila. The bronchus, blood vessels, nerves and lymphatics enter and leave through the hilum of each lung, forming stalks attaching the lungs to the mediastinum, the central structure of the thoracic cavity which contains the heart, etc. The mechanical properties of this system determine how much force must be applied, and when, to produce an adequate pattern of ventilation of the lung.

The lungs change considerably in volume during breathing, and so must be very elastic.

The outer surface of the lungs, the visceral pleura, is not physically attached to the chest wall, which is lined by the parietal pleura. There is a thin layer of fluid – the pleural fluid – between these two smooth surfaces which allows the lungs to slide inside the chest wall. If the lungs are removed from the thorax, they collapse to a volume less than that ever achieved during the breathing cycle, so in life they are always stretched, even in full expiration. The normal tendency of the lungs to collapse generates a negative pressure in the thin film of fluid between the pleural surfaces which balances the tendency of the lungs to collapse by their own elastic recoil. The intrapleural pressure normally varies with the phases of breathing (Fig. 7.1.2) being between 5 and 10 cm of water less than atmospheric pressure. This also generates a small collapsing pressure difference on the rib cage. However, the chest wall is fairly rigid so only small changes in chest diameter are generated. The diaphragm is more elastic, and it is pushed up into the thorax by the pressure difference between the intrapleural space and the abdominal pressure. In a resting expiratory position, with no muscular activity, the whole system is stable until additional forces are applied.

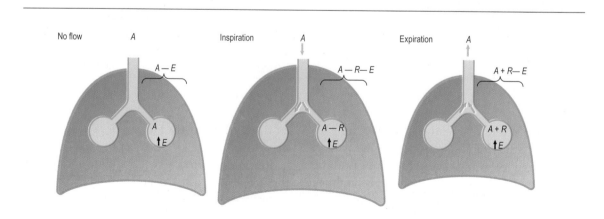

Fig. 7.1.2 Pressures in alveoli and intrapleural space during breathing. See text for details.

When there is no airflow into or out of the lungs the pressure in alveoli is atmospheric (A) (see Fig. 7.1.2). The lungs recoil with pressure (E). Relative to atmospheric pressure the intrapleural pressure is therefore ($A - E$). During inspiration this equilibrium is upset by the diaphragm descending, which makes the intrapleural pressure more negative. This extra negative pressure is used to draw air along the airways against what is known as airway resistance. Overcoming this resistance requires a pressure of (R). During expiration the diaphragm relaxes and intrapleural pressure becomes less negative. This cannot therefore keep the alveoli stretched and they tend to get smaller, driving air out of the lungs along the airways. Airway resistance opposes this and tends to maintain pressure within the alveoli.

Thus, during inspiration, elastic recoil opposes inflation of the lungs and intrapleural pressure has to be *more* negative than at rest to achieve inspiration. Intrapleural pressure in relation to atmospheric pressure is ($A - R - E$) where A is atmospheric pressure, R is the pressure to overcome airway resistance to flow and E is elastic recoil pressure.

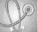

Clinical Example

'Pink puffers' and 'blue bloaters'

These picturesque piscine terms are used to differentiate between two major types of respiratory patient with chronic obstructive pulmonary disease (COPD) and represent the two extremes of a spectrum between pure bronchitis and pure emphysema, two conditions which very rarely exist in their pure state.

Pink puffer

This patient (sometimes referred to as Type A COPD) appears to be 'fighting his disease'. He is tachypnoeic, dyspnoeic and frequently breathes with pursed lips. Blood analysis reveals a mild hypoxaemia, if any, and a normal haematocrit. This patient is predominantly suffering from emphysema.

Blue bloater

On the other hand, this patient (Type B COPD) appears to be 'not fighting his disease'. He provides a history of cough producing sputum on most days for at least 3 months of the year for

more than 1 year. He is cyanotic secondary to hypoxaemia. Blood analysis also reveals hypercapnia and increased haematocrit. His legs are swollen, and distended neck veins point to right-sided heart failure. This patient is primarily suffering from chronic bronchitis.

In the vast majority of patients, chronic bronchitis and emphysema coexist and the clinical presentation is mixed. Lung function tests, of course, reveal airway obstruction and there will be an increase in lung volumes where emphysema predominates. In this case, transfer factor will be markedly decreased. The chest X-ray of the predominantly emphysematous patient shows overexpanded lungs pushing down and flattening the diaphragm, with lung fields lacking the usual markings and vessels because of tissue destruction.

It is fortunate that an exact quantification of the proportions of chronic bronchitis and emphysema is not important in practical terms for treatment and management of these patients, for whom the most important aspect of management is stopping smoking, the most important factor in the aetiology of the disease.

During expiration, elastic recoil assists expiratory flow and intrapleural pressure becomes *less* negative than if there were no flow. Intrapleural pressure in relation to atmospheric pressure is $(A + R - E)$.

During both inspiration and expiration, airway resistance opposes the change of lung volume, and so in inspiration intrapleural pressure is more negative the greater the resistance and in expiration it is less negative the greater the resistance.

Pneumothorax

A pneumothorax occurs when perforation of the lung or chest wall brings the intrapleural pressure towards atmospheric and, because of elastic recoil, the lung collapses leaving an air-filled pleural space.

- An open pneumothorax occurs when the chest wall is penetrated, leaving an opening which allows the elastic recoil to collapse the lung (Fig. 7.1.3). Air moves into and out of the pneumothorax as the patient breathes.
- In a closed pneumothorax air enters from the lung, usually through a tear in its pleural surface.

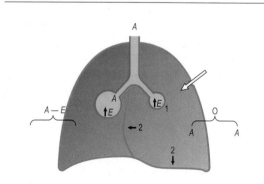

Fig. 7.1.3 A pneumothorax. If the thoracic wall is breached on one side, thus allowing the intrapleural pressure on that side to rise towards atmospheric:

1. the elastic recoil of the lung is unopposed and the lung collapses
2. the increased intrapleural pressure pushes the diaphragm down on that side and the mediastinum across to the side opposite the injury.

In both instances, if the hole seals, air which had entered the intrapleural space will be absorbed within 1–2 weeks. During this time lung function will be impaired. Because the mediastinum in humans is fairly rigid and divides the thorax into right and left sides, the lung collapse due to a pneumothorax is to some degree restricted to one side.

On the collapsed side, the alveoli will be poorly ventilated and blood perfusing them will not be properly oxygenated; consequently it will retain its venous character. A physiological veno-arterial shunt (see p. 672) will occur. Ventilation of the healthy lung will also be impaired as the raised pressure of the affected side will push the mediastinum across, minimizing possible increase in volume during inspiration and reducing the tidal volume of the lung. Because intrathoracic pressure is raised, the return of blood to the great veins in the thorax will be impeded, thus reducing the cardiac output.

These effects on ventilation and cardiac output can become life-threatening if, as in a closed pneumothorax, a flap of lung forms a valve which allows entry but not exit of air from the pleural space. The pressure in the pleural space can then progressively increase and become greater than atmospheric pressure.

Resolution of a pneumothorax

Air in any closed space within the body will be absorbed in 1 or 2 weeks. This air can be the result of a pneumothorax, air trapped in alveolar regions of the lung because of airway collapse, bubbles of air in an injection, or bubbles forming in the blood of a diver, causing 'the bends'. All these situations are hazardous mainly because of the mechanical problems this air causes.

In working out how this air is disposed of by absorption into the body fluids, we must remember two important points:

- Partial pressure of a gas in a mixture of gases = Total pressure × % (concentration).

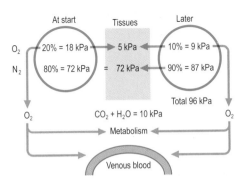

Fig. 7.1.4 The partial pressures of the most important gases in a bubble of air trapped in the tissues (a pneumothorax, a collapsed area of lung or injected air) at the start and later in its absorption.

 Summary

Mechanical properties

- The lungs are separated from the chest wall by a small amount of fluid.
- Intrapleural pressure – the pressure in this fluid – is negative with respect to the atmosphere.
- Reduction in intrapleural pressure stretches (inflates) the lungs.
- Elastic recoil opposes inspiration and aids expiration.
- A pneumothorax is absorbed by the same mechanisms that absorb any bubble of air in the tissue – diffusion down concentration gradients.

- Diffusion of a gas in a mixture of gases is independent of the other gases and dependent on its own concentration gradient.

Now, considering an injected volume of air, we can first dispose of CO_2. There is virtually none in fresh air and there is no metabolism going on in the bubble to make any. However, CO_2 is a great diffuser and CO_2 equilibrium will be set up with CO_2 dissolved in the tissues as the bubble shrinks by mechanisms we will now consider.

O_2 and N_2 are the most important gases in this phenomenon. CO_2 and water vapour exert a combined partial pressure of about 10 kPa in the bubble which, because it is surrounded by flexible tissue, cannot have a total pressure very different from atmospheric pressure (100 kPa). So we have approximately 20% O_2 and 80% N_2 in a bubble at 100 kPa total pressure. Subtracting the partial pressures of CO_2 and water vapour, the pressure exerted by $O_2 + N_2 = 90$ kPa (18 kPa, O_2; 72 kPa, N_2). But this bubble is surrounded by tissue with very different gas tensions (5 kPa, O_2; 72 kPa, N_2) (Fig. 7.1.4).

Oxygen presents no problem. It is soon used up by metabolism or removed in venous blood. Nitrogen, on the other hand, is inert and only removed by diffusion down its concentration gradient. The metabolic removal of O_2 provides the conditions for this. Initially, the bubble contains approximately 20% O_2 and 80% N_2. This provides a steep gradient for removal of O_2 and about a balance for N_2. But as O_2 is removed, the percentage, and therefore partial pressure, of N_2 increases and provides a gradient driving it into the tissues. The removal of O_2, therefore, provides the driving force for the removal of N_2. An extreme example of this mechanism is seen in a patient who is breathing 100% O_2. If an airway leading to a section of lung collapses sealing off that section, the whole part will quickly collapse as the 100% O_2 it contains is absorbed.

The phases of breathing

The changes in volume of the lungs that make up what we know as breathing can be recorded in a number of ways – by directly recording the volume of air breathed in and out using an instrument called a **spirometer**, by integrating airflow in and out, by recording changes in

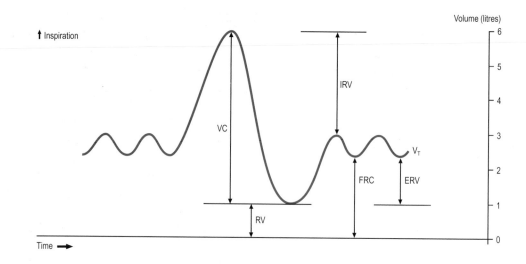

Fig. 7.1.5 Some lung volumes. VC = vital capacity; RV = residual volume; FRC = functional residual capacity; IRV = inspiratory reserve volume; ERV = expiratory reserve volume; V_T = tidal volume. Because we cannot breathe out the last residue of air from our lungs, the residual volume and functional residual capacity cannot be measured directly.

volume of the chest, and several other methods. However the record is obtained, there is a well-established nomenclature which describes the lung volumes that make up the phases of breathing (Fig. 7.1.5).

In order to inhale, the lung volume has to be increased from the functional residual capacity (FRC; the resting volume) by the application of force to displace the equilibrium. Importantly, once that force is removed, the system will return to its original equilibrium position by passive elastic recoil.

- Breathing in from functional residual capacity requires muscular effort, but breathing out to functional residual capacity can be achieved by passive recoil.
- Breathing out below functional residual capacity requires muscular effort, but the subsequent inspiration back to functional residual capacity is passive.

Breathing in from the functional residual capacity

Inspiration from functional residual capacity is brought about by the increase in intrathoracic

volume created as the diaphragm, the most important inspiratory muscle, contracts and moves down into the abdomen, and the intercostal muscles contract raising the ribs and increasing thoracic diameter. During quiet breathing, the main inspiratory effect comes from the movement of the diaphragm. During forced or heavy breathing, accessory muscles including the pectoral muscles are progressively brought into play to raise the ribs more forcefully.

Expiration

When inspiratory effort ends, passive recoil ensures that the system reverts to its resting equilibrium position. An expiration beyond FRC cannot be achieved by passive recoil, or by action of the diaphragm, an inspiratory muscle. Under these circumstances expiration is brought about by contraction of the muscles of the abdominal wall. Their contraction pulls down the ribs, narrowing the thoracic cavity, and, by raising the intra-abdominal pressure, pushes the diaphragm upwards. During such a forced expiration the intrapleural pressure may rise above atmospheric.

Artificial ventilation

It is sometimes necessary to take over a patient's breathing, because we wish to paralyse him for surgery or because he is unable to ventilate his lungs adequately for himself. We usually impose artificial ventilation on a patient by blowing air into his lungs under positive pressure, as in mouth-to-mouth resuscitation. This produces unhelpful changes in intrapleural pressure which have significant physiological consequences. We have seen that inspiration is normally brought about by the pressure around the lungs being reduced so they expand and air is sucked into them. This cycling negative pressure within the thorax has the additional useful function of sucking blood into the great veins supplying the heart from the thorax. This is called the respiratory pump. During positive-pressure artificial ventilation this effect is absent. In fact – and worse – inflation of the lungs, far from making intrapleural pressure more negative, makes it positive. This embarrasses the heart and circulation. One way out of this problem is to use negative pressure ventilation with a cabinet or tank ventilator, sometimes called an 'iron lung'. In these machines, the patient's chest is surrounded by an airtight box from which the head protrudes. By reducing the pressure in the box, air is sucked into the lungs by negative pressure just as in normal life, but with both the lungs and chest wall expanding together under the reduced pressure just as the lungs do normally.

Clinical Example

Poliomyelitis

Poliomyelitis is now rare in the developed world but occurs when an individual succumbs to poliovirus type I, II or III (picornaviruses). These viruses attack the nervous system and, in particular, the anterior horn cells of the spinal cord, producing any degree of respiratory involvement up to total paralysis of all respiratory muscles.

Under these circumstances, ventilation of the patient's lungs must be taken over for him. This can be achieved by applying an intermittent positive-pressure supply of air to the patient's airway (IPPV). Although the consequences of withholding ventilation from the patient are, of course, disastrous, there is considerable concern about the effects of long-term tracheostomy, necessary to provide a good seal for inflation and to prevent food and other material being forced into the lungs, and the undesirable effects of positive pressure in the chest on the output of the heart.

The circulatory problems were overcome by ventilators of the 'iron lung' type (see above), but this did not address the problem of aspiration of material into the lungs and, because the machine is unaware when that has happened, horrific accidents have occurred.

A more convenient version of the iron lung, which is also more acceptable to the patient, is the cuirass ventilator where negative pressure is only applied to the anterior abdominal wall. This technique may be sufficient when the patient has inadequate spontaneous ventilation and reduces but does not solve the problem of accidental uncontrolled aspiration.

Basic Science 7.1.1

Some laws

There are four physical laws which help explain the physiology of respiration described in this section.

Hooke's law

This tells us that the ratio of the increased weight (ΔW) hanging on a spring to the increase in length of a spring (ΔL) is a constant:

$$\frac{\Delta L}{\Delta W} = K .$$

The spring increases in only one dimension, length, so applied to a three-dimensional system like the lungs this law tells us that, over a reasonable range at least, the increase in volume of the lungs (ΔV) is proportional to the increase in the pressure inflating them (ΔP):

$$\frac{\Delta V}{\Delta P} = K .$$

Laplace's law

Because the molecules in the surface of a liquid are attracted to each other, there is tension in that surface and, hence, a tendency for such a surface to shrink. This is called surface tension.

If the surface is flat, all the forces act only along the surface. In a curved surface part of the force is directed (resolved) toward the centre of curvature; the greater the curvature the greater the proportion of the force resolved toward its centre. Physicists work out the magnitude and direction of this force using what is known as the rule of the triangle of forces: two forces acting on an object can be represented by a single resultant force if the two forces can be represented in magnitude and direction by two sides of a triangle; the third side which

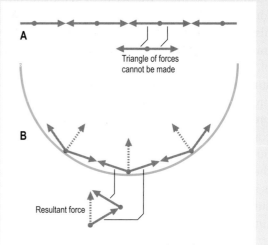

Fig. BS7.1.1 Molecules in liquid surfaces.
A. Flat surface. **B.** Curved surface (why there is pressure in a bubble).

completes the triangle represents the resultant force in magnitude and direction. So we see that in a flat surface (Fig. BS7.1.1A) there is no way of making a triangle out of the forces acting on a molecule. In a curved surface (Fig. BS7.1.1B) the rule of the triangle of forces enables us to calculate the force resolved towards the centre of curvature.

In a closed volume like a bubble this surface tension (T) produces a pressure (P) which is related to the radius (r) of the bubble by the expression $P = 4T/r$. In the case of a drop of liquid, or the liquid lining of the spherical alveoli of the lungs, there is only one air–liquid surface (a bubble has two) and this expression becomes:

$$P = \frac{2T}{r} .$$

This expression makes the rather surprising statement that the pressure in a large bubble is less than that in a small one.

Basic Science *(Continued)*

Poiseuille's law

The physics of the flow of fluids, such as air, in tubes can be incredibly complicated. The simplest situation is laminar flow where the molecules progress in an orderly streamlined fashion in the direction of flow. In quiet breathing we can make the bold approximation that flow in the lungs is laminar and apply Poiseuille's law:

$$\text{Airflow} = \frac{P \times \pi \times r^4}{8\eta l}$$

(where P = driving pressure; r = radius of tube; η = viscosity of fluid; l = length of tube).

Dalton's law of partial pressures

Dalton's law of partial pressures states that the pressure exerted by each component of a mixture of gases is the pressure it would exert if it alone occupied the volume of the mixture. This law is made clear by considering a gas cylinder whose contents exert a pressure of 100 kPa. If the cylinder contains pure N_2, then obviously all the pressure comes from N_2 molecules and the partial pressure of N_2 is 100 kPa. If the cylinder contains 50% N_2 and 50% O_2, 50% (50 kPa) of the total pressure comes from N_2 and 50% (50 kPa) comes from O_2. Similarly, when the mixture is 50% N_2, 30% O_2 and 20% CO_2, the partial pressures are 50, 30 and 20 kPa. Vapours of liquids exert partial pressures which depend on temperature; thus water vapour at body temperature exerts a pressure of 6.1 kPa (47 mmHg).

Factors influencing the effort required to inspire from functional residual capacity

As the thoracic volume increases during inspiration, the force required to continue the movement depends on several factors:

- the force required to inflate the lungs
- the force required to move the thoracic cage and to overcome any impediment to the movement of the diaphragm into the abdominal space
- the force required to overcome the resistance of the airways to gas flowing through them.

The first force, related to inflation of the lungs, is usually the most significant but the second component can become significant if, for example, the abdomen is occupied by a full-term uterus, and airway resistance can become limiting in asthma-like obstructive diseases. When disease makes breathing difficult for any reason, patients are more comfortable in bed propped up rather than lying supine when intra-abdominal pressure can hinder movement of the diaphragm.

Compliance

Under normal circumstances the force required to inspire is determined mainly by the physical properties of the lungs. Resistance to inflation comes from two sources: the stretching of the fabric of the lungs and the moving of the air into the lung. The measure of ease of stretching the lungs is known as lung compliance. Compliance is a description of the distensibility (elasticity) of the lung and is expressed as the change in volume per unit change in applied pressure.

Highly compliant tissues distend readily; less compliant tissues are less easily distended:

$$\text{Compliance} = \frac{\text{Change in volume}}{\text{Change in pressure}}.$$

Static compliance

Static compliance is usually not measured in life under totally static conditions but rather by relating the pressure inflating the lungs to their volume during very slow inspiration. The lungs are stretched slowly, so that airway resistance (see below) will not significantly affect the process. Changes in lung volume are measured with a spirometer. The inflating pressure is the pressure difference between the atmosphere and the pleural cavity. Intrapleural pressure may be estimated by measuring the pressure in the thoracic part of the oesophagus with a balloon or via a **whole body plethysmograph**. A plot of volume change against pressure change yields a slope defining compliance. The more compliant lungs are, the easier they are to stretch. A normal compliance is 0.2 litres/cmH$_2$O.

Specific compliance

One problem of measuring compliance is that the measured value of compliance depends on the amount of lung tissue present. To take an extreme example, the compliance of the remaining lung of a patient who has had one lung removed will be very low, although the elastic properties of the remaining lung may be normal. The low value is arrived at because there is not much tissue to expand. This difficulty is often overcome by dividing the measured compliance by the starting lung volume to yield 'specific compliance', which is a measure of lung elasticity independent of lung volume.

Surface tension

Several factors are important in determining lung compliance. Lungs removed from the body are easier to inflate with saline solution than with air. Inflating with saline fills the air spaces, obliterates the air–fluid interface which lines the lung, and stretches only the elastic elements in the lung tissues, so the presence of elastic tissue cannot completely explain lung recoil. The fact that inflation with air within the lungs is harder suggests that some process adds an additional element of recoil. This is not due to the air itself, but occurs because the thin fluid lining of the alveoli forms a fluid–air interface. Such an interface will have surface tension; that is to say the intermolecular forces within it will tend to reduce its surface area. This is why soap bubbles collapse. The millions of alveoli are the equivalent of millions of bubbles all tending to collapse. At mid-range lung volumes about half of the force needed to stretch the lungs is required to stretch elastic tissues in the walls of the airways, and about half to overcome surface tension forces in the fluid film lining them.

It is possible to predict the contribution of surface tension forces to lung recoil. If it is assumed that surface tension is constant and about equal to that of tissue fluids irrespective of the volume of the lungs, this calculation yields values close to those measured at the largest lung volumes in the physiological range, but grossly overestimates the force required to stretch lungs at lower volumes. It follows that something must be reducing surface tension in the lungs under most circumstances.

Substances which reduce surface tension are known as detergents, and it has become clear that the fluid lining the lungs contains a mixture of detergent-like substances, known in this case as surfactants. By reducing surface tension forces at most lung volumes, surfactant makes lungs easier to inflate, thus greatly decreasing the work of breathing. However, the surface tension of a film of water, or indeed solutions of common detergents such as those in washing powder, does not change as the area of the surface is altered. Surfactant has the additional, and important property of changing its effect on surface tension as the area of the fluid film changes.

Surfactant is secreted by cells in the walls of the alveoli and small airways, known as type II cells. Samples of surfactant can be obtained by washing fluid from the lungs. Its major component is phosphatidylcholine, which is very hydrophobic. It therefore accumulates in high concentration at the air–water interface.

Surfactant is present in very high concentration in the alveolar membranes. Its tendency to pack the air–water interface creates a surface pressure that counteracts the aqueous surface tension. When the surface area is reduced, as in deflation of the lung, the surfactant molecules are packed closer together, raising the surface pressure and further reducing the surface tension. The effect of pulmonary surfactants upon surface tension, therefore, is not the same at all lung volumes. You will recall that at small lung volumes a given increase in volume requires very much less force than at large lung volumes.

An additional complication of surfactant is that its surface-tension-reducing effect depends not only upon the area of the film containing it, but also on the direction in which that area is changing. This effect is known as **hysteresis** (Fig. 7.1.6). When the surface is expanded from a small area, the effects of surfactant dissipate rapidly, so surface tension increases rapidly with area before stabilizing. When the surface is compressed from a large area to a small one, the surface tension initially decreases rapidly then stabilizes.

A

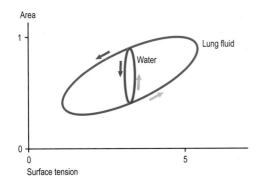

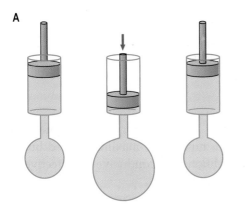
B

C

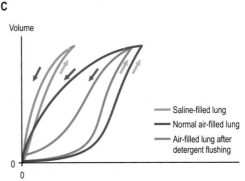

Fig. 7.1.6 The measurement of the effects of surfactant.
A. If a bubble is varied in size cyclically the surface tension in the film can be calculated from the pressure generated. **B.** If the surface area is plotted against surface tension a 'hysteresis curve' results. The arrows on the curves represent the direction of movement (inflation or deflation). The larger the area enclosed within the loop the more work is lost with each cycle. **C.** If a plain water bubble or a saline-filled lung were to be cycled then, as with a simple detergent bubble, little energy would be lost – that put into the surface as it is expanded is recovered when it shrinks. If surfactant is present, then the curve encloses a large area – much of the energy put into the expanding surface is not recovered as it shrinks. This effect is physiologically useful in resisting collapse of the lung but can be removed experimentally by washing out the lung with detergent.

The effects of this on inspiration and expiration at large tidal volumes are twofold:

1. Mechanical work has been done in stretching the lungs which is not recovered during passive recoil.
2. As the lungs are expanded from a small starting volume it becomes progressively harder to expand them further as the surface-tension-reducing effects of surfactant decrease, although they are never completely lost. Large inspirations are much harder work than small ones.

Surfactant has another important effect. It stabilizes the structure of the lungs. To understand why, we must consider briefly the physics of bubbles. A bubble is a quantity of gas contained within a film of fluid. Surface tension forces will cause the fluid to reduce to minimum surface area. This causes the bubble to assume a spherical form. Further reduction in the surface area can only be achieved by reducing the radius of the sphere. As this occurs, the gas within the bubble is compressed causing an increase in bubble pressure. When the pressure on the bubble wall matches that of the surface tension, the bubble becomes stable. At this equilibrium point, the pressure in the bubble is described by Laplace's law: $P = 2T/r$, where T is the surface tension of the fluid, and r the radius of the bubble (see Basic Science 7.1.1).

Thus pressure in a bubble is inversely proportional to its radius. Strange as it may seem, small bubbles will have a larger pressure within them than large bubbles.

If a small bubble is connected to a large one, since gas flows from high pressure to low pressure, gas in the smaller bubble will pass to the larger one. The contents of the smaller bubble pass into the larger bubble, which will thus get bigger (Fig. 7.1.7).

The lungs consist, in essence, of millions of small interconnected bubbles, or alveoli, of varying size. In the absence of any other factors, larger bubbles will contain a lower pressure, and so expand at the expense of their smaller

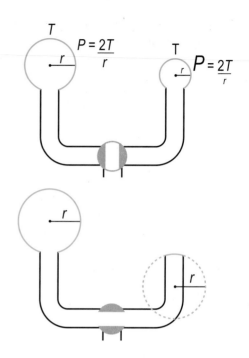

Fig. 7.1.7 The effect of surface tension on two interconnected bubbles. When a connection is made the smaller collapses into the larger until the radii of curvature of the surfaces of both, and hence their internal pressures, are equal (lower diagram).

neighbours. Such a lung would reduce to a minimum number of maximum-sized bubbles – a condition not conducive to effective gas exchange (see p. 671).

However, the presence of surfactant causes an area-dependent surface tension, T, which increases as radius increases, so that the pressure in a large bubble will be much higher than otherwise, allowing it to coexist with smaller bubbles, i.e. the pressure effects which could have been caused by differences in diameter are compensated for by differences in surface tension.

Respiratory distress syndrome. If surfactant is absent, altered or for some reason ineffective, then the unwanted collapse of small alveoli takes place exactly as predicted. Surfactant appears in the lung relatively late in gestation, around the end of the second trimester. Babies born very prematurely, therefore, often suffer a condition known as respiratory distress syndrome, where ventilation and gas exchange in the lung is greatly affected by change in lung structure due to the absence of surfactant (see also Ch. 10.4, p. 935).

Airway resistance

The pressure gradients generated by changes in lung volume create the flow of air through the airways. The pressure gradient required for a given flow is determined by the resistance of the airways.

The resistance to flow offered by an airway depends largely upon its diameter, but also on the nature of the gas flowing, and the way in which it is flowing. As airways get smaller, their individual resistance per unit length increases dramatically. The resistance of each airway depends inversely on the fourth power of its radius (Poiseuille's law; see Basic Science 7.1.1).

Under most conditions in the airways, the flow of air is laminar, that is to say there is a smooth gradient of velocity from the edge to the middle of the airways (see also Ch. 6.1, p. 510). During laminar flow, the rate of flow is linearly related to the pressure gradient. However, laminar flow breaks down under some conditions into 'turbulent flow'. This can occur at branch points in larger airways, and, at high rates of ventilation, in the largest airways such as the trachea and major bronchi. The resistance to flow is increased when flow becomes turbulent. Turbulent flow is noisy. If you breathe out hard, the gasp you hear is clearly in your throat and comes from your larynx and trachea where turbulent flow is taking place.

The airways form a branching structure where, at each branch, a larger airway feeds two smaller 'daughter' airways. Each bronchus divides in this way some 20–30 times forming smaller conducting airways, the bronchioles, leading into about 10^6 respiratory bronchioles, followed by three generations of alveolar ducts, each duct of which gives rise to about 30 alveoli.

At each branch point the diameter of the 'daughter' bronchioles decreases by about 15% to 0.85 of the diameter of the 'mother'. This progressively reduces the diameter of each individual airway from 25 mm in the trachea down to the 1 mm terminal bronchiole. At each branch point the total cross-sectional area of the system increases by a factor of about 1.4 (2×0.85^2) owing to the effect of the increasing numbers of bronchioles more than cancelling out the reduction of individual diameter. This behaviour is not a chance phenomenon. Such a branching pattern minimizes the work of breathing. Decreasing the diameter more rapidly would greatly increase the work done against the resistance of the system; a smaller decrease would

Summary

The work of breathing

- Inspiration must overcome opposing properties of the lung (recoil and airway resistance) and opposition to descent of the diaphragm by the contents of the abdomen.
- Compliance describes the distensibility (elasticity) of the lungs.
- The greater the compliance, the less the elastic recoil of the lungs.
- About half the recoil of the lungs is due to the liquid lining of the alveoli acting like tiny bubbles.
- Surfactant in the liquid lining reduces recoil and, because its surface tension changes with area, equalizes pressure in large and small alveoli. This counteracts collapse of the lung.
- Airway resistance describes the resistance to flow of air through the conducting airways of the lungs. It therefore only exists when flow is taking place.

reduce this work but increase, by a greater amount, the work done ventilating the increased 'dead space' thus created. A further important point is that the region of highest resistance in the bronchial tree is not that of the smallest most numerous airways but that of the fewer medium-sized bronchioles. These airways have a lot of smooth muscle in their walls and its contraction increases resistance enormously in conditions such as asthma.

Flow–volume relationships in the lung

At most lung volumes above functional residual capacity, and in particular during inspiration, when a healthy subject is breathing quietly the contribution of airway resistance to the work of breathing is negligible. Most of the work is done against the elastic recoil of the lungs and chest walls.

At larger tidal volumes, during inspiration, air flows easily through the airways. During expiration, and in particular forced expiration, the situation can be quite different. Most of the airways in the lungs are not rigid tubes. Although the walls of the trachea and bronchi are reinforced with cartilage, bronchioles have elastic walls, so their diameter may change passively during breathing.

During inspiration, the stretch of the lungs is translated to the walls of the airways, so that the smaller bronchioles in particular are expanded. By Poiseuille's law small changes in radius produce large reductions in resistance, so airway resistance falls. In a disease like chronic asthma where the airway resistance is raised, making breathing hard work, sufferers try to make breathing easier by breathing from a greater resting lung volume, thus increasing their FRC, and thus develop a 'barrel chest'.

During an expiration into the expiratory reserve, the lung volume is reduced beyond the resting expiratory level by external compression using the accessory muscles of ventilation. The diameter of the small airways is reduced,

and, as a result, resistance will increase, moving the site of highest resistance to flow down into the lower reaches of the airways.

The mechanism of airway compression

During a vigorous expiration after a large inspiration, the effect of the raised intrathoracic pressure upon airway diameter is complex. Air flows out of the alveoli along the airways to the atmosphere down a pressure gradient from the highest pressure in the alveoli and the smaller bronchi. This pressure gradient is generated by the expiratory effort and the elastic recoil of the lung.

Just before the beginning of an expiration made after a maximal inspiration there is no flow in the airways and the airway pressure is uniformly atmospheric (Fig. 7.1.8). The intrapleural pressure is negative at about $-10\ \mathrm{cmH_2O}$ (1 kPa). The effect of this pressure difference across the wall of the airway is to hold the airway open. The onset of vigorous expiratory effort raises the intrapleural pressure to about $+30\ \mathrm{cmH_2O}$ (3 kPa) tending to compress both the alveoli and the airways. The intra-alveolar pressure remains higher than intrapleural because of the elastic recoil of the lung. Air flows out of the lung down the pressure gradient thus produced into the atmosphere. The pressure in the airways within the chest decreases as they approach the trachea, pressure having been used up to produce flow. The pressure difference holding the airway open thus decreases until at some point the difference becomes zero. This is termed the equal pressure point. At all points nearer the trachea than this the pressure across the airway wall is reversed and tends to close the airway.

You should note that:

- This effect is greater the greater the expiratory effort, with the result that maximal expiratory flow is attained with an expiratory effort well below the maximum effort possible.

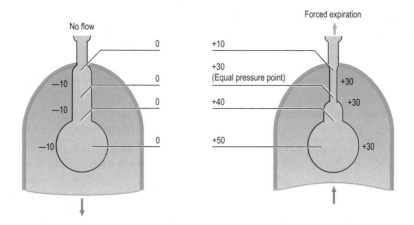

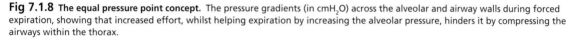

Fig 7.1.8 The equal pressure point concept. The pressure gradients (in cmH₂O) across the alveolar and airway walls during forced expiration, showing that increased effort, whilst helping expiration by increasing the alveolar pressure, hinders it by compressing the airways within the thorax.

- The maximal flow rate is heavily dependent upon the elastic recoil of the lung because this is the only force tending to keep alveolar–intrapleural pressure difference positive, thus holding the small airways open.

The importance of lung recoil is clear when it is reduced, as in the disease of **emphysema**.

In this condition the alveolar–intrapleural pressure difference is reduced because of a lack of elastic recoil so that the equal pressure point moves deeper into the lung and closer to the alveoli. The 'wheeze' so characteristic of the emphysematous patient is the sound of the trapped air escaping through the collapsed airways. Further expiratory effort by the patient is not helpful and only leads to greater distress.

Clinical Example

Obstructive sleep apnoea and snoring

The phenomenon of snoring although considered humorous is far from trivial for those who suffer from it. As we have seen in this section, inspiration is brought about by expansion of the lungs producing a negative pressure within the airways, which draws air into the lungs. This negative pressure tends to cause the airways to collapse, particularly the extrathoracic airways which are not surrounded by negative intrapleural pressure. Of the extrathoracic airways, the nose is surrounded by bone and the

trachea supported by cartilaginous rings. The pharynx, however, is bounded anteriorly by the genioglossus muscle of the tongue and the soft palate and laterally by muscular walls.

During REM (rapid eye movement) sleep there is a general relaxation of muscle tone which may be sufficient to allow the negative intraluminal pressure to collapse the pharynx. The characteristic rattling sound of snoring is the subject dragging air through this collapsed section of airway.

It is thus an encouraging sound, signalling success in ventilation. The snorer falling silent,

Clinical Example *(Continued)*

far from being a cause for joy, can have sinister implications. He, and it is most frequently he, may have been momentarily awakened by the obstruction, and this cycle of falling into REM sleep, airways collapse and awakening may occur literally hundreds of times each night. These awakenings are too brief for the patient to be aware of them but they deprive him of essential REM sleep. He suffers personality changes due to this deprivation and may take 'micro-sleeps' during the day, with possible fatal consequences if he is driving or operating machinery.

Alternatively, the snorer's silence may signal a total cessation of breathing. Under these circumstances desaturation of the blood can embarrass the myocardium to a degree that is eventually fatal. The problem of obstructive sleep apnoea can be so serious that patients have resorted to surgery to tighten up the muscles of the pharynx or even to a tracheostomy to bypass the pharynx altogether. A modern, less traumatic, equally effective form of treatment consists of pressurizing the air in the pharynx with air from a blower administered via tubes in the nostrils or by a face-mask. A pressure of 1 kPa is all that is required and it is not yet known whether the therapeutic effect is a simple inflation of the pharynx or whether there is a reflex stimulation of pharyngeal muscle tone.

Asthma

Obstruction to expiration is also the obvious problem in asthma. The fundamental cause is the inappropriate contraction of the smooth muscle of the bronchioles. Not only does this increase the work of breathing by increasing small airway resistance, which increases the pressure gradient along the airways during inspiration, it moves the equal pressure point deeper into the lung, causing collapse of the larger airways during expiration. In this disease also, further expiratory effort only leads to greater distress. Unlike emphysema, however, the obstruction in asthma is reversible and disappears when the contraction of the smooth muscle relaxes.

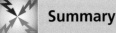

Summary

Airflow in the lungs

- In quiet breathing with healthy lungs, most work is done against the elasticity of lungs and chest wall.
- Airway diameter changes through each cycle of breathing.
- In asthma, reduced airway diameter increases work of breathing in inspiration and expiration.

- During expiration, intrapleural pressure becomes less negative, providing less support to the airways.
- During forced expiration, intrapleural pressure becomes positive, collapsing the airways.
- Elastic recoil of the alveoli makes pressure in the airways more positive than intrapleural pressure. This expands the airways.
- In emphysema, elastic recoil is lost and the airways tend to collapse.

Work involved in different patterns of breathing

Quiet breathing

During quiet breathing, inspiration starts from FRC and tidal volume is less than 1 litre. Work of breathing is at its minimum. Muscular effort is required only during inspiration; expiration will occur spontaneously by recoil and some of the energy used in inspiration is regained. The area of the lung surfaces is not greatly expanded, so the surface tension of the alveolar fluid stays low as pulmonary surfactant remains effective throughout the breathing cycle. Because the lungs are not actively compressed, the radius of the small airways remains large enough to ensure that the maximum resistance to airflow stays in the upper airways, whose resistance is not great because the velocity of flow is not high enough to generate significant turbulence. Airway resistance is therefore not limiting to ventilation. Dead space ventilation of the non-respiratory 'conducting' airways is about 25% of the tidal volume. The size of the dead space is minimized by autonomic bronchoconstriction which is greatest during inspiration when the inspiratory effort tends to open up the airway.

During exercise

Increased ventilation, as in exercise, can be achieved by increasing the number of breaths taken and by increasing the tidal volume. Increases in tidal volume are achieved by expiring to below the FRC and inspiring into the inspiratory reserve. Passive recoil will return lung volume to FRC. Further expiration requires contraction of expiratory muscles, particularly those in the abdomen. If the lungs are expanded towards vital capacity, not only does the effort increase with increasing volume but also the work to be done against the surface tension of the alveoli increases more steeply. As the area of the surfaces increases, the effects of surfactant in reducing surface tension becomes much less.

Breathing in becomes progressively harder as inspiration continues.

Deep breathing

During deep breathing airway diameter becomes important. Expiring beyond FRC tends to compress the airways. During deeper inspiration the airways are expanded. There is a greater difference, during increased ventilation, between the autonomic drive to the bronchiolar smooth muscle during inspiration and expiration. With larger gas flows through the airways, their resistance becomes important and contributes significantly to the work of breathing. The optimum airway diameter that minimizes the total work (the sum of the work of ventilating the dead space and of ventilating the alveoli) is now greater and the mean airway diameter is set at a larger value by the autonomic drive.

The limits to tidal volume increase

Clearly, individuals with larger thoraxes can breathe in more, but in any individual inspiration stops when the inspiratory muscles cannot stretch the lungs any further. This point is affected by:

- the strength of the muscles – weakness will limit maximum inspiration
- the compliance of the lung – less compliant lungs will stretch less for the same maximum muscular effort.

Expiration is limited by the collapse of the airways and this determines the residual volume.

For a normal individual of given size, therefore, maximum inspiration is determined by the compliance of the lungs; maximum expiration by the diameter of the airways, and therefore the airway resistance. Diseases affecting principally lung compliance affect maximum inspiration, producing 'restrictive deficits'; those affecting the diameter of small airways affect maximum expiration, producing 'obstructive deficits'.

A test of lung function (FEV₁)

A common screening test of lung function requires a subject to inspire maximally, and then breathe out as fast and as far as possible (usually with much encouragement from bystanders) through a spirometer, which produces a plot of volume expired against time (Fig. 7.1.9).

Most of the air is expelled from the lungs in the first second, initially at a high flow rate (i.e. a steep slope of curve relating volume to time). Towards the end of expiration, as the small airways are compressed, the resistance to flow increases, and so the flow rate (slope of the trace) decreases, until eventually no more air can be expelled. The total volume expired is known as the forced vital capacity or FVC. The volume expired in the first second, usually expressed as a percentage of forced vital capacity, is known as the forced expiratory volume in 1 second or FEV_1.

We can predict how this curve will change in different pathological conditions.

Consider first patients with a pure restrictive deficit, i.e. they cannot fill their lungs as much as normal, because of some restricting mechanical change (e.g. fibrosis).

They will start the expiratory manoeuvre with less air in their lungs, but as they have normal airways will be able to expire it normally. The initial part of the curve will therefore be as normal, but the plateau will be achieved at a lower volume. Forced vital capacity will be reduced. With these two changes (reduced FEV_1 and reduced forced vital capacity) comes a potential source of error. Because we usually express FEV_1 as a percentage of FVC, if both are reduced as in a patient with a restrictive disease, the percentage calculated may be normal. The reduced absolute value of both gives the clue to the problem.

In patients having an obstructive deficit, their narrowed airways will not much affect maximum inspiration; because the lungs are stretched open in inspiration they will fill slowly but to a normal maximum. As the air is expired, however, the increased resistance of the small airways will become significant. Total resistance determines total rate of flow, so the rate of flow (i.e. volume per unit time – the slope of the curve) will be lower than normal. The more the lungs are compressed, the greater the deficit in flow rate – producing the curve shown in Figure 7.1.9. Expiration will be prolonged and the FEV_1 will be a smaller fraction of FVC.

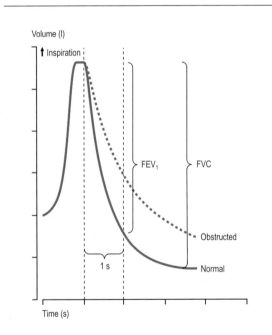

Fig. 7.1.9 A spirometer trace. The subject breathes out as fast as possible from a maximum inspiration. The volume expelled is related to the lung capacity. The volume expelled in the first second (FEV₁) is usually expressed as a percentage of FVC and is normally more than 80% of the total forced vital capacity. Any decrease in this fraction, as shown by the broken line, indicates some airway obstruction.

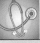

Summary

Efficiency of breathing

- During quiet breathing, much of the energy put into inspiration is returned to expiration by elastic recoil. Surfactant is at its most efficient and there is little turbulence in the airways.
- During exercise and deep breathing, inspiratory lung volumes exceed the range where surfactant is most efficient and

expiration is below FRC, which requires activation of abdominal muscles.
- Inspiration is limited by inspiration muscle strength and lung compliance, expiration by airways collapse.
- A forced expired volume trace from a spirometer can expose pathological, obstructive and restrictive changes.

Clinical Example

The Vitalograph

A useful instrument for testing lung function and one almost universally found in lung function laboratories is the Vitalograph.

This consists of a bellows-type spirometer which is used to measure only expiratory volume, i.e. the subject first breathes in, then puts his mouth over the Vitalograph mouthpiece and breathes out as fast and as far as he can.

The bellows pushes a pen in the vertical direction across a sheet of paper calibrated for volume. As soon as the instrument detects the start of expiration, it moves the paper at a fixed speed in a horizontal direction under the pen, producing a plot of volume against time.

The traces one might expect for normal subjects, and patients with obstructive and restrictive disease are shown in Figure CE7.1.1.

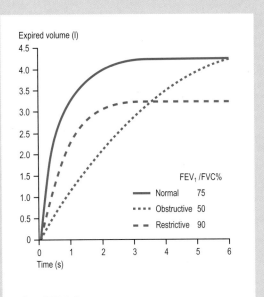

Fig. CE7.1.1 A Vitalograph trace.

Ventilation and perfusion

Ventilation

We have so far referred to ventilation ($\dot{V}$) of the lungs as if all of the approximately 7 litres/min we breathe at rest contributes equally to the exchange of gases with the blood. This is not so. Because evolution has resulted in the human respiratory surface being taken inside the body, a system of **conducting airways** exists to carry air to and from the respiratory surface in a tidal fashion. We have already noted that this is called the tidal volume of breathing. The connecting airways do not have a sufficiently good blood supply, and their walls are too thick, for efficient gas exchange to take place across them. They are to all intents 'dead' to the respiratory exchange process and the air space they contain is referred to as **anatomical dead space**, because it relates to the normal anatomy of the lungs. A person's anatomical dead space in millilitres is approximately numerically equal to his weight in pounds. Figure 7.2.1 shows how at the end of expiration dead space fills with 'used' air, which must be inhaled before fresh air can be taken into the lungs. To a small extent in health, and to a greater extent in lung disease, there are also other regions of the lung that are not adequately perfused to function as gas exchange regions. The sum of the volume of these regions and the anatomical dead space is called the **physiological dead space**.

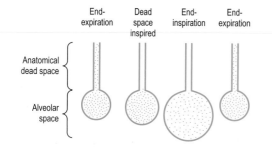

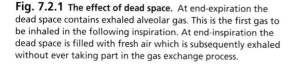

Fig. 7.2.1 The effect of dead space. At end-expiration the dead space contains exhaled alveolar gas. This is the first gas to be inhaled in the following inspiration. At end-inspiration the dead space is filled with fresh air which is subsequently exhaled without ever taking part in the gas exchange process.

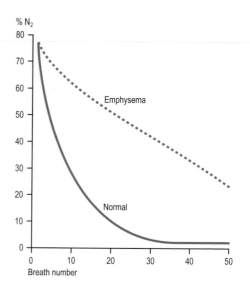

Fig. 7.2.2 Concentration of nitrogen in expired air of sequential breaths of a healthy subject and a patient with emphysema while breathing pure oxygen. The nitrogen from pre-oxygen breathing is more slowly washed from the emphysematous lungs because of less uniform distribution of ventilation.

Ventilation of any space or of the lungs is measured as the number of changes of air per minute that take place. The action of these changes of air (breathing in the case of lungs) is to wash out old, residual, air. If all parts of the lungs are uniformly ventilated, then all parts will be flushed out at the same rate by breathing – an efficient process. If some parts of the lung are not as well ventilated as others, then they will not be as efficiently flushed out and the gas they contain will continue to appear in the exhaled air after the better-ventilated regions have been flushed clean.

A clinical test of the degree of this inefficient, uneven, ventilation is the **multiple breath washout**. In this, the patient begins to breathe pure oxygen and the fraction of nitrogen in each expired breath is plotted against the breath number from starting breathing oxygen (Fig. 7.2.2). This nitrogen comes from the air the patient was breathing before the switch to pure oxygen. If the lungs are reasonably efficiently, uniformly ventilated, the graph will be as shown in the 'Normal' line. If inefficient, non-uniform, ventilation exists, nitrogen in poorly ventilated regions will be more slowly washed out and the graph will fall more slowly.

As well as disease, gravity, smooth muscle control of airway diameter and age all influence distribution of ventilation in the lungs.

Perfusion

It is important for efficient functioning, that regional perfusion (blood flow, $\dot{Q}$) in the lungs should match ventilation. Good blood flow should not be wasted on regions of poor ventilation containing little oxygen and with little capacity for removing carbon dioxide. Alternatively, poor blood flow obviously has little capacity for transporting respiratory gases. We have seen that poor blood flow gives rise to dead space in the lung. Conversely, blood passing through regions of poor ventilation is called **shunting** and is equally inefficient.

Gravity has a profound effect on lung perfusion, causing it to be greater at the base of the lungs than at the apex (see later). Smooth muscle in the pulmonary arterioles changes their diameter to regulate blood flow locally. Vasoconstriction in response to oxygen lack (hypoxia) directs blood away from poorly ventilated areas. Although there is relatively little

![Summary icon]

Summary

Ventilation and perfusion

- The conducting airways, which connect the respiratory surface of the lungs to the atmosphere, contain the anatomical dead space.
- Physiological dead space is anatomical dead space plus those regions of the lung that are ventilated but not perfused.
- Ventilation can be measured as the number of changes of air or rate of flow of air through a region of the lungs per minute.
- Uniformity of ventilation is measured by 'washout' tests.
- A shunt is a region of the lung with a blood supply but no ventilation.
- Gravity affects distribution of ventilation in the lung and affects perfusion even more because blood is denser than air.
- Smooth muscle in the airways and pulmonary arterioles also regulates the distribution of ventilation and perfusion.

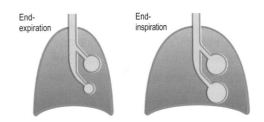

Fig. 7.2.3 Effects of intrapleural pressure differences. Differences in alveolar volumes from end-expiration to end-inspiration resulting from the differences in intrapleural pressure at the apex and base of the lungs. (The effect is, of course, exaggerated for clarity.)

smooth muscle in the walls of pulmonary blood vessels, it is sufficient to affect regulation of blood flow because the pressure in the system is relatively low.

The effects of gravity

The lungs are surrounded by negative pressure, the changes of which bring about the lung inflation and deflation that constitute ventilation. This apparently simple situation is complicated by the fact that the contents of the thorax behave as a semi-liquid contained within the vessel of the thoracic walls. Just like any liquid, its internal pressure increases as we descend into the body of the liquid, and this effect is due

to gravity. Because of this effect, the intrapleural pressure at the base of the lungs of a standing subject is less negative (more positive) than at the top because of the weight of tissue bearing down. This gradient of pleural pressure has, not entirely expected, effects on ventilation and perfusion of the lungs.

Ventilation

At end-expiration the lungs are filled with 'used' air which has been in contact with the respiratory surface, and if we could look at the alveoli at the apices and bases of the lungs we would find those at the top expanded to a considerable fraction of the volume they will reach at end-inspiration. Alveoli at the base of the lungs on the other hand are only expanded to a small fraction of their potential volume owing to the weight of overlying lung 'crushing' them. During inspiration therefore the alveoli at the base of the lungs have a greater potential for expansion than those at the top (Fig. 7.2.3).

Ventilation can be expressed as the *change* of volume of the lungs and, therefore, because the alveoli at the base take up their potential for expansion, the bases of the lungs are better ventilated than their apices. This difference in ventilation results in different dilutions by inspired air of the 'used' alveolar gas remaining in the lungs, and this is further modified by different blood flows at the apex and base of the lungs removing O_2 and adding CO_2 at different rates.

Distribution of ventilation becomes increasingly non-uniform with age, and lung disease can produce gross inequalities.

Perfusion

The pulmonary circulation, which perfuses the lungs, has several unique features. Many of these are related to the fact that the lungs are the only place in the body where blood capillaries come into contact with the atmosphere. For such a situation to be viable, the blood pressure in the circulation must be low. This is achieved by a system of blood vessels which are short and, owing to an enormous number of parallel vessels, have an enormous total cross-sectional area. Low pulmonary capillary pressure is maintained during exercise by normally closed capillaries opening and those already open distending. The properties of the pulmonary circulation are such that blood flow through it is extremely pulsatile, increasing with every contraction of the right ventricle of the heart. A large part of this effect is due to the blood leaving the right heart having to pass from regions of negative intrapleural pressure into thin-walled capillaries which are surrounded by alveoli containing air at near atmospheric pressure (Fig. 7.2.4).

During diastole, the alveoli around the capillaries at the top of the lung clamp them shut because the pressure in the alveoli is greater than the pressure in the blood vessels (made negative by negative intrapleural pressure). As you descend the lung, intrapleural pressure becomes less negative and the pressure in the capillaries may become sufficient to force blood through the capillaries which are clamped by the alveoli. This increase in blood pressure as one descends the lung is simply hydrostatic pressure developed in the column of blood in the upright lung. This situation during diastole thus closely represents the simple physical

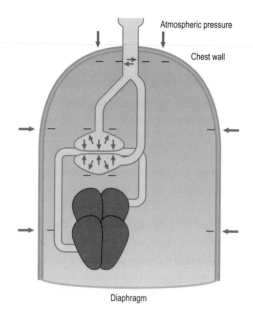

Fig. 7.2.4 The alveolar clamp. When we measure pressure (gas pressure or liquid pressure) it must be compared to some baseline 'reference pressure'. This can be an absolute vacuum (when the pressure is called an absolute pressure) or more usually the pressure is compared to atmospheric pressure.

If we compare the pressure in the pulmonary circulation with the *intrapleural pressure* as our reference pressure you can see one of the problems the body is faced with in providing lung perfusion. The blood in the vessels in the chest takes on the intrapleural pressure surrounding them, which is negative to atmospheric pressure. When it comes to be forced through the pulmonary capillaries (surrounded by alveoli at atmospheric pressure) it has to be pumped 'uphill' against this higher atmospheric pressure.

situation one would find in a vertical tube of water where pressure increases as one descends below the surface. When systole takes place, the effect of the right heart injecting blood into the pulmonary circulation is to add extra pressure to that due to hydrostatic pressure and force open capillaries higher in the lung (Fig. 7.2.5). The overall effects of these factors are:

- highly pulsatile blood flow through the pulmonary circulation
- a matching and increasing of ventilation and blood flow from apex to base of the lungs.

Diastole   Systole

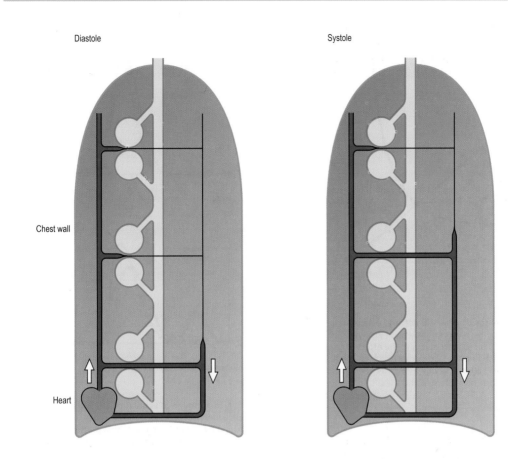

Chest wall

Heart

Fig. 7.2.5 The effect of gravity on blood flow through the upright lung. During diastole only the hydrostatic pressure of the column of blood is available to force blood through the capillaries pinched between the alveoli. During systole, extra pressure is available to open capillaries higher in the lung.

Ventilation–perfusion ratios ($\dot{V}/\dot{Q}$)

The importance of matching ventilation and blood flow (perfusion) in the lungs cannot be overemphasized.

When standing upright, both ventilation and perfusion increase from apex to base in the lungs. This increase is due to gravity and, because blood is denser than air, the effect on perfusion is greater than the effect on ventilation. Consequently, the ratio of perfusion to ventilation changes from apex to base of the lungs (Fig. 7.2.6).

If a mathematical model of an ideal lung is constructed in which ventilation and perfusion are ideally matched, it only exchanges 2–3% more gas than a normal lung. So you could say that the normal lung is doing a 97–98% perfect job of matching. In diseased lungs, however, mismatch creates great problems.

Mathematical models of the lung have been constructed in which there are three 'compartments':

1. Normal with $\dot{V}/\dot{Q} = 1$
2. Physiological shunt with $\dot{V}/\dot{Q} = 0$
3. Physiological dead space with $\dot{V}/\dot{Q} = \infty$.

675

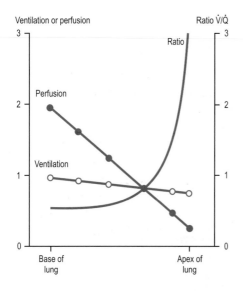

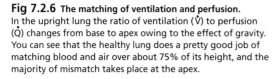

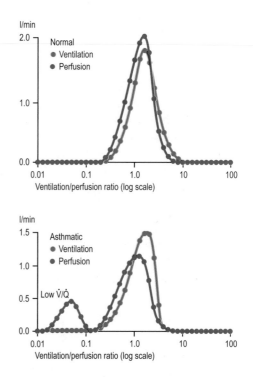

Fig 7.2.6 The matching of ventilation and perfusion. In the upright lung the ratio of ventilation ($\dot{V}$) to perfusion ($\dot{Q}$) changes from base to apex owing to the effect of gravity. You can see that the healthy lung does a pretty good job of matching blood and air over about 75% of its height, and the majority of mismatch takes place at the apex.

Fig. 7.2.7 Distribution of ventilation ($\dot{V}$) and perfusion ($\dot{Q}$). The multiple inert gas technique shows us how much ventilation and perfusion is going to a region with a particular $\dot{V}/\dot{Q}$ ratio. In the normal lung most of both are going to regions with a ratio of 1.0. In the asthmatic lung, about 25% of total perfusion is going to regions with a ratio less than 0.1 (low $\dot{V}/\dot{Q}$) owing to airway obstruction. Note that the ratio is a log scale so the spread is greater than the diagram suggests.

This model has been used to calculate what happens when there is a combination of different degrees of mismatch in the lung. This is all very well theoretically, but there is a whole range of ventilation–perfusion ratios in the lung and these can be revealed by an investigation known as the **multiple inert gas technique**.

The results of this technique are plotted as the amount of ventilation and the amount of perfusion against ventilation–perfusion ratio, i.e. it tells us how much blood (or air) is coming from a region with a particular ratio (Fig. 7.2.7).

You can see that in a healthy lung, perfusion and ventilation are clustered about the ratio 1. In a disease like asthma, a peak of low $\dot{V}/\dot{Q}$ results from alveoli whose airways are narrowed or blocked.

Finally, we must not forget that the dissociation curves for O_2 and CO_2 affect the exchange of these gases between blood and air in regions of different $\dot{V}/\dot{Q}$ ratios. This effect can be briefly and boldly summarized by the observation that, because of the different shapes of these curves, overventilated/underperfused regions blow off extra CO_2 but do not absorb much more O_2, whereas underventilated/overperfused regions excrete less CO_2 but still absorb quite a lot of O_2 because of the steepness of the oxygen–haemoglobin dissociation curve for blood returning to the lungs; $\dot{V}/\dot{Q}$ mismatch thus affects O_2 uptake more than CO_2 loss Dissociation curves are considered in greater detail in the next chapter.

Summary

Gravity and matching

- The contents of the thorax behave like a liquid, exerting more pressure on the base of the upright lung than on the apex. This effect is due to gravity.
- The excess pressure empties the alveoli at the base of the lungs more effectively than those at the apex.
- Because it is more completely emptied at the beginning of inspiration, the base of the lung is better ventilated than the apex.
- Gravity also produces greater perfusion at the base of the upright lung than at its apex.

- Pulmonary perfusion pressure is low and blood flow is pulsatile, depending on hydrostatic and pulsatile arterial pressure to overcome the 'alveolar clamp'.
- Matching of ventilation to perfusion is very important for the efficiency of the lung and is carried out effectively in healthy lungs.
- The different shapes of the dissociation curves of O_2 and CO_2 cause the exchange of these gases to be affected differently by ventilation–perfusion mismatch.

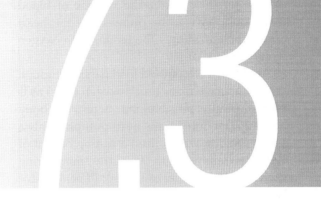

Blood gas carriage

Introduction

One of the main functions of the circulation is to deliver oxygen to the tissues and to remove carbon dioxide from them. Even at rest, an adult uses about 0.25 litres/min of oxygen. In exercise, O$_2$ consumption can increase many fold. CO$_2$ production is similarly increased. Large amounts of gases therefore have to be transported by the circulation. If these gases can be transported by a relatively small volume of blood, the work required of the heart is minimized. Evolution has produced very special adaptations to increase the capacity of the blood to transport these gases.

Transport of oxygen

Part of the problem of oxygen transport is that oxygen is not very soluble in water. The amount of a gas which dissolves in a liquid is determined by:

- the temperature
- the partial pressure of the gas in the gas mixture to which the liquid is exposed
- the solubility of the gas in the liquid.

At a constant temperature there is a straight-line relationship between the partial pressure of oxygen in the gaseous phase and the amount of oxygen which dissolves in water. At the conditions found in the alveoli of the lungs, 1 litre of water will dissolve 2 ml of oxygen.

If the tissues had to rely upon this dissolved oxygen for their needs, the volume of blood that would have to be pumped by the heart each minute to supply the tissues with oxygen would be very large.

Assuming each litre of blood passing through the tissues gave up as much oxygen (75%) as is physiologically possible and at rest the body needs 250 ml/min O_2, the heart pumping only a saline solution would need a resting output of 120 litres/min rising to 6000 litres/min during exercise. These values can be put in perspective by remembering that the volume of the whole body of an adult man is only 75 litres.

Most species have evolved means of increasing the amount of oxygen transported by the blood. The more oxygen the blood can pick up in the lungs and lose in the tissues, the less blood the heart needs to pump.

The solution to this problem is to supplement the dissolving of oxygen in the aqueous component of blood by a reversible chemical reaction of oxygen with a specialized **respiratory pigment**. Such a chemical reaction would increase the amount of oxygen absorbed in the lungs, but this oxygen can only be supplied to the tissues if the reaction is readily reversible in the tissues. The requirements of cellular survival are similar throughout the body, so the conditions in the lungs and tissues cannot be very different. This requires a reaction which ensures that the pigment avidly takes up oxygen at alveolar air P_{O_2} and readily releases the amount required at tissue P_{O_2}.

The chemical combination of oxygen with a pigment takes place in quite a different way from simple dissolution in water. First, the amount of oxygen which can react with a given amount of pigment is limited. That is to say the pigment can be saturated. There is a partial pressure of oxygen beyond which no more oxygen can be taken up. Second, the amount of oxygen taken up does not bear a straight-line relationship to P_{O_2}. There is a complex relationship, or oxygen dissociation curve, describing the relationship between the amount of O_2 taken up and the P_{O_2}. Its shape depends upon factors controlling the affinity of the pigment for oxygen.

There are a large number of respiratory pigments found in mammals, but for humans, we need consider only two:

- myoglobin (Mb), which is found in metabolically active cells, such as muscle, but not in blood
- haemoglobin (Hb), the oxygen-transporting pigment found in red blood cells.

Respiratory pigments

Oxygen transport and storage on these pigments is known as oxygenation (not oxidation because the valency of the carrier molecule does not change). An oxygen molecule (O_2) combines with a metallic ion bound into an organic molecule. In myoglobin and haemoglobin, oxygen is bound to an Fe^{2+} ion within a group known as haem. The haem is itself bound into a protein – globin. This binding greatly modifies how the Fe^{2+} reacts with oxygen. Binding to the protein prevents oxidation, but allows oxygenation – a relatively loose bond of an oxygen molecule to the haem. Changes in the protein surrounding the haem take place with the addition of each O_2 and modify the ease with which the next oxygen binds, i.e. they modify the affinity of the molecule for oxygen.

The pigment myoglobin is made up of a single haem and globin part. Haemoglobin is made up of four subunits, each comprising a haem and globin element. All the haems are the same, but in the adult, two of the four globin molecules are of one type, 'α-chains', and two of another, 'β-chains'.

As with most proteins there is variation between species, and even between individuals, in the precise structure of the protein molecules. As the proteins affect the affinity of haem for oxygen, these differences may be physiologically significant. One example in humans is 'fetal haemoglobin', which is present in babies at the end of gestation and for the first few weeks of independent life. This is made up of two α-chains, and two chains of a different type – γ-chains.

The binding sites of oxygen to myoglobin can be saturated. The relationship between the amount of oxygen bound and the Po_2 is hyperbolic (see Fig. 7.3.1A). Myoglobin saturates with oxygen at a Po_2 well below that in the alveoli of the lungs. The shape of this curve means that myoglobin is 50% saturated even when the Po_2 is only 1 kPa. (The terms oxygen **saturation** and oxygen **content** have very specific and different meanings which should be noted, see Fig. 7.3.1.) This allows the myoglobin to capture O_2 from the blood even when the blood Po_2 is low. Myoglobin would be quite unsuitable as an oxygen transporter in the blood as it will not give up O_2 until the surrounding partial pressure is relatively low. It is, however, well suited for the storage of oxygen within cells that are likely to experience sudden increases in oxygen demand – such as muscle cells.

Haemoglobin, on the other hand, is made up of four subunits. This structure of haemoglobin leads to a quite different relationship between Po_2 and the amount of oxygen bound, because changes in the structure of one subunit brought about by its reaction with oxygen can induce changes in the structure of the other subunits of the molecule, changing their affinity for oxygen. Like myoglobin, haemoglobin saturates with oxygen below the Po_2 normally found in the alveoli, though of course, each haemoglobin molecule binds four oxygen molecules, not one. 1 mol of pure haemoglobin will bind a maximum of 4 mol or 4×22.4 litres of O_2.

The effect of the presence of haemoglobin on the oxygen-carrying capacity of blood is enormous. A typical haemoglobin concentration for an adult is 140 g/litre which can bind 195 ml O_2. Compare this with the amount of 2 ml/litre calculated above to be in simple solution.

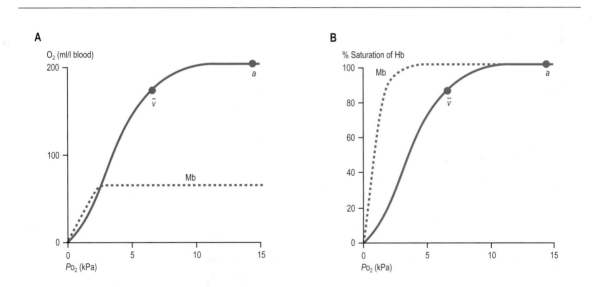

Fig. 7.3.1 The oxygen–haemoglobin dissociation curve for adult haemoglobin at arterial pH and temperature. **A.** Oxygen content (the amount of O_2 carried by 1 litre of blood). **B.** Oxygen saturation (the percentage of potential O_2-carrying sites occupied by O_2). *a* and $\bar{v}$ represent the Po_2 in arterial and mixed venous blood. The dissociation curve for myoglobin (Mb) is shown as a broken line. A molecule of Mb carries a maximum of one molecule of O_2, wheras a molecule of Hb carries a maximum of four. The O_2 capacities of equimolar solutions of these pigments reflect this ratio.

Summary

Respiratory pigments

- Respiratory pigments store O_2 at a fixed site (myoglobin) or moving round the circulation (haemoglobin).
- Carrying O_2 by the process of oxygenation (not oxidation), haemoglobin improves the carrying capacity of blood 100 times.
- Because they bind O_2 only at specific molecular sites, respiratory pigments can become fully loaded, e.g. in normal lungs blood picks up the maximum amount of O_2 and can carry very little more.
- Saturation is measured as the percentage of a pigment's total capacity that is being used. Content is the amount of O_2 carried by a specific amount of pigment.
- Myoglobin is more saturated than haemoglobin at most physiological PO_2.

Changes in the affinity of haemoglobin for oxygen

The haemoglobin molecule can exist in two different structural forms, the tense (T) form and the relaxed (R) form. The difference between these forms is small, the transition being produced by a slight rotation of one pair of subunits with respect to the other. The effects of the transition upon the binding of oxygen are large. Oxygen binds about 70 times more easily to a haem in the relaxed form than in the tense form.

In any given solution, haemoglobin molecules are constantly changing between the two states. The proportion of molecules in each affects the affinity of the solution for oxygen. If the transition from tense to relaxed state becomes more probable than the reverse transition, then affinity will rise, and vice versa.

These probabilities are affected by many factors. One very important influence is the binding of oxygen to haem. As more haems bind oxygen, the transition to the relaxed state becomes more likely and the affinity for oxygen rises.

Thus at low PO_2 (as in active tissues) the affinity of haemoglobin for oxygen is low and at high PO_2 (as in the lungs) the affinity is high.

As haemoglobin takes up oxygen, the binding of further oxygen becomes easier until four oxygens have been bound, when the haemoglobin is saturated.

A graph of the relationship between PO_2 and amount of oxygen bound is therefore initially shallow, then steep, then shallow again, an S-shaped or sigmoid curve.

Compare this relationship with that of myoglobin. As myoglobin binds only one oxygen per molecule, the maximum amount of oxygen bound at the same concentration is of course less, but if we express binding as a percentage of the maximum possible, or as percentage saturation, the curves may be compared (Fig. 7.3.1B).

Both haemoglobin and myoglobin are saturated at the normal alveolar PO_2 of 13.2 kPa, but as PO_2 falls, haemoglobin gives up much more oxygen at a higher PO_2. Reducing the PO_2 to 3.7 kPa will cause haemoglobin to give up half its oxygen load while myoglobin remains 95% saturated. Saturation at a given PO_2 can be considered as the molecule's 'appetite' for oxygen. Thus a substance with a high saturation of O_2 at a particular partial pressure is more 'hungry' for O_2 than a substance with a low saturation.

As the red cells containing haemoglobin reach the tissues, therefore, they are able to give up a large fraction of their oxygen to myoglobin.

The lower limit of capillary PO_2 compatible with life is determined by several factors. The cells need a minimum intracellular PO_2 to survive, but this is surprisingly low (well under 1 kPa). Oxygen must diffuse out of the capillaries to the metabolically active cells which consume it. Thus a gradient of PO_2 is required between the capillary (the supplier) and the cell (the consumer). The magnitude of the gradient depends on the diffusion resistance between the capillary and the most remote cell. If capillaries are sparse, and cells highly active and a long way from them, the capillary P_{O_2} must be quite high to maintain cell P_{O_2}. If capillaries are dense, then the capillary P_{O_2} can fall, because a lower gradient is required to supply the cells, which are on average nearer to the capillaries.

At rest, mixed venous blood is still 75% saturated. On average the tissues do not remove a large fraction of oxygen from the arterial blood. Some tissues, however, are much more demanding than others.

The fraction of oxygen given up by haemoglobin is increased if the capillary P_{O_2} falls. Some tissues are adapted to lower intracapillary P_{O_2} by an increase in capillary density. The most obvious examples are skeletal and cardiac muscle. Here the capillary P_{O_2} can fall dramatically while still maintaining the muscle cell O_2 supply by allowing a much larger fraction of the oxygen to be given up. The presence in muscle cells of myoglobin, whose affinity for oxygen is very much higher than haemoglobin, also tends to 'facilitate' the diffusion of oxygen to the cells. The usual minimum intracapillary P_{O_2} corresponds to about 30% saturation of haemoglobin.

Some tissues, most notably the heart and exercising skeletal muscle, extract more than 70% of the oxygen from the blood passing through them and this unloading is facilitated by the effects of temperature and pH.

Effects of pH and temperature on haemoglobin

The structure of haemoglobin is affected by a number of factors in addition to oxygen binding. The two most important influences are hydrogen ions and temperature. Haemoglobin molecules bear a negative charge and will react with hydrogen ions. This reaction changes the haemoglobin structure, so that oxygen will not bind so easily and affinity is reduced. At any given P_{O_2} below 100% saturation, low pH

causes haemoglobin to bind less oxygen – the dissociation curve is shifted along the P_{O_2} axis to the right, a change known as the Bohr shift and illustrated in Figure 7.3.2.

Tissue pH decreases during activity. Metabolism produces acids – in the form of both dissolved volatile CO_2 and non-volatile acids such as lactic acid. If the blood pH falls from 7.4 to 7.2 as it enters exercising muscle with a P_{O_2} of 4 kPa, the fraction of oxygen given up increases. At a constant pH of 7.4, the blood would give up about 45% of its oxygen (i.e. saturation will fall to 55%). But as pH falls to 7.2, the dissociation curve changes to the blue line on Figure 7.3.2, so saturation now falls to 40%, i.e. the blood now gives up 60% of its oxygen (one-third more that it would at a fixed pH of 7.4).

Working tissues also generate heat. The temperature within working muscle may be a degree or more higher than in the rest of the body. This affects haemoglobin. As temperature rises the oxygen–haemoglobin dissociation curve shifts to the right along the P_{O_2} axis. It changes in the same way as when pH falls, i.e. more oxygen will be given up at any given P_{O_2} (see Fig. 7.3.2).

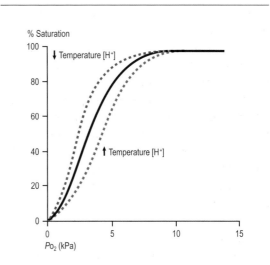

Fig. 7.3.2 The effects of changes in temperature and [H⁺] on the oxygen–haemoglobin dissociation curve.

The conditions within metabolically active tissues therefore favour the release of oxygen from haemoglobin by reducing its affinity for oxygen. It is important to realize, however, that these changes are reversed when the blood returns to the lungs. The conditions in the alveolar capillaries increase the affinity of haemoglobin for oxygen, moving the oxygen–haemoglobin dissociation curve to the left along the P_{O_2} axis. These properties of haemoglobin therefore optimize both the loading of haemoglobin with oxygen in the lungs and the unloading of oxygen in the tissues.

In exercise, oxygen consumption can increase more than 10-fold, but cardiac output increases only fivefold at maximum. The extra oxygen required is provided by greater extraction of oxygen from the blood by the active muscles now removing up to 70% of the oxygen from the blood perfusing them rather than the 30% at rest (see above).

This greater extraction is facilitated by:

- lower tissue pH – producing the Bohr shift
- higher temperatures in the tissues
- a fall in P_{O_2} in the tissues.

Long-term changes

Under some conditions oxygen supply to the tissues is chronically threatened. This occurs if the alveolar P_{O_2} is lower than normal (hypoxia) either because of disease of the lungs or because the inspired P_{O_2} is low (e.g. at high altitude).

Under these conditions the oxygen content of arterial blood can be increased by increasing the haemoglobin concentration. In chronic hypoxia, increased red cell production leads to a polycythaemia (increased number of red cells), and haemoglobin concentration may rise by up to 40%. Another way is to extract more oxygen at the tissues. In chronic hypoxia the affinity of haemoglobin for oxygen is reduced by an increase in the intra-red cell concentration of **2,3-diphosphoglycerate (2,3-DPG)**, which acts on haemoglobin to reduce oxygen affinity.

Unlike the Bohr shift, however, the effects of 2,3-DPG are not reversed in the lungs, and oxygen loading may be compromised slightly. However, because of the shape of the oxygen–haemoglobin dissociation curve, the reduction in uptake in the lungs produced by 2,3-DPG, which takes place on the flat upper part of the curve, is less than the increase in unloading in the tissues, which takes place on the sloping part of the curve.

The oxygen-carrying capacity of the blood is thus increased by the reversible oxygenation of the pigment haemoglobin. The relationship

Summary

Oxygen–haemoglobin dissociation curve

- Oxygen binds 70 times more readily to the relaxed form of haemoglobin than to the tense form.
- The changing fractions of tense and relaxed forms in a quantity of haemoglobin as it picks up O_2 give the oxygen–haemoglobin dissociation curve its S shape.
- A fall in tissue P_{O_2} increases O_2 extraction from the blood.
- The loading and unloading of O_2 onto haemoglobin is facilitated by the movement of the dissociation curve to the right at the tissues (unloading) and left at the lungs (loading).
- Movement of the oxygen–haemoglobin dissociation curve is largely brought about by changes in the hydrogen ion concentration and temperature.
- In chronic hypoxia, 2,3-diphosphoglycerate increases in the red blood corpuscles and reduces the affinity of haemoglobin for O_2. It therefore releases O_2 more readily and the dissociation curve moves to the right.

between P_{O_2} and the amount of oxygen bound to haemoglobin (the oxygen–haemoglobin dissociation curve) is sigmoid. At the P_{O_2} in the lung each haemoglobin molecule saturates by binding four oxygen molecules. At the P_{O_2} in the tissues, most of this oxygen can be given up. Unloading is progressively facilitated by falling P_{O_2} and by effects of low pH and increased temperature, which reduce the affinity of haemoglobin for oxygen. In extreme conditions, up to 85% of the oxygen in blood can be unloaded to the tissues, but normally (at rest) less than one-third is given up.

Carbon dioxide in blood

Carbon dioxide crosses cell membranes much more readily than O_2. It is produced by metabolism, and must be transported from the tissues to the lungs. Carbon dioxide also plays a vital part in maintaining the body fluids at their correct pH – mechanisms of acid–base balance. It is not possible to consider CO_2 transport in isolation from these mechanisms, so we will first examine the reactions that carbon dioxide undergoes in relation to pH of plasma before considering the CO_2 transport.

Clinical Example

Carbon monoxide poisoning

Since natural gas has replaced coal gas (which contains carbon monoxide) as a domestic fuel, accidental and suicidal poisoning from this source has declined dramatically. However, incomplete combustion of any hydrocarbon because of inadequate ventilation can result in carbon monoxide (CO) rather than dioxide formation and there are many deaths due to the use of combustion heaters when ventilation has been restricted in an attempt to conserve warmth. In addition, suicides achieve their aim by inhaling exhaust fumes (petrol cars without a catalytic converter emit about 4% CO while those with one emit 0.03%).

The clinical features of CO poisoning include headache, nausea, mental impairment and, in severe cases, coma. The patient's skin has a deceptively healthy looking and characteristic 'cherry pink' colour due to carboxyhaemoglobin formation. Sufficient exposure leads to myocardial damage and respiratory arrest.

Carbon monoxide exerts its effects by binding to haemoglobin on its oxygen-binding sites, but with more than 200 times the affinity and, therefore, to the exclusion of oxygen. The detrimental effects of CO determine the treatment of the condition.

1. The oxygen-carrying capacity of blood is reduced; therefore, the highest concentrations of oxygen possible are given to occupy all available sites and increase the dissociation of carboxyhaemoglobin.
2. CO shifts the oxygen–haemoglobin dissociation curve to the left, reducing the amount of oxygen released at any particular partial pressure. This makes CO poisoning one of the few clear indications for the administration of carbon dioxide to a patient. Carbon dioxide will not only stimulate ventilation, it will move the dissociation curve of the remaining oxyhaemoglobin to the right, as well as improving perfusion of certain organs.

The rationale of both these treatments is combined in the commercially available gas mixture 'Carbogen' which contains 5% carbon dioxide in oxygen.

CO$_2$ in plasma

Blood leaving the alveoli is in equilibrium with alveolar gas and contains CO$_2$ at a partial pressure of 5.3 kPa. Carbon dioxide is more soluble than oxygen in water. At a PCO$_2$ of 5.3 kPa and 37°C, the dissolved CO$_2$ concentration is 1.2 mmol/litre. The amount in simple solution increases linearly with the PCO$_2$. Unlike oxygen, however, carbon dioxide reacts with water. This reaction produces carbonic acid which then dissociates into its ions, H$^+$ and HCO$_3^-$. The reaction and dissociation are reversible. The amount of CO$_2$ in the plasma is therefore determined solely by the PCO$_2$, but the form it is in depends upon what fraction dissociates:

$$(CO_2)_{gaseous} \rightleftharpoons (CO_2)_{aqueous} + H_2O$$
$$\rightleftharpoons H_2CO_3 \rightleftharpoons H^+ + HCO_3^-.$$

If PCO$_2$ increases, more CO$_2$ dissolves and the concentration of H$^+$ and HCO$_3^-$ will rise. If on the other hand the concentration of H$^+$ or HCO$_3^-$ is raised, then the reaction will be driven back towards CO$_2$, and the dissolved CO$_2$ will be given up to the gaseous phase.

Like all equilibria, the proportions on either side of the reaction are governed by the chemical law of mass action, which states that the ratios of the active masses of the reactants are related thus:

$$[H_2CO_3] \rightleftharpoons [H^+] \times [HCO_3^-].$$

This can be rearranged to provide the dissociation constant (K_A):

$$K_A = \frac{[H^+] \times [HCO_3^-]}{[H_2CO_3]}.$$

(Square brackets [ ] round a substance indicate its 'active mass'; roughly its concentration.)

Taking logs of the above equation, we can write it as:

$$\log K_A = \log[H^+] + \log\frac{[HCO_3^-]}{[H_2CO_3]}.$$

In physical chemistry the term 'p' is known as an operator and represents taking the negative logarithm of a number. Thus, pH is $-\log$ [H$^+$] and is the chemical notation for acidity.

Rearranging the above equation and using 'p' instead of $-\log$, we get:

$$pH = pK_A + \log\frac{[HCO_3^-]}{[H_2CO_3]}.$$

This is known as the Henderson–Hasselbalch equation.

The value of pK_A for the carbonic acid/bicarbonate system is 6.1. Therefore:

$$pH = 6.1 + \log\frac{[HCO_3^-]}{[H_2CO_3]}.$$

As [H$_2$CO$_3$] bears a straight-line relationship to PCO$_2$, it may be replaced by the product of CO$_2$ solubility (0.225) and PCO$_2$:

$$pH = 6.1 + \log\frac{[HCO_3^-]}{P\text{CO}_2 \times 0.225}.$$

If the PCO$_2$ in plasma rises, pH will fall. It is important to remember that in the blood, the reaction:

$$H_2O + CO_2 \rightleftharpoons H^+ + HCO_3^-$$

is not a closed system. PCO$_2$ can be modified by breathing, [H$^+$] can be modified by buffers and HCO$_3^-$ can be added to or subtracted from the plasma by the kidney. The plasma pH effectively depends upon the relationship between dissolved CO$_2$ and the bicarbonate ions in plasma.

Changes in PCO$_2$ can be seen to have a large effect on plasma pH. The other factor in this expression is [HCO$_3^-$]. The factors affecting [HCO$_3^-$] will be considered when we turn our attention to the other component of blood – the red cell.

Carriage of CO$_2$ in the blood

Reactions of CO$_2$ in the red cell

CO$_2$ diffuses easily into the red cell, where it dissolves in the intracellular fluid. Just as in the plasma, the dissolved CO$_2$ can dissociate into

H⁺ and HCO_3^-. Unlike in the plasma, however, the reaction is not slow, but is catalysed by the enzyme **carbonic anhydrase**, present at high concentrations within the red cell.

In plasma the dissociation of dissolved CO_2 is limited by the presence of its products. In the red cell the removal of one of the products leads to more and more CO_2 dissociating, allowing more CO_2 to dissolve. The key to this process is haemoglobin. The haemoglobin molecules have negative charges, and so can act as buffers by reacting with positively charged hydrogen ions. As the hydrogen ions are removed in this way, more CO_2 will dissolve.

The uptake of CO_2 into the red cell is not therefore limited by the solubility of CO_2, as is the case in plasma. The reaction will be limited by the buffering capacity of haemoglobin.

In arterial blood this capacity is considerable. A fully oxygenated haemoglobin molecule can bind about eight hydrogen ions, leading to the reaction, within the red cell, of about 200 ml of CO_2 per litre of whole blood.

As the hydrogen ions are removed, HCO_3^- ions accumulate within the red cell, eventually rising to a concentration which drives them out through the cell membrane into the plasma.

The movement of negatively charged ions will tend to make the membrane positive inside. This will resist the further movement of ions unless it is compensated for, either by the outward movement of a positively charged ion (cation), or the inward movement of a negatively charged ion (anion). In this situation an anion, Cl⁻ moves into the cell – a movement known as the 'chloride' or 'Hamburger' shift.

The net effect of CO_2 reacting within the red cell, therefore, is to replace Cl⁻ ions in the plasma with HCO_3^- ions. The products of carbon dioxide dissociation (H⁺, HCO_3^-) are carried in the blood, partly as protonated haemoglobin in the red cell (Hb-H⁺) and as sodium bicarbonate in the plasma.

Figure 7.3.3 is a diagram of the whole process.

Put another way, the negative charges, or 'buffering capacity', of haemoglobin are used up

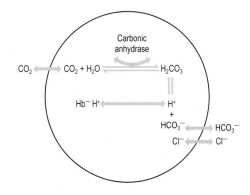

Fig. 7.3.3 The loading or unloading of the plasma with CO_2 in the form of HCO_3^- via the red blood corpuscle. Electrical neutrality is maintained by the chloride shift.

to allow the formation of plasma bicarbonate. This, of course, is the bicarbonate referred to above, which modulates the dissociation of dissolved CO_2 in plasma, and therefore controls plasma pH. Haemoglobin therefore exerts influence on the pH of plasma by modulating its concentration of bicarbonate.

We could therefore rewrite the Henderson–Hasselbalch equation as:

$$pH = K + \log \frac{\text{Reaction of } CO_2 \text{ in red cell}}{\text{Dissolution of } CO_2 \text{ in plasma}}.$$

The reaction of CO_2 in the red cell is determined principally by the properties of haemoglobin, with only minor influence of P_{CO_2}. The concentration of CO_2 in plasma is dependent only upon the P_{CO_2}.

Buffering within the body therefore represents the maintenance of the ratio of $[HCO_3^-]$ to H_2CO_3. $[H_2CO_3]$ is in turn proportional to P_{CO_2}. The organs which maintain HCO_3^- and P_{CO_2} levels by retaining or excreting these substances are the kidneys and lungs respectively. It has been suggested that the equation:

$$pH = K + \log \frac{[HCO_3^-]}{[H_2CO_3]}$$

(remembering that $[H_2CO_3]$ is proportional to P_{CO_2}) can be rewritten:

$$pH = \frac{\text{Kidney activity}}{\text{Respiratory activity}}.$$

CO_2 undergoes another reaction within the red cell. It can react directly with $-NH_2$ groups on the protein subunits of haemoglobin to form **carbamino compounds**. This accounts for the reaction of about 1.1 mmol of CO_2 per litre of whole blood. It does not affect plasma pH.

The effect of these mechanisms is that if the P_{CO_2} of whole arterial blood rises, the concentration of CO_2 dissolved in plasma will rise, but the $[HCO_3^-]$ in plasma will also rise as more HCO_3^- is formed in the red cell and exported. Thus, by maintaining the ratio of HCO_3^- to dissolved CO_2 more nearly constant, the formation of extra bicarbonate in the red cell reduces the pH change produced by the dissolution of CO_2 in plasma.

This reduction is even greater if, as in the tissues, the blood both takes up CO_2 and gives up oxygen. As haemoglobin loses oxygen, its affinity for hydrogen ion increases. It can now buffer more H^+, allowing more CO_2 to react with water, forming HCO_3^- which diffuses into the plasma.

In the plasma, therefore, both the P_{CO_2} and $[HCO_3^-]$ will rise, and so their ratio, which determines the pH, will not change very much at all.

Removing oxygen from haemoglobin allows blood to absorb more CO_2 in a way which minimizes the change in plasma pH.

Haemoglobin, as it loses oxygen, is also more able to react with CO_2 to form carbamino compounds. This decrease in the carrying capacity for CO_2 by blood when it becomes oxygenated, and the increase when it becomes deoxygenated, mirrors the Bohr effect for oxygen (p. 683) and is known as the Haldane effect. This effect results in a shift of the dissociation curve shown in Figure 7.3.4. This shift means that the functional CO_2 dissociation curve, over the physiological range, is very steep, which enhances the loading and unloading of CO_2.

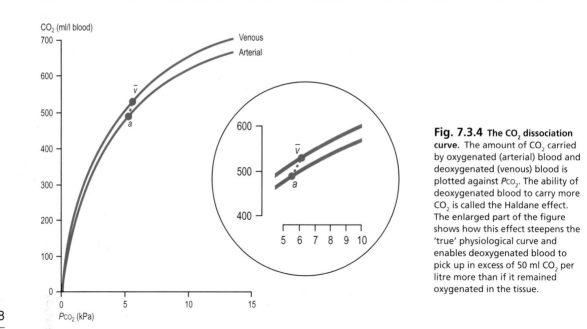

Fig. 7.3.4 The CO_2 dissociation curve. The amount of CO_2 carried by oxygenated (arterial) blood and deoxygenated (venous) blood is plotted against P_{CO_2}. The ability of deoxygenated blood to carry more CO_2 is called the Haldane effect. The enlarged part of the figure shows how this effect steepens the 'true' physiological curve and enables deoxygenated blood to pick up in excess of 50 ml CO_2 per litre more than if it remained oxygenated in the tissue.

We are now in a position to spell out the reaction of CO_2 in blood as it passes from lungs to tissues and back again. This can be expressed in terms of the differences in composition between arterial and venous blood (Table 7.3.1).

In terms of mmol/litre therefore, blood at the tissues gains 0.2 mmol/litre of dissolved CO_2 because of the increase in P_{CO_2}, 1.6 mmol/litre HCO_3^- mainly because of increased buffering capacity of haemoglobin, with a small effect of increased P_{CO_2}, and 0.2 mmol/litre of carbamino compounds.

When the blood returns to the lungs P_{CO_2} falls, so the dissolved CO_2 falls, and haemoglobin becomes oxygenated and its affinity for H^+ falls; H^+ is thus given up, converting HCO_3^- back to CO_2 which is lost via the lungs. Carbamino compound also dissociates because of the oxygenation of haemoglobin.

Haemoglobin therefore plays a central role in the transport of both oxygen and CO_2 because of its ability to bind both oxygen and hydrogen ions.

Thus, as well as being a continuous product of metabolism which must eventually be removed from the body, CO_2 is important in the control of acid–base balance. CO_2 reacts in both plasma and red cell. It dissolves in plasma, and some dissolved CO_2 dissociates to form hydrogen ions, which determine the extracellular pH of the body. The extent of dissociation, and therefore the pH, is also controlled by the plasma bicarbonate concentration. CO_2 reacts in the red cell to form hydrogen ions, which are mopped up by haemoglobin, and HCO_3^-, which is exported to the plasma. The formation of HCO_3^- depends upon the capacity of haemoglobin to bind hydrogen ions – its buffering capacity. Haemoglobin therefore indirectly controls plasma pH. Some CO_2 reacts directly with haemoglobin to form carbamino compounds.

At the tissues, P_{CO_2} rises, so more CO_2 dissolves; but as haemoglobin loses oxygen it binds more H^+ ions, so more bicarbonate is formed from CO_2 in the red cell.

At the lungs, the oxygenation of haemoglobin and fall in P_{CO_2} reverse the reactions, so the extra CO_2 is given up. Of the CO_2 in venous blood being transported from tissues to lungs, 80% travels as bicarbonate, 10% as dissolved CO_2 and 10% as carbamino compounds.

Table 7.3.1 The composition of arterial and venous blood

	Blood gas values	
	Arterial blood	Mixed venous blood
Oxygen		
Partial pressure (mmHg/kPa)	100/13	40/5.5
Content (ml/l)	200	150
Saturation %	98	75
Carbon dioxide		
Partial pressure (mmHg/kPa)	40/5.5	46/6.1
Content (whole blood)* (ml/l)	490	530
Content (plasma) (ml/l)	600	640
Plasma acidity		
pH	7.40	7.39
[H⁺] (nM)	40	42

* The carbon dioxide content per litre of whole blood is less than that per litre of pure plasma because approximately half the volume of whole blood is made up of red blood cells, which contain only half the content of carbon dioxide per litre of pure plasma.

Summary

CO_2 in the blood

- CO_2 is an acid product of metabolism which must be removed. It is a major determinant of blood pH.
- In solution it forms carbonic acid H_2CO_3.
- CO_2 is mainly transported as plasma HCO_3^-.
- The majority of plasma HCO_3^- is formed in the red blood corpuscles where the reaction $H_2CO_3 \rightleftharpoons H^+ + HCO_3^-$ is accelerated by carbonic anhydrase.

- Formation of HCO_3^- is limited by haemoglobin's ability to 'mop-up' H^+.
- Plasma pH is controlled by the ratio of H_2CO_3 (determined by the effect of respiration on CO_2) to HCO_3^- (determined by the action of the kidney).
- Removing O_2 from haemoglobin at the tissues enables it to pick up more H^+ and allow the formation of more HCO_3^-. At the lungs the reverse reaction forms CO_2 for excretion.

Control of breathing

Introduction

Homeostatic systems such as respiration must be able to change their level of activity in response to the changing levels of activity of the organism. In ourselves we see this most clearly in the way that breathing responds to exercise. To respond constructively to change, a system must have sensors (receptors) to monitor the variables being regulated and control mechanisms to regulate the system in an appropriate way. Although control of breathing normally proceeds as a seamless whole, it is possible, for ease of study, to divide it into chemical and neural control of breathing.

Chemical control of breathing

Respiration is particularly concerned with the chemical composition of the blood in terms of O_2 and CO_2 – closely related to $[H^+]$. The sensors of this composition are called chemoreceptors and can be divided into central (within the central nervous system) and peripheral (outside the central nervous system). Chemical control of breathing can be further divided into control of oxygen lack (the peripheral receptors only) and carbon dioxide excess (the central and peripheral receptors). Chemoreceptors control the **minute ventilation** of a subject – the volume of air breathed in or out in 1 minute. The neural control of breathing (see later) is more to do with pattern of breathing.

Oxygen lack – hypoxia

Hypoxia is the general term for oxygen deficiency or lack. Receptors of oxygen lack in the circulation are specifically concerned with the arterial blood, where low P_{O_2} is known as **hypoxaemia**. These receptors are the peripheral chemoreceptors and are unique in being the only tissues of the body that are stimulated by O_2 lack. The peripheral chemoreceptors comprise:

- the **carotid bodies**, situated close to the bifurcation of the common carotid artery on either side of the neck, which are served by the glossopharyngeal nerves
- the **aortic bodies**, situated close to the aortic arch, which are served by the vagus nerves.

These peripheral receptors are tiny nodules of glomus tissue (4 mm diameter). A characteristic which gives us a clue to the way they work is the fact that, for their size, they have an enormous blood supply, and this is matched by a high metabolic rate. This supports the idea that the specific stimulus to peripheral receptors is a build-up of anaerobic metabolites, which takes place when their oxygen supply, the product of blood flow and oxygen content, is insufficient for their metabolic needs. Peripheral chemoreceptors therefore respond to hypotension, which reduces blood flow, and hypoventilation, which reduces the O_2 content of the blood.

Ventilation and hypoxia

The ventilatory response to low alveolar or arterial P_{O_2} is remarkably insensitive (Fig. 7.4.1). Arterial P_{O_2} ($P_{a_{O_2}}$) has to fall to about half normal before breathing begins to be stimulated. Part of this insensitivity is due to 'the hypocapnic brake'. This is the effect that increased ventilation resulting from hypoxia has on arterial P_{CO_2}. As ventilation increases it washes CO_2 (a potent drive to breathe) out of the blood. If it were not for this effect, hypoxia would be 10 times more powerful as a stimulus to breathing.

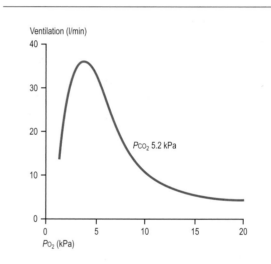

Fig. 7.4.1 Response of minute ventilation to changes in arterial P_{O_2}.

Summary

Hypoxia

- The sensors involved in chemical control of breathing are chemoreceptors (central and peripheral).
- Oxygen lack (hypoxia) stimulates only peripheral receptors – the aortic and carotid bodies.

- The specific stimulus to peripheral chemoreceptors is a build-up of anaerobic metabolites.
- The response to hypoxia is relatively insensitive; this is due in part to the 'hypocapnic brake'.

Clinical Example

Types of hypoxia

Hypoxia means low oxygen content or tension. Frequently the terms anoxia, which means totally without oxygen, and hypoxaemia, which means low oxygen content or tension in the arterial *blood*, are used synonymously and incorrectly.

Hypoxia is functionally important to the tissues. It is the consequence of their oxygen requirement exceeding their supply and is usually due to one or more of three causes.

Anaemic hypoxia

This is due to a reduction in the oxygen-carrying capacity of the blood. There may have been a frank reduction in the amount of haemoglobin in a litre of blood or a reduction in the ability of the blood to carry oxygen, as in carbon monoxide poisoning.

Anoxic hypoxia

This type of hypoxia is due to reduced arterial oxygen saturation, which in turn is due to one or more physiological causes (other causes such as high altitude or deficient ventilating apparatus are not considered here).

- Hypoventilation – insufficient fresh air reaching the lungs per minute. This is often the result of failure of systems outside the lungs (diseases of the respiratory central pattern generator of the brain or upper airway obstruction for example) and is always accompanied by hypercapnia, which is a useful diagnostic pointer.
- Impairment of diffusion. Equilibrium between alveolar air and capillary blood does not take place, because of thickening of the respiratory membrane between air and blood, as in pulmonary fibrosis.
- Ventilation–perfusion inequality. This is always present to a certain degree but is seen in the extreme case as dead space or shunt.

Stagnant hypoxia

Stagnant hypoxia occurs when regional blood flow or total cardiac output is reduced in conditions such as shock. Under these conditions, priority of perfusion is given to the brain and myocardium and other organs such as the kidneys may suffer from being deprived of blood.

Carbon dioxide excess – hypercapnia

Arterial carbon dioxide is the major chemical factor regulating minute ventilation. Even small increases in inhaled CO_2 will stimulate breathing. Unlike O_2 there is very little CO_2 in the surrounding air (0.04%) and voluntary or artificial overventilation, if sufficiently severe, can wash CO_2 out of the blood and suppress breathing, owing to hypocapnia. However, this effect is very minor because the shape of the ventilation–$Paco_2$ curve (Fig. 7.4.2) is flat over the normal range of breathing, so that reduced $Paco_2$ has little effect on breathing. Respiratory arrest after hyperventilation is usually restricted to those who know a little respiratory physiology and think they should stop breathing.

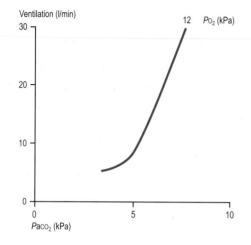

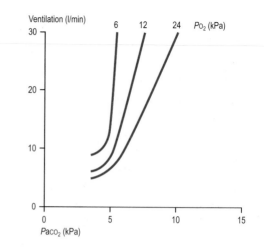

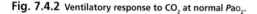

Fig. 7.4.2 Ventilatory response to CO_2 at normal Pao_2.

Fig. 7.4.3 The effect of asphyxia on ventilation.

Ventilation and hypercapnia

The rapid response (within 30 s) followed by about 5 minutes to reach equilibrium in response to a step increase in inhaled CO_2 can be explained in terms of the two sites where CO_2 acts to stimulate breathing. The peripheral receptors respond within seconds. The central receptors, which are situated about 0.2 mm below the surface of the ventrolateral medulla of the brain, and are responsible for about 80% of the increase in breathing, take longer. A large part of the effect of CO_2 is due to its formation of hydrogen ions. Figure 7.4.2 shows the equilibrium response to changes in arterial Pco_2.

Asphyxia

Hypoxia and hypercapnia as have been described here rarely occur in isolation. They usually occur together, as when one swims under water. The actions of the two stimuli are synergistic, being more than the simple sum of their individual effects – as illustrated by the

steepening of the $Paco_2$–ventilation graphs in Figure 7.4.3 when progressive hypoxia is added to the response to CO_2 shown in Figure 7.4.2.

Chronic responses

Going to high altitude for several weeks or contracting chronic bronchitis both result in hypoxaemia. At altitude CO_2 is washed out of the blood and in disease CO_2 may be retained. Arterial blood is separated from the cerebrospinal fluid which surrounds the central chemoreceptors by the **blood–brain barrier**. It is the business of this barrier to maintain the constancy of composition of the cerebrospinal fluid, and after a few days this is what happens. While this is happening, the subject at high altitude may suffer from acute mountain sickness. In the case of chronic lung disease, the patient adapts to the high levels of CO_2 and the major drive to breathe comes from O_2 lack. This can result in disastrous consequences if the patient is given high partial pressures of O_2, which remove the major drive to breathe.

⚡ Summary

Hypercapnia and asphyxia

- Increased levels of arterial P_{CO_2} (hypercapnia) stimulate both central and peripheral chemoreceptors.
- Unlike oxygen lack, the smallest increase in Pa_{CO_2} stimulates breathing.
- CO_2 forms hydrogen ions which are the specific stimulus of the receptors.

- Asphyxia is a combination of hypoxia and hypercapnia and the ventilatory response to it is greater than the response to the sum of its component parts.
- Response to chronic hypercapnia reduces with time because the environment of the central chemoreceptors is actively restored to normal.

Neural control of breathing

All control of breathing can be considered neural, because the chemoreceptors we have described are nervous tissue. However, it is convenient to deal with those neural mechanisms which are involved in reflexly determining patterns of breathing under a separate heading. It appears that, in some animals at least, the reflexes arising from mechanoreceptors in the lungs and airways, interacting with a central pattern generator in the brain, develop the most efficient pattern in terms of energy to provide a particular minute ventilation. This can be demonstrated by cutting the vagus nerves, which carry activity from the mechanoreceptors to the pattern generator in the pons and medulla of the brain. The central pattern generator produces a basic 'rough and ready' pattern of breathing. This pattern is modified and refined by other regions of the brain and afferent neural activity.

In the vagotomized condition when the central pattern generator is deprived of information about the lungs, breathing becomes slow, deep and inefficient. Most of the neural control of breathing can be explained in terms of the activity of three types of receptors in the lungs. Two types – slowly adapting pulmonary stretch receptors and rapidly adapting (irritant) receptors – send their information to the brain in myelinated fibres in the vagi, while the third C-fibre (or J) receptors send their information in unmyelinated fibres.

Slowly adapting pulmonary stretch receptors

Being slowly adapting these receptors maintain their rate of discharge in response to a sustained specific stimulus – which in this case is inflation of the lungs. They signal to the brain the volume of the lungs at any moment. Slowly adapting receptors are situated in the smooth muscles of the bronchi and trachea and are stimulated by stretch of these muscles. Their reflex effects, in experimental animals at least, are to inhibit inspiration, lengthen expiration, and cause bronchodilatation and tachycardia. Although there is considerable dispute about the importance of stretch receptors in the control of quiet breathing in man, inhibition of inspiration by lung inflation (the Hering–Breuer reflex) is present during sleep.

Rapidly adapting receptors

These receptors have previously been called irritant or deflation receptors, mainly because of the stimuli used by investigators to activate them. The natural stimulus of those found in the lungs is rate of change of volume of the lungs. Rapidly adapting receptors are found in the airways of the lungs, where their activity accelerates breathing by shortening expiration, and in the trachea and larynx where their activity promotes cough.

The augmented breath or sigh we take every 15 minutes or so originates from rapidly adapting receptors stimulated by gradual collapse of the lungs (atelectasis). The purpose of a sigh appears to be to reinflate the collapsed areas. This action is probably implicated in the deep first breaths of the newborn.

C-fibre (J) receptors

The majority of afferent fibres in the pulmonary vagus are non-myelinated C-fibres. Some of these terminate as free nerve endings in the walls of the trachea and bronchi. Others end close to the pulmonary capillaries and hence their alternative name of J-receptors (juxta-pulmonary capillary receptors). Although a role for C-fibre receptors in normal breathing has not been demonstrated, experimental stimulation results in apnoea or rapid shallow breathing accompanied by a fall in heart rate and blood pressure.

Reflexes from upper parts of the respiratory tract, including the sneeze, cough and swallowing reflexes, are protective. They prevent foreign bodies and noxious substances entering the airways. These reflexes are mainly associated with superficial free nerve endings in the airway epithelium. Of the automatic systems of the body associated with homeostasis, the respiratory system in man is unique in the degree to which it is under voluntary control, and the automatic and voluntary systems have separate pathways that control the respiratory muscles. The automatic systems in the brainstem send their pathways down the anterior part of the spinal cord while the voluntary pathways from the cerebral cortex descend separately in the pyramidal tracts and the lateral areas of the spinal cord.

It seems that control of breathing in man differs more profoundly from that of other animals than almost any physiological control system. This is probably because breathing is intimately involved with our unique facility for speech.

Summary

Neural control of breathing

- Neural control makes breathing more energy efficient.
- The basic pattern of breathing is generated in the brainstem.
- Mechanoreceptors in the lungs send impulses to the brain to make the pattern of breathing energy efficient.
- Slowly adapting receptors signal lung volume. They switch off inspiration.
- Rapidly adapting receptors signal rate of change of volume of the lung. They shorten expiration and cause 'sighs'.
- C-fibre receptors are found close to pulmonary capillaries and their stimulation causes a halt in breathing or rapid shallow breathing.
- Reflexes from the upper airways (coughs and sneezes) protect the respiratory tract.

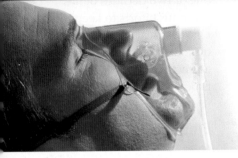

75

Chronic obstructive pulmonary disease

Introduction – patterns and causes

'Chronic obstructive pulmonary disease' refers to the commoner of the two main types of generalized disease of the lungs – restrictive and obstructive. In restrictive disease the volume available for gas exchange is reduced but the flow of air along the airways is not impeded. In obstructive pulmonary disease, also referred to as obstructive airways disease, the volume of the lungs is not reduced but the flow of air along the airways is impeded in a variety of ways. There are four main mechanisms which produce narrowing of the airways, especially the smaller and medium-sized bronchioles and bronchi:

1. spasm of the circular muscle of the airways
2. inflammatory swelling of the mucosa of the airways
3. excessive secretions, particularly mucus
4. loss of elastic tissue which normally holds open smaller airways.

Combinations of these mechanisms give rise to three main varieties of obstructive pulmonary disease: asthma, chronic bronchitis and emphysema.

Asthma

Here a major feature is intermittent spasm of the

697

smooth muscle in the walls of the airways. The prevalence of this condition has increased markedly in recent decades, for reasons which are not clear, but which may include certain forms of atmospheric pollution, allergies and changing patterns of exposure to microorganisms. Many people, particularly children and young adults, suffer from a relatively mild form, which is well controlled by inhaled aerosol drugs, but in severe cases asthma is a medical emergency requiring urgent and energetic therapy. Particularly in these more severe attacks, and when the condition has become well established, the condition also includes inflammation and swelling of the mucosa and excessive secretion, often of tenacious mucus.

Chronic bronchitis

As the name implies, this condition is characterized by persistent inflammation of the bronchial walls. Sufferers produce excessive mucus leading to a chronic cough with sputum. The airway mucosa is swollen and secretion of excessive mucus is a major cause of obstruction of the airways. Because the chronic inflammation damages the cilia of the airways, patients sometimes require postural drainage to clear the secretions. This means lying in positions, e.g. head down, where the excessive secretions drain from the lungs by gravity.

Severe atmospheric pollution (smoky fog or 'smog') has been a major cause of chronic bronchitis, but nowadays much of the blame lies with cigarette smoke, which contains a mixture of irritants well calculated to damage the airways. As well as causing excessive secretion of mucus, chronic bronchitis also obstructs airways by inducing smooth muscle spasm – chronic *wheezy* bronchitis – and in some cases there is also damage to pulmonary elastic tissue. This damage increases the tendency to airway narrowing and collapse, or closure. The condition is then referred to as 'chronic bronchitis and emphysema'. Emphysema is considered below.

A condition related to chronic bronchitis is *fibrocystic disease*, or *mucoviscidosis*. Here also the airways are blocked by mucus. However, in this case the cause is a genetic abnormality so that secretions are excessively tenacious, viscous and difficult to clear – hence the term mucoviscidosis. The trapped secretions favour chronic inflammation and infection. A similar state exists in the pancreatic ducts (fibrocystic disease of the pancreas, which impairs secretion of digestive enzymes) and abnormalities can also be detected in the sweat. However, while pancreatic digestive enzymes can be replaced orally, the pulmonary damage has, until recently, usually proved fatal in the first one or two decades of life. Vigorous efforts to keep the airways clear can improve the outlook, and genetic therapy to correct the abnormal secretions is being tested.

Emphysema

This term can be confusing as it has more than one meaning. In relation to histological sections of the lung it refers to distension and confluence of the alveoli into larger air sacs inefficient for gas exchange. However, in relation to obstructive pulmonary disease it refers to loss of pulmonary elastic tissue, leading to airway collapse. In thinking of this condition, it is useful to bear in mind that the lungs are traversed by a network of elastic fibres and that these are normally in a state of tension. This state of tension is demonstrated when an opening is made in the chest wall or when a pneumothorax is present. The lung collapses down to a small fraction of its usual volume. In a severe case the X-ray will show a shrunken lung near the hilum, with the rest of the hemithorax devoid of lung markings. So the normal lung is greatly stretched even in expiration. The stretched elastic fibres attached to the airways hold them open, so when these fibres are damaged the small airways are liable to collapse, particularly during forced expiration, when intrapulmonary pressure rises above atmospheric pressure.

In the pathophysiological state of isolated emphysema, the patient shows the signs of obstructive pulmonary disease without excessive sputum. It has been found that this state does not correlate well with histological emphysema in the patient's lungs.

Many patients show a combination of chronic bronchitis and emphysema, which is not surprising since cigarette smoking is a major cause of both bronchial irritation and damage to pulmonary elastic tissue.

The umbrella term of chronic obstructive pulmonary disease covers all of the above conditions, and is particularly useful for the large group of patients who have multiple mechanisms of airway narrowing.

Effects

The lungs have a considerable reserve of function and we rarely call on our full ventilatory ability even in severe exercise. Thus a patient may be unaware of early pulmonary disease if there is no associated cough, though serial respiratory function tests (discussed below) would pick it up. As the disease progresses, the patient begins

to notice *dyspnoea* and *exercise intolerance* and in some cases *respiratory failure* will eventually appear.

Dyspnoea

Dyspnoea refers to an unpleasant awareness of breathing. It is normal to be aware of laboured breathing during severe exertion, when normal speech is impossible. However, the dyspnoea of chronic pulmonary disease is recognized as inappropriately severe for the level of exertion. It may hamper speech when a companion walking at the same speed has no such difficulty. In obstructive pulmonary disease it is due to the increased effort demanded of the ventilatory muscles to provide adequate alveolar ventilation. This effort is related to the increased work required to force the required tidal volume through the increased resistance of the narrowed airways. With airways as with blood vessels, resistance is inversely related to the fourth power of the radius, so that halving the radius would increase resistance 16-fold and reducing it to a third would increase resistance 81-fold.

In such circumstances the airway narrowing associated with pulmonary compression during expiration is often associated with an audible wheeze. It is tempting to assume that such patients find

expiration more difficult than inspiration. However, when asked, many will state that they find inspiration more difficult than expiration. The reason is probably related to an increased *functional residual capacity*.

This is the volume of air left in the lungs at the end of a quiet expiration (conventionally two or more lung *volumes* added together are termed a lung *capacity*). The functional residual capacity equals expiratory reserve volume plus residual volume. The increased functional residual capacity in obstructive disease can be explained as follows. When these patients breathe out, their airways start to close before they have expelled the tidal volume. Air is trapped distal to the collapsed airways. When they breathe in their end inspiratory volume is higher than normal and with the passage of time the functional residual capacity may rise to more than two-thirds the total lung capacity (rather than less than half). Thus the patient is faced with the increasingly difficult task of constantly expanding an already overdistended thorax – the barrel chest of obstructive disease.

Exercise intolerance

Because of the hugely increased work of breathing and the correspondingly reduced rate of airflow into and out of the alveoli, patients reach the end of their ability to ventilate the lungs at relatively low rates of activity. A healthy adult would normally be able to increase activity to a level requiring an oxygen uptake 10 or more times the resting level, but the maximal oxygen uptake declines as obstructive pulmonary disease progresses so that walking at a normal speed or climbing stairs normally may be impossible. A patient who can no longer double the resting oxygen uptake cannot leave the house for normal working or social activities and is regarded as 100% disabled, the term 'respiratory cripple' being sometimes applied.

Respiratory failure

Despite the incapacitating dyspnoea just described, the typical patient maintains arterial oxygen and carbon dioxide levels close to the normal values and does not appear blue (cyanosed). This is the state described as the *pink puffer* in Chapter 7.1 and it implies an essentially normal response by the central pattern generator to the enormously increased burden of ventilation. However, in a minority of patients it appears that the central pattern generator gives up the attempt to maintain normal blood gas pressures, leading to the *blue bloater* state – blue

because of the cyanosis due to considerable amount of nonoxygenated haemoglobin in small blood vessels in the skin and mucosa, and bloater because of the bloated state due to secondary heart failure (cor pulmonale) considered below.

This type of respiratory failure is characterized by both a fall in arterial oxygen pressure (hypoxia) and a rise in the carbon dioxide pressure (hypercapnia) and is due to inadequate ventilation of the lungs. When such patients are asked to hyperventilate voluntarily they may be able to relieve the cyanosis temporarily but with their normal breathing pattern and during sleep the blue discoloration of central cyanosis (reduced oxygenation of arterial blood) returns. Features of the condition can be explained by a combination of hypoxia of respiratory origin (*hypoxic hypoxia*) and *hypercapnia*.

Hypoxic hypoxia

Hypoxic hypoxia produces direct and compensatory effects.

Direct effects. The main direct effect is to interfere with aerobic metabolism in the mitochondria and increase anaerobic metabolism with production of lactic acid. Cellular function throughout the body declines and this is particularly noticeable in the brain so that the patient may

appear confused, uncooperative and drowsy. If the hypoxia becomes more severe, coma and death can result.

Compensatory effects. These are polycythaemia, which may be helpful, and pulmonary vasoconstriction, which is harmful and can lead to heart failure. Polycythaemia results because the reduced arterial content of oxygen is detected by renal tubular cells, which respond by increasing the level of erythropoietin so that bone marrow activity increases and the number of circulating erythrocytes rises. This favours transport of oxygen but increases cardiac work by increasing blood viscosity.

Normally, local pulmonary vasoconstriction in response to local hypoxia diverts blood away from poorly ventilated regions of lung, beneficially maintaining a normal overall ventilatory–perfusion match. However, when pulmonary hypoxia is generalized because of generalized alveolar underventilation, the overall pulmonary vascular resistance rises. Since pulmonary blood flow must be maintained to maintain cardiac output, the result is pulmonary hypertension – [normal flow] × [increased resistance] = [increased pressure]. This increases right ventricular afterload and hence the workload of the right ventricle. Pulmonary artery pressure may more than double.

Initially, this leads to right ventricular hypertrophy in response to the increased work, but ultimately the ventricle fails and dilates. This *right-sided cardiac failure* shows the usual features of a raised central venous pressure and swelling (oedema) of the dependent parts (usually mainly ankles). This state has been described as 'cor pulmonale' since it is a heart (cor) problem secondary to a pulmonary problem.

Hypercapnia

Hypercapnia adds to the depression of cellular function produced by hypoxia. In addition it causes a *respiratory acidosis*, i.e. the hydrogen ion content of the body increases owing to the inadequate respiratory excretion of carbon dioxide. In the simplest version of the Henderson–Hasselbalch relationship (see p. 686) it can be stated that [hydrogen ion concentration] = [carbon dioxide pressure]/[bicarbonate ion concentration]. Thus the hypercapnia causes acidosis. The relationship also predicts that if the bicarbonate ion concentration is subsequently raised, the ratio and hence the hydrogen ion concentration will move towards normal. This is the basis of a *compensated respiratory acidosis* – renal excretion of hydrogen ions is associated with accumulation of bicarbonate ions in the body. The level may rise by a quarter or more and the blood pH may return close to normal. Particularly before compensation, the acidosis, combined with the hypoxia is extremely dangerous and may contribute to the death of the patient in coma.

Investigations

These are used to confirm the diagnosis, to quantify the severity of the condition and to monitor progress.

Confirming the diagnosis

Confirmation of the diagnosis is suggested by a low *peak expiratory flow rate* and established by *timed spirometry* which measures the *forced expiratory volume in the first second* (FEV_1)and the *vital capacity*. In all cases results are compared with the normal expected in relation to the three major factors that affect respiratory volumes: size as indicated by height or normal weight (since increasing weight by increasing fat stores does not increase expected lung volumes), sex and age of the patient. As a rough guide, values are about 20% lower in small compared with large people, in females compared with males and in people of 70 compared with people of 20 (Fig. 7.5.1A,B).

A low to very low peak expiratory flow rate makes obstructive disease very likely, though severe restrictive disease is a much rarer possibility. An obstructive pattern can be confirmed by finding a reduced FEV_1, combined with a reduced percentage when this is compared with the vital capacity. By its nature, the main effect of obstructive disease is to slow expiration – it is likely to be present if it takes a person longer than 5–6 seconds to expire the vital capacity – so the peak flow rate is severely reduced and the percentage of the vital capacity which can be expired in the first second drops from around 70–80% to, typically, around 40–50% (Fig. 7.5.1C).

Estimating the severity

In terms of severity, the peak expiratory flow rate is quite sensitive. Thus in moderate disturbance it falls to around half and in severe cases to around one-fifth. Severity can also be judged quite precisely by the fall in the FEV_1, and similar criteria apply. Thus if somone's normal value is 4.0 litres in the first second (with a vital capacity of 5.0 litres), a value of 2.0 litres would indicate moderate disease and 0.8 litres severe disease. At around the level of 0.8 litres the patient would be severely disabled in everyday life, major surgery and anaesthesia would be extremely hazardous and the removal of a lung (e.g. for cancer) would be likely to leave the patient without sufficient lung function to sustain life. Removal of a lung usually leads to loss of just over half of the previous lung function. With very low levels of forced expiratory volume, the vital capacity is usually also much reduced since the residual volume increases greatly and the total lung capacity increases relatively little (Fig. 7.5.1C).

Monitoring progress

This is most effectively done by serial measurements of timed spirometry, with the FEV_1 the most sensitive guide. However, peak expiratory flow rate is

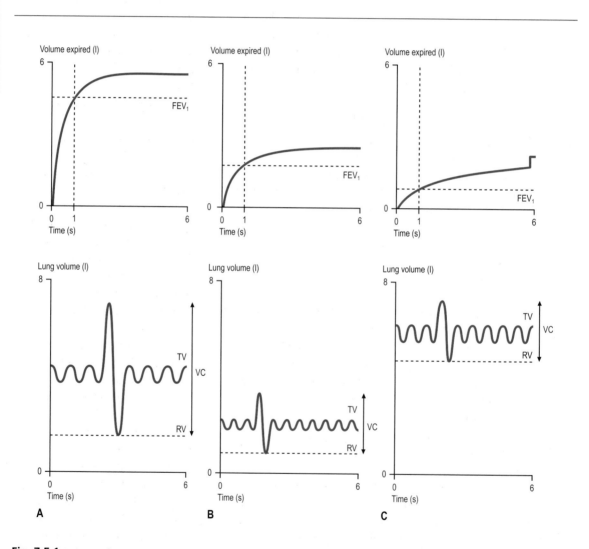

Fig. 7.5.1 Patterns of respiratory function. The three upper panels show examples of *dynamic lung volume* tests (timed spirometry). The three lower panels show corresponding *static lung volumes*. **A.** Normal traces for a tall young man with a vital capacity (VC) of 5.5 litres and a FEV_1 of 4.5 litres (ratio about 80%). **B.** Traces for the same individual as in (A) with severe restrictive disease, or for a normal small, elderly woman. **C.** Traces for the same individual as in (A) with severe obstructive disease. Note that he has taken longer than 6 seconds to expire the vital capacity, as indicated by the terminal upward deflection. FEV_1 is about a third of the greatly reduced vital capacity. The lower panel indicates the enormous increase in the residual volume (RV) (and hence functional residual capacity, which equals expiratory reserve volume plus residual volume). Total lung capacity is little affected. TV = tidal volume.

almost as useful and, with moderately accurate devices for its measurement now extremely cheap, it is widely used for home monitoring by patients, including children with asthma. A sudden drop in the value, often accompanied by symptoms, is an indication to seek medical advice. Although not so often measured, the static lung volumes, including residual volume, help to complete the picture. Some examples of these, together with timed (dynamic) spirometry are given in Figure 7.5.1.

When respiratory failure is suspected, *arterial blood gases* are measured for accurate diagnosis and management. Although referred to as blood gases (oxygen and carbon dioxide partial pressures), the measurements include pH and bicarbonate content. A sample can be taken from any artery but usually the radial artery is used. Venous blood varies enormously, particularly in oxygen content, so is generally unsuitable for such measurements. However, by promoting a very high skin flow the venous blood is said to be 'arterialized' and may then give an estimate of the arterial values. Capillary blood from a warmed earlobe can also be used. However, arterial puncture is the standard method and is widely and safely used. In the intensive care situation a tiny plastic tube (catheter, line) is placed in an artery for a variety of purposes, including taking samples for blood gas measurements.

In respiratory failure these measurements on the arterial sample quantify the twin problems of hypoxic hypoxia and respiratory acidosis as discussed above. Broadly speaking, an arterial blood Po_2 half normal indicates a serious problem and need for intervention, and a pH of 7.25 has the same connotations. Lower values carry an increasing risk of imminent death. The physiological principles involved in managing such patients with oxygen are considered below.

Treatment

Treatment is related to relieving airway obstruction caused by the first three of the four underlying problems mentioned at the beginning of this chapter, and to the amelioration of respiratory failure.

Treatment of airway narrowing

Spasm of airway muscle is the mechanism most amenable to treatment. Such treatment is widely available in the form of portable nebulizers, which allow small particles of active agent to be inhaled into the airways. Airway muscle may be relaxed either by stimulating receptors which mediate relaxation – β_2-*adrenoceptor stimulants* – or by blocking transmitters which mediate contraction, i.e. *blocking the action of acetylcholine* released by parasympathetic (vagal) nerve fibres supplying the airways.

Many inflammatory/allergic mediators such as histamine and leukotrienes play a part in obstructive disease, particularly asthma, and treatment is increasingly directed at them, since such treatment can potentially reverse not only muscle spasm but also inflammatory swelling of the mucosa and excessive secretions. Most fundamentally, *glucocorticoids* related to cortisol can control most of these manifestations. They probably do so by diverting metabolism away from the synthesis of proteins involved in such effects. These agents are also given by aerosols, with particle size around 1–2 μm so that they reach the smallest bronchi and can act locally, rather than being deposited in larger airways and absorbed. Blocking agents for leukotrienes have been developed recently.

Physical methods are used to help the drainage of excessive secretions. These include aerosol inhalations to make secretions less viscous and adherent, especially in mucoviscidosis, and postural drainage as described earlier.

703

Treatment of respiratory failure

This mainly involves dealing with the hypoxia since, given time, the body can largely compensate for the respiratory acidosis of carbon dioxide retention. However, a major problem is that oxygen therapy can seriously inhibit ventilation with the potential to cause a sudden rise in carbon dioxide levels and death from coma due to the associated acidosis (carbon dioxide narcosis).

Figure 7.5.2 indicates the principles and pitfalls of oxygen treatment in respiratory failure. In phase I, a patient has been admitted with an exacerbation of chronic obstructive pulmonary disease. The oxygen partial pressure is dangerously low and there is an incompletely compensated respiratory acidosis. At this stage the patient is likely to be drowsy and perhaps confused and uncooperative. Cyanosis is likely to be marked. This is *central cyanosis* because it is due to the bluish colour of the arterial blood leaving the heart, rather than to low blood flow in the peripheries. Cyanosis is caused by the desaturated haemoglobin visible in the superficial blood vessels of the skin and mouth. The amount of such haemoglobin is increased by secondary polycythaemia (increased haemoglobin secondary to

chronic hypoxia) and a high output state (increased peripheral blood flow due to vasodilator 'metabolites' such as hypoxia and hypercapnia)

bringing increased amounts of blood to the skin.

It is natural, and necessary to give supplemental oxygen in this state, but phase II of

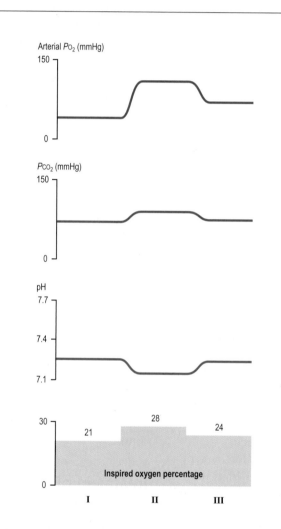

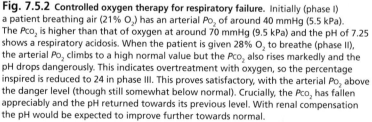

Fig. 7.5.2 Controlled oxygen therapy for respiratory failure. Initially (phase I) a patient breathing air (21% O_2) has an arterial Po_2 of around 40 mmHg (5.5 kPa). The Pco_2 is higher than that of oxygen at around 70 mmHg (9.5 kPa) and the pH of 7.25 shows a respiratory acidosis. When the patient is given 28% O_2 to breathe (phase II), the arterial Po_2 climbs to a high normal value but the Pco_2 also rises markedly and the pH drops dangerously. This indicates overtreatment with oxygen, so the percentage inspired is reduced to 24 in phase III. This proves satisfactory, with the arterial Po_2 above the danger level (though still somewhat below normal). Crucially, the Pco_2 has fallen appreciably and the pH returned towards its previous level. With renal compensation the pH would be expected to improve further towards normal.

the diagram shows that when the inspiratory oxygen concentration is increased from 21% in room air to 28%, the hypoxia has been relieved, but the pH has fallen precipitously. The patient's level of consciousness has probably fallen also. The reason for this is that patients in chronic respiratory failure show little response to increasing levels of carbon dioxide. Their central respiratory drive has become insensitive and it can be shown that the response to carbon dioxide is greatly blunted or absent. In this situation their ventilation is sustained by *hypoxic drive*. If this is totally removed ventilation is liable to fall calamitously.

In order to improve the situation, the inspired oxygen concentration is reduced to 24% (phase III). This oxygen concentration has lowered the patient's arterial oxygen, but it is still above the danger level. The pH has risen; it is a little lower than in phase I, but not seriously so.

This method of administering oxygen is referred to as *controlled oxygen therapy*, because the oxygen percentage is controlled carefully by administering a mixture of air and a precisely controlled flow rate of supplemental oxygen. Usually the optimal value is between 24–28% inspired oxygen. The aim is to achieve an arterial oxygen level around 75% of the normal value. This level of oxygen should restore haemoglobin saturation to values around 90–95% and this can be confirmed using a pulse oximeter applied to a digit or earlobe.

It is interesting that the principle of adjusting inspired oxygen percentage to achieve normal arterial partial pressures is also used in relation to abnormal atmospheric pressures. At a diving depth of 90 metres where the pressure is 10 atmospheres the correct inspired oxygen concentration is 2%, whereas at an altitude where the barometric pressure is half normal, supplemental oxygen to 40% would give normal saturation of the blood with oxygen.

As well as relieving dangerous hypoxia in the short term, it has been found that prolonged administration of modestly increased oxygen concentrations in their own homes to patients with persistent hypoxia can relieve the pulmonary vasoconstriction responsible for pulmonary hypertension and right heart failure. The modestly elevated oxygen is administered for as much as possible of the day and night – this is known as *domiciliary oxygen therapy*.

Further reading

Cotes J E, Leathart G L 1993 *Lung function,* 5th edn. Blackwell Science, Oxford.

A classic treatise on methods of measuring lung function. Should be looked at by undergraduates who are interested in how the measurements mentioned in this section are made.

Grippi M A 1995 *Pulmonary pathophysiology.* Lippincott Williams and Wilkins, Philadelphia.

Although not strictly a textbook of physiology, this book provides studies of the pathophysiology of many interesting clinical situations.

Lumb A B 1999 *Nunn's applied respiratory physiology*, 5th edn. Butterworth-Heinemann, Oxford.

This outstanding work has been revised and lost nothing of the original author's brilliant presentation. A must for the serious student of respiratory physiology applied to medicine.

Staub N C 1991 *Basic respiratory physiology.* Churchill Livingstone, Edinburgh.

A focused and precise textbook for undergraduates.

West J B 1999 *Respiratory physiology*, 6th edn. Lippincott Williams and Wilkins, Philadelphia.

A well organised and concise introductory text by one of the leaders in this field.

Widdicombe J G, Davies A 1991. *Respiratory physiology*, 2nd edn. Edward Arnold, London.

A concise textbook with a pleasant didactic style.

Questions

Answer true or false to the following statements:

7.1

During quiet inspiration:
A. The intrapleural pressure becomes more negative.
B. The intra-alveolar pressure is lower than the atmospheric pressure.
C. Intra-abdominal pressure rises.
D. The diaphragm contracts.
E. Surfactant deficiency is associated with a more negative intra-alveolar pressure than normal.

7.2

Expiration:
A. Is associated with a positive intra-alveolar pressure during quiet breathing.
B. Is associated with a positive intrapleural pressure during quiet breathing.
C. Is driven by elastic recoil of the lungs during quiet breathing.
D. May be accelerated by actively increasing the intra-abdominal pressure.
E. Causes an increase in intravascular pressure within the thorax.

7.3

The work of breathing:
A. Is increased by an increase in lung compliance.
B. Is increased by an increase in airways resistance.
C. Is decreased by the surface tension of the alveolar fluid.
D. Is decreased by the action of surfactant.
E. Is increased by turbulent airflow in the airways.

7.4

In lung function tests:
A. A reduction in FEV_1 relative to the expected value for height, sex and age is diagnostic of obstructive airways disease.
B. A reduction in FVC relative to the expected value for height, sex and age is diagnostic of restrictive airways disease.
C. Alveolar ventilation = tidal volume × respiratory rate.
D. Passive recoil returns the lungs to their residual volume.
E. Loss of pulmonary elastic tissue leads to a decrease in lung compliance.

7.5

The ventilation–perfusion ratio:
A. Is decreased in areas of physiological shunting within the lungs.
B. Is increased in areas contributing to physiological dead space within the lungs.
C. Decreases between the apex and the base of the lungs in the standing position.
D. Averages closer to 1.0 than 0.5 in healthy lungs.
E. Tends to have a greater effect on the content of O_2 than CO_2 in systemic arterial blood when it is abnormally high in some parts of the lung and abnormally low in others.

7.6

The oxygen dissociation curve for blood:
A. Reaches a plateau when the Po_2 is adequate to cause saturation of the O_2-binding sites.
B. Is independent of haemoglobin concentration when plotted in terms of haemoglobin saturation.
C. Is independent of haemoglobin concentration when plotted in terms of O_2 concentration.
D. Curves upwards at low Po_2 because O_2 binding at one site on haemoglobin increases the molecule's affinity for O_2.
E. Lies to the left of the equivalent curve for myoglobin.

(Answers overleaf →)

7.7

Release of O_2 from the blood in metabolizing tissues:

A. Is increased by an increase in local pH.
B. Is increased by an increase in local P_{CO_2}.
C. Is increased by a decrease in tissue temperature.
D. Is increased by a fall in tissue P_{O_2}.
E. Is increased by any factor which decreases the O_2 affinity of haemoglobin.

7.8

CO_2 transport in the blood:

A. Is saturated at a P_{CO_2} of approximately 6 kPa.
B. Is promoted by an increase in the O_2 content of the blood.
C. Mainly occurs in the form of HCO_3^-.
D. Is promoted by carbonic anhydrase within the erythrocytes.
E. Leads to an increase in plasma Cl^- levels.

7.9

Chemoreceptors:

A. Stimulate an increase in ventilation when the arterial P_{O_2} falls by 10%.
B. Stimulate an increase in ventilation when the arterial P_{CO_2} increases by 10%.
C. In the carotid body provide the main drive to ventilation under normal circumstances.
D. Can lead to an increase in ventilation when the arterial pH falls.
E. In the brain are responsive to changes in arterial P_{CO_2}.

7.10

At an altitude of 3000 m (9750 feet):

A. Systemic arterial P_{O_2} is reduced.
B. Systemic arterial P_{CO_2} is increased.
C. Systemic arterial pH is increased.
D. The red cell count tends to increase.
E. The O_2 affinity of haemoglobin is likely to be increased.

Answers

7.1

A. **True.** This provides a distending force causing expansion of the lungs.
B. **True.** This provides a pressure gradient driving airflow through the resistance of the airways into the alveoli.
C. **True.** This is a passive consequence of descent of the diaphragm.
D. **True.** This pulls the diaphragm downwards providing the main contractile effort for quiet inspiration.
E. **False.** The intra-alveolar pressure required to generate normal airflow will not be affected unless airway resistance is increased; however, surfactant deficiency will mean that a more highly negative intrapleural pressure is required to cause inflation of the lungs, since compliance will be decreased.

7.2

A. **True.** This means that there is a pressure gradient driving air out to the atmosphere through the airways.
B. **False.** The intrapleural pressure becomes less negative but does not become positive unless there is forced expiration.
C. **True.** Expiration is passive during quiet breathing.
D. **True.** This helps force the diaphragm upwards and is achieved by contraction of the abdominal muscles.
E. **True.** The increase in pulmonary pressures during expiration is transmitted to the compressible blood vessels. This may impede venous return to the heart during forced expiration.

7.3

A. **False.** This would decrease the work required to overcome the elastic recoil of the lungs during inspiration.
B. **True.** This increases the work necessary to move air through the airways, e.g. in asthma.
C. **False.** Surface tension increases the work of breathing by decreasing lung compliance.
D. **True.** Surfactant decreases the effective surface tension.
E. **True.** Airways resistance is effectively increased if airflow is turbulent rather than laminar.

7.4

A. **False.** FEV_1 will be reduced if FVC is reduced, even in the absence of airways obstruction. For this reason the ratio of FEV_1/FVC is regarded as more informative; it should be greater than 0.8 in normal individuals.
B. **False.** FVC may also be reduced in obstructive disease (see Fig. 7.5.1C, p. 702)
C. **False.** Alveolar ventilation = (tidal volume – dead space) × respiratory rate.
D. **False.** Residual volume is the volume left after maximal, forced expiration; the volume left after passive expiration is called the functional residual capacity.
E. **False.** This tends to increase compliance by increasing lung distensibility.

7.5

A. **True.** These are areas which are perfused but poorly ventilated.

B. **True.** These are areas which are ventilated but poorly perfused.

C. **True.** Both ventilation and perfusion increase on moving from the apex to the base of the lung when upright. The effect of gravity on perfusion is greater than its effect on ventilation, however, so the ventilation–perfusion ratio decreases.

D. **True.**

E. **True.** Regions of the lung operating at partial pressures off the plateau of the O_2 dissociation curve cannot be compensated for in terms of O_2, but can be in terms of CO_2 (see pp. 681 and 688).

7.6

A. **True.**

B. **True.**

C. **False.** The O_2 concentration or content of blood will depend on both the concentration and the saturation of haemoglobin.

D. **True.** This means that the increase in saturation for a given increase in PO_2 is greater than it would otherwise have been.

E. **False.** Myoglobin has a greater affinity than haemoglobin for O_2, so the dissociation curve for haemoglobin lies to the right of that for myoglobin.

7.7

A. **False.** This would reduce extraction by increasing the O_2 affinity of haemoglobin; pH tends to decrease in active tissues, however, and this does increase O_2 extraction – the Bohr effect.

B. **True.** This is the Bohr effect, with reduced O_2 affinity and a shift in the oxyhaemoglobin dissociation curve to the right.

C. **False.** An increase in tissue temperature promotes O_2 extraction by the Bohr effect.

D. **True.** The resulting shift along the oxyhaemoglobin dissociation curve greatly reduces the O_2 saturation of the blood, the additional O_2 being released to the tissues. This effect is quantitatively much more important than the Bohr effect in exercising muscles, for example.

E. **True.** Decreasing the O_2 affinity of haemoglobin increases the release of O_2 to the tissues.

7.8

A. **False.** CO_2 transport does not saturate in the way O_2 transport does; also the PCO_2 in mixed venous blood does not usually rise much above 6.1 kPa.

B. **False.** It is promoted by a decrease in the O_2 content of the blood because deoxyhaemoglobin is better able to buffer the protons released from carbonic acid than is the oxygenated form. The shift in the CO_2 dissociation curve associated with changes in O_2 content is referred to as the Haldane shift.

C. **True.** This accounts for about 80% of the total CO_2 transport.

D. **True.** This catalyses the reaction of CO_2 with H_2O; it does not change the amount of CO_2 transported at equilibrium but allows this equilibrium to be achieved within the time available when blood is passing through the capillaries.

E. **False.** It tends to decrease plasma Cl^-, owing to the exchange of Cl^- for HCO_3^- from erythrocytes.

7.9

A. **False.** The peripheral chemoreceptors do respond to hypoxia but only when the arterial Po_2 falls by 40–50%.
B. **True.** Ventilation is regulated to maintain a normal arterial Pco_2.
C. **False.** Ventilation is driven by spontaneously active respiratory neurones in the medulla. The main chemoreceptor input comes from the central chemoreceptors, not the peripheral receptors.
D. **True.** This is the basis of the respiratory compensation for metabolic acidosis.
E. **True.** These are the central chemoreceptors.

7.10

A. **True.** This is because of the reduced atmospheric pressure, which causes a reduction in atmospheric and alveolar Po_2.
B. **False.** If anything, Pco_2 is likely to be decreased, since the hypoxic drive to ventilation blows off CO_2.
C. **True.** This respiratory alkalosis is due to the reduced Pco_2.
D. **True.** Hypoxia leads to renal production of erythropoietin, which stimulates marrow activity. This compensatory effect takes several weeks to develop fully.
E. **False.** Chronic hypoxia leads to accumulation of 2,3-diphosphoglycerate in the erythrocytes and this decreases the O_2 affinity of haemoglobin.

The renal system

8

production of red blood corpuscles and regulating blood-pressure.

The importance of our kidneys is seen in those unfortunate people whose kidneys have ceased to function, and who depend on dialysis machines to maintain the composition of their blood; they can only live normally for a few days while their bodies accumulate wastes before having to make use of an 'artificial kidney'.

Introduction

Our cells are surrounded by a watery environment that is probably similar in composition to the primordial sea in which life originated. The constancy of this 'internal environment' of extracellular fluid is a requirement of life, and the process of maintaining this constancy is called homeostasis. The kidneys, together with the lungs, are the most important organs ensuring a constant chemical composition of our extracellular fluid.

The kidneys' importance can be gauged from the fact that they receive one-fifth of the cardiac output of blood, i.e. 1 litre per minute.

The major role of the kidneys is to 'purify' blood by extracting waste products of metabolism; they must also help to control the osmolality, volume, acid–base status and ionic composition of the extracellular environment by modifying the composition of that part of the extracellular fluid (the blood plasma) that passes through them. The waste products extracted by the kidneys must be ejected from the body and, of course, this is done in the urine, a watery solution. However, the kidneys have a limited water budget with which to do this. We can not afford to use unlimited amounts of water, even to carry out this important task, and the wastes are concentrated by reabsorbing 99% of the water that enters the millions of functional units (nephrons) which make up our kidneys.

As if this were not enough, our kidneys play important roles in controlling the

Section overview

This section outlines:

- The kidney's regulation of volume and composition of extracellular fluid by the processes of filtration, reabsorption and secretion

- The gross structure of the kidney, which is a cortex surrounding a medulla containing an inner cavity, the pelvis

- The functional unit of the kidney – the microscopic nephron (1 million in each kidney)

- How about 180 litres of plasma filters into the nephrons each day and how most of it is reabsorbed

- Autoregulation of renal blood flow which, along with renal nerves and the renin–angiotensin system, influences the rate of filtration

- Active reabsorption of substances from the nephrons, and how water follows passively

- Regulation of absorption by endocrine factors including prostaglandins, the renin–angiotensin–aldosterone system, atrial natriuretic peptide and antidiuretic hormone

- The effect of the shape of the loop of Henle enabling countercurrent multiplication to produce hyperosmotic extracellular fluid in the medulla. This effect is reinforced by movement of urea

- The excretion of fixed acids formed and absorbed by the body

- The control of acid–base balance by the kidneys in conjunction with the lungs

- Passage of urine from the kidney to the bladder and micturition.

General functions of the kidney

8.1

Introduction

The main function of the kidneys is to regulate the volume and composition of the extracellular fluid. This they do by filtering large volumes of plasma, retaining only plasma proteins, and then selectively reabsorbing from or secreting into the filtrate. The urine therefore contains 'unwanted' solutes in water. The processes of filtration, absorption and secretion are regulated homeostatically so as to minimize changes in extracellular fluid composition; in achieving this, urine of appropriate volume and composition is produced.

The kidneys also:

- excrete metabolic waste products including creatinine, urea, uric acid and some end products of haemoglobin breakdown
- excrete foreign substances and their derivatives, including drugs, and food additives – such substances are therefore excreted less efficiently when kidney function is impaired
- synthesize prostaglandins and kinins that act within the kidney
- function as endocrine organs, producing the hormones renin, erythropoietin and calcitriol, the active form of vitamin D.

Basic Science 8.1.1

Filtration and osmosis

Filtration

At a molecular level, filtration is the bulk flow of fluid through a membrane or other barrier that selectively impedes the movement of some molecules, the largest being impeded most. This process is sometimes called **ultrafiltration**. The movement is driven by a hydrostatic pressure difference across the barrier. The volume of fluid filtered per unit time is proportional to the hydrostatic pressure difference, the surface area of the barrier and its permeability. Those molecules that are too large to pass through the pores of the membrane are concentrated on the high-pressure side of the barrier. The concentration of freely filtered solutes in the filtrate is the same as in the filtered fluid.

Osmosis

When two aqueous solutions are separated by a semipermeable membrane that is permeable to the solvent (water), but not to the solute, and if the concentration of solute is higher on one side of the membrane than on the other, then solvent will move from the less concentrated solution to the greater. Thus, water will move across a semipermeable membrane down its own concentration gradient. This process is known as **osmosis**. Any solutes to which the membrane is permeable will move with the osmotic flow of water. Their concentrations will not be changed by osmosis.

The tendency for water to move to the region of high solute concentration can be prevented by applying a pressure to the concentrated solution (Fig. BS8.1.1). The pressure needed to completely prevent movement is termed the osmotic

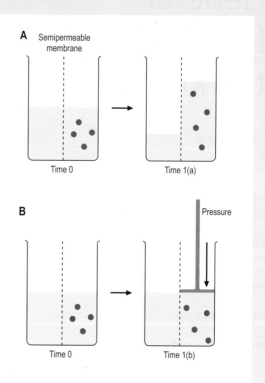

Fig. BS8.1.1 Osmosis. A. At 'Time 0', water is placed on the left of a semipermeable membrane and an equal volume of water containing solute molecules (the dots) is placed on the right. The membrane is permeable to water but not solute so that by 'Time 1(a)' water molecules will have moved down their concentration gradient to increase the volume of solution. **B.** If sufficient pressure is applied to the solution this movement can be prevented – 'Time 1(b)'. This pressure is the osmotic pressure.

pressure of the fluid. Osmotic pressure is expressed in the same units as hydrostatic pressure. You should note that the solution can only exert an osmotic pressure when it is in contact with another solution via a membrane that is permeable to the solvent and not to the solute.

Structure of the kidneys

The kidneys are paired, bean-shaped organs that lie behind the peritoneal lining of the abdominal cavity (Fig. 8.1.1). Each kidney is surrounded by a thin capsule, which is usually removed when the kidney is used for culinary purposes. The capsule resists stretch and limits swelling. This has important consequences for the renal circulation. The renal artery and the renal vein, renal lymphatics and ureter enter and leave the kidney through its concave surface, at the **hilum**.

When the kidney is cut in half longitudinally, an outer layer, the **cortex**, can be seen surrounding the **medulla**, which is made up of a series of conically shaped **pyramids**. The apical end of each pyramid, the **papilla**, opens into a space,

the renal **pelvis**, which is continuous with the **ureter**. The ureter drains into the bladder.

Structure of the nephron

The basic unit of the kidney is the nephron (Fig. 8.1.2), which is a blind-ended tubule running from **Bowman's capsule** into the ureter at the renal pelvis. There are about one million of them in each human kidney.

Each nephron begins at the **glomerulus**, which comprises a tuft of glomerular capillaries contained within Bowman's capsule, which is the blind end of the nephron. The capillaries are derived from an afferent arteriole and drain into an efferent arteriole. The many branches of the capillaries form a cluster that invaginates

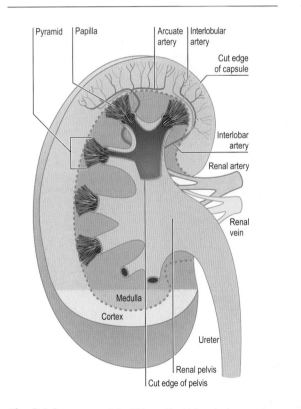

Fig. 8.1.1 Structure of the kidney. The kidney is shown cut across so that the hollow pelvis, which empties into the ureter, is partially opened. Into the pelvis project the papillae which are made up of the apices of two or more pyramids. The pyramids make up most of the medulla of the kidney.

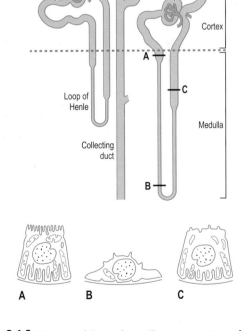

Fig. 8.1.2 Structure of the nephron. There are two types of nephron (see text) in which the proportions of their parts are different. The structure of the epithelium of the tube in these parts is shown.

into Bowman's capsule, like a fist pushed into a partially inflated balloon. All glomeruli are found in the cortex. The glomerulus produces a more or less protein-free filtrate of plasma.

Fluid from Bowman's capsule flows into a coiled segment, the **proximal convoluted tubule**, and then into the **loop of Henle**, which courses down into the medulla forming a hairpin shape. Two different populations of nephrons exist:

- **cortical nephrons** that have glomeruli in the outer two-thirds of the cortex and short loops of Henle that just dip into the outer medulla

- **juxtamedullary nephrons** that have glomeruli in the inner cortex and long loops of Henle that plunge deep into the medulla, as far as the tips of the papillae.

The terms descending and ascending are used to describe the two limbs of the loop of Henle. The nephron first descends into the medulla and then ascends back into the cortex. The ascending limb of the loop of Henle leads into a second coiled section, the **distal convoluted tubule**. The distal convoluted tubule begins at a specialized structure known as the juxtaglomerular apparatus (Fig. 8.1.3). Here the tubule passes between the afferent and efferent

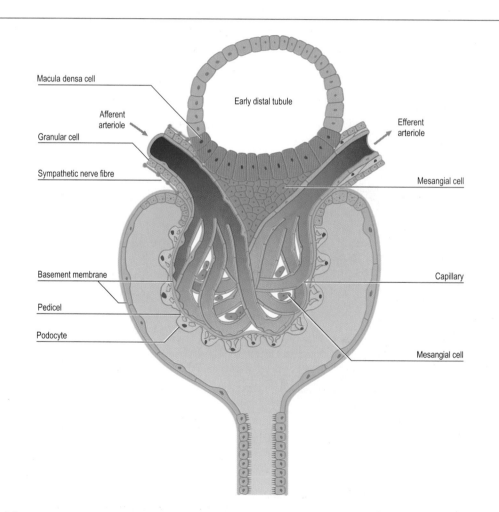

Fig. 8.1.3 The glomerulus and juxtaglomerular apparatus. The early distal tubule lies very close to the afferent and efferent arterioles of the glomerulus. Cells of all three structures are modified as described in the text and there is a rich supply of sympathetic nerves.

arterioles that supply the tubule's own glomerulus. This short section of tubule is known as the **macula densa** and senses the flow and composition of tubular fluid. It abuts onto a specialized region of the afferent arteriole whose granular cells secrete renin.

The distal tubules of several different nephrons join to form a **collecting duct** that passes through the medulla to the papilla.

Throughout its length, the nephron is composed of a single layer of epithelial cells resting on a basement membrane. There are characteristic differences in the structure of the cells along the length, which reflect their different functions (see below). The cells form a selectively permeable barrier to diffusion into or out of the tubule; they are joined together to form the barrier by specialized tight junctions that limit diffusion between the cells.

Structure of the glomerulus

In the glomerulus, the filtrate of plasma has to pass through three layers:

- The fenestrated (perforated; from the Latin *fenestra* – a window) endothelium of the capillary which is the filtering membrane.
- The basement membrane of the Bowman's capsule (Fig. 8.1.4) which is mainly composed of connective tissue, but also contains mesangial cells that are both phagocytic and contractile. By contracting they are thought to be able to actively reduce glomerular filtration by reducing the area available for filtration.
- The epithelial cells of the capsule. These are known as podocytes because they have numerous foot-like projections (pedicels) that clasp the tubes of capillary endothelium. Substances that pass through the filtration

⚡ Summary

Structure of the kidney

- The kidney is composed of an outer cortex and an inner medulla, which reflect the position and arrangement of the renal tubules (nephrons).
- Each tubule consists of a glomerulus, proximal convoluted tubule, loop of Henle and distal convoluted tubule.
- Distal convoluted tubules join to form collecting ducts which drain into the renal pelvis and ureter.
- All glomeruli are found in the cortex; cortical nephrons have short loops of Henle which just dip into the outer medulla, whereas juxtamedullary nephrons have long loops of Henle that reach deep into the medulla.
- The renal artery and vein, renal lymphatics and ureter enter and leave the kidney via its concave surface – the hilum.

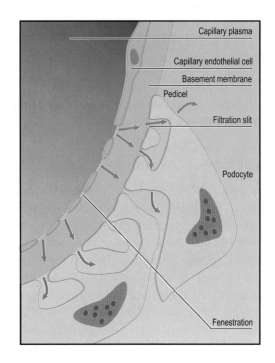

Fig. 8.1.4 Glomerular filtration. The structures that renal filtrate passes through from the glomerular capillary to the lumen of the Bowman's capsule.

719

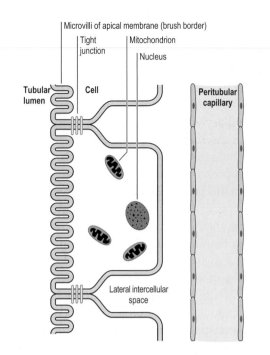

Fig. 8.1.5 **Tubular cells and peritubular capillaries.** The microvilli, tight junctions and intercellular spaces provide the anatomical basis for the absorptive mechanisms of the tubule described in the text.

Summary

The nephron

- Each nephron begins at Bowman's capsule – the blind end of the tubule.
- Bowman's capsule contains a knot of capillaries which is supplied by an afferent arteriole and drained by an efferent arteriole. This whole structure is known as a glomerulus and it filters plasma.
- Fluid passes from Bowman's capsule to the proximal tubule, to the descending and ascending limbs of the loop of Henle and thence to the distal convoluted tubule which begins at a specialized structure known as the juxtaglomerular apparatus.
- In the juxtaglomerular apparatus, the tubule passes between the afferent and efferent arteriole of its own glomerulus. This section of the tubule is known as the macula densa and it abuts onto a specialized region of the afferent arteriole which secretes renin.

slits (or pores) between the pedicels therefore pass close to the cell surface of the podocytes (see Fig. 8.1.4).

Structure of the tubule

The epithelial cells of the proximal tubules contain many mitochondria and have many microvilli at their luminal surface, called a **brush border**, which increase the surface area (Fig. 8.1.5). Adjacent cells are joined together at their luminal (apical) ends by tight junctions (see p. 60). At their basal ends, there are gaps between them, known as lateral intercellular spaces.

The descending limb of the loop of Henle and the first part of the ascending limb are thin walled: the epithelial cells contain relatively few mitochondria and are flattened with few microvilli. The ascending limb becomes thick walled as it enters the cortex; there are many mitochondria and microvilli, but fewer than in the proximal tubule. Along the length of the distal tubule and collecting ducts, the numbers of mitochondria and microvilli decrease. In the late part of the distal tubule and collecting duct there are two specialized types of cells (**principal** and **intercalated**) that are involved in Na^+–K^+ balance and H^+ balance (see Ch. 8.4).

Renal blood supply

As it enters the kidney, at its hilum, the renal artery branches to form interlobar arteries which radiate out towards the cortex (Fig. 8.1.6).

A

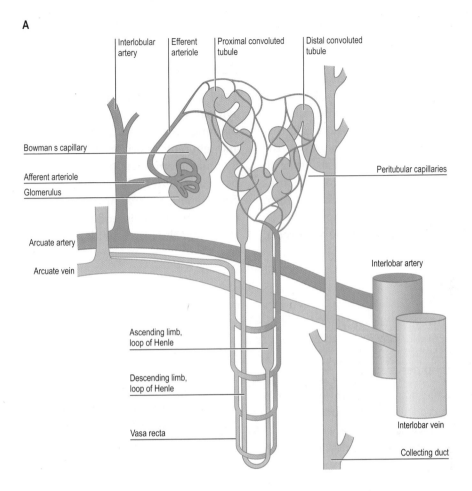

Interlobular artery

Efferent arteriole

Proximal convoluted tubule

Distal convoluted tubule

Bowman s capillary

Afferent arteriole

Glomerulus

Peritubular capillaries

Arcuate artery

Arcuate vein

Interlobar artery

Ascending limb, loop of Henle

Descending limb, loop of Henle

Interlobar vein

Vasa recta

Collecting duct

B

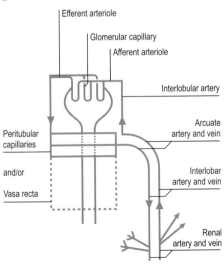

Efferent arteriole

Glomerular capillary

Afferent arteriole

Interlobular artery

Arcuate artery and vein

Peritubular capillaries

Interlobar artery and vein

and/or

Vasa recta

Renal artery and vein

Fig. 8.1.6 Renal blood supply. A. The blood supply to a juxtamedullary nephron is shown. Cortical nephrons, having a much shorter loop of Henle, lack the vasa recta. **B.** A generalized 'vascular circuit' from the renal artery through a single glomerular tuft of capillaries back to the renal vein.

At the boundary between the cortex and medulla, arcuate arteries branch off at right angles and from these arise the interlobular and afferent arterioles that supply the glomeruli. The efferent arterioles that drain the glomeruli branch to form a secondary capillary, or a portal system. Those from the cortical glomeruli give rise to a peritubular capillary network that supplies the renal tubules. Those from the juxtamedullary glomeruli give rise either to similar peritubular capillaries, or to capillaries which plunge deep into the medulla and form hairpin loops parallel with the loops of Henle. These vascular loops are called the **vasa recta**.

All the capillaries drain into a cortical venous system and then into the renal vein.

Renal nerve supply

The kidney is richly innervated. Postganglionic **sympathetic** noradrenergic nerve fibres supply the renal artery and its branches. The afferent and efferent arterioles of the glomeruli and the juxtaglomerular renin-secreting cells are particularly densely innervated. Sympathetic noradrenergic fibres also supply the proximal tubules, the thick ascending limb of the loop of Henle and the distal tubule.

Summary

Renal blood and nerve supply

- The renal artery branches to form interlobar arteries that radiate out to the cortex.
- At the corticomedullary boundary, arcuate arteries branch off at right angles, giving rise to interlobular arteries. These in turn give rise to the afferent arterioles that supply the glomerular capillaries.
- Efferent arterioles which drain the glomerular capillaries, branch to form a second, or portal, capillary system.

- Efferent arterioles from cortical glomeruli give rise to the peritubular capillaries. Those from juxtamedullary glomeruli form either peritubular capillaries or the vasa recta, which are capillary loops that run parallel with the loops of Henle.
- The kidney has a rich sympathetic noradrenergic innervation, which supplies the renal artery and its branches, the juxtaglomerular renin-secreting cells and the renal tubules, particularly the proximal tubule.

Glomerular function

8.2

Introduction

By the process of ultrafiltration (filtration at a molecular level) of blood plasma, the glomerulus produces enormous amounts of tubular fluid, the volume and composition of which is modified by absorption, or secretion, according to the requirements of the body to retain, or excrete, specific substances. The process of filtration is so intimately associated with renal blood flow and pressure that they can all be considered together.

Glomerular filtration

In the glomeruli, blood is exposed to a filtering membrane of about 1 m^2 in area, equal to over half of the external surface of the body. As described in Chapter 8.1, the filtering membrane is composed of three layers. The capillary endothelium, being fenestrated, is about 50 times more permeable than, for example, the capillary endothelium of skeletal muscle. The filtration barrier only allows substances of up to a molecular weight of 10 000 to pass freely. Larger molecules are increasingly restricted, those of molecular weight of 100 000 and above usually being unable to pass through at all. An additional barrier is formed by fixed negative charges, probably on the basement membrane but possibly on the podocyte cell membrane as well, which repel negatively charged anions.

723

Thus, haemoglobin from lysed red blood cells passes into the tubule far more easily than albumin, even though they both have a molecular weight of about 70 000, simply because albumin has more negative charges.

The fluid that filters into Bowman's capsule is therefore more or less protein-free and contains all other substances that are present in plasma in virtually the same concentrations as they are found free in the plasma. The exceptions that are not immediately obvious are low molecular weight substances that bind to plasma proteins and are therefore not filtered. These include some hormones (e.g. thyroxine), much of the plasma calcium and almost all plasma fatty acids.

Glomerular filtration rate

Glomerular filtration rate is determined by the difference between the hydrostatic pressure and osmotic pressures in the glomerular capillaries and in the lumen of the Bowman's capsule (Fig. 8.2.1).

The hydrostatic pressure in the glomerular capillary is higher than in other capillaries in the body because:

- renal **afferent arterioles** are usually wider than most other arterioles and offer less resistance
- renal **efferent arterioles** offer a substantial postcapillary resistance.

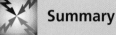

Summary

Glomerular filtration

- Fluid passes into Bowman's capsule by a process known as ultrafiltration through three layers:
  - the fenestrated endothelium of the glomerular capillary
  - the basement membrane of Bowman's capsule
  - the epithelial cells (podocytes) of Bowman's capsule.
- This filtration barrier generally allows substances of <10 000 molecular weight to pass. However, negatively charged ions are restricted more because the barrier has a negative charge which repels anions.
- Low molecular weight substances (e.g. thyroxine) and ions (e.g. Ca^{2+}) that are bound to plasma proteins do not pass.

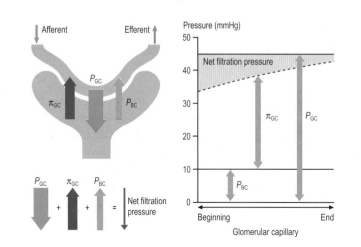

Fig. 8.2.1 Glomerular filtration. The pressures involved in glomerular filtration are shown on the left, and plotted against position in the glomerular capillary on the right. The glomerular capillary hydrostatic pressure (P_{GC}), the back pressure built up in the Bowman's capsule (P_{BC}) and the colloid osmotic pressure of the glomerular capillary plasma (π_{GC}) result in a net filtration pressure – the shaded area of the graph. The situation when there is a vigorous capillary blood flow is shown. At low flow rates there may be insufficient net pressure to bring about filtration at the end of the capillary but whether that is so is still open to debate.

The presence of efferent arterioles (unique to the renal circulation) and the fact that the glomerular capillaries are relatively short and wide explains another difference between glomerular and other capillaries; that is, the hydrostatic pressure does not fall significantly along the length of the glomerular capillary and is about 45 mmHg.

The hydrostatic pressure of the tubular fluid in Bowman's capsule is about 10 mmHg. Therefore, there is a hydrostatic difference of 45 – 10 mmHg (35 mmHg) between the capillary and the fluid in Bowman's capsule. This is the net **hydrostatic filtration pressure**. Because the barrier between the glomerular capillary and Bowman's capsule acts as a semipermeable membrane that is impermeable to protein, the protein in the plasma exerts an osmotic pressure that tends to draw water back into the capillary (see Ch. 8.1). An osmotic pressure that is due to protein is known as **oncotic pressure**. It is about 25 mmHg at the arteriolar end of the capillary. By contrast, the oncotic pressure in Bowman's capsule is negligible and can be regarded as zero. Therefore, there is an osmotic pressure difference between the capillary and Bowman's capsule which by itself would cause an osmotic flow of water into the capillary. The hydrostatic pressure difference is greater than, and opposed to, the osmotic pressure difference so there is a net outward filtration of fluid into Bowman's capsule.

The net outward movement of water from the capillary leads to a gradual increase in the plasma protein concentration as the blood passes along the capillary. Because fenestrated capillaries are so much more permeable to water than, for example, continuous capillaries in skeletal muscle, outward movement of water has a much greater effect on the plasma protein concentration in glomerular capillaries than in muscle capillaries. When the plasma oncotic pressure in the glomerular capillary reaches 35 mmHg, the hydrostatic and osmotic forces are in equilibrium and filtration ceases. (This equilibrium is reached towards the end of the capillary in the rat, but in man it may not be reached at all.)

Summarizing, we can write:

Hydrostatic pressure difference across filtration barrier $= P_{GC} - P_{BC}$

and

Osmotic pressure difference across filtration barrier $= \pi_{GC} - \pi_{BC}$

where P_{GC} and P_{BC} are hydrostatic pressures in the glomerular capillary and Bowman's capsule respectively and π_{GC} and π_{BC} are mean oncotic pressures in the glomerular capillary and Bowman's capsule respectively. (π_{BC} is included for completeness but is usually zero, as noted above.)

Therefore,

$$\text{GFR} \propto (P_{GC} - P_{BC}) - (\pi_{GC} - \pi_{BC})$$

where GFR (glomerular filtration rate) is the filtration volume per unit time.

GFR is also dependent on the permeability of the filtration barrier and on the surface area available for filtration. If K_F (the **filtration coefficient**) is the product of these two factors we can write:

$$\text{GFR} = K_F(P_{GC} - P_{BC}) - (\pi_{GC} - \pi_{BC}).$$

Clearly, if any of the factors that determine GFR change, then the GFR would be expected to change. Pathologically, GFR can be reduced by disease processes that reduce the number of functioning nephrons. Measurement of GFR is therefore important in renal physiology and in assessment of renal function in patients.

Measurement of GFR

GFR is not measured directly, but by measurement of the excretion of a marker substance.

If a substance has the same concentration in the glomerular filtrate as in plasma and if that substance is neither added to the urine nor taken away from it by the tubules, then the amount of that substance filtered per minute must equal the amount excreted per minute:

$$P_X \times \text{GFR} = U_X \times V$$

where P_X and U_X are the concentrations of the substance, X, in plasma and urine respectively and V is urine flow as a volume per unit time.

Therefore

$$\text{GFR} = \frac{U_X \times V}{P_X}.$$

GFR can be measured by using **inulin**, a polymer of fructose, which is freely filtered and neither secreted nor reabsorbed by the nephron. Inulin does not occur naturally in the body and must be given as a continuous intravenous infusion to achieve a constant plasma concentration.

In an average human adult, GFR is approximately 125 ml/min (180 l/24 h). As the total volume of plasma is about 3 litres, the entire plasma volume is filtered about 60 times every 24 hours.

Clinically, **creatinine** is often used for the measurement of GFR. It is naturally occurring and is released into plasma at a fairly constant rate by skeletal muscle. Therefore there is no need to give an infusion. Although it is freely filtered, some additional creatinine is secreted by the nephron. However, the methods available for measuring creatine concentration tend to overestimate its concentration in plasma. Thus, the errors tend to cancel out and GFR values estimated with creatinine agree well with those measured with inulin.

Renal clearance

The method just described for measuring GFR is one of several 'clearance methods'. Clearance is a concept, rather than an actual physiological process. The clearance of a substance is the rate at which plasma would have to be completely cleared of that substance in order to yield the substance at the rate at which it appears in the urine:

$$\text{Clearance} = \frac{U \times V}{P}.$$

Because inulin is neither secreted nor reabsorbed, its clearance is equivalent to the volume of filtrate produced in the glomerulus per unit time (GFR). If a substance has a clearance greater than that of inulin, then it must have been secreted into the tubular fluid by the nephron epithelium. If it has a clearance lower than that of inulin, either it was not filtered freely at the glomerulus, or it must have been reabsorbed from the tubular fluid.

Summary

Glomerular filtration rate (GFR)

- GFR is the filtration volume per unit time.
- It is determined by the difference between the hydrostatic pressures in the glomerular capillaries and Bowman's capsule (P_{GC} and P_{BC}) and the osmotic pressures in the glomerular capillaries and Bowman's capsule (π_{GC} and π_{BC}):

$$\text{GFR} \; \alpha \; (P_{GC} - P_{BC}) - (\pi_{GC} - \pi_{BC}).$$

- It is also dependent on the permeability of the filtration barrier and the filtration surface area – the filtration coefficient (K_F):

$$\text{GFR} = K_F \, (P_{GC} - P_{BC}) - (\pi_{GC} - \pi_{BC}).$$

- It can be measured indirectly via the 'clearance method' by administering a marker substance (e.g. inulin) which is neither reabsorbed nor added to the urine.
- For such a substance (X) the amount filtered must equal the amount excreted, i.e.:

$$P_X \times \text{GFR} = U_X \times V$$

or

$$\text{GFR} = \frac{U_X \times V}{P_X}$$

where P_X and U_X are the concentrations of X in plasma and urine and V is urine volume per unit time.
- GFR can be measured clinically, but with a small error, by using the naturally occurring substance, creatinine.

Regulation of GFR

A change in any of the hydrostatic or osmotic forces within the glomerulus can produce a change in GFR.

It might be expected that changes in capillary hydrostatic pressure, GFR and renal blood flow would be produced by changes in systemic arterial pressure. However, capillary pressure, GFR and renal blood flow (see below) are held nearly constant over the systemic mean arterial pressure range 90–200 mmHg (Fig. 8.2.2). This is known as **autoregulation**. Autoregulation of blood flow and GFR can occur in denervated kidneys (e.g. transplanted kidneys) and in isolated, perfused kidneys. Thus, it is not dependent on the nerve supply, nor on blood-borne substances. Autoregulation can be explained in part by an intrinsic or myogenic property of vascular smooth muscle; when pressure within the afferent arteriole increases, it stretches the vessel wall and triggers contraction of its smooth muscle, so leading to arteriolar constriction. This increase in afferent arteriolar resistance prevents an increase in systemic arterial pressure from reaching the capillaries.

The opposite happens when systemic arterial pressure falls.

Another process that plays a part in autoregulation of GFR is **tubular glomerular feedback**; within each individual nephron, the rate at which filtered fluid arrives at the distal tubule regulates the GFR of that nephron. It seems that the sensors controlling this process are the cells of the macula densa, but the mechanisms are still controversial.

One explanation is that the macula densa cells are sensitive to sodium chloride concentration. When flow rate in the tubule increases, more NaCl arrives at the macula densa. This causes release of substances at the glomerulus that reduce GFR. Recent evidence suggests that one of these substances is **adenosine**, which constricts afferent arterioles and dilates efferent arterioles, so reducing glomerular capillary hydrostatic pressure. Adenosine may also inhibit renin secretion and thereby reduce the concentration of angiotensin II, whose preferential constrictor action is on efferent arterioles (see Ch. 8.5).

A decrease in the flow rate at the macula densa would produce opposite effects, so tending to increase GFR.

GFR is also maintained constant when there is a moderate increase in sympathetic noradrenergic activity to the kidney. This causes balanced constriction of both afferent and efferent arterioles, so that hydrostatic pressure in the glomerular capillaries does not change, even though renal blood flow is reduced (see below).

Circumstances in which GFR does not remain constant

A large increase in sympathetic activity, as occurs after a major haemorrhage, causes greater constriction of the afferent than of the efferent arteriole and GFR falls. On the other hand, an increase in GFR can be produced by a decrease in plasma oncotic pressure. This can happen when plasma protein concentration is reduced, for example in liver disease or malnutrition.

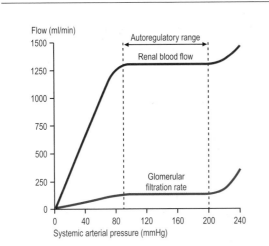

Fig. 8.2.2 Autoregulation. The effects of changing arterial blood pressure on total renal blood flow and glomerular filtration rate in the absence of any extrinsic influences on the kidney.

Although it is not immediately obvious from looking at the hydrostatic and osmotic forces that determine GFR, GFR can be decreased by a decrease in renal blood flow and increased by an increase in renal blood flow. The reason for this is that, if renal blood flow is reduced, plasma spends longer traversing the glomerular capillary. This allows a greater time for filtration of solvent out of any given volume of plasma. Thus, the capillary oncotic pressure will rise more for a given distance along the capillary and the point at which equilibrium is reached between the outwardly directed filtration force and the inwardly directed osmotic force occurs earlier. Therefore, less of the length of the glomerular capillary takes part in filtration (Fig. 8.2.1). The opposite occurs when blood flow is increased.

If the filtration coefficient (K_F) is reduced, this can also reduce GFR. This can be brought about by contraction of the mesangial cells, which probably reduces the capillary surface area available for filtration by causing twisting and occlusion of some capillary loops. Mesangial cells can be contracted by a number of substances including angiotensin II, vasopressin and noradrenaline. Pathologically, K_F is most often reduced by a loss of filtration surface area as a result of disease or damage of the glomeruli.

Summary

Regulation of GFR

- GFR can be held constant over the systemic mean arterial pressure range (90–200 mmHg) because glomerular capillary pressure (P_{GC}) is kept constant. This is known as autoregulation.
- Autoregulation is achieved by:
  - the myogenic response of the afferent arteriole, which constricts when systemic arterial pressure rises, so stretching the blood vessel wall
  - tubular glomerular feedback, such that an increase in the flow rate of fluid in the distal tubule causes constriction of the afferent arteriole of that tubule.
- GFR can be changed. For example:
  - a large increase in renal sympathetic activity constricts the afferent arteriole and thereby reduces P_{CG} and GFR
  - a decrease in plasma oncotic pressure reduces π_{GC} and thereby increases GFR
  - a decrease in K_F produced by a decrease in the permeability or surface area of the filtration barrier can decrease GFR.

Clinical Example

Glomerulonephritis

As the name implies, this is a condition where there is inflammation of the glomeruli of the kidneys. A complex condition which has been recognized for some two centuries, it takes many possible forms with varied effects. Some of these illustrate glomerular function by demonstrating what happens when normal function is lost. Inflammation, swelling and subsequent damage interfere with the normal functions of the glomerulus. In the early stages, swelling of tissues in the glomeruli can cause a reduced glomerular filtratation rate. In the later stages, damage can lead to serious loss of protein in the urine, which is normally protein-free.

Clinical Example *(Continued)*

The *reduced glomerular filtration rate* leads to scanty urine (oliguria) and an accumulation of extracellular fluid (oedema). The accumulated fluid leads to a puffy appearance and to circulatory overload with venous congestion in both the systemic and pulmonary circulations. In the systemic circulation this is manifested by venous engorgement, with the back pressure transmitted to the hepatic sinusoids causing enlargement of the liver. In the pulmonary circulation there is increased fluid in the lungs, leading to an uncomfortable awareness of breathing (dyspnoea). The heart is also enlarged.

When the acute stage has passed, some patients develop *loss of protein* as a result of damage to the glomerular membrane (nephrotic syndrome). Although protein is normally absent from the urine, a small amount is filtered at the glomeruli, and completely reabsorbed by cells in the proximal convoluted tubules. With damage to the glomerular membrane, protein, largely albumin, can be lost in large amounts, e.g. 10 g or more per day (*proteinuria*, or more precisely, *albuminuria*). This steady loss of protein eventually leads to a serious fall in the albumin level in the blood (*hypoalbuminaemia*).

The balance sheet of protein handling by the glomeruli in normal circumstances and in someone with severe albuminuria (20 g per day lost in the urine) illustrates the precision of normal renal retention of plasma albumin and the effect of a relatively small derangement of function. If we assume a glomerular filtrate of 125 ml/min, this equals 7.5 litres per hour or 180 litres per day. If each litre of plasma contains 45 g of albumin, then the plasma filtered per day originally contained some 8100 g of albumin. Since the retention of albumin within the glomerular capillaries is not 100% complete, some passes through the glomerular membrane with the filtrate. Of some 45 g of albumin per litre, only about 0.2 g is filtered and this is completely reabsorbed by a mechanism which is nearly saturated by this amount. Thus about 36 g/day are filtered and reabsorbed, the tubular maximum for albumin being about 45 g/day. The balance sheet of renal protein handling in health and in a severe case of the nephrotic syndrome would then be approximately as shown in Table 8.2.1.

This albuminuria and consequent hypoalbuminaemia cause an appreciable drop in the plasma colloid osmotic pressure which is normally a major force retaining fluid in the capillaries throughout the body, opposing the outward hydrostatic pressure gradient. As a result, fluid leaks from the circulation into the interstitial spaces and results in oedema in the dependent parts of the body, usually the ankles, or over the sacrum in someone spending much of the time lying flat.

As with oedema due to raised capillary hydrostatic pressure in heart failure, a vicious circle of positive feedback tends to develop. Fluid loss from the circulation leads to a fall in circulating blood volume. The body responds to this by increasing aldosterone secretion which causes salt retention in the kidney (see p. 755).

Table 8.2.1 Renal protein handling in health and disease

	Normal	Nephrotic syndrome
Albumin in plasma to be filtered (g)	8000	8000
Albumin actually filtered (g)	36	65
Albumin reabsorbed (g)	36	45
Albumin lost in urine (g)	0	20

Renal blood flow

Measurement of renal blood flow

Renal blood flow can be measured directly by placing an electromagnetic or ultrasonic flow probe around the renal artery. Renal plasma flow (RPF) can be measured indirectly using the clearance technique (see above). Thus, if a substance is completely removed from the plasma passing through the kidney, leaving none in the plasma in the renal vein, then the clearance of that substance is equal to renal plasma flow. **Para-aminohippuric acid** (PAH) is a substance that approaches this ideal. PAH is not normally present in the blood, but can be infused intravenously to achieve a low stable plasma concentration. Almost all PAH is extracted in one passage through the kidney; some is filtered at the glomerulus and the remainder is secreted into the lumen by the proximal tubules (see Transport mechanisms, p. 734). However, remember that not all renal artery blood flow passes through vessels supplying the proximal tubule, some passes from the efferent arterioles into the vasa recta (see Ch. 8.1). This means that some PAH (less than 10% of the total) in the renal artery escapes excretion and appears in renal venous blood. It is possible to correct for this. However, usually the uncorrected value obtained from the clearance of PAH is taken as the **effective renal plasma flow** (ERPF).

$$ERPF = \frac{U_{PAH} \times V}{P_{PAH}}$$

where U_{PAH} and P_{PAH} are urine and plasma concentration of PAH respectively, and V is urine flow in ml/min. P_{PAH} is usually measured in a sample taken from a limb vein where the concentration of PAH is equal to that in arteries supplying the limb and the kidney.

In a normal adult man, ERPF averages 630 ml/min. Assuming the extraction of PAH from arterial blood is 90%, then actual RPF could be estimated as:

$$RPF = \frac{ERPF}{0.9} = \frac{630}{0.9} = 700 \text{ ml/min.}$$

If the packed cell volume (PCV), the fraction of whole blood occupied by red blood cells, is 0.44, then the fraction occupied by plasma is:

$$1 - 0.44 = 0.56.$$

Therefore:

$$\text{Total renal blood flow (RBF)} = \frac{700}{0.56} = 1250 \text{ ml/min.}$$

Thus, the two kidneys, which represent about 0.5% of body weight, receive about 20% of the resting cardiac output.

Regulation of renal blood flow

Renal blood flow, like GFR (see above), shows autoregulation in response to changes in systemic arterial pressure (Fig. 8.2.2). Since blood flow and GFR are autoregulated simultaneously, it seems that the myogenic behaviour of the afferent arteriole must be more important than the myogenic behaviour of the efferent arteriole. For example, myogenic constriction of the afferent arteriole would reduce both renal blood flow and GFR, whereas myogenic constriction of the efferent arteriole would reduce renal blood flow, but increase GFR, by increasing capillary hydrostatic pressure.

The function of autoregulation of renal blood flow is that it tends to stabilize renal function. However, changes in renal blood flow and renal vascular resistance do occur in many circumstances in which renal blood perfusion is sacrificed to maintain systemic arterial blood pressure and to redistribute blood flow to other vital tissues.

Such changes are achieved mainly by the **sympathetic noradrenergic fibres**. Moderate increases in renal sympathetic activity in response to a change in body position from supine to standing, mild exercise or mild emotion, reduce renal blood flow and increase renal vascular resistance, but have no effect on GFR because there is balanced constriction of afferent and efferent arterioles. Larger increases in renal sympathetic activity occurring in heavy exercise, strong emotion or severe haemorrhage, increase renal vascular resistance even more, but decrease both renal blood flow and GFR because the afferent arterioles are constricted more than the efferent arterioles.

Summary

Renal blood flow

- Renal plasma flow can be measured indirectly via the clearance method and by using a marker substance which is completely removed from plasma by one passage through the kidney. PAH is a suitable substance.
- Renal blood flow can be calculated from renal plasma flow and the fraction of whole blood that is occupied by plasma (1 – packed cell volume).
- Renal blood flow (like GFR) can show autoregulation over the mean arterial pressure range of 90–200 mmHg.
- Renal blood flow can be decreased by an increase in renal sympathetic activity.

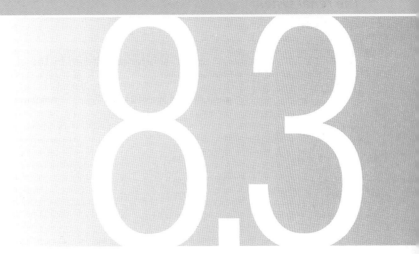

Tubular function

Introduction

Glomerular filtration rate (GFR) in the normal adult is relatively fixed, at about 120 ml/min. Urine production can vary from 0.5% of this during water deprivation to up to 10% during maximal diuresis, showing that water reabsorption is a major tubular function. Flexibility in the reabsorption of the components of the filtrate allows the kidney to rapidly adjust the body's fluid and salt balances.

Once a substance (X) has been filtered at the glomerulus into the tubule, the tubular epithelial cells progressively modify its concentration as the fluid flows through the nephron. They may remove some of it (**reabsorption**), or they may add to the tubular fluid (**secretion**). They may do both. Net reabsorption or secretion can be shown by measurement of clearance (see Ch. 8.2).

As indicated in Chapter 8.2, if the clearance of a substance is smaller than GFR, then there has been net reabsorption, and if it is greater than GFR, then there has been net secretion. This is the same as saying that the net amount of X that is transported by the tubule (T_X) is equal to the filtered load of X (which is the product of GFR and the plasma concentration of X (P_X)) minus the amount of X that appears in the urine (which is the product of urine concentration of X (U_X) and urine flow rate (V)), i.e.:

$$T_X = (P_X \times GFR) - (U_X \times V).$$

Table 8.3.1 Amounts of various substances filtered by the glomeruli and excreted in the urine by a healthy adult on an average diet

	Amount filtered (mmol/24 h)	Amount excreted (mmol/24 h)
Sodium	2550	150
Potassium	700	100
Calcium	550	10
Bicarbonate	4500	2
Chloride	18500	180
Glucose	1000	0.5
Urea	900	450
Water	180 litre/24 h	1.5 litre/24 h

If T_X is positive, then reabsorption exceeds secretion. If T_X is negative, then secretion exceeds reabsorption.

Table 8.3.1 shows filtered loads and excretion rates per day for a normal adult on an average diet. It is clear that the filtered loads are very large, that the reabsorption of some physiologically useful substances like water and sodium is very efficient and that reabsorption of waste products like urea is relatively incomplete. Some substances, like potassium, are both reabsorbed and secreted.

Transport mechanisms

Substances can be reabsorbed or secreted by passing either:

- across the tubular epithelial cells (**transcellular** route), or
- between the cells via the tight junctions and lateral intercellular spaces (**paracellular** route) (see Fig. 8.1.5, p. 720).

Substances move passively between the interstitial space and the blood in the peritubular capillaries. Most substances that are secreted come from the plasma of the peritubular capillaries. Ammonia is an important exception; it is synthesized and secreted by the tubular cells (see Ch. 8.7).

Transcellular transport usually involves active transport across either the luminal or basolateral membrane of the tubular epithelial cell. Transport across the other membrane (i.e. the luminal membrane if active transport is across the basolateral membrane, and vice versa) and paracellular transport occur by diffusion. Transport from the interstitial space into the peritubular capillaries occurs by a combination of bulk flow, when water and solutes move together, and diffusion. The small amount of albumin and the small proteins that filter into the tubule at the glomerulus, including unbound hormones like angiotensin and insulin, are reabsorbed, mostly in the proximal tubule, by pinocytosis.

Active transport is transport of a substance up an electrochemical gradient. This transport requires energy and is often directly coupled to, and dependent on, ATP-hydrolysis. This is called **primary active transport** to distinguish it from **secondary active transport**, when the movement of a substance by primary active transport creates a gradient across a cell membrane that drives the movement of a second substance. If, during the linked movement, the second substance moves in the same direction as the first, the process is termed **cotransport** or a **symport**. If they move in opposite directions, the process is termed **countertransport** or an **antiport**.

Sodium is an example of a substance that is reabsorbed by primary active transport in the cells of walls of the proximal and distal tubules and collecting ducts. Other substances, including glucose, phosphate and amino acids, are cotransported with sodium into the cells.

Summary

Transport mechanisms

- Substances can be reabsorbed or secreted across tubular epithelial cells (transcellular) or between the cells via tight junctions and lateral intercellular spaces (paracellular).
- Transcellular transport usually involves active transport across either the luminal or basolateral membrane of the epithelial cells. Transport across the other membrane is by diffusion.
- Primary active transport is movement of a substance up an electrochemical gradient which is directly dependent on ATP hydrolysis.
- Primary active transport can create a gradient for the movement of a second substance by secondary active transport; this can be cotransport (symport) or countertransport (antiport).
- Most substances that are actively secreted come from the plasma of the peritubular capillaries. Ammonia is an exception; it is synthesized by the tubular cells.
- Substances move passively between the interstitial space and peritubular capillaries by bulk flow (of water and solutes), which is dependent on osmotic and hydrostatic pressure differences, and by diffusion (of solutes).

A

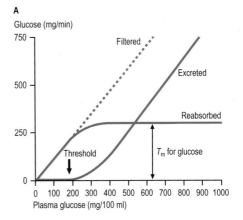

B

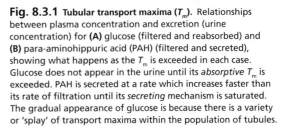

Fig. 8.3.1 Tubular transport maxima (T_m). Relationships between plasma concentration and excretion (urine concentration) for **(A)** glucose (filtered and reabsorbed) and **(B)** para-aminohippuric acid (PAH) (filtered and secreted), showing what happens as the T_m is exceeded in each case. Glucose does not appear in the urine until its *absorptive T_m* is exceeded. PAH is secreted at a rate which increases faster than its rate of filtration until its *secreting* mechanism is saturated. The gradual appearance of glucose is because there is a variety or 'splay' of transport maxima within the population of tubules.

Tubular transport maximum

All active transport systems have a **transport maximum (T_m)**, i.e. a limit for the amount of the substance they can transport per unit time. This is because the membrane proteins responsible for transport become saturated. Glucose is normally entirely reabsorbed from the tubular fluid so that none appears in the urine (Table 8.3.1). When the concentration of glucose in plasma is increased, glucose is presented to the tubule at increasing rates. Glucose is absent from urine until the transport process is saturated, i.e. the T_m for glucose reabsorption is reached (Fig. 8.3.1A). From then on glucose appears in urine at a rate which increases linearly with the filtered load.

The **renal threshold** for glucose is the plasma concentration at which glucose first appears in the urine. Note that the rate at which glucose appears in the urine increases slowly at first, while the absorption curve flattens off gradually. This deviation from the ideal curve is called **splay**. This reflects the fact that different tubules have different T_m values.

Active secretion shows similar characteristics to active reabsorption. Using PAH as an example, when the plasma concentration of

PAH increases, there is a linear increase in the filtered load of PAH, but there is a steeper increase in the rate of excretion of PAH, because it is secreted into the tubule until the T_m for PAH secretion is reached (Fig. 8.3.1B). From then on, PAH excretion increases at the same rate as the filtered load.

The proximal tubule

In the proximal tubule, about 60–70% of the filtered load of sodium, water and urea is reabsorbed. In addition, there is almost complete reabsorption of chloride, bicarbonate, phosphate, potassium, glucose, amino acids and protein. Hydrogen ions, ammonia and organic acids are secreted into the tubule.

Sodium reabsorption

Sodium reabsorption (Fig. 8.3.2) in the proximal tubule is important because it conserves total body sodium and because the reabsorption of many other substances (chloride, water, glucose, amino acids) depend upon it. The proximal tubular cells have an **Na⁺/K⁺ ATPase pump** on the basolateral membrane which pumps sodium out of the cell into the interstitial fluid.

Summary

Tubular transport maximum (T_m)

- All active transport systems have a T_m
  – an upper limit for the amount of the substance they can transport per unit time.
- A substance (e.g. glucose) that is actively reabsorbed appears in urine when the T_m is exceeded.
- The plasma concentration at which this occurs is called the renal threshold.

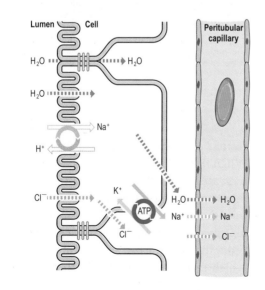

Fig. 8.3.2 Sodium, chloride and water reabsorption in the proximal tubule. This figure shows only an outline of mechanisms operating in the proximal tubule; these vary from the early to late tubule. The key element throughout is the ATP-driven Na⁺/K⁺ exchange mechanism on the basolateral membrane.

This keeps the intracellular concentration of sodium low relative to the lumen. The cell interior also has a membrane potential of −70 mV relative to the lumen. Thus, sodium ions move passively from the lumen into the cell, down concentration and electrical gradients and are actively pumped out of the cell, in exchange for potassium ions at the basolateral membrane (Fig. 8.3.2). Much of the sodium is pumped into the lateral spaces between the epithelial cells. Three Na^+ leave for every two K^+ that enter the cell. These K^+ can leave the cells passively via K^+ channels that are mainly on the basolateral, rather than the luminal membrane. Thus, the intracellular concentration of K^+, which is high, as in the majority of cells in the body, is not changed by the Na^+/K^+ pump.

Chloride reabsorption

In the early part of the proximal tubule, sodium entry into the cells is accompanied by H^+ secretion (see Fig. 8.3.4) which maintains electrical neutrality within the cell and leads to bicarbonate reabsorption as CO_2 (see Fig. 8.3.4). Sodium reabsorption is, most importantly, accompanied by water (see below). This results in chloride concentration in the tubular lumen increasing along the length of the proximal tubule. In the final two-thirds of the proximal tubule the chloride gradient generated is so large that chloride moves passively into the cell and thence into the interstitial fluid (Fig. 8.3.2). This movement of chloride makes the interstitial fluid negative relative to the lumen and so, in turn, some sodium moves passively into the interstitial fluid from the lumen.

Water reabsorption

The movement of sodium, bicarbonate and chloride from the cells into the interstitial space, particularly the **lateral spaces**, reduces the osmolality of the tubular fluid and increases the osmolality in the lateral spaces. The lateral spaces are particularly affected because they are long, tortuous and narrow and have restricted access to the rest of the interstitial space. This causes net osmotic flow of water from the lumen into the lateral space by transcellular and paracellular routes (Fig. 8.3.2).

Reabsorption into peritubular capillaries

The movement of water into the lateral spaces raises the interstitial fluid hydrostatic pressure and thus increases the hydrostatic pressure gradient both between the lateral space and the tubular lumen and between the lateral space and the peritubular capillaries. Since the tight junctions between the epithelial cells are very permeable to water and salts, some of the water and solutes leak back into the lumen. However, much of the water and solutes are driven into the peritubular capillaries by both the osmotic and hydrostatic pressure gradients. Thus, because the filtrate at the glomerulus is essentially protein-free, the fluid that remains in the glomerular capillaries and which then circulates to the peritubular capillaries has a high protein concentration and therefore a high oncotic pressure. Water and solute reabsorption in the peritubular capillaries is also facilitated by the low capillary hydrostatic pressure resulting from the resistance of the efferent arterioles.

The volume of water that is reabsorbed is dependent partly on the **filtration fraction**, i.e. the ratio of GFR to renal plasma flow. For example, if the filtration fraction increases, then more water and solutes will be filtered at the glomerulus leaving a higher concentration of protein in the glomerular capillary. This means that the oncotic pressure in the peritubular capillaries is also raised and, consequently, reabsorption from the lateral spaces is increased. The opposite happens if the filtration fraction decreases.

In this way proximal tubular reabsorption matches GFR very closely over a wide range of GFR values. This is known as **glomerular–tubular balance**. Since an increase in GFR leads to an increase in the amount of sodium filtered, glomerular tubular balance means that there is an automatic, compensatory increase in sodium reabsorption. Thus, sodium is conserved. In fact, the percentage of filtrate and therefore sodium that is reabsorbed in the proximal tubule, is fixed over a wide range of GFR.

Glucose reabsorption

At normal levels of plasma glucose, all glucose in the filtrate is reabsorbed in the proximal tubule. It is **cotransported** with sodium at the luminal membrane, when sodium moves down its electrochemical gradient using the sodium gradient as a source of energy. Glucose then diffuses from the cell into the interstitial fluid and thence to the peritubular capillaries (Fig. 8.3.3).

The normal plasma concentration of glucose is between 0.6 and 1 mg/ml (3.3–5.5 mmol/litre). So, if we take 0.8 mg/ml as an example and assume GFR is 125 ml/min then glucose is filtered at 100 mg/min. The transport maximum for glucose is about 375 mg/min in men. (It is lower, 350 mg/min, in women and even lower in pregnancy.) Thus, the renal threshold for glucose (the plasma concentration at which glucose first appears in urine) is about 375 mg/min divided by 125 ml/min (GFR), i.e. 0.3 mg/ml for men. In fact, the renal threshold is about 0.2 mg/ml (11 mmol/l). The difference is accounted for by the splay of individual transport maxima (see above). Glucose appears in the urine (glycosuria) in diabetes mellitus when plasma glucose concentration is characteristically high.

Bicarbonate reabsorption

In the proximal tubule, hydrogen ions that enter the lumen in exchange for sodium or are secreted by H^+ ATPase (see below), combine with the bicarbonate ions that were filtered at the glomerulus and form H_2CO_3 (Fig. 8.3.4). This leads to the formation of H_2O and CO_2, so raising the luminal P_{CO_2}. This reaction is catalysed by **carbonic anhydrase** present in the luminal brush border. The CO_2 diffuses into the cell and, by the reverse reaction, forms H^+ and HCO_3^-. These hydrogen ions replace those that entered the lumen. HCO_3^- then diffuses across the basolateral cell membrane, in association with Na^+, into the interstitial space, to be reabsorbed into the peritubular capillaries.

The normal plasma concentration of bicarbonate is about 25 mmol/litre and, as it is freely filtered at the glomerulus, the same concentration is present in the filtrate. Although there is no active transport of bicarbonate, the processes involved in reabsorption behave as if there were a T_m for bicarbonate, with a value very close to the amount filtered at normal GFR and normal plasma concentration. Not surprisingly, the T_m can be varied by changes in H^+ secretion and Na^+ reabsorption. However, the close correspondence of the T_m for bicarbonate to the normal filtered load means that if plasma bicarbonate concentration rises, then T_m tends to be exceeded and the excess excreted. This is considered further in the section on acid–base balance (Ch. 8.7).

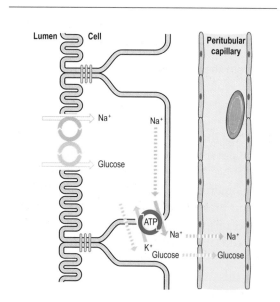

Fig. 8.3.3 Glucose reabsorption. Glucose, and many other metabolically useful substances, are reabsorbed by 'cotransport' with sodium. The movement of sodium down its concentration gradient into the cell powers the mechanism that absorbs glucose.

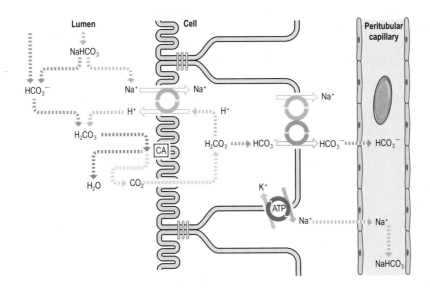

Fig. 8.3.4 Reabsorption of bicarbonate. Carbonic anhydrase (CA) on the brush border of tubular cells accelerates the equilibrium between carbon dioxide, water and carbonic acid. Carbonic acid within the cells dissociates to form bicarbonate which is largely removed via a symport with sodium on the basolateral margins of the cells.

Amino acids

Amino acids are freely filtered at the glomerulus and so occur in the filtrate at the same concentration as in plasma, approximately 3 mmol/litre. They are reabsorbed by **cotransport** with sodium at the luminal membrane, using the sodium gradient as the source of energy. Several carrier systems are involved, each with its own T_m. There is one each for the acidic (such as glutamic and aspartic acid), basic (such as cysteine, ornithine, arginine and lysine), and neutral amino acids, one for imino acids (e.g. proline) and a separate one for glycine.

Phosphate

Phosphate occurs in plasma at a concentration of 1 mmol/litre, as a breakdown product of protein metabolism. It is freely filtered at the glomerulus and is **cotransported** with sodium at the luminal border of the proximal tubules. The T_m for its reabsorption is very close to the

normal filtered load. Thus, any increase in plasma phosphate concentration can automatically lead to an increase in phosphate excretion. The rate of phosphate reabsorption is regulated hormonally; it is decreased by **parathyroid hormone** and increased by **calcitriol**, the active form of vitamin D.

Sulphate

Sulphate is also a breakdown product of protein metabolism. Like phosphate, it is reabsorbed by **cotransport** with sodium. The T_m for sulphate is normally exceeded, so that sulphate appears in the urine and the plasma concentration is held at 1–1.5 mmol/litre.

Urea

Urea is a product of protein metabolism. It is present in plasma at a concentration of 2.5–7.5 mmol/litre. It is freely filtered and about 50% is reabsorbed by the end of the proximal tubule. This occurs because reabsorption of water and ions increases urea concentration in the tubule lumen. Thus, urea **diffuses** out of the tubule down its concentration gradient. The overall movement of these solutes and water results in the concentration of urea in the fluid that leaves the proximal tubule being approximately the same as in plasma.

Potassium

The proximal tubule reabsorbs about 80% of filtered potassium, but the mechanisms responsible are not fully understood. Potassium is freely filtered at the glomerulus and so is present in the filtrate at a concentration equal to that in plasma (4–5 mmol/litre). It appears to be reabsorbed **passively** into the cells of the proximal tubule. The reabsorption of sodium and water into the lateral spaces also tends to cause an increase in potassium concentration in the lumen so that some potassium probably diffuses passively through paracellular pathways. In addition, it seems that there is an active transport mechanism for potassium at the luminal border.

Calcium

Plasma normally has a calcium concentration of about 2.5 mmol/litre. 40–50% of plasma in calcium is **bound** to protein and cannot be filtered by the glomerulus. The remainder is ionized Ca^{2+}, and is freely filtered by the glomerulus. Ca^{2+} is reabsorbed from the proximal tubule in parallel with sodium and water so that its concentration in the tubule stays more or less constant. Ca^{2+} enters tubule cells passively, down concentration and electrical gradients, but probably leaves the cell by a Ca^{2+}/Na^+ **countertransport** mechanism or via a Ca^{2+} ATPase mechanism.

Hydrogen

Hydrogen ions formed in the proximal tubule cells from the dissociation of H_2CO_3 (see Fig. 8.3.4) are secreted into the lumen. Most of this H^+ secretion takes place late in the proximal tubule and is associated with Na^+ reabsorption via a **countertransport** process, but some may be mediated by a H^+ ATPase.

Organic cations and anions

The proximal tubule secretes organic cations and anions, some of which are end products of metabolism that circulate in plasma, e.g. bile salts, oxalate, urate, prostaglandins, creatinine, adrenaline, noradrenaline. The proximal tubule also secretes exogenous organic compounds, e.g. PAH which is used to determine renal plasma flow (see above) and drugs such as penicillin, aspirin, morphine and quinine. Because many of these substances are bound to plasma proteins, they are not freely filtered at the glomerulus. Therefore, secretion into the lumen provides an extremely important means of eliminating these potentially toxic substances from the body.

Taking PAH as an example, at plasma concentrations of up to 0.10–0.12 mg/ml the PAH-secreting process can completely remove PAH from the tubular capillaries, but at plasma concentrations above this level, significant concentrations of PAH begin to appear in the renal vein. In other words, there is a T_m for PAH, of about 80 mg/min. Therefore, if PAH is to be used to measure renal plasma flow (see Measurement of renal blood flow, p. 730), the plasma concentration of PAH must be below 0.12 mg/ml so that the T_m is not exceeded. There is competition for the secreting transport process between all organic anions so that at raised plasma levels, PAH can compete with, for example, secretion of penicillin. The organic cations use a different secreting process, but also compete with one another.

Summary

The proximal tubule

- 60–70% of filtered Na^+ is reabsorbed by primary active transport across the basolateral membrane into the lateral intercellular spaces.
- The reabsorption of Cl^- is dependent on Na^+ transport, into the lateral intercellular spaces.
- Transport of Na^+ and Cl^- into the lateral intercellular spaces causes an osmotic flow of water from the lumen into the same space.
- Water and solutes are driven from the lateral intercellular spaces primarily into the peritubular capillaries by osmotic and hydrostatic pressure gradients.

Some water and solutes may leak back into the tubular lumen.

- Glucose is cotransported with Na^+ up to a T_m of 350–375 mg/min, the renal threshold being ~2 mg/ml (11 mmol/litre).
- H^+ is countertransported (secreted) with Na^+ into the lumen and combines with filtered HCO_3^- to form H_2CO_3. This leads by a sequence of reactions to reabsorption of HCO_3^-.
- Amino acids, urea, phosphate, calcium and sulphate ions are cotransported with Na^+. K^+ reabsorption also seems to be dependent on Na^+ transport.

Loop of Henle, distal tubule and collecting duct

Introduction

The part of the nephron after the proximal tubule can be divided into the thin descending and ascending limbs of the loop of Henle, the thick ascending limb, the early and late parts of the distal tubule and the collecting duct (Fig. 8.1.2, p. 717). The functional characteristics of these sections are very different. However, it is convenient to consider them together since they have a common role: concentrating the urine. Briefly, the descending limb has a high water permeability and a low solute permeability, which means water moves across the descending limb into the interstitium until osmotic equilibrium is reached between the tubular fluid and interstitial fluid. By contrast, the thin and thick ascending limbs have a low permeability to water and the thick ascending limb actively reabsorbs sodium from the tubular fluid. Since the thick ascending limb has a large transport capacity, it plays a major role in diluting the tubular fluid and is often known as the diluting segment of the kidney.

The distal tubule and collecting duct also reabsorb sodium. In the absence of antidiuretic hormone (ADH), they are impermeable to water. However, in the presence of ADH, the later part of the distal tubule and the collecting duct become very permeable to water. This allows water to move out until the tubular fluid and interstitial fluid reach osmotic equilibrium.

Since urea also plays an important role in the concentrating process, as is discussed below, it is important to consider the urea permeability of individual parts of the nephron. The highest urea permeability is found in the inner, medullary part of the collecting duct and can be increased by ADH. The thick ascending limb, distal tubule and cortical parts of the collecting duct have very low, or no, permeability to urea, but the thin descending and ascending limbs of the loop of Henle are both permeable to urea. Urea moves passively down its concentration gradient and recycles from the medullary collecting duct to the medullary interstitium, where it raises the urea concentration of the interstitial fluid, and from there it passes to the thin limbs of the loop of Henle.

Finally, it should be noted that the late distal tubule and collecting duct are important in secreting K^+ and H^+ and in reabsorbing K^+ and HCO_3^-.

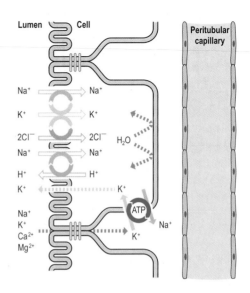

Fig. 8.4.1 Transport mechanisms in the thick ascending tubule. The positive charge within the tubule is probably due to the to the return of K^+ to the lumen via a K^+ channel. This charge is largely responsible for the paracellular reabsorption of cations, which accounts for 50% of total reabsorption in the thick ascending tubule.

Transport processes

The active reabsorption of Na^+ that occurs in the thick ascending limb, the distal tubule and collecting duct is dependent on the **Na^+/K^+ ATPase pump** in the basolateral membrane, just as it is in the proximal tubule. This maintains a low concentration of Na^+ in the cell, so favouring movement of Na^+ into the cell from the tubular fluid. In the thick ascending limb, this mainly occurs via an $Na^+/Cl^-/K^+$ symporter, which couples the movement of these three ions in the ratios $1:2:1$. In addition, some Na^+ also moves in via an Na^+/H^+ antiporter, thereby leading to **H^+ secretion** (Fig. 8.4.1) and HCO_3^- reabsorption (as shown in Fig. 8.3.4, p. 739). The Cl^-, HCO_3^- and some of the K^+ leave the cell via the basolateral membrane, but much of the K^+ that enters the cell leaves again via a K^+ channel in the luminal membrane. This K^+ is probably responsible for generating a positive charge in the lumen of the thick ascending limb which drives the movement of Na^+, K^+, Ca^{2+} and Mg^{2+} out of the tubule via the paracellular route.

In the early distal tubule, Na^+ moves into the cell via an Na^+/Cl^- symporter and the Cl^- leaves the cell again via the basolateral membrane.

In both the thick ascending limb and early distal tubule, water cannot follow the movement of solute from the lumen to the interstitium, so the luminal fluid is diluted.

In the collecting duct there are two types of cells:

- the **principal cells**, which actively reabsorb Na^+ and secrete K^+ and, in the presence of ADH, also absorb water
- the **intercalated cells** whose important function is to secrete H^+ (and reabsorb HCO_3^-).

In the principal cells, the Na^+/K^+ ATPase on the basolateral membrane is responsible for the reabsorption of Na^+ and for producing a high concentration of K^+ in the cell, which then causes K^+ to diffuse out of the cell, through K^+ channels, into the luminal fluid where the K^+

concentration is low (Fig. 8.5.1, p. 755). The fact that the permeability of the luminal membrane to K^+ is higher than that of the basolateral membrane favours the movement of K^+ into the lumen. Both the reabsorption of Na^+ and the secretion of K^+ in this segment of the tubule are affected by **aldosterone** (see Ch. 8.5).

In the presence of **ADH**, water channels are incorporated into the luminal membrane of the principal cells (see Ch. 8.5). The basolateral membrane is freely permeable to water. Therefore in the presence of ADH, water passes through the cell, from the lumen to the interstitial fluid down the osmotic gradient caused by the high osmotic concentration of the interstitial fluid.

In the intercalated cells, H^+ is generated from the dissociation of H_2CO_3 and, as in the proximal tubule, the formation of H_2CO_3 is facilitated by carbonic anhydrase. However, in contrast to the proximal tubule, it is thought that all of the H^+ leaves the intercalated cells via an H^+ ATPase

pump in the luminal membrane, rather than via countertransport with Na^+. The HCO_3^- that is formed from the dissociation of H_2CO_3 diffuses out of the intercalated cells across the basolateral membrane. These cells also reabsorb K^+ from the tubule, but the mechanism is not known.

In the thick part of the ascending limb of the loop of Henle and in the distal tubule there is also reabsorption of Ca^{2+} and these are the major sites at which much excretion of Ca^{2+} is regulated. Entry of Ca^{2+} into the cells is passive, as in the proximal tubule. Exit from the cells at the basolateral membrane is by an Na^+/Ca^{2+} countertransport mechanism and, more importantly, by an active Ca^{2+} ATPase. The regulation of Ca^{2+} absorption is dealt with in Chapter 8.5.

Countercurrent multiplication by the loop of Henle

The kidney can excrete urine that is either hypo-osmotic or hyperosmotic relative to plasma. This requires that water be separated from solute. Hypo-osmotic urine can be formed simply by reabsorbing solute from the tubule without allowing water to follow. The formation of hyperosmotic urine is more difficult to understand because it means that water must be removed from the tubular fluid leaving solute behind and because water can only move **passively** from a region of low osmotic pressure to one of high osmotic pressure. Thus, in order to remove water from the tubular fluid, the kidney must create an area of high osmotic pressure *outside* of the nephron. This is done by the loop of Henle.

The loop of Henle consists of two parallel limbs arranged so that tubular fluid flows into the medulla in the descending limb and out of the medulla in the ascending limb, i.e. the flow in the two limbs is in opposite directions, or **countercurrent**. The fluid that enters the descending limb from the proximal tubule has an osmotic concentration approximately equal to that of plasma (300 mOsm/kg H_2O for numerical simplicity; Fig. 8.4.2). As indicated

⚡ **Summary**

Important features of the concentrating process

- The descending limb of the loop of Henle has a high permeability to water and a low permeability to solutes.
- The ascending limb of the loop of Henle has a low permeability to water, but actively reabsorbs Na^+.
- The distal tubule and collecting duct also actively reabsorb Na^+. In the presence of ADH they are permeable to water.
- The descending and thin ascending limbs of the loop of Henle are permeable to urea. The thick ascending limb and cortical part of the collecting duct have low permeability to urea. The medullary part of the collecting duct has a high permeability to urea that can be increased by ADH.

above, the ascending limb is **impermeable** to water but reabsorbs solutes, principally NaCl, from the tubular fluid. Thus, the tubular fluid becomes more dilute as it passes up the ascending limb, while solute accumulates in the interstitial fluid around the loop, raising its osmolality. On the other hand, the descending limb is freely **permeable** to water. Thus, the hyperosmotic interstitial fluid causes water to move out of the descending limb into the interstitium. This 'single effect' of the counter-current system creates an osmotic gradient between the tubular fluid in the ascending limb and descending limb, limited to 200 mOsm/kg H_2O because this is the maximum gradient that the cells of the ascending limb can sustain across their walls.

This 'single effect' is multiplied – the **countercurrent multiplication process** – because new fluid is continually entering the descending limb, pushing fluid from the descending limb around the loop to the ascending limb. This means that hyperosmotic fluid enters the bottom of the ascending limb, and hypo-osmotic fluid is pushed out of the ascending limb. Solute is again removed from the ascending limb and water again moves osmotically from the descending limb into the interstitial space until there is a gradient of 200 mOsm/kg H_2O between the two limbs at each point along their lengths. As seen in Figure 8.4.2, this has the effect of increasing the osmotic concentration of the interstitial fluid and luminal fluid at the tip of the loop and reducing the osmolality of the fluid that leaves the ascending limb, so creating an osmotic gradient from the junction of the medulla and cortex to the tip of the loop.

This countercurrent multiplication process continues with the help of **urea** (see below) until the osmolality of the tubular and interstitial fluid at the tip is 1200–1400 mOsm/kg H_2O which is four to five times that of plasma. This is very energy efficient since this considerable longitudinal osmotic gradient is achieved by using only the energy required to create an osmotic gradient between the two limbs of

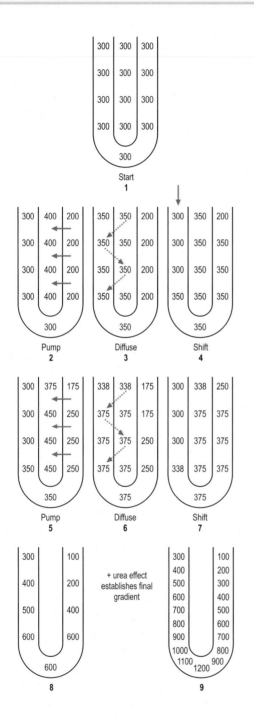

Fig. 8.4.2 Countercurrent multiplication. In steps 1–8 the effect of Na+ pumping is shown. The final osmolality can be as high as 1200–1400 mOsm/kg owing to the additional effects of urea, which is shown in the step from 8 to 9. Note that although the difference in osmolality between the incoming fluid and the tip is more than 1000 mOsm/kg, the difference between the two limbs is never more than 200.

200 mOsm/kg H_2O. About 15% of nephrons have long loops of Henle that dip down into the medulla. The osmotic gradient is produced by this 15%. Nephrons with short loops do not contribute significantly to the gradient, but their collecting ducts do pass through the medulla and therefore use the gradient to concentrate urine (see below).

Fluid that leaves the ascending limb of the loop of Henle is **hypo-osmotic** with respect to plasma and has an osmolality of only 100 mOsm/kg H_2O (Fig. 8.4.2). The distal tubule and cortical part of the collecting duct are impermeable to water except in the presence of ADH, which increases their water permeability (see Ch. 8.5). In the presence of ADH, water begins to diffuse out of the tubule into the interstitium where the osmotic concentration is higher; this begins the process of urine concentration. The maximum osmolality that the tubular fluid can reach by the end of the cortical collecting duct is 300 mOsm/kg H_2O. This is the same as the osmolality of the plasma and interstitium at this point and the same as the osmolality of the fluid that entered the descending limb of the loop of Henle, but the composition is very different. The fluid entering the medullary collecting duct contains much less NaCl, because NaCl has been actively reabsorbed, and it contains a higher concentration of urea, because urea has been added to the tubular fluid as it passes through the loop of Henle (see below).

In the medullary part of the collecting duct, water continues to diffuse out of the tubule into the interstitium along an osmotic gradient, particularly if ADH is present to increase the collecting duct's water permeability. This increases the osmotic concentration of the tubular fluid. The maximum osmotic concentration that can be reached in the tubule in the presence of ADH is therefore ~1200 mOsm/kg H_2O, equal to the osmolality of the interstitium at the tip of the loop of Henle. This process of concentrating the urine is facilitated by the fact that ADH also increases the permeability of the medullary

collecting duct to urea. Urea makes a major contribution to the total osmolality of the interstitium (see below).

In the absence of ADH, urine osmolality may be less than 100 mOsm/kg H_2O because solute is still reabsorbed from the distal tubule and collecting duct, but water cannot follow.

The role of urea

Although the countercurrent multiplication process is very important in establishing an osmotic gradient from the cortex to the tip of the loop of Henle (by actively transporting NaCl at the tip of the loop of Henle), NaCl only accounts for about *half* (600 mOsm/kg H_2O) of the total osmolality of the interstitial fluid. The remaining 600 mOsm/kg H_2O is due to urea.

Urea is freely filtered at the glomerulus; 50% of it is reabsorbed as the fluid passes through the proximal tubule. Since more than 50% of filtered water is reabsorbed in the proximal tubule, the concentration of urea in the fluid that enters the descending limb of the loop of Henle is slightly greater than in plasma. The loop of Henle and the cortical part of the collecting duct have relatively low permeability to urea. However, the medullary part of the collecting duct has a high permeability to urea, which can be further increased by ADH (see above). Thus, most of the urea remains trapped in the tubule until it reaches the medullary collecting duct.

By then, reabsorption of water has concentrated urea in the tubule. Urea diffuses out of the collecting duct into the interstitium, down its concentration gradient, so adding to the osmolality of the interstitium (Fig. 8.4.3). Urea tends to re-enter the loop of Henle. Thus, there is some **recycling of urea**, from the medullary collecting duct to the loop of Henle and through the tubule to the collecting duct. Since the permeability of the loop of Henle to urea is relatively low, the urea in the interstitial fluid around the loop acts as a very effective osmotic agent, playing a major role, with sodium

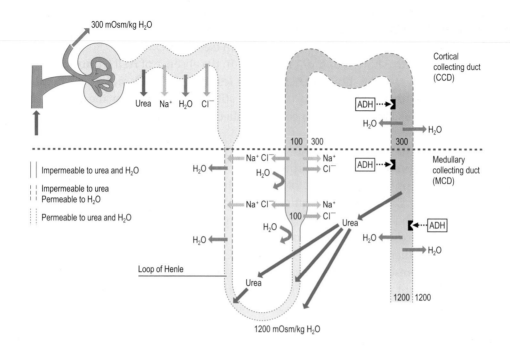

Fig. 8.4.3 Role of urea in concentration of urine. Because the loop of Henle has a relatively low permeability to urea, urea remains trapped in the interstitium of the medulla where it exerts about half of the kidney's concentrating effect on the tubular fluid.

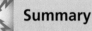

Summary

Countercurrent multiplication; urea

- Fluid enters the loop of Henle at an osmotic concentration of ~300 mOsm/kg H_2O.
- At each level of the loop of Henle, the ascending limb actively reabsorbs solutes, mainly NaCl, from the tubular fluid into the interstitial fluid. Water cannot follow because the ascending limb is impermeable to water.
- The hyperosmotic solution in the interstitial fluid causes water to move from the descending limb to the interstitium.
- This process creates an osmolality gradient of 200 mOsm/kg H_2O between the ascending and descending limbs.

- The fluid in the ascending limb flows in the opposite direction (countercurrent) to that in the descending limb.
- Therefore the osmotic difference at a single level of the loop of Henle is multiplied (the countercurrent multiplication process) many times over as new fluid continually enters the descending limb.
- Urea that diffuses out of the collecting duct into the interstitium adds to the osmolality of the interstitium around the loop of Henle.
- The final outcome is that the osmotic concentration of the interstitium at the tip of the loop of Henle is 1200–1400 mOsm/kg H_2O. The fluid leaving the ascending limb has an osmolality of ~100 mOsm/kg H_2O.

chloride, in dragging water out of the descending limb of the loop of Henle along an osmotic gradient (see above).

ADH increases water permeability of the cortical and medullary collecting ducts and urea permeability of the medullary collecting duct.

The importance of urea in concentrating the urine is illustrated by the fact that people who are chronically malnourished and in whom there is a low rate of protein catabolism and therefore a low concentration of urea in plasma, do not concentrate urine as well as normal individuals.

The vasa recta

The vasa recta supply blood to the medulla. They are capillary loops in parallel with the loop of Henle. The fact that they are arranged in loops allows them to remove the water that is reabsorbed from the tubules without dissipating the longitudinal osmotic gradient from cortex to medulla that is built up by the loop of Henle. They act as **countercurrent exchangers**. Capillaries are freely permeable to solute and water and equilibrate with the surrounding interstitial fluid. Therefore, plasma flowing down the descending limb of the vasa recta, will be coming from a region of *lower* osmolality and it will be passing plasma in the ascending limb that is coming from a region of *higher* osmolality. It follows that, at any level, the osmolality of the ascending limb will be higher than that of the descending limb and water will pass from the descending to the ascending limb so bypassing the deeper medulla (Fig. 8.4.4). On the other hand, at any level, the solute concentration, including NaCl and urea, will be higher in the ascending limb than in the descending limb and solute will tend to diffuse from the ascending to the descending limb. This traps solute in the medulla. However, for these same reasons, the vasa recta are inefficient in supplying oxygen and removing carbon dioxide from the deeper regions of the medulla. Thus, oxygen tends to diffuse from the descending limb to the

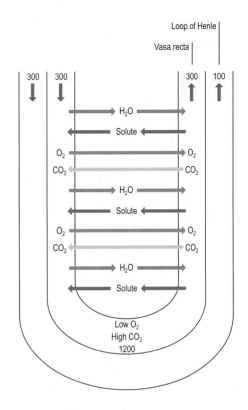

Fig. 8.4.4 Solute trapping by the vasa recta. Exchange of water and solutes between the two limbs of the vasa recta avoids dissipation of the osmotic concentration gradient, provided the blood flow in the vasa is not too great.

ascending limb down its concentration gradient so that less oxygen is available to be taken to the deeper medulla. On the other hand, carbon dioxide diffuses from the ascending limb to the descending limb so the blood that reaches the deeper medulla already has a high carbon dioxide concentration.

Although the anatomical arrangement of the vasa recta is effective in maintaining the osmotic gradient, changes in the blood flow can affect that gradient. If the blood flow in the vasa recta is increased, then solutes *are* washed out of the medulla and its interstitial osmolality *is* decreased. If blood flow is decreased, the opposite happens. The latter happens when ADH (also known as vasopressin because of its vasoconstrictor effect) constricts the renal arterioles

Summary

The vasa recta

- The anatomical arrangement of these blood vessels means that they do not dissipate the interstitial osmotic gradient created by the loop of Henle.
- However, they are inefficient in exchanging O_2 and CO_2 with the cells in the deeper medulla.
- Large changes in blood flow in the vasa recta can reduce or increase the medullary interstitial osmolality beyond its normal value.

and reduces blood flow. This helps to maintain the highest possible osmolality in the medullary interstitium and so allows maximal osmolalities to be reached in the tubular fluid.

Potassium excretion

Potassium is vital for the normal functioning of many cells, particularly excitable cells. Most K^+ is intracellular, its concentration being about 140 mmol/litre. The normal extracellular and plasma concentration of K^+ is 4 mmol/litre and this large concentration gradient between the extracellular and intracellular space is important in maintaining the potential difference across resting cell membranes. The normal diet contains 40–100 mmol K^+/day which is far more than the body needs. In fact, 40–50 mmol of K^+ may be absorbed at a single meal which would increase plasma K^+ concentrations to a potentially lethal value of 7–8 mmol/litre if all of this K^+ were to remain in plasma. Such a rise in plasma K^+ is normally prevented in the short term (minutes) because K^+ is removed from the plasma under the influence of several hormones (adrenaline, insulin and aldosterone) that promote K^+ uptake into liver, skeletal muscle, bone and red blood cells. However, in the longer term (over hours), the K^+ ingested must be excreted from the body by the kidneys to maintain K^+ balance. The kidneys excrete over 90% of the K^+ that is ingested; only 5–10% is lost in faeces and sweat.

The **proximal tubule** reabsorbs about 80% of the filtered K^+. There is further reabsorption of K^+ in the thick ascending limb but much of this probably leaks back from the interstitium into the descending limb, i.e. it is recycled rather like urea. Thus, it is the process of K^+ secretion by the **distal tubule** and **collecting duct** that is predominantly responsible for the K^+ that appears in the urine. Alterations in the balance of K^+ reabsorption and K^+ secretion by the distal tubule and collecting duct are responsible for changes in the urinary excretion of K^+. The rate of secretion of K^+ is determined by:

- the activity of Na^+/K^+ ATPase in the basolateral membrane of the principal cells (see Fig. 8.5.1, p. 755)
- the electrochemical gradient for K^+ efflux across the luminal membrane into the lumen
- the permeability of the luminal membrane to K^+.

An increase in plasma K^+ stimulates Na^+/K^+ ATPase, so increasing K^+ uptake across the basolateral membrane and increasing the driving force for K^+ efflux into the lumen. This effect is facilitated because an increase in plasma K^+ stimulates aldosterone secretion by the adrenal cortex (see p. 434), which acts synergistically with K^+. **Aldosterone** increases the activity of Na^+/K^+ ATPase and so increases the intracellular concentration of K^+ (as well as pumping Na^+ out of the cell). It also increases the permeability of the luminal membrane to K^+. On the other hand, if plasma K^+ is decreased, then K^+ secretion is decreased by effects that are opposite to those just described. Indeed, if plasma K^+ becomes very low, there is net reabsorption

![Summary icon] **Summary**

Excretion of K⁺

- The proximal tubule reabsorbs ~80% of the filtered K⁺.
- K⁺ secretion by the principal cells of the distal tubule and collecting duct is mainly responsible for the K⁺ in urine.
- An increase in K⁺ in plasma stimulates the Na^+/K^+ ATPase on the basolateral membrane of the principal cell, so increasing K⁺ uptake into the cell. This increases the driving force for K⁺ efflux into the lumen.
- This process is facilitated because an increase in plasma K⁺ stimulates aldosterone secretion, which increases the Na^+/K^+ ATPase pump activity and increases the permeability of the luminal membrane to K⁺.
- A decrease in plasma K⁺ has exactly opposite effects, so minimizing K⁺ loss in urine.

of K⁺ all along the nephron, and K⁺ loss in urine is minimized.

K⁺ secretion is also regulated by the flow rate of tubular fluid and changes in acid–base balance. An increase in flow rate as might be produced by an increase in circulating blood volume, or by diuretics, increases K⁺ secretion. This is because the K⁺ that is secreted into the lumen is carried downstream more quickly, minimizing the increase in the lumen concentration and preserving the driving force for K⁺ efflux across the luminal membrane. A decrease in tubular flow rate has the opposite effect.

Increased plasma hydrogen ion concentration (acidosis) reduces K⁺ excretion, at least in the short term, probably because acidosis inhibits Na^+/K^+ ATPase and reduces the permeability of the luminal membrane to K⁺. Alkalosis has the opposite effect.

Hydrogen ion secretion

The mechanism for hydrogen ion secretion was described above (p. 738). Regulation of hydrogen ion and ammonia secretion is dealt with in Chapter 8.7 (p. 773).

Renal regulation

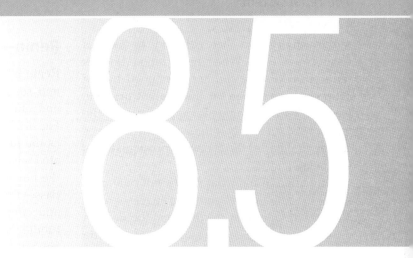

Introduction

Renal function is regulated by **neural** and **hormonal** influences. The most important of these are:

- renal sympathetic nerves
- renin–angiotensin system
- aldosterone
- atrial natriuretic peptide
- antidiuretic hormone
- prostaglandins
- parathyroid hormone and vitamin D.

Renal nerves

The afferent and efferent renal arterioles and the tubules are supplied by **sympathetic** noradrenergic fibres. Although the kidney can autoregulate in response to changes in arterial pressure so that renal blood flow remains constant, this does not mean that renal blood flow is always constant. When arterial pressure falls slightly as during a mild haemorrhage, the kidney shows autoregulation (see p. 727). However, during a more severe haemorrhage, the renal arterioles respond to the increase in renal sympathetic activity caused by the baroreceptor reflex: they show vasoconstriction and renal blood flow falls. During moderate and severe exercise and during emotional stress, renal sympathetic nerve activity also increases and so reduces renal blood flow. When renal blood flow is reduced, GRF may still be maintained by the action of angiotensin on the efferent arteriole (see below). You should also appreciate that the vasoconstrictor effects of the sympathetic nerves can be limited by the action of prostaglandins (see below).

Activation of the renal nerves not only constricts the blood vessels, but also increases reabsorption of sodium by the proximal tubule with a consequent increase in absorption of chloride and water. In addition, activation of the renal nerves also stimulates renin release.

Qualitatively similar effects to those produced by activation of the renal nerves can be produced when plasma levels of noradrenaline and adrenaline are raised by secretion of these hormones by the *adrenal medulla*. On the other hand, a fall in renal sympathetic nerve activity or in plasma catecholamine levels produces the opposite effects.

Summary

The actions of the renal nerves

- A strong increase in renal sympathetic nerve activity can reduce renal blood flow. Meanwhile, GFR may be maintained by autoregulation, but may fall.
- An increase in renal sympathetic activity also:
  – directly increases reabsorption of Na$^+$ by the proximal tubule
  – directly stimulates renin release and thereby angiotensin II production.
- The effects of an increase in renal sympathetic activity can be limited by locally released prostaglandins.

Renin–angiotensin system

Renin is an **enzyme** that is synthesized, stored and secreted by granular cells of the afferent and efferent arterioles of the glomerulus (see Fig. 8.1.3, p. 718) in a specialized region known as the **juxtaglomerular apparatus**. This is situated where the distal tubule comes very close to the Bowman's capsule of its own nephron and passes through the angle formed by the afferent and efferent arterioles. The cells of the distal tubule that are closest to the afferent and efferent arterioles and Bowman's capsule are morphologically distinct and are known as **macula densa** cells. They respond to changes in the composition of the tubular fluid.

Renin secretion is stimulated by three factors:

- Increased renal sympathetic nerve activity.
- Reduced renal perfusion pressure. The actual stimulus seems to be a reduction in the pressure within the afferent arteriole and the resulting reduction in the wall tension in this arteriole. This can occur as a direct result of a reduction in systemic arterial blood pressure. It may be reinforced by constriction caused by an increase in sympathetic activity to the kidney, since the site of afferent arteriolar constriction is upstream of the renin-secreting cells.
- Decreased NaCl delivery to the macula densa. It is not clear whether it is Na$^+$, or Cl$^-$ concentration, or NaCl concentration or NaCl content that is actually sensed.

However, renin secretion is stimulated by the macula densa mechanism under conditions which would be expected to decrease NaCl delivery to the distal tubule, for example when blood volume is reduced and Na$^+$ reabsorption by the proximal tubule is increased.

Renin secretion caused by the renal nerves is mediated by **β_1-adrenoceptors**. Renin secretion that is caused by the macula densa is mediated by prostaglandins, particularly **prostacyclin**. Prostacyclin is released by the macula densa and acts on the renin-secreting cells.

Once formed, renin cleaves the decapeptide **angiotensin I** from **angiotensinogen**, which is an α-globulin. Angiotensin I is then converted into the octapeptide **angiotensin II** by **angiotensin-converting enzyme** (ACE). Angiotensinogen is produced by the liver and circulates in the blood. ACE is found in high concentrations in vascular endothelium. Therefore, much of the angiotensin II that circulates in the blood is formed in the lungs where there is a large surface area of vascular endothelium. However, angiotensin II can also be produced locally within the kidney itself from intrarenal angiotensinogen, without activation of the systemic renin–angiotensin system. This locally generated angiotensin II may reach a concentration within the kidney that is 1000 times higher than that in the systemic circulation and is very important in the regulation of GFR and sodium excretion.

Angiotensin II has the following effects:

- It causes **vasoconstriction**. Within the systemic circulation as a whole this increases arterial blood pressure. Within the kidney, angiotensin II preferentially constricts the efferent arterioles. This raises pressure in the glomerular capillaries and helps to maintain GFR constant when renal perfusion pressure is reduced (autoregulation, see p. 727).
- It stimulates **sodium reabsorption** by the proximal tubule, and chloride and water follow passively.
- It stimulates **aldosterone secretion** by the adrenal cortex.
- It stimulates **antidiuretic hormone** (ADH) secretion from the posterior pituitary gland.
- It stimulates **thirst** by an action on the brain.

Angiotensin II also has a negative-feedback effect on renin secretion by the granular cells of the juxtaglomerular apparatus.

Aldosterone

Aldosterone is synthesized and released by the glomerular cells of the **adrenal cortex**. The most important stimuli for its release are an increase in the concentration of angiotensin II and an increase in plasma K^+ concentration. Aldosterone acts within the kidney to stimulate Na^+ absorption and K^+ secretion by the principal cells of the distal tubule and collecting duct (Fig. 8.5.1).

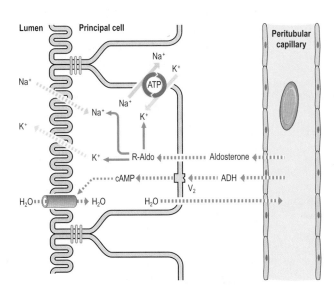

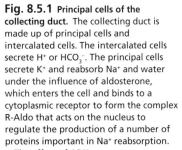

Fig. 8.5.1 Principal cells of the collecting duct. The collecting duct is made up of principal cells and intercalated cells. The intercalated cells secrete H^+ or HCO_3^-. The principal cells secrete K^+ and reabsorb Na^+ and water under the influence of aldosterone, which enters the cell and binds to a cytoplasmic receptor to form the complex R-Aldo that acts on the nucleus to regulate the production of a number of proteins important in Na^+ reabsorption.

The effect of ADH on water reabsorption shown in this figure is dealt with later in the text.

Clinical Example

Renal hypertension

The concept of a 'normal' blood pressure is a purely statistical one in that it is a blood pressure that falls within a 'normal' range on either side of the mean of that of the population. However, complications that are characteristic of hypertension are clearly related to the value of diastolic pressure. The World Health Organization recommends that a diastolic pressure of >90–95 mmHg be regarded as hypertensive. About 20% of the adult population of the UK have blood pressures above 160/95. Hypertension is the most important risk factor in strokes and heart failure. In ischaemic heart disease it is as important as hypercholesterolaemia, obesity or smoking.

Arterial blood pressure is the product of cardiac output and peripheral vascular resistance. Because the kidneys receive 20% of the cardiac output, it is little wonder they can have a profound effect on arterial pressure or be profoundly damaged by it. In fact, it is often difficult clinically to decide whether the kidneys are the origin or victims of hypertension.

Both kidneys, or in a small percentage of cases one kidney, may be diseased sufficiently to cause hypertension. The mechanisms involved are:

- *Renal artery stenosis*. This exerts a direct haemodynamic effect of increasing peripheral resistance, but more importantly, it reduces renal perfusion pressure, which in turn affects the renin–angiotensin system.
- *The renin–angiotensin–aldosterone system*. Decreased perfusion pressure leads to activation of the juxtaglomerular apparatus of the nephrons, which, via the production of renin, produce angiotensin II, the most potent hypertensive agent in the body. Angiotensin II stimulates the release of aldosterone, which in turn stimulates sodium reabsorption. Sodium reabsorption is also favoured by reduced perfusion pressure, which in turn reduces the hydrostatic pressure in the peritubular capillaries, so increasing sodium reabsorption from the proximal tubule.
- *Retention of sodium*. Sodium retention by the mechanisms described above, together with reduced excretory ability, results in increased blood volume and hence blood pressure.

Hypertension has its most profound effect in glomerulonephritis (see Clinical Example, p. 728), and control of hypertension is essential in this condition to prevent further deterioration of renal function secondary to the vascular damage produced by the excess pressure itself.

Hypertension due to renal artery stenosis is the result of a purely physical condition that, in about 50% of cases, is amenable to surgical correction by angioplasty to dilate the lumen. On the other hand, if unilateral renal disease has destroyed most of the useful excretory function of a kidney, which is therefore doing more harm than good, unilateral nephrectomy is indicated.

In the management of hypertension it is important to first establish whether the hypertension is primary, called *essential hypertension*, or secondary as a result of disease in another system, for example the kidneys. These secondary causes should be excluded before essential hypertension (for which no single factor is found responsible) is treated. Medical management of renal hypertension is generally directed to improving the excretory function of the kidneys and their perfusion, which, if successful, brings about a reduction in blood pressure.

It achieves these effects by entering the cells, binding to a receptor and inducing the synthesis of a number of proteins. These, in turn are involved in increasing the number of Na^+ and K^+ channels in the luminal membrane and in increasing the activity of Na^+/K^+ ATPase in the basolateral membrane.

Atrial natriuretic peptide (ANP)

ANP is synthesized and released by myocardial cells of the **atrium**. It is released by stretch of the atrium. In heart failure, it is released by the ventricles as well. Myocytes contain granules of the precursor (prohormone) of ANP which has 126 amino acids. The ANP that is released has 28 amino acids. ANP has several actions that are not yet fully understood. In general, they tend to oppose the actions of the renin–angiotensin system and include the following:

- vasodilatation within the kidney
- inhibition of renin secretion by the granular cells of the afferent and efferent arterioles
- inhibition of aldosterone secretion by the adrenal cortex
- inhibition of ADH secretion by the posterior pituitary and of the actions of ADH on water transport in the collecting duct
- an increase in sodium and water excretion.

The inhibition of aldosterone secretion caused by ANP is, in part, secondary to inhibition of renin secretion, but also reflects a direct action of ANP on the renin-secreting cells. The increase in sodium and water excretion is partly explained by the other actions of ANP. However, ANP may also act directly on the cells of the collecting tubule to close Na^+ channels on the luminal membrane.

The physiological importance of ANP is not yet clear.

Clinical Example

Atrial natriuretic peptide and heart failure

Measuring the level of hormones can be a useful way of assessing body function in health and disease. Thus after the menopause when ovarian hormonal function declines, the level of the controlling hormones, follicle-stimulating hormone (FSH) and luteinizing hormone (LH), rise dramatically. These high levels indicate that the body itself has evaluated ovarian hormonal function and declared it severely reduced. Similarly, in hypothyroidism, the pituitary 'diagnoses' an inadequate level of thyroid hormones and increases the level of thyroid-stimulating hormone (TSH) to stimulate the flagging thyroid, at the same time providing a useful diagnostic aid for the condition. In atrophic gastritis, when the stomach cannot produce an acid secretion, the controlling hormone gastrin rises to very high levels. In the same way the level of atrial natriuretic peptide (ANP) provides a diagnostic aid for the presence and severity of congestive heart failure.

Atrial muscle fibres contain granules of this peptide and, when stretched beyond a certain point, they release the peptide hormone into the circulation. This occurs in normal people when the extracellular fluid volume increases. An increase in extracellular volume is reflected in a rise in plasma volume and hence blood volume. Since the bulk of the blood is contained in the venous system, a surplus volume leads to increased stretching of the atria. The released ANP plays a role, albeit probably a minor one, in returning the volume to normal by favouring excretion of salt and water.

In heart failure the increase in extracellular volume exceeds normal variations and the atria become very distended by the heart's inability to keep up with the venous return. Even in early heart failure there is quite severe stretching of the atria and this causes massive release of natriuretic peptide so that the circulating blood level exceeds the normal limits and, and in severe cases, can rise five- to tenfold. As well as opposing to some extent the increase in extracellular volume, the hormone provides a useful marker, confirming the presence of heart failure and indicating its severity and progress. This is a very 'physiological' assessment, as the secretion of peptide is related directly to the stretching strain on the heart.

Until recently the use of atrial natriuretic peptide in the diagnosis and monitoring of heart failure was confined mainly to research studies, but development of the assays used in its

measurement should make it increasingly practical for routine use. In this connection it can be noted that, in fact, more than one natriuretic peptide is released from the atria, including confusingly named brain natriuretic peptide (BNP), so called because it was initially identified in the brain. However, the circulating level of this related natriuretic peptide seems to be determined by its release from overdistended atria just as with ANP and its stability may avoid the necessity for the rapid analysis needed for its less stable relative.

These assays are particularly important at a time when treatment of heart failure is improving markedly, thanks to treatment aimed at decreasing the load on the failing heart. An assay which can accurately diagnose heart failure and monitor its progress is very valuable in a condition whose effects are often insidious and hard to quantify.

Antidiuretic hormone (ADH)

ADH is released from the posterior pituitary gland (see Ch. 5.2). The major stimuli for ADH secretion (Fig. 8.5.2) are an increase in **plasma osmolality** (by stimulation of osmoreceptors in the hypothalamus) and a decrease in arterial blood pressure or blood volume (via the afferent pathways from the arterial baroreceptors and volume receptors; see p. 600).

ADH has two main effects:

- It causes **vasoconstriction** of arterioles of the systemic circulation, including the kidney, by acting on vasopressin V_1 receptors.
- It increases **water reabsorption** by the kidney, primarily by increasing water permeability of the collecting duct.

ADH binds to V_2 receptors on the basolateral membrane of the principal cells, which stimulates adenylyl cyclase activity and increases the intracellular concentration of cAMP. This results in the insertion of water channels into the luminal membrane of the cell (Fig. 8.5.1). Any water that enters the cells through these channels can leave through the basolateral membrane which is freely permeable to water. ADH also increases the urea permeability of the medullary portion of the collecting duct by activating specific urea transporters in the membrane. This increase in urea permeability contributes to the ability of the kidney to concentrate the urine.

A

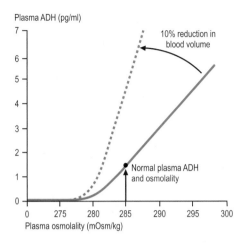

B

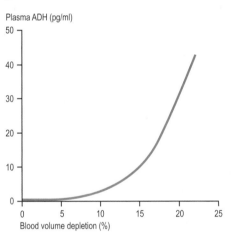

Fig. 8.5.2 Control of ADH secretion. A. Control of ADH (antidiuretic hormone) secretion by plasma osmolality is potentiated by blood volume reduction. **B.** Blood volume reduction alone exerts a powerful effect on plasma ADH level.

Prostaglandins

Prostaglandins are lipid molecules synthesized from arachidonic acid and can be produced by most tissues of the body. They do not generally function as circulating hormones, but **act locally**. Within the kidney, their synthesis is increased by renal sympathetic nerve activity, when angiotensin II levels are high and when

renin release is stimulated, i.e. under circumstances of renal vasoconstriction when renal blood flow might be impaired. Renal prostaglandins are **vasodilator** and help to prevent excessive reductions in renal blood flow and renal ischaemia. Renal prostaglandins are important clinically because many patients are taking non-steroidal anti-inflammatory drugs to treat such conditions as arthritis. These drugs inhibit prostaglandin synthesis. They can therefore produce a large fall in renal blood flow and GFR in patients who have raised levels of sympathetic activity and angiotensin II resulting from blood volume depletion or cardiac failure.

Parathyroid hormone (PTH) and vitamin D

PTH is secreted by the parathyroid gland (Ch. 5.6). Its secretion is stimulated by a reduction in the plasma concentration of ionized calcium. PTH stimulates the production of **calcitriol**, which increases Ca^{2+} and phosphate absorption from the gastrointestinal tract (see below) and stimulates bone resorption. In the kidney, PTH stimulates Ca^{2+} reabsorption by the thick ascending limb of the loop of Henle and the distal tubule. Since all of these effects of PTH tend to increase the plasma Ca^{2+} concentration, the filtered load of Ca^{2+} may increase. Thus, Ca^{2+} excretion may actually increase despite the increase in renal reabsorption.

The kidney is important in the production of calcitriol. Vitamin D_3 (cholecalciferol) is a fat-soluble steroid that is normally present in the diet and that can be synthesized in the skin in the presence of ultraviolet light. Vitamin D_3 is converted to 25-hydroxycholecalciferol in the liver and thence to the active metabolite calcitriol in the kidney (mainly in the proximal tubule). The conversion to calcitriol is stimulated by PTH and is therefore indirectly stimulated by a reduction in Ca^{2+}. Calcitriol increases Ca^{2+} and phosphate absorption by the gut and it enhances bone resorption. The effects of calcitriol on the kidney are not fully understood.

Clinical Example

Renal stones and hyperparathyroidism

Stones in the renal tract, often no more than a few millimetres across, can cause excruciating pain known as *renal colic*. This pain is produced when the stone passes down the ureter by peristalsis, just as our urine normally passes quite painlessly. The problem with the unyielding stone is that it severely stretches the smooth muscle wall of the ureter, thereby powerfully stimulating pain endings there – just like the parallel situation when spasm of the gut wall causes intestinal colic.

As at other sites (parotid gland, gall bladder), stones in the urinary tract have varying compositions, but calcium is often an important component (such stones are often referred to as *renal calculi*). The causes of these stones are often obscure and multifactorial. However, in a relatively small number of patients, their renal tract stones can be clearly related to overactivity of the parathyroid gland. The reason is that in *hyperparathyroidism* the urine is unusually rich in both calcium and phosphate ions so that the product of their concentrations – [calcium] × [phosphate] – can exceed the value up to which the ions are soluble (the *solubility product*) and calcium phosphate comes out of solution.

The parathyroid glands mobilize calcium from bone through their hormone, parathormone, which stimulates osteoclasts to digest bone matrix and releases calcium and phosphate into the extracellular fluid. Excessive amounts of the hormone are usually produced by an autonomous tumour. Unlike normal parathyroid tissue, the tumour is not suppressed by the high level of circulating calcium ions produced by its activity. (About half the circulating plasma calcium is normally bound to plasma proteins, but it is the level of ionized calcium that influences physiological functions such as nerve conduction.)

The excess calcium ions are freely filterable at the glomeruli and so the amount of calcium in the filtrate rises sharply. Although much of this is reabsorbed, the net effect is that the urinary calcium concentration rises.

A second action of parathormone is to impair the renal reabsorption of filtered phosphate ions (the logic of this normal action is that it helps to maintain the level of circulating calcium by lowering the level of circulating phosphate and hence reducing the [calcium] [phosphate] solubility product). The consequence is that a high level of parathormone greatly increases the phosphate content of the urine. Thus overactivity of the parathyroids leads to very high levels of both calcium and phosphate ions, exceeding the solubility product, and crystals of calcium phosphate are formed in the urinary tract, often in the renal pelvis just above the start of the ureter. Over time these crystals can grow into calculi, and the very severe pain (said to resemble the unrelieved pain of childbirth) produced as they are passed by peristalsis down the ureter may be the first symptom of the underlying hyperparathyroidism.

It is therefore good practice to confirm or exclude hyperparathyroidism in people with renal calculi. A tumour is suggested by an increased level of calcium ions and a reduced level of phosphate ions in the blood, and there may be X-ray signs of bone erosion. If a parathyroid tumour (adenoma) is indeed present, then its removal is part of the treatment of the renal calculi.

Regulation of
body fluids

8.6

Introduction

Water balance in the normal individual is regulated by mechanisms that are able to prevent large changes in plasma osmolality, which is itself primarily determined by the plasma sodium concentration. On the other hand, sodium balance in the normal individual is regulated by mechanisms that are able to prevent large changes in extracellular fluid volume. In practice, the important component of extracellular fluid volume is plasma volume, since this perfuses the tissues. Further, it is plasma volume, or more precisely blood volume (i.e. plasma volume plus red and white cells), that is regulated, in that there are receptors that are sensitive to the 'fullness' or 'pressure' within the blood vascular system.

Because of the relationship between plasma osmolality and plasma sodium concentration, it might be thought that an abnormal plasma concentration of Na^+ in an individual can be explained by an abnormality in sodium balance. However, this is not the case; it actually reflects an abnormality in water balance. Changes in Na^+ balance lead to changes in the volume of extracellular fluid, not in its osmolality. Put briefly, plasma osmolality is regulated by changes in water intake and excretion, whereas sodium balance is regulated by changes in sodium excretion.

Regulation of body fluid osmolality

Water is lost from the body via the lungs during breathing, from the skin by sweating, from the gastrointestinal tract in faeces and via the kidneys as urine. Of these, the **kidneys** are the most important route because water excretion can be controlled independently of solutes, to keep plasma osmolality constant. Water is provided for the body by drinking, by the water content in food and by metabolism. Of these, the volume of fluid ingested by drinking regulated by the sensation of thirst is most important. **Osmoreceptors** that are sensitive to changes in osmolality play a major role in the regulation of water excretion by the kidneys and in thirst. **ADH** is the major factor involved in regulating water excretion and thereby osmolality.

Osmoreceptors in the supraoptic and paraventricular nuclei of the anterior hypothalamus respond to changes in the osmolality of the plasma that perfuses them from the carotid artery. They sense changes in osmolality by shrinking or swelling and this changes the output of ADH from the neurohypophysis (posterior pituitary gland). Osmoreceptors in the same region, which may or may not be the same cells as those that regulate ADH output, induce the sensation of thirst.

If excessive water is lost from the body by sweating or in faeces, or if water intake is severely restricted, plasma osmolality is increased and the osmoreceptors stimulate the secretion of ADH and cause the sensation of thirst. The actions of ADH upon the kidney then conserve water, so that a small volume of urine is produced which is hyperosmotic to plasma. In addition, the individual will actively seek water or fluid to drink. As plasma osmolality returns towards normal by these mechanisms, so the secretion of ADH and the sensation of thirst are reduced. On the other hand, if a large water load is consumed and plasma osmolality falls below normal, osmoreceptors will decrease the release of ADH and remove the sensation of thirst. ADH secretion will rise again as the plasma osmolality returns towards normal.

The osmoreceptors are extremely sensitive. They respond to changes in osmolality of as little as 1%, or 3 mOsm/kg H_2O from the normal plasma osmolality of ~285 mOsm/kg H_2O. The relationship between plasma osmolality and ADH production is steep (Fig. 8.5.2A, p. 759) as is the relationship between plasma ADH concentration and urine osmolality. Thus, the sensitivity of the system that regulates osmolality is very high. Further, because ADH is rapidly degraded in plasma, circulating levels of ADH can be reduced to zero within minutes of ADH secretion being inhibited. Thus, the system can respond very rapidly to changes in plasma osmolality.

Normally, ADH is far more important than thirst in regulating plasma osmolality because most of our drinking is habitual or social and not regulated by osmoreceptors. Also, the osmotic regulation of thirst is far from perfect; the sensation of thirst can be satisfied by the act of drinking before sufficient water has been absorbed from the gastrointestinal tract to reduce the plasma osmolality to normal. This is probably due to the input from receptors in the oropharyngeal regions and upper gastrointestinal tract.

Regulation of extracellular fluid volume

We have seen that **extracellular fluid volume** (EFV) is dependent upon Na^+. Thus, if a hyperosmotic solution of NaCl were added to the extracellular fluid, then both the Na^+ concentration and the osmolality of the extracellular fluid would increase and, via the osmoreceptors, this would stimulate ADH secretion and thirst. The resulting decrease in water excretion by the kidneys and the increased drinking of water would restore the osmolality of plasma and other extracellular fluid to normal. However, the volume of the extracellular fluid would show a parallel increase.

On the other hand, if NaCl were to be lost from the extracellular fluid, then the volume of the extracellular fluid would decrease.

The EFV is regulated by regulating Na$^+$ excretion, and in the normal individual this works well. However, problems arise in certain disease states. For example, in congestive heart failure, cardiac output is decreased, but the EFV, including plasma volume, is increased. This occurs because the reduction in cardiac output leads to retention of Na$^+$ by the kidney. (This is considered further, below.)

Of the various mechanisms that regulate EFV in the normal individual, it should first be stated that maintenance of a normal EFV depends upon there being adequate Na$^+$ in the diet. If this is the case, then **Na$^+$ excretion** by the kidneys regulates EFV.

If EFV falls, then the following occur:

1. Reduction in blood volume *reduces the pressure in the venous part of the systemic circulation*. This change is transmitted back into the kidney so that hydrostatic pressure in the peritubular capillaries that supply the proximal tubules is reduced. The reabsorption of Na$^+$ and fluid by the proximal tubule is therefore automatically increased, since it is dependent upon the balance of hydrostatic forces between the lateral intercellular spaces and the capillaries.

2. The decrease in venous pressure also *reduces the stimulus to* (i.e. unloads) the volume or stretch receptors in the great veins and atria. This results in a reflex increase in the sympathetic activity to the kidney.

3. If the reduction in EFV and blood volume is sufficiently large to produce a *reduction in arterial blood pressure*, this will reduce the stimulus to (i.e. unload) the baroreceptors in the carotid sinuses and aortic arch. Even if mean arterial pressure does not fall, a small decrease in blood volume normally reduces arterial pulse pressure and this will unload the arterial baroreceptors. A reduction in baroreceptor

afferent activity results in a reflex increase in sympathetic activity.

4. An increase in sympathetic activity in the kidney, if sufficiently pronounced (see Ch. 8.5), causes *renal vasoconstriction*. This decreases renal blood flow and can, in turn, decrease capillary hydrostatic pressure in the glomerulus and GFR.

5. The increase in renal sympathetic activity also directly stimulates *renin* release, this being augmented by the decrease in pressure in the afferent arteriole caused by vasoconstriction proximal to the afferent arteriole (see Ch. 8.5) and by any fall in mean arterial pressure or in pulse pressure.

6. The increase in renin activity stimulates the production of *angiotensin II*.

7. The constriction of the afferent and efferent arterioles caused by increased sympathetic activity and angiotensin II may further reduce hydrostatic pressure in the peritubular capillaries, so augmenting Na$^+$ and fluid reabsorption. The increase in renal sympathetic activity and angiotensin II also directly stimulate Na$^+$ reabsorption by the proximal tubule.

8. The increase in the plasma concentration of angiotensin II stimulates the *release of aldosterone*. This increases the reabsorption of Na$^+$ by the late part of the distal tubule and collecting duct.

9. A reduction in venous pressure and thereby atrial pressure reduces the stimulus to atrial cells that secrete ANP. Since ANP promotes Na$^+$ and water excretion by the kidney by various mechanisms (see Ch. 8.5) a reduction in plasma ANP would tend to support the other effects described above.

10. As Na$^+$ excretion begins to fall as a result of the above mechanisms, so *plasma osmolality* may begin to increase. This stimulates the secretion of ADH. ADH secretion is also stimulated by a reduction in the activity of the volume receptors and arterial baroreceptors (see p. 600). ADH reduces water excretion. It should be noted that if

the initial fall in EFV causes a large enough decrease in the activity of the volume receptors and arterial baroreceptors, this will stimulate the secretion of ADH from the outset (see below).

11. *Thirst* is stimulated. This probably occurs by the action of angiotensin II on the brain.

Thus, these integrated effects upon the kidney mean that Na^+ and water are retained by the kidneys such that EFV is restored and plasma osmolality remains constant.

If EFV increases, exactly the opposite changes occur. Na^+ and water excretion by the kidneys are increased so that EFV decreases towards normal, while osmolality remains constant.

Summary

Principles of regulation of plasma osmolality and plasma sodium

- Plasma osmolality is largely determined by plasma sodium concentration.
- A change in plasma sodium normally leads to an osmotic flux of water between extracellular and intracellular space and thence to a change in plasma volume. Therefore, an abnormal plasma Na^+ concentration reflects an abnormality in water balance, rather than an abnormality in sodium balance.
- Plasma osmolality is largely regulated by changes in water intake and excretion via changes in the secretion of ADH that are mediated by hypothalamic osmoreceptors.
- Plasma volume is largely regulated by changes in sodium excretion via direct effects on the kidney and via reflex mechanisms involving:
  - stretch receptors in the atria and great veins
  - arterial baroreceptors.

Interaction between osmoregulatory and volume regulatory influences upon ADH

We have seen that secretion of ADH is regulated by the osmoreceptors, which respond to changes in plasma osmolality, and that this regulatory mechanism is very sensitive. Secretion of ADH is also regulated by **volume receptors** and **arterial baroreceptors**. The sensitivity of the influence of these receptors upon ADH release is less than that of the osmoreceptors; blood volume or arterial pressure has to decrease by 5–10% before ADH secretion is stimulated (Fig. 8.5.2B, p. 759). However, changes in blood volume and arterial pressure do affect the relationship between plasma osmolality and ADH secretion (see Fig. 8.5.2A, p. 759). The importance of this effect is seen particularly when blood volume is decreased. The relationship between osmolality and ADH is shifted to the left and the slope of the relationship is increased. This means that if blood volume falls substantially, ADH secretion can be maximal or near maximal even when plasma osmolality is substantially below normal. In other words, faced with a life-threatening reduction in blood volume and arterial pressure, the influence of the volume receptors and baroreceptors over ADH secretion predominates over the influence of the osmoreceptors. Thus, the kidneys retain water and defend **blood volume** even though the penalty is a reduction in plasma osmolality.

Regulation of EFV in pathological states

Chronic heart failure

In chronic heart failure, impairment of myocardial contractility, usually of the left ventricle, results in a reduction in cardiac output and consequently a reduction in arterial pressure and in renal perfusion pressure. These factors lead to the retention of NaCl and water by the kidney. This fluid retention results in an increase in the volume of blood held within the venous vessels of the systemic circulation, since these are the distensible vessels of the systemic circulation. As a consequence, central venous pressure will rise when the venous vessels have reached the limit of their distensibility and capillary hydrostatic pressure may also rise. A rise in capillary hydrostatic pressure together with the fall in plasma oncotic pressure that is caused by water retention favours the movement of fluid out of the capillaries into the interstitial fluid and peripheral **oedema** – the accumulation of excess fluid in the interstitial space. The increase in central venous pressure, the filling pressure for the right side of the heart, will help to increase right ventricular output, by Starling's law of the heart (Fig. 8.6.1). This, in turn, will increase filling pressure for the left side of the heart.

If the disease of the ventricle is mild, then the increase in filling pressure and therefore volume may improve left ventricular performance, according to Starling's law of the heart, so that stroke volume and cardiac output move towards normal. A new, **compensated** state can therefore be reached when arterial pressure, renal perfusion pressure and thereby sodium excretion return to normal, but at the expense of a raised plasma volume and oedema.

On the other hand, if the disease is severe, then the increase in left ventricular filling pressure may not improve its performance significantly (Fig. 8.6.1). In fact, stroke volume and thereby cardiac output remain below normal in this situation; the rise in left ventricular filling pressure will be transmitted back to the pulmonary circulation, so producing pulmonary oedema. Moreover, the reduced left ventricular output leads to further retention of NaCl and water by the kidney and a further rise in capillary hydrostatic pressure and oedema formation. In untreated cardiac failure, this positive feedback in the systemic circulation can eventually be limited because the accumulation of fluid in the tissues spaces will cause tissue hydrostatic pressure to rise, so neutralizing the effect of the rise in capillary hydrostatic

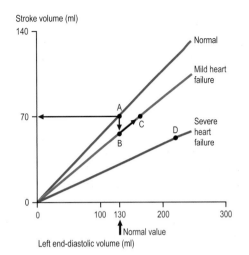

Fig. 8.6.1 Heart failure. Mild heart failure (A to B) can be compensated for by an increase in filling pressure and thereby in left end-diastolic volume (LEDV) and stroke volume (SV) (B to C). In severe heart failure the filling pressure and end-diastolic volume are already greatly increased (D) but the heart is working on a lower function curve; a further increase in filling pressure and LEDV cannot improve the situation.

pressure. However, the pulmonary oedema is potentially life-threatening because it impairs alveolar gas exchange.

Peripheral oedema cannot be detected clinically until 2–3 litres of excess fluid have accumulated in the interstitial fluid compartment. Therefore, patients with chronic heart failure and peripheral oedema have a greatly increased interstitial fluid volume and an increased plasma volume, i.e. a greatly expanded EFV and yet they behave as if they are volume depleted. The problem from the regulatory point of view is that they have a reduced circulating blood volume and the compensatory mechanisms that are brought into play make the condition worse.

Liver disease

Regulation of EFV may also be disturbed in liver disease. In liver disease there is commonly a rise in hydrostatic pressure in the hepatic portal vein, because of:

- obstruction within the liver, and
- vasodilatation of the splanchnic circulation.

There is a consequent rise in pressure in the capillaries of the intestine which forces fluid out into the abdominal cavity. This causes oedema formation in the abdominal cavity, known as **ascites**. The splanchnic vasodilatation, whose cause is unclear, together with the loss of plasma fluid into the abdominal cavity cause systemic arterial pressure to fall. This fall may be exacerbated because of the development of anatomical arteriovenous fistulae (shunts) throughout the body, which causes total peripheral resistance to fall further. As a compensatory response to the fall in systemic arterial pressure, cardiac output may be raised above normal via the baroreceptor reflex, contrasting with the low cardiac output of congestive heart failure. However, this increase in cardiac output is not sufficient to raise the arterial pressure in the face of reduced total peripheral resistance and loss of plasma volume into the interstitial space. Thus, as in congestive heart failure, patients with liver disease behave as if they are volume depleted; the kidneys retain sodium and water, even though the EFV is raised above normal.

Summary

Interactions between the regulation of plasma osmolality and plasma volume

- ADH secretion is regulated by osmoreceptors.
- ADH secretion is also regulated by volume receptors and arterial baroreceptors.
- The sensitivity of the influence of volume receptors and arterial baroreceptors on ADH secretion is less than that of the osmoreceptors.
- However, a decrease in blood volume greatly increases the sensitivity of the relationship between osmolality and ADH and shifts it to the left.
- Thus, if blood volume falls substantially, ADH secretion can be maximal even when plasma osmolality is below normal; plasma volume is defended at the expense of plasma osmolality.

Clinical Example

Diuretics

In broadest terms a diuretic is something that produces a diuresis or increased urine formation. Thus 1 litre of water drunk surplus to normal requirements is a powerful diuretic, as demonstrated by generations of students in their physiology practical classes. However, in medical terms a diuretic usually refers to a drug which causes a diuresis in someone who would otherwise pass much less urine. In practice the definition is even more restricted since, in general, diuretics act by causing a loss of excess sodium, chloride and water (though other ions are often lost in excess too) thereby *reducing the extracellular fluid volume*, which is the dominant site of sodium and chloride.

Sodium has been described as the skeleton of the extracellular fluid. The intracellular sodium level is relatively low and fixed, so extra sodium taken into the body is added to the extracellular fluid, and sodium lost from the body is lost from the extracellular fluid. Given a certain amount of sodium in the extracellular fluid, electrical neutrality demands an equal amount of anion. Thus chloride is retained to balance the

Clinical Example *(Continued)*

sodium ions. To maintain normal osmolality, an equivalent amount of water is retained. Thus the extracellular fluid clothes the sodium skeleton.

In normal circumstances the body tolerates moderate fluctuations in extracellular fluid volume. When we eat a salty meal and are compelled by the accompanying thirst to drink more fluid, our extracellular volume may go up by a litre or more without disturbing body function. The extra fluid is excreted in a leisurely fashion over a day or two under the influence of reduced aldosterone and increased natriuretic hormone. Both these hormones act primarily by regulating body sodium.

However, in some diseases there are gross changes in body sodium and consequently extracellular fluid. In heart failure the volume may rise from around 10–15 litres (depending on body size) by several litres in mild cases and by 5–10 litres in severe cases. Similar changes can occur in liver and renal failure. The excessive extracellular fluid is distributed between the interstitial compartment, where several extra litres are manifested as oedema, and the intravascular compartment, where increased blood volume leads to venous congestion and cardiac strain. In these circumstances, diuretics can improve the situation dramatically.

Essentially diuretics are selective poisons of the kidney's ability to reabsorb sodium from the glomerular filtrate. They do not affect the obligatory reabsorption in the proximal convoluted tubule, but act on the distal convoluted tubule, and in the case of the highly potent loop diuretics on the cells of the ascending limb of the loop of Henle. By reducing sodium reabsorption, diuretics increase sodium loss in the urine, and this is accompanied by loss of chloride and of water. The benefits can be immediate and dramatic in the case of heart failure. In advanced heart failure excessive extracellular fluid leads to severe dependent oedema (which is mainly an inconvenience), and an increased intravascular volume which places a severe burden on the failing heart and favours the development of life-threatening pulmonary oedema. Intravenous administration of a powerful diuretic can relieve the pulmonary oedema and improve the cardiac state within the hour, with continuing improvement in the next few days. The loss of fluid is apparent in the huge quantities of urine passed, e.g. 5 litres in the first few hours. It can also be monitored by the simple measure of weighing the patient. Loss of, say, 7 litres of surplus extracellular fluid in a week results in a loss of weight of 7 kg, since each litre of urine or extracellular fluid weighs very close to 1 kg. Nutritional changes over this period of time would normally produce little change in weight.

Diuretics are also used in the treatment of hypertension, particularly as an initial treatment of mild hypertension. Their action is complex, but at least part of the effect is due to loss of extracellular fluid, leading to a reduced plasma volume, a fall in stroke volume and hence a fall in arterial blood pressure. Excessive diuretic therapy can sometimes lead to inappropriately low blood pressure, by excessively reducing circulating blood volume.

Diuretics vary in their effects on electrolytes other than sodium and chloride. In general, a diuresis tends to reduce the opportunity for reabsorption of other ions such as potassium, and so potassium depletion is a risk, requiring in some cases potassium supplements. In contrast, diuretics which antagonize the actions of aldosterone tend to raise body potassium by antagonizing aldosterone's promotion of potassium excretion in exchange for sodium reabsorption.

Regulation of acid–base balance

8.7

Introduction

It is very important that the H^+ concentration of the body fluids is kept relatively constant because the activities of many of the body's enzymes are critically dependent on H^+ concentration; they only function normally within a narrow range. The normal plasma concentration of H^+ is 40 nmol/litre or 0.00004 mmol/litre, which is very low relative to the concentration of, for example, Na^+ (140 mmol/litre or 140 000 000 nmol/litre). Because the H^+ concentration is so low, it is often expressed as the negative logarithm to base 10 of the H^+ concentration in mol/litre, i.e. $-\log [H^+]$ or $\log 1/[H^+]$ or pH. Thus, 40 nmol/litre equals 0.00000004 mol/litre which is equivalent to pH 7.4. The pH range 7.8–6.8 (16–160 nmol/litre) can be tolerated, but in healthy individuals pH is generally kept between 7.36 and 7.44 (36–44 nmol/litre).

Hydrogen ions are generated by the normal metabolism of food.

1. The metabolism of carbohydrates and fats produces large quantities of CO_2. This combines with water to form H_2CO_3 which generates H^+ by the following reaction the first part of which is catalysed by carbonic anhydrase:

$$CO_2 + H_2O \rightleftharpoons H_2CO_3 \rightleftharpoons H^+ + HCO_3^-.$$

This CO_2 does not normally result in a net increase in H^+ concentration in plasma because the CO_2 can be excreted from the body via the lungs. The H_2CO_3 is therefore known as a **volatile acid**.

2. The metabolism of proteins generates **non-volatile acids** that cannot be excreted via the lungs. Thus, sulphuric acid is formed from the metabolism of the amino acids cysteine and methionine, and hydrochloric acid is formed from the metabolism of lysine, arginine and histidine. In addition, certain organic acids, such as $H_2PO_4^-$ are simply consumed in the diet. This gain of H^+ is partly offset by the metabolism of aspartate, glutamate and citrate which results in the production of HCO_3^- which can then buffer the H^+ (see below). Nevertheless, there is a net gain of H^+ of 65–74 mmol/day in an individual who has a normal western diet. These H^+ must be dealt with if the pH is to remain normal.

The astute student will remember that we have already touched upon the effect of CO_2 on plasma pH in the section on respiration. The chemistry that follows here is a detailed description of what was outlined there; and reinforces the fact that the kidneys and respiratory system are inextricably entwined in the control of body fluid pH.

Buffering in body fluids

If the H^+ gained by ingestion and metabolism were to be freely distributed in total body water (about 40 litres), then a net gain of say 70 mmol H^+ in a day would increase the H^+ concentration in body water by 17.5 mM, i.e. to almost 1 million times normal. This does not happen because the rise in H^+ concentration is limited by various buffer systems. Two factors determine the capacity of a buffer system to stabilize pH:

- the pK of the buffer system in relation to the ambient pH (see Basic Science 8.7.1), and
- the quantity of the buffer present.

In the intracellular fluid, the major buffers are *phosphates* and *proteins*, including the

haemoglobin in red blood cells. The reactions may be written as:

$$H^+ + HPO_4^{2-} \rightleftharpoons H_2PO_4^-$$

$$H^+ + Protein^- \rightleftharpoons H\,Protein.$$

In the extracellular fluid, proteins, phosphate and bicarbonate are important, and in bone, carbonate (CO_3^{2-}).

In plasma, the bicarbonate–carbon dioxide system is of major importance:

$$CO_2 + H_2O \rightleftharpoons H_2CO_3 \rightleftharpoons H^+ + HCO_3^-.$$

Since the H_2CO_3 concentration is very small, H_2CO_3 can be ignored and the reactions can be simplified to:

$$CO_2 + H_2O \rightleftharpoons H^+ + HCO_3^-.$$

The Henderson–Hasselbalch equation for this buffer system can then be written as:

$$pH = pK + \log \frac{[HCO_3^-]}{[CO_2]}.$$

Since the concentration of CO_2 depends on its partial pressure (P_{CO_2} in mmHg) and on its solubility in plasma (0.03 mmol/litre·mmHg^{-1}), we can write:

$$pH = pK + \log \frac{[HCO_3^-]}{0.03 \times P_{CO_2}}.$$

The pK of this system is 6.1, the pH at which the buffer is most effective (which is more than 1 pH unit from the normal plasma pH of 7.4). On this basis, the bicarbonate system is not a very effective buffer in plasma. However, physiologically, it is very important because:

- $[HCO_3^-]$ is relatively high
- $[HCO_3^-]$ and P_{CO_2} are controlled independently, by the kidneys and lungs respectively.

In the normal individual who is in acid–base balance, $[HCO_3^-]$ is 24 mM and P_{CO_2} is 40 mmHg. Therefore the equation can be written as:

$$pH = 6.1 + \log \frac{24}{0.03 \times 40} = 6.1 + \log \frac{24}{1.2} = 7.4.$$

Basic Science 8.7.1

Buffers

A buffer solution is one which minimizes, or resists, changes in H^+ concentration. The general form of a buffering reaction is:

$$Buffer^- + H^+ \rightleftharpoons H\ Buffer.$$

$Buffer^-$ is known as a base – it can accept H^+; whereas H Buffer is an acid – it can donate H^+.

Therefore, we can rewrite the equation above as:

$$Base + H^+ \rightleftharpoons Acid. \tag{1}$$

The H^+ concentration (pH) of the solution changes little when H^+ is added to the base because the acid generated is a **weak acid** which means it does not dissociate very readily. In other words, the added hydrogen ions are 'mopped up'; they do not appear as free H^+.

The equilibrium or dissociation constant K for Equation 1 can be expressed as:

$$K = \frac{[H^+]\ [Base]}{[Acid]} \tag{2}$$

or solving for H^+, this can be rearranged as:

$$[H^+] = \frac{K \times [Acid]}{[Base]}. \tag{3}$$

The constant, K, has the dimensions of concentration and is a measure of the strength of the acid. The larger the K, the stronger the acid, i.e. the more completely it dissociates. Since K is usually a very small number, it is usually expressed as the negative logarithm to base 10 (pK), in analogy with the relationship between H^+ concentration and pH.

If we take the negative logarithm of both sides of Equation 3, then we get:

$$pH = pK + \log \frac{[Base]}{[Acid]}. \tag{4}$$

This is the **Henderson–Hasselbalch equation** (see also Ch. 7.3). It follows from this equation that if we know the ratio of the base to acid concentrations and the pK of a given buffer system, then the pH can be calculated. It also follows, since pK is the equilibrium constant of the reactions of Equation 1, that buffer solutions most strongly resist changes in pH near the point of half dissociation of the acid, i.e. when the concentrations of the base and acid are equal and therefore pH = pK and the equilibrium has the greatest 'room to move' in either direction. The range over which a buffer is effective is about 1 pH unit on either side of the pK.

Buffering of blood by the bicarbonate–carbonic acid system is illustrated in Figure BS8.7.1.

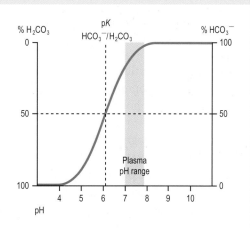

Fig. BS8.7.1 Blood buffering. An important buffer in the blood is the bicarbonate (HCO_3^-)–carbonic acid (H_2CO_3) system. The ratio of this weak acid to its base (bicarbonate) determines the pH of a solution containing them (plasma). This buffer would be chemically most effective at its pK, a pH of 6.1, where the line is steepest and changes in the concentration of the two components would produce the smallest changes in pH. However, plasma has a pH of 7.4. This system is nevertheless a very important buffer of the blood for reasons which are explained in the section on Respiration (see p. 686).

The ratio of $[HCO_3^-]$ to $[CO_2]$ is therefore 24 : 1.2, i.e. 20 : 1. This means that if either the nominator or denominator is changed, the pH can be brought back to 7.4, when this ratio is brought back to 20 : 1.

Having considered the principles of buffering, we can now consider how the body deals with the *volatile* and *non-volatile* acids that are the products of metabolism. The hydrogen ions that are generated from the volatile acid H_2CO_3, are very effectively buffered during their transit in the blood from tissues to lungs, mainly by the **haemoglobin** (protein) in the red blood cells (see p. 680). The non-volatile acids H_2SO_4 and HCl are predominantly buffered by the **bicarbonate** in plasma, which circulates combined with the major cation in plasma, Na^+.

Thus:

$$H_2SO_4 + 2NaHCO_3 \rightleftharpoons Na_2SO_4 + 2CO_2 + 2H_2O$$

$$HCl + NaHCO_3 \rightleftharpoons NaCl + CO_2 + H_2O .$$

These reactions are backed up by the other buffer systems of plasma, interstitial fluid, intracellular fluid and bone. The reactions that occur in extracellular fluid occur in minutes, whereas those that operate within cells, or involve bone, can take hours.

The important consequences of this buffering is that free hydrogen ions have become hydrogen atoms in water, while HCO_3^- has been removed from the plasma to produce CO_2, which in normal individuals can be excreted from the body via the lungs. A normal acid load can therefore be buffered very effectively.

The buffering is made more efficient because even a small increase in $[H^+]$ (fall in pH) stimulates respiration via the peripheral chemoreceptors (see p. 691), so tending to reduce P_{CO_2} below normal. The buffer reactions shown above are therefore driven further to the right, reducing $[H^+]$ but at the expense of losing more HCO_3^- from plasma. In this way, the ratio $[HCO_3^-]$ to $[CO_2]$ in the Henderson–Hasselbalch equation can return to normal and the pH returns to normal.

The consequence of this is that the absolute concentration of HCO_3^- is reduced. Therefore, to ensure enough HCO_3^- to maintain acid–base balance in the future, the $[HCO_3^-]$ must be restored. This is done by the kidney. The filtered load of HCO_3^- at the kidney is very large, ~24 mmol/litre in 180 litres per day, i.e. 4320 mmol/day. Thus, not only must all of the filtered HCO_3^- be reabsorbed, but an *additional* amount must be reabsorbed equal to that lost by buffering H^+. The reabsorption of HCO_3^- and the generation of new HCO_3^- depend upon the secretion of H^+ by the nephrons.

Bicarbonate reabsorption, hydrogen secretion and buffering

The majority (85%) of bicarbonate filtered is reabsorbed in the **proximal tubule**. The remaining 15% is reabsorbed by the **distal tubule** and **collecting duct**. (The processes involved have been described in previous chapters, and are summarized in Fig. 8.3.4, p. 739.) In both regions, bicarbonate reabsorption is linked to H^+ secretion, but in the proximal tubule, H^+ secretion mainly occurs via the Na^+/H^+ countertransporter, whereas in the later parts of the nephrons, H^+ secretion is mainly mediated by the H^+-ATPase pump. Although the hydrogen ions are buffered in the lumen, $[H^+]$ does rise substantially; pH falls from 7.4 to about 7 in the proximal tubule and to as low as 4.5 in the collecting duct. The H^+-ATPase in the later parts of the nephron is therefore very important in allowing H^+ to be secreted against a substantial $[H^+]$ gradient.

The H^+ that is secreted by the proximal tubule is predominantly buffered by HCO_3^- that was filtered at the glomerulus, to form H_2CO_3. This is converted to CO_2 and H_2O in a reaction catalysed by **carbonic anhydrase** in the brush border of the luminal membrane. The CO_2 and H_2O rapidly diffuse into the cell where HCO_3^- formation is again catalysed by the action of carbonic anhydrase, and this HCO_3^- is reabsorbed into the blood. Thus, this process allows one HCO_3^- to be reabsorbed for each H^+ that is secreted.

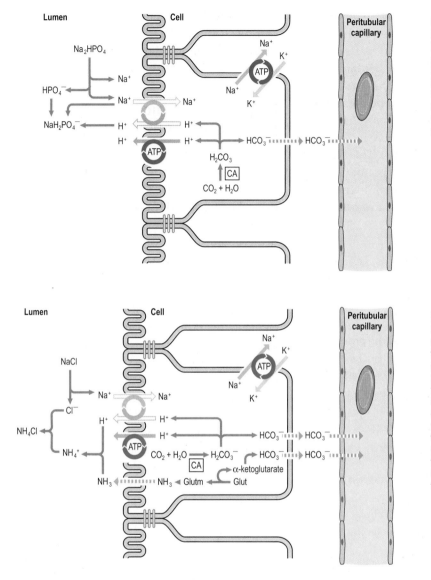

Fig. 8.7.1 Tubular fluid buffering by phosphate. Because it is operating near its pK of 6.8, the phosphate system is chemically very efficient as a buffer in the tubular lumen and is the primary urinary buffer. However, its effect is limited by the amount of phosphate present.

Fig. 8.7.2 Formation of NH_3 in the distal tubule. Glutamine (Glut) is converted to α-ketoglutarate, which generates bicarbonate, and glutamic acid (Glutm) with the formation of NH_3. The NH_3 diffuses into the lumen and captures an H^+ to form NH_4^+, which cannot diffuse back into the body. This mechanism generates HCO_3^- which enters the blood. NH_4^+ formation becomes important at low tubular pH (<6.0).

Buffers other than bicarbonate

Phosphate

H^+ that is secreted into the lumen can also be buffered by HPO_4^{2-} that is filtered at the glomerulus, so as to form $H_2PO_4^-$ (Fig. 8.7.1). As the H^+ secreted is formed within the tubule cell from the dissociation of H_2CO_3, this process allows additional HCO_3^- to be generated, over and above the amount that is reabsorbed from the tubule lumen as an indirect consequence of urinary buffering by HCO_3^-. The phosphate reaction is very effective at buffering H^+ in the tubular fluid because its pK is 6.8. However, its importance is limited because the concentration of $H_2PO_4^-$ in the filtrate is low and much of it is reabsorbed in the proximal tubule.

Ammonia

It is the production of ammonia by the kidney that is of major importance both in excreting

H⁺ and in generating new bicarbonate for the plasma (Fig. 8.7.2). Ammonia is produced in the cells of the proximal and distal parts of the nephron by the conversion of **glutamine** to glutamic acid and α-ketoglutarate. The further metabolism of α-ketoglutarate generates HCO_3^- that is reabsorbed into plasma. The NH_3 diffuses out of the cell into the lumen where it combines with secreted H⁺ to form **NH₄⁺**. The NH_4^+ is trapped in the lumen because the tubule cells are relatively impermeable to it. The excretion of NH_4^+ normally amounts to 30–50 mmol/day, so

allowing an equivalent production of HCO_3^-. During acidosis, NH_4^+ excretion can increase to over 300 mmol/day with a corresponding increase in HCO_3^- reabsorption.

Regulation of bicarbonate reabsorption and hydrogen secretion

The kidney behaves as if there is a transport maximum (T_m) for HCO_3^- excretion. This means that when plasma $[HCO_3^-]$ is normal (24 mmol/litre) or below, there is virtually no HCO_3^- in urine because it is reabsorbed, whereas when $[HCO_3^-]$ in plasma is above normal, then HCO_3^- is readily excreted.

Since HCO_3^- is dependent on H⁺ secretion, as explained above, HCO_3^- reabsorption is changed by factors that change H⁺ secretion. Thus the T_m for HCO_3^- can be increased, i.e. more HCO_3^- is reabsorbed when H⁺ secretion is increased. When H⁺ secretion decreases, the opposite occurs.

A major determinant of H⁺ secretion is plasma pH. When plasma pH falls, either because of addition of H⁺ or a decrease in $[HCO_3^-]$, then H⁺ secretion increases (as does HCO_3^- reabsorption). This is believed to be the result of an increase in intracellular $[H^+]$, which has several effects:

- the **gradient** for H⁺ excretion between tubule cell and lumen is increased with a consequent increase in Na⁺–H⁺ exchange via the countertransporter
- there is an increase in activity of the H⁺-ATPase **pump** owing to the insertion of new pumps in the membrane
- there is stimulation of the production of **ammonia**.

When plasma pH rises, exactly the opposite happens and H⁺ secretion is decreased (as is HCO_3^- reabsorption).

Since H⁺ secretion and Na⁺ reabsorption are linked, H⁺ secretion is affected by factors that influence Na⁺ reabsorption. Thus, a decrease in

Summary

H⁺ buffering in the renal tubule

- H⁺ secreted into the lumen by the proximal tubule is primarily buffered by HCO_3^- that is filtered at the glomerulus. The H⁺ that is secreted originates from the dissociation of H_2CO_3 within the cell. One HCO_3^- is reabsorbed for every H⁺ secreted.
- H⁺ secreted into the tubular lumen can also be buffered by:
  - HPO_4^{2-} that is filtered at the glomerulus, so forming $H_2PO_4^-$
  - NH_3 that is produced by the tubular cells and secreted into the lumen, so forming NH_4^+.
- Buffering by HPO_4^{2-} and by NH_3 both allow an additional HCO_3^- ion to be generated over and above that reabsorbed as an indirect consequence of H⁺ buffering by filtered HCO_3^-.
- Buffering by HPO_4^{2-} is relatively unimportant because the concentration of HPO_4^{2-} in tubular fluid is low.
- Buffering by NH_3 can become very important: in acidosis, NH_4^+ excretion can be >300 mmol/day and there is a corresponding increase in circulating HCO_3^-, which is then available to buffer plasma H⁺.

effective circulating volume, which results in an increase in Na$^+$ reabsorption by the proximal tubule (see Ch. 8.6), also increases H$^+$ secretion (and HCO$_3^-$ reabsorption). In addition, stimulation of Na$^+$ reabsorption by the action of aldosterone on the distal tubule and collecting duct, increases H$^+$ secretion (and HCO$_3^-$ reabsorption). This is thought to be because the reabsorption of Na$^+$ into the tubule cell creates a positive charge which improves the gradient for H$^+$ secretion into the lumen. Conversely, a decrease in Na$^+$ reabsorption leads to a reduction in H$^+$ secretion (and HCO$_3^-$ reabsorption).

Acidosis and alkalosis can affect K$^+$ excretion by the kidney (see Ch. 8.4). It is also the case that changes in plasma [K$^+$] can affect acid–base balance, H$^+$ secretion (and HCO$_3^-$ reabsorption). Thus, if plasma [K$^+$] falls, for example as a consequence of hyperaldosteronism (see p. 442), then K$^+$ tends to diffuse out of cells down its concentration gradient and electroneutrality is maintained by movement of H$^+$ (and Na$^+$) into the cells. Thus, plasma pH tends to rise. In the kidney, the movement of H$^+$ into tubule cells increases H$^+$ secretion (and HCO$_3^-$ reabsorption), so augmenting the alkalosis. An increase in plasma [K$^+$] to above normal has the opposite effects, resulting in acidosis.

Disturbances of acid–base balance

Normal plasma pH is 7.4. Acidosis exists if arterial plasma pH is below 7.4. Alkalosis exists when pH is greater than 7.4. If the disturbance is caused by the respiratory system, it is called a **respiratory acidosis** or **respiratory alkalosis**. If it is caused by a factor other than the respiratory system, it is called a **metabolic acidosis** or **metabolic alkalosis**. In the equations:

$$CO_2 + H_2O \rightleftharpoons H_2CO_3 \rightleftharpoons H^+ + HCO_3^-$$

and:

$$pH = pK + \log \frac{[HCO_3^-]}{CO_2} = pK + \log \frac{20}{1}$$

respiratory disorders primarily affect CO$_2$, whereas metabolic disorders primarily affect [HCO$_3^-$]. When a change in pH occurs, the buffer systems of the body, the kidney and the respiratory system act to restore pH to normal, the respiratory system controlling CO$_2$ and the kidney controlling HCO$_3^-$.

Respiratory acidosis

This disorder is characterized by raised PCO$_2$ and reduced pH. The raised PCO$_2$ can be caused by a reduction in ventilation due to the actions of drugs such as anaesthetics and barbiturates on the respiratory neurones in the brain or to central neural lesions. More commonly it is caused by chronic bronchitis or emphysema

![Summary icon] **Summary**

Regulation of HCO$_3^-$ reabsorption and H$^+$ secretion

- There is an apparent T_m for HCO$_3^-$ excretion. If plasma [HCO$_3^-$] is normal (24 mM), HCO$_3^-$ is reabsorbed, but when plasma [HCO$_3^-$] is >24 mM, the excess is excreted.
- However, the T_m for HCO$_3^-$ can be increased when H$^+$ secretion is increased, or decreased when H$^+$ secretion falls.
- H$^+$ secretion is dependent on plasma [H$^+$]; an increase in plasma [H$^+$] increases H$^+$ secretion and vice versa.
- Since H$^+$ secretion and Na$^+$ reabsorption are linked, an increase in Na$^+$ reabsorption can increase H$^+$ secretion into the tubule.
- A decrease in plasma [K$^+$] can also increase H$^+$ secretion into the tubule; K$^+$ diffuses out of all cells down its concentration gradient and H$^+$ moves in, down the electrical gradient. The movement of H$^+$ into the renal tubule cells leads to H$^+$ secretion, so augmenting the fall in plasma [H$^+$] (and increasing plasma pH).

which impairs the removal of CO_2 from the lungs. The reaction:

$$CO_2 + H_2O \rightleftharpoons H_2CO_3 \rightleftharpoons H^+ + HCO_3^-$$

is therefore shifted to the right and $[H^+]$ and $[HCO_3^-]$ rise (Fig. 8.7.3). In fact, because CO_2 diffuses easily into body cells, and because cells contain carbonic anhydrase, this reaction occurs most quickly within the cells and the $[H^+]$ of all cells including those of the kidney tends to increase. This H^+ is mainly buffered by **proteins** and HCO_3^- diffuses out, so raising plasma $[HCO_3^-]$. This occurs *within hours*, but the return of pH towards normal is limited by the efficiency of the available buffers to buffer the H^+. This, in turn, limits the extent to which the reaction can shift to the right and limits the rise in HCO_3^-. Thus, the rise in $[HCO_3^-]$ is actually rather modest. Therefore, the ratio $[HCO_3^-]$ to

$[CO_2]$ in the Henderson–Hasselbalch equation stays less than 20, the P_{CO_2} remains high and, consequently, the pH is low ($[H^+]$ is high).

In the kidney, the rise in intracellular $[H^+]$ stimulates H^+ secretion and HCO_3^- reabsorption, as explained above. This provides additional HCO_3^- for the plasma, which is used to buffer the H^+ generated from CO_2 and, at the same time, additional H^+ is excreted by the kidney. The kidney can therefore compensate *over several days* for respiratory acidosis and return the pH towards normal by increasing $[HCO_3^-]$ and bringing the ratio $[HCO_3^-]$ to $[CO_2]$ closer to $20:1$ (Fig. 8.7.3).

However, clearly all is not normal; the plasma $[HCO_3^-]$ was increased as a primary effect of the rise in CO_2 and has been increased further as a secondary consequence of the actions of the kidney. Thus, the other characteristic of a

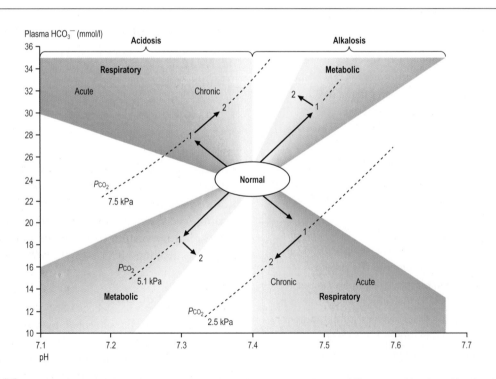

Fig. 8.7.3 Acid–base abnormalities. The relationship between plasma HCO_3^- and pH at different P_{CO_2} (the dotted lines) is shown in this diagram, which is sometimes known as a Davenport diagram. It allows us to illustrate what happens to the acid–base situation in respiratory disturbances (blue) and metabolic disturbances (pink). The primary disturbance moves the situation to the acute position 1. The body then *compensates* by using the intact, undisturbed, system (lungs or kidney) to restore pH to as near normal as possible – position 2.

chronic respiratory acidosis, apart from raised P_{CO_2} and reduced pH, is a raised $[HCO_3^-]$. The only way acid–base balance can be restored completely to normal is by correction of the primary respiratory disorder.

Respiratory alkalosis

This is caused by **hyperventilation** when the individual ventilates more than is necessary to remove the CO_2 generated by metabolism. Excess CO_2 is therefore 'blown off' and plasma P_{CO_2} falls (Fig. 8.7.3). This can be induced voluntarily (experimentally) and it can occur in anxiety states or emotional stress (hyperventilation syndrome). Hyperventilation also occurs at high altitude when respiration is stimulated by hypoxia (see p. 692).

The reaction:

$$CO_2 + H_2O \rightleftharpoons H_2CO_3 \rightleftharpoons H^+ + HCO_3^-$$

is therefore shifted to the left, resulting in a decrease in $[H^+]$ and $[HCO_3^-]$. What happens is essentially the opposite of what happens in respiratory acidosis. Less CO_2 diffuses into the cells and less HCO_3^- diffuses out into the plasma so that $[HCO_3^-]$ is reduced. This fall in $[HCO_3^-]$ tends to decrease the ratio of $[HCO_3^-]$ to $[CO_2]$, but it is not sufficient to reduce it to 20:1 and the pH therefore stays high ($[H^+]$ is low). The decrease in $[H^+]$ in the tubule cells reduces H^+ secretion and decreases HCO_3^- reabsorption. Thus, over days, this renal compensation alters the ratio of $[HCO_3^-]$ to $[CO_2]$ so that it falls closer to 20:1 and the pH returns towards normal. The plasma $[HCO_3^-]$ fell as a consequence of the primary disturbance and falls again as a secondary consequence of renal compensation (Fig. 8.7.3). For the acid–base disturbance to be completely corrected, ventilation must return to normal.

Metabolic acidosis

This can occur because of the ingestion of abnormally large quantities of acids, or because of the excess generation of acids. The latter occurs in severe **exercise** when lactic acid is produced and in diabetes when keto acids are formed. Acidosis also occurs when excess bicarbonate is lost from the gastrointestinal tract by diarrhoea and in renal failure when the kidney fails to excrete H^+. Clearly, the reaction:

$$CO_2 + H_2O \rightleftharpoons H_2CO_3 \rightleftharpoons H^+ + HCO_3^-$$

is shifted to the left if the primary change is a rise in $[H^+]$. If the primary change is a fall in $[HCO_3^-]$, then there will be less buffer available to buffer H^+, the free $[H^+]$ rises and again the reaction shifts to the left. Thus, in all cases there is a reduction in $[HCO_3^-]$, the ratio $[HCO_3^-]$ to $[CO_2]$ falls and the pH falls ($[H^+]$ rises; Fig. 8.7.3).

Assuming there is no respiratory disorder, the rise in $[H^+]$ stimulates respiration, by acting on the peripheral chemoreceptors. Thus, more CO_2 is blown off, the reaction is driven further to the left, the P_{CO_2} falls and the $[HCO_3^-]$ falls further (Fig 8.7.3). This **respiratory compensation** allows the pH to return towards normal because the ratio $[HCO_3^-]$ to $[CO_2]$ rises towards 20:1.

However, because the buffering and hyperventilation are not fully effective in preventing a rise in $[H^+]$, the $[H^+]$ remains raised throughout the body. In the kidney, this stimulates H^+ secretion and HCO_3^- reabsorption. Over days, the kidney (except in renal failure) may be able to correct the disturbance by excreting the excess H^+ and adding to the plasma the HCO_3^- that was lost both as a direct consequence of the primary disturbance and as a secondary consequence of the respiratory compensation. Once this has happened, plasma $[H^+]$ returns to normal and ventilation is also normalized.

Metabolic alkalosis

The most common explanation for this disturbance is the loss of H^+ from the gastrointestinal tract by **vomiting** because gastric secretions are highly acidic. It can also be induced by ingestion of $NaHCO_3$-containing, alkaline antacid indigestion mixtures. In addition, metabolic alkalosis is frequently associated with **volume depletion** because avid reabsorption of Na^+ leads to H^+ secretion and HCO_3^- reabsorption by the kidney (see above). It is also associated with **K^+ depletion** such as can be caused by hyperaldosteronism (see above).

Because metabolic acidosis can be regarded as the addition of a base (or any kind of H^+ acceptor) to the plasma, the reaction:

$$CO_2 + H_2O \rightleftharpoons H_2CO_3 \rightleftharpoons H^+ + HCO_3$$

shifts to the right. What happens is essentially the opposite of what happens in metabolic acidosis (Fig. 8.7.3). The fall in $[H^+]$ reduces the stimulation of the peripheral chemoreceptors, ventilation is reduced and therefore less CO_2 is blown off ($[CO_2]$ rises). This **respiratory compensation** therefore drives the reaction further to the right so that more H^+ is generated and $[HCO_3^-]$ rises further (Fig. 8.7.3). Thus, pH returns towards normal because the ratio $[HCO_3^-]$ to $[CO_2]$ falls towards $20:1$.

As in metabolic acidosis, the kidney may correct the disturbance over several days. The rise in pH (fall in $[H^+]$) in renal tubule cells reduces H^+ secretion (and HCO_3^- reabsorption) so allowing plasma $[H^+]$ to rise, reducing plasma (HCO_3^-) and finally removing the inhibitory effect on ventilation. However, it should be noted that this cannot occur in metabolic alkalosis resulting from volume depletion. In this case, HCO_3^- reabsorption (and H^+ secretion) continues in association with increased Na^+ reabsorption. The acid–base disturbance can only be corrected if the volume depletion is corrected.

Identification of acid–base disturbances

In the clinical setting, it is important not only to be able to recognize that an acid–base

Table 8.7.1 Changes in arterial blood composition in acid–base disturbances

Disturbance	pH	$[HCO_3^-]$	CO_2
Respiratory alkalosis	↑	↓	↓
Metabolic alkalosis	↑	↑	—
Respiratory acidosis	↓	↑	↑
Metabolic acidosis	↓	↓	—

Key: ↑ = above normal; ↓ = below normal; — = normal

disturbance is present, but to be able to identify the cause of the disturbance so that it can be treated appropriately. A simple key is provided in Table 8.7.1. (The degree of these changes depends on the amount of compensation that has taken place.)

The first step is to look at the plasma pH. The buffering, compensatory and corrective mechanisms described above cannot fully correct an acid–base disturbance. Therefore, the pH will still indicate the direction of the original disorder. If pH is >7.4 the disturbance is an alkalosis; if it is < 7.4, it is an acidosis.

Next the $[HCO_3^-]$ and P_{CO_2} must be studied (see Fig. 8.7.3). An uncompensated **respiratory** alkalosis would be associated with P_{CO_2} <40 mmHg and $[HCO_3^-]$ <24 mM. A **metabolic** alkalosis would initially be associated with $[HCO_3^-]$ >24 mM. When renal and respiratory compensation occur for respiratory and metabolic alkalosis respectively, then the pH moves nearer to normal, but $[HCO_3^-]$ falls even further *below* normal in respiratory alkalosis, whereas $[HCO_3^-]$ rises even further *above* normal in metabolic alkalosis. Moreover, in compensated respiratory alkalosis, P_{CO_2} remains low, whereas in compensated metabolic alkalosis P_{CO_2} is high.

On the other hand, respiratory acidosis can be recognized by P_{CO_2} >40 mmHg and $[HCO_3^-]$ >24 mM, the $[HCO_3^-]$ rising even further as a consequence of renal compensation. Metabolic acidosis can be recognized by $[HCO_3^-]$ <24 mmol/litre and P_{CO_2} <40 mmHg.

If the pattern of the pH, $[HCO_3^-]$ and P_{CO_2} disturbance does not correspond with one of these four categories, then a mixed disorder is present, which means that there are two or more underlying causes for the disturbance. An example would be an individual who has chronic bronchitis with a consequent compensated respiratory acidosis who then develops a gastrointestinal infection that leads to vomiting. Metabolic alkalosis will then be superimposed upon the original disorder.

Summary

The structure and functions of the kidney

- The function of the kidneys is to regulate volume and composition of the extracellular fluid. This they do by the processes of filtration, reabsorption and secretion.
- The gross structure of the kidney is a cortex surrounding a medulla and an innermost cavity, the pelvis.
- The functional unit of the kidney is the microscopic nephron (1 million in each kidney).
- Fluid filters into the nephrons at a rate of about 180 litres/day; the vast majority is reabsorbed.
- Filtration is influenced by renal blood flow, which is subject to a high degree of autoregulation, and to control by renal nerves and the renin–angiotensin system.
- There is active reabsorption of substances from the nephron while water flows passively.

- Regulation of absorption is by endocrine factors including prostaglandins, the renin–angiotensin–aldosterone system, atrial natriuretic peptide and the antidiuretic hormone.
- The shape of the loop of Henle enables a process called countercurrent multiplication to produce a hyperosmotic extracellular fluid in the medulla. This is reinforced by movement of urea.
- The kidneys excrete the fixed acids formed and absorbed by the body.
- They control the acid–base balance of the body by reabsorbing bicarbonate, secreting hydrogen ions and forming ammonia at variable rates.
- In disturbances of acid–base balance, the kidneys and lungs act together to restore normality.

Recent Advances

Recombinant erythropoietin and its use in renal failure

Renal failure is characterized by a substantial reduction in GFR, usually to less than 20% of normal, which results in an increase in plasma concentrations of urea and creatinine, substances that are normally cleared by the kidney. Approximately 8000 people die annually in the UK of chronic renal failure and almost 40% of them are in the prime of life. The most common causes of chronic renal failure are diabetes, atherosclerosis that affects the renal artery and damage to the glomeruli secondary to infections of the urinary tract and to congenital renal abnormalities such as polycystic kidney disease. In all cases the number of functioning glomeruli is reduced. This eventually results in an inability to regulate electrolytes and water balance and to excrete organic solutes that include not only urea and creatinine which are non-toxic, but other protein metabolites that are toxic. Thus, oedema, low plasma sodium, high plasma potassium and phosphate, and metabolic acidosis are generally present in patients with untreated renal failure. Dialysis can be used very effectively to remove fluid, regulate electrolyte balance and remove organic solutes, providing the patient is also willing to control the dietary intake of fluid, protein and certain ions. However, even when these factors are well controlled, patients with renal failure are still likely to develop bone disease as a consequence of reduced production of calcitriol, and anaemia as a consequence of reduced production of erythropoietin (EPO) by the kidney.

In the 1980s the gene for EPO was identified on chromosome 7 and, since 1986, human recombinant EPO has been available and has been used increasingly in the treatment of patients with renal failure. It would not be an exaggeration to state that the recombinant EPO has revolutionized the management of these patients. Indeed, it has become apparent that anaemia, rather than a build-up of toxins, is largely responsible for their general feeling of malaise, muscle weakness and fatiguability, cold intolerance, mental sluggishness and loss of appetite. Treatment with EPO not only greatly improves their quality of life, but reduces their tendency to develop left ventricular hypertrophy, a secondary consequence of anaemia that is an independent risk factor for early death.

In parallel with the use of recombinant EPO, our understanding of the synthesis and actions of EPO has been greatly improved by extensive studies on laboratory animals and human tissues, some of which have involved the techniques of molecular biology. The site of production of EPO had been elusive, but it has become clear that the mRNA for EPO is present in the interstitial cells of the renal cortex, near the basal membrane of the proximal tubule cells. Since the proximal tubule cells have a very high O_2 consumption associated with their active transport mechanisms, they are in an ideal position to sense a reduction in O_2 availability. It seems that the O_2 sensor is a haem-containing protein. A reduction in local Po_2 causes a conformational change in the haem protein in much the same way as the haem moiety of haemoglobin in the red blood cell is changed when O_2 is given up by haemoglobin. The conformational change in turn causes the production of a protein named hypoxia-inducible factor (HIF), which increases the rate of transcription of the EPO gene, thereby increasing the synthesis of EPO. EPO has been shown to act, via a specific transmembrane receptor, on the progenitor cells of the bone marrow to potentiate their proliferation, and to be

Recent Advances *(Continued)*

essential for the transformation of progenitor cells into precursor cells. The proliferation and maturation of these cells into erythrocytes is apparently not dependent on EPO.

Therefore, it is clear that in individuals with normal renal function, the kidney plays a pivotal role in determining the O_2 supply to all body tissues. The synthesis of EPO by the kidney is dependent on the supply of O_2 to the kidney, which is itself dependent on the haematocrit as well as on the arterial Po_2. In a normal individual, plasma EPO levels are high enough to keep the haematocrit stable and within the normal range, and EPO synthesis by kidney is increased in anaemia, following haemorrhage and in systemic hypoxia such as occurs in respiratory disease and at high altitude. EPO is also produced by macrophages and the liver, but this extrarenal production contributes less than 20% of the total and cannot compensate for loss of renal production in renal failure.

In fact, many studies have shown that in patients with renal failure there may be such a gross impairment of O_2 sensing and EPO production that the haematocrit is less than 30%

of normal and EPO production fails to show the normal increase in response to acute exacerbation of the anaemic hypoxia. In such patients, administration of human recombinant EPO produces a dose-dependent increase in the plasma concentration of EPO and in the haematocrit, but the sensitivity of this relationship varies between individuals. The cause of this variability has not yet been established; it may be that varying concentrations of an inhibitor of EPO are present in different individuals. The only serious complication associated with the use of EPO is the development of arterial hypertension, which has been reported in about 30% of individuals in some clinical studies. This is thought to be associated with the increase in blood viscosity that results from the increase in haematocrit. It seems that this can be avoided if the upper target for the haematocrit is limited to 30–35% and providing fluid gain is well controlled between periods of analysis. The patient then receives the benefits of amelioration of the anaemia without incurring the risks of hypertension.

Urine collection and micturition

8.8

Passage of urine from kidney to bladder

Urine passes from the collecting ducts of the renal tubules into the renal **pelvis**. Contraction of the smooth muscle of the pelvis aids the movement of urine into the **ureter**. When distended, the smooth muscle of the ureter, which is arranged circularly, contracts. This contraction closes the junction between the pelvis and the ureter and pushes urine further into the ureter, causing distension and subsequent contraction of the next section of the ureter, and so on. Thus a peristaltic wave is initiated, which propagates along the length of the ureter and propels urine into the **bladder**. Peristaltic waves are initiated about five times per minute from the renal pelvis.

Each ureter joins the bladder at an oblique angle, passing between the epithelium and smooth muscle for a short distance before it opens into the bladder. This arrangement helps to ensure that when pressure within the bladder rises, the ureters are compressed, so preventing reflux of urine up into the ureters. If the ureter is blocked by a kidney stone, then the pressure in the ureter rises sharply because of continuing peristaltic contraction. This causes considerable pain (renal colic) but may help to dislodge the stone and push it into the bladder.

⚡ Summary

Passage of urine from kidney to bladder

- Urine passes from the renal pelvis into the ureters, aided by contraction of the smooth muscle of the pelvis.
- Contraction of the smooth muscle of the distended ureter initiates a wave of peristalsis that propels urine into the bladder.
- When pressure within the bladder rises, reflux of urine is prevented by pressure on the ureters as they pass through the bladder wall.

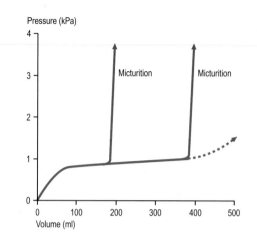

Fig. 8.8.1 Pressure changes in the bladder. Pressure increases a little on initial filling from empty. However, filling from 50–400 ml occurs with very little increase in pressure. When micturition occurs, from a small or larger bladder volume, pressure rises very steeply; the dotted line shows the pressure change that would have occurred, had micturition not happened.

Micturition

Micturition is the act of emptying the urinary bladder – urination. Urine is formed continuously at a rate of about 1 ml per minute in normally hydrated subjects. It is stored and released, by adult humans, when it is socially acceptable and convenient to do so. Storage and controlled release is the function of the urinary bladder and its associated sphincters.

The bladder

The bladder lies in the pelvis, below the peritoneum. The bladder can be almost empty or contain up to 400 ml without much increase in pressure (Fig. 8.8.1). This feature is a result of its structure. Because the bladder is essentially spherical, the relationship between pressure in the bladder, its radius and wall tension follows the law of Laplace (see p. 658) which states that lumen pressure is equal to twice the wall tension divided by the radius. Thus, even though the wall tension may increase as the bladder fills, so does the radius and the increase in lumen pressure is small, at least until bladder volume becomes large. Importantly, the mucosal lining of the bladder is **transitional epithelium**, well capable of stretch without damage, and thrown into ridges that flatten out as the bladder fills. This epithelium has unique properties: it is very impermeable to salts and water, which means that there is no exchange between the urine and the capillaries of the bladder wall.

The muscle coat around the lining epithelium is made up of bundles of smooth muscle, interlacing, running in all directions and stimulated to contract by **parasympathetic** fibres that run in the pelvic nerves. These layers of muscle are best considered as a single structure, the **detrusor muscle**. The mucosal lining is generally loosely attached to the underlying muscle, except at the base of the bladder where the entrance of the two ureters and the exit of the urethra form a triangle – the **trigone** – where the mucosa is firmly attached. This forms the thickest and least distensible part of the bladder. The outlet of the bladder into the urethra is guarded by two sphincters: internal and external.

The internal sphincter

The internal sphincter is formed by a loop of muscle that is an extension of the detrusor muscle: it is not under voluntary control. When the detrusor muscle contracts, the fibres forming this loop shorten, so shortening and widening the proximal part of the urethra and opening the sphincter.

The external sphincter

The external sphincter, which is composed of skeletal muscle, is continuous with the **levator ani**: it is under conscious, voluntary control by somatic motor nerves that run in the **pudendal nerve**. These muscles are kept contracted by tonic stimulation from the brain and they are responsible for continence. In women, the structures round this neck are the end of the system and the point of exit of urine from the body. The external sphincter muscle is rather poorly developed and women are more prone to become incontinent, particularly after childbirth. In men, the urethra continues through the penis: urine remaining in the urethra can be expelled by contractions of the bulbocavernosus muscle. These different arrangements mean that men and women tend to develop different pathologies (see below).

Filling and emptying

The muscular wall of the bladder contains **stretch receptors** that measure tension and transmit the sensation of fullness to the spinal cord via the pelvic nerves; from there the information is transmitted to the brain. Filling of the bladder excites the stretch receptors, increasing the afferent activity in the pelvic nerve and causing a reflex increase in the activity of the

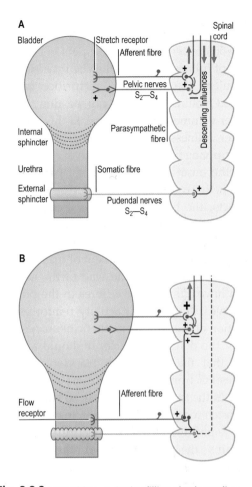

Fig. 8.8.2 Micturition. A. During filling, the descending inhibitory influence on the parasympathetic supply to the detrusor muscle and the descending excitatory influence on the somatic supply to the external sphincter *inhibit* micturition (– and + signs indicate inhibitory and excitatory influences respectively). **B.** During emptying, *activation* of the parasympathetic supply to the detrusor muscle causes its contraction, and *removal* of the tonic excitatory influence on the somatic supply to the external sphincter causes its opening. Emptying of the bladder is facilitated by the input from the flow receptors in the urethra, which reinforces the contraction of the detrusor muscle and the relaxation of the external sphincter.

parasympathetic fibres in the pelvic nerve. This, in turn, causes contraction of the detrusor muscle and micturition. The sensitivity of this reflex is determined by descending influences from the brain (Fig. 8.8.2A). There is a dominant tonic inhibitory influence over this reflex such that the bladder is allowed to fill until it contains ~300 ml, even though the person becomes aware of fullness at ~150 ml. When it is socially convenient, the process of micturition can be initiated voluntarily. This can be done at all bladder volumes up to ~600 ml: at this volume, bladder fullness causes the sensation of pain and emptying becomes imperative.

At the onset of micturition the parasympathetic activity increases, the detrusor muscle contracts, the bladder pressure increases, the internal sphincter opens and urine passes through the internal sphincter into the urethra (see Fig. 8.8.2B). This movement of urine stimulates **flow receptors** in the wall of the urethra which have afferent nerve fibres in the pudendal nerves. This afferent activity reinforces the excitation of the parasympathetic neurones that supply the detrusor muscle. It should also be noted that the increase in bladder pressure that results from detrusor muscle contraction increases the tension in the wall, so stimulating the stretch receptors and reinforcing the reflex. Thus, a positive-feedback cycle develops that maintains the contraction of the detrusor muscle.

The afferent activity from the flow receptors also exerts an inhibitory influence over the **somatic neurones** that supply the external sphincter and the strong descending voluntary control over these neurones is also removed (Fig. 8.8.2B). Thus, the external sphincter opens and urine is forced out of the body. Once initiated, micturition normally proceeds until the bladder is emptied. The process is aided by contraction of the abdominal muscles and lowering of the diaphragm. However, micturition can be halted, particularly in men, by voluntary contraction of the external sphincter. This is followed by inhibition of the reflex contraction of the detrusor muscle.

The detrusor muscle also receives a sympathetic nerve supply that originates in the upper lumbar segments of the spinal cord and is carried to the bladder in the **hypogastric nerve**. Stimulation of these fibres causes relaxation of the detrusor muscle and because the internal sphincter is formed by an extension of the detrusor muscle (see above) they also tend to close this sphincter. These fibres may exert a tonic inhibitory influence upon the detrusor muscle that facilitates bladder filling. However, they play no part in micturition. It is thought that they are activated during **ejaculation**: the sympathetic fibres that supply the seminal vesicles and vas deferens via the hypogastric nerves are activated, so propelling semen into the urethra, and the activation of the sympathetic fibres that supply the detrusor muscle closes the internal sphincter, preventing semen from entering the bladder.

Voluntary control of urination normally develops over the first few years of life when the child learns to control the external sphincter and levator muscles. It is thought that voluntary initiation of micturition involves relaxation of the levator ani and external sphincter muscles. Because contraction of these muscles not only closes the external sphincter but compresses the ureters towards the bladder, their relaxation allows the pelvic floor to drop and causes a downward tug on the urethra and bladder. This additional stretch on the detrusor muscle is sufficient to cause reflex contraction of the detrusor muscle via the parasympathetic nerves. This process may be aided by voluntary contraction of the diaphragm and abdominal muscles, which helps to increase the pressure in the bladder.

Disruption of the descending influences or of the pathways involved in the spinal reflexes disturbs normal micturition, for example following spinal transection (see Clinical Example).

Summary

Micturition

- Emptying the bladder (micturition) is a reflex process, which is usually under conscious control.
- The bladder distends as urine flows into it but because of its structure the increase in lumen pressure is small until bladder volume becomes large.
- Micturition can be initiated voluntarily up to bladder volumes of ~600 ml, above which emptying becomes imperative.
- Stretch receptors in the bladder wall are stimulated by distension of the bladder and cause it to contract via a spinal reflex and activation of the parasympathetic supply to the detrusor muscle. This increases pressure in the bladder and the internal sphincter opens.
- Concomitantly the inhibitory influence from the brain over the somatic nerves that contract the external sphincter is removed, allowing urine to pass through into the urethra.
- Stimulation by the urine of flow receptors in the urethral wall provides input that reinforces contraction of the bladder and relaxation of the external sphincter.
- The process of micturition is aided by contraction of the abdominal muscles and lowering of the diaphragm.

Clinical Example

Bladder function in the paraplegic patient

Acute paraplegia results from severing of the spinal cord, often in the lower cervical region, owing to a diving, sporting or road traffic injury. For reasons which are not clear, the sudden withdrawal of an input from the brain causes the spinal reflexes to fail, typically for several weeks, so there is an early *spinal shock* and a later *brisk reflex* stage. Bladder emptying is a spinal stretch reflex and behaves like other such reflexes (e.g. knee and ankle jerks) in the paraplegic patient.

Failure, in the spinal shock phase, of the bladder emptying reflex, whose coordinating centre lies in the sacral spinal cord, means that stretching of the bladder as it fills with urine fails to elicit reflex emptying. Without intervention, the bladder would continue to distend until overfilling resulted in a slow trickle of urine (overflow incontinence). Constant overdistension for several weeks would lead to damage to the bladder and, to avoid this, a tube (bladder catheter) is passed into it so that drainage can take place and overdistension is avoided.

In the recovery phase after the spinal shock phase, the spinal reflexes, including bladder emptying, return. For the bladder this means that input to the sacral segments of the spinal cord from stretch receptors in the bladder wall leads to reflex activation of coordinated bladder emptying. This is brought about mainly by parasympathetic nerves activating the detrusor muscle of the bladder, with accompanying relaxation of the sphincter muscles.

Clinical Example *(Continued)*

Because of the severing of connections between the brain and the sacral cord, the patient is unaware of the state of the bladder and cannot by volition alone initiate or inhibit micturition. The micturition reflex is now autonomous, with the sacral cord behaving as a small accessory brain, sensing filling of the bladder and deciding when it is to be emptied.

This state of affairs provides satisfactory emptying of the bladder but the time of emptying cannot be predicted with any accuracy. To avoid incontinence, the patient needs a method of initiating the reflex at an appropriate time. This can be provided in several ways. At an appropriate interval from the last emptying, when the bladder can be expected to be approaching the threshold volume for automatic emptying, the patient may be able to apply pressure to the abdomen to raise bladder pressure and trigger the micturition reflex by stretching the bladder wall. Alternatively, this may be done by an attendant, and the reflex can sometimes also be elicited by stimulation of the perineal area or adjoining thigh.

Another reflex which is centred in the sacral spinal cord and behaves similarly in the paraplegic patient is the defecation reflex. In the spinal shock phase the reflex is lost so that the rectum would distend and eventually semisolid faeces would leak out (faecal incontinence). The solution at this stage is to wash out the rectum regularly by using an enema. Later on, automatic emptying develops and the aim is to develop strategies to ensure that this occurs at a convenient time.

The prostate

The differences in structure between the urinary tracts of men and women result in different incidence of pathologies. Women have much shorter urethras than men and are therefore much more susceptible to bacterial invasion of the bladder. In men, the urethra penetrates the **prostate gland**, which in about half the men over 60 undergoes **benign hyperplasia**. This enlargement only presents a problem when the prostate compresses the urethra to such a degree that the bladder cannot empty properly. In the early stages, the detrusor muscle hypertrophies, so helping to force urine out against the increased resistance. As the condition progresses, the discomfort of a constantly overfilled bladder and the damage to bladder and kidneys that retention can cause require treatment of the condition. This can be by drugs that shrink the prostate by interrupting the action of hormones that stimulate it or by surgical removal of the gland.

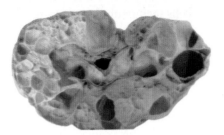

Applied physiology

8.9

Renal failure

Introduction – patterns and causes

Renal failure is present when the normal functions of the kidneys, e.g. regulation of the extracellular levels of electrolytes and waste products, are shown to be quantitatively deficient. Often the first indication is a raised blood level of urea and creatinine. For precise diagnosis, the blood creatinine level and the 24-hour creatinine excretion can be combined to measure creatinine clearance and hence demonstrate a *reduced glomerular filtration rate.* (Clearance = [urinary concentration] × [urinary flow ml/min]/[plasma concentration].)

Renal failure is described in terms of its time-course and cause. *Acute renal failure* manifests itself in the course of days, and sometimes is recognized within hours, as when a patient fails to pass any urine (anuria) postoperatively owing to complete loss of renal function as a result of processes operating during the anaesthetic and surgery. It may show rapid recovery when a treatable cause is addressed. *Chronic renal failure* in contrast often unfolds over a period of months or years. Causes of renal failure can be grouped as prerenal, renal and postrenal, referring to the flow of fluid from the circulation, through the kidneys and from the kidneys into the lower renal tract.

Prerenal renal failure

This is due to a failure of renal perfusion. The normal resting renal blood flow of about a fifth of the cardiac output

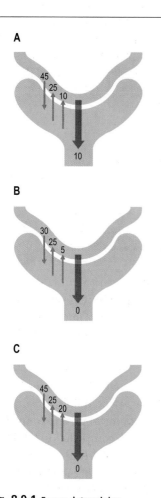

Fig. 8.9.1 Forces determining glomerular filtration, and mechanisms of pre- and postrenal renal failure. **A.** The pressures involved in glomerular filtration are from left to right, glomerular capillary hydrostatic pressure (P_{GC}) and the opposing plasma oncotic pressure (π_{GC}) and Bowman's capsular hydrostatic pressure (P_{BC}). The net filtration pressure (broad arrow) equals $45 - (25 + 10) = 10$ mmHg. **B.** A fall in glomerular capillary hydrostatic pressure results in a zero filtration pressure and cessation of filtration. **C.** A rise in Bowman's capsular hydrostatic pressure results in a zero filtration pressure and abolishes filtration.

provides an important buffer to protect the vital cerebral and coronary circulations in times of circulatory stress. Thus, when a patient suffers a serious haemorrhage, e.g. 20% of the blood volume, non-vital circulations are reduced by the vasoconstrictor action of sympathetic nerves. Such vasoconstriction takes place in the skin initially and as the situation deteriorates, i.e. the blood volume continues to decrease, the vasoconstriction spreads to the viscera, including the kidneys. The combination of a fall in general arterial pressure and compensatory vasoconstriction of the renal resistance vessels (glomerular afferent arterioles) leads to a fall in glomerular capillary hydrostatic pressure (P_{GC}), so that eventually it no longer exceeds the combined opposing pressures of the plasma oncotic pressure (π_{GC}) and the hydrostatic pressure in the Bowman's capsule (P_{BC}). Filtration and formation of urine then cease (Fig. 8.9.1B).

'Renal' renal failure

Here the cause of the renal failure lies within the kidneys themselves. Firstly, following on from the prerenal circulatory cause just mentioned, an even more severe failure of the renal circulation may, in addition to abolishing the filtration pressure gradient, lead to a blood flow so low that it is

inadequate for the metabolic needs of the renal cells. This typically leads to serious damage or death (necrosis) of the highly active renal tubular cells (acute tubular necrosis) and hence acute (potentially reversible) renal failure.

A great variety of diseases can lead to gradual destruction of the kidneys. These include infectious and other inflammatory causes, the deposition of toxic material and in some cases overstretching when there is raised pressure due to obstruction of the urinary tract (this overlaps with the postrenal renal failure considered below). The end result of all these varied diseases is that the normal finely structured architecture of the kidney, on which normal function relies, is replaced by tiny scarred organs, or by abnormal material, or by thin-walled expanded sacs. Since structure and function are complexly and intimately related in the kidneys, it is not surprising that these abnormal organs steadily decline in their capacity to maintain homeostasis of the body fluids and eventually become worse than useless. Removal is often carried out when the kidneys are actually harming the body, e.g. by causing hypertension.

Postrenal renal failure

In this case the cause of the problem lies distal to the kidneys. Obstruction to the renal tract can occur in one ureter and lead to loss of function of the corresponding kidney, but to cause renal failure, both kidneys must be affected, so the obstruction is usually in the urethra. Most commonly this is in the male and due to obstruction by an enlarged prostate gland. In this case (Fig. 8.9.1C), glomerular filtration is reduced and eventually abolished by back pressure which elevates the glomerular capsular pressure to cancel out the normal reserve of the glomerular capillary pressure over the opposing plasma protein oncotic pressure. At this stage renal failure develops, but if the obstruction is promptly relieved the kidneys may recover.

Effects

The effects of renal failure are due to impairment of the range of normal functions, which can be grouped under the headings: (a) fluid and electrolyte balance; (b) excretion; and (c) endocrine functions. The distinction between (a) and (b) is that balance is maintained by great variation in the amounts of various substances lost in the urine, whereas excretion refers particularly to unwanted substances which, as far as possible, are totally eliminated from the body.

Failure of fluid and electrolyte balance

Balance is maintained in terms of sodium chloride, which determines extracellular fluid volume, osmolality, which determines total body water, potassium, and hydrogen ions (acid–base balance).

Sodium chloride

Sodium chloride has been called the skeleton of the extracellular fluid. The reason is that its ions constitute the great bulk of the dissolved particles in extracellular fluid. Osmoregulation will determine that these ions are dissolved in an appropriate volume of water, thereby determining extracellular fluid volume. Extracellular fluid volume tends to rise in renal failure because most people take more salt than they need in their diet and the kidney can no longer excrete the surplus. The extracellular volume may increase until the body is seriously waterlogged, with massive dependent oedema and the risk of circulatory overload (blood plasma volume rises and falls with extracellular volume) and fatal pulmonary oedema. Less commonly, the body may lose extracellular fluid, e.g. with diarrhoea or vomiting, and in this case the kidney may make matters worse by failing to conserve salt.

Osmolality

Osmolality of the urine varies widely in the healthy young adult – from around four times the normal body value of 285 mOsm/kg H_2O to around one-third of this (Fig. 8.9.2). The negative feedback system involved has detectors in the region of the hypothalamus. When extracellular osmolality rises, e.g. by the ingestion of salt in the diet, water is drawn out of the detector cells, which shrink. Signals are sent from the hypothalamus down the axons of the pituitary stalk and vasopressin (antidiuretic hormone) is released from the posterior pituitary into the circulation. This acts on the cells of the renal collecting ducts to induce water channels so that most of the water remaining in the glomerular filtrate is reabsorbed owing to the increasing osmolality of the interstitium of the renal medulla as the collecting ducts pass towards the renal pelvis.

In renal failure the whole architecture of the kidney is damaged so that the delicate structure with its countercurrent mechanism, which allows water reabsorption, steadily falls in efficiency. The cells that create the osmotic gradient from renal cortex (osmolality around 300 mOsm/kg H_2O) to inner medulla (around 1200 mOsm/kg H_2O) and that lead to a filtrate osmolality of around 100 mOsm/kg H_2O as

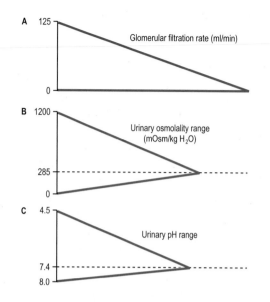

Fig. 8.9.2 Progression of renal failure. The condition worsens from left to right as shown by the decline in the glomerular filtration rate. Meanwhile, the ability to vary urinary composition declines (over a 12-range for osmolality). Eventually, urine of constant tonicity cannot correct errors in body fluid osmolality. The same applies to the ability to produce strongly acid or alkaline urine. The initial values would apply to a healthy young adult.

the fluid leaves the distal convoluted tubules and enters the collecting ducts, decrease in number and the essential structure is disrupted. The remaining nephrons have no power to modify the osmolality of their contents from that of the filtrate so the urine has a fixed osmolality similar to that of the body fluids. Figure 8.9.2B indicates this situation where, as renal failure progresses, the range of urinary osmolality contracts, so that eventually the urine is of fixed composition ('isosthenuria' or 'same strength urine') and cannot correct disturbances in body osmolality.

Potassium

Potassium is normally secreted in the urine in accordance with body needs, by a pump which exchanges absorbed sodium for secreted potassium or hydrogen ions. As the system fails, the body is at the mercy of the amount of ingested ion for its content of that ion. Potentially, either deficiency or excess of potassium could result, but in practice an excess of potassium is much more common, especially in diets which restrict salt and protein in order to minimize accumulation of salt and the toxic products of protein. Potassium can rise quickly,

particularly if there is breakdown of body cells as in acute renal tubular necrosis due to ischaemia. Major cardiac problems are a serious risk and are often preceded by increasingly high T waves in the electrocardiogram.

Hydrogen ions

Hydrogen ion accumulation is one of the most serious problems of renal failure. The degree of accumulation approaches that in diabetic ketoacidosis. In both these examples of non-respiratory acidosis, or *metabolic acidosis*, involuntary hyperventilation (Kussmaul respiration) provides *respiratory compensation*, which limits the fall in pH (see Fig. 8.7.3, p. 776). The Henderson–Hasselbalch relationship indicates that hydrogen ion content is proportional to the ratio: [carbon dioxide concentration]/[bicarbonate ion concentration]. Hydrogen ion accumulation reduces the bicarbonate concentration because of buffering. Reducing the carbon dioxide concentration then helps to restore the ratio, and hence the hydrogen ion concentration, to normal. However, despite this compensation, in severe renal failure, a seriously low pH contributes to coma and death. Figure 8.9.2C indicates how the ability to vary urinary pH is lost as renal failure progresses. Remember that the normal range of pH (4.5–8) indicates a variation in hydrogen ion excretion of about 3000-fold. In addition, the normal kidney has the ability (again lost in renal failure) to synthesize and secrete ammonia to buffer secreted hydrogen ions.

Failure of excretion

Many toxins are steadily cleared from the body by mechanisms that transport them into the tubular fluid, similarly but in the reverse direction to the transport of glucose out of the tubular fluid. Like the glucose transport mechanism, they have a tubular maximum above which no more can be excreted, but in normal life there is considerable reserve. However, as renal tissue is lost, the capacity to excrete falls below the required level and the toxins accumulate. Many of these toxins are protein-related. The major protein excretory product urea, is not, however, a major toxin. Infusions of urea which raise the level well above normal do not harm normal people, though an osmotic diuresis is likely to be produced as the urea molecules retain water in the tubular fluid. Thus it is assumed that other protein-derived toxins (not fully defined) are responsible for the depression of body function, including drowsiness and impairment of consciousness, associated with renal failure.

Such effects are reduced by restricting protein intake, which also reduces the acid residue of metabolized proteins.

An important consequence of failure of secretion is that *drugs* may accumulate excessively in the body. When a patient with severe renal failure is given the normal daily dose of, for example, antibiotics, the levels may build up over a few days to seriously toxic levels. This can be allowed for if the glomerular filtration rate is known. If it is half normal, then the clearance of the drug will be around half normal; if filtration rate is a quarter normal, then clearance will be correspondingly slowed. A normal loading dose can be given for prompt action and the maintenance dose is reduced in relation to the glomerular filtration rate. This applies to drugs whose elimination is mainly or entirely due to renal excretion. The situation is different for drugs whose elimination is due mainly to metabolic breakdown, e.g. morphine in the liver.

Failure of endocrine functions

Major endocrine functions of the kidney include control of red cell formation via erythropoietin and control of arterial blood pressure via the renin–angiotensin system. Renal failure can lead to anaemia and hypertension.

Anaemia

Anaemia in renal failure, particularly severe renal failure, is related mainly to deficiency of *erythropoietin*. This is evidenced by the dramatic improvement in anaemia in these patients when they are given the hormone therapeutically (a currently very expensive form of treatment produced by genetically modified bacteria, see Recent Advances, p. 780). Erythropoietin is believed to be formed in the renal cortex, in metabolically very active cells able to sense the hypoxia due to anaemia (or arterial desaturation, see p. 693). The patient with renal failure produces less and less of the hormone and in some cases the haemoglobin level falls well below half normal. Treatment with erythropoietin can then double the red blood cell and haemoglobin level, greatly increasing the potential for physical activity by doubling the total available oxygen in the circulation. In fact care has to be taken to avoid the red blood cell concentration becoming too high, as this can increase the risk of vascular occlusion.

Hypertension

Hypertension has long been recognized as a complication of renal disease, including renal failure. The mechanisms involved are complex and have been studied for many decades

793

without complete elucidation. However, major causes are likely to be secretion of inappropriately large amounts of renin and inability to excrete adequate amounts of salt and water. Particularly in early renal failure, parts of the kidney may suffer from inadequate circulation (ischaemia) and secrete *renin* from the juxtaglomerular cells. The renin activates a circulating peptide to angiotensin I and this is converted in the circulation, particularly the pulmonary capillaries, to angiotensin II with its dual actions of vasoconstriction and stimulation of the salt- and water-retaining hormone aldosterone from the zona glomerulosa of the adrenal cortex. This would account for the hypertension in early renal failure. Later in renal failure, retention of salt and water probably plays a role – the patient's blood pressure can be reduced during dialysis by the removal of salt and water from the circulation.

Investigations

The diagnosis of renal failure may be suggested in a number of clinical situations, e.g. failure to pass urine postoperatively, or gradual development of weakness and drowsiness in someone with recurrent urinary infections. Biochemical studies, however are needed for confirmation.

Quantitative confirmation of failure and assessment of its severity are obtained by measuring the glomerular filtration rate. While inulin clearance is regarded as the gold standard, *creatinine clearance* is also useful and is much easier to measure. Instead of requiring infusion of inulin, use is made of a naturally occurring blood component and clearance can be measured by combining the plasma creatinine level (measured routinely) with measurement of the volume and creatinine level in a 24-hour collection of urine. Glomerular filtration rate equals creatinine clearance, which equals [urinary creatinine concentration] × [urinary volume/minute]/ [plasma creatinine concentration]. The average adult value is around 120–150 ml/minute, so a value below 100 suggests possible early impairment, a value below 50 definite failure and a value around 5–10 ml/minute indicates severe failure, requiring dialysis. Normal values, like lung volumes, vary with body size, sex and age, with much smaller values in infants and young children. As usual, *serial measurements* are particularly helpful in deciding whether the condition is getting worse or improving.

Once the diagnosis is established, and particularly in severe failure, details of the condition and guidance to treatment can be obtained from plasma measurements of various electrolytes, including sodium and potassium, together with acid–base assessment by measuring arterial blood pH and blood gases, and bicarbonate levels. Haemoglobin levels will indicate whether anaemia is present, and, if so, its severity. In appropriate cases, X-ray studies may be used to detect abnormalities of the kidneys. If required, the function of each kidney can be assessed separately by collecting its urine from a ureteric catheter and measuring creatinine clearance.

Finally, a simple but fundamental test, not often used in view of more precise measurements, is to assess the *range of urinary concentration*. This can be done by depriving a person of fluids for up to 24 hours to assess maximal concentration (normally sparse dark-yellow urine with a high specific gravity, around 1.030 or more, and an osmolality around 1000 mOsm/kg H_2O) and then obtaining a urinary sample when the person has taken a surplus litre of fluid when already fully hydrated, to assess minimal concentration (copious clear urine with a specific gravity around 1.001 and an osmolality around 100 mOsm/kg H_2O). In everyday life we can observe these variations. Someone whose urine varies from deep yellow to clear is unlikely to have renal failure, lying well to the left in Figure 8.9.2.

Treatment

Treatment can be in four forms:

- conservative
- haemodialysis
- peritoneal dialysis
- renal transplantation.

These treatments deal with the problem in very different ways.

Conservative treatment

This refers to the adjustment of food and fluid intake to minimize the load on the kidneys. Because protein provides the bulk of dietary toxins, it is restricted to around a quarter of normal. Because the patient's energy requirements must be met to prevent breakdown of the tissues (releasing amino acids) the carbohydrate and fat content must be fairly high. Fluids should be adjusted to balance the patient's urinary output, and electrolytes adjusted according to the plasma levels. Usually this means a low sodium content. Overall this diet is difficult to maintain, unpalatable and of limited effectiveness, but the general principles are applied, in a rather more relaxed manner, during long-term dialysis as a back-up to this therapy.

Haemodialysis

Introduction of this treatment has dramatically extended life in patients with severe renal failure. The principle is simple. The patient's blood is withdrawn from the circulation and passed through tubing surrounded by a dialysate fluid. The tubing is permeable to water and to the smaller particles in the blood, including ions, glucose, urea and creatinine, but the tubing does not allow plasma proteins and cellular elements to be lost from the blood. The dialysate fluid is free of unwanted items such as urea and contains appropriate amounts of various ions. Thus, if there is need to lose sodium, the dialysate will have a low sodium content. The dialysate should also be free of unwanted materials and care is needed to avoid infection. The patient's 'purified' blood is then returned to the circulation.

Advancing technology has led to increasingly efficient systems which, rather like the kidney, contain multiple fine tubes in a very small space. However, the simple principle of equilibration with a dialysate is much different from the sophistication of normal renal function with its filtration, reabsorption, excretion, medullary osmotic gradient, complex vasculature and hormonal control.

For early 'artificial kidney' treatment, the patient's blood was drawn from an artery and returned to a vein. However, with dialysis required two or three times per week for an indefinite period, this led to serious problems with arteries damaged by repeated punctures. Then the concept of an *arteriovenous shunt* was developed. Initially a tube connected a forearm artery and vein. The tube rather than the artery and vein could then be punctured for dialysis. However, this tubing was uncomfortable and there was a considerable risk of bleeding. Finally, a *surgical arteriovenous fistula* was devised. An opening, usually in the radial artery, was connected to a nearby vein so that the forearm veins draining the fistula became dilated and carried an adequate flow for dialysis. Haemodialysis using such 'arterialized' veins can maintain health for long periods, provided there are no complications with thrombosis or infection.

Peritoneal dialysis

This is an alternative to haemodialysis – it uses the capillaries of the peritoneal cavity as the tubing, and fluid passed into the peritoneal cavity and withdrawn after an equilibration period as the dialysate. The dialysate is supplied in plastic bags and is passed into the peritoneal cavity under the influence of gravity by raising the bag above the level of the patient's abdomen. The peritoneal cavity is capable of holding several litres of fluid without any difficulty. In practice, fluid is kept in the peritoneal cavity almost continuously. About four times a day, the patient drains as much fluid as possible by connecting an empty bag to the peritoneal cavity and placing the bag on the floor. When drainage has ceased, a fresh 2-litre bag is hung up well above the patient's abdomen and the fluid run in. Thus solute exchange can proceed throughout the day and night by a procedure analogous in slow motion to gas exchange in the alveolar air, replenished by the tidal ventilation. This process has the advantage of relative simplicity compared with haemodialysis but it is laborious for the patient and still carries the risk of infection.

Treatment with erythropoietin has already been mentioned in relation to endocrine disturbances of renal failure. It is, of course, not required with successful renal transplantation and this is now the definitive treatment which can liberate patients from the onerous demands of either form of dialysis treatment.

Renal transplantation

Renal transplantation is now well established. The requirements are:

1. connection of the renal artery of the transplanted organ to any convenient artery in the recipient
2. a corresponding venous connection
3. connection of the donor ureter to the patient's bladder, and
4. prevention of rejection of the kidney.

In practice, the donor kidney is usually placed in one of the iliac fossae, with attachments to the neighbouring major blood vessels. Prevention of rejection is achieved by as close a match as possible for cellular antigens (identical twins have provided a perfect match on rare occasions) and by drugs, including glucocorticoids, which suppress immune responses. The donor organ may come from a relative, friend, or from the body of someone who has died in circumstances where the kidney can be removed prior to post-mortem deterioration. The organ must then be preserved prior to transplantation, sometimes during a considerable journey,

to a well-matched recipient. It is kept in isotonic solution at around 4–5°C. This temperature is high enough to avoid freezing, with the disastrous formation of destructive ice crystals, and low enough to reduce the metabolic rate of the renal cells to ensure survival for several hours.

Once the organ has been 'plumbed in', it will begin to function and produce urine. While various blood tests may give clues about transplant rejection, measurements of glomerular filtration rate by creatinine clearance provide the definitive indication of function. A substantial and gradually rising clearance indicates good function, whereas a falling clearance suggests that rejection has begun. Prior to transplantation, the kidney had provided half the renal function and the initial glomerular filtration rate of the transplanted kidney will be about half normal. However, as the sole kidney in the recipient, the organ will undergo gradual hypertrophy with an increase in glomerular filtration rate over the next 2–3 months. All functions of the kidney, including appropriate formation of erythropoietin, can be expected to be normal.

Further reading

Holmes O 1993 *Human acid-base physiology.* Arnold, London

Of all aspects of renal physiology, this subject gives students most trouble. This book will help them overcome their problems. It very usefully provides the physical chemistry to understand the principles of the physiology and a substantial glossary of terms. Revision is aided by collecting key material into tables and providing self-tests.

Koeppen B M, Stanton B A 2000 *Renal physiology,* 3rd edn. Mosby, St Louis.

This book focuses on essential points in a concise way. The end of chapter summaries and self-test exams are a great help to learning.

Lote C J 1994 *Principles of renal physiology,* 4th edn. Kluwer Academic Publishers, Dortrecht, Netherlands.

A first-class concise book for undergraduates, written in a very clear style and suitable for systems-based courses. The author has the ability to make complex concepts clear.

Seldin D W, Giebisch G 2000 *The kidney.* Lippincott Williams and Wilkins, Philadelphia.

This comprehensive work in two volumes provides a first line of reference on the subject of renal physiology and pathophysiology.

Questions

Answer true or false to the following
statements:

8.1

Glomerular filtration rate:
A. Can be measured using a substance that is
   completely cleared from the plasma.
B. Tends to increase in hypoalbuminaemia.
C. Tends to increase when the efferent
   arteriole is constricted.
D. Increases during strenuous exercise.
E. Is normally closer to 40% than 20% of the
   renal plasma flow.

8.2

**When renal clearance of a substance X is
measured in a normal individual:**
A. If the clearance is 250 ml/min, then X must
   be secreted by the nephron.
B. If the clearance is 60 ml/min, then X must
   be reabsorbed from the nephron.
C. If the clearance is zero, then X may be
   glucose.
D. The clearance of X may be calculated from
   the arterial–venous concentration difference
   in the renal vessels.
E. If the clearance rises linearly with plasma
   concentration, then it is likely that X is
   freely filtered but is neither secreted nor
   reabsorbed in the nephron.

8.3

In the proximal convoluted tubule:
A. The epithelium is flat and contains few
   mitochondria.
B. Reabsorption of water increases the
   osmolality of the tubular fluid which enters
   the loop of Henle.
C. The rate of water absorption increases as
   the glomerular filtration fraction increases.
D. Bicarbonate reabsorption is coupled to
   H^+ secretion.
E. The T_m for phosphate reabsorption is
   increased by parathormone (PTH).

8.4

The loop of Henle:
A. Actively pumps ions across the epithelium
   of the descending limb.
B. Has a low permeability to water in the thick
   portion of the ascending limb.
C. Makes use of countercurrent exchange to
   amplify the ionic concentration gradients
   generated by active pumps.
D. Is responsible for the high osmolality in the
   renal medulla.
E. Returns a fluid of high osmolality to the
   distal convoluted tubule.

8.5

Renal sympathetic nerves:
A. Are adrenergic.
B. Preferentially constrict the efferent arteriole,
   helping to maintain GFR.
C. Reduce renal blood flow during maximal
   exercise.
D. Stimulate renin production.
E. Inhibit Na^+ reabsorption from the
   convoluted tubules.

8.6

In heart failure:

A. The levels of circulating renin are likely to be high.
B. The levels of angiotensin II are likely to be high.
C. The levels of aldosterone are likely to be high.
D. Treatment with an inhibitor of angiotensin-converting enzyme (ACE) may help reduce oedema.
E. Plasma osmolality is usually reduced because of water retention.

8.7

Antidiuretic hormone:

A. Is released from the anterior pituitary in response to a rise in plasma osmolality.
B. Is a vasoconstrictor.
C. Increases water permeability in the loop of Henle.
D. Increases urea reabsorption from the medullary portion of the collecting duct.
E. Is a steroid hormone.

8.8

If a young man, found in a semiconscious state, is dehydrated, has glucose in his urine and the following results on analysis of an arterial blood sample: pH 7.0; Po_2 13.0 kPa (100 mmHg); Pco_2 3.0 kPa (22 mmHg); $[HCO_3^-]$ 4.5 mmol/litre:

A. He is likely to have been hyperventilating.
B. He has a metabolic acidosis.
C. There has been no respiratory compensation in this patient.
D. He has lost HCO_3^- in his urine.
E. He is dehydrated because of an osmotic diuresis.

8.9

Following ingestion of 700 ml of water by a normal adult:

A. Urinary volume increases.
B. The rate of urinary salt excretion increases.
C. Antidiuretic hormone levels fall.
D. The permeability of the collecting ducts to water increase.
E. There is little or no change in the intracellular fluid volume.

8.10

Aldosterone:

A. Secretion is stimulated by circulating renin.
B. Secretion is stimulated by low levels of plasma $[K^+]$.
C. Increases the permeability of the collecting ducts to water.
D. Stimulates Na^+/K^+-ATPase activity in the proximal convoluted tubule.
E. Promotes loss of Na^+ and H_2O from the body.

(Answers overleaf →)

Answers

8.1

A. **False.** Such a substance would provide a measure of renal plasma flow, not GFR.

B. **True.** This reduces the plasma oncotic pressure in the glomerulus, increasing the net filtration pressure.

C. **True.** This increases the hydrostatic pressure in the glomerular capillaries.

D. **False.** Although GFR is autoregulated, there will be a tendency for it to fall in very strenuous exercise because of sympathetic constriction of the renal vasculature.

E. **False.** If GFR is about 125 ml/min and renal plasma flow, or RPF, is approximately 700 ml/min, then GFR/RPF is about 18%. This is referred to as the filtration fraction.

8.2

A. **True.** If the renal clearance exceeds GFR, then X must be being secreted within the nephron. The high clearance tells us that more of the substance is appearing in the urine than can be accounted for by filtration.

B. **False.** This would only be true if one knew for certain that X was freely filtered in the nephron. Any substance which is only poorly filtered, as well as one which is reabsorbed, will have a clearance below the GFR.

C. **True.** All of the filtered glucose is normally reabsorbed, up to plasma concentrations which exceed the renal threshold, i.e. about 11 mmol/litre.

D. **False.** One would also need to know the renal plasma flow rate. Clearance would then equal (A–V concentration difference) × Plasma flow rate/Arterial plasma concentration.

E. **False.** Clearance is independent of plasma concentration for such a substance; it is always equal to the GFR.

8.3

A. **False.** It is tall, mitochondria rich and has a brush border of microvilli. These features reflect its high transport capacity.

B. **False.** NaCl, urea and H_2O are all absorbed in similar proportion to their concentrations in the filtrate, and plasma, and so there is a large decrease in fluid volume along the length of the proximal tubule, with little change in osmolality.

C. **True.** This helps maintain glomerular–tubular balance, in which a large and fixed fraction of the filtered Na^+ and H_2O is reabsorbed in the proximal tubule. Part of the mechanism is increased plasma oncotic pressure in the peritubular capillaries due to upstream filtration of a greater fraction of the available plasma volume.

D. **True.** There is a one-to-one relationship.

E. **False.** PTH promotes phosphate excretion by the kidney by inhibiting reabsorption.

8.4

A. **False.** Movement of ions and H_2O is passive in this region, with water being drawn out into the medulla and ions diffusing in.

B. **True.** This means that as ions are pumped out in this region, H_2O is trapped within the lumen.

C. **True.** This increases the osmolality achieved within both tubular fluid and interstitium as the loop of Henle descends into the medulla.

D. **True.**

E. **False.** The fluid which enters the distal convoluted tubule has a low osmolality due to the diluting effect achieved by ion absorption with H_2O retention in the thick ascending limb.

8.5

A. **True.**
B. **False.** They constrict both afferent and efferent arterioles, decreasing renal blood flow and GFR. This effect may, however, be counterbalanced by the actions of angiotensin and prostaglandins.
C. **True.** This can fall by as much as 70%.
D. **True.** They have a direct action on the renin-secreting cells.
E. **False.** They tend to increase reabsorption of Na^+, Cl^- and H_2O.

8.6

A. **True.** Reduced cardiac output leads to reduced renal perfusion, a stimulus to renin release from the juxtaglomerular apparatus.
B. **True.** This is due to the action of renin on angiotensinogen, which produces angiotensin I, which is converted to angiotensin II by angiotensin-converting enzyme in vascular capillaries, especially in the lungs.
C. **True.** Aldosterone release is stimulated by angiotensin II.
D. **True.** Treatment with an ACE inhibitor reduces angiotensin II, and thus aldosterone production, so limiting renal reabsorption of Na^+ and H_2O in the distal convoluted tubule.
E. **False.** The water retention in heart failure is driven by secondary hyperaldosteronism, as described above. This primarily promotes Na^+ reabsorption, so plasma osmolality is unlikely to be changed.

8.7

A. **False.** ADH is released from the posterior pituitary.
B. **True.** It is also known as vasopressin.
C. **False.** It acts on the collecting ducts and the distal convoluted tubule.
D. **True.** ADH increases the permeability to urea and H_2O in this region of the nephron.
E. **False.** It is a peptide hormone. Aldosterone is a steroid.

8.8

A. **True.** The low P_{CO_2} indicates this.
B. **True.** The low pH indicates an acidosis. The very low bicarbonate tells us that it is metabolic.
C. **False.** The low P_{CO_2} will partly offset the acidosis by helping to raise the $[HCO_3^-]:P_{CO_2}$ ratio. This is classical respiratory compensation for a metabolic acidosis.
D. **False.** The patient would in fact be reabsorbing all of the filtered HCO_3^- in exchange for secreted H^+ and excreting a highly acid urine. $[HCO_3^-]$ is low because it is being used up to buffer the additional metabolic acid load.
E. **True.** This is driven by retained glucose within the tubules which hold H_2O osmotically, preventing its reabsorption. This does not normally occur because all the filtered glucose is reabsorbed. At very high plasma [glucose], however, the T_m for reabsorption is exceeded. This, and the other features of the case, are typical of a diabetic ketoacidosis.

8.9

A. **True.** There is a diuresis.

B. **False.** There is usually no change in the rate at which salt is excreted. Since urinary volume is increased, this means that urinary osmolality falls.

C. **True.** This is a response to the reduction in plasma osmolality and increase in plasma volume. The fall in ADH causes the rapid diuresis.

D. **False.** Reduced ADH causes reduced H_2O permeability, with less reabsorption into the medulla.

E. **False.** The reduced osmolality in extracellular fluid leads to an initial osmotic uptake of H_2O by cells. As water is cleared by the kidneys, raising the $[Na^+]$ towards normal, this fluid is distributed back into the extracellular space, until volume and osmolality have returned to normal throughout the body.

8.10

A. **False.** Angiotensin II is the direct stimulant.

B. **False.** High $[K^+]$ levels stimulate aldosterone, which promotes the secretion of K^+ in the distal convoluted tubule.

C. **False.** This is an action of ADH.

D. **False.** Na^+/K^+-ATPase activity in the proximal convoluted tubule is not modulated by aldosterone. Aldosterone-sensitive Na^+ and H_2O reabsorption occurs only in the distal part of the distal convoluted tubule.

E. **False.** It promotes reabsorption of Na^+ and H_2O.

The gastrointestinal system

9

Introduction

Human beings, like all animals, are heterotrophs – they build their own bodies from components of other living organisms that they have ingested. Plants are autotrophs, building up macromolecules from simple inorganic precursors. The human gastrointestinal tract (GIT) performs various essential functions in relation to this heterotrophic activity:

- food and water are *captured* and held enclosed by the body
- the food is *digested* into smaller absorbable components
- water and the products of digestion are *absorbed* into the body
- the remaining undigested remnants of food are *removed* from the body.

These functions are unevenly distributed along the length of the gastrointestinal tract. Food is held in the stomach and digestion is begun. Digestion and most of the absorption takes place in the small intestine. In the large intestine these processes are completed and the undigested remnants are concentrated as faeces for voiding.

Problems with gastrointestinal tract function are several and common. The digestive process must not affect the tract itself. If the GIT lining is eroded, ulcers are formed. This ulceration is both painful and dangerous.

Surgical removal of parts of the GIT produces problems for the individual which relate to the normal function of the lost part. Total removal of the stomach leads to vitamin B_{12} deficiency (pernicious anaemia, see p. 856) as the stomach is the source of intrinsic factor, which is essential for the vitamin's absorption by the small intestine.

The processes of digestion involve the secretion of large volumes of fluid into the GIT.

If these are not reabsorbed, the loss of water caused can be fatal within hours. Cholera and dysentery, infections of the GIT, are dangerous for this reason.

It is clearly important to understand the functions of the different parts of the GIT, which involve the movement of GIT contents and water and electrolyte secretions which are then reabsorbed, in order to appreciate the basis of diagnosis and treatment of gastrointestinal disease.

Section overview

This section covers:

- The common structure of the gut and how this is modified in specific regions
- The 'local' and 'distant' neural and endocrine control of the GIT
- The function, composition, origin, mechanisms of production and control of secretions of the GIT
- Defences of the stomach against abrasion and digestion
- Concentration of bile
- Enterohepatic circulation of bile acids
- Endocrine activity of the GIT
- Properties of intestinal smooth muscle
- The importance of chewing
- The coordination of swallowing
- Characteristics and control of motility in the small and large intestine
- Defecation
- Transport processes and structure that aid absorption
- Absorption of water, electrolytes and nutrients.

Digestion

9.1

Introduction

All cells in the body require a supply of nutrients in the form of small, easily metabolized molecules. These must come from food, where they are present as carbohydrates, fats, proteins, etc. (see Basic Science 9.1.1, page 806). These complex molecules are broken down by the process of digestion and then absorbed into the bloodstream. Digestion requires the food to be acted upon by *enzymes* and *cofactors* whose activity has to be facilitated by mechanical agitation of the gut contents. Absorption is a relatively slow process that requires controlled movement of material through the absorptive sections of the gut. There are, therefore, three basic processes that take place in the gut:

- secretion – adding enzymes and cofactors necessary for digestion
- absorption – taking up the products of digestion
- motility – controlled agitation and movement of material through the system.

The structure of food

The food on which the gut acts can be classified into three main groups: carbohydrates, fats and proteins.

Carbohydrates

These have the general formula $C_x(H_2O)_y$ and it is because of this equivalence to 'hydrated carbon' that this group have received their name. The principal carbohydrates in food can be divided into:

- polysaccharides, e.g. starch $(C_6H_{10}O_5)_n$
- disaccharides, e.g. sucrose, lactose, maltose $(C_{12}H_{22}O_{11})$
- monosaccharides, e.g. glucose, fructose $(C_6H_{12}O_6)$.

The overall pattern of carbohydrate digestion is:

Carbohydrate	Enzyme	Product
Starch	Amylase	Maltose
Maltose	Maltase	Glucose
Sucrose	Sucrase	Glucose + Fructose
Lactose	Lactase	Glucose + Galactose

Galactose and fructose are then converted into glucose – galactose by the liver, and fructose by the liver and many other cells. The end product of carbohydrate digestion is therefore glucose, which has the structure shown in Figure BS9.1.1.

The six carbon atoms of glucose are numbered as shown in the figure. Glucose is stored as glycogen, which is made up of many hundreds of glucose molecules from which the elements of water have been removed to form linkages between carbon atoms 1 and 4 (α 1–4 linkage) or 1 and 6 (α 1–6 linkage) to join separate molecules of glucose. This numbering convention is used to show at what point enzymes act on a molecule.

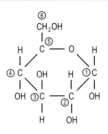

Fig. BS9.1.1 The structure of glucose.

Fats

The fat of food is mainly neutral fat with small amounts of free fatty acid. Neutral fats are triglycerides (glycerol esters of fatty acids).

Lipase in the gut hydrolyses triglycerides in stages, splitting off each fatty acid molecule in turn. The end products are undigested triglyceride, di- and monoglycerides, fatty acids and glycerol (Fig. BS9.1.2).

Proteins

These have a complex molecular structure in which their three-dimensional properties are very important in determining the way they behave. They are constructed of alpha- (right-hand twist) amino acids joined into chains called polypeptides by peptide bonds. Cross-links between specific amino acids join several polypeptides to form proteins.

Amino acids have the general formula:

$R \cdot CH(NH_2) \cdot COOH$

where R can be any one of a variety of organic groupings.

Peptide bonds are of the type shown in Figure BS9.1.3.

Digestion of protein consists of breaking more and more of the peptide bonds until amino acids are formed.

Basic Science *(Continued)*

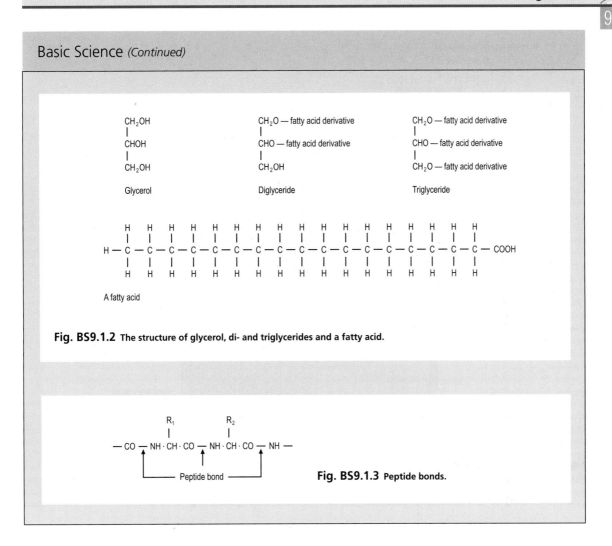

Fig. BS9.1.2 The structure of glycerol, di- and triglycerides and a fatty acid.

Fig. BS9.1.3 Peptide bonds.

Structure of the gut

The structure and function of the gut varies between different mammalian species depending upon the diet, but the human gut is a fairly typical example of that found in omnivores – species who live on a mixed diet of animal and vegetable material.

The gut is a long tube divided into recognizably distinct regions. The walls of the tube have the same basic structure of concentric layers along most of its length, though this is greatly modified to facilitate function.

The structure is illustrated in Figure 9.1.1. Starting from the lumen and working outwards the layers are:

- the mucosa – made up of **epithelial** cells
- the lamina propria – consisting mainly of **loose connective tissue** rich in collagen and elastin, but also containing blood vessels and lymph tissue
- the muscularis mucosae – a thin layer of **smooth muscle** whose contraction throws the mucosa into folds and ridges

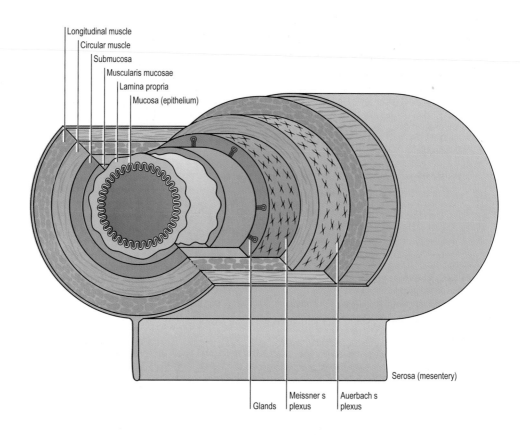

Fig. 9.1.1 General organization of the layers of the gastrointestinal tract (GIT). This figure most closely approximates to the structure of the small intestine. Considerable variation relates the structure of other specialized parts of the GIT to their functions.

- the submucosa – like the lamina propria mostly **connective tissue**, but also contains larger blood vessels and, in some parts of the gut, submucosal glands
- the submucosal nerve plexus (Meissner's plexus) – a dense network of nerve cells innervated by the **autonomic nervous system** which, when isolated, function as an independent nervous system in their own right – the enteric nervous system (see p. 146)
- a thick 'circular layer' of smooth muscle – bundles of smooth muscle cells arranged circumferentially or helically around the gut, whose contraction tends to constrict the lumen
- a 'myenteric' nerve plexus (Auerbach's plexus) – a second dense network of nerve cells similar to the submucosal plexus and also part of the enteric nervous system
- an outer longitudinal layer of smooth muscle – bundles of smooth muscle cells arranged along the gut, which is shortened by their contraction
- the serosa – or outermost layer of connective tissue covered with a layer of squamous mesothelial cells.

The major compartments of the gut are illustrated in Figure 9.1.2.

In addition to the main tube of the gut, there are a number of **ducted exocrine glands** which supply secretions necessary for digestion. Three pairs of salivary glands produce saliva, and the pancreas and liver empty secretions into the intestines.

The oesophagus passes from the pharynx, posteriorly to the trachea, through the thorax and diaphragm to the stomach. The stomach is in contact with the underside of the diaphragm, and is divided by the pylorus from the first part of the small intestine – the duodenum. The duodenum is about 30 cm long, receives ducts from the liver and pancreas and connects with the next part of the small intestine – the jejunum. The jejunum and the rest of the small intestine, the ileum, have a length which is variable depending on their state of activity of between 4 and 7 metres. There is a gradual change in structure along the length of the small intestine, but no obvious junction between jejunum and ileum.

The ileum ends at the ileocaecal junction. The caecum is the first part of the large intestine. It connects to the ascending, transverse and then descending colon, which connects in the pelvis to the sigmoid colon and then the rectum, which ends in the anus.

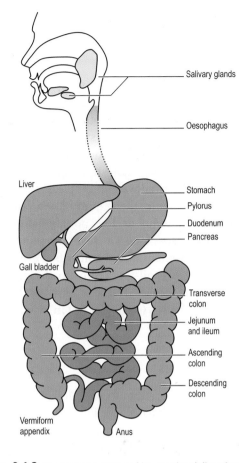

Fig. 9.1.2 The digestive tract and its associated digestive organs. The location of the major regions of the gut and associated glandular structures is illustrated (not to scale). The oesophagus and small intestine have been shortened for clarity.

Summary

Basic functions and structure of the gut

- The gut functions by the basic processes of secretion, absorption and motility.

- Working outwards, the layers of the gut are mucosa, lamina propria, muscularis mucosae, submucosa, Meissner's plexus, circular muscle, Auerbach's plexus, longitudinal muscle, serosa.

Neuroendocrine control mechanisms

Extrinsic nerves

The gut is innervated by the **sympathetic** and **parasympathetic** branches of the autonomic nervous system. Whilst both branches have important effects, the parasympathetic vagal innervation is the most important during digestion and absorption. Vagal stimulation increases tone of the intestinal wall and increases the rate of peristalsis. Sympathetic stimulation reduces peristalsis and tone but does not abolish them. It also increases tone in several sphincters, delaying movement of gut contents. Peristalsis continues even if all the nerves to the gut are cut and only ceases if the submucosal and myenteric plexuses (see Fig. 9.1.1) in its wall are paralysed.

Enteric nerves

The two plexuses, submucosal (Meissner's) and myenteric (Auerbach's) (see Fig. 9.1.1) can exert considerable control even when separated from the CNS. This independence of function is possible because of the complexity of neural processing which can take place. Whilst many of its neurones, like postganglionic parasympathetic neurones, release acetylcholine as their transmitter, there is a whole variety of different transmitter substances present (see p. 158).

Gut hormones

An enormous number of putative gut hormones have been identified; this chapter deals with those generally recognized to be most important.

The first hormone discovered – secretin – is a gut hormone. The gut has a well-developed endocrine system, but does not have anatomically discrete endocrine glands. Gut hormones are secreted from groups of cells, known as **APUD** (amine precursor uptake and decarboxylation) cells scattered along its length, though there are major concentrations in the pyloric antrum of the stomach, the duodenum, and the upper part of the jejunum.

All identified gut hormones are peptides and many other peptides have been suggested to be hormones but for only a few has this role been confirmed. Gut hormones seem to be organized into two, structurally related, families – gastrins and secretins.

Gastrins

Gastrin is secreted by cells in the pyloric antrum of the stomach and the duodenum in several different forms containing different numbers of amino acids. The most active form, in relation to acid secretion, contains 17 amino acids.

Gastrin promotes acid secretion in the stomach, and also has growth-promoting (trophic) effects in the gut as a whole.

The second member of the family is **cholecystokinin** (CCK), a hormone secreted from the duodenum, whose release is stimulated by hypertonicity, fats and amino acids. It acts on the pancreas to promote secretion of enzymes, and on the gall bladder. It has much of its amino acid sequence in common with gastrin, including the terminal five amino acids. In the absence of the other, gastrin and CCK can stimulate one another's receptors, but when both are present each can competitively inhibit the other.

Secretins

The second family of hormones is typified by **secretin**. This polypeptide is released from cells in the duodenum and jejunum by acidity in their lumen. It acts on the pancreas and liver to stimulate secretion of alkaline juice.

The other member of the group which has full gut hormone status is **gastric inhibitory polypeptide** (GIP), which is produced by the physical filling of the intestines and acts to reduce the rate of emptying of the stomach. It also acts on the endocrine β-cells of the pancreas to promote the secretion of **insulin**.

Local mediators

There are many other peptides – the secretin family also contains the important substance vasoactive intestinal peptide (VIP), which is not strictly a hormone, as it is not released into the bloodstream, but does act as a local **paracrine** substance (and as a neurotransmitter in the CNS). Hyperacidity in the small intestine stimulates local VIP release. It is a vasodilator and inhibits gastric acid secretion. Another polypeptide – somatostatin – may also be important as a paracrine substance whose most obvious effect is to inhibit the actions of most other gut hormones.

Another paracrine substance (which is not a peptide) is **histamine**, which is particularly important in the stomach (see p. 826).

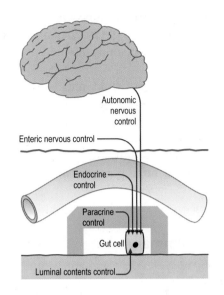

Fig. 9.1.3 Gut control. Layers of control of an effector cell (e.g. muscle or secretory cell) in the gut.

The control of GIT function

Any given function in the gut is controlled at a number of levels. Many cells are directly sensitive to the luminal contents of their part of the gut, and control their own activity accordingly. They may also be controlled from nearby cells by diffusion of local mediators. Parts of the gut that are further afield may also exert control by means of hormones travelling in the bloodstream, or by impulses travelling along the enteric nervous system. Finally, operating over the whole, there is the extrinsic innervation by the autonomic nervous system, through which the central nervous system modulates gut function. These complex 'layers' of control are illustrated in Figure 9.1.3.

Gut 'balance sheet'

A typical individual consumes a few hundred grams of food each day, which, together with normal drinking, yields a total volume ingested of around 2 litres. The salivary glands add 1.5 litres of saliva each day to facilitate the ingestion of food. Each day therefore, about 3.5 litres of fluid enters the stomach. The stomach adds

another 2 litres of secretions. These contain acid and enzymes to begin the processes of digestion. The churning action of the stomach, and the digesting effects of its secretions convert solid food particles into a semi-liquid **chyme**. About 5.5 litres of chyme empties each day from the stomach into the duodenum. Chyme is acidic, but also, as digestion in the stomach has started to break macromolecules down into smaller molecules, it contains more osmotically active particles than the body fluids – it is hypertonic.

Chyme is neutralized and made isotonic by the addition of 3.5 litres of fluid, secretions from the pancreas and liver, and water that is drawn by osmosis into the duodenum across its wall, which, unlike that of the stomach, is permeable to water.

About 9 litres of fluid therefore enter the small intestine per day – over four times the volume that is actually consumed.

Most of the fluid is then absorbed in the small intestine, which normally removes about 8.4 litres per day, leaving around 0.5 litres per day to enter the large intestine where most of the remaining water and electrolytes are removed to leave faeces containing about 0.1 litres of water.

Huge volumes of fluid must be added to what we eat in order to digest it, and then be removed. The gut is a very sophisticated 'flow reactor' with substances being added and removed in a highly controlled way. There is obviously a huge potential for problems in the system. Very small excess of secretion over absorption can lead to large changes in the amounts of water and electrolytes lost in the faeces and upset the body's fluid balance dangerously.

It is clear that the gut must be subject to highly sophisticated control by the autonomic nervous system, hormones in the blood and paracrine substances which diffuse locally in the gut wall.

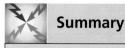

Summary

Control of the gastrointestinal tract

- Control of the gastrointestinal tract can be considered in 'layers' of command.
- Peristalsis is independent of extrinsic drive.
- Of the gut's dual innervation, the parasympathetic (vagal) supply is most important, stimulating digestion and absorption.
- Sympathetic nervous activity increases the tone of several sphincters, delaying movement of gut contents.

- Gut hormones are secreted by APUD (amine precursor uptake and decarboxylation) cells scattered throughout its length.
- Gut hormones mainly fall into the secretin and gastrin families, with many other peptides exerting important actions.
- About 2 litres of water are consumed per day; to this, 7 litres of secretions are added by the time it reaches the small intestine. Absorption by the small and large intestines removes all but 0.1 litre.

Digestive secretions

9.2

Introduction

In order to digest and absorb nutrients from our daily food intake, we produce several litres of secretions, each containing a variety of components that contribute to different stages in the digestive process. The final outcome is a large volume of neutral, isotonic juice containing small nutrient molecules suitable for absorption in the small intestine. There are a number of questions that may be asked about any digestive secretion, and we will consider these questions in turn. They are:

- what are the *functions* of the secretion?
- what does it *contain* to fulfil these functions?
- what is the *origin* of each component of the secretion?
- what is the *mechanism* of secretion of each component?
- how is the secretion *controlled*?

We will consider in turn, secretions from the salivary glands, the stomach, the pancreas, and the liver.

Salivary glands

Three pairs of salivary glands (Fig. 9.2.1) produce around 1.5 litres of saliva per day in a normal adult.

Functions of saliva

The functions of saliva are mouth health, easing swallowing, and digestion of starches.

Mouth health

Saliva protects the mouth, and facilitates the swallowing of food. The epithelium lining the mouth must be kept constantly wet and lubricated if ulceration and infection are to be avoided. This warm, wet environment, often containing residues of food, is a good environment for the growth of microorganisms. Growth of pathogenic organisms needs to be controlled. In part, this is achieved by a protective flora which develops in the mouth. Even the normal buccal flora, however, produce acid by their

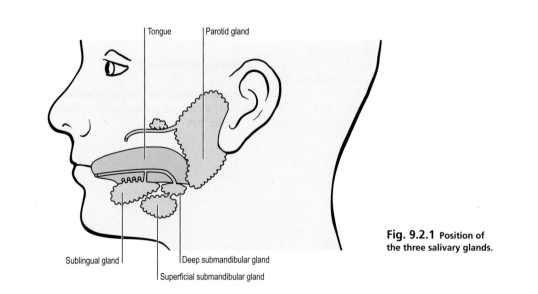

Tongue | Parotid gland

Sublingual gland | Deep submandibular gland
Superficial submandibular gland

Fig. 9.2.1 Position of the three salivary glands.

metabolism. If this acidity is unchecked the teeth will be attacked. Saliva therefore contains substances which limit and regulate bacterial growth, and alkali which neutralizes acid, thus protecting the teeth. Saliva also contains sufficient calcium to prevent tooth calcium salts dissolving passively.

Easing swallowing

Mucus in saliva facilitates ingestion of food, though it is not essential for normal digestion. For swallowing to occur easily, food must be moistened and lubricated, so that it can be broken down by chewing before being swallowed. Moistening the food can largely replace this role of saliva.

Digestion of starches

Some digestion of starches begins in the mouth. Eating is also made more pleasant by saliva as the dissolution of substances responsible for taste and flavour allows them to reach the appropriate sensory receptors.

Inadequate salivation

Inadequate production of saliva may occur for a variety of reasons ranging from fear to trauma. If this continues for long, a condition known as **xerostomia** (dry mouth) develops and damage occurs. After a few weeks there is rapid tooth decay and the development of buccal ulceration. Ulcers become infected by unchecked bacterial growth. Washing the mouth with an artificial saliva is essential in this condition.

Composition of saliva

The most important property of saliva, for both protecting the mouth and facilitating eating, is that it should be wet. Its principal component therefore is water, and, under all circumstances, saliva is a more dilute solution than the body fluids – it is hypotonic and contains a complex mixture of inorganic and organic constituents.

The main inorganic components (electrolytes) are Na^+, K^+, Cl^- and, importantly, bicarbonate (HCO_3^-), which is generally present at higher concentrations than in the body fluids, making saliva alkaline. K^+ is sometimes present at higher concentrations than in body fluids, but most other ions are invariably present at much lower concentrations. Table 9.2.1 shows the composition of saliva produced at rest, and whilst consuming food (stimulated saliva). The reasons for the differences in composition between these two conditions will be explained below.

Saliva also contains an unusually high concentration of iodide (I^-), which may help in controlling the bacterial population of the mouth.

The main organic constituents of saliva are mucus and the enzyme salivary **amylase**. Amylase catalyses the first stage in the breakdown of polysaccharide starches into mono- and disaccharides. There are, however, many minor components, including various immune substances such as IgA and IgM which, again, are particularly important in controlling the buccal flora. Blood group antigens are also present in the saliva, with some individuals, known as secretors, producing larger amounts, and a greater variety of antigens than others.

Table 9.2.1 Composition of saliva: outline of the changes in flow and composition of parotid saliva at rest and when flow is stimulated by chewing

	Resting	Stimulated
Flow (ml/min)	0.02	1.0
Na^+ (mmol/l)	2.6	56.7
K^+ (mmol/l)	37.2	17.6
Cl^- (mmol/l)	8.0	18.0
HCO_3^- (mmol/l)	0.6	29.7
Ca^{2+} (mmol/l)	4.2	3.3
Amylase (mmol/l)	0.6	1.2
Total protein (g/l)	2.6	3.2
Osmolality (mOsmol/kg)	85	127

Values compiled from data of Shannon et al in a number of studies from 1960 to 1972

Sources of saliva

There are three pairs of salivary glands (see Fig. 9.2.1), which are ducted exocrine glands.

- The **parotid** glands, the biggest, lie below and anterior to the ear, their ducts opening into the mouth on the inner surface of the cheek, opposite the second upper molar teeth.
- The **submandibular** glands lie under cover of the mandible, their ducts opening on the floor of the mouth beneath the tongue.
- The **sublingual** glands, which are the smallest, lie on the floor of the mouth just posterior to the midline part of the mandible, opening by many small ducts both into the buccal cavity directly and into the submandibular duct.

Some mucus is also produced by small glands in the mouth, particularly on the tongue.

The secretions of the main pairs of glands can be collected separately as each has a distinct duct. Parotid glands secrete a watery solution, which makes up about 25% of the daily salivary production. It contains electrolytes and enzymes, but little mucus. Submandibular glands secrete the main component (70%) of the daily salivary flow, which contains all constituents, including mucus. Sublingual glands secrete only a small volume each day, about 5% of the total flow, but this is particularly rich in mucus, and may also be a major source of secreted antibodies and antigens.

The solution produced by the parotid glands is known as **serous** saliva. That produced by the sublingual glands is **mucus**-rich saliva, while the submandibular glands produce a mixed type of saliva. The different compositions result from the different cellular populations of the glands.

All three glands have the same basic histological structure. Blind-ended acini connect with ducts which drain via a branching network into the main ducts. The cells surrounding the acini (acinar cells) are histologically distinct from those surrounding the ducts (see Fig. 9.2.2). Serous cells in the parotid glands also stain differently from those in the sublingual glands, so there are distinct mucous and serous cell and gland types. Histological examination of the submandibular gland reveals an intermediate structure; some acini are serous and others are mucous.

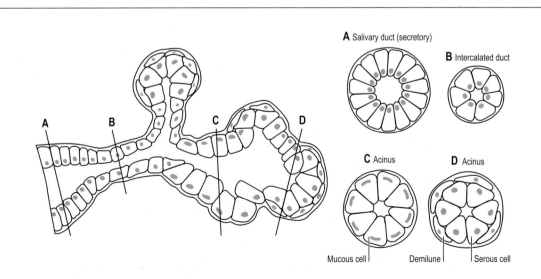

A Salivary duct (secretory)

B Intercalated duct

C Acinus

D Acinus

Mucous cell   Demilune   Serous cell

Fig. 9.2.2 Structure of the salivary gland. The proportion of serous and mucous cells varies. In the parotid gland, the secreting cells are mainly serous; in the sublingual gland, mucous cells predominate.

Broadly speaking, fluid from serous acini contains electrolytes and enzymes, mucous acini secrete mucus and immune proteins.

The submandibular gland secretion is mixed because the gland has both types of acini, not because it has a different mechanism of secretion.

Mechanisms of secretion of saliva

Mucous and serous acini secrete by different mechanisms.

Mucus is a complex mixture of mucoproteins and mucopolysaccharides synthesized within the acinar cells and secreted together with a small volume of fluid which is probably similar in composition to an ultrafiltrate of extracellular fluid. Relatively little is known about the production mechanisms of mucous saliva. The mechanisms by which proteins are secreted are described in the sections on the pancreas (p. 829) and exocytosis (p. 33).

Serous secretion has been studied in much greater detail and is well understood at the cellular level.

The main challenge faced in the production of saliva is its hypotonicity. There are no mechanisms for moving water across epithelia directly, and so it is not possible to produce dilute secretions such as saliva or sweat by adding water to them. Electrolytes can, however, be moved across cell membranes actively against their concentration gradients; osmotic forces can then cause water movement. Thus, the mechanism of production of a dilute solution is first to produce an isotonic primary secretion whose composition is similar to extracellular fluid and then to remove solute from it by **active transport**. These two functions, production of a primary secretion and its subsequent modification, are served by different cell types at different places within the gland.

By collecting minute samples of fluid from within the salivary glands, using the technique of micropuncture with tiny glass pipettes, it has been shown that the acinar cells produce a primary secretion which is then modified by the duct cells as it passes through the ducts towards the mouth (see Fig. 9.2.3).

The primary secretion is isotonic, or even slightly hypertonic (i.e. less water) when compared with extracellular fluid. The concentration of most ions is similar to that in extracellular fluid, though chloride has been reduced, replaced by bicarbonate.

The primary secretion is not produced by ultrafiltration, such as occurs in the kidney. It is produced by active transport across the acinar cells. The precise cellular mechanism is not certain, but the current view is that both Cl^- and HCO_3^- are actively transported into the acini, and that other constituents follow electrochemical and osmotic gradients produced by this active transport. ATP is required for secretion to occur, and the rate of production of primary secretion (Fig. 9.2.4) may be controlled by intracellular messengers which modify the rate at which chloride ions may leave the cell into the acinar lumen.

Once the primary secretion enters the ducts it is modified (Fig. 9.2.5). The main change is the removal of Na^+ and Cl^- by mechanisms

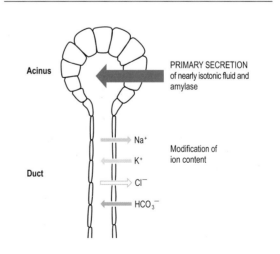

Fig. 9.2.3 Mechanism of saliva production. Saliva is not produced with the composition it has when secreted into the mouth. A primary secretion made by the acinus is modified by the duct of the gland.

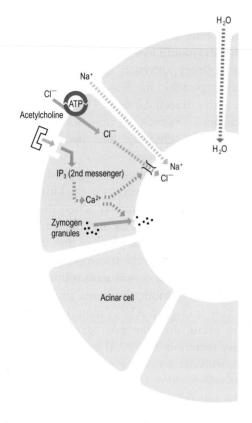

Fig. 9.2.4 Production of a primary salivary secretion. This is an isotonic solution similar to extracellular fluid, produced by active transport, probably of both Cl⁻ and HCO₃⁻.

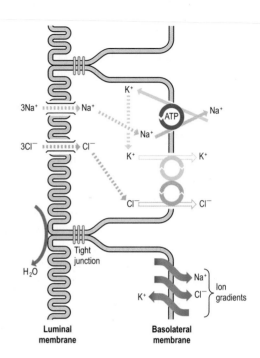

Fig. 9.2.5 Modification of primary serous saliva. This is mainly by the removal of Na⁺ and Cl⁻ by active transport mechanisms like those found in other parts of the gut and kidney.

similar to those operating elsewhere in the gut and in the kidney.

Duct cells have ion pumps in their basolateral membranes (i.e. those facing away from the lumen and into the extracellular fluid). The main pump is the Na^+/K^+ $ATPase$ type, described elsewhere (see p. 30), which expels $3Na^+$ from the cell in exchange for the inward movement of $2K^+$. Both movements are against concentration gradients. Energy is supplied by the hydrolysis of ATP. Like all cells, therefore, the concentration of Na^+ in the intracellular fluid is much lower than in the extracellular fluid. The rate of expulsion of Na^+ (and therefore also, of course, the rate of influx of K^+) is controlled mainly by the intracellular Na^+ concentration.

As the K^+ is moving back down its concentration gradient, i.e. on diffusing out of the cell, the energy released can be used to move a second ion up a concentration gradient by **co-** or **countertransport** through linking their movements via a channel protein. In the case of the salivary duct cells, the transporter protein is a *symport* and, as K^+ leaves the cell, Cl^- is also expelled up its concentration gradient (see p. 28).

The end result is that $3Na^+$ and $2Cl^-$ are transported from the lumen to the extracellular fluid. This imbalance of charge movement results in an electrical gradient being set up with the lumen becoming negative to the body fluids.

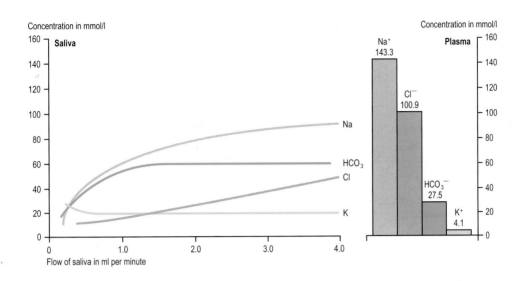

Fig. 9.2.6 **Composition of saliva compared with extracellular fluid (plasma), and how it changes with salivary flow.** Saliva is always hypotonic and its composition departs most from that of extracellular fluid, from which it is made, when its rate of flow is low and the tubular cells have more time to act on it.

The duct cells also add small amounts of some other substances, such as iodide and amino acids to saliva.

Because the duct cells are joined by water-impermeable **tight junctions** of their luminal membranes, water does not follow the electrolytes and an osmotic gradient between lumen and body fluids is set up. As the primary secretion passes along the ducts, it becomes progressively more hypotonic. Each duct cell can only transport ions up to a maximum rate. At high rates of saliva flow, this rate is reached and the final secretion comes close in composition to the primary secretion (i.e. less hypotonic). Even at maximum flow rate, however, the final product is always hypotonic to plasma.

The variation of composition of serous saliva with flow rate is shown in Figure 9.2.6.

Control of salivary secretion

From what has been said above, it will be realized that the volume of saliva produced is determined by the activity of acinar cells; duct cells affect the composition of saliva but have less effect on the volume.

Control of saliva flow must therefore be exerted at the acinar cells. The ion movements associated with serous production, and presumably the exocytotic events of mucus secretion, are stimulated by rises in the concentration of intracellular **second messengers**, themselves produced by the binding of agonists to cell surface receptors.

The principal agonists are neurotransmitters released from postganglionic neurones of the autonomic nervous system. Both sympathetic and parasympathetic divisions are involved, though major control is exerted via the parasympathetic fibres (Fig. 9.2.7). Their activity is controlled by a variety of reflexes. The presence of food in the mouth, the smell or sight of food, or learned reflexes relating to stimuli associated with food all result in increased parasympathetic activity and increased salivation.

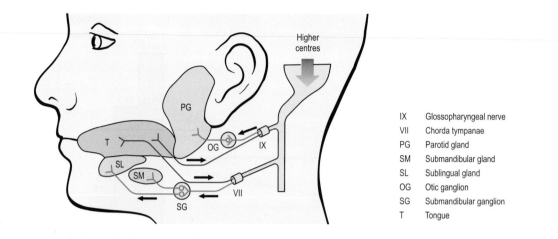

Fig. 9.2.7 Control of the salivary glands by the parasympathetic system. Both sympathetic and parasympathetic divisions of the autonomic nervous system control the salivary glands. Unlike their opposing actions in other parts of the gut, both promote secretion, but with different timescales.

Parasympathetic activity also greatly increases blood flow through the salivary gland, providing the resources required for the energy-demanding processes of salivary secretion and modification. Vasodilatation is probably due to the local release of vasoactive intestinal peptide (VIP).

The salivary acini and ducts are surrounded by smooth muscle cells – **myoepithelial cells** – whose contraction ejects enzyme-rich preformed saliva from the glands and supports the fragile secretory epithelium during periods of high secretion. These myoepithelial cells are stimulated to contract by both parasympathetic and sympathetic activity.

The dry mouth associated with fear is due to the unopposed actions of sympathetic nerves. However, activity in the sympathetic innervation of the glands has several effects upon salivation.

Noradrenaline released from sympathetic nerves stimulates the release of an enzyme-rich saliva, and also contracts myoepithelial cells. Although sympathetic stimulation acting alone will vasoconstrict salivary blood vessels, which tends to reduce secretion, this vasoconstriction

may be overcome by local vasodilator influences if the gland is active. A peptidase, **kallikrein**, released from active cells acts on plasma kininogen, producing powerful vasodilator kinins.

It is interesting that the reabsorption of sodium in the ducts may be increased by aldosterone during sodium deprivation. The action of the hormone in the salivary gland, as in the renal tubule, is to promote the synthesis of the Na^+ pump protein.

Overall, saliva is a complex secretion whose volume and composition are controlled to meet the requirements of the moment.

Excessive loss of saliva

Saliva is normally swallowed and its constituents are not lost to the body. Occasionally, because of either trauma exteriorizing a duct or neuronal damage preventing swallowing, the dribbling of saliva from the mouth can result in ion imbalances. As saliva's composition is near that of extracellular fluid the main deficit will be loss of Na^+.

Summary

Saliva

- Normal adults produce 1.5 litres of saliva per day.
- Saliva is bacteriostatic, alkaline and prevents passive tooth erosion.
- Mucus in saliva aids swallowing; amylase begins the digestion of starch.
- Mucous and serous acini secrete by different mechanisms.
- Serous acini produce isotonic primary saliva which is rendered hypotonic by duct cell absorption of ions by active transport.
- Control of volume and composition of saliva is by autonomic (mainly parasympathetic) transmitters stimulating the production of intracellular second messengers.

Gastric secretions

Human feeding usually takes the form of a few large meals. Food is stored in the stomach after a meal. It is then slowly delivered into the intestines at a rate at which it can be processed. In the stomach it is subjected to preliminary digestion and liquefaction to form **chyme**. The stomach secretions both liquefy the food and begin its digestion.

Functions of gastric secretions

The conversion of a wide variety of foodstuffs from solid to semi-liquid chyme requires a non-selective, but powerful process of digestion. In a test tube most foodstuffs can be disrupted by the addition of a strong acid. Low pH also has the ability to disinfect food by killing many, if not all, of the contaminating microorganisms. Acid hydrolyses fat and starch. Proteins, which are more resistant to acid hydrolysis, are broken down in the stomach by proteolytic enzymes to yield a mixture of polypeptides.

The combination of acid and these enzymes is capable of breaking down most biological material into its constituent parts in a short time.

The stomach itself is susceptible to mechanical damage by food fragments and to digestion by its own secretions. It must protect itself. Thus another function of the stomach secretions is to protect the organ from autodigestion.

Composition of gastric secretions

The major component of stomach secretions is hydrochloric acid (HCl), secreted to a concentration of about 150 mmol/l. Because of the limited buffering capacity of the contents of the stomach, this produces a stomach lumen pH between 1 and 2.

In addition, the stomach secretes **pepsins**, proteolytic enzymes which are endopeptidases, cleaving proteins by hydrolysing peptide bonds. These enzymes are secreted in an inactive form, as proenzyme pepsinogens. In the stomach lumen, away from the stomach lining, these proenzymes are activated to form pepsins by low pH (<5.0) and the action of active proteolytic enzyme already present.

The stomach protects itself from mechanical damage and digestion by secretion of two substances – mucus and alkali. The alkali is in the form of bicarbonate (HCO_3^-). Their combined effect is to provide a lubricated, buffered, *unstirred layer* of viscous fluid over the stomach mucosa in which the pH is kept high and where the stomach's proteolytic enzymes are not active (see p. 823).

Mucus is made up of water and a glycoprotein, **mucin**. A major sugar in the glycoprotein is *N*-acetylglucosamine, a basic sugar. Mucin exists as a tetramer of four subunits of molecular weight c. 500 000 linked by disulphide bonds. Even in concentrations as low as 50 g/l these tetramers form a stiff gel.

Intrinsic factor

The stomach also secretes **intrinsic factor**, which is essential for the absorption of **vitamin B$_{12}$** in the intestines. One of the life-threatening consequences of removal of, or damage to, the stomach is reduced absorption of vitamin B$_{12}$, which if untreated will lead to anaemia. Intrinsic factor production is the only indispensable function of the stomach.

Sources of gastric secretions

The various components of gastric secretions are produced in various proportions from different parts of the stomach. By forming pouches from different regions of the organ, early investigators showed that most acid and enzymes are secreted from the body (or corpus) of the stomach (Fig. 9.2.8), whereas the area around the base of the oesophagus – the cardia – secretes relatively more bicarbonate, as do the pyloric antrum and pylorus. Mucus is secreted throughout the stomach.

Histological examination of the mucosa has revealed four main cell types that contribute to the secretory process and are present in different proportions in different areas. This suggests that specific cells might be responsible for the components of the gastric secretion.

The surface of the gastric mucosa is largely populated by two types of cells – surface epithelial cells and goblet cells. The staining characteristics of the goblet cells clearly indicates that they produce and secrete mucus. Surface epithelial cells secrete bicarbonate.

In the body of the stomach there are numerous shallow depressions in the mucosa, known as **gastric pits** (Fig. 9.2.9), which lead to shallow ducts lined with three cell types arranged in three zones. Moving from the surface inwards there are:

- the neck cells, which secrete mucus
- the parietal (oxyntic) cells, which secrete acid
- lastly, in the base of the pits, the chief cells, which secrete proteolytic enzyme precursors – the pepsinogens.

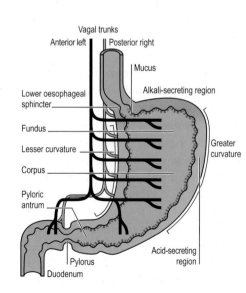

Fig. 9.2.8 Innervation and regional activity of the stomach. Neural control of gastric secretion is almost exclusively by the vagus. The secretion varies in composition from region to region.

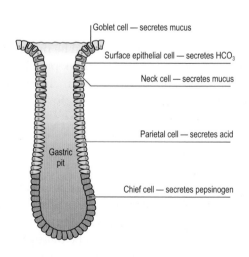

Fig. 9.2.9 Structure of a gastric mucosal pit. The different proportions of the three cell types present almost divides the gland into three regions.

Each of the major components of stomach secretions therefore comes from a different cell type. Intrinsic factor is secreted with acid by the parietal cells.

Defences of the stomach against abrasion and digestion

The luminal contents of the stomach, at a pH often below 2 and with active proteolytic enzymes, are a hostile environment for living tissue, and, to prevent damage, the stomach's own mucosa must be protected. Mucus is a major part of this protection. It is a mixture of mucoproteins and mucopolysaccharides, which is viscous and sticky. It adheres very closely to the mucosal surface, forming a layer of up to 200 μm thick. By adhering, it also protects the stomach wall against mechanical damage. The mucus layer is pliant, so it can cope with the powerful contractions occurring during stomach motility, and it flows readily over the surface so that if mechanical abrasion removes part of the mucus layer it rapidly heals, with mucus flowing in from surrounding areas.

Mucin is not immune to attack by the stomach secretions. Its thickness and viscosity create a local microenvironment which is different from that in the main stomach lumen – this is known as an unstirred layer. Molecules diffuse into this layer from the lumen or from the mucosa, so the local concentrations can be controlled independently of the rest of the stomach by local chemical reactions.

The mucin molecule has many basic side-chains, so hydrogen ions diffusing into it will react and the pH will rise. This alkalinity is further bolstered by the secretion of HCO_3^- from the surface epithelial cells of the stomach, which diffuses towards the lumen (Fig. 9.2.10). The viscosity of the mucus layer ensures that it remains unstirred, which prevents it from mixing with the acid in the stomach. The two do react but the rate is limited by their rates of diffusion. Over a distance of 200 μm mixing times are measured in seconds. As hydrogen

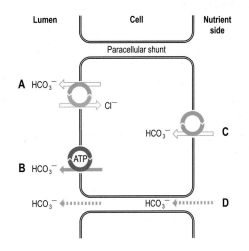

Fig. 9.2.10 **Proposed mechanisms for gastroduodenal HCO_3^- transport.** This involves (A) electroneutral Cl^-/HCO_3^- exchange; (B) active electrogenic transport; (C) anion carrier; and (D) passive migration.

ions diffuse into the mucus therefore, they react with HCO_3^- to produce CO_2, and so the pH does not fall. This mechanism allows the pH on the surface of the stomach under the mucus to be maintained close to 7.0, a hydrogen ion concentration 10^5 times less than in the stomach itself.

The surface cells are therefore protected against attack by acid and, additionally, as pepsins will only work at pH below 5.0, the cells and most of the mucus layer also are protected against proteolytic attack.

These defences must be continuously renewed, otherwise acid attack will produce local inflammation and damage – known as gastritis or acid indigestion – and, if the attack is prolonged, sufficient damage to produce ulceration which may be very reluctant to heal.

The control of secretion of defences is in part local and in part related to the need for defence, i.e. dependent on the amount of acid being secreted.

Any local irritation to mucosa stimulates the production of local mediators such as

prostaglandins, which increase production of mucus and bicarbonate, and also other tissue changes that promote healing of local damage.

Stimuli that increase acid secretion (see below) also promote secretion of defence agents, so that the defensive capability of the stomach is at its maximum when the acid secretion is highest. The turnover of the cells of the stomach lining is very rapid with a high rate of cell division. Cells constantly migrate up from the pits and old cells are sloughed off and digested. The repair of damage is an extension of this process and is usually very rapid.

How might the stomach defences be breached?

Alcohol abuse is often associated with damage to the stomach mucosa. Alcohol initially leads to an increase in acid secretion by local stimulation of secretion, by a mechanism involving histamine, and reflexly via the vagus. If this occurs on an empty stomach with little buffering present, the unstirred mucus layer may be inadequate protection. About one-third of heavy drinkers have a chronic gastritis which eventually leads to destruction of the mucosal integrity and an inability to secrete acid, **achlorhydria**.

Many anti-inflammatory drugs have as their most important side-effect the induction of gastric bleeding. This is related to their interference with the production of local prostaglandins, which normally stimulate mucus and bicarbonate secretion in the presence of acid or damage.

Mechanisms of secretion of acid

Acid is secreted by the **parietal cells**. Production of acid from body fluids which are slightly alkaline requires hydrogen ion (H^+) to be secreted against its concentration gradient by active transport. Hydrogen ions are produced from carbon dioxide and water, and then secreted by the action of an H^+/K^+-stimulated ATPase pump.

The parietal cell has a highly specialized structure. Figure 9.2.11A shows that the cells have a truncated pyramidal shape with the apex oriented towards the stomach lumen. There are extensive invaginations of the luminal membrane, forming canaliculi whose membranes are lined with protein molecules, the ion pumps.

The cytoplasm surrounding these canaliculi is packed with mitochondria. Their presence allows these cells to sustain the high metabolic rate needed to support the active secretory processes of this cell type.

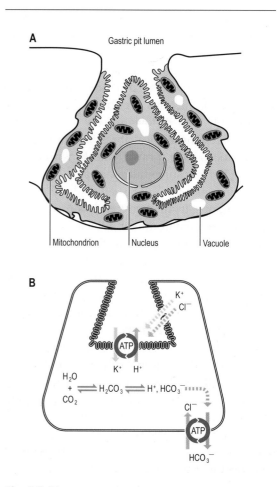

Fig. 9.2.11 The parietal (oxyntic) cell. A. Structure of a typical parietal cell. Note the invagination of its inner surface by many canaliculi that connect to the gland lumen, which in turn opens into the lumen of the stomach. **B.** The process of acid production and secretion by the parietal cell.

The lumen of the canaliculi is normally some −70 mV with respect to the extracellular fluid bathing the basolateral aspect of the parietal cell. Acid secretion causes this potential difference to reduce to some −40 mV.

The production of hydrogen ions from CO_2 and water is catalysed by **carbonic anhydrase** and the H^+ is secreted by ion pumps located in the canalicular membranes. These pumps export hydrogen ions against a considerable concentration gradient, producing a luminal $[H^+]$ around 150 mmol/l. The pump involved in this process is a unique H^+/K^+ ATPase, which moves hydrogen ions out of the cell in exchange for inward movement of K^+; both are movements against concentration gradients. Energy is supplied by hydrolysis of ATP. The effect of these steps is to increase $[HCO_3^-]_i$ and $[K^+]_i$. However, bicarbonate moves out of the cell across the basolateral cell membrane via an antiport with Cl^-, raising $[Cl^-]_i$. At the luminal membrane Cl^- diffuses passively out of the cell through a Cl^- channel. K^+ also moves down its concentration gradient into the lumen through a K^+ channel, providing luminal K^+ for the H^+ pump. High $[K^+]_i$ and low $[Na^+]_i$ are maintained by a Na^+/K^+ ATPase in the basolateral membrane.

Potassium ions therefore cycle to and fro across the membrane, being pumped in and then leaking out again accompanied by Cl^-.

The end result is a high concentration of H^+ and Cl^-, i.e. hydrochloric acid, in the lumen of the canaliculi.

The alkali inevitably produced by making acid from a neutral solution therefore remains in the cell as HCO_3^-. This is exported from the cell via the basolateral membranes to the extracellular fluid, in exchange for inward movement of Cl^-. The resulting increase in $[HCO_3^-]$ in the blood is known as the **alkaline tide**. For every mole of acid secreted into the stomach, one mole of bicarbonate enters the blood. Each day the stomach secretes about 350 mmol of acid and equivalent amounts of alkali enter the blood.

The whole process of acid secretion is shown in Figure 9.2.11B.

Control of acid secretion by the stomach

Many factors influence the secretion of acid from the stomach, but all are dependent eventually on the intracellular mechanisms for producing acid described above. The activity of these mechanisms is influenced by intracellular second messengers, released as a consequence of the binding of agonists to cell surface receptors on the basolateral membrane of the cells.

The principal intracellular messenger is the calcium ion. If the intracellular concentration of free calcium ions rises, then the activity of the canalicular H^+/K^+ exchange pump is increased and more acid is secreted. A rise in $[Ca^{2+}]_i$ may be triggered by the release of inositol 1,4,5-trisphosphate from the cell membrane after binding of agonists to receptors.

Stimulation of at least three receptors can lead to an increase in acid secretion:

- a receptor for the polypeptide hormone **gastrin**
- a receptor of the H_2 subtype for the local mediator **histamine**, and
- a muscarinic receptor for the neurotransmitter **acetylcholine**.

Binding of each specific agonist to any of these receptors leads to a rise in intracellular calcium concentration, leading to a rise in acid secretion. It is believed that binding of histamine may also trigger a rise in another intracellular messenger – cyclic AMP – as a result of stimulation of an adenylate cyclase enzyme. This also increases acid production.

There is some cooperation between the three receptors, so that simultaneous activation of more than one will lead to a greater gastric acid secretion than the sum of each acting alone.

The agonists to these receptors, gastrin, histamine and acetylcholine, are derived from different cells.

Histamine

Histamine is secreted from **enterochromaffin-like (ECL) cells** which are scattered throughout the gastric mucosa, close to the parietal cells. Histamine diffuses through the extracellular fluid to the parietal cell, and so the agonist is a local mediator, a paracrine substance. ECL cells are stimulated to release histamine by a variety of stimuli, the most important being gastrin and acetylcholine. Each agonist, therefore, stimulates acid secretion by two routes – directly by binding to parietal cell receptors and indirectly by promoting histamine release. The latter route amplifies their effects.

Histamine, however, has another important action. As elsewhere in the body, it acts upon the smooth muscle in the walls of arterioles, causing a local vasodilatation and increased blood flow. This increase in blood flow is essential to support the massive increase in metabolism associated with acid secretion.

The H_2-type receptors for histamine on the parietal cells are found in very few other places in the body, and so provide a specific target for a drug, cimetidine, the H_2 antagonist used to reduce acid secretion in the stomach (see below).

Gastrin

Gastrin is secreted from **G cells**, found in two areas. The first is the pyloric antrum where they are located in the mucosa sufficiently close to the lumen to be affected by substances present in the stomach. A second population of G cells is found in the mucosa of the duodenum. These cells secrete a different form of the hormone, which has more amino acids. It has the same action on parietal cells as gastrin from the antrum, but has a more persistent action as it survives for longer.

Gastrin travels in the bloodstream to the parietal cells, and is therefore a true hormone. Indeed it was one of the first hormones to be discovered.

The release of gastrin is triggered by a variety of stimuli. If the stomach contains amino acids or peptides, more gastrin is released. Alcohol stimulates gastrin release, as do organic acids such as acetic acid or butyric acid. Gastric contents of low pH, however, inhibit gastrin release, so between meals, for example, when luminal pH is low and there are no other stimuli, gastrin secretion is greatly reduced.

Acetylcholine

The secretion of parietal cells is also affected by neurotransmitters released from postganglionic parasympathetic nerves. Acetylcholine acts on muscarinic, M_2, receptors blocked by atropine. Their stimulation opens Ca^{2+} channels allowing Ca^{2+} to move into the cell. The effect of vagal stimulation is partly atropine resistant and there is evidence that the vagus releases not only acetylcholine, but also a peptide, known as **gastrin-releasing peptide** (GRP).

The action of GRP is complex. It can act directly upon G cells to promote release of gastrin, but may also act by inhibiting release of somatostatin from nearby D cells, which acts as a paracrine substance inhibiting release of gastrin.

Thus increased activity in the parasympathetic nerves, resulting from the activation of *stretch* receptors in the stomach wall, or efferent (outflow) activity in the vagus nerves from the central nervous system, will lead to increased gastrin release and more acid secretion.

The enteric nervous system can also affect the parietal cells directly by release of acetylcholine from nerve endings close to them, which acts on the muscarinic receptors on the cells. This nervous activity also results from activation of local stretch receptors or efferent activity in the vagus. Vagal activity therefore promotes acid secretion in two ways:

- by release of acetylcholine from nerve endings in the body of the stomach close to the parietal cells – they are stimulated directly, as are mast cells which release the powerful secretagogue histamine

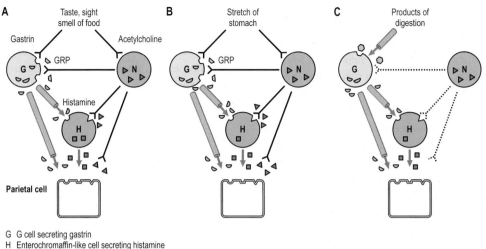

G G cell secreting gastrin
H Enterochromaffin-like cell secreting histamine
N Parasympathetic nerve cell secreting acetylcholine and GRP

Fig. 9.2.12 **Control of the parietal (oxyntic) cell.** **A.** Cephalic; **B.** gastric; and **C.** intestinal phases of control of gastric secretions which, by endocrine and neural mechanisms, initiate and terminate secretion by the parietal cells.

- by release of GRP from nerve endings in the pyloric antrum, which acts upon G cells to promote the release of gastrin, which passes via the bloodstream to the parietal cells.

The control of parietal cell activity is summarized in Figure 9.2.12.

Control of acid secretion evoked by a meal

Cephalic phase of acid secretion

The mechanisms described are activated in a well-defined sequence by a meal. When food is first detected by sight or smell, or other signals normally associated with food, the cephalic phase of secretion begins. There is no food in the stomach at this stage and acid secretion is stimulated by reflex activation of the vagus. If the vagus is cut, then the cephalic phase of secretion does not occur. The vagus acts both directly on the parietal cells and indirectly via gastrin.

Gastric phase of acid secretion

Once food is swallowed, the gastric phase of secretion begins. The arrival of food in the stomach has two initial effects. First, the volume of the stomach increases. This distension is detected by stretch receptors in the stomach walls, and increases activity in the enteric nervous system, which stimulates parietal cells both directly and indirectly via gastrin and histamine. If there was no food in the stomach before the meal, then luminal pH is low, inhibiting gastrin release. Then, as the first food arrives in the stomach it reacts with and buffers many of the hydrogen ions, so the pH rises. This relieves the inhibition on gastrin secretion, and more is therefore released to act upon the parietal cells and increase acid secretion.

Both of these initial effects of food are transient. Stretch receptors adapt, and as more acid is secreted the pH of the lumen falls again. The gastric phase of secretion is then maintained by the action of the luminal contents upon gastrin secretion as more amino acids and peptides are produced by digestion.

Intestinal phase of acid secretion

As soon as chyme begins to empty from the stomach, the third, intestinal, phase of secretion, occurs. Initially there is increased acid secretion as the duodenal G cells secrete their gastrin, but later, as acid chyme moves down the duodenum other hormones (enterogastrones) are released, which reduce acid secretion.

Secretin, besides causing secretion of an alkaline pancreatic juice, also inhibits gastric acid secretion by both inhibiting gastrin release from G cells and reducing its effect on the parietal cells. The presence of fatty acids in the duodenum releases the polypeptide hormones **gastric inhibitory peptide** (GIP) and **cholecystokinin** (CCK).

CCK has a very similar structure to gastrin and competitively antagonizes its effects at the gastrin receptors on the parietal cell. CCK and GIP, like secretin, suppress gastrin release. CCK was named because of its first recognized effect – contraction of the gall bladder.

Control of pepsinogen release

Pepsinogen release from **zymogen granules** of the chief cells is controlled by similar mechanisms to those controlling acid secretion but a major control is by the vagus nerves. An exception to this is that secretin and CCK both stimulate pepsinogen release.

Clinical Example

Reduction of gastric acid production for therapeutic reasons

The most readily pharmacologically influenced of the mechanisms controlling gastric acid production is histamine. The H_2 histamine receptor is uncommon elsewhere in the body, and antagonists to it have few unwanted side-effects. The H_2-selective antagonist **cimetidine** is commonly used to reduce acid secretion in patients suffering from peptic ulceration of the stomach or duodenum.

An alternative method of therapeutically treating excess acid secretion, and one of growing importance, is the use of drugs such as omeprazole, which blocks the final step in the acid secretory pathway, the (H^+/K^+ ATPase) proton pump.

It is also possible surgically to interrupt the vagus (vagotomy) and reduce acid secretion. As the vagus mediates many functions, including motility of the stomach, cutting the whole vagus will have undesirable side-effects. It is, however, possible to cut the small branch of the nerve which runs to the main acid-secreting area of the stomach – an operation known as **proximal selective vagotomy**. Finally, the part of the stomach containing the G cells can be removed (partial gastrectomy), so eliminating a source of gastrin. The pyloric sphincter is also cut (pyloroplasty) to promote gastric emptying.

⚡ Summary

Gastric secretions

- Gastric secretions amount to about 2 litres per day.
- The stomach's secretions have a uniquely low pH, which disinfects and disrupts food, and contain endopeptidases (pepsins).
- The wall of the stomach is protected from the acid contents by mucus forming a microenvironment over its mucosa.
- Hydrochloric acid is secreted by parietal (oxyntic) cells under the control of gastrin (a hormone from G cells), histamine (a local mediator) and acetylcholine (the vagal parasympathetic neurotransmitter).
- Pepsin is released from zymogen granules in chief cells as a precursor, pepsinogen, by vagal activity, secretin and cholecystokinin.
- The stomach's secretions are controlled in three distinct phases – cephalic, gastric and intestinal – activated by a meal.
- Intrinsic factor, secreted by the stomach, is essential for vitamin B_{12} absorption.

Pancreas

Functions of pancreatic secretions

The chyme which empties from the stomach is very acidic, very hypertonic and, although some digestion has started, the nutrients formed cannot be absorbed. Hypertonicity is corrected by the osmotic movement of water across the duodenal wall, which is freely permeable to water. Acidity is corrected by the addition of alkali, and digestion completed by the addition of a cocktail of enzymes and other substances. Alkali and enzymes come from three sources: first, the exocrine pancreas; second, the exocrine liver; and third the intestines themselves.

Composition of pancreatic juice

The exocrine pancreas secretes alkali and enzymes. The alkali is bicarbonate (HCO_3^-). The concentration of HCO_3^- in pancreatic juice varies from around 30 mmol/l in the resting gland up to 140–150 mmol/l when the gland is secreting at a maximal rate. The solution is isotonic and, like extracellular fluid, the principal cation (positively charged ion) is Na^+.

The enzymes form a complex mixture. Each component digests a particular component of the diet. The enzymes are:

- Trypsin – a proteolytic enzyme released as inactive trypsinogen. Trypsinogen is activated by the enzyme enterokinase. Trypsin is an endopeptidase, which hydrolyses peptide bonds between amino acids within polypeptide chains.
- Chymotrypsin – another proteolytic enzyme secreted in an inactive form, chymotrypsinogen. Chymotrypsin is also an endopeptidase but with different amino acid selectivity.
- Carboxypeptidase – yet another proteolytic enzyme. It is an ectopeptidase which removes single amino acids from the terminal end of the polypeptides produced by the action of pepsin, trypsin and chymotrypsin.
- Pancreatic amylase. This breaks down the polysaccharide chains of starches by hydrolysing 1,4 glycosidic bonds.
- Lipases. Several enzymes in pancreatic juice break down fats into fatty acids and monoglycerides.

- Other enzymes. There are various other enzymes, including ribonucleases and deoxyribonucleases which attack RNA and DNA, and elastase which breaks down elastic tissues.

Origin of pancreatic secretions

The endocrine part of the pancreas, the islets of Langerhans, are scattered between the acini. Their function as secretors of insulin and glucagon is described on page 451. The exocrine pancreas is structured in a similar fashion to other ducted glands. Blind-ended acini are connected to a network of ducts draining eventually into the duodenum. There are two major secretory cell types – the acinar cells and the duct cells.

Their functions have been studied by using drugs which destroy each type selectively. If the acinar cells are destroyed, the pancreas remains capable of secreting alkaline juice in large quantities, but does not produce enzymes. When the duct cells are destroyed, then the gland no longer secretes alkali, but does produce a normal complement of enzymes, dissolved in a small quantity of isotonic juice whose electrolyte composition is similar to extracellular fluid.

The *enzymes* are therefore secreted by the acinar cells, and the *alkali* by the duct cells. These two components are mixed together to form the final output of the gland.

The histological structure of the pancreas is illustrated in Figure 9.2.13.

Mechanisms of pancreatic secretion

Enzymes

The acinar cells produce all the enzymes secreted by the pancreas (Fig. 9.2.14). As with other protein-secreting cells, the enzymes are created upon ribosomes attached to rough endoplasmic reticulum, of which the acinar cells have a large amount. Once synthesized, the proteins are then packaged into zymogen granules. These pass first to the Golgi apparatus,

where they are coated with a layer of lipid membrane, before entering condensing vacuoles and being formed into dense, membrane-bound granules. The membranes surrounding the zymogen granules will, on receipt of an appropriate intracellular signal, fuse with the cell membrane and open outwards, releasing the proteins by a process of **exocytosis**.

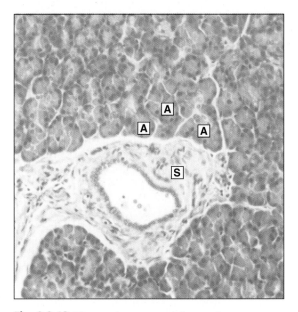

Fig. 9.2.13 Microscopic structure of the exocrine pancreas. The acini (A) form the blind-ended intercalated ducts which drain into the interlobular ducts, which in turn drain into the interlobular ducts supported by sheaths (S) of connective tissue. (From Young B, Heath JW 2000 *Wheater's Functional Histology*, 4th edn. Churchill Livingstone, Edinburgh.)

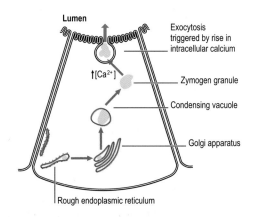

Fig. 9.2.14 Secretion of enzyme precursors by the pancreatic acinar cells.

Alkaline juice

The duct cells secrete a variable volume of juice rich in bicarbonate, which is almost always present at a higher concentration in the juice than in extracellular fluid. There is, however, a high concentration of HCO_3^- in the interstitial fluid, which is increased further by the 'alkaline tide' from the stomach during digestion of a meal, so the duct cells merely have to transport bicarbonate ion into the tubular fluid.

As in the kidney tubule, the movement of HCO_3^- is an indirect process involving pumping of hydrogen ions, illustrated in Figure 9.2.15.

A transporter protein in the basolateral membrane of the cells expels H^+ ions in exchange for the inward movement of Na^+. The sodium ions are moving down their concentration gradient, and so give up energy which can be used to move H^+ ions up a concentration gradient out of the cell. As the ions move in opposite directions this transporter is an antiport.

The gradient of Na^+, which would otherwise be degraded, is maintained by Na^+/K^+ exchange pumps which utilize ATP in the normal way.

H^+ ions ejected from the cell react with HCO_3^- to form CO_2 and H_2O. CO_2 can easily cross cell membranes, so it enters duct cells, where, assisted by the enzyme carbonic anhydrase, it reacts with water to form H^+ and HCO_3^-.

The HCO_3^- formed within the cell then diffuses into the duct lumen with the aid of another transporter protein which exchanges Cl^- for HCO_3^-. The inward movement of Cl^- down its concentration gradient provides the means of expelling HCO_3^- to the region of higher concentration in the pancreatic juice.

Chloride ion that has entered the cell then leaves via the basolateral membrane, associated with the outward movement of the K^+ which has entered the cell as a result of the Na^+/K^+ ATPase activity. The end result of the whole process is that for each molecule of ATP hydrolysed $3Na^+$ and $3HCO_3^-$ cross from the extracellular fluid to the pancreatic juice. The resulting **osmotic gradient** draws water into the ducts through their permeable walls, increasing the volume of the solution and maintaining isotonicity.

The alkalinity of the juice is essential for the release of the proenzymes and their subsequent activation in the small intestine.

Control of pancreatic secretion

Pancreatic secretion of enzymes and alkaline juice are separately controlled (Fig. 9.2.16).

Enzymes

The fusion of zymogen granules with the cell membrane, and the consequent exocytosis of enzymes, is triggered by a rise in the intracellular concentration of calcium ions. This is itself triggered by a cascade of biochemical events initiated by the binding of agonists to cell surface receptors. In the case of acinar cells, it is believed that agonist binding increases the

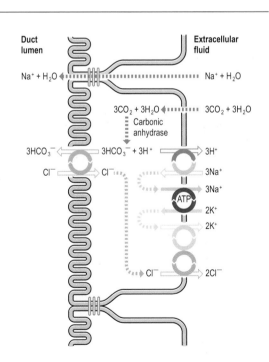

Fig. 9.2.15 **Secretion of bicarbonate by the pancreatic duct cells.** The primary mechanism is acidification of the blood by pumping H^+ in exchange for Na^+.

831

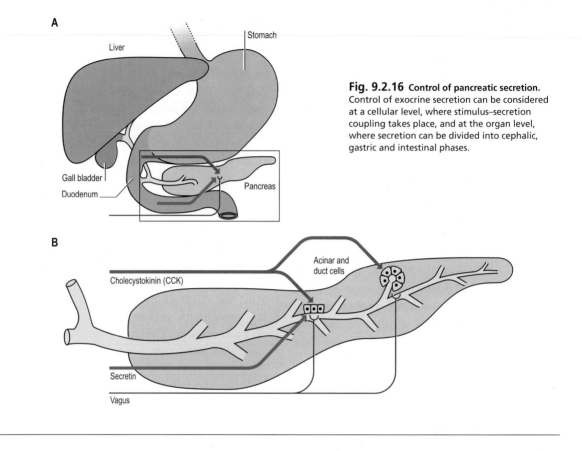

Fig. 9.2.16 Control of pancreatic secretion.
Control of exocrine secretion can be considered at a cellular level, where stimulus–secretion coupling takes place, and at the organ level, where secretion can be divided into cephalic, gastric and intestinal phases.

activity of a membrane-bound enzyme that cleaves membrane phospholipids into **inositol 1,4,5-trisphosphate** (IP_3) and **diacylglycerol** (DAG). A rise in the IP_3 concentration then releases calcium ions from intracellular stores, so triggering the release of zymogen granules.

Two agonists are particularly important triggers. The first is acetylcholine, which binds to muscarinic receptors. Acetylcholine is released from parasympathetic, postganglionic neurones of the vagus nerve. This nerve activity is triggered in several ways: by the taste and smell of food and other stimuli associated with eating (via a vagal reflex) and by signals from the stomach and duodenum. The second trigger is a polypeptide hormone, *cholecystokinin* (CCK), released from cells in the wall of the duodenum. Release is stimulated by:

- the hypertonicity of the chyme entering from the stomach
- the presence in the chyme of fats, particularly long chain fatty acids such as palmitic and stearic acid
- certain amino acids, particularly the essential amino acids, phenylalanine and methionine.

Alkaline juice

The main influence upon the pancreatic duct cells is a polypeptide hormone, *secretin*, though its action is modulated by several other factors.

Secretin is released from S cells, located mainly in the jejunum. These cells are stimulated by low pH in the intestinal lumen. The hormone then passes in the bloodstream to the duct cells of the pancreas, where it stimulates bicarbonate secretion. One of the long-standing puzzles of pancreatic control is that the pH in the jejunum rarely falls low enough to stimulate the release of large amounts of secretin; and indeed, circulating concentrations of the hormone after a meal are very low. Some factor or factors must render the duct cells exquisitely sensitive to the hormone. It now seems likely that two influences are important:

- CCK. This hormone does not itself stimulate secretion of alkaline juice, but will potentiate the action of low concentrations of injected secretin.
- Acetylcholine. There is a fairly constant vagal discharge – vagal tone – which releases acetylcholine. Like CCK this is not in itself adequate to stimulate alkaline secretion, but potentiates the action of secretin.

As with the secretion of acid by the stomach, the secretion of the pancreas is controlled in distinct phases during the digestion of a meal:

- When food is first detected and tasted, increased vagal activity leads to the release of acetylcholine, promoting the secretion of enzymes in the cephalic phase of secretion.
- When food reaches the stomach there is a gastric phase. This is, in part, due to increased vagal activity to the pancreas as a result of afferent signals from the stomach, but also because of the release of gastrin, which is structurally similar to CCK and, like CCK, can stimulate acinar cells.
- The main phase of secretion of the pancreas is, however, the intestinal phase, when the arrival of acid chyme in the duodenum stimulates massive release of CCK and also of secretin.

The mix of enzymes secreted by the pancreas is not always the same. There is evidence that long-term changes in diet are associated with alterations in the balance of the enzymes to suit the new mix of nutrients. The mechanisms of this process of adaptation are unknown.

Summary

Pancreatic exocrine secretions

- Pancreatic secretions average about 2 litres per day.
- The secretions' major roles are neutralization of gastric acid with bicarbonate and addition of amylase, proteases and lipases.
- The bicarbonate solution is secreted by the duct cells; the enzymes by the acinar cells.
- Enzymes are released as proenzymes in zymogen granules by exocytosis.
- There is separate phasic control of the exocrine pancreas's secretion of enzymes, by acetylcholine and cholecystokinin (CCK), and of the bicarbonate, mainly by secretin.

Liver

The liver produces an important digestive secretion, the **bile**. The organ has many other functions which will not be considered here. Note that this exocrine secretion of the liver is also an important vehicle for the excretion of products of metabolism produced in the liver and elsewhere. About 0.7–1.2 litres of bile per day are produced by the liver. A major role of bile is to provide alkali required to neutralize gastric juice. It also contains several substances which facilitate the absorption of fats.

Formation of bile

The liver has a very distinctive histological structure. It is organized into polygonal segments, each surrounding a central vein (Fig. 9.2.17). At the points of the polygon there are three vessels:

- an artery, which supplies capillaries around the liver cells

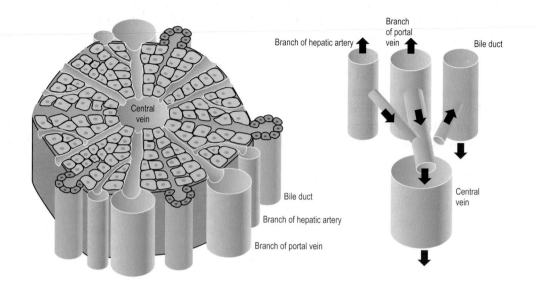

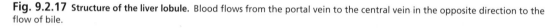

Fig. 9.2.17 **Structure of the liver lobule.** Blood flows from the portal vein to the central vein in the opposite direction to the flow of bile.

- a vein receiving blood from the hepatic portal vein, which drains the intestines
- a branch of the bile duct.

Blood enters sinusoids (liver capillaries) from the portal vein. The sinusoids carry it from the periphery of the polygon towards the central vein. The sinusoids are lined with hepatocytes – liver cells which fulfil the functions of the organ related to homeostasis of the body fluids.

Other spaces, canaliculi, begin as blind-ended structures near the central vein, and then drain from the centre towards the periphery of the polygon, where they run into bile ducts, which then drain into the main bile duct from the liver to the duodenum. The cells lining these canaliculi contribute to the production of bile, as do the duct cells which line the bile ducts. The close relationship between the canalicular cells and the hepatocytes means that both cell types can act upon the blood returning from the gut, which flows in the opposite direction along

the sinusoids to that of secretions formed in the canaliculi. The gall bladder is a blind diverticulum off the bile duct which stores and concentrates bile.

Mechanism of bile secretion

Bile is made up of two, distinct fractions. One fraction is only produced if sufficient bile acids are available from the blood. This bile-acid-dependent fraction is produced by the canalicular cells. The production of the other fraction is independent of bile acid availability. This bile-acid-independent fraction is produced by the duct cells.

Bile-acid-dependent fraction

Bile acids are secreted only when they are available in the blood. The production of the bile-acid-dependent fraction of the bile does not occur when a meal is consumed, but in the final stages of digestion of a meal.

Most of the constituents of bile are secreted by the canalicular cells into the bile-acid-dependent fraction. One of the most important constituents is the **bile acids**. These acids are water-soluble derivatives of **cholesterol**. Two main bile acids are produced in the liver: cholic acid, and chenodeoxycholic acid (Fig. 9.2.18). The first is produced at twice the rate of the second. Both acids are conjugated completely with glycine or taurine, making them more water soluble. The fate of the bile acids in the intestine is crucial to their rate of synthesis in the liver.

After performing their function in the absorption of fats (see p. 856), they are released back into the intestinal lumen, and progress along the ileum to its terminal portion. As they do so, about 25% are deconjugated by the action of bacteria. The conjugated bile acids are then completely reabsorbed in the terminal ileum and return to the liver in the hepatic portal vein. Much of the unconjugated bile acid is also reabsorbed, but some is converted by bacterial action into lithocholic acid, which cannot be absorbed and is excreted in the faeces. The majority of the bile acids, however, return in one form or another to the liver. As they pass through the blood sinusoids they are removed by hepatocytes and pumped by the canalicular cells back to the canaliculi.

This continuous 'recycling' of the bile acids is known as the **enterohepatic circulation** (Fig. 9.2.19). The rate of circulation of bile acids is such that even though the total amount in circulation at any one time is around 1.8–3.2 g (the 'total bile acid pool'), 19–72 g are secreted into the bile each day. The small losses incurred on each cycle of the enterohepatic circulation are made up by synthesis of new bile acids within the liver. If for some reason reabsorption is impaired, then the liver can compensate and synthesize bile acids at quite a high rate.

As the conjugated bile acids, which are anionic, are secreted into the canaliculi they take with them the cation Na^+ and, because of

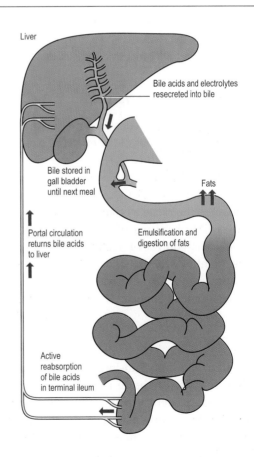

Fig. 9.2.19 The circulation of bile. Bile acids are secreted and continuously reabsorbed for reuse – the enterohepatic circulation.

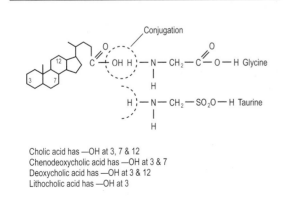

Cholic acid has —OH at 3, 7 & 12
Chenodeoxycholic acid has —OH at 3 & 7
Deoxycholic acid has —OH at 3 & 12
Lithocholic acid has —OH at 3

Fig. 9.2.18 Structure of the common bile acids. Conjugation with glycine or taurine increases their water solubility, which is essential for their role in digestion of fats.

the osmotic gradient so produced, substantial quantities of water.

Most components of bile are stored until they are needed for the next meal. This is the function of the gall bladder.

The bile-acid-dependent fraction of bile also contains the bile pigments, which are excretory products being disposed of by the liver via the gut. The main bile pigment is **bilirubin**, which is formed from the breakdown of haem. Haem is converted to bilirubin mostly in the spleen and bone marrow, and the bilirubin then travels in the bloodstream bound to plasma proteins such as albumin, as it is very insoluble in water, which is why it cannot be eliminated via the kidney. The hepatocytes remove bilirubin from the blood very effectively, and the pigment is bound to intracellular cytoplasmic proteins. It is then conjugated to form a polar, water-soluble, molecule before being exported by a carrier-mediated, energy-dependent process into the bile.

Bile-acid-independent fraction

The intrahepatic duct cells are functionally very similar to the duct cells of the exocrine pancreas, and appear to produce the same secretion – an alkaline juice isotonic with body fluids in which the main anion is HCO_3^-. The mechanism of secretion is the same as that of pancreatic duct cells (see Mechanisms of pancreatic secretion, p. 830). The control of secretion also appears to be identical, in that the hormone **secretin**, potentiated by *CCK*, stimulates the production of large volumes of juice.

Gall bladder

Although the bile-acid-independent fraction of bile is made at the time it is required, the bile-acid-dependent fraction has to be produced when the raw materials return from the gut to the liver, and then stored until needed. This fraction flows down the bile duct and, as the sphincter into the duodenum is normally closed, is diverted into the gall bladder.

Concentration of bile

When produced, the bile-acid-dependent fraction is isotonic with body fluids, as the walls of both canaliculi and ducts are permeable to water. The gall bladder concentrates the stored bile by the removal of non-essential solutes and water, leaving the bile acids and bile pigments.

This process of concentration operates in part by the active transport of sodium ions into clefts between the cells lining the gall bladder. There are tight junctions between them, which have a low permeability to water.

The process is illustrated in Figure 9.2.20. The intercellular clefts are long, narrow channels closed at the luminal end. Membrane pumps transport solute, principally NaCl, into these clefts, and it diffuses out through the

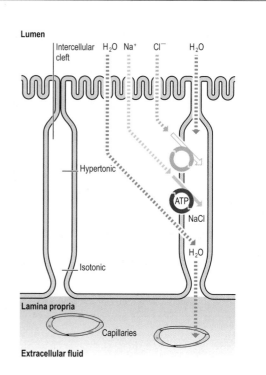

Fig. 9.2.20 Concentration of bile in the gall bladder.
Pumping of Na$^+$ into the long intercellular spaces sets up an osmotic gradient, which is highest at the luminal end. This draws water from the bile through adjacent cells.

open end into the extracellular fluid. Within the clefts, however, the osmotic pressure is high at the luminal end and declines to isotonicity at the basolateral end – a standing gradient. The contents of the gall bladder are therefore exposed to a fluid which is hypertonic, and water moves into it, not at a sufficient rate to destroy the gradient, but sufficient to allow the contents of the gall bladder to be concentrated. When this theory was first proposed it was thought that the luminal and intercellular fluids were separated by tight junctions which were, as their name implies, tight or impermeable to the passage of water. It is now clear that the junctions are more leaky than first thought and a modification of the theory suggests that a non-selective barrier exists at the base of the cells that has to be overcome by hydrostatic pressure before fluid flows out of the clefts between the cells. This barrier can be thought of as acting like a 'flap valve' isolating the clefts from the extracellular fluid. Solute is pumped into the clefts, water follows through the 'tight junctions' and when pressure builds up this solution escapes via the valve into the extra-cellular space.

This process of concentration can cause problems. The bile acids and cholesterol present in bile can, under some circumstances, particularly if calcium concentration is high, precipitate out and form stones – **gallstones**. These grow large by gradual accretion of solute.

Contraction of the gall bladder

The gall bladder has a muscular coat. This is partly contracted all the time, but contracts vigorously when chyme arrives in the duodenum, delivering a slug of concentrated bile into the duodenum to aid the digestion and absorption of fats. The mechanism of this contraction is endocrine.

Cholecystokinin (CCK) released from the duodenum contracts the muscle of the gall bladder and relaxes the sphincter on the bile duct to allow the secretions into the duodenum.

Summary

Bile

- The liver produces about 1 litre of bile per day.
- The digestive roles of bile are to neutralize gastric acid and facilitate absorption of fat.
- There are two distinct fractions of bile formed, one bile acid dependent, the other bile acid independent.
- Bile acids are recirculated via the bloodstream – the enterohepatic circulation.
- Bile is stored in the gall bladder and ejected in response to cholecystokinin (CCK).
- The insoluble breakdown product of haemoglobin – bilirubin – is excreted in the bile.
- The GIT is an endocrine organ whose secretions form part of its own control system.

Intestinal secretions

In the duodenum, secretions are produced by **Brunner's glands** in the mucosa. This secretion is a viscous, mucus-rich alkaline fluid. One of the main functions is to protect the duodenum from stomach acid until it can be neutralized by pancreatic and hepatic secretions. Mucus secretion is also present throughout the rest of the intestine.

In the jejunum and ileum there are many cells which secrete enzymes critical to the final stages of digestion and for the absorption of nutrients. These are considered in Chapter 9.4.

The gastrointestinal tract as an endocrine organ

The gastrointestinal tract secretes many different hormones to control the processes of digestion.

These hormones and related peptides are located in endocrine cells dispersed in various concentrations throughout the gut. The cells producing these hormones are part of a widely distributed system of amine precursor uptake and decarboxylation (APUD) cells. The distribution of gastrointestinal hormones and peptides is shown in Figure 9.2.21.

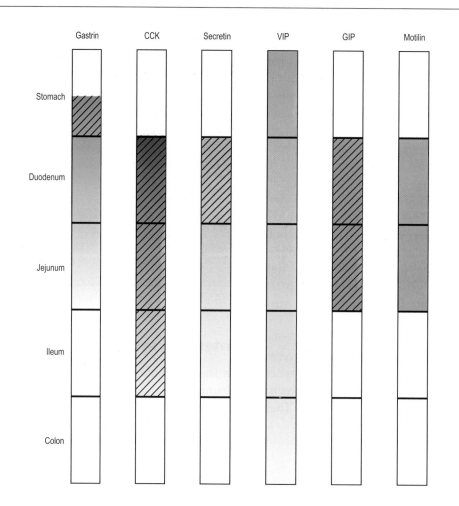

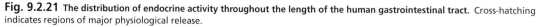

Fig. 9.2.21 **The distribution of endocrine activity throughout the length of the human gastrointestinal tract.** Cross-hatching indicates regions of major physiological release.

Recent Advances

Helicobacter pylori and peptic ulcers

Peptic ulcers occur in any part of the gastrointestinal tract exposed to the action of acid gastric juice, but principally in the duodenum and stomach. Up to 15% of Europeans suffer from peptic ulcers during their lifetime. There is twice the incidence in men over women and the most common age of onset is 20–40 years with a familial tendency for duodenal but not gastric ulcers.

Recently the bacterium *Helicobacter pylori* has been implicated in the pathogenesis of peptic ulcers and gastric adenocarcinoma. This organism is spiral shaped and was identified on the gastric mucosa more than a century ago. It was previously known as *Campylobacter pylori* but later differentiated from campylobacter by, among other properties, its multiple flagellae. It is found in the upper gastrointestinal tract, particularly in the pyloric antrum, under the mucus layer attached to the cells by pedicels. It does not colonize the epithelial cells. The familial tendency of duodenal ulcers suggests a person-to-person spread by an

oro-oral or faeco-oral route. Infection occurs in childhood, mainly under 5 years, with higher prevalence associated with low socioeconomic status and overcrowding.

There is a 95% association between the organism and chronic gastritis and the gastritis is healed by treatment which eradicates the organism. Experimental ingestion of *H. pylori* by healthy volunteers results in dyspepsia and gastritis. The organism is almost inevitably found at the site of duodenal ulceration. In 1994 *H. pylori* was defined as a Grade 1 carcinogen and in 1997 its eradication in all patients with gastric and duodenal ulceration was recommended.

The exact role of the bacterium in the pathogenesis of peptic ulcers is still unclear but it may in some way make the mucosa more susceptible to the acid and pepsin which are secreted in excess in these cases. Whether *H. pylori* is implicated in this hypersecretion is also not yet known.

The organism is particularly good at avoiding the host's immune defences and attempts to develop a vaccine are continuing.

Gastrointestinal motility

Introduction

Although the unitary nature of the gut should always be borne in mind, the fact remains that it is made up of parts of very different structure and function. An important part of digestion is therefore the movement of food from one part to the next in a controlled manner. This movement is brought about by gut motility. In this chapter we answer a number of questions about gut motility.

- How important is *chewing* food?
- In what way does *swallowing* prevent food entering the respiratory tract?
- By what method does motility of the *stomach* prepare solid food for subsequent digestion and prevent large particles from entering the duodenum?
- How does motility of the *small intestine* aid digestion?
- What are the characteristics of *large intestine* motility?
- How is *defecation* brought about?
- What are the common mechanisms that *control* motility of the GIT?

The motility of the stomach and large intestine differs in some important ways from the basic rhythmic activity of the small intestine, which consists of peristalsis – contraction of rings of circular muscle moving caudally at about 2–3 cm/s – and segmentation, where rings of circular muscle contract, dividing the intestine into segments and assisting in the mixing of gut contents. The longitudinal muscles also contract to assist in this mixing. These movements are **intrinsic** – independent of external activity – but can be modified by the autonomic nervous system.

In vomiting, the movement of the contents of the intestine is reversed by a retrograde peristaltic contraction. In the stomach, activity in the fundus is inhibited and dividing rings of contraction drive stomach contents toward the pylorus. At the onset of vomiting a deep breath is taken and the diaphragm descends; this, together with the abdominal muscles, compresses the stomach and ejects its contents in a well-coordinated reflex originating in a vomiting centre in the brain.

The gut is a sophisticated flow reactor, whose function depends on precise control of the movement of material within and between its compartments. Apart from the processes of swallowing and defecation, this control is exerted by means of the smooth muscle coats within its walls. The properties of intestinal smooth muscle determine the patterns of motility that are observed, so we will begin by considering intestinal smooth muscle in general, before going on to consider the specific patterns of motility of various parts of the gut.

Intestinal smooth muscle

The gut has two main layers of smooth muscle in its walls, an outer layer in which the cells are oriented along the length of the gut – the longitudinal layer – and an inner layer whose cells are organized around the circumference – the circular layer. The nerve plexuses which are vital for the control of motility lie between and beneath these layers.

Most intestinal smooth muscle cells are stimulated to depolarize, and therefore contract, by being connected to other cells that are already firing an action potential. If one cell within a bundle fires an action potential, therefore, all

will as the activity spreads. Activity spreads between bundles, either by simple conduction or via the nerve plexuses.

This still leaves the question of what starts the first action potential. There are two mechanisms. First neurotransmitters released from the nerve plexuses may depolarize the muscle cell to threshold. Second, some smooth muscle cells within the gut depolarize spontaneously. These cells have a resting membrane potential which is not stable. It oscillates over a relatively long period of time, becoming depolarized for a few seconds before repolarizing again. This is illustrated in Figure 9.3.1 and is known as the **basic electrical rhythm** or slow wave. Its mechanism is not known but the membrane potential moves spontaneously above threshold for a short time every few seconds. This means that each depolarization will produce a prolonged burst of action potentials, making these pacemakers different from that in the heart which generates only one action potential each time it depolarizes.

The frequency of the basic electrical rhythm is different in different parts of the gut, which is

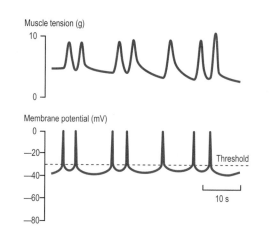

Fig. 9.3.1 Basic electrical activity of the gastrointestinal tract. A series of slow waves initiated by the myogenic pacemaker develop into spikes when they pass a critical threshold. Contractions occur as a result of spikes.

an important determinant of the pattern of motility in each part of the gut.

A more detailed description of the properties of smooth muscle is given in Section 2.

We can now examine how these basic properties of gut smooth muscle are exploited to produce the different patterns of motility of the different parts of the gut.

Summary

Basic gut motility

- A basic electric rhythm of inner circular and outer longitudinal muscle layers brings about the basic motility of the gut.
- Basic gut motility is modified by the activity of nerve plexuses between and beneath the muscle layers.

Mastication

Mastication breaks up food into pieces that are easily swallowed and adds to the pleasure of eating. Although under voluntary control, it is also reflex in nature, set in motion by the presence of food in the mouth. **Deglutition**, the process of swallowing, automatically follows. It is a very complicated series of movements carried out in a short time to deliver a bolus of food to the oesophagus.

Swallowing and oesophageal motility

The first stage of gastrointestinal motility, the transfer of food from the mouth to the stomach occurs very quickly, in a few seconds. There are three phases. First, under *voluntary* control, a 'bolus' of food is formed by chewing movements and the tongue, and this is propelled into the pharynx by the tongue moving backwards and upwards (Fig. 9.3.2A). Once this voluntary

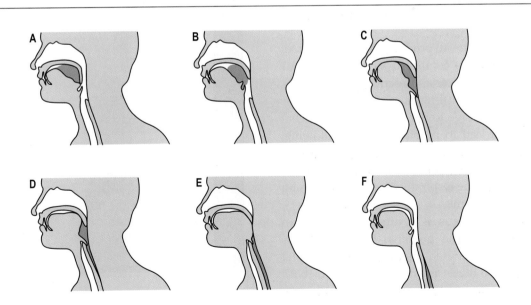

Fig. 9.3.2 **Sequence of events during swallowing. A.** Formation of a bolus of food. **B.** and **C.** The soft palate and epiglottis (backed up by the glottis, not shown) move to protect the nasopharynx and airway respectively from entrance of food. **D.** and **E.** The tongue pistons back pushing the bolus over the epiglottis. There is a slight delay at the hypopharyngeal sphincter before the soft palate relaxes (**F**), the epiglottis ascends and the bolus moves down the oesophagus. The whole beautifully coordinated voluntary and reflex movement takes about 1 second.

phase has occurred the remaining stages of swallowing are reflex. The arrival of the bolus in the pharynx stimulates mechanoreceptors. Impulses are conveyed via the glossopharyngeal (IX) and vagus (X) cranial nerves to the medulla and pons, where a group of neurones known as the 'swallowing centre' coordinates a complex sequence of contraction of the skeletal muscles, which delivers the bolus of food to the oesophagus whilst preventing it from entering the larynx:

1. The soft palate elevates, so food does not enter the nasopharynx (Fig. 9.3.2B).
2. Respiration is inhibited.
3. The muscles attached to the hyoid bone pull it forward and upward, which opens the laryngopharynx (Fig. 9.3.2C).
4. The bolus of food passes onward, pushing the tip of the epiglottis over the glottis deflecting food away from the airway (Fig. 9.3.2D and E).
5. As the bolus of food enters the oesophagus these changes are reversed, the epiglottis becomes vertical once more and the larynx opens prior to resumption of respiration (Fig. 9.3.2F).

The events are all produced by contraction of striated muscles controlled by neuromuscular transmission processes described on page 173. The nervous outflow is coordinated by the medulla. Damage to the neural control mechanisms can lead to problems with swallowing, and increased risk of choking. General anaesthetics and alcohol can lead to entry of food or vomitus into the respiratory tract by depressing these mechanisms.

The oesophagus is a tube about 250 mm long. In man, the proximal (upper) third is composed of striated muscle, whilst the distal (lower) two-thirds is smooth muscle. In both parts there is an outer, longitudinal layer and an inner, circular layer, with nerve plexuses between them. There are sphincters at both ends which are normally closed. The cricopharyngeal

or upper oesophageal sphincter prevents entry of air into the oesophagus during respiration, whereas the gastro-oesophageal ('cardiac') or lower oesophageal sphincter prevents reflux of gastric contents. Incompetence of this sphincter, as in **hiatus hernia**, leads to reflux of gastric contents and damage to the oesophagus.

Both sphincters relax to allow passage of food to the stomach. A bolus is propelled rapidly between them by a wave of peristalsis which lasts up to 7 seconds, and sweeps from the oral to the gastric end of the tube (Fig. 9.3.3).

Peristalsis is a coordinated, travelling pattern of contraction of circular and longitudinal muscle layers. The circular layer is contracted behind the bolus of food, and the 'ring' so

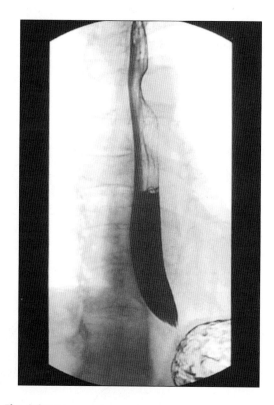

Fig. 9.3.3 The oesophagus. Swallowing a drink containing radio-opaque barium shows up the structure of the oesophagus in X-ray with the drink being held at cardiac sphincter at its lower end. The 'knuckle' of the aorta making a dent in the oesophagus can be seen clearly. (Courtesy of Dr Margaret Jones.)

formed pulled in a forward direction by contraction of the longitudinal muscles around the bolus. The longitudinal muscle then relaxes, followed by the circular muscle, and a new ring of circular muscle further along the tube then contracts to begin the whole process again.

In effect, the bolus of food is swept along the oesophagus by a travelling constriction behind it. The peristaltic wave of the oesophagus is entirely under reflex nervous control. The oesophageal smooth muscle has no pacemakers and does not contract spontaneously. The swallowing centres in the medulla produce a burst of efferent activity in the vagus nerve, which generates the peristaltic wave, though there is almost certainly a high degree of coordination of the activity within the nerve plexuses of the oesophagus itself.

As the peristaltic waves arrive at the lower oesophageal sphincter, the structure relaxes. The contraction of the sphincter at rest is believed to be largely a myogenic property of the muscle itself, though it may be increased by a variety of factors, including gastrin from the stomach, which is, of course, secreted in large quantities when acid secretion in the stomach is greatest and reflux into the oesophagus needs to be prevented.

The sphincter is relaxed by activity in the vagus nerve, though the transmitter is not identified for certain. **Vasoactive intestinal peptide** (VIP) is a strong candidate.

Overall, the medullary centres coordinate a smooth transfer of a bolus of food between the mouth and the stomach in 2–5 seconds.

Motility of the stomach

The stomach serves to store food, which we ingest faster than it can be digested. It also subjects food to physical and chemical disruption by attack with acid and enzymes, and delivers the resulting chyme to the intestines at a rate they can handle. These functions require a complex pattern of motility.

Like the rest of the gut, the stomach has longitudinal and circular muscle layers in its wall, and complex nerve plexuses between them. It also has an oblique muscle layer with the fibres set in horseshoe bands below the circular layer. Unlike the oesophagus, it also has groups of cells which act as **pacemakers**, producing bursts of action potentials every 20 seconds or so. In between meals, the firing of the pacemaker cells produces only feeble contractions which flutter over the surface of the organ on top of a tonic contraction, with little or no effect.

Receptive relaxation

Once food is consumed, the first pattern of 'motility' of the stomach is a relaxation of the resting tone in the muscle coats, which allows the volume of the organ to increase with a negligible rise in intragastric pressure. This change, known as **receptive relaxation**, is essential if reflux of gastric contents into the oesophagus and excessively rapid gastric emptying of chyme are to be avoided, as both will be produced by any large rises in intragastric pressure.

Receptive relaxation is mediated by the **vagus** nerve, and can be regarded as a part of the swallowing reflex. The transmitter released is not acetylcholine, which would normally contract smooth muscle. Likely candidates are ATP and vasoactive intestinal peptide (VIP). If the vagus is damaged, receptive relaxation does not occur and patients complain of **heartburn**, produced by acid entering the relatively unprotected oesophagus, and **dumping**, a complex of effects, including fullness and cardiovascular and blood glucose changes, produced by too rapid stomach emptying into the duodenum.

Mixing

Once the stomach begins to fill, periodic, strong contractions of the smooth muscle begin. These contractions agitate the contents of the stomach, facilitating the action of the acid and enzymes, and are also an important part of the mechanism which controls the rate of stomach emptying. When the pH in the region of the pylorus falls, it relaxes allowing chyme into the duodenum.

Cells in the longitudinal muscle layer act as pacemakers, generating bursts of action potentials three times a minute. This activity originates on the upper part of the greater curvature (see Fig. 9.2.8, p. 822), and then spreads over the fundus and the main body of the stomach towards the pyloric antrum and pylorus. As it propagates away from the pacemaker, the force of contraction and speed of propagation change.

The upper part of the stomach – the fundus, and the upper part of the corpus – contracts weakly and the wave propagates quite slowly. This part of the stomach, where most large lumps of undigested food are stored, is therefore subject to agitation as the whole contents are moved back and forth with each wave.

When the contraction wave reaches the remainder of the body of the stomach, it becomes more forceful and propagates more rapidly. The stomach can often appear to be almost divided into two by such powerful contractions. This contraction serves to retain larger, undigested lumps of food in the upper, storage, part of the stomach, whilst in effect 'decanting' the semi-liquid chyme. This is then propelled towards the pyloric antrum.

Emptying

The terminal part of the stomach, before the pyloric sphincter, is the **pyloric antrum**, a region of marked thickening of the muscle layers. The antrum and sphincter control exit from the stomach. Increase in volume of chyme in the pyloric antrum induces antral contractions and opening of the sphincter. A small amount of chyme is ejected into the duodenum. After a short time the pyloric sphincter contracts, preventing further release of chyme. The combined action of the fundus and **antral 'mill'** macerates the gastric contents, exposing them to early enzymic action preparatory to release

as semi-fluid chyme into the duodenum. The rate of stomach emptying is very precisely controlled by a number of factors acting on the contractions of the pyloric sphincter and antrum. These include the state of the gastric contents and events in the upper duodenum. Rate of emptying is increased by increased volume and decrease in pH of the stomach contents. Gastric emptying is reduced by filling of the duodenum and increased pH and osmolality of its contents. Composition of a meal can affect the rate of stomach emptying, which is, for example, reduced by fats.

Mechanisms involved in this emptying may be partly neural. The enterogastric reflex, mediated by the vagus nerve, has an inhibitory action on gastric motility. An endocrine component of this control is derived from the action

Summary

From mouth to stomach

- Swallowing, like defecation, has voluntary and involuntary components.
- Oesophageal peristalsis is entirely under nervous control; oesophageal smooth muscle has no pacemakers.
- Receptive relaxation of the stomach allows increase in volume on feeding without much increase in pressure.
- Pacemakers in the longitudinal muscle of a full stomach generate about three strong contractions per minute.
- The pyloric antrum 'mills' food before its sphincter releases the food in small amounts into the duodenum.
- Stomach emptying is neurally and endocrinologically controlled to match the nutritional composition of the stomach contents.

of secretin released by increased acidity in the upper small intestine. Similar inhibition of gastric emptying by fat and amino acids in the small intestine results from the action of cholecystokinin (CCK).

Overall, the regulation of gastric emptying is normally precise, so that chyme is supplied to the intestines at an appropriate rate for them to process it.

Motility of the small intestine

The small intestine is the major site of absorption of nutrients and reabsorption of secretions added to the gut. Its pattern of motility reflects its function. The mucosa lining the small intestine has a structure which provides an enormous area for exchange (see p. 852), and the chyme within it needs to be gently agitated and propelled slowly from the duodenum to the terminal ileum.

Gentle agitation and propulsion are produced by a motility pattern known as **segmenting**. The rate at which segmental contractions occur varies along the length of the intestine. It is highest in the duodenum, at 10–12 per minute in man, and lowest in the terminal ileum, at around six per minute. This decline in the frequency of segmenting is known as the **intestinal gradient**.

The precise mechanism by which segmenting occurs is unknown, but involves pacemaker cells within the muscle layers and nerve plexuses. In general terms, each section of intestine seems to be driven by a single pacemaker at its oral end. The bursts of action potentials generated by this pacemaker propagate in a caudal direction, presumably via the nerve plexuses, and every few centimetres or so they 'escape' to stimulate a short contraction in nearby muscle. When the next wave of activity propagates, those areas of muscle which have just contracted do not do so again and some other areas respond.

Chyme will tend to move slowly from a section segmenting at a high rate to one segmenting at a lower rate, thus gradually moving in a caudal direction. Any given particle of chyme, however, is not propelled linearly from duodenum to terminal ileum, but moves backwards and forwards constantly, so the total distance travelled is many times the length of the intestine, ensuring efficient mixing.

Peristaltic contractions, more dependent on longitudinal than circular (segmenting) muscles, are concerned with propulsion over only a few centimetres and then die out.

Whilst segmenting is the principal pattern of small intestinal motility, other patterns appear occasionally. If one part of the intestine is distended – because of, say, a minor obstruction or a gas bubble – then this will induce a local vigorous peristaltic wave like that described above in the oesophagus, which propagates for just a few centimetres and generally clears the obstruction. If the obstruction persists, the contractions persist, becoming painful, as colic.

Less painful, if more frequent, is a form of contraction known as the **migrating myoelectric complex** (MMC). About 10 times each day, between digestive episodes associated with meals, human intestine shows bursts of electrical and contracting activity which sweep from the stomach to the terminal ileum. The waves start at a speed of about 10 cm/minute, slowing down to 1 cm/minute in the terminal ileum, which it takes about 2 hours to reach from the duodenum. During these episodes, the ileum segments about every 5 seconds and these contractions advance down the gut one after the other.

This activity can be reduced by distending the stomach with air or milk. It is thought that the MMC acts as an 'interdigestive housekeeper', keeping the lumen of the intestine 'clean and tidy', because these powerful contractions remove undigested food particles, cell debris and even bacteria from the surface of the villi and propel them along the gut.

Summary

Small intestine motility

- Motility in the small intestine has a 'segmenting' pattern.
- Rate of segmenting decreases from 10–12/minute in the duodenum to 6/minute in the terminal ileum – the 'intestinal gradient'.
- The pattern of segmenting shuffles chyme backward and forward and gradually moves it caudally.

Motility of the large intestine

About 1.5 litres of chyme per day enter the large intestine. This progresses slowly through the organ and is desiccated to a few hundred grams of faeces. At appropriate moments, the faeces must be disposed of by **defecation**. The contents of the ascending colon and most of the transverse colon are liquid, but by the time the descending colon is reached, the contents become more solid as they are formed into faeces.

The arrangement of muscle layers in the large intestine is somewhat different from that in the rest of the gut. Whilst it retains a powerful circular muscle layer, its longitudinal muscle layer is reduced to three bands distributed around its circumference – the taeniae coli.

The patterns of motility vary along the length of the colon. In the ascending and transverse colon, the main pattern of motility is similar to segmenting in the small intestine. Throughout the large intestine, however, the constrictions produced by muscular contraction are greater and longer lasting, which divides the colon into compartments which are known as **haustra**.

Pacemakers in the colonic wall, located in the submucosal muscle rather than the longitudinal muscle as elsewhere in the gut, fire bursts of action potentials four to six times a minute. This produces segmenting-like contractions which move the contents repeatedly backwards and forwards between haustra – a process known as **haustral shuttling**. Contents move forwards and backwards to increase exposure to the mucosal surfaces and facilitate reabsorption of water and salts.

In the distal colon (transverse, descending and sigmoid colon) the contractions are normally less propulsive, and serve to knead the faeces into their final form.

Over the whole colon the contents are propelled very slowly in the anal direction, at about 5 cm/hour on average. This produces a gradual accumulation of faeces in the descending colon.

Several times a day the colon exhibits another pattern of motility – a form of peristalsis known as a **mass movement** which propels the contents in an anal direction at an increased rate, about 5 cm/minute.

The mechanisms controlling colonic motility are complex. The organ is capable of generating coordinated motility if its extrinsic nerves are cut. But for some patterns of motility the intrinsic nerve plexuses are essential. In **Hirschsprung's disease** the neurones of the nerve plexuses are congenitally absent from part of the colon, which, unrestricted by the myenteric plexus, produces constant (tonic) contraction of the circular muscles and consequent obstruction. The colon oral to the obstruction becomes distended with faeces.

Some patterns of motility are clearly dependent upon extrinsic innervation. Mass movements, in particular, are triggered at particular times of day, or by stimuli associated with eating – the so-called **gastrocolic reflex**. We are all aware that in many individuals colonic activity is enhanced by anxiety.

Normally the colon presents a load of faeces to the rectum, producing an urge to defecate.

Clinical Example

Hirschsprung's disease

Hirschsprung's disease is a good example of how disease can demonstrate physiological mechanisms; in this case the neural mechanisms which control how material is propelled through the intestine. Hirschsprung's is one of several diseases known as megacolon and has the alternative name of congenital megacolon. The term megacolon describes a number of congenital and acquired conditions where the colon is dilated, frequently secondarily to chronic constipation. The disease is caused by the failure to develop of ganglion cells in the myenteric and submucosal plexuses of the colon. In many cases the absence of ganglia, which usually starts at the anorectal junction, is restricted to the rectum, but in exceptional cases the entire rectum and colon are affected.

Without ganglia, the affected segment cannot carry out peristalsis and remains narrow and spastic, acting as a functional intestinal obstruction. The contents of the gut pile up proximal to the obstruction, distending the colon. Frequently on X-ray the non-functional segment appears normal compared to the grossly distended segment.

Most children with this problem present soon after birth with a distended abdomen and a history of vomiting after failing to pass the meconium plug which represents their first bowel movement. Newborn children are very susceptible to fluid and electrolyte imbalance and, without treatment, those suffering from this disease would soon die from this imbalance or from frank perforation of their dilated caecum. Occasionally the disease is missed in children in whom only a short segment of the gut is involved, and all young patients presenting with megacolon should have Hirschsprung's disease excluded.

Diagnosis is made by staining histological sections of a biopsy of the rectal wall for cholinesterase, an enzyme associated with cholinergic transmission. Absence of this enzyme suggests absence of ganglia. The diagnosis is supported by pressure tests which demonstrate failure of the internal anal sphincter to relax.

The condition can be effectively treated by surgical removal of the aganglionic segment, provided it is not too extensive.

A similar condition caused by infection with *Trypanosoma cruzi* is known as Chagas' disease and is prevalent in South America. The organisms live in the wall of the gut and destroy the intramural ganglia. The situation is more difficult than in Hirschsprung's disease because the destruction may be more extensive and reinfection is common.

Defecation

Most of the time the rectum is empty and exhibits segmental-like contractions which tend to propel any contents back into the sigmoid colon.

When a mass movement occurs in the descending and sigmoid colon, however, faeces are propelled into the rectum and distend it, leading to an urge to defecate and an accompanying relaxation of the smooth muscle of the internal anal sphincter.

At this stage the striated muscle of the external anal sphincter remains contracted, until, under normal circumstances, it is relaxed under voluntary control if defecation is appropriate. At the same time, a squatting position is adopted to align the rectum and the anal canal, and intra-abdominal pressure is increased by contraction of abdominal muscles. In this way the faeces are eliminated. Faeces moving into the rectum stretch its wall and provoke the defecation reflex, which consists of peristaltic waves in the descending and sigmoid colon and rectum and contraction of the abdominal muscles. This reflex can take place in the absence of CNS modification but is usually fortified by reflex activity in the sacral spinal cord and parasympathetic fibres in the nervi erigentes. The reflex is used in the management of paraplegic defecation.

If voluntary defecation does not take place, the urge to defecate initially goes away, the internal sphincter contracts and reverse peristalsis empties the contents of the rectum back into the colon until the next mass movement.

Summary

Large intestine motility and defecation

- About 1.5 litres of liquid chyme entering the ascending and then transverse colon is desiccated to a few hundred grams of faeces by the time the descending colon is reached.
- Contraction of its circular muscle divides the colon into haustra, between which the contents slowly shuffle to and fro.
- A few times a day, mass movement propels the faeces into the normally empty rectum.
- Voluntary relaxation of the external anal sphincter in response to mass movement results in defecation.

Intestinal absorption

9.4

Introduction

The processes of digestion yield a variety of
small ions and molecules that must be absorbed,
together with the large quantities of water and
electrolytes added by the gut for digestion.
Most absorption takes place in the small intestine, with some further absorption of water and
ions in the large intestine. The small intestine
absorbs water; electrolytes such as Na^+, K^+, Cl^-;
sugars such as glucose, galactose and fructose;
amino acids and dipeptides; vitamins and minerals; and fats.

Transport processes in absorption

Substances move from the lumen of the intestine into the extracellular fluid by a variety of
mechanisms. First, any substance which is present at a higher concentration in the gut than in
the body fluids can move by diffusion down its
concentration gradient. How rapidly it moves
depends upon the concentration gradient and
the nature of the substance. Molecules which
pass readily through cell membranes move
quickly, sometimes from parts of the gut which
do not normally absorb, such as the stomach.
Alcohol is a good example. It can be absorbed
by passive diffusion from all parts of the gut.

   Molecules which are more hydrophilic (i.e.
polar molecules, which are more soluble in
water and do not readily cross cell membranes)

will only move down a concentration gradient if some means of transport is provided. Diffusion must be facilitated by providing either an aqueous route through a membrane channel – as happens with many ions – or a transporter protein in the cell membrane, known as facilitated diffusion.

Whatever the route of absorption, however, a major factor affecting the rate of movement is the area available for exchange.

Substances present at a higher concentration in the body fluids than in the intestine, or at the same concentration, will not move by passive diffusion, facilitated or otherwise. In this case, energy must be supplied to move them up concentration gradients by processes of active transport. The energy is usually supplied by hydrolysis of ATP, which drives the movement either directly or indirectly. Often one substance is moved up its concentration gradient by linking that movement to another substance travelling down a concentration gradient, with the latter gradient often having been established by ion pumping using ATP.

Again, however, a major factor influencing the rate of exchange is the area over which it occurs.

Structure of the small intestinal mucosa

The lining of the small intestine is specialized for exchange. The area available is greatly increased by huge numbers of finger-like villi, projecting into the lumen (Fig. 9.4.1).

The intestinal villi make the luminal surface look like velvet. Their form changes along the length of the intestine. The duodenum has broad, ridge-like villi, whereas there are tall structures in the jejunum, slowly modifying to shorter, finger-like processes throughout the ileum.

Each villus is composed of a layer of columnar epithelial cells on a basement membrane, a lymph vessel, blood vessels, a few smooth muscle fibres and some connective tissue. The height of a normal villus is up to 1 mm and

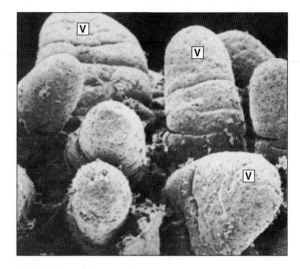

Fig. 9.4.1 **Intestinal villi and crypts of Lieberkühn.** Pore-like openings of goblet cells are seen to cover the surface of these villi (V). The crypts lie at the base of the villi. (From Young B, Heath JW 2000 *Wheater's Functional Histology*, 4th edn. Churchill Livingstone, Edinburgh.)

the villi vary in density from 10–40/mm². The presence of villi increases the area available for exchange in the intestine by about 600 times. The area available is, however, increased still further by the structure of the epithelial cells on the sides and tops of the villi. Their luminal surfaces are covered with huge numbers of **microvilli**, which are about 1 µm long and 0.1 µm in diameter. These structures constitute the **brush border**.

In between the villi are found the **crypts of Lieberkühn**, which are simple tubular glands secreting a variety of substances. There are a few mucus-secreting goblet cells, but mostly the cells are undifferentiated structures, which proliferate continuously to provide replacements for the cells covering the villus. In humans the entire epithelial cell population of the small intestine is replaced about every 6 days. Cells produced in the crypt move up the villi, and are then lost from 'extrusion zones' at their tips. The rate of proliferation of cells can be affected by a number of factors. It is greatly reduced during starvation, and if one part of the intestine is exposed to unusual concentrations of nutrients there may be increased proliferation.

Absorption takes place via the cells on the sides and tips of the villi – the cells in the crypts produce secretions.

Absorption of water and electrolytes in the small intestine

The intestinal contents are isotonic with body fluids and generally have similar concentrations of the major electrolytes, so this absorption must be active. Water cannot be moved directly, but will follow osmotic gradients, so the driving force for reabsorption will be active transport of ions. The majority of reabsorption is of water which has been secreted into the gut and comprises several litres per day.

The key to the whole process is the sodium pump – and Na^+/K^+ ATPase located on the basolateral (blood side) membrane of the intestinal epithelial cell. The hydrolysis of one molecule of ATP to ADP leads to the expulsion of $3Na^+$ from the cell in exchange for the inward movement $2K^+$. Both ion movements are against concentration gradients. As a result, the concentration of sodium ions within the cell is kept very low.

As in all other cells of the body, the rate at which the sodium pump operates is determined by the intracellular concentration of sodium ions. Should this rise, the pump will work harder and more Na^+ will be expelled.

The low intracellular concentration of Na^+ ensures that there is always a concentration gradient favouring the movement of Na^+ from the intestinal contents into the cell across the luminal membrane. This inward movement of sodium occurs by a variety of routes, including both **membrane channels** and **transporter proteins** which link its movement to that of other substances. Sodium which enters the cell by any of these routes is rapidly expelled via the basolateral membrane sodium pumps.

K^+ leaves the cell down its concentration gradient, via the basolateral membrane. This outward movement down a concentration gradient is linked to the outward movement of another ion, Cl^-, against its concentration gradient, as it is present in the cell at a lower concentration than outside.

Each 'turn' of the sodium pump, therefore, in effect ejects $3Na^+$ and $2Cl^-$ from the basolateral membrane. The Na^+ has entered via the luminal membrane, as has the Cl^-, down their concentration gradients. The imbalance of charge moved ($3Na^+$ to $2Cl^-$) leads to a small potential difference between lumen and extracellular fluid, which tends to drag a third Cl^- across the epithelium, so $3NaCl$ moves in practice.

As solute is moved across the cell in this way, an osmotic gradient is developed between the lumen and the blood, which will tend to make water follow the salt. This indeed happens, as water passes, probably via channels between the cells, to follow the NaCl. Any factor which increases the absorption of salt will therefore also increase the absorption of water, which is the basis of a very common treatment for diarrhoea – oral rehydration therapy (see below).

Summary

Absorption from the small intestine

- Absorption from the small intestine is by diffusion, facilitated diffusion and active transport, activities enhanced by the structure of the mucosa.
- The intestine only absorbs small molecules (except in young infants; see below).
- Absorption of water follows Na^+ pumped by the basolateral membrane of the intestinal epithelium.
- Villi increase the surface area of the intestine 600 times. This is further increased by microvilli on the epithelial cells of the villi.
- Intestinal epithelium is replaced about every 6 days.

Absorption of carbohydrates

The intestine can only absorb single sugar molecules (**monosaccharides**) and possibly some disaccharides, so any polysaccharides must first be broken down by digestion.

Brush border enzymes include:

- maltases
- isomaltases
- sucrase
- lactase.

The end products of the activity of these enzymes are the monosaccharides, glucose, fructose and galactose, which must then be absorbed.

It has been known for many years that sugars are absorbed by active transport mechanisms. Their absorption is dependent upon continued metabolic activity of the epithelial cells and can occur against a concentration gradient. Several sugars also compete with one another for what is obviously a saturable uptake process.

It is now becoming clear how sugars are absorbed. Figure 9.4.2 shows the model for glucose. Glucose enters the epithelial cell through the luminal membrane by means of a **cotransporter** molecule that links the inward movement of glucose with inward movement of Na$^+$ down its concentration gradient, which, of course, provides the energy to drive glucose up its concentration gradient.

There may be more than one transporter molecule with different affinities for glucose and different stoichiometry between glucose and Na$^+$ movement. Glucose and galactose share the same cotransporter, and so will compete with one another for absorption.

At the basolateral membrane, glucose leaves the cell by both simple diffusion and carrier-mediated facilitated diffusion down its concentration gradient.

Fructose, a ketohexose, is absorbed at a slower rate than glucose or galactose, but probably has its own Na$^+$-independent carrier mechanism providing facilitated diffusion, as it

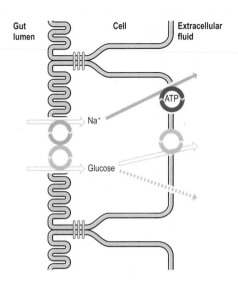

Fig. 9.4.2 Absorption of glucose. Glucose is absorbed into the epithelial cell via a cotransporter of Na$^+$ (which it shares with galactose). This is powered by the movement of Na$^+$ down a concentration gradient produced by the active transport of Na$^+$ out of the basolateral membranes of the cell. Glucose moves out of the cell and into the blood by diffusion and facilitated diffusion.

is transported faster than would be expected by simple diffusion, but cannot be transported against a concentration gradient.

Because there is cotransport of sodium and glucose from the gut, glucose enhances sodium and therefore water uptake. This is the basis of **oral rehydration therapy**. Patients who are suffering from diarrhoea are given an isotonic solution of sodium chloride and glucose to stimulate extra water uptake and prevent severe dehydration.

Absorption of amino acids

The digestion of proteins begins in the stomach, when the endopeptidase, pepsin, breaks them down into polypeptides. These polypeptides are cleaved into oligopeptides by the pancreatic endopeptidases, trypsin and chymotrypsin, from which amino acids are liberated by carboxypeptidase. Like the carbohydrates, however, the final stage of conversion to molecules suitable for absorption occurs in the brush border of the villus epithelial cells, where other enzymes act to produce amino acids and dipeptides.

The transport of amino acids into the epithelial cells can operate against a concentration gradient and, like the absorption of glucose, requires sodium ions to be present in the lumen. It is now clear that amino acids also cross the luminal membrane by means of a cotransporter which links their movement to the inward movement of sodium down its concentration gradient, providing the energy to move amino acids up their concentration gradient if necessary. There are, however, a number of cotransporters specific for different groups of amino acids. In all cases only the L-forms of the amino acids are transported. Three transporters are known to exist:

- the neutral brush border system, which transports most neutral amino acids
- the IMINO system, which transports proline and hydroxyproline
- the PHE system, which transports phenylalanine and methionine.

(IMINO stands for imino acids, as proline is strictly an imino rather than an amino acid. PHE is the biochemical abbreviation for phenylalanine.)

Two others have been described. One transports basic amino acids (e.g. lysine) and the other dicarboxylic acids such as glutamic. All amino acids then leave the cell into the extracellular fluid, via the basolateral membrane, by a mechanism which does not involve the movement of sodium ions.

There is also evidence that the epithelial cells can absorb dipeptides by different mechanisms. It could be that dipeptides are absorbed on a cotransporter which links their inward movement to that of H^+ ions, which have themselves been expelled from the luminal membrane by a mechanism linking H^+ with outward movement of Na^+.

There is one time in life when whole proteins are absorbed in the intestine – that is just after birth. In most mammalian species immune proteins are secreted into the first-produced milk – **colostrum**. The neonate absorbs these proteins without digestion, thus transferring immunity from mother to child.

At all ages, however, there is secretion of **immune proteins** (particularly IgA) onto the mucosal surfaces of the gut to protect against infection.

Absorption of minerals and water-soluble vitamins

A variety of minerals are absorbed from the diet. Two of particular importance are calcium and iron. Water-soluble vitamins are also absorbed, and vitamin B_{12} is of particular significance.

Calcium

Only a small fraction of ingested calcium is absorbed, and many factors influence how much absorption can occur. In the neutral conditions of the intestine, calcium will attach to many substances that may limit its absorption, but there is generally sufficient available for absorption across the intestinal wall to occur.

Intracellular calcium concentration is very low; there is, therefore, a steep concentration gradient tending to drive calcium into epithelial cells across the luminal membrane, as in other cells. Calcium crosses the membrane by a carrier or by a channel. Once in the cell it binds to calcium-binding protein, which may be involved in carrying it to the basolateral membrane, across which it is exported by active transport against a concentration gradient. Two mechanisms are involved:

- a Ca^{2+} ATPase which transports calcium with hydrolysis of ATP
- an Na^+/Ca^{2+} exchanger which links the movement of Na^+ down its concentration gradient into the cell to remove the Ca^{2+} from it.

All steps within the absorption process are stimulated by the substance **1,25-dihydroxy-cholecalciferol** ($1,25(OH_2)D_3$; calcitriol), which is the active product of vitamin D.

Vitamin D is present in certain foods such as cod liver oil, but may also be made from 7-dehydrocholesterol in the skin if it is exposed to sunlight. It is converted to its active form in the liver and kidney, particularly when parathyroid hormone levels are elevated because of a fall in extracellular calcium concentration.

Iron

Like calcium, iron in the ferrous form can bind to various substances in the gut which limit its absorption. Most dietary iron is in the inabsorbable ferric form. The absorbable ferrous form can be produced by the action of gastric secretions. This forms soluble complexes with ascorbate and other substances. Ferrous salts are more soluble at the pH of the intestinal contents and are therefore more easily absorbed. It seems that only certain cells can absorb iron. It crosses the luminal membrane on a carrier protein. In the cell it binds to a variety of substances, including ferritin and various binding proteins. It is then transported across the basolateral membrane via a second carrier protein.

Vitamin B$_{12}$

Vitamin B$_{12}$ (cobalamin) is released from food by the action of pepsins and acid in the stomach. It then binds immediately to a protein secreted by the salivary glands and stomach – R protein. The R protein–vitamin B$_{12}$ complex then enters the duodenum, together with another protein secreted by the stomach – **intrinsic factor**. In the duodenum and jejunum the pancreatic enzymes break down R protein, releasing the vitamin B$_{12}$, which then binds to intrinsic factor, which is essential for its absorption.

It is believed that the intrinsic factor–vitamin B$_{12}$ complex then passes unchanged to the terminal ileum, where it is absorbed by a receptor-mediated endocytosis. The vitamin B$_{12}$ is then released within the epithelial cell.

Patients with damage to their stomach from chronic gastritis (e.g. alcoholics) or who have had parts of their stomach surgically removed cannot secrete intrinsic factor and, as a result, have poor absorption of vitamin B$_{12}$, leading to **pernicious anaemia**.

Absorption of fat

The handling of fat in the gut poses problems that are quite different from those associated with the absorption of the water-soluble substances we have considered so far. Fats will, of course, cross fat-based cell membranes with ease, provided they can be got to them in the right form. The trick is to convey fats in very small particles which, by virtue of incorporation of other substances, are sufficiently water soluble to remain in solution in the gut lumen, and provide a large surface area for water-soluble, fat-digesting enzymes to work on.

Fat digestion occurs mainly in the small intestine. The acid and churning action of the stomach break dietary fats into very small particles, which are delivered at a controlled rate into the duodenum. There they mix with emulsifying agents which produce stable particles, 0.5–1.0 μm in diameter.

The main emulsifying agents are the bile acids – cholic acid and chenodeoxycholic acid (see Ch. 9.2), which, together with polar lipids such as lecithin and cholesterol, are incorporated into the liquid droplets.

These droplets are then acted upon by lipases, mostly of pancreatic origin, which produces 2-monoglycerides and free fatty acids – only about 30% of fats are completely hydrolysed to fatty acids and glycerol.

The free fatty acids and monoglycerides are then incorporated into tiny particles known as **micelles**, formed from bile acids. These micelles are 4–5 nm in diameter and are formed when the concentration of bile acids exceeds a critical value. Bile acids aggregate into polymolecular units arranged so that hydrophilic parts of the molecule face out towards the surrounding solution, while the hydrophobic parts of the molecule form a core into which fatty acids and monoglycerides can migrate and be transported in what is known as a 'mixed micelle'. These then diffuse into an *'unstirred layer'* next to the surface of the epithelial cells, and the fatty acids and monoglycerides can then diffuse into the cell membrane. The bile acids remain in the gut and are reabsorbed.

Once in the cell, the fatty acids and monoglycerides are reassembled by a number of metabolic pathways into fats. Triglyceride droplets so formed migrate to the Golgi apparatus of the cells, where they are coated and enclosed within vesicles. The coat is made up of protein, phospholipid and cholesterol. The particles produced are known as **chylomicrons**, and have diameters ranging from 75–600 nm. These chylomicrons are then exported across the basolateral membrane of the cell, and leave the villus via its lymph vessel, eventually passing into the venous side of the circulation via the lymphatic system.

Intestinal secretion

In addition to its main function of absorption, the intestine is also able to produce large volumes of secretions under some circumstances. It seems that when secretion occurs it is the immature cells in the crypts of Lieberkühn which are responsible. When appropriately stimulated, these cells seem capable of actively transporting large amounts of Cl^- into the gut lumen. This may be achieved by means of a $Na^+/K^+/Cl^-$ cotransporter protein in the basolateral membrane of the cells. The result is the movement of NaCl into the intestinal lumen, which generates an osmotic gradient leading to movement of water into the intestines.

Why should such a process occur in an organ where normal function is to absorb water and electrolytes? One possible reason why secretion is required in normal individuals is to provide a source of Na^+ for the absorption of those substances, such as glucose and amino acids, which are absorbed by cotransport with Na^+. Intestinal secretion is in part under control of the enteric nervous system and may increase following sympathetic stimulation. There may also be local reflexes originating from the mucosa, presumably in response to some property of the luminal contents.

An important clinical consequence of the intestine's ability to secrete huge quantities of water and electrolytes is its ability to respond to the toxin produced by *Vibrio cholerae*. In this disease there is massive diarrhoea which cannot be explained just by failure of intestinal reabsorption (see Clinical Example: Cholera, p. 67).

Absorption from the large intestine

The large intestine absorbs water and electrolytes by slightly different mechanisms from those of the small intestine. The chyme which leaves the ileum, though greatly reduced in volume by absorption of water and electrolytes, is still isotonic with body fluids. In the colon more water is absorbed than electrolytes, so the water movement occurs against a concentration gradient.

As in the small intestine, however, the whole process is driven by Na^+/K^+ ATPases, in this case located both in the basolateral membrane of the cells and in the lateral membranes. The activity of these lateral membrane pumps extrudes Na^+ into the spaces between the cells, which are bounded at the luminal end by a form of tight junction which prevents NaCl from diffusing into the lumen. The intercellular spaces therefore develop a **standing gradient** of sodium ion concentration, so that the fluid nearest the lumen is hypertonic to body fluids. (NB: This is a similar process to that occurring in the gall bladder.) This standing gradient allows more water to be absorbed, leaving the luminal contents hypertonic to the body fluids.

As in the small intestine, electrolytes enter the luminal membrane by a variety of mechanisms. Sodium can enter via sodium channels. The entry of sodium is linked to an outward movement of hydrogen ions by means of an Na^+/H^+ cotransporter. This leaves a high concentration of HCO_3^- within the cells, which can then pass out down its concentration gradient via a transporter that links the movement to the influx of Cl^-. The Cl^- then leaves the cell at the basolateral membrane by a cotransporter which links movement to the efflux of the K^+ that has been pumped into the cell by the basolateral Na^+/K^+ ATPase. There is an asymmetry in the absorption of Na^+ and Cl^-, because the sodium pump exports $3Na^+$ from the cell, but only imports $2K^+$, so only $2Cl^-$ leave. This leaves the lumen negative with respect to the body fluids. This potential gradient draws extra Cl^- across the cells, and the potential difference draws K^+ out into the lumen. This is why, in severe diarrhoea, there can be considerable loss of K^+ from the body.

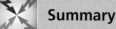

Summary

Carbohydrates, proteins, vitamins, minerals and the final residues

- Glucose and amino acids are cotransported with Na^+.
- The intestinal brush border contains fixed enzymes essential for the final conversion of many carbohydrates and proteins into absorbable forms of monosaccharides and amino acids.
- For a short time after birth babies can absorb whole proteins (immune proteins) from their mothers' milk.
- Calcium is absorbed by diffusion into the intestinal epithelium and active transport across the basolateral membrane, all steps in the processes stimulated by vitamin D.

- Only ferrous iron is absorbed, by a carrier protein.
- Vitamin B_{12} depends on intrinsic factor, secreted by the stomach, for its absorption.
- The key to fat absorption is its reduction to tiny particles (emulsification) to increase its surface area for enzyme action.
- The production of intestinal secretions is probably to provide a source of Na^+ for its absorptive activities.
- The final absorption of residual water in the large intestine is the result of 'standing gradients' of Na^+ between the cells.

Clinical Example

Starvation

Even when doing no physical work, a human being needs about 8500 kJ of energy per day to maintain life. Starvation is the abstinence from food because of either scarcity or pathologically being unable to benefit from food, owing to chronic malabsorption or cancer for example. Under these circumstances the victim has to use the tissues of his own body to provide the energy for life.

For 4–6 hours after the last meal, energy requirements of the body are met by glucose from ingested carbohydrates. Once that source has been exhausted, glycogen in the liver is converted into glucose (glycogenolysis). This process peaks within about 8 hours and since there are only a few hundred grams of liver glycogen cannot continue for more than a few days.

Next blood glucose, which is maintained at a steady level almost to the end of life, is supplemented by the production of glucose from non-carbohydrate sources (gluconeogenesis). These sources are lactate, pyruvate, amino acids and most importantly glycerol from fats. The fat which is used is neutral fat found in adipose tissue, which is taken to the liver where it is completely metabolized or changed into ketone bodies which are oxidized in the tissues. Remarkably, while the fat from adipose tissue is being used, the lipids which make up the cell membranes are spared.

Fatty acids and ketone bodies can provide most of the energy need of the cells, with ketones supplying most of the needs of the brain, supplemented with a small amount of glucose, but the high levels of acidic ketones which are now appearing in the blood produce acidaemia, which is compensated for by increased pulmonary ventilation and acidity of the urine.

In starvation, tissue protein is treated like dietary protein and hydrolysed to amino acids. Breakdown of tissue protein is controlled by the adrenal cortex and is not uniform throughout the body. The muscles, liver and spleen will lose 50% of their mass before the heart and brain lose 5%. The priority use of amino acids from tissue breakdown is to maintain the supply of enzymes and hormones; the next priority is the use of the carbon portion of the amino acids to maintain blood glucose.

When fat stores are exhausted, the breakdown of protein is the last process to supply energy for life. This breakdown liberates nitrogen, which is excreted as urea, and a rapid rise in urinary nitrogen indicates that the end is near.

Death usually occurs after about 8 weeks as a result of severe alterations in electrolyte balance and loss of renal, pulmonary and cardiac function. Body weight will be reduced by 50%.

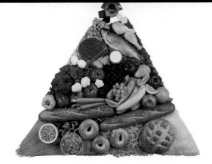

9.5

Good diet

Introduction

Chacun à son goût. The vast variety of foods eaten by different societies with their different cultural and religious prohibitions makes it a wonder that any definitive statements about human nutrition are possible.

In fact, although nutrition is a rapidly developing science, we can make several clear statements about what we need to eat to maintain good health.

The science of nutrition can be divided into what we may term **micronutrition**, the study of those essential substances we need in very small amounts of less than a gram per day, and what we may term **macronutrition**, which is the study of those substances that we need to eat in amounts measured in a gram or more per day. The micronutrients include vitamins, some minerals, and trace elements, which are dealt with in those sections of this book that describe the systems to which they are essential. Here we deal with the substances that are present in macroscopic amounts in our diet.

These macronutrients are built up into the structure of our bodies and provide the energy for homeostasis, which maintains that structure.

The chemical energy contained in the food we eat is converted by the body into mechanical work (muscular contraction), electrical work (maintenance of ionic gradients) and chemical work (synthesis of new macromolecules). The food we eat is the only source of energy for the body and is provided by the macronutrients, which are carbohydrates, lipids and proteins.

Carbohydrates

Carbohydrates are, arguably, the most important of the macronutrients since they should account for at least 50–55% of the macronutrient contribution to the overall diet, not only in the UK but also for most of the world. In the UK, however, the carbohydrate content of the diet is typically around 40%, with the 'missing' 10–15% being provided by fat. This is one of the reasons for the prevalence of the dietary related chronic diseases, including heart disease, cancer and obesity.

Definition

Carbohydrates are hydrates of carbon, i.e. compounds that contain carbon together with hydrogen and oxygen in the same proportion as water. The basic unit of a carbohydrate is the monosaccharide. The most abundant monosaccharides in the diet are glucose, fructose and galactose. They all have the same chemical composition $(C_6H_{12}O_6)$ but are structurally different, as shown in Figure 9.5.1.

Two monosaccharides joined together form a disaccharide. Common dietary disaccharides include sucrose (glucose and fructose), maltose (glucose and glucose), and lactose (glucose and galactose).

Carbohydrates may be classified as simple or complex according to their level of structural organisation. Mono- and disaccharides are known as simple carbohydrates; complex carbohydrates consist of chains of glucose bound together to form polysaccharides, such as in the most abundant plant polysaccharide – starch. The most abundant human polysaccharide is the storage compound glycogen found in muscle and liver, while starch is the storage form of carbohydrate in plants.

Starch is digested by enzymes called amylases, beginning in the mouth with salivary amylase and continuing with the secretion of pancreatic amylase in the lumen of the jejunum. The action of amylase yields disaccharides, which are further hydrolysed to their constituent monosaccharides by the brush border enzymes, maltase, sucrase, and lactase. Glucose and galactose are actively absorbed with the aid of specific carrier molecules which are indirectly powered by ATP, while fructose is absorbed more slowly by a process of facilitated diffusion.

Dietary fibre

Starch that is resistant to digestion and other non-starch polysaccharides were formerly

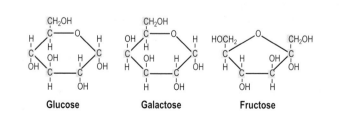

Fig. 9.5.1 Common dietary monosaccharides.

known under the umbrella term dietary fibre. These compounds, which have escaped digestion and absorption in the small intestine, undergo bacterial fermentation in the large intestine into short-chain fatty acids and gas. Soluble fibres are more readily fermented, whereas insoluble fibres are largely unfermented and add 'bulk' to stools.

Why do we need carbohydrate?

The major function of carbohydrates in vivo is as an energy source, providing approximately 3.75 kcal per gram. The main source of this energy is glucose. Glucose is the primary fuel of all cells and is the only fuel that the brain can use, excluding ketone bodies in the case of starvation or pathology. The cells of the body receive a constant supply of glucose, delivered in the bloodstream from the liver. Additionally, since the stores of glycogen are finite (approximately 200–500 g in a well-fed, rested human), some of the glucose is used to metabolise fat. This is because fatty acids are broken down into acetyl-coenzyme A (AcCoA), which is used to produce energy in the form of ATP from the citric acid cycle. AcCoA can only be used to produce energy via the citric acid cycle if it can combine with a 4-carbon oxaloacetate molecule derived from carbohydrate metabolism.

What happens if we have too much carbohydrate in the diet?

The answer to this question is largely dependent upon the type of carbohydrate. The biggest problem with too much simple dietary carbohydrate is dental caries. Different carbohydrate-rich foods have different cariogenic potential. Sticky sweets eaten on their own, without other food, have the greatest cariogenic potential, whereas the same sweets eaten with meals and drinks seem to have their cariogenic potential blunted. Thus, mode and frequency of consumption influence the potential of simple carbohydrates to cause dental caries. Additionally, however, over-consumption of simple carbohydrates may influence development of obesity and can thus have an indirect effect on health, influencing the development of coronary heart disease and type II diabetes.

Over-consumption of non-starch polysaccharide or dietary fibre may also have adverse effects. Over-consumption of insoluble fibre combined with a relatively low fluid intake may lead to constipation and haemorrhoids, while over-consumption of soluble fibre may lead to loose stools and excess flatus.

What happens if we have too little carbohydrate in the diet?

The beneficial effects of high-carbohydrate diets are quite well understood, especially those high in non-starch polysaccharides. However, the effects of too little carbohydrate are not so well understood and assumptions are made on the basis of disease prevalence in populations that consume too little carbohydrate, such as the average person following an average UK diet. The problems lie with the fact that the 'missing' energy that should normally be provided by carbohydrate-containing foods is made up by consumption of high-fat foods. This leads to obesity, coronary heart disease, various cancers and type II diabetes.

Dietary sources of carbohydrate

Good sources of both starch and non-starch polysaccharide include the following:

- potatoes
- cereals (including breakfast cereals such as porridge and wheat-based cereals)
- bread
- fruit
- vegetables.

Simple carbohydrates are found in sweet foods such as sweets, biscuits, cakes, sweetened drinks, e.g. squashes and fizzy drinks, and table sugar.

Lipids

Lipids, also known as fats, are a group of compounds that are insoluble in water but soluble in organic solvents such as chloroform and methanol. This is virtually the complete opposite of carbohydrates. The most obvious difference between types of lipid is their physical state at room temperature. Some lipids are solid at room temperature whereas others, such as oils, are liquid. This is the result of the different chemical composition of the fats, and it is important because this apparently simple difference can have serious consequences for human health. Generally, those lipids that are solid at room temperature, such as lard and the visible fat around meat, have high concentrations of saturated fats in their make-up, whereas liquid oils contain large concentrations of unsaturated fats.

Definition

Lipids are, chemically speaking, composed of fatty acids and glycerides. A fatty acid is a chain of carbon atoms linked together by chemical bonds with a methyl (CH_3) group at one end and a carboxyl (COOH) group at the other. Chain lengths can vary considerably, as can the number of double bonds in the chain, and hence give rise to different fatty acids and classifications. The most common lipid in the diet and in the body is a triglyceride. Triglycerides are three fatty acids bound to a single molecule of glycerol (Fig. 9.5.2) and comprise approximately 95% of dietary lipids.

Classification of fatty acids

Fatty acids are categorized by the number of carbon atoms in their chain and also the location and type of bonds between these atoms. Fatty acids always have even numbers of carbon atoms with hydrogen atoms attached. The carbon atom of the end methyl group is known as the omega (ω) carbon atom, and the carbon atoms are counted from the carboxyl end. It is the structural features of these molecules that influence their physical properties and which in turn influence their capacity to affect human health. Saturated fatty acids have no double bonds between their carbon atoms, e.g. stearic acid (C18:0) found in lard. Unsaturated fatty acids have a single double bond between two carbon atoms and are known as mono-unsaturated fatty acids, e.g. oleic acid (C18:1ω-9) found in olive oil. Polyunsaturated fatty acids have two or more double

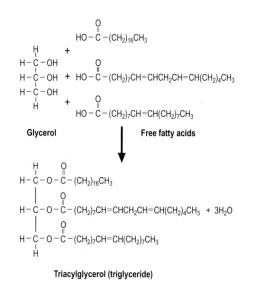

Fig. 9.5.2 The formation of a triglyceride.

bonds separated by a methylene (CH_2) group, e.g. linoleic acid (C18:2ω-6) found in sunflower oil and eicosapentaenoic acid (C20:5ω-3) found in oily fish such as sardines.

The nomenclature used above describes the molecular structure of these fatty acids. Thus:

- C18:0 tells us stearic acid has 18 carbon atoms and no double bonds (it is saturated).
- C18:1ω-9 tells us that oleic acid has 18 carbon atoms and 1 double bond (it is mono-unsaturated) that is situated 9 carbons away from the terminal ω carbon.
- C18:2ω-6 tells us that linoleic acid has 18 carbon atoms and 2 double bonds (it is polyunsaturated) the first of which is 6 carbons away from the terminal ω carbon.

Why do we need lipids?

Lipids have several important functions in the body. Dietary lipids provide a concentrated source of energy, yielding 9 kcal per gram. Fatty acids may be used directly for energy as AcCoA in the citric acid cycle or reassembled upon absorption and stored in the adipose tissue as triglycerides. They are also important from a structural point of view, forming a large proportion of cell membranes. In addition, dietary fats provide essential fatty acids and fat-soluble vitamins. Many of the flavours and aromas of foods are fat-soluble and contribute to the enjoyment of food. This may be one of the reasons for non-compliance with low-fat diets where food is thought to taste bland.

Certain fatty acids such as arachidonic acid (20:4ω6) act as precursors to important biochemical compounds – the eicosanoids. Eicosanoids may be subclassified into prostaglandins, thromboxanes and leukotrienes, which are all produced by the enzymatic peroxidation of arachidonic acid – prostaglandins and thromboxanes via cyclo-oxygenase, and leukotrienes via lipoxygenase. Non-enzymatic peroxidation of arachidonic acid leads to formation of lipid hydroperoxides, which can oxidize cell membrane fatty acids leading to apoptosis.

What happens if we have too much fat in the diet?

Again the answer to this question is not straightforward and depends upon the type of fat consumed. Over-consumption of saturated fat is linked to atherosclerosis and coronary heart disease; it is also linked to increases in blood cholesterol, specifically low-density lipoprotein (LDL) cholesterol. Over-consumption of polyunsaturated fatty acids (PUFAs) can lead to increased levels of peroxides in the blood simply as a result of increased substrate availability. Thus high intakes of PUFAs are associated with increased requirement for the lipid-soluble antioxidant vitamin E. However, high intakes of the omega-3 fats, the fish triglycerides (eicosapentaenoic and docosahexaenoic acid), have been associated with decreased risk of coronary heart disease and myocardial infarction.

What happens if we have too little fat in the diet?

Too low consumption of fat can result in deficiency of the essential fatty acids (linoleic and α-linolenic acid), although this is very rare in the UK. Deficiency of the fat-soluble vitamin E may occur with low intakes, though again this is rare in the UK. Generally, the main problem with dietary fat in the UK is one of over-consumption.

Dietary sources of fat

Dietary sources of fat include the visible fats and oils that are used in cooking and appear around meat; also, 'hidden' fats are found in processed foods such as cakes and biscuits and ready meals. One consequence for human health of the processing of fat by the food industry is the increased intake of hydrogenated fats.

Hydrogenation of fats increases the melting point, making them solid at room temperature, but also alters some of the double bonds to the *trans* configuration. This change in configuration causes the hydrogenated fats to behave in the body as saturated fats and carry the attendant risks associated with their over-consumption. The over-consumption of *trans* fatty acids has been linked to increased risk of coronary heart disease.

Proteins

Proteins are extremely important in physiology and nutrition. They are fundamental structural and functional elements within every cell. After water, protein is the next most abundant chemical compound in the healthy individual. A 70-kg well-fed, healthy male will have approximately 16% of his total body weight composed of protein, and 50% of that protein is present as four proteins: actin, myosin, haemoglobin and collagen.

Definition

Proteins consist of large units with molecular weights ranging from 1000 to >1 000 000 daltons and can be hydrolysed to their constituent units – the amino acids. Amino acids are linked together in proteins by peptide bonds where the amino group (NH_2) of one amino acid is linked to the carboxyl group (COOH) of another with the elimination of water. A further defining feature of protein when compared to either carbohydrate or fat is the presence of the element nitrogen.

Why do we need protein?

Dietary protein provides the raw material to make all the various types of proteins that the body needs, which then perform their respective structural and regulatory functions. In some circumstances protein can be used as energy, yielding approximately 4 kcal per gram. Dietary protein also provides the amino acids that cannot be synthesised by the body, and which are therefore 'essential' in the diet. The essential amino acids in humans are:

1. leucine
2. isoleucine
3. valine
4. methionine
5. phenylalanine
6. threonine
7. tryptophan
8. lysine.

Histidine is also considered an essential amino acid, since it is required by infants for growth and is needed to maintain nitrogen balance over the first 2 or 3 weeks postpartum.

Proteins undergo hydrolysis by several proteolytic enzymes in the gastrointestinal tract, releasing peptides and amino acids. The peptic cells of the stomach secrete pepsin, which is most effective in an acidic environment – this, of course, is provided by gastric hydrochloric acid. The action of pepsin brings about the initial partial digestion of protein to polypeptides. The most important proteolytic enzyme is trypsin, which is found in the pancreatic juice and is most effective in the alkaline environment of the small intestine; thus the pancreatic juice is the most important means of digesting protein. The digestion of protein continues until all bonds are broken down and the constituent amino acids are then absorbed in the small intestine.

Any residue of protein entering the colon or shed by colonic mucosa undergoes bacterial metabolism and is ultimately excreted in the faeces. Patients with obstructive pancreatic disease or with the genetic defect cystinuria are unable to absorb cysteine, arginine, and lysine fully. Unabsorbed amino acids are metabolized by colonic bacteria and passed as foul-smelling stools and flatus.

Traditionally, it is believed that 6.25 g of dietary protein yields 1 g of nitrogen incorporated into polypeptides and amino acids. The amount of protein synthesized daily is dependent upon requirements for growth, manufacture of enzymes and replacement of proteins used in the cells of the various tissues. The tissues of the body are under continual repair and are virtually in constant flux. For example, the mucosa of the small intestine is renewed virtually every 2 days, while erythrocytes have a life span of approximately 120 days. Amino acids that are surplus to requirements are deaminated in the bloodstream, producing a carbohydrate molecule and ammonia, which is excreted as urea by the kidneys.

It is extremely difficult to measure protein turnover or synthesis, i.e. protein status. Traditionally, nitrogen balance studies employed the following equation:

$$I = U + F + S$$

where I = dietary intake; U = output in urine; F = output in faeces; and S = output in sweat. The subject is said to be in nitrogen balance when the equation balances, and nutritionists use the relationship to determine protein requirements in man.

Modern technology has seen the use of radioactive labelled leucine (^{13}C-leucine) as the method of choice for measuring protein turnover, although there is still considerable debate as to actual protein requirement determined by this method.

Current UK dietary guidelines suggest a basic protein intake of 0.75 g/kg body weight per day for all adults over 19 years of age.

What happens if we have too much protein in the diet?

It is unlikely that over-consumption of protein will cause harm in a healthy individual. Its most likely consequence is obesity, since protein-containing foods typical of the UK diet usually contain fats and the extra energy thus consumed will be stored, leading to weight gain. The situation is different in individuals with pre-existing renal disease, since protein exerts a renal load that may be detrimental to normal renal function.

What happens if we have too little protein in the diet?

Low protein intake can lead to the deficiency disease kwashiorkor, although this is extremely unlikely in the UK. Typically, this is a paediatric disorder, occurring in children who have been fed on a low-protein diet, although distinguishing between kwashiorkor and the protein–energy deficiency disorder marasmus is often difficult. However, the child with kwashiorkor may not be underweight, whereas the child

with marasmus will almost certainly, by definition, be underweight.

So what is a 'good diet'?

Apart from air and water, which are frequently ignored but present in surprising amounts in our food, the bulk of our 'diet' is usually considered to consist of the three groups of substances we have already described as macronutrients: proteins, carbohydrates and fats.

These are present in different proportions in the four main classes of foods:

- meats (or their substitutes)
- cereals (including breads)
- milk and milk products
- fruits and vegetables.

A combination of these foods supplies us with the essential amino acids and fatty acids, 13 vitamins and the 18 or so elements that, interestingly, are clustered about carbon in the upper, lighter half of the periodic table. We carbon-based creatures seem to shun the heavier elements, many of which are poisonous to us.

The four classes of foods contain macronutrients in different proportions, and a good diet contains sufficient of one sort of food to make up for deficiencies of nutrients in the others, bearing in mind that the requirements of individuals change with their condition,

867

for example during infancy, sedentary occupation, pregnancy and old age.

The dietary guidelines for most healthy adults are generally agreed and well set out in the US National Research Council's prescription:

• *Reduce total fat to 30% or less of calories and saturated fat to less than 10% of calories and dietary cholesterol to less than 300 mg/day. Polyunsaturated fatty acid optimal intake 7% to 8% of calories (not over 10%). Omega-3 polyunsaturates from regular fish consumption. (Concentrated fish oil supplements not recommended for general public.)*
• *Eat five or more servings of vegetables or fruits daily, especially green and yellow vegetables and citrus fruits, and six or more daily servings of bread, cereals, and legumes. Do not increase intake of added sugars.*
• *Maintain a moderate protein intake, not more than twice the RDA [recommended dietary allowance].*
• *Balance food intake and physical activity to maintain appropriate body weight.*
• *If you drink alcohol limit it to no more than two standard drinks a day. Women who are pregnant or attempting to conceive should avoid alcoholic beverages.*
• *Limit total salt intake to 6 g a day sodium chloride.*
• *Maintain adequate calcium intake.*
• *Avoid eating nutrient supplements with dose above the RDA (i.e. avoid megavitamin supplements).*
• *Maintain an optimal intake of fluoride, particularly during the years of primary and secondary tooth formation and growth.*

This advice is not quantitative and does not address the major dietary problem of developed countries – obesity.

Make less thy body hence, and more thy grace;
Leave gourmandizing; know, the grave doth gape
For thee thrice wider than for other men.

Henry IV Part II, V.v.

In developed countries, except in exceptional circumstances, society attempts to ensure that no-one need go short of food. In this case, protein–carbohydrate malnutrition is almost always associated with disease, except in the case of some old people who may neglect their diet because of apathy or difficult social conditions. Obesity, on the other hand, is almost endemic with 8% of men and 12% of women in Great Britain having a body mass index (BMI) greater than 30 (BMI = Weight (kg) /Height^2 (m^2)). The acceptable BMI range is generally considered to be 20–25 and those with a BMI >40 are classed as grossly obese. These people are at risk of premature death from a variety of causes, but not quite to the extent that Shakespeare prophesied. For them, the grave gapes about twice as wide as for other men. The cure for obesity can on occasion be worse than the complaint, and a number of 'diets' peddled by the unscientific or unscrupulous to the gullible have proved damaging, particularly to the fetuses of pregnant women, and in some cases even fatal.

As in so many other things, the human body is resistant to changes in the proportions of its diet. There is a range of amounts of a nutrient required for health and the recommended daily intake (RDI) of a substance quoted by most authorities is usually at the lower end of the range required to ensure good health.

Further reading

Bender DA 1997 *Introduction to nutrition and metabolism*, 2nd edn. Taylor and Francis, London.

Primarily for students of health sciences and nursing, this text helpfully provides the basic chemistry and biochemistry necessary to the understanding of nutrition and metabolism. Metabolic pathways are well illustrated with diagrams in this useful book.

Johnson L R 2001 *Gastrointestinal physiology*, 6th edn. Mosby, St Louis.

That this book has arrived at its 6th edition demonstrates how popular it has been with students. Concise and well illustrated, its summaries, review questions and mini-exam are all aids to learning.

Sandford P A 1992 *Digestive system physiology*, 4th edn. Edward Arnold, London

One of the 'Physiological principles' series, this book strikes just the right level for Honours students in physiology. Despite his comments on bibliographies in his introduction the ones that the author offers in his very readable book are excellent .

Smith M, Morton D 2001 *The digestive system*. Churchill Livingstone, Edinburgh.

One of the 'Systems of the body' series this book provides an integrated approach to the digestive system emphasizing the basic science underlying the physiology and pathology of the system.

Stipanuk, M H 2000 *Biochemical and physiological aspects of human nutrition*. W B Saunders, Philadelphia.

Suitable as a textbook and reference book for students of nutrition, biological sciences and medicine.

Truswell A S 1999 *ABC of nutrition*, 3rd edn. BMJ Books, London.

One of the excellent ABC series published by the BMJ primarily for clinicians, this slim volume makes interesting reading for all.

Questions

Answer true or false to the following statements:

9.1

Within the gastrointestinal tract:

A. There are many enzyme-secreting endocrine cells.
B. Parasympathetic nerves promote motility and digestion.
C. There are layers of circular and longitudinal striated muscle throughout its length.
D. Mechanical activity depends on extrinsic nervous control.
E. The surface area of the small intestine is greatly increased by epithelial microvilli.

9.2

Saliva:

A. Secreted by the parotid glands is mainly mucous in nature.
B. Secretion is stimulated by acetylcholine.
C. Becomes hypertonic following ion transport within the salivary ducts.
D. Is more alkaline when saliva flow rates are high.
E. Contains amylase which can digest carbohydrate.

9.3

Acid secretion in the stomach:

A. Can be inhibited by atropine.
B. Can be inhibited by antihistamines.
C. Is stimulated by gastrin.
D. Is a function of the chief cells.
E. Produces a metabolic alkalosis during a meal.

9.4

Gastric secretion:

A. Of bicarbonate helps protect the mucosa from acid digestion.
B. Of pepsinogen occurs within the gastric pits.
C. Of intrinsic factor allows vitamin B_{12} to be absorbed by the stomach.
D. Of mucus occurs mainly from the parietal cells.
E. Of acid depends on secondary active transport of protons via an antiport carrier mechanism.

9.5

The pancreas:

A. Secretes a range of active proteases into the duodenum.
B. Secretes alkali into the lumen of the pancreatic ducts.
C. Has both exocrine and endocrine functions.
D. Produces enzymes which digest carbohydrates, releasing monosaccharides.
E. Secretes enzymes which can digest all the major nutritional molecules in our diet.

9.6

Pancreatic secretion:

A. Of bicarbonate-rich fluid is strongly stimulated by secretin.
B. Of bicarbonate-rich fluid is strongly stimulated by the vagus.
C. Of digestive enzymes is strongly stimulated by cholecystokinin.
D. Of digestive enzymes depends on endocytosis.
E. Of digestive enzymes is stimulated by intracellular production of inositol 1,4,5-trisphosphate.

9.7

Bile:

A. Contains a high proportion of unconjugated bile pigment.
B. Contains HCO_3^- most of which is secreted by the bile canaliculi.
C. Contains conjugated bile acids which are mostly manufactured on demand immediately prior to secretion.
D. Release from the gall bladder is stimulated by the steroid hormone cholecystokinin.
E. Plays an important role in lipid digestion and absorption.

9.8

Swallowing:

A. Is a reflex coordinated at the level of the spinal cord.
B. Is associated with active closure of the epiglottis over the opening of the larynx.
C. Relies on both somatic and parasympathetic nerves.
D. Leads to relaxation of the oesophageal sphincters.
E. Is assisted by the presence of salivary mucus.

9.9

In the small intestine:

A. Mucosal enzymes complete the digestion of some food types.
B. Glucose is absorbed by a primary active transport system.
C. Absorbed lipids are taken to the liver within the portal vein.
D. Peristalsis is the dominant type of mechanical activity.
E. Only conjugated bile acids are reabsorbed.

9.10

In the large intestine:

A. Water is absorbed from the intestinal contents by a mechanism which relies on the Na^+/K^+ ATPase ion pump.
B. The defecation reflex is coordinated within the spinal cord.
C. The internal anal sphincter is stimulated to contract by parasympathetic nerves.
D. The external anal sphincter is stimulated to contract by somatic nerves.
E. Control of defecation depends on ascending sensory and descending motor pathways, to and from the brain.

(*Answers overleaf* →)

Answers

9.1

A. **False.** The enzyme-secreting cells are exocrine, rather than endocrine.
B. **True.** Parasympathetic nerves are both motor and secretomotor within the gastrointestinal tract.
C. **False.** These muscle layers consist of smooth muscle. Striated muscle is only found in the upper part of the oesophagus, which is also controlled by somatic motoneurones rather than autonomic nerves.
D. **False.** Contractile activity can be observed in isolated segments of gut.
E. **True.** This is very important in the digestive/absorptive activities of the small intestine.

9.2

A. **False.** Parotid secretions are serous; sublingual secretions are mucous and submandibular are mixed.
B. **True.** This is the parasympathetic transmitter and acts on muscarinic receptors.
C. **False.** Ion transport mechanisms in the salivary ducts make saliva hypotonic.
D. **True.** This reflects a higher HCO_3^- concentration.
E. **True.** Salivary amylase probably is of little physiological significance because it requires near neutral pH and ceases to act when food enters the stomach.

9.3

A. **True.** Atropine inhibits the action of parasympathetic stimulation via muscarinic receptors.

B. **False.** Histamine from the enterochromaffin-like cells is an important stimulus to acid secretion. It acts on H_2 receptors, however, and is blocked by H_2 receptor blockers. The term antihistamines has come to refer exclusively to the H_1 receptor antagonists used in the treatment of allergies.
C. **True.** Gastrin is a peptide hormone mainly secreted by the G cells in the gastric antral mucosa, with some secretion from the duodenum and upper jejunum.
D. **False.** It is a function of parietal cells; chief cells secrete pepsinogen.
E. **True.** The loss of acid from the extracellular fluid raises the arterial pH and causes production of alkaline urine. This effect is limited by the subsequent secretion of HCO_3^- from the small intestine.

9.4

A. **True.** This combines with secretion of mucus to provide a crucial protective barrier.
B. **True.** Pepsinogen is secreted by the chief cells. The gastric pits are also the sites of acid and intrinsic factor secretion by the parietal cells.
C. **False.** B_{12} absorption does require gastric intrinsic factor but absorption actually occurs in the terminal ileum.
D. **False.** This is a function of cells on the surface of the gastric mucosa and in the neck region of the gastric pits.
E. **False.** There is a primary active transport system in which an ATPase links breakdown of ATP to H^+ secretion and K^+ uptake from the gastric lumen. Cl^- uptake from the interstitial fluid by the parietal cell occurs by an antiport mechanism, HCO_3^- being exchanged.

9.5

A. **False.** Proteases are secreted in an inactive form. They are activated within the duodenum; enterokinase on the epithelial brush border activates trypsinogen to trypsin, which can activate both trypsinogen and chymotrypsinogen.
B. **True.** This alkali neutralizes gastric acid within the duodenum.
C. **True.** The pancreatic acini and ducts have an exocrine function, whereas the islets of Langerhans are endocrine.
D. **False.** Pancreatic amylase digests starches to produce disaccharides which are further digested by brush border disaccharidases.
E. **True.** Food can be quite adequately digested in the absence of salivary or gastric enzymes.

9.6

A. **True.** Secretin is released into the blood from the duodenum and small intestine, particularly in response to acid chyme from the stomach; the resulting increase in alkaline pancreatic secretions helps neutralize this.
B. **False.** Vagal stimulation of the pancreas leads to the release of a small volume of enzyme-rich secretion.
C. **True.** CCK is another peptide hormone from the upper small intestine; its secretion is stimulated by the presence of the proteins and lipids which will be further digested by the pancreatic enzymes.
D. **False.** The process whereby membrane-bound enzyme granules fuse with the luminal membrane to release their contents is exocytosis.
E. **True.** CCK activates pancreatic phospholipase C producing inositol 1,4,5-trisphosphate (IP_3) and diacylglycerol. The IP_3 releases Ca^{2+} from intracellular stores and this stimulates exocytosis of digestive enzymes.

9.7

A. **False.** Bilirubin is conjugated prior to its secretion into bile.
B. **False.** HCO_3^- is mainly secreted by the intrahepatic bile ducts. Like the pancreatic ducts, these are stimulated to release large volumes of alkaline fluid by secretin.
C. **False.** Most of the conjugated bile acids are actually recovered from the intestine and secreted into the bile following a meal after fat absorption is completed – enterohepatic recirculation. They are then stored in the gall bladder to be released during the next meal.
D. **False.** Cholecystokinin is a peptide hormone.
E. **True.** It allows for the emulsification of lipids prior to digestion and the formation of micelles containing the products of lipid digestion. These present a large surface area for absorption of fatty acids and monoglycerides released by lipase activity.

9.8

A. **False.** It is coordinated within the medulla oblongata and pons.
B. **False.** The epiglottis does protect the larynx but it is depressed passively by the food bolus, rather than actively contracting.
C. **True.** Somatic nerves supply the striated muscle in the upper oesophagus; parasympathetic nerves supply the smooth muscle along the rest of its length.
D. **True.**
E. **True.** Mucus has important lubricant actions.

9.9

A. **True.** Oligosaccharidases are particularly important, completing carbohydrate digestion.

B. **False.** Glucose absorption depends on secondary active transport in which Na^+ diffusion is linked to glucose uptake in a symport system.

C. **False.** Lipids, in the form of chylomicrons, pass through the lymphatics to the systemic veins, initially bypassing the liver. Other absorbed nutrients, however, are carried in the hepatic portal vein.

D. **False.** Segmentation is more common, although there is some localized peristalsis.

E. **False.** Deconjugated bile acids are also reabsorbed, although not so completely.

9.10

A. **True.** This pump builds up a standing gradient of hypertonic fluid within the paracellular spaces because of the presence of tight junctions between the epithelial cells. Water is absorbed osmotically. This seems to be the general mechanism of water absorption within the intestine.

B. **True.** The reflex is coordinated at the sacral level.

C. **False.** Although parasympathetic nerves increase contractile activity in most of the smooth muscle along the length of the gastrointestinal tract, they relax the associated sphincter muscle, including that of the internal anal sphincter. Sympathetic nerves contract the sphincters, while relaxing the rest of the circular and longitudinal muscle.

D. **True.** These are classical motoneurones controlling the striated muscle in the external sphincter.

E. **True.** Faecal continence relies on sensory awareness of the urge to defecate, and motor outputs which inhibit the reflex if required. In spinal injuries the reflex remains but the sufferer will be incontinent.

The reproductive system and neonatal physiology

Introduction

'The survival of the fittest' is a phrase which has permeated almost every field of human knowledge, from economics to the biology in which it was originally coined. It implies that in any population of individuals there are differences which provide advantages to some that improve their chances of survival. Equally important is the biblical observation that 'Like begets like'. This is important for two reasons: first it focuses on the fact that there is something that determines the adult form of an individual that is present even before birth (elephants do not give birth to gazelle), which we now know as genes. Secondly, it describes the fact that the survivors of the struggle for life will produce offspring with their parents' improved chances of surviving for long enough to produce still more survivors. However, these survivors are only 'like' their parents; they are not identical to them. They are not identical to their parents for a number of reasons, the most important of which is the arrival in the biological world some many millions of years ago of the process known as sexual reproduction.

The process of natural selection of winners in the survival race means that there must be a variety of competitors to select from. Variety arises randomly as a result of a number of factors such as mutation, but random design is an expensive way to construct a winner because most of the variations which arise by chance are lethal and very, very few individuals are blessed with an advantageous mutation.

So, until the advent of sexual reproduction, evolution within the living world was relatively slow, involving a single type of individual the occasional mutation of whose offspring usually brought about change which was lethal to its carrier.

Sexual reproduction revolutionized this process by involving two individuals in contributing genes of different characteristics which mixed to produce more varied offspring. That is not to say that the dread process of selection was any kinder; the losers were as inexorably weeded out, but there was a more rapid production of variety and hence an increased chance of a very successful winner turning up.

In addition to this purely mechanical operation of the process of gene mixing came the new process of individual selection. A winner could select another individual with genes for survival to mate and mix its genes with, increasing the chances of the offspring being blessed with a double portion of genes for success. Alternatively, the successful individual might distribute its genes amongst a large number of partners, again rapidly increasing the variety of individuals and the chance of a successful survivor turning up.

The definition of 'winners' and 'losers' is open to much debate beyond the realms of a textbook of systems physiology but the importance of sexual reproduction, as described in this section in relation to human beings, is undeniable.

Section overview

This section covers:

- How chromosomal differentiation determines gonadal sex, which in turn determines phenotypic (genital) sex
- Production of sex steroids and protein hormones and their levels through life
- Structure of the testis, regulation of spermatogenesis and production of testosterone
- Control of oogenesis and ovulation to produce the ovarian cycle
- Changes in the uterus, consequent on the ovarian cycle, that produce the menstrual cycle
- Changes in the structure of a sperm to ready it for fertilization
- Formation and functions of the placenta, its secretions of chorionic gonadotrophin, oestrogens, progesterone and chorionic somatomammotrophin
- Changes in the myometrium and cervix in preparation for parturition
- The oestrogen : progesterone ratio and its effect on the onset of parturition
- Hormonal control of breast growth, milk production and release
- Placental role in transfer of respiratory gases, nutrients and waste products
- How the fetal circulation differs from that of the adult, and how this changes at birth
- Thermoregulatory, gut, renal and endocrinological problems after birth.

Reproductive function and its control

Introduction

The survival of most species depends on effective sexual reproduction, involving as the starting point the formation of a zygote from an oocyte, produced by the female, and a spermatozoon, produced by the male. This process is known as fertilization. The zygote carries the genes which define the unique set of characteristics expressed by an individual. Half of these genes come from the oocyte, and half from the sperm. The oocytes and sperm are known as germ cells (gametes) and differ in their mature form from every other cell in the body in that they contain only half the normal number of chromosomes, the haploid number (Fig. 10.1.1). The reduction in chromosome number is achieved by a process of cell division called meiosis (see Basic Science 10.1.1, p. 879).

At fertilization, the two haploid sets of chromosomes come together in the zygote to form a cell containing the normal complement of chromosomes, the diploid number. Two of these chromosomes, X and Y, are responsible for defining the sex of an individual. Germ cells produced by the female contain only X chromosomes, while sperm may contain X or Y chromosomes. Chromosomes carry genes which convey genetic characteristics from one generation to the next. These genes constantly change slightly (mutation) and this in part is why no two individuals are identical (except 'identical'

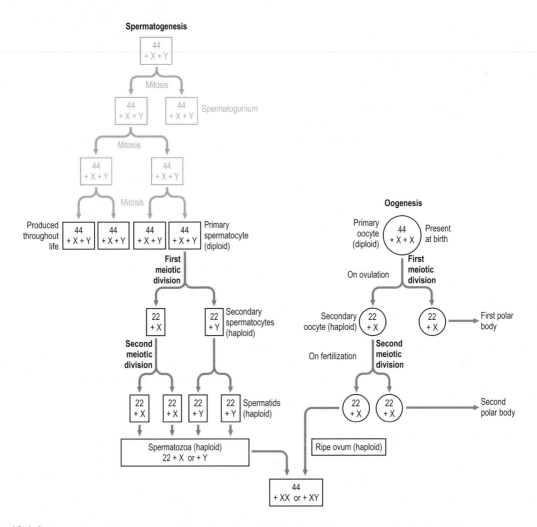

Fig. 10.1.1 **Spermatogenesis and oogenesis.** Somatic cells contain 22 *pairs* of chromosomes + 1 pair of sex chromosomes (X + X = female; X + Y = male). These cells are said to be diploid. Gametes contain 22 *single* chromosomes and a single X or Y sex chromosome. They are haploid. Two gametes come together to form the normal diploid number of 22 *pairs* + 1 pair of sex chromosomes in the zygote.

monozygotic twins), even though they may have the same parents.

In order to produce a male and female gamete, different reproductive apparatuses are required, which has resulted in the evolution of males and females. The main structure is the gonad, which produces the gamete, together with the reproductive tract, which in the male is modified to transfer the sperm into the female tract. The female tract is modified to receive the sperm, to allow implantation of the zygote and

to provide an appropriate environment for the subsequent development of the embryo during pregnancy. The gonads (the male testis and female ovary) also produce a number of hormones of which the principal ones are known generically as sex steroids. These are vital for the formation of the gametes and maintenance of the reproductive tract. They also influence the physiology of the individual, resulting in the characteristic male and female appearance and behaviour patterns, called the sexual phenotype.

Cell division

For cells to function they require a basic set of 'instructions' on how to work. These instructions are written in the genes of the chromosomes. A specific instruction is found at the same place on the same chromosome in all cells of an organism. The matter is somewhat complicated by the fact that the message is actually in two parts because chromosomes come in homologous pairs, one from the father and one from the mother.

As an organism grows or worn-out cells are replaced, the new cells must contain the same instructions as the original ones or chaos will result; similarly, the gametes (reproductive cells) from two parents must be produced by a process which allows their fusion to result in an offspring with the correct genetic message. Both these requirements are met by different processes of cell division.

There are two types of normal cell division:

- The first is the everyday replication of general body cells to replace those that are worn out, or to bring about growth, and is called mitosis.
- The second type is involved in the production of gametes for sexual reproduction; it involves halving the genetic material in the cell so that when two gametes fuse to form the new individual the correct complement of genetic material is restored. The reduction division of cells to form gametes is called meiosis.

Mitosis

Cells reproduce at different rates but they all go through the same cycle of events to provide for tissue growth and cell replacement. The daughter cells must have the same genetic composition as the original cell, and because

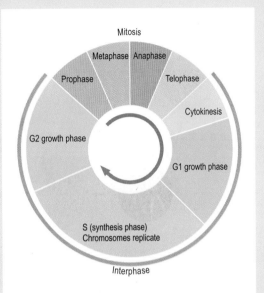

Fig. BS10.1.1 The cell cycle. The time for a cell to complete the cycle varies with cell type.

chromosomes in ordinary somatic (body) cells come in pairs we say a somatic cell has 2n chromosomes, n pairs, where n depends on the species from which the cell comes and is called the haploid number. The number of chromosomes doubles or halves at definite points in the cell cycle (Fig. BS10.1.1) and is normally 23 pairs in man.

In the longest phase of the cell cycle (the interphase) the genetic material in the form of chromosomes is not visible to light microscopes and so we do not observe a most important fact – each chromosome doubles to form two chromatids, in preparation for mitosis.

During the prophase of mitosis the two chromatids link together at the centriole and become visible (Fig. BS10.1.2). The individual sister chromatids (each pair is called a bivalent) are then separated and drawn one to each end of the cell during the metaphase and anaphase.

Basic Science *(Continued)*

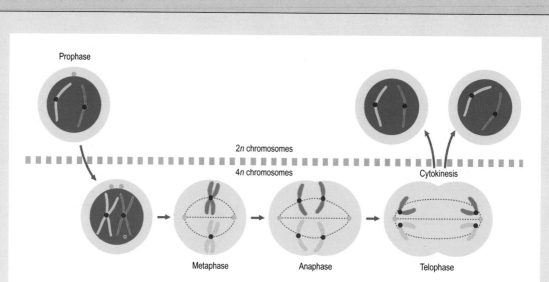

Prophase

2*n* chromosomes

4*n* chromosomes

Cytokinesis

Metaphase   Anaphase   Telophase

Fig. BS10.1.2 Mitosis. The chromosomes of an homologous pair are shown; one chromosome comes from the mother, the other from the father.

During telophase new nuclear membranes form round the two new sets of chromosomes, which are identical with each other and those in the original cell (before they doubled).

The cytoplasm of the cell then divides (cytokinesis) to form two new cells.

Meiosis (Fig. BS10.1.3)

The number of chromosomes in a human cell (before it has doubled in preparation for division) is called the diploid number (22 pairs + a pair of sex chromosomes: XX – female; XY – male). This must be reduced to half, the haploid number, when gametes are produced.

As in mitosis, the cell first doubles its chromosomes during the interphase to produce chromatids. There are at this point 23 *pairs* of bivalents, each bivalent made up of two chromatids. In preparation for the first meiotic division, the bivalents line up on the equator

of the cell and at this time there is crossing over of genetic material between chromatids. The *first meiotic division* takes place with bivalents being randomly assigned to either of the two daughter cells. This mixing and random division results in many millions of genetic combinations being possible in these two daughter cells. The daughter cells undergo a *second meiotic division* in which each bivalent splits and each daughter cell, now a gamete, randomly receives a chromatid containing half the genetic material (23 *unpaired* chromosomes) of a normal somatic cell.

In men, each spermatogonium yields 16 spermatids by a series of mitotic followed by meiotic divisions (see Fig. 10.1.1), all equally viable. In women, half the daughter cells produced at each meiotic division are small 'polar bodies' which degenerate, so each oogonium yields one ovum.

Basic Science *(Continued)*

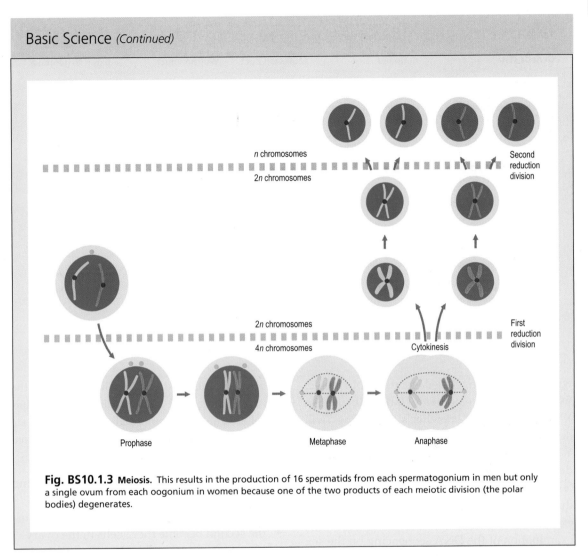

Fig. BS10.1.3 **Meiosis.** This results in the production of 16 spermatids from each spermatogonium in men but only a single ovum from each oogonium in women because one of the two products of each meiotic division (the polar bodies) degenerates.

Sexual differentiation

Genetic sex

The X and Y chromosomes are known as the **sex chromosomes** and are only 1 of 23 *single* chromosomes present in each gamete (the other 22 chromosomes determine non-sexual characteristics and are called **autosomes**). At fertilization, when two gametes fuse, 23 *pairs* of chromosomes are formed, of which one pair will be sex chromosomes. A female zygote contains two X chromosomes, one from each gamete, while a male contains an X and a Y. The Y chromosome is responsible for the development of the male gonads and genitalia. Whenever a Y chromosome is present testes and associated structures develop; when it is absent ovaries develop. Thus the Y chromosome is responsible for initiating sexual **dimorphism** (two different sexual forms, male and female, of the same animal).

Occasionally, abnormalities occur in the complement of X and Y chromosomes. For example, in Turner's syndrome there is only a single X chromosome (XO); the individual is a female

Table 10.1.1 Examples of abnormal development of the reproductive system

Genetic state	Gonad	Müllerian duct	Wolffian duct	External genitalia
XY, normal male	Testis	Regressed	Developed	Male
XX, normal female	Ovary	Developed	Regressed	Female
XO, Turner's syndrome	Streak devoid of germ cells	Developed	Regressed	Female
XY, loss of X-linked gene for androgen receptor	Testis	Regressed	Regressed	Female
XY, deficient testosterone synthesis	Testis	Regressed	Regressed to variably developed	Male/female
XY, deficient 5α-reductase	Testis	Regressed	Developed	Male/female
XXY, Klinefelter's syndrome	Dysgenetic testis	Regressed	Developed	Male
XX, adrenal 21- or 11-hydroxylase deficiency	Ovary	Developed	Regressed	Male/female

with normally developed genitalia but defective ovarian development (Table 10.1.1). An XXY individual (Klinefelter's syndrome) will develop testes because of the presence of the Y chromosome; however, sperm formation is deficient. Superfemales (XXX) develop fully as females but frequently have shortened reproductive lives, while supermales (XYY) often exhibit deficient spermatogenesis. Extensive examination of the DNA sequencing on the sex chromosomes of these and normal individuals has shown that one region on the Y chromosome is critical if normal sex determination is to take place. This region is described as containing a controller gene called SRY – the sex-determining region of the Y chromosome.

Gonadal sex

For the first few weeks of embryonic life, gonad development is identical in males and females and at this stage is described as indifferent. Primordial germ cells (PGCs) differentiate as early as 5 days after fertilization, and after 3 weeks will be found in the epithelium of the yolk sac. By this time a tissue which will form the matrix of the gonad, the gonadal primordia, has developed and the primordial germ cells migrate into this tissue to form the gametes. The stromal tissue of the gonad comprises two cell types:

- the first develop into the oestrogen-secreting granulosa cells in the ovary or the Sertoli cells in the seminiferous tubules in the testis
- the second become theca cells in the ovary or testosterone-secreting Leydig cells in the testis.

In a normal male embryo at 6–7 weeks, following the primordial germ cell migration, because of the presence of the Y chromosome containing the SRY gene, Sertoli cells differentiate and enclose the primordial germ cells, and seminiferous tubules start to form. The interstitial cells of Leydig, which will secrete the male sex steroid testosterone, develop at 8 or 9 weeks. In the normal female, differentiation of the indifferent gonad into an ovary does not occur until 9 weeks, when the X chromosomes are activated. This results in mitotic proliferation of the primordial germ cells, which subsequently

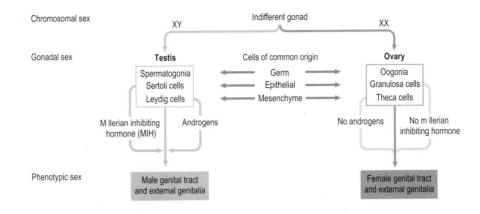

Fig. 10.1.2 **Development of sex.** Sexual characteristics exist at several levels, expressed at different times as the individual develops. The fertilized embryo has male (XY) or female (XX) chromosomal sex. This causes the indifferent gonad to develop into an ovary or testis (gonadal sex). The testis secretes testosterone, which is largely responsible for the development of male phenotypic sex. Absence of testosterone leads to development of female phenotypic sex (hence the aphorism: 'Add testosterone get a male, add nothing get a female').

undergo meiotic division to form primary oocytes. The meiosis stops at the late prophase stage, and the primary oocytes remain in this state until possible ovulation, which will not occur until many years later. At about 9 weeks, the ovary starts to secrete oestrogens, the principal female sex steroids. An overview of these processes is illustrated in Figure 10.1.2.

Genital (phenotypic) sex

Gonadal development up to 9 weeks of fetal life has been independent of hormonal regulation; however, the normal development of the genital ducts and external genitalia is hormone dependent. Unlike the differentiation of the male gonad, differentiation of the male genital tract requires positive hormonal involvement, its absence resulting in the formation of a female genital tract.

During the period of gonadal development, two genital ducts develop on each side, one set (the wolffian ducts) having the potential to develop into the male tract, the other (the müllerian ducts) into the female tract. Each set

of ducts is described as being unipotential in that it can only develop into the tract system associated with the genetic sex of the fetus.

In the male fetus, at 9 weeks, the Leydig cells under the influence of chorionic gonadotrophin from the placenta, start to secrete testosterone, which stimulates the growth and development of the wolffian ducts to form the epididymis, vas deferens, seminal vesicles and ejaculatory duct (Fig. 10.1.3). Transplantation and implantation experiments have shown this to result from each testis acting unilaterally on its own wolffian duct. In addition, at about 7 weeks, the testes secrete a second hormone (müllerian inhibiting hormone; MIH) which causes active regression of the müllerian ducts.

In the female, because there is no testicular secretion of MIH or testosterone, the müllerian ducts mature to form the oviducts, uterus, cervix and part of the vagina. In the absence of testosterone, the wolffian duct system regresses (Fig. 10.1.4). Transplantation of testicular material into a female fetus at this critical stage results in development of the male duct system and regression of the müllerian duct.

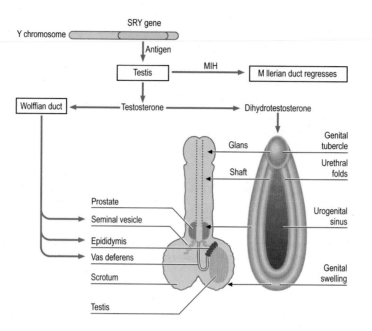

Fig. 10.1.3 **Development of male reproductive tract.** Showing how testosterone and müllerian inhibiting hormone (MIH) affect the indifferent structures.

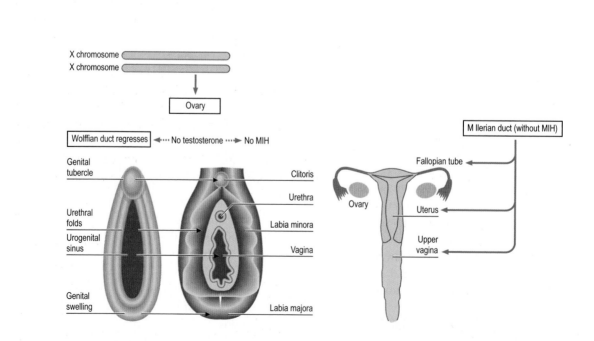

Fig. 10.1.4 **Development of female reproductive tract.** Showing how the absence of testosterone and absence of inhibition of the müllerian ducts affects development.

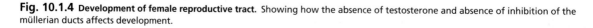

By contrast with the internal genital ducts, the primordia of the external genitalia are bipotential and development is dependent on the hormonal environment. In the female, in the absence of testicular testosterone, the female system develops with the urethral folds and genital swellings forming the labia minor and majora and the genital tubercle becoming the clitoris (Fig. 10.1.4). These changes do not require hormonal regulation, and occur quite normally in the absence of ovarian hormones. Conversely, testosterone, which must first be converted to **dihydrotestosterone** (DHT), is required for the normal development of the male genitalia with the urethral folds fusing and, together with the genital swellings, forming the shaft of the penis (Fig. 10.1.3). In addition, fusion of the genital swellings in the midline results in formation of the scrotum (which later houses the testes) and the genital tubercle becomes the glans penis. Pituitary

luteinizing hormone (LH) is required to stimulate Leydig cell secretion at this stage because of the higher amounts of androgen required. Hormonal influence can be demonstrated by exposing female fetuses to androgens, in which case their genitalia become masculinized, while castration of male fetuses results in feminization of their genitalia. Other characteristics associated with phenotypic sexual differentiation take place long after birth, mainly at puberty, and will be discussed at the appropriate point in this chapter.

Reproductive hormones

Gonadal steroid synthesis

Biosynthesis of the sex steroids in the gonads of both sexes is essentially the same as for all steroid hormones (see Ch. 5.4). The starting compound is cholesterol, a lipid, and this can be either taken up from the plasma or manufactured in situ from acetyl CoA, with the latter source likely to be quantitatively more important in the gonads. Testosterone is the major secretory product of the testis, with only small quantities undergoing conversion to dihydrotestosterone, or further conversion to 5α-androstenediol within the testis (these are known generically as androgens). Oestradiol-17β and progesterone are the major secretory products of the ovary, with androgens being obligatory precursors in both pathways (Fig. 10.1.5). Other oestrogens secreted in the female are oestrone and oestriol.

Another group of lipid-based reproductive hormones are the **eicosanoids**, principally the prostaglandins (PGs), with the **leukotrienes** playing a relatively minor reproductive role. Usually manufactured from the essential polyunsaturated fatty acid, arachidonic acid, PGs are synthesized in most tissues of the body, including uterine myometrium, cervix, ovary, placenta and fetal membranes. They have a very short half-life and mainly act as paracrines.

Summary

Differentiation

- Gametes (oocytes or sperm) contain half (i.e. the haploid number, 23) of the chromosomes of general somatic cells (which contain 23 *pairs*).
- Two chromosomes, X and Y, determine an individual's sex (XY = male, XX = female).
- Male and female embryos have an initial common (indifferent) development of gonads. At 6 weeks in the male or 9 weeks in the female the gonads take on their sexual characteristics.
- Development of the male genital tract requires testosterone; in its absence a female tract develops.

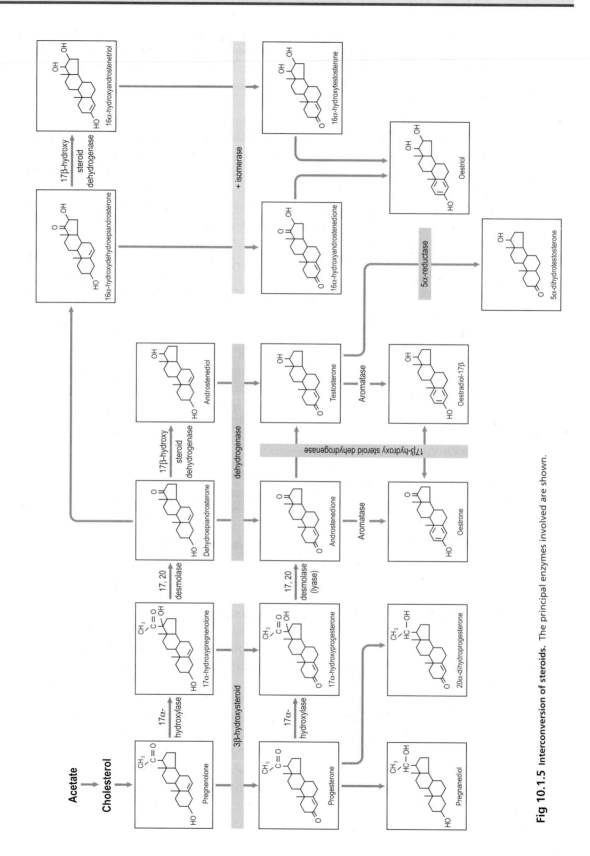

Fig 10.1.5 Interconversion of steroids. The principal enzymes involved are shown.

Protein hormones

There are several subgroups of these.

Gonadotrophic glycoproteins

The **gonadotrophic glycoproteins** stimulate gonadal activity and comprise follicle-stimulating hormone (FSH) and luteinizing hormone (LH) from the anterior pituitary, and human chorionic gonadotrophin (hCG) secreted by the placenta. The hypothalamic–pituitary–gonadal axis changes at significant points in the human life span, and this is reflected in the pattern of gonadotrophin secretion (Fig. 10.1.6). Changes in the pattern of gonadotrophin secretion are mirrored by fluctuations in the secretion of the male and female sex steroids.

Somatomammotrophic polypeptides

A second group, the **somatomammotrophic polypeptides**, are so called because of their widespread effects on tissue growth and function, including the mammary glands. There are three main ones: prolactin (PRL) and growth hormone (GH; also called somatotrophin) secreted by the anterior pituitary, and placental lactogen (PL; also called placental somatomammotrophin). PRL and PL are directly involved with lactation, while GH exerts its main effects during puberty. In addition, all three hormones provide a permissive role by assisting other hormones to act optimally.

Cytokines

Cytokines are a third group of proteins that are not classical hormones but often modulate or mediate the actions of reproductive hormones, and so deserve mention as they demonstrate the close relationship between the immune and endocrine systems. They are polypeptides and commonly act in autocrine, paracrine or juxtacrine mode, with an endocrine mode being less common. Three cytokines produced in the gonads are activins, inhibins and MIH. Inhibin inhibits gonadotrophin-releasing hormone (GnRH) stimulated FSH secretion by the anterior pituitary, while activin stimulates FSH secretion.

Small peptides

The fourth group of protein hormones comprises small peptides, of which there are four with particular reproductive significance. Gonadotrophin-releasing hormone is a decapeptide neurosecretory product of the hypothalamus involved with the regulation of FSH and LH secretion from the anterior pituitary.

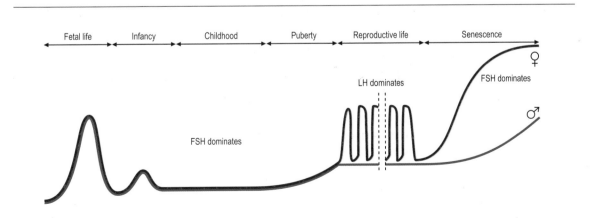

Fig 10.1.6 Gonadotrophin secretion throughout life. The ratio of LH to FSH changes at different times in life. Male gonadotrophin levels do not show the female cycles.

Oxytocin, a nonapeptide, is a another hypothalamic neurosecretory hormone released from the posterior pituitary with actions in the uterus and mammary gland. The other important peptides are β-endorphin, which has an intrahypothalamic role, and vasoactive intestinal peptide (VIP), which has been implicated in prolactin release from the anterior pituitary. Their roles will be discussed at the appropriate point.

Age-related reproductive hormone secretion

In both sexes the pattern of gonadotrophin secretion changes at significant points during the life cycle.

Gestation and childhood

Throughout gestation and childhood the male and female pattern of gonadotrophin secretion is similar. GnRH can be detected in the embryonic hypothalamus from 4 weeks, followed by the appearance of FSH and LH in the pituitary by week 10. There is a peak of gonadotrophin secretion during the mid-gestation phase; this declines to low levels before birth, but exhibits a transient rise at about 2 months after birth (Fig. 10.1.6). Levels of FSH and LH then remain low throughout childhood. Gonadal hormone secretion in both sexes mirrors the pattern of gonadotrophin secretion.

Puberty

Puberty is the stage during the life cycle when the individual moves from being non-reproductive to reproductively active. For this to occur, a major change in the pattern of reproductive hormone secretion is needed. During puberty, the adrenal glands begin to secrete adrenal androgens, a process described as **adrenarche**. Paradoxically, during childhood, FSH and LH concentrations are low despite the apparent lack of negative feedback by the gonadal steroids and inhibin. Two theories have been suggested to account for this.

- The first, the **gonadostat** theory, is that the hypothalamus is so sensitive during this period that its set point responds to the very low levels of circulating gonadal hormones, and this set point then increases to become less sensitive as puberty progresses.
- The second, the **hypothalamic maturation** theory, says that the hypothalamus simply does not work during childhood, but that maturation of the CNS during this time results in the adult secretion pattern of GnRH gradually becoming established.

Although it is not yet known what causes the change in the CNS, there is an expanding body of evidence indicating that the CNS/hypothalamic maturation theory is more likely to be correct.

During puberty the gonadotrophin levels gradually increase towards adult levels. This is associated with a marked nightly increase in the size, and possibly the frequency, of LH pulses, known as **sleep-augmented LH secretion**. Once puberty is complete, and adulthood has been achieved, the daily variation in gonadotrophin secretion disappears. There is a marked difference in the gonadotrophin secretion patterns in adult males and females. In the female, while she is reproductively active, gonadotrophin secretion exhibits a monthly rhythmicity associated with the ovarian cycle. This pattern is established about 2 years into puberty and is marked by the onset of menstruation (the **menarche**), which often takes some time to settle into a regular cycle length. By contrast, relatively stable plasma gonadotrophin levels are seen in the male.

Climacteric and menopause

The **climacteric** describes the time later in life when the gonads begin to lose their responsiveness to gonadotrophins. This is a slower process in the male, associated with a gradual rise in gonadotrophin levels, and with reproductive capacity reducing over the years, but often continuing well into the eighth decade. In females reproductive activity is lost more abruptly, usually during the fifth decade, when the **menopause** occurs and the ovarian cycle stops. The menopause is accompanied by much higher increases in gonadotrophin levels than are seen in the male (Fig. 10.1.6). The loss of ovarian follicles results in a fall in plasma oestrogen concentrations, and subsequent oestrogen synthesis is dependent on peripheral conversion of adrenal androgen. The dominant oestrogen is now oestrone rather than oestradiol. Oestrogen withdrawal causes a range of symptoms in menopausal women including insomnia and 'hot flushes'. The fall in plasma oestrogen is also associated with a decrease in bone density and, if this bone loss is excessive, osteoporosis may develop, leaving the woman prone to bone fractures.

Summary

Reproductive hormones and age-related reproductive hormones

- Reproductive hormones are steroid or protein hormones.
- The steroid hormones are: in the male testosterone and its products; in the female mainly oestradiol-17β and progesterone.
- The protein hormones are gonadotrophic glycoproteins, somatomammotrophic polypeptides, cytokines and small peptides.
- During childhood, gonadotrophin levels are low and fluctuating, slowly rising to adult levels at puberty.
- Climacteric, the loss of sensitivity of the gonads to gonadotrophins, is signalled in women by the menopause.

Clinical Example

Hormone replacement therapy

Menopause is a universal experience of women at an average age of 50–51 years. It is not significantly affected by age of menarche, childbearing, or race. Present-day life expectancy means that women can now expect to survive for one-third of their lives after their last period.

For up to 10 years before menopause the majority of women report irregularity of menstruation. These changes are primarily the result of declining ovarian function. Primary follicles are present but are becoming more and more resistant to gonadotrophin stimulation. The hypothalamus and pituitary function normally and in fact increase their output of FSH and LH as a result of the decreasing production of oestradiol and progesterone by the ovaries. Oestrone (a form of oestrogen) continues to be produced in increasing amounts and this is associated with an increased risk of endometrial cancer.

As ovarian function decreases, breast tissue involutes. Vasomotor changes cause hot flushes – dilatation of blood vessels of the head and neck in particular, which are accompanied by nausea, dizziness and palpitations. About 75% of menopausal women suffer these symptoms.

Loss of bone mass and increased brittleness of bone (osteoporosis) predispose some women to bone fracture and the premenopausal protection against heart disease enjoyed by women when compared to men is lost. Hormone replacement therapy (HRT) has proved effective in counteracting many of the problems of the menopause.

The rationale of replacing the products of a failing ovary seems exemplary, and the reduction of symptoms, heart disease, cerebrovascular accidents and blood pressure generally outweighs the risks from the oestrogen therapy (migraine, thrombosis) unless there are clear contraindications in individual patients.

In hormone replacement therapy the oestrogen should be given cyclically with a progestogen (a drug with a progesterone-like action) to reduce the risk of endometrial carcinoma that results from administering oestrogen alone.

Testicular structure and function

Male reproductive activity is continuous, exhibiting no cyclical events. The human testes develop in the abdomen and about 2 months before birth, under the influence of testosterone, descend into the scrotum where the lower temperature provides the correct environment for normal sperm development. Failure of the testes to descend is known as cryptorchidism and, if not corrected, results in infertility and a higher susceptibility to develop testicular cancer. Each testis weighs about 40 g and 80% of the testis comprises some 900 seminiferous tubules containing germ cells (spermatogonia), sperm in various stages of development and Sertoli cells. The remaining 20% is supportive connective tissue containing testosterone-secreting Leydig cells, blood vessels and lymphatics (Fig. 10.1.7). Spermatozoa are transferred from the seminiferous tubules via ducts called *tubuli recti* to the epididymis where they are stored. From here they are transferred via the vas deferens to the ejaculatory duct for emission.

Each seminiferous tubule is bounded by a basement membrane on which are sited the germ cells and the Sertoli cells (Fig. 10.1.7C). Between the Sertoli cells, spermatozoa in various stages of development can be seen, with the most mature being near the luminal surface of the Sertoli cells. Tight junctions between the Sertoli cells provide an effective barrier to the blood, which prevents sperm products getting into the bloodstream where they might evoke an immune response. The cytoplasm of the Sertoli cells also effectively filters circulating substances, preventing them from reaching the developing sperm.

Spermatogenesis

Spermatogenesis continues throughout reproductive life with some 200–400 million sperm being produced daily. The production of mature spermatozoa can be divided into three distinct phases, the first being mitotic division of the spermatogonia. Several mitotic divisions are followed by two meiotic divisions during which the diploid number of chromosomes is halved to the haploid number (see Fig. 10.1.1). During development, the intermediate spermatocytes are linked together by thin cytoplasmic bridges, separation occurring only during the final stages of spermatogenesis. Each primary spermatogonium produces 16 spermatids.

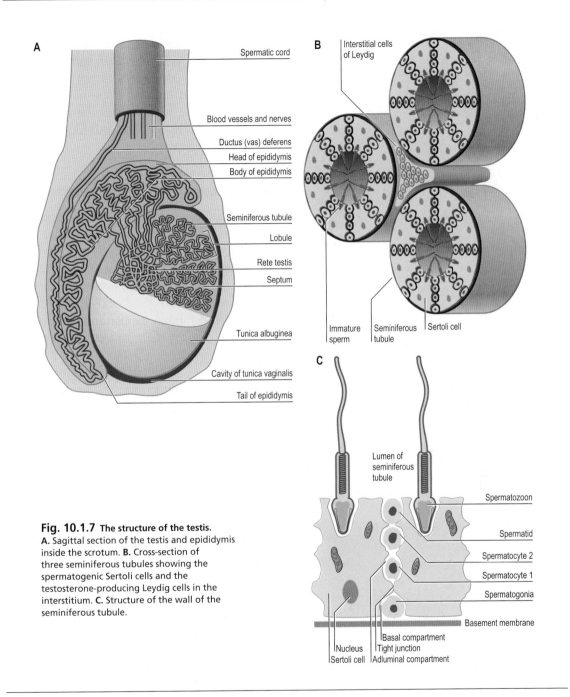

Fig. 10.1.7 The structure of the testis.
A. Sagittal section of the testis and epididymis inside the scrotum. **B.** Cross-section of three seminiferous tubules showing the spermatogenic Sertoli cells and the testosterone-producing Leydig cells in the interstitium. **C.** Structure of the wall of the seminiferous tubule.

Finally, each spermatid undergoes extensive structural change (**spermiogenesis**) to produce a spermatozoon (Fig. 10.1.8) which is capable of effectively delivering the chromosomes to the oocyte within the female reproductive tract.

During spermiogenesis a tail develops to confer motility to the sperm. A midpiece containing energy-providing mitochondria forms. The head is made up of the nuclear envelope containing the haploid chromosomes, the acrosome which

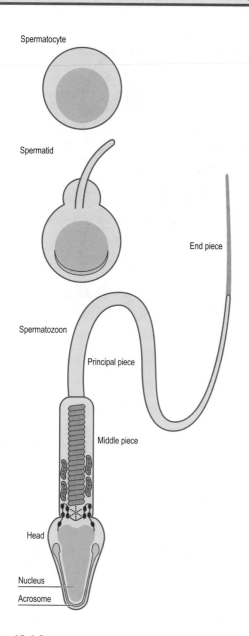

Spermatocyte

Spermatid

End piece

Spermatozoon

Principal piece

Middle piece

Head

Nucleus

Acrosome

Fig. 10.1.8 Development of a spermatozoon. The morphological changes that take place from spermatocyte to spermatozoon.

releases enzymes to penetrate the oocyte, and the equatorial and post-acrosomal cap region which plays an important part in sperm–oocyte fusion.

Following spermiogenesis the spermatozoa are released into the lumen by a process of

spermiation (see Ch. 10.2). From the first mitotic division of the spermatogonia to the production of mature spermatozoa takes some 64 days. However, spermatogenesis is not an entirely random activity; rather it appears to be regulated to occur in regular cycles at intervals of about 16 days. The nature of this regulation has yet to be fully explained.

Hormonal regulation of spermatogenesis

Several hormones play an essential role in spermatogenesis and these act sequentially. First, stimulated by anterior pituitary LH, the interstitial cells of Leydig secrete testosterone, which then diffuses across the basement membrane into the seminiferous tubules (Fig. 10.1.9). Both prolactin and inhibin facilitate the stimulation of Leydig cells by LH. Testosterone, most of which is converted to the more active dihydrotestosterone, is essential for the growth and division of spermatogonia. The testicular concentration of testosterone is some 100 times that found in plasma and is essential for the successful completion of the later stages of spermatogenesis. Testosterone also stimulates the formation of FSH receptors in Sertoli cells. Once these are established, FSH stimulates the Sertoli cells whose functions are required to support spermatogenesis, including early mitoses, meiosis and spermiogenesis. Next, FSH and testosterone synergistically stimulate the synthesis of an **androgen-binding protein** (ABP) which transports oestrogens and testosterone into the seminiferous tubular fluid to support spermatogenesis.

FSH also stimulates the Sertoli cells to convert testosterone to oestrogens, which are thought to be necessary for spermiogenesis. Finally, growth hormone from the anterior pituitary helps provide a stable metabolic background for normal testicular function and, more specifically, promotes early mitotic division of the spermatogonia.

The growth factors inhibin and activin are also synthesized in Sertoli cells and they have

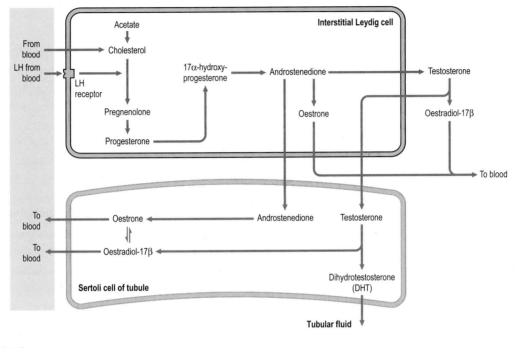

Fig. 10.1.9 Testicular steroidogenesis.

an endocrine role in regulating gonadotrophin secretion by the anterior pituitary. Oxytocin produced by Leydig cells has been shown to stimulate the motility of both seminiferous tubules and the epididymis.

Secretion and metabolism of androgens

The biosynthesis of the principal androgen, testosterone, by the Leydig cells has already been described (Fig. 10.1.9). Because of the pulsatile nature of the release of LH, which stimulates testosterone synthesis, plasma testosterone levels also exhibit small pulses. Superimposed on these is a diurnal trend whereby plasma testosterone levels are some 25% lower in the evening. Over the life span of an individual there is a marked variation in Leydig cell function and hence in testosterone secretion (Fig. 10.1.10). The high testosterone levels seen in late fetal life (4 ng/ml) are necessary for

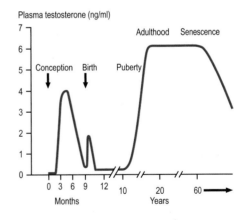

Fig. 10.1.10 Male plasma testosterone concentration. The change in plasma testosterone concentration during the life span of a normal human male.

development of the external genitalia. Levels are low during prepuberty owing to the absence of Leydig cells. Following its reappearance at about age 11, testosterone levels rise

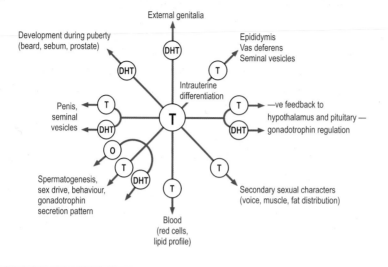

External genitalia

Development during puberty
(beard, sebum, prostate)

Epididymis
Vas deferens
Seminal vesicles

Intrauterine
differentiation

Penis,
seminal
vesicles

—ve feedback to
hypothalamus and pituitary —
gonadotrophin regulation

Spermatogenesis,
sex drive, behaviour,
gonadotrophin
secretion pattern

Secondary sexual characters
(voice, muscle, fat distribution)

Blood
(red cells,
lipid profile)

Fig. 10.1.11 Androgenic
effects of testosterone in the male.
DHT = dihydrotestosterone;
O = oestradiol-17β; T = testosterone.

throughout puberty reaching an adult plateau level (6 ng/ml) which is maintained for some 50 years (Fig. 10.1.10). The decline in concentration observed in later years is probably due to decreased responsiveness of Leydig cells to LH.

Approximately 98% of plasma testosterone is bound to a plasma protein, **sex steroid-binding globulin** (SSBG), and only the free portion is biologically active, since it is this free hormone which is able to leave the circulation and enter cells. In peripheral tissues testosterone is converted to potent alternative androgens, dihydrotestosterone (DHT) and 5α-androstenediol. The extratesticular effects of androgens fall into two main areas:

- those associated with reproductive functions and secondary sexual characteristics
- those more generally associated with growth and maturation of tissues.

The involvement of the two main androgens, testosterone and DHT, in relation to these various functions is summarized in Figure 10.1.11.

The mechanism of action of androgens follows the typical steroid hormone model. Once inside most target cells, testosterone is rapidly converted to DHT, which is biologically more potent in some androgenic actions. In some cells, testosterone is converted to 5α-androstenediol by the enzyme 5α-reductase. While testosterone is the major circulating androgen, it is largely considered to serve as a prohormone for the other two. Testosterone exhibits intrinsic activity in those tissues lacking 5α-reductase, and is directly implicated in male genital tract development, stimulation of the pubertal growth spurt, enlargement of the larynx, and closure of epiphyseal plates in bone.

Summary

Testicular function

- The testes must descend out of the abdomen to function properly.
- Spermatozoa are produced by mitosis followed by meiosis followed by spermiogenesis.
- The main hormones of spermatogenesis are LH, testosterone, and FSH, together with several ancillary hormones.

Ovarian structure and function

Female reproductive function falls into two major phases: preparation for conception and gestation; and the period of gestation which is usually referred to as pregnancy. The reproductive organs of the female lie in the pelvis and comprise the ovaries, fallopian tubes (oviducts) and the uterus, which is connected to the exterior via the cervix and vagina (see Fig. 10.1.4). Female reproductive activity differs from that of the male in that it exhibits a definite monthly sexual cycle, normally referred to as the **menstrual cycle**. The first half of this cycle is oestrogen dominated and is concerned with follicular development, preparing the female tract for receipt of the spermatozoa and fertilization of the oocyte which is released midcycle. The progesterone-dominated second half of the cycle prepares the uterus for **implantation** of a fertilized oocyte and its subsequent nurture. If implantation does not take place, the monthly cycle is repeated.

Each ovary weighs approximately 15 g and ovarian tissue is made up of stromal tissue containing the primordial follicles, and the interstitial glandular tissue which is equivalent to testicular Leydig cells (Fig. 10.1.12). A major

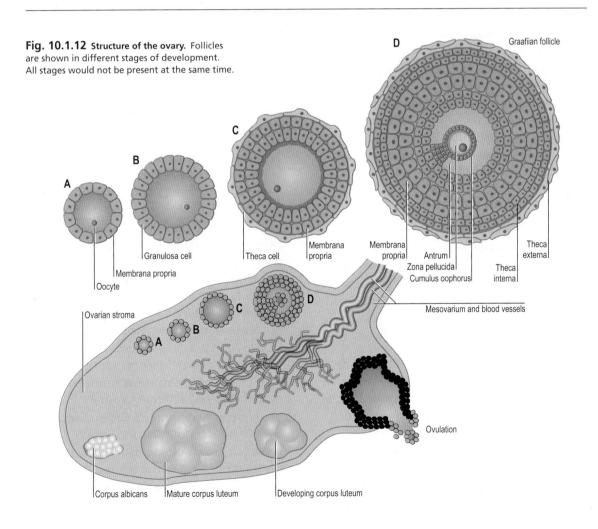

Fig. 10.1.12 Structure of the ovary. Follicles are shown in different stages of development. All stages would not be present at the same time.

difference from the male is that the adult female ovary is not able to make new oogonia, and the primary oocytes present at birth represent an already declining population, from a maximum of some 7 million at 24 weeks' gestation, down to 2 million at birth, with a further decline to around 400 000 at puberty. The germ cells present at birth are primary oocytes (equivalent to primary spermatocytes) with a potential life span of 50 years. The meiotic division is suspended in prophase, with the first meiotic division being completed only at ovulation. The primary oocytes are contained in primordial follicles which are formed as a result of a single layer of mesonephric spindle cells from the stroma being induced to surround the oocyte. These spindle cells are precursors of the granulosa cells and they secrete a basement membrane, the *membrana propria*, to surround the primordial follicle. Further development of some primordial follicles will occur before puberty, and a number of follicles in various stages of early development are visible in the ovaries at any point in time, but regular follicular development is seen only after puberty when a few follicles will start to develop further each day.

Oogenesis and ovulation (the ovarian cycle)

Each month a series of events associated with the maturation of an ovum occurs. In the adult female this ovarian cycle has an average length of 28 days, although there is significant individual variation from 21–33 days. Physiologically the cycle can be divided into three phases:

- The **follicular phase**, during which follicle growth takes place, is timed from the start of the menstrual blood flow which signifies the end of the previous cycle. This phase is of variable length, ranging from 9–23 days, although it tends to be reasonably constant for each individual.
- The **ovulatory phase** is 1–3 days in length and ends with ovulation.

- The final **luteal phase**, when the corpus luteum is active, is more consistent in length, averaging 14 days and ending with the menstrual bleed.

Follicular phase

During each cycle, a number of oocytes start to develop slowly over the subsequent two cycles. Some 20 follicles will have grown to about 2–4 mm by this stage, and will be responsive to the increase in FSH which will occur in the third cycle. 1 week into the follicular phase one follicle tends to be larger (11 mm) than the others and will become dominant, probably owing to its ability to produce more oestradiol than its counterparts because of its greater size. A higher FSH receptor density in this follicle may also make it more able to cope with the declining level of FSH which is occurring at this time. The other follicles become **atretic** and disappear.

Primordial follicles pass through three developmental stages prior to ovulation (see Fig. 10.1.12).

- The first stage is the formation of a primary, or preantral, follicle characterized by an increase in size from 20 µm to larger than 200 µm, with most of the increase being associated with growth of the oocyte. During this period a translucent zone, the *zona pellucida*, forms around the oocyte separating it from the surrounding granulosa cells, which themselves proliferate to become several layers thick. Ovarian stromal cells condense around the *membrana propria* at this time to form the *theca*, which subsequently proliferates into an inner glandular and highly vascular *theca interna* surrounded by the *theca externa*, a fibrous capsule.
- The secondary, or antral, follicle is formed when follicular fluid starts to appear between the granulosa cells. Follicular fluid is a mixture of granulosa cell secretions and serum transudate. The drops of fluid gradually come together to form a single

antrum and further increase in follicular size is associated mainly with the accumulation of follicular fluid. During this period the oocyte, surrounded by some granulosa cells (the *cumulus oophorus*), becomes suspended in the follicular fluid.

- The antral follicle is frequently called a **graafian follicle** and, when mature, is ready to enter the third and final preovulatory phase.

Effective follicle maturation is dependent on hormonal support, principally by pituitary gonadotrophins. LH and FSH receptors appear during the late preantral and early antral stages of development, with LH receptors being found in theca interna cells and FSH receptors in granulosa cells. Under the influence of these hormones the two cell types synthesize steroid hormones (Fig. 10.1.13). In vitro incubation experiments have demonstrated that LH stimulates thecal cells to convert acetate and cholesterol to androgens, and follicular androgens account for up to 70% of all circulating androgens in the female. Thecal cells are also capable of synthesizing limited amounts of oestrogens. Following diffusion of some of the androgen into the granulosa cells, the presence of FSH stimulates its aromatization to oestrogens. The main oestrogens produced are oestradiol-17β and oestrone. Granulosa cells contain oestrogen receptors to which the oestrogens bind, resulting

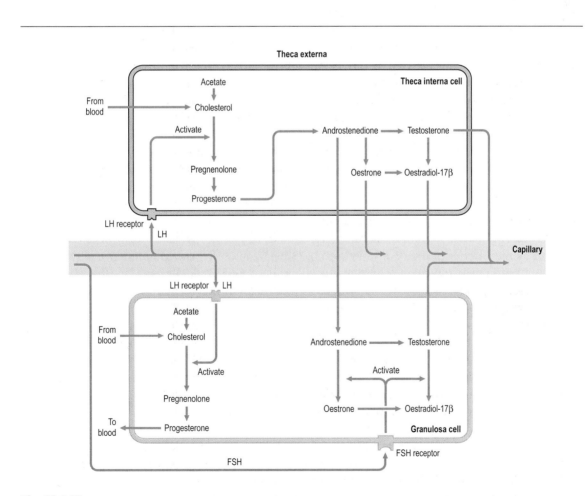

Fig. 10.1.13 Steroidogenesis in the human ovary.

in further granulosa cell proliferation and further oestrogen receptor synthesis. More granulosa cells means yet more aromatization of androgens to oestrogens, so oestrogen is stimulating the production of more oestrogen, an example of positive feedback. This escalating oestrogen synthesis ends with a surge in the level of circulating oestrogen. A further role of the oestrogens, together with FSH, is to stimulate the appearance of LH receptors on granulosa cells, which is a critical precursor of the antral follicle moving on to the preovulatory phase of follicular development.

Ovarian cytokines also have important functions in the developing follicles. **Activin** is produced early in the antral phase and performs the dual role of suppressing thecal androgen output while stimulating granulosa cells to increase aromatizing capacity. **Inhibin**, which is produced later, stimulates androgen output and reduces aromatizing activity. It has been suggested that these cytokines serve to maintain a balance between androgen production and conversion to oestrogens, while avoiding the production of inappropriately high levels of androgen.

Ovulatory phase

The ovulatory stage of follicular development now occurs. It is dependent on a surge of LH secretion by the anterior pituitary. Within hours of the LH binding to follicular cells, the suspended first meiotic division moves to completion. A secondary oocyte containing the haploid number of chromosomes is formed, with the other chromosomes being lost via the formation of a polar body, which rapidly disintegrates. While the LH surge is necessary for the completion of meiosis, it must exert its effect indirectly because LH receptors are not found in the oocyte.

Immediately prior to ovulation, LH stimulates a further increase in follicular size through rapid accumulation of more follicular fluid and increased blood flow. This causes the granulosa

and thecal cells to form a relatively thin wall to the follicle, which in turn tends to bulge under the epithelial surface of the ovary with only a thin epithelial layer separating the follicle wall from the peritoneal cavity. Close observation of this stage shows cells in the area degenerating, owing to local synthesis and action of prostaglandins, thromboxanes and leukotrienes, resulting in rupture of the follicle and expulsion of the oocyte and the cumulus oophorus. Changes in the levels of FSH, LH and local enzymes are also involved in this process. Cilia on the fimbriae (finger-like projections at the end of the fallopian tube) waft the oocyte into the oviduct.

Luteal phase

During the luteal phase of follicular development, the granulosa cells, stimulated by LH, begin to synthesize progesterone. Following ovulation, a fibrin clot forms within the cavity left after expulsion of the oocyte, granulosa cells collapse into the space, and the whole is surrounded by a capsule of thecal tissue. This structure becomes the **corpus luteum** whose main function is the secretion of progesterone during the postovulatory, or luteal, phase of the menstrual cycle. In addition, the corpus luteum secretes small amounts of oestradiol-17β, inhibin to stimulate further progesterone synthesis, and oxytocin. Maintenance of the corpus luteum is LH dependent. In the absence of fertilization the corpus luteum survives up to 14 days and its regression after this time is thought to be due to the reduction in luteotrophic support as LH levels fall. The resulting avascular scar is known as the **corpus albicans**.

Hormonal patterns during the ovarian cycle

Each of the phases described above is dependent on hormonal regulation, and the hormones involved exhibit characteristic secretion patterns during the cycle (Fig. 10.1.14). The cyclic changes observed in the secretion of gonadal steroids

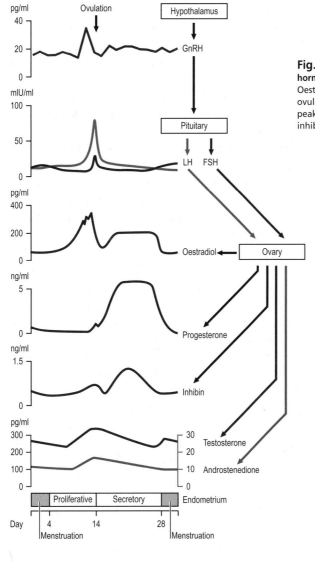

Fig. 10.1.14 Menstrual cycle: plasma hormone levels in relation to ovulation. Oestradiol and GnRH surges precede the ovulatory surges of LH and FSH. The broad peaks of progesterone, oestradiol and inhibin are produced by the corpus luteum.

and inhibin are regulated by the monthly cyclic pattern of pituitary FSH and LH secretion, which are in turn dependent on changes in hypothalamic GnRH secretion and in sensitivity of the pituitary to GnRH. It should also be remembered that GnRH secretion is itself regulated by both positive and negative feedback control by gonadal steroids and inhibin.

FSH and LH levels are at their lowest at the end of the luteal phase of the previous cycle. At this point LH secretion just exceeds that of FSH, but just prior to the start of the menstrual bleed FSH levels begin to rise, stimulating follicle growth and oestrogen secretion, followed by a rise in LH levels a few days later. Progesterone levels remain low throughout the follicular phase. In the second half of the follicular phase FSH levels decrease while LH secretion continues to increase, and LH level again exceeds FSH. The increasing LH levels result in a sharp

899

increase in oestradiol and oestrone secretion, with levels peaking immediately prior to the start of the ovulatory phase. The oestradiol comes from the maturing follicle while the oestrone is produced by peripheral conversion of oestradiol and androstenedione. Under the influence of the rising oestrogen secretion, progesterone levels also begin to rise at the end of the follicular phase. At this point the high levels of oestrogen, combined with increasing levels of inhibin, depress FSH secretion by negative feedback. The high level of oestrogen, acting in both the hypothalamus and the pituitary, provides a positive feedback effect on LH. During the second half of the follicular phase, increases in testosterone and androstenedione levels are seen.

Successful ovulation during the short ovulatory phase is dependent on a sharp, transient peak in gonadotrophin secretion, with LH secretion far exceeding that of FSH (the so-called **LH surge**; Fig. 10.1.15). This peak of gonadotrophin secretion can be broadly divided into three phases, with secretion increasing over 15 hours to a plateau, which is maintained for a further 15 hours, then declining over the subsequent 20 hours. During this declining phase oestrogen levels fall sharply, and a small rise in progesterone level occurs.

The luteal phase is characterized by the large increase in progesterone secretion by luteal cells. Also observed during the luteal phase are broad second peaks in oestrogen, oestrone and inhibin secreted by the corpus luteum. Throughout the luteal phase the levels of testosterone and androstenedione decline. In the absence of fertilization, at the end of the ovarian cycle, there is a sharp fall in oestrogen, progesterone and inhibin levels. This removes the negative feedback on FSH, whose level begins to rise, and the whole sequence is repeated. The withdrawal of gonadal hormone support from the uterus results in the start of the next menstrual bleed.

A considerable body of evidence now exists which indicates that the determination of the LH surge described above arises from the ovary rather than the central nervous system. Experimental evidence supporting this conclusion includes lack of cyclic gonadotrophic secretion in women with non-functioning ovaries, no LH surge until the dominant follicle has achieved a critical size, and mimicking of the preovulatory oestradiol profile resulting in the LH surge (even in postmenopausal women). While the GnRH pulse generator is necessary to initiate follicular development, it appears to be the critical nature of the ovarian secretions which in turn condition the pulse generator, and subsequently the gonadotrophs, to produce the LH surge. It is also important to note that factors other than ovarian feedback can influence the secretion of GnRH and gonadotrophins. Emotional, caloric, thermal, photic and inflammatory factors are all well documented as affecting reproductive activity, further illustrating the close integration with the behavioural and vegetative functions of the hypothalamus.

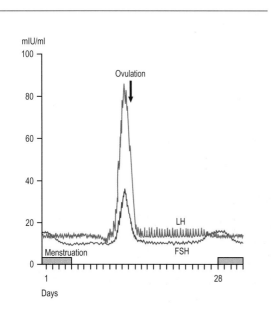

Fig. 10.1.15 Menstrual cycle: plasma LH and FSH levels in relation to ovulation. Note the hourly pulses whose amplitude increases after the ovulatory surge.

The uterine (menstrual) cycle

Equally important to ovulation resulting in pregnancy is the assurance that at the appropriate point in each cycle all parts of reproductive tract are in optimal condition to undertake their role in the reproductive process. The uterine lining, or endometrium, itself undergoes cyclic changes each month in response to the changing levels of ovarian hormones in the blood (Fig. 10.1.16). There are three phases in the uterine cycle:

- menstrual
- proliferative
- secretory.

The first, or **menstrual**, phase is the menstrual bleed which occurs at the end of an ovarian cycle when fertilization and implantation have not occurred. Menstruation is the shedding of endometrial lining.

The second and third phases of the uterine cycle describe the rebuilding of the endometrium ready for a possible implantation during the next ovarian cycle.

The **proliferative** phase coincides with the follicular and ovulatory phases of the ovarian cycle, when the rising level of oestrogen in the blood causes the uterine endometrium to thicken, glands to increase in size and become

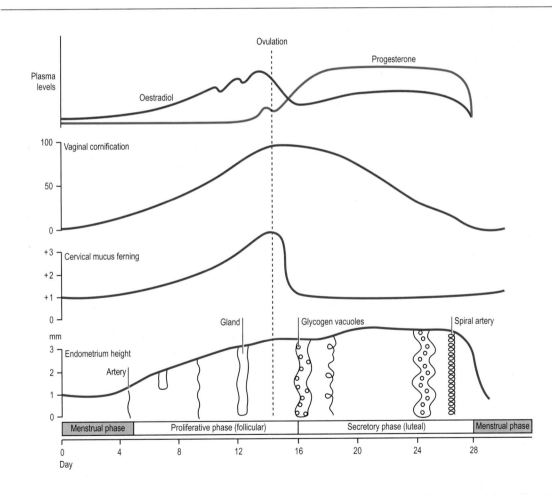

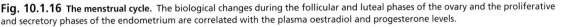

Fig. 10.1.16 The menstrual cycle. The biological changes during the follicular and luteal phases of the ovary and the proliferative and secretory phases of the endometrium are correlated with the plasma oestradiol and progesterone levels.

tortuous, and spiral arteries within the tissue to elongate. Under the influence of rising oestrogen levels the cervical mucus secretion becomes copious and more watery and conducive to sperm motility.

The **secretory** phase begins immediately following ovulation, when the rising progesterone level, along with the oestrogen, causes the uterine glands to become secretory. The glycogen, glycoproteins and glycolipids contained in this secretion both sustain the fertilized ovum and assist in its attachment to the uterine wall. Simultaneously the uterine stroma becomes oedematous and the spiral arteries become coiled. Under the influence of progesterone the cervical mucus becomes scant, thick, viscous and inelastic, and inhospitable to sperm.

If pregnancy does not occur, the corpus luteum degenerates and oestrogen and progesterone levels fall. Deprived of hormonal support, the spiral arteries and uterine muscles go into spasm causing ischaemia and necrosis and the subsequent menstrual bleed.

Other actions of female sex steroids

The **fallopian tubes** are also dependent on gonadal hormones to ensure that they are in optimal condition to receive the ovum at ovulation. During the follicular phase, rising oestrogen causes both an increase in the number of cilia and their rate of beating, and an increase in epithelial secretory cells and production of a mucus which aids sperm transport. As ovulation approaches, the contractions of the tubes and movements of the fimbriae at the end of the fallopian tubes both increase to draw the ovum into the tube. The progesterone secreted during the luteal phase further increases ciliary beating and stimulates an epithelial secretion which provides nutrition for the ovum, any sperm present in the fallopian tube, and the zygote formed as a result of fertilization.

Rising oestrogen levels during the follicular phase cause the vaginal epithelium to thicken,

become rich in glycogen and cornify, and vaginal secretions to increase. As progesterone levels rise during the luteal phase, the number of cornified cells falls.

The breasts, or mammary glands, also exhibit cyclical changes as gonadal hormone levels fluctuate throughout the menstrual cycle. The effect of these hormones on breast development and during pregnancy are discussed in Chapter 10.3. During the menstrual cycle, oestrogen stimulates further proliferation of lobular tissue, causing noticeable swelling and tenderness in some women, which disappears by the end of the luteal phase.

In addition to their effects on the reproductive tract, gonadal hormones have effects on other body tissues which are equivalent to the effects of testosterone and DHT in males. Oestradiol is responsible for most of the body changes which bring about the normal female phenotype. These changes include the maturation of the external genitalia, breast development, skeletal growth, development of wider hips to cope with childbirth, and increased adiposity compared with males, coupled with a lower muscle and bone mass.

Secretion and metabolism of gonadal steroids

The main oestrogen is oestradiol, and in menstruating women the ovary is the main source, with small amounts being derived from the aromatization of testosterone in adipose tissue and liver. A second oestrogen, oestrone, is produced by peripheral conversion from oestradiol. Oestrone becomes the dominant oestrogen following the menopause, when it is derived from adrenal and ovarian androgens. Both molecules are carried in the blood loosely bound to SSBG, but with a much lower affinity than seen in relation to androgen binding to SSBG in males. Much of the oestrogen is carried loosely bound to albumin. During pregnancy a third oestrogen, oestriol, is produced in significant amounts.

Progesterone in the non-menstruating female is derived in similar amounts from the adrenal glands and ovary, whereas during the luteal phase in menstruating women the majority is secreted by the ovary. Transport in the blood is mainly by low affinity binding to albumin.

Females also produce testosterone, most of which is derived from the peripheral conversion of other androgens produced by the adrenal glands and ovary. Overproduction of testosterone in females results in varying degrees of virilization.

Summary

Ovarian function

- The first half of the ovarian cycle involves follicular development and is oestrogen dominated and separated by a short ovulatory phase from the progesterone-dominated second half which prepares the uterus for implantation.
- All a woman's primary oocytes (2 million) are present at birth; no more are made.
- The ovarian cycle consists of one of several follicles developing into a primary, then graafian follicle, than a corpus luteum under the influence of FSH and LH.
- Ovulation is triggered by a powerful surge of gonadotrophins.
- The ovarian cycle is 'shadowed' by the menstrual cycle during which the uterine endometrium is first proliferative (due to oestrogen) then secretory (due to oestrogen and progesterone).
- Decline in progesterone and oestrogen when the corpus luteum degenerates precipitates menstruation.

Pregnancy

Introduction

In the previous chapter we explored the genetic basis of the sexes and the development and function of the male and female gonadal apparatus. These are all necessary to allow sexual reproduction to take place, which, in turn, ensures the continuation of the species. Sexual activity between a male and female, called copulation or sexual intercourse, results in the transfer of sperm into the female reproductive tract. If this happens around the time of ovulation, fertilization may occur and, if the resulting zygote implants in the endometrial wall, pregnancy will ensue. Human pregnancy is clinically calculated as 40 weeks from the first day of the last menstrual bleed; as the ovum which is fertilized to produce the pregnancy is in fact released 2 weeks after that date (in midcycle) the true gestational period for women is approximately 38 weeks. Pregnancy is conventionally divided into three trimesters at the end of which the mother is said to have 'come to **term**'.

Sexual functioning

In Chapter 10.1, the process of spermatogenesis was described up to the stage of spermiation, when the spermatozoa are released into the lumen of the seminiferous tubules. From here they travel to the epididymis, a journey taking up to 24 hours. During this period there is further maturation of the sperm, involving the loss of the remainder of their cytoplasm, and they become more motile. The sperm movement into the epididymis is assisted by a mixture of tubular fluid currents and contractions of the testicular capsule. As the sperm move through the epididymis they are exposed to a tubular fluid of changing composition. Several different proteins that act to increase the efficacy of the sperm are present in the tubular fluid and bind to the sperm membrane as they pass through the epididymis. These proteins include a forward-mobility protein, an acrosome-stabilizing factor and a zona pellucida-binding protein. A further protein, oscillin, has been identified and is believed to cause the oscillations in Ca^{2+} responsible for activating the development of the egg.

At any one time, approximately 1 day's sperm production is stored in the epididymis, sufficient for one ejaculation, with a volume of 3–4 ml and containing 200–400 million sperm.

In order for the ejaculate to be delivered effectively into the female tract, the penis is required to become firm and erect so that it can be introduced into the female's vagina. This is achieved by parasympathetic stimulation causing the engorging of venous sinuses within the penis with blood, which is effectively trapped in the penis by a combination of arteriolar dilatation and venous constriction (see p. 628).

As the ejaculate passes through the vas deferens, further substances are added to it, first from the prostate and second from the seminal vesicles. The alkaline prostate fluid helps to neutralize the acid pH of the semen, and vaginal and cervical secretions. In addition, it contains calcium, zinc, citrate and acid phosphate. The secretions of the seminal vesicle make up the majority of the later portion of the ejaculate and contain fructose, an energy substrate for the spermatozoa, and prostaglandins which probably cause uterine and fallopian tube contractions to aid sperm transport through the female tract.

Sexual arousal in the female is also important in achieving effective copulation. Parasympathetic activity causes vascular tissue to become erect and vaginal glands to produce a copious secretion which lubricates the movement of the penis within the vagina. Most of the ejaculate is trapped in the cervical mucus where sperm capacitation takes place. From here, the sperm escape into the uterus over 48 hours following sexual intercourse. Approximately 1 per 100 000 of the many millions of sperm contained in the ejaculate make it as far as the fallopian tubes.

Fertilization and implantation

Fertilization

Sperm transport through the female reproductive tract is facilitated during the follicular phase of the ovarian cycle when the tract is oestrogen dominated. At this time, and especially just prior to ovulation, the cervical mucus is watery, profuse and elastic. If a sample is allowed to dry on a microscope slide, a characteristic ferning pattern is observed. Sperm have been found in the fallopian tubes within minutes of copulation, much faster than can be predicted by the sperms' own motility. There is evidence to suggest that the release of oxytocin and/or prostaglandins during sexual intercourse stimulates mild contractions of the uterine muscle which serve to draw the sperm through the uterus. However, these sperm are unlikely to have undergone capacitation and are incapable of causing fertilization. Following ejaculation, sperm survive for several days; however, the oocyte is viable for a maximum of some 24 hours after ovulation. The timing of copulation therefore greatly influences the chances of fertilization. In ideal circumstances, fertilization should also take place in the fallopian tube, since this increases the possibility of the **zygote** implanting in a favourable site in the uterus, ideally in the rear wall at the top.

Before an ejaculated sperm can fertilize an ovum it needs to pass through a process of capitation, which involves the removal of seminal fluid. This occurs naturally within the female tract, and usually while the sperm are trapped in the cervical mucus, but the seminal fluid has to be washed off sperm if they are to be used for in vitro fertilization. During capacitation, motility becomes whip-like, and there is a withdrawal of cholesterol from the sperm membrane resulting in a redistribution of membrane proteins. Finally, there is an influx of calcium into the sperm resulting in the **acrosomal reaction** during which the acrosomal membrane fuses with the outer sperm membrane, creating pores through which acrosomal enzymes are able to pass. These enzymes, acrosin (proteolytic), a neuraminidase and hyaluronidases, digest the intercellular cement between granulosa cells in the *cumulus oophorus*, forming a path for the sperm through to the *zona pellucida* of the oocyte. Penetration of the zona by a sperm causes an influx of calcium which results in the release of substances from the ovum which change the nature of the zona surface and inhibit the penetration by further sperm (Fig. 10.2.1).

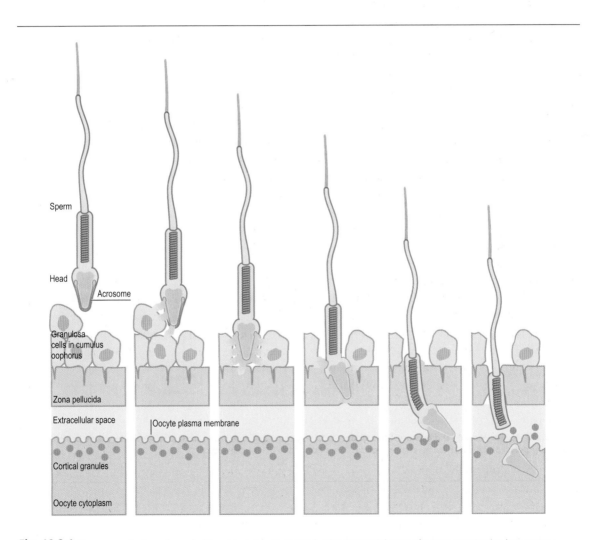

Fig. 10.2.1 Sperm penetration of oocyte (slow block to polyspermy). The sequential steps of oocyte penetration by a sperm. Many sperm are needed to release enough acrosomal enzyme to enable one of them to penetrate the zona radiata and zona pellucida to fuse with the oocyte membrane. This fusion provokes the zonal reaction, which releases the oocyte's cortical granules into the extracellular space, preventing the penetration of more sperm.

This is known as the **zonal reaction**, and ensures that the ovum is fertilized by one sperm only.

At this point the second polar body, resulting from the second stage of meiosis, is released from the ovum leaving it with the haploid number of chromosomes. The pro-nuclei of the ovum and sperm come together to form the metaphase spindle with the two haploid sets of chromosomes at its equator. Syngamy (sexual reproduction) has occurred, fertilization is complete, and a zygote containing the full diploid complement of chromosomes is formed.

Ideally this process has occurred in the fallopian tube, which still has to be traversed before implantation takes place, a process which normally takes about 3 days. Occasionally implantation occurs in the fallopian tube resulting in an **ectopic pregnancy**. This is potentially very dangerous for the mother because the growing fetus and placenta stretch the fallopian tube to such an extent that it eventually ruptures and, if not diagnosed rapidly,

can result in the death of the mother because of haemorrhage.

Immediately the zygote has formed the embryo starts to develop, with five mitotic divisions taking place to form a 32-celled **morula** before implantation occurs (Fig. 10.2.2). The morula develops into a **blastocyst** with a fluid-filled cavity and the cells differentiate into two distinct groups, the eccentrically placed **inner cell mass** (which will develop into the fetus) and the **trophectoderm** cells, which form the placenta. The *zona pellucida* has been present to this point, but 'peels off' about 6 days after zygote formation. This occurs in part due to the blastocyst undergoing expansion and contraction cycles, and is aided by lytic substances present in the uterine secretions. The blastocyst is now ready for implantation into the uterine wall. During this period the zygote receives nutrients secreted by uterine tubal and endometrial glands under progesterone stimulation.

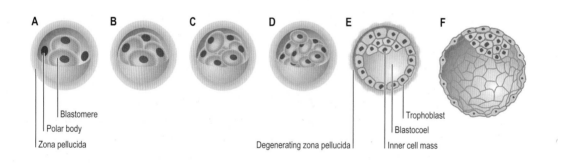

| A | B | C | D | E | F |

Blastomere
Polar body
Zona pellucida

Degenerating zona pellucida

Trophoblast
Blastocoel
Inner cell mass

Fig. 10.2.2 **Zygote cleavage and blastocyst formation. A–C.** Progressive cell divisions to form **(D)** the morula, a solid ball of 32 cells. As cleavage proceeds the cells become smaller. **E** and **F.** Formation of the hollow blastocyst.

Clinical Example

Contraception

There are wide variations in fertility and even wider differences in mortality in different human societies. Levels of fertility alter slowly, while mortality may change suddenly. For most of human history, population has increased at less than 1% per annum. Mortality has shown fluctuations resulting from war, famine and pestilence. In the 20th century, population growth rates reached a very high level – in some countries more than 3% per annum – a rate that cannot be sustained for many generations (Fig. CE10.2.1).

The accelerated growth of population in some countries was not the result of more children being born but of more surviving to be adults.

Control of human fertility is a difficult undertaking complicated by cultural attitudes which are often irrational. The path from coition to pregnancy can be interrupted at a number of places. These include the behavioural methods such as coitus interruptus and rhythm methods, which prevent the introduction of sperm into the female tract, and intercourse during infertile periods respectively (see Recent Advances: Electronic rhythm, p. 917).

Mechanical 'barrier' methods – condoms, vaginal diaphragms and sponges, cervical caps – prevent sperm reaching the ovum, and chemical spermicides inserted into the vagina kill sperm or reduce their motility.

The 'pill' consists of various combinations of sex steroids. The combined oestrogen–progestogen type mimics the positive feedback of the woman's own oestrogen and progesterone and prevents ovulation. The 'progestogen-only' type disrupts a number

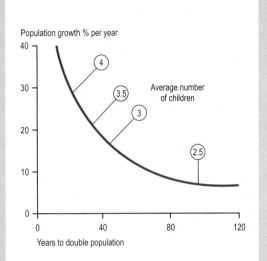

Fig. CE10.2.1 Population growth (with western levels of mortality) related to average number of children per family.

of aspects of the delicate process from ovulation to implantation, including in some women preventing ovulation. In most women, progestogen-only contraceptives disrupt endometrial secretory patterns, make cervical mucus thicker and more hostile to sperm and accelerate tubular transport of ova which results in the ova arriving in the uterus and being lost before they are sufficiently mature to implant. The 'pill' can be prescribed to be taken orally in the conventional manner for a certain number of days during each menstrual cycle or be given as depot injections, which can act for up to 5 years.

Intrauterine contraceptive devices (IUCDs) are inserted into the cavity of the uterus where they interfere with implantation of the fertilized ovum by increasing tubular transport and altering the biochemical environment within the uterus. Some types of IUCD contain copper which interferes with the enzyme activity necessary for implantation. These copper-bearing devices have to be replaced every 2–8 years when the copper has been eluted. Other types of device can be left in place almost indefinitely.

Fallopian tube ligation and vasectomy surgically interrupt the tubes carrying gametes from the ovaries and seminiferous tubules. These procedures are the most effective forms of contraception but, because of the difficulty of reversing the surgical damage, should in most cases be considered as permanent sterilization.

The effectiveness of a number of methods of contraception are given in Table 10.2.1.

Table 10.2.1 Pregnancies occurring per year in 100 normally sexually active fertile women using different methods of contraception*

Method	Effectiveness
Fallopian tube ligation	0.006
Vasectomy	0.15
Oestrogen–progesterone pill	4–10
Progestogen-only pill	5–10
Condom + spermicide	5
Condom alone	10
Intrauterine device	0.5–4
Vaginal diaphragm + spermicide	2–20
Cervical cap	2–20
Spermicide alone	2–30
Vaginal sponge	13–16
Coitus interruptus	20–25
Rhythm	21–40
No contraception	90

*Data from Vessey M, Lawless M, Yeates D 1982 Efficacy of different contraceptive methods. *Lancet* I(8276): 841–842. The wide range of success of some of these methods probably reflects the wide range of behaviour and motivation of the users.

Implantation

Implantation ideally takes place about halfway through the luteal phase of the ovarian cycle when the endometrium is under sufficient progesterone influence. It occurs when the blastocyst makes contact with the wall of the uterus, usually in the upper posterior region. Within an hour, modification of the uterine stromal tissue begins in a process described as **decidualization** which is dependent on oestrogen and progesterone. The changes observed are an increase in vascular permeability leading to tissue oedema, accompanied by a change in the composition of the intercellular matrix and the structure of stromal cells, and an increase in the permeability of capillaries. The trophoblast cells of the blastocyst are then able to invade the uterine wall and continue to do so until the blastocyst has completely penetrated into the wall, described as **interstitial implantation** (Fig. 10.2.3).

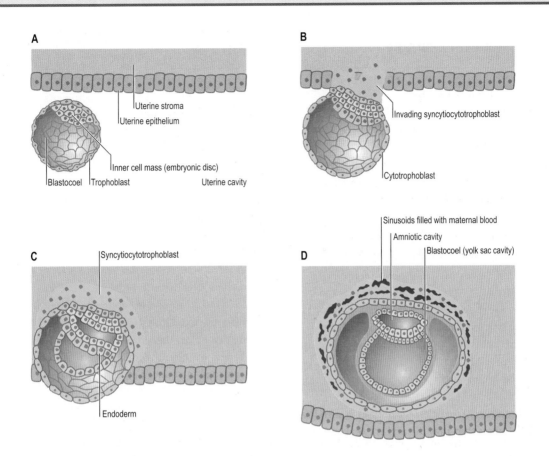

Fig. 10.2.3 **Implantation.** **A.** The blastocyst free in the uterine cavity. **B.** The trophoblast crossing the epithelium and invading the stroma. **C.** Development of an amniotic cavity. **D.** Growth of uterine tissue over the implantation site.

Summary

Pregnancy

- Human pregnancy lasts 40 weeks, conventionally divided into three trimesters.
- Only 1 per 100 000 sperm of the 200–400 million contained in the 3–4 ml of ejaculate deposited near the cervix, where capacitation takes place, reach the fallopian tubes where fertilization ideally occurs.

- Enzymes from the acrosomes of many sperms digest the intercellular cement between the cumulus cells, allowing a single sperm to penetrate.
- On penetration by the first sperm, the ovum becomes impervious to other sperm. A second polar body is released at this time, leaving the haploid number of chromosomes.
- About 6 days after fertilization, the zygote (now a blastocyst) implants.

Clinical Example

Assisted reproduction

There are many causes of infertility due to problems of the man, the woman or both. Many of these problems can be resolved. It may be that the would-be father suffers from azoospermia (total lack of sperm in the ejaculate). Such men can be divided into two major groups:

1. Men who produce sperm but, owing to either blockage or absence of the connecting tubes from the testes, these sperm cannot be ejaculated. The main causes are blockage due to previous infection of the reproductive tract, previous vasectomy or failure of the connecting tubes (usually the vas deferens) to develop.
2. This group comprises men who suffer from azoospermia because the testicles do not produce sperm or produce them in such low numbers that they die and are reabsorbed before they are ejaculated.

It is now possible to aspirate sperm from the epididymis or testis by inserting a hypodermic needle through the skin of the scrotum. If no sperm can be obtained by these methods, a testicular biopsy (a small piece of testicular tissue containing seminiferous tubules) is taken and cultured in vitro when, hopefully, the spermatogonia will produce spermatozoa.

Spermatozoa so obtained can be frozen almost indefinitely in liquid nitrogen until other preparations for fertilization have been made.

In the case of the would-be mother, the environment of her uterus may be inhospitable to sperm owing to increased viscosity of the mucus, acidity or the presence of antibodies to sperm.

Blockage of the fallopian tubes as a result of pelvic inflammatory disease, sexually transmitted disease, endometriosis or other factors may prevent a perfectly good ovum from reaching the uterus or fallopian tubes for fertilization.

If the impediment to fertility is difficulty in effecting the physical union between the ovum and sperm it may be possible to harvest ova from the woman and unite them outside the body with sperm obtained by the methods described.

The woman is treated with gonadotrophins to induce the maturation of several follicles at the same time. The maturing follicles are regularly imaged by ultrasound to judge when they are sufficiently ripe. Close to maturity, a small slit is made just below the woman's umbilicus, where there are few blood-vessels, and a fibreoptic laparoscope introduced into the abdomen, which has been inflated with carbon dioxide to give the surgeon space to work. The laparoscope is like a telescope through which the surgeon can view the ovaries and, using a device like a hypodermic needle, suck up the ova developing within the follicles. This procedure is sufficiently minor to be carried out under local anaesthetic in a day clinic.

The ova can then be placed in contact with the sperm, which have been washed with culture medium, which capacitates them by simulating the trip through the cervix, uterus and fallopian tubes.

If the sperm are very few in number and therefore too precious to be left to carry out the risky process of fertilization themselves, or if the sperm are incapable of penetrating the ovum, they can even be relieved of that responsibility by the technique of intracytoplasmic sperm injection (ICSI). A sperm is taken up in a tiny hypodermic needle and bodily injected into the cytoplasm of the ovum. This results in a better than 70% chance of fertilization.

The ovum is watched under a microscope and, if developing normally, can be transferred to its mother's uterus where, hopefully, it will implant. Because this implantation is another risky process, several fertilized ova are transferred at the same time in the hope that at least one will survive. If things go better than expected this can result in several fetuses developing.

Because every step in this procedure involves risk to the sperm or ova, several ova are fertilized at the same time and allowed to develop to a level suitable for implantation. The unused embryos can be frozen and introduced into the mother's uterus at a much later date.

The fate of these embryos and the fact that the woman who is implanted with them does not have to be the same woman who provided the ovum present ethical problems that are beyond a standard textbook of physiology.

The placenta

Functions of the placenta

As the invasion by the embryo continues, the maternal blood vessels are eroded such that developing fetal blood vessels are sitting in a lake of maternal blood, described as a **haemochorial placenta**. It is important to note, and of paramount importance to the success of the pregnancy, that throughout pregnancy the fetal and maternal bloods are always separated by at least one cell layer. The placenta is a site of selective exchange in both directions between mother and fetus, although cells and large molecules such as proteins are normally excluded. A successful pregnancy is wholly dependent on the integrity of the placenta being maintained throughout. It undertakes a number of physiological functions on behalf of the fetus, namely the roles of respiratory gas exchange, supply of nutrients and regulation of fluid balance and metabolic excretion (see Ch. 10.4). During pregnancy the organ systems that carry out these functions are non-functional in the fetus. Equally important is the placenta's role as an endocrine organ, synthesizing steroid, peptide and protein hormones which act to maintain the pregnancy, influence maternal and fetal metabolism, and prepare the mammary glands for lactation. With regard to some endocrine functions, the placenta and fetus act together in hormone synthesis, giving rise to the term **fetoplacental unit**. The trophoblast cells differentiate into two lines, cytotrophoblasts and syncytiocytotrophoblasts, with both cell types secreting protein and peptide hormones and the steroid hormones being synthesized by the syncytiocytotrophoblasts.

Placental hormones

Human chorionic gonadotrophin

Secretion of **human chorionic gonadotrophin** (hCG or HCG) early in the pregnancy is essential for its continuation. In an ovarian cycle when conception does not take place, luteal progesterone and oestrogen inhibit LH secretion, maintenance of the corpus luteum ceases, and progesterone and oestrogen levels fall removing hormonal maintenance of the endometrium, which breaks down as a menstrual bleed. For pregnancy to become established the oestrogen and progesterone levels must be maintained in order to support the endometrium. This is achieved by hCG acting as a placental gonadotrophin and taking over from LH in maintaining the corpus luteum, thus ensuring a continued supply of progesterone and oestrogen. hCG, a protein, is detectable in urine within 9 days of conception and levels then rise rapidly during the first trimester, peaking at 9–12 weeks (Fig. 10.2.4). The presence of hCG in the urine is used to test for pregnancy, and pregnancy testing kits based on a one-stage radioimmunoassay will reliably detect pregnancy within days of a period being missed.

By the start of the second trimester the placenta is synthesizing sufficient progesterone and oestrogen to maintain the endometrium independently of the corpus luteum. hCG declines to a low level which is maintained for the remainder of the pregnancy, and the corpus luteum ceases to function in the absence of hCG support. Since hCG synthesis continues throughout pregnancy, it is likely that it subserves other functions and possible roles attributed to it include the stimulation of fetal Leydig cells to secrete testosterone and stimulation of fetal adrenal cells to secrete dehydroepiandrosterone sulphate (DHEA-S).

Oestrogens

Throughout pregnancy oestrogen levels increase steadily. During the first trimester the initial source is the corpus luteum, with the placenta producing increasing quantities as pregnancy progresses (Fig. 10.2.4). At the start of the second trimester, when the corpus luteum ceases to function, the placenta becomes the source of both **oestrogens** and **progesterone**. Optimal synthesis of oestrogen requires efficient functioning of the fetal adrenals. Both maternal and fetal adrenals synthesize DHEA-S, which circulates to the placenta where it is deconjugated and aromatized to oestrogens (Fig. 10.2.5). Approximately 50% of the DHEA-S is fetal in origin.

The principal oestrogen produced by the placenta is **oestriol**, together with smaller amounts of oestradiol-17β and oestrone-17β. This contrasts with the menstrual cycle when oestradiol-17β is the principal oestrogen secreted. Placental synthesis of oestriol requires 16α-hydroxy-DHEA which is derived solely from the fetus, whereas oestradiol and oestrone depend equally on maternal and fetal supply of DHEA-S. By late pregnancy plasma oestriol levels are 400 nmol/1 as compared with 50 nmol/1 for

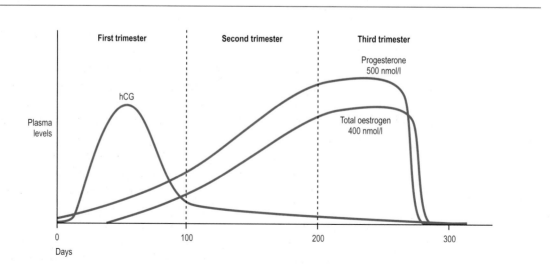

Fig. 10.2.4 Plasma hormone levels during pregnancy.

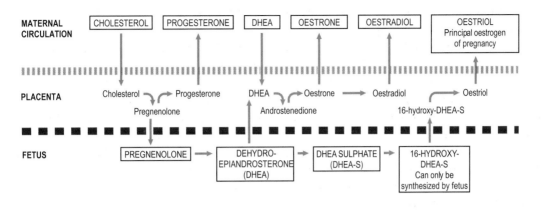

Fig. 10.2.5 Fetoplacental steroid production. The placenta also produces protein hormones.

oestradiol. Urinary oestrogen levels are used to assess the efficiency with which the fetoplacental unit is functioning. If fetal function is impaired, there is a greater fall in oestriol than in total oestrogen excretion.

Progesterone

This is sometimes called the hormone of pregnancy because it is the most important hormone in relation to establishing and sustaining the fetus while in the uterine cavity. Levels increase steadily throughout pregnancy, reaching some 500 nmol/l during the second and third trimesters, and like oestrogens the site of synthesis switches from the corpus luteum to the placental syncytiocytotrophoblasts at about 12 weeks' gestation (Fig. 10.2.4). Synthesis is dependent on the availability of cholesterol, which is usually maternal in origin. The higher plasma concentration of progesterone as compared with oestrogens means that throughout pregnancy the uterine smooth muscle is progesterone dominated, which renders it quiescent and less likely to contract inappropriately. This is achieved by the progesterone inhibiting prostaglandin production and decreasing muscle sensitivity to oxytocin. Placental progesterone

is also used to provide substrate for the fetal adrenals to synthesize cortisol and aldosterone. In the mother, progesterone acts synergistically with oestrogens in mammary gland development in readiness for lactation.

Human chorionic somatomammotrophin

Human chorionic somatomammotrophin (HCS) is the other main protein hormone produced by the placenta. It is similar in structure to pituitary growth hormone and prolactin and is sometimes referred to as **human placental lactogen** (HPL). As hCG levels fall, HCS levels increase and continue to rise throughout pregnancy, plateauing towards term. There is a close relationship between placental weight and HCS concentration, which in turn is taken as an indication of fetal well-being. A sudden fall in HCS production indicates that placental function is impaired. If this occurs early in the pregnancy, spontaneous abortion of the fetus may result; late in the pregnancy it is an indicator of placental insufficiency. Although the daily production of HCS exceeds that of any other protein hormone, its precise functions during pregnancy remain unclear, although they are likely to include lactogenic and anabolic functions in the mother. Another role may be related to its lipolytic actions which could provide an alternative energy source for the mother other than glycogenolysis. HCS's anti-insulin effect will also help to maintain blood glucose levels. Certainly, fasting by the mother stimulates HCS secretion, followed by a rise in plasma glucose.

Other hormones

Prolactin

Secretion of **prolactin** by the maternal pituitary increases linearly throughout pregnancy, by term achieving levels up to 10 times those seen in the non-pregnant female. The prolactin functions in concert with oestrogens and progesterone in mammary gland development, acting particularly on lobule development. During pregnancy, milk production is inhibited by high levels of oestrogen and progesterone, although the mammary glands are capable of milk production from about 5 months' gestation. Following parturition, when oestrogen and progesterone levels have fallen dramatically, prolactin adopts its lactogenic role of stimulating milk production. The elevated levels of prolactin present in lactating mothers help to suppress the return of the ovarian cycle, acting as a natural contraceptive. However, this contraceptive action is reliable only during the early postpartum period.

Relaxin

Relaxin is secreted during the first trimester by the corpus luteum, and in the later stages of pregnancy by the decidual cells of the endometrium. Although secreted throughout pregnancy, its main role is during parturition when it causes relaxation of the pelvic bones and ligaments, and softens the cervix. Its ability to inhibit myometrial contractions may be significant during pregnancy.

Other maternal hormone changes

As pregnancy develops, characteristic changes occur in a number of maternal hormone systems. The pituitary is noticeably enlarged and this is accompanied by elevated secretion of ACTH, TSH and prolactin. Gonadotrophin secretion is inhibited by the high circulating levels of oestrogen and progesterone, and GH actions are largely replaced by HCS. The ACTH stimulates cortisol secretion, and although the total plasma cortisol level is increased, free cortisol rises only slightly because oestrogen has enhanced the binding capacity present in the plasma by stimulating cortisol-binding globulin production. Whether the elevated cortisol serves any specific function is unclear, although it may contribute to mammary gland development and the increased adiposity associated with pregnancy.

Aldosterone levels rise throughout pregnancy, stimulated by the effects of oestrogen on the renin–angiotensin system. This results in the mother being in positive sodium balance, which is necessary to maintain the increase required in maternal plasma volume and to provide adequate fluids for the developing fetus. Some mothers develop significant fluid retention towards term, which is likely to be related to this sodium retention.

The thyroid gland can increase in size by as much as 50% in response to the elevated TSH. As with cortisol, there is an elevated total T_3/T_4 and again this is largely due to increased plasma protein increasing the available binding capacity. Free hormone levels remain normal, and hyperthyroidism is not normally observed.

Calcium is required for the development of the fetus and this is achieved through enhanced intestinal absorption of calcium due to elevated synthesis of 25-OH-vitamin D and 1,25-(OH_2)-vitamin D. As a result of this action, maternal plasma calcium levels are maintained despite the constant drain on supplies by the fetus, largely for skeletal development.

Summary

The placenta

- The human haemochorial placenta allows the mother's organ systems to function for the fetus and also exercises endocrine control.
- Fetus and placenta act together as a fetoplacental unit, but maternal and fetal blood must be kept separate.
- Placental human chorionic gonadotrophin takes over the maintenance of the corpus luteum from LH.
- The placenta takes over the production of oestrogen and progesterone from the corpus luteum after the first trimester of pregnancy.

- Placental synthesis of oestriol depends on activity of the fetus and is used to assess function of the fetoplacental unit.
- Placental progesterone inhibits inappropriate contractions of the myometrium.
- Human chorionic somatomammotrophin acts as an alternative to maternal pituitary growth hormone on the fetus and stimulates lactogenic and anabolic activity in the mother.
- Prolactin from the pituitary and relaxin from the corpus luteum and endometrium increase during pregnancy.

Recent Advances

Electronic rhythm

The fact that human conception can only take place during a limited part of the menstrual cycle has been known for a very long time. The physiological basis for this is that ovulation usually occurs 14 days prior to menstruation and that the ovum survives for approximately 2 days after ovulation. Sperm in the female reproductive tract are capable of fertilization for only a little longer.

Outside the few days around ovulation a 'safe period' exists during which coitus can take place with reduced risk of pregnancy. Abstaining from sex during the period around ovulation suggests itself as a safe method of contraception that involves no physical barriers or drug interventions. The fly in the physiological ointment of this method is the difficulty in predicting or even detecting ovulation. The importance of prediction rather than detection is clear, since detection of ovulation immediately after coitus is of little use as a contraceptive method. Prediction is made difficult by the notoriously irregular length of some women's periods. There is also the suggestion by some scientists that some women may (like rabbits and ferrets) ovulate in response to coitus near to the predicted ovulatory date, which means that a greater latitude should be allowed before the predicted date.

Several methods have been used to predict ovulation and hence the safe period:

- A woman may record her menstrual cycle over 6 months and then calculate the safe period from these dates. This is laborious and compliance by patients is low. This 'calendar' method has been largely superseded by 'temperature' and 'mucus' methods.
- In the temperature method the woman takes her basal body temperature each morning immediately on wakening. The progesterone surge on ovulation causes a rise of about 0.5°C (Fig. RA10.2.1).

Recent Advances (Continued)

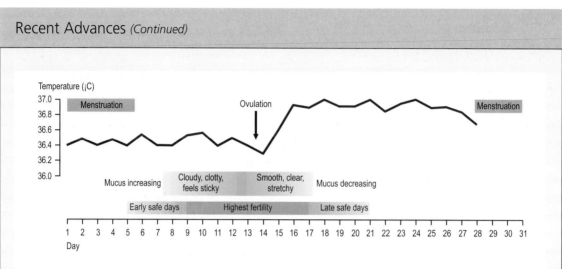

Fig. RA10.2.1 Detecting ovulation. Charting body temperature or changes in the texture of cervical mucus are used to detect ovulation.

- The mucus method utilizes the fact that, prior to ovulation, oestrogens make mucus secretions of the uterine cervix cloudy and sticky, whereas the rise in progesterone on ovulation causes the mucus to become clear and slippery (Fig. RA10.2.1). The woman is instructed how to feel the texture of this mucus, and the ability to draw it out between finger and thumb into threads longer than 10 cm (*spinnbarkeit*, German – fit for spinning) is taken as indication of the ovulatory phase.

The problem with these methods of controlling fertility is that they are better at detecting ovulation than predicting it, and even the detection of ovulation depends on mainly subjective signs and symptoms. The problem of predicting ovulation involves at least two components – recording the event in a number of cycles and from this predicting the next time the event will occur.

An electronic device has recently been developed which enables a woman to monitor the rise in the urinary metabolite of oestradiol (oestrone-3-glucuronide) which accompanies the development of the dominant follicle in the ovary, and the surge of luteinizing hormone which precedes ovulation by less than 48 hours. These objective measurements of hormone levels are clearly superior to subjective methods of estimating the time of ovulation. The machine also utilizes electronic memory to 'remember' when previous ovulations occurred in previous cycles and so improve prediction of future ovulations.

The device is about the size of a pocket calculator and comes with a supply of chemically treated paper strips which are dipped into the woman's early morning urine and inserted into the machine. This is done eight times per month and the machine builds up a 'memory' of the monthly hormone profile over the previous 6 months and predicts which days are safe for coitus.

The manufacturers claim an efficiency of 6 pregnancies per 100 woman years (about twice as efficient as the temperature or mucus methods), which is on a par with mechanical methods of contraception.

The initial expense of the device and the compliance necessary to build up the hormone cycle program probably mean that the instrument will appeal most to a fairly sophisticated population.

Parturition and lactation

Parturition

Parturition, or labour, is the term used to describe the process at the end of pregnancy during which the fetus is expelled from the uterus. The onset of parturition in women is still poorly understood and much of the experimental data used to explain the process have been derived from other species, mainly the sheep and goat. These data indicate that the hormonal basis of parturition is likely to be identical in all species studied, even though the way in which parturition starts may vary between species. Two processes are required for the successful expulsion of the fetus:

- coordinated contractions of the **myometrium**
- relaxation of the **cervix**.

Myometrium

The myometrium is the musculature within the uterus wall; it consists mainly of single-unit smooth (non-striated) muscle fibres, and has a rich blood supply, together with nerves and lymph tissue. As pregnancy proceeds, the mass of the myometrium increases markedly in response to oestrogen stimulation; this hypertrophy is largely due to the increase in size of individual muscle cells (up to 500 μm), rather than an increase in muscle cell number. Uterine muscle cells are able to function as a syncytium (similar to cardiac muscle) because of the electrical coupling between cells provided by the so-called gap junctions or nexuses. The presence of this electrical coupling allows depolarizing electrical current to flow rapidly through the tissue in such a way as to produce coordinated contractions. However, such activity is not required throughout pregnancy, only during parturition, and so is closely controlled by the hormonal environment of the myometrium at each stage of pregnancy.

Mechanism of contraction

In common with all muscle types, the mechanism of contraction in the myometrium requires the interaction of actin and myosin by the sliding filament mechanism, triggered by a rise in the concentration of intracellular calcium ions, with the whole process being energized by ATP. The intracellular calcium is in part released from intracellular stores and in part derived from extracellular fluid, the increase in calcium being triggered by the action potential in the muscle cell membrane. Each muscle cell is capable of generating spontaneous pacemaker potentials and, when the magnitude of these exceeds a critical threshold, a burst of action potentials is superimposed on the pacemaker potentials, resulting in a sharp rise in intracellular calcium levels, followed by contraction. The contraction process in smooth muscle differs from that in other muscle types, with the calcium interacting with a regulatory molecule, calmodulin, and myosin light-chain kinase, which acts on the thick myosin filaments (see p. 120). The thin actin filaments do not contain the troponin complex found in striated muscle, and so are always ready for contraction. Following contraction, relaxation occurs when intracellular calcium levels fall as a result of calcium being pumped back into intracellular stores and out of the cell.

Characteristically, contraction in uterine smooth muscle is slow, sustained and resistant to fatigue, and can maintain the same tension of contraction for prolonged periods at much lower energy costs than in striated muscle.

Hormonal control of contractility

How is variation in the contractility of the myometrium achieved? A number of hormones affect the contractility of uterine muscle. During the pregnancy the high levels of **oestrogen** are responsible for stimulating the hypertrophy of the myometrium, while the high levels of **progesterone** tend to hyperpolarize the membranes of the muscle cell, making them quiescent and unlikely to contract. Towards the end of pregnancy the production of progesterone falls off, removing this 'braking' effect on contraction. Simultaneously the oestrogen concentration is at its highest, and stimulates the myometrial cell membranes to manufacture receptors to a third hormone, **oxytocin**. Oxytocin has two effects on the myometrium:

- it lowers the excitation threshold in the muscle cells
- it stimulates the release of a fourth hormone, prostaglandin $PGF_{2\alpha}$, which enhances the release of calcium from intracellular stores.

Cervix

During pregnancy the high connective tissue content, consisting mainly of **collagen** fibres in a proteoglycan matrix, of the cervix makes it very resistant to stretch and enables it to help retain the developing fetus within the uterus. Birth cannot occur unless the cervix is able to dilate sufficiently to allow the passage of the fetus through the birth canal. This dilatation process requires that the very nature of the cervix must change so that the appropriate relaxation of the structure can occur. This softening process involves a reduction in the collagen content of the cervix, and a loosening of the remaining collagen bundles. **Prostaglandins** have been shown to be capable of increasing the distensibility of the cervix, and the softening of the cervix is thought to be another important action of this group of hormones during the parturition process. Increased production towards term of a further hormone, **relaxin**, by the corpus luteum, is also thought to aid enlargement of the birth canal by causing relaxation of the cervix, pelvic ligaments and pubic symphysis.

Hormonal changes and the onset of parturition

Throughout pregnancy the concentrations of oestrogen and progesterone rise, reaching a plateau during the third trimester, and it is possible to talk about the oestrogen : progesterone ratio. This ratio shows a progesterone dominance during pregnancy, resulting in overall quiescence of the myometrium; it is likely that this progesterone dominance has other endocrine effects as well. Towards term the production of progesterone declines before that of oestrogen, resulting in oestrogen dominance. We have already described the effect this has on the contractility of the myometrium. In addition, the change in the oestrogen : progesterone ratio has been shown to affect both the synthesis and release of prostaglandins.

Prostaglandins are synthesized in most tissues in the body, but during pregnancy the endometrium is the most important site; it is likely that the myometrium, cervix, placenta and fetal membranes also synthesize prostaglandins. There is an inhibition of prostaglandin synthesis during pregnancy, possibly owing to the stabilizing effect of progesterone on lysosomal membranes preventing the release of phospholipase A_2, an enzyme required for the production of arachidonic acid, a precursor of prostaglandin synthesis. Oestrogen, dominant at term, has the opposite effect, thus stimulating prostaglandin production.

The increase in prostaglandin release is achieved via the oxytocin-dependent mechanism

mentioned earlier; by increasing the number of myometrial oxytocin receptors it is possible to stimulate the release of prostaglandin without increasing the amount of oxytocin in the system.

Oxytocin release is an example of a neuroendocrine reflex (described in detail in Chapter 5.1, p. 374) requiring tactile stimulation of the reproductive tract, and particularly the cervix (Fig. 10.3.1). This stimulation activates sensory afferent nerves which pass up the somatosensory pathways in the anterolateral columns of the spinal cord. The detail of the connections through the brainstem is unknown, but the magnocellular cells producing the oxytocin (mainly in the paraventricular nucleus) are ultimately stimulated, with the oxytocin being released from the terminals of these neurosecretory cells by the passage of action potentials along their axons. The oxytocin released into the blood provides the efferent endocrine limb of the reflex, travelling to the uterus where it produces the effects described earlier.

Since it is widely hypothesized that prostaglandins are central to the parturition process, it is necessary to try to establish what influences the timing of the increase in prostaglandin synthesis and release. Extensive animal studies show a wide variety of mechanisms, but common to all, both fetal and maternal endocrine changes are critical. Indeed, it has been postulated that maturational changes in the fetal hypothalamo-pituitary–adrenal axis, resulting in increased production of **cortisol**, may be critical to the whole process of parturition by producing the increasing oestrogen : progesterone ratio.

Phases of labour

The process of labour is traditionally divided into three phases:

- The *first stage*, usually the longest, describes the onset of labour and is characterized by regular, painful contractions. During this

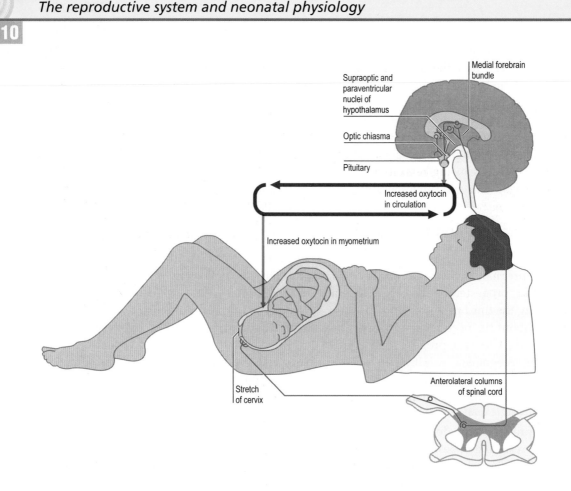

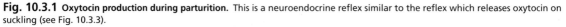

Fig. 10.3.1 **Oxytocin production during parturition.** This is a neuroendocrine reflex similar to the reflex which releases oxytocin on suckling (see Fig. 10.3.3).

stage the relaxation of the cervix also occurs, the full dilatation of which signals the end of the first stage. It tends to be longer for first pregnancies, often exceeding 15 hours, reducing to an average of 8 hours for subsequent pregnancies.

- The *second stage*, lasting about 1 hour, is the period between achieving full dilatation of the cervix and delivery of the fetus.
- The *third stage* is relatively quick and ends with the expulsion of the placenta. This final stage is often aided by the administration of oxytocic drugs, which both speed the

expulsion of the placenta by increasing the strength of uterine contractions, and help to reduce postpartum bleeding.

Prolonged labour can result in fetal distress and/or hypoxia, and when this is detected, by monitoring the fetal heart rate or, increasingly, fetal blood pH, the decision may be taken to deliver the fetus by caesarean section. Following delivery, under natural biological conditions, the neonate is totally dependent on the mother to provide for its well-being and, in particular, its nutritional requirements.

![Summary icon] **Summary**

Parturition

- Parturition depends on contraction of the myometrium and relaxation of the cervix.
- At the end of pregnancy, falling progesterone levels remove its inhibition of myometrial contractions and increased oestrogen sensitizes the myometrium to the excitatory effects of oxytocin.
- Near term, prostaglandins soften the cervix by reducing and loosening its collagen fibres, while relaxin relaxes the cervix, pelvic ligaments and pubic symphysis.

- At parturition, the oestrogen : progesterone ratio is reversed, with oestrogen now dominating, favouring prostaglandin production, which sharply peaks under other influences.
- These influences on prostaglandin production include a surge of oxytocin produced by a neuroendocrine reflex, and maturation of the fetal hypothalamo-pituitary axis.
- Labour is divided into three phases: first – from onset of contractions to full dilatation of the cervix; second – to delivery of the fetus; third – the expulsion of the placenta.

Lactation

Throughout pregnancy the bilateral mammary glands undergo development such that following parturition they are functional and able to provide adequate nutrition for the neonate. Developmentally, the mammary glands are modified **sweat glands** contained within a rounded skin-covered breast. Just below the centre of each breast is a ring of pigmented skin (the areola) which surrounds a protruding nipple. Secretions of sebaceous glands in the areolar area prevent suckling causing cracking of the nipples. The presence of smooth muscle fibres in the areola and nipple cause them to become erect following tactile stimulation.

By the third trimester of pregnancy each mammary gland is made up of some 15–25 lobes; each lobe consists of lobules containing the glandular **alveoli** that produce the milk, which drains via lactiferous ducts opening at the nipple (Fig. 10.3.2). In non-pregnant women the glandular structure of the breast is largely undeveloped, the duct system is rudimentary, and the size of the breast is mainly dictated by the degree of adipose tissue present.

The development of the mammary glands during pregnancy is regulated by hormones. During early pregnancy, considerable hypertrophy of the ducts, lobes and alveoli occurs, principally under the influence of **oestradiol** and **progesterone**. Prolactin and insulin may contribute to this stimulation of growth. In addition, specific growth factors contributing to mammary gland development have been identified and localized in mammary tissue: they are epidermal growth factor and transforming growth factor α.

The mammary glands are capable of milk production by the fourth month of pregnancy. Differentiation of the alveoli largely occurs when duct and lobule development is complete. The alveoli consist of a single layer of cuboidal/columnar cells responsible for milk synthesis

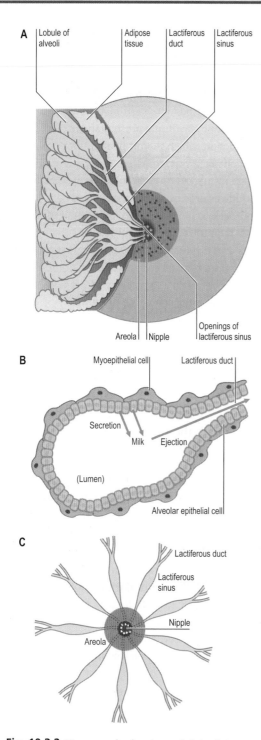

and secretion, with contractile **myoepithelial** cells situated between the alveolar cells and the basement membrane being responsible for moving the milk from the alveoli into the duct system, an effect known as 'let down' of milk, produced by oxytocin released in a neuro-endocrine reflex stimulation of the nipple (Fig. 10.3.3).

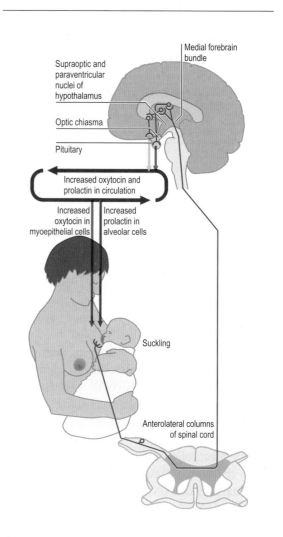

Fig. 10.3.2 Mammary gland anatomy. A. Lateral structure of right breast of a pregnant woman. Alveoli open into milk-collecting ducts which unite to form lactiferous ducts, each draining one lobe of the gland. The ducts dilate into sinuses which form small milk reservoirs beneath the areola. **B.** Structure of an alveolus. **C.** Arrangement of the lactiferous sinuses beneath the nipple.

Fig. 10.3.3 Prolactin and oxytocin production during **suckling.** This is a neuroendocrine reflex similar to the reflex which releases oxytocin during parturition (see Fig. 10.3.1).

Summary

Lactation

- During pregnancy, the breasts hypertrophy under the action of oestradiol and progesterone, with contributions from prolactin, insulin and local growth factors.
- Suckling maintains prolactin stimulation of milk production and, because of oxytocin release, causes an immediate 'let down' of milk.

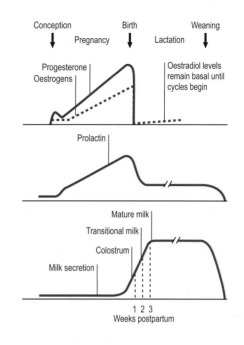

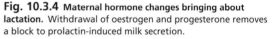

Fig. 10.3.4 Maternal hormone changes bringing about lactation. Withdrawal of oestrogen and progesterone removes a block to prolactin-induced milk secretion.

Regulation and maintenance of milk secretion

Despite the presence prior to parturition of high levels of prolactin, the hormone mainly responsible for stimulating synthesis and secretion of milk by the alveolar cells and present at its highest concentration at term, milk secretion is inhibited by the high levels of maternal steroids, particularly progesterone. Following parturition, prolactin levels fall, but not as abruptly as oestrogen and progesterone, and plateau at a lower level which is still significantly higher than that in the non-pregnant female (Fig. 10.3.4). This level of production of prolactin will be maintained for some 3–4 weeks in the absence of suckling, and will support some milk production. However, the copious milk production required to satisfy the nutritional requirements of the neonate demands regular suckling to maintain prolactin secretion to support full lactation.

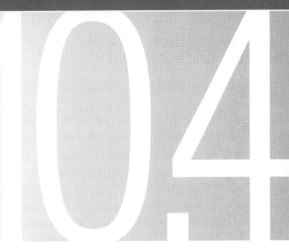

Maternal, fetal and neonatal physiology

Introduction

The transition from fetus to newborn baby, or **neonate**, is possibly one of the greatest physiological challenges encountered during life. While in the uterus, the fetus is dependent on the mother for maintaining its oxygen supply, nutrition, excretion and temperature regulation. In addition, because fetal development occurs in a fluid medium, fluid balance poses no problems. From the moment of birth, these maternal support systems are removed and the neonate's respiratory, gastrointestinal and renal systems are required to function independently. Fluid balance and temperature regulation also become the responsibility of the neonate.

During gestation, there are modifications in the physiology of the mother and in the anatomy and physiology of the fetus to enable optimal development of the fetus. During the first half of a pregnancy the mother is in a state of anabolism, during which significant growth occurs in the breasts, uterus and musculature, and energy stores accumulate in the form of adipose tissue and glycogen. These changes enable the mother to withstand the later stages of pregnancy, when the fetus and placenta are growing rapidly and are a huge metabolic drain on her.

Anatomical modifications are seen in the fetal circulatory system, where a series of shunts ensures that blood is delivered preferentially to those tissues in the fetus that need it most.

Placental function in fetal nutrition and excretion

The placenta is unique in being an organ which develops solely to support pregnancy, and which has a limited life span. It grows throughout pregnancy, achieving a weight of some 700 g by parturition, with a daily blood flow of 285 litres, about 10% of total maternal blood flow. Throughout fetal life the placenta functions to supply the fetus with oxygen and nutrients, remove carbon dioxide and metabolic waste, and maintain ionic and fluid balance. As described in Chapter 10.2, the placenta, in conjunction with the fetus, synthesizes the hormones on which the overall maintenance of the pregnancy depends. Prior to implantation, nutrition of the embryo is derived from secretions of the fallopian tubes and endometrium. Following implantation, all fetal vital body functions are supported via the maternal circulation and placenta. Optimal development of the fetus is also dependent on the efficient functioning of the placenta throughout pregnancy, when the placenta functions as the lungs, gastrointestinal tract and kidneys of the developing fetus.

The structure of the human placenta differs from that seen in most other mammals and is described as **haemochorial**. It consists of finger-like projections of placental tissue and fetal blood vessels which are bathed in maternal blood (Fig. 10.4.1). A physical separation is always maintained between maternal and fetal blood. At the start of pregnancy this barrier is some 25 μm thick, reducing to 2 μm towards term, thus facilitating transfer between mother and fetus as the latter grows and its requirements increase.

Gas exchange

The fetus, surrounded by **amniotic fluid**, develops within the amniotic sac in the uterine cavity. In this state it does not have access to atmospheric air and so is dependent on the

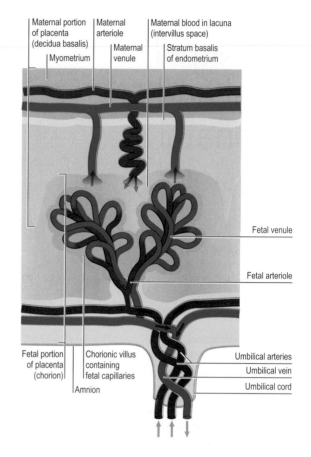

Fig. 10.4.1 The human placenta. The relationship between maternal and fetal blood systems.

placenta for the delivery of oxygen and removal of carbon dioxide.

As with the alveolocapillary membranes in the lungs, gases cross the placental and fetal membranes by diffusion, driven by the partial pressure of the gas on either side of the barrier. Similarly, the placenta is less permeable to oxygen than to carbon dioxide, necessitating a greater partial pressure gradient for oxygen in order to transfer similar amounts of oxygen and carbon dioxide per unit of time. Maternal P_{O_2} is about 90 mmHg (12 kPa) compared with umbilical vein P_{O_2} ranging from 23–38 mmHg (3–5 kPa). Should fetal P_{O_2} rise above this level,

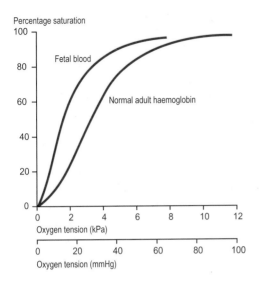

Fetal blood

Normal adult haemoglobin

Fig. 10.4.2 Fetal and maternal oxygen–haemoglobin dissociation curves.

normally in the range 40–44 mmHg (5–5.5 kPa) compared with 40 mmHg (5 kPa) in maternal blood.

Of other gases which might be present in the mother's blood, two non-physiological gases are of particular significance for the well-being of the fetus. Gaseous anaesthetics, which may be used during delivery, can cross the placenta and affect the fetus; so too can carbon monoxide. CO is present in the blood of smoking mothers, and may also accumulate there as a result of passive smoking. It will diffuse into the fetus and be preferentially taken up by the HbF, thus compromising its oxygen-carrying capacity. There is now convincing evidence that the babies of smoking mothers are of lower birth weight than those of non-smoking mothers, and these babies have an increased incidence of birth abnormalities.

constriction occurs in the umbilical vessels, which in turn will limit oxygen transfer to the fetus. This means that the fetus has to obtain its oxygen at low PO_2 values, but this situation is made easier by the presence in the fetal blood of a form of haemoglobin (HbF) which saturates at much lower PO_2 values than adult haemoglobin (HbA) and is also insensitive to 2,3-diphospho-glycerate (2,3-DPG), an inhibitor of oxygen binding in HbA (Fig. 10.4.2) and explained in detail in Section 7 (p. 684). The globin chains in HbF comprise two α- and two δ-chains, com-pared with the two α- and two β-chains seen in HbA. HbF reaches about 80% saturation at the PO_2 levels seen in the umbilical veins, and ensures a level of oxygen transfer into the fetus which is adequate to support normal develop-ment. Oxygen transfer is also helped by the existence of the Bohr effect, whereby the pres-ence of carbon dioxide facilitates the dissocia-tion of oxygen from oxyhaemoglobin.

Carbon dioxide passes across the placenta by simple diffusion, the rate being dependent on the size of the partial pressure gradient existing across the membrane. Fetal PCO_2 values are

Nutrient and ionic transfer

During the later stages of pregnancy, when the fetus requires larger amounts of glucose, the mother becomes insulin resistant with the effect that plasma levels of carbohydrate, protein and fat all remain elevated following a meal, result-ing in increased placental transfer to the fetus. Between meals, plasma glucose and amino acid levels fall faster in pregnant than non-pregnant women because of the continued placental transfer to the fetus. However, the mother is assured of a supply of energy substrate through increased lipolysis of the adipose stores laid down during the anabolic phase of pregnancy. **Human chorionic somatotrophin** is thought to be an important mediator of these changes.

The major carbohydrate used by the fetus is glucose, and because D-glucose is transferred in preference to L-glucose, a carrier-mediated mechanism is likely to be used. Amino acids are transferred using active transport carrier mechanisms, with higher concentrations being achieved in fetal blood compared with that of the mother. Short-chain fatty acids and glycerol diffuse freely across the placenta, with more complex lipids being synthesized either by the fetus or in the placenta.

The free diffusion of fatty acids supports the diffusion across the placenta of fat-soluble vitamins, whereas water-soluble vitamins require active transport. Proteins, including maternal protein and peptide hormones, are not normally able to cross the placenta, a major exception being the transfer of the immunoglobulin IgG, which is thought to have a specific transfer mechanism.

The growing fetus requires a constant and increasing supply of minerals to maintain it in positive mineral balance. Although most minerals are able to diffuse freely across placental membranes, there is evidence that specific ion pumps are also involved. Some toxic heavy metals are able to cross the placenta, in particular lead and mercury.

Summary

Placental functions for the fetus

- During the first half of pregnancy, a mother is strongly anabolic, laying down stores for later use.
- Humans have a haemochorial placenta with finger-like projections dipping into pools of maternal blood.
- Oxygen transfer to the fetus is helped by the special properties of fetal haemoglobin.
- During pregnancy, a mother's plasma nutrient levels are elevated because of insulin resistance, which helps transfer to the fetus.
- Much transfer across the placenta is carrier mediated.
- Proteins do not cross the placenta, except the immunoglobulin IgG.

The fetal circulation

The fetus has an extra dimension to its circulatory system in the form of the umbilical vessels which pass deoxygenated blood from the fetus, through the placenta where gaseous and metabolic exchanges take place, and back into the fetus via the umbilical veins, which contain oxygenated blood. The arrangement of these umbilical vessels means that oxygenated blood is entering the right heart of the fetus, as compared with the left heart in the adult. In addition, the lungs in the fetus are collapsed and non-functional. **Shunts** exist in the fetal circulation to ensure that the inactive lungs are largely bypassed, and that blood containing higher levels of oxygen is directed to the areas of the fetus most in need, namely the head and upper body.

Blood, in which the haemoglobin is about 80% saturated with oxygen, travels from the placenta to the liver in the umbilical vein. During fetal development the liver is itself developing and not required to undertake the metabolic functions it serves in the adult, and its requirement for oxygen is consequently modest. In order to conserve oxygen levels in the blood entering the heart, about 60% of the blood in the umbilical vein bypasses the liver by passing through the first of the three shunts present in the fetal circulation, the **ductus venosus** (Fig. 10.4.3). This shunt links the umbilical vein with the inferior vena cava, which is carrying deoxygenated blood from the lower trunk and limbs of the fetus back to the heart. Within this vessel there is a valve, which largely maintains separation of the two streams of blood as they enter the heart (Fig. 10.4.4) and directs them on to the **crista dividens**.

The stream of oxygenated blood is thus directed through the **foramen ovale**, which connects the right and left atria, thus shunting blood with higher oxygen content directly into the left heart. The presence of the foramen ovale means that the two sides of the fetal heart are

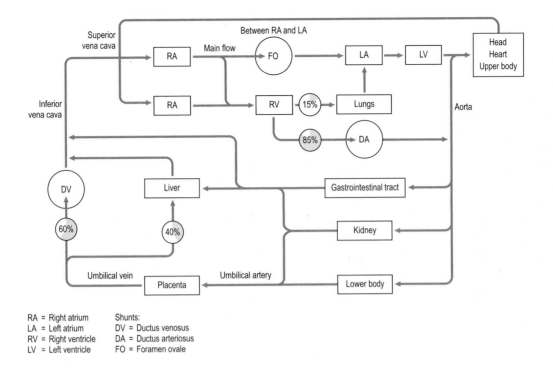

Shunts:
RA = Right atrium
LA = Left atrium   DV = Ductus venosus
RV = Right ventricle DA = Ductus arteriosus
LV = Left ventricle   FO = Foramen ovale

Fig. 10.4.3 The fetal cardiovascular system. The diagram illustrates the division of blood flow at shunts that exist only in the fetus.

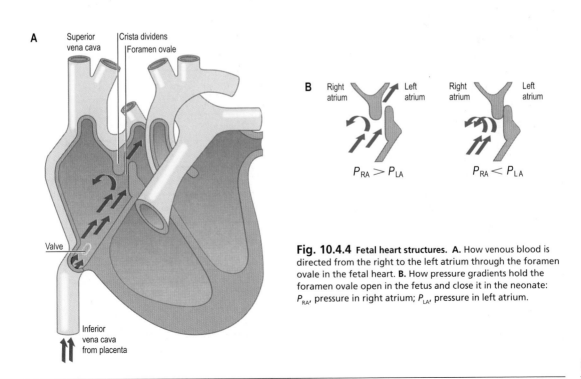

Fig. 10.4.4 Fetal heart structures. A. How venous blood is directed from the right to the left atrium through the foramen ovale in the fetal heart. **B.** How pressure gradients hold the foramen ovale open in the fetus and close it in the neonate: P_{RA}, pressure in right atrium; P_{LA}, pressure in left atrium.

operating in parallel, rather than in series as in the adult. The foramen ovale is a flap valve whose patency is maintained by the higher pressure existing in the right side of the heart because of the greater volume of blood being returned to the right atrium as compared with the left. Deoxygenated blood from the inferior and superior vena cavae passes from the right atrium through the tricuspid valve into the right ventricle.

From the right ventricle, blood passes into the pulmonary artery and travels towards the lungs. In the adult, all the blood in this vessel would pass through the lungs for oxygenation, but because the fetal lungs are functionally inactive, about 85% of the pulmonary arterial blood is passed through the third shunt, the **ductus arteriosus**, which diverts the blood into the aorta below the point at which arteries to the head and upper limbs have already left the aorta, thus ensuring delivery of blood rich in oxygen to these regions (Fig. 10.4.5). Peripheral resistance in the fetus is low compared with in the adult and so the amount of muscle in the walls of the right and left ventricles is similar; this changes over time postnatally when the left heart has to contract against an increased peripheral resistance. The blood passes easily into the ductus arteriosus because the pulmonary vessels in the unexpanded lungs of the fetus offer a high resistance to blood flow. This is in direct contrast with the adult where the pulmonary vessels are low resistance, capacitance vessels.

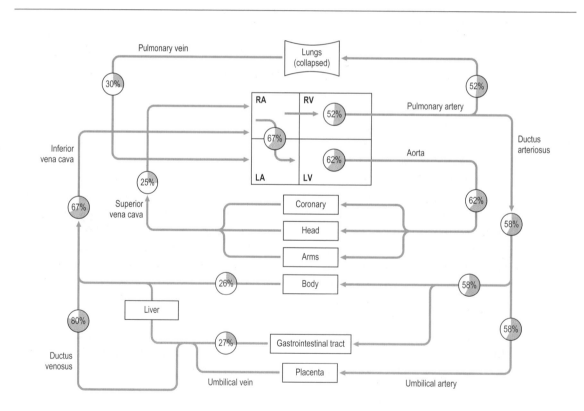

Fig. 10.4.5 **Percentage saturation of haemoglobin with oxygen in blood in the fetal circulation.** There is a priority of supply to the head and upper body. RA, right atrium; LA, left atrium; RV right ventricle; LV, left ventricle.

Neonatal systems

Cardiovascular system

Circulatory changes occurring at birth

At birth, the lungs become inflated with atmospheric air and this is accompanied by a large fall in the resistance of the pulmonary vessels. This fall in resistance is in part due to the pulmonary capillaries being stretched open by the inflating alveoli, and partly a result of the dilating effect on the musculature of the pulmonary vessels of the sudden increase in Po_2 in the lungs. The consequence is a sudden increase in blood flow to the lungs, and consequently in blood flowing back from the lungs to the heart via the pulmonary veins, which empty into the left atrium, resulting in a rise in pressure in the left atrium.

The sudden fall in the resistance to flow in the pulmonary artery results in a fall in pressure in this vessel, which causes a reversal in the pressure gradient across the ductus arteriosus, with the effect that flow through this shunt is reversed. Within minutes the ductus arteriosus starts to constrict and 10–15 hours after birth is functionally closed. This is achieved in part by the response of the ductus musculature to the sudden increase in Po_2, which may be acting directly or causing the release of local constrictor agents such as prostaglandins.

Following parturition in humans the umbilical vessels are traditionally tied and severed. Even when this does not happen, the thick musculature in the vessel walls responds to trauma, local agents and changes in oxygen tension by undergoing constriction to prevent haemorrhage in the neonate. The net effect of this contraction in the fetal circulation is an increase in total peripheral resistance, and hence of blood pressure. Constriction in the umbilical vessels results in a sharp reduction in flow through the ductus venosus, which starts to close, but the mechanisms underlying this response are not known.

Absence of blood returning to the fetal circulation from the umbilical vessels causes a fall in right atrial pressure. When this is combined with the increased pressure in the left atrium, described above, the pressure in the left atrium now exceeds that in the right and the foramen ovale flap valve is functionally closed, separating the two sides of the heart and converting it to the adult state of acting as two pumps in series.

Within hours of birth all three shunts are functionally closed, with the ductus venosus becoming the **ligamentum venosum**, the ductus arteriosus the **ligamentum arteriosum** and the foramen ovale the **fossa ovalis**. Permanent closure takes longer, but problems occur in the neonate if one or more of the shunts fail to close properly and significant blood flow through the shunt persists. When appropriate, these situations are corrected surgically.

Blood pressure and cardiac output

At birth, distribution of muscle in the walls of the ventricles and pulmonary vessels differs from that in the adult. In the ventricles the fetal right ventricular wall is slightly more muscular than the left. In the months following birth, the right ventricular wall becomes thinner and the amount of muscle in the left ventricular wall increases substantially to enable the left heart to pump blood against the high peripheral resistance present in the aorta. As the amount of muscle increases, systolic pressure rises from the 70–80 mmHg (9.5–10.5 kPa) observed in the neonate to 90–100 mmHg (12–13 kPa) at about 6 weeks, with adult levels being achieved during puberty (Fig. 10.4.6). Cardiac output per kilogram body weight in the neonate is two to three times that of the adult, being about 180 ml/kg per minute.

Heart rate in the neonate is higher than in the adult, varying from 95–145 beats per minute, rising to about 170 during the first few months, and gradually reducing until the adult rate of

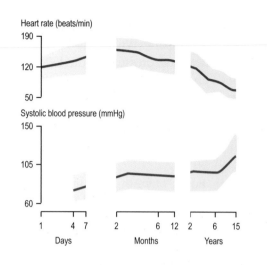

Heart rate (beats/min)

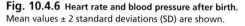

Fig. 10.4.6 **Heart rate and blood pressure after birth.**
Mean values ± 2 standard deviations (SD) are shown.

55–100 beats per minute is achieved in the adolescent (Fig. 10.4.6). These changes in part reflect the different rates of development of the sympathetic and parasympathetic nervous systems, with parasympathetic control dominating at birth and again in the adult.

Pulmonary blood flow

Pulmonary blood vessels are very sensitive to Po_2 and in the fetus are constricted because oxygen levels in lung fluid are very low. This situation is maintained in part by the increased amount of smooth muscle in the pulmonary vessel walls as compared with that in the adult. Following the first inspiration and the rise in alveolar Po_2, the pulmonary vessels dilate, and the resistance to flow through these vessels falls. Over the succeeding months, as the pulmonary vessels develop, the proportion of muscle in their walls approaches adult values.

Respiratory system

Fetal respiratory movements

Fetal monitoring has shown that respiratory movements occur throughout pregnancy, and become more regular as gestation proceeds. By birth these movements can be occurring up to 90% of the time. Why these movements should take place is not fully understood, since no gaseous exchange is occurring across the fetal lung alveolocapillary membranes during gestation. During development, the lungs are filled with a mixture of viscous alveolar secretion and amniotic fluid to about 40% of total lung capacity, and minor movement of this fluid is all that will be achieved by activity in the respiratory muscles. It has been suggested that these movements are simply an indication that the part of the brain controlling the respiratory muscles is developing and becoming active, and ensuring that the muscles are fully functional when needed immediately following parturition. The respiratory movements may also play a role in lung development and growth.

Surfactant production

Ventilation in the adult is made easier by the secretion of **surfactant** in the lungs. This reduces the surface tension of the fluid lining the alveoli, thus decreasing the work of breathing. In the fetus the cells responsible for surfactant secretion, **type II pneumocytes**, develop at about 24 weeks' gestation, and surfactant secretion becomes significant from about 32 weeks. A fetus delivered before 32 weeks is unlikely to be able to breathe by itself, and will require assistance in the form of positive-pressure ventilation until producing sufficient surfactant to breathe independently, a situation described as **respiratory distress syndrome** (RDS).

Clinical Example

Respiratory distress syndrome of the newborn

Respiratory distress syndrome of the newborn (RDS) causes more neonatal deaths than any other condition in this age group. It is alternatively known as idiopathic respiratory distress syndrome and hyaline membrane disease (HMD). Respiratory distress syndrome affects about 0.1% of all neonates and up to 10% of premature infants. Its complications are responsible for up to 50% of all neonatal deaths and 70% of deaths in premature infants.

The condition is twice as common in males as in females. It frequently follows delivery by caesarean section, and infants of diabetic mothers are five times more likely to develop RDS. The chief predisposing factor, however, is premature birth.

Atelectasis (collapse of areas of the lung) is the primary problem with RDS. Three interrelated developmental problems exist in these infants. They have:

- small alveoli which are difficult to inflate
- an excessively compliant chest wall
- insufficient pulmonary surfactant to reduce surface tension within the lung and ease inflation.

Of these, the lack of surfactant is perhaps the most important.

Surfactant can normally be detected in the amniotic fluid at 28–38 weeks' gestation. This large variation explains why some infants delivered before 30 weeks do not present with RDS. Without surfactant, each breath requires much more effort than normal, resulting in exhaustion and decreased ability to maintain lung inflation. This in turn leads to atelectasis. With increasing atelectasis, pulmonary vascular resistance increases. This causes return to the fetal form of circulation with right-to left-shunting through the ductus arteriosus and foramen ovale. Hypoxaemia and hypercapnia result, which cause pulmonary vasoconstriction, further increasing pulmonary vascular resistance. As the condition worsens, capillary leakage deposits fibrin in the interstitium and anaerobic glycolysis produces increased amounts of lactic acid. These changes deprive the alveoli of the materials needed for the production of surfactant and a vicious cycle is set up.

Clinical manifestations of the disease include tachypnoea, with respiratory rates over 40 per minute, expiratory grunting, intercostal and subcostal retraction, nasal flaring and duskiness of the skin. The characteristics of hypoxaemia and dyspnoea develop and apnoea and irregular respiration occur as the infant tires. Respiratory distress syndrome can progress to death in severe cases but in milder cases the condition reaches a peak within 3 days, after which there is usually a gradual improvement. Death is rare after this time.

Supportive treatment to maintain oxygenation and circulation of the blood dramatically alters the outcome of RDS. Mechanical ventilation and the administration of exogenous surfactant can play a part in treatment. Even in severe cases, recovery can be complete within 14 days with an excellent prognosis for normal pulmonary function.

Establishing lung function

At birth, once the umbilical cord has been severed, respiratory gas exchange can no longer occur across the placenta and the lungs must start to function immediately. Failure of this transition can result in irreversible brain damage due to lack of adequate oxygen supply. During gestation the lungs and airways are filled with fluid. The small amount of fluid present in the lungs will be absorbed across the alveolar membranes into the lymphatic system in the hours following birth. If there is significant retention of this fluid, it can easily be sucked from the airway by the midwife.

At birth, the neonate normally gasps, takes a deep breath and begins to cry, and a respiratory rhythm is established within minutes. It is not clear what causes this sequence of events but it has been suggested that the heightened sensory stimulation caused to the baby by the birth process results in enhanced nervous activity in the brain involving stimulation of the respiratory neurones in the brainstem. It is also possible that following the loss of placental oxygen a mild acidosis develops, stimulating the respiratory chemoreceptors, which are already functional.

The neonate's lungs are small and the first inspiration is of the order of 30–40 ml, associated with an intrathoracic pressure 40–100 cmH$_2$O (4–10 kPa) below atmospheric pressure. This high intrathoracic pressure is required to overcome the low compliance of the lung when it is fully collapsed. Once the lungs have been expanded by the first inspiration, the surfactant prevents full collapse of the lungs on expiration, and a lower inflationary pressure is required for all subsequent ventilatory cycles. Lung compliance increases steadily over the next 24 hours, accompanied by a fall in resistance. The neonate is more dependent on gaseous exchange occurring in the respiratory bronchioles than is the adult, a reflection of there being insufficient alveoli in the newborn to support the amount of gaseous exchange that is required.

Lung volumes in the neonate are necessarily much lower than those of the adult, with a tidal volume of the order of 20 ml and total minute volume some 500–600 ml, produced as a result of the higher respiratory rate of about 30 per minute. The fractional physiological dead space is of the same order as that seen in the adult, being between 30 and 35%. Oxygen consumption per unit mass is approximately double that of the adult, with higher values still if the neonate is exposed to thermoregulatory stress requiring activation of the brown adipose tissue (see below).

Once fetal blood is involved in gaseous exchange with alveolar air rather than maternal blood, the P_{O_2} rises and there is a subsequent increase in the percentage saturation of haemoglobin from the 40–50% observed in the fetus to 80–90% in the neonate.

Changes in blood

Production of blood cells in the fetus occurs in various sites depending on the stage of development. Initially the **liver** is the main site, with production transferring to the bone marrow when the skeleton is sufficiently developed. As already described, during pregnancy the fetal haemoglobin (HbF) produced differs from that in the adult (HbA). Immediately following birth there is a significant rise in both the haematocrit and haemoglobin concentration. This is thought to be due to the movement into the fetus of blood previously held in the umbilical vessels. This process is known as '**placental transfer**' and has been estimated to be as much as 35% of the neonate's blood volume. The fluid component of this blood will be redistributed in the fetus or lost through the kidney, resulting in the observed increase in haematocrit and haemoglobin concentration.

Within a few days of birth, haemoglobin concentration starts to fall. Kidney erythropoietin secretion in the fetus is high in response to the low P_{O_2} levels. In the neonate the P_{O_2} levels rise and erythropoietin production is inhibited, followed by a fall in erythropoiesis. This situation is maintained for upwards of 4 weeks, when erythropoietin secretion increases again, followed by increased red cell production. This is accompanied by a transition from production of HbF to HbA.

Thermoregulation

While in the uterus, the fetus is maintained in a thermoneutral environment and experiences no thermoregulatory stress. Following birth it is immediately exposed to an environmental temperature that will be at least 10°C below that in the uterus, and below its thermoneutral zone. The thermoneutral zone for neonates, the temperature range in which a naked individual can maintain body temperature without active heat production, is significantly above that of adults, being 32–36°C as compared to 27–31°C. Immediately following birth, the neonate will also lose body heat faster than an adult, partly because of its higher surface area to volume ratio, and partly through evaporation because its skin will be covered in amniotic fluid. Adults have heat conservation and heat production processes which enable them to withstand thermoregulatory stress, but the neonate is unable to do so because these processes are not sufficiently well developed at this stage in the baby's life. The neonate also lacks the insulation normally provided by subcutaneous fat in the adult.

The neonate's main problem is excessive heat loss that cannot be matched by its limited heat production via cellular metabolism. Heat production cannot be boosted by normal muscular activity or shivering because these systems are not developed. Compensation exists in the form of **brown adipose tissue** (BAT), a special type of fat cell distributed over the neonate's body, which is capable of high levels of heat production when stimulated by adrenaline, a process described as **non-shivering thermogenesis**.

BAT is found across the shoulders, down the spine and sternum, and around the kidneys and constitutes some 2–6% of the neonate's body weight. Because it is laid down during the later stages of gestation, premature babies have an even greater problem of maintaining body temperature than full-term neonates. The baby becomes less dependent on non-shivering thermogenesis after 6 months, once other heat production and conservation processes begin to develop.

Other systems

Gastrointestinal tract (GIT)

During gestation all nutrients have been supplied to the fetus via the placenta, with metabolic waste being lost via the same route. This pathway is lost immediately after birth, and neonates do not normally start to feed for several hours. Current practice is not to feed neonates for 24 hours following birth. Towards the end of gestation energy stores begin to accumulate, mainly in the form of glycogen in the liver, and these sustain the neonate while a feeding pattern is established. Maternal glucose has been the main source of carbohydrate in utero, but once feeding is established the lactose contained in either maternal milk or proprietary feeds predominates.

Although not functional, there is good evidence to show that all aspects of gastrointestinal activity are sufficiently developed to support oral nutrition of the neonate before birth. The swallowing reflex is operational, and glands throughout the tract (salivary, gastric and pancreatic, and GIT hormone-secreting cells) are all functional. Motility in the fetal GIT is rare, and when it does occur results in release of **meconium**, which fills the tract during gestation, into the amniotic fluid. This can be dangerous for the fetus if it is ingested, and meconium release is used as an indicator of fetal distress. Babies normally defecate far more frequently than children or adults, and can pass stools as often as 10–12 times a day. It takes several years before control of defecation is fully achieved.

Kidney function and fluid balance

The kidneys develop throughout pregnancy and become increasingly functional towards term, with the urine produced forming a significant proportion of the amniotic fluid. However, the kidneys are not fully mature at birth and it takes several years to achieve adult functionality. In the fetus, any excessive loss of fluid through the kidney is automatically compensated by placental transfer. In the neonate, fluid intake and loss need to be matched and this is normally achieved some 7–10 days after parturition. Fluid balance can pose a problem for babies because they are not able to communicate when they are thirsty rather than hungry. Water loss can be excessive, particularly in warm weather when insensible water loss from the skin increases, and babies need to be given water rather than a traditional feed. Vomiting and diarrhoea also pose particular problems, in part because oral replenishment of fluid may not be possible, and in part because of the loss of essential electrolytes. In severe cases intravenous rehydration may become necessary.

Neonatal endocrinology

Throughout pregnancy the fetus has provided essential endocrine support for the optimal production of oestrogens by the placenta. Within the fetus all other endocrine glands are active by about 10 weeks' gestation, and there is no reliance on the transfer of maternal hormones. For many hormone systems, a gradual development profile is seen. However, normal development of the fetus is dependent on an adequate supply of certain hormones, particularly in the perinatal period.

The **adrenal** gland, through its secretion of cortisol and adrenaline, is essential for optimal adaptation to extrauterine life. Both hormones stimulate processes within the lungs, heart, liver, pancreas and gastrointestinal tract which ensure that these systems function efficiently in the new environment. In addition, cortisol stimulates the adrenal medulla to produce more noradrenaline, thus ensuring an adequate supply of adrenaline, and adrenaline is essential for the stimulation of brown adipose tissue to generate heat.

Thyroid hormones, particularly thyroxine (T_4), are critical in the perinatal period for normal development of the CNS and bone. Deficiency at this stage results in behavioural retardation and reduced development of the skeleton causing the condition known as **cretinism**, when the individual is mentally slow and of small stature. Neonates are routinely screened for hypothyroidism, because thyroid hormone replacement during this critical period prevents cretinism.

Summary

Fetal and neonatal systems

- In the fetal circulation the lungs are largely excluded from the circulation by modifications which are reversed at birth.
- The presence of surfactant is very important to ease and stabilize the first few breaths after birth.
- About one-third of the neonate's blood volume has come from the umbilical vessels.
- Neonates rely heavily on non-shivering thermogenesis of brown adipose tissue for thermoregulation.
- Neonatal systems are at different degrees of maturity at birth. Thyroid function is particularly critical to prevent cretinism.

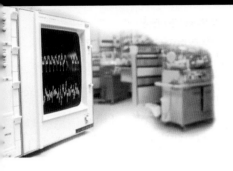

10.5

Congenital defects in the neonate

Introduction

Although the vast majority of neonates are born without significant anatomical defects, there is a wide spectrum of congenital defects that may be present and the physiological disturbance that they can cause is very variable. In this chapter, just some of the commoner congenital defects are considered in relation to their effects on neonatal physiology and the extent to which they can be corrected.

Congenital cardiac defects

Congenital cardiac disease is present in about 7 per 1000 live births and represents the commonest form of congenital abnormality. Traditionally, congenital cardiac defects are divided into cyanotic and acyanotic defects. Cyanotic defects result in deoxygenated blood bypassing the lungs and entering the arterial circulation, resulting in central cyanosis. This can be distinguished from cyanosis due to lung disease because it does not respond to oxygen therapy.

Acyanotic heart disease does not result in significant amounts of deoxygenated blood entering the arterial circulation, and cyanosis is not an early feature of this condition. If severe, it may nevertheless result in cardiac failure.

Cyanotic heart disease

Transposition of the great vessels

In this rare condition, the aorta arises from the right ventricle and the pulmonary artery arises from the left ventricle. However, the great veins remain in the usual configuration. In other words, blood draining from the lungs is pumped back into the lungs, and blood from the systemic circulation is pumped straight back into the systemic circulation without passing through the lungs. The infant's pulmonary and systemic circulations would therefore be effectively isolated from each other, a condition incompatible with life were it not for some mixing of the two circulations through the foramen ovale and the ductus arteriosus, which are patent at birth but begin to close soon thereafter.

Affected infants quickly become cyanotic. Initial treatment may involve making an artificial hole in the atrial septum. This is usually done under radiological control by passing a balloon-ended catheter through the venous circulation, and through the foramen ovale. A balloon on the end of the catheter is inflated to make a large artificial connection between the atria, which allows blood to flow between the two circulations. Definitive treatment involves surgically reimplanting the great vessels into the correct ventricles.

Tetralogy of Fallot

In this condition there is a hole in the ventricular septum immediately adjacent to the aorta. The aorta is incorrectly situated directly over this septal defect instead of lying to one side of an intact septum and connecting to the left ventricle as normal. In addition to this, there is stenosis of the pulmonary artery, as a result of which the right ventricle becomes hypertrophied. Deoxygenated blood flows from the right ventricle into the misplaced aorta, resulting in cyanosis which is particularly noticeable when the infant exerts itself, for example when crying. The severity of the condition is variable; at its worst there is almost complete obstruction of the pulmonary artery. Surgical correction of the defect is generally necessary.

Acyanotic heart disease

Acyanotic congenital heart disease is often the result of a connection between the atria, the ventricles or the great vessels. The clinical consequences depend upon the site of the connection and the amount of blood that flows between the two sides of the circulation. In these defects, blood flows from the left side of the heart, where the pressure is higher, to the right side. Because there is no blood bypassing the lungs, central cyanosis is not usually a feature of these conditions unless they are complicated by cardiac failure.

Defects in the interventricular septum

This is the commonest form of congenital heart disease. The defect (a hole) usually lies in the upper part of the interventricular septum, close to the atrioventricular valves. Small holes are usually asymptomatic and are detected as a murmur; they may either close spontaneously or remain the same absolute size. As the child grows, the defect becomes relatively smaller in comparison with the rest of the heart. Larger defects may result in heart failure and require surgical closure.

Defects in the atrial septum

Defects in the atrial septum are usually divided into ostium primum and ostium secundum defects.

Ostium secundum defects are usually found in the fossa ovale, the remnant of the foramen ovale. They are therefore high in the atrial septum. They are usually noticed because of the heart murmur that they cause and do not generally produce symptoms until later in life when heart failure may occur. They can be corrected surgically.

Ostium primum defects are rarer than ostium secundum and are generally more serious. The defect occurs low down in the atrial septum, close to the atrioventricular valves and is often complicated by incompetence of the mitral valve. The defect usually produces symptoms of cardiac failure in infancy or childhood, and surgical repair of the septum and, if necessary, the mitral valve is required.

Patent ductus arteriosus

The ductus arteriosus is a vessel that connects the fetal aorta to the pulmonary artery. In utero, blood flows in the vessel from the pulmonary artery to the aorta, bypassing the fetal pulmonary circulation (see p. 932). At birth, the increase in arterial oxygen tension usually triggers the closure of the ductus arteriosus, but in some cases it inappropriately remains patent. Blood flows through a patent ductus arteriosus from the aorta to the pulmonary artery after birth, i.e. it flows in the opposite direction to that in which it flowed in utero. This is because at birth the pressure in the pulmonary circulation falls as the lungs expand and so the pressure in the aorta is higher than that in the pulmonary artery. A small patent ductus may produce few symptoms, but a larger patent ductus may require to be surgically ligated.

Obstructive lesions

A number of congenital lesions may result in obstruction to blood flow. Stenosis of the aortic or pulmonary valves, usually associated with anatomical defects of the valves, may result in cardiac failure requiring surgery. Coarctation of the aorta is a short area of narrowing in the descending aorta, usually just past the left subclavian artery, causing an obstruction to blood flow. Blood is usually able to reach the lower part of the body via collateral vessels, but the coarctation usually results in high blood pressure in the upper part of the body. Surgery is usually necessary to prevent heart failure.

Congenital defects of the gastrointestinal tract

Congenital diaphragmatic hernia

This condition is due to a hole in one side of the diaphragm, usually the left. Abdominal contents pass into the chest cavity, compressing the lungs and shifting the mediastinum. The infant may become increasingly distressed as it swallows air, inflating its stomach and further compressing its lungs. Initial treatment involves insertion of a nasogastric tube to deflate the stomach, and in severe cases endotracheal intubation and ventilation may be required. Although it is often possible to repair the diaphragm surgically, the condition may be associated with congenital pulmonary or cardiac defects that may themselves limit survival.

Tracheo-oesophageal fistulae and oesophageal atresia

This condition is caused by abnormal development of the trachea and oesophagus. In the majority of cases, the upper oesophagus ends in a blind pouch and the lower part of the oesophagus communicates with the trachea, forming a tracheo-oesophageal fistula. The affected infant is clearly unable to swallow and so dribbles saliva profusely. Furthermore, the infant may aspirate saliva or feed, which may result in choking. As the lower end of the oesophagus is connected to the trachea, the stomach is frequently distended with air. The condition is often associated with other congenital defects, which limits the success of surgical repair.

Exomphalos and gastroschisis

These conditions are congenital herniations of the gut contents through the abdominal wall. During normal embryonic development, the developing intestines herniate into the umbilical cord.

In exomphalos, the intestines fail to pass back into the abdomen, and in severe cases a large mass containing loops of intestine may be present on the abdominal wall of the neonate. The contents of the exomphalos are covered with a membrane consisting of peritoneum and amnion. The condition is very often associated with other defects and is frequently fatal.

In gastroschisis, there is a full-thickness hole in the anterior abdominal wall, through which pass intestines and other abdominal contents. The condition is not often associated with other congenital defects, and can often be repaired surgically with good results.

Intestinal obstruction

There are a variety of conditions that may lead to partial obstruction (stenosis) or complete obstruction (atresia) of the large or small intestine.

Small bowel obstruction

Pyloric stenosis, due to hypertrophy of the circular muscle at the gastric pylorus, is relatively common, resulting in persistent vomiting. The loss of hydrochloric acid from the stomach may results in hypovolaemia combined with a hypochloraemic alkalosis, which may require treatment prior to surgery. The condition is easily treated surgically by division of the muscle fibres, and the prognosis is excellent. Other causes of small bowel obstruction include:

- missing segments of intestine
- diaphragms across the lumen of the bowel
- twisted loops of bowel.

These may be repaired surgically.

Large bowel obstruction

The two most important causes of large bowel obstruction are Hirschsprung's disease and imperforate anus.

Hirschsprung's disease (see Clinical Example, p. 849) is characterized by a lack of neuronal ganglia in the wall of part of the large bowel. There is no peristalsis in the aganglionic part of the large bowel, and this leads to obstruction. Treatment ultimately involves removing the aganglionic part of the large bowel.

Imperforate anus is characterized by a large bowel that is either blind ended or fails to perforate the perineum in the normal position but which communicates with another pelvic organ such as the urethra or vagina. Although these defects may be associated with other congenital intestinal defects, they are usually correctable surgically.

Congenital defects of the nervous system

The spinal cord, brain and meninges form early in uterine life. The spinal cord is formed by a folding of two longitudinal ridges of the outer layer (ectoderm) of the embryo to form a tube, the neural tube. This folding of the two sides of the dorsal surface of the embryo towards the midline continues until the neural tube is enclosed within the embryo. The folding that forms the neural tube starts in the mid part of the embryo and spreads towards its head and tail. By 23 days old, folding should be complete and a neural tube should be formed that is entirely contained within the body of the embryo.

Failure of the process can lead to a wide spectrum of neurological defects in the newborn. The most severe of these defects is anencephaly, a complete failure of the cerebral hemispheres to develop. Affected fetuses are stillborn or die within a few hours of birth.

Failure of complete enclosure of the neural tube leads to spina bifida. Spina bifida defects are broadly divided into two groups, spina bifida occulta and spina bifida cystica.

Spina bifida occulta defects

Spina bifida occulta is associated with small defects in the vertebrae overlying the spinal cord. The majority of cases are associated with a birthmark or other lesion on the skin overlying the defect. Usually, spinal bifida occulta defects are not associated with neurological defects, although a few individuals suffer bladder problems or neurological problems in the lower limbs.

Spina bifida cystica defects

In these defects, there is failure of closure of vertebrae around the spinal cord, usually in the lumbar or sacral regions. In its mildest form, spina bifida cystica defects consist of a sac of cerebrospinal fluid (meningocele) which herniates through a gap in the overlying vertebra and which may or may not be covered by a layer of skin. In a meningocele, the neural tissue is normally positioned and neurological problems in the lower limbs are present in a minority of infants.

In a myelomeningocele, neural tissue is abnormally placed and in the severest cases there may be widespread exposure of neural tissue over a large area of the back. Myelomeningoceles are very often associated with severe neurological defects in the lower limbs and are also associated with hydrocephalus.

Spina bifida can be a very disabling condition, but fortunately its incidence in the UK is falling as a result of prenatal screening for the condition by measurement of the concentration of α-fetoprotein in the maternal plasma or in amniotic fluid.

Further reading

FitzGerald M J T, FitzGerald M 1994 *Human embryology*. Baillière Tindall, London.

Organized on a regional basis rather than the usual systems approach, this book provides a clear account of the development of the human fetus from fertilization to birth. The line drawings which make up the majority of the illustrations are particularly clear.

Ferin M, Jewelewicz R, Warren M 1993 *The menstrual cycle*. Oxford University Press Inc, USA.

Synthesizing information from many sources, this book presents the state of knowledge at its time of publishing in a detailed and authoritative fashion. Pathophysiology and clinical presentations of common menstrual disorders are presented in this reference work.

Johnson M H, Everitt B J 1999 *Essential reproduction*, 5th edn. Blackwell Science (UK), Oxford

One of the 'Essential' series, this book covers the core content of a course in mammalian reproduction.

Tanner J M 1989 *Foetus into man*, 2nd edn. Castlemead Publications, Ware, Herefordshire

A fascinating book which takes a broad look at physical growth from conception to adulthood. A jolly good read.

Thorburn G D, Harding R 1994 *Textbook of fetal physiology*. Oxford Medical Publications, Oxford.

A substantial description of the foundations of fetal development covering all the major systems and the maternal adaptation to pregnancy.

Questions

Answer true or false to the following statements:

10.1

In humans:

A. The normal karyotype consists of 46 chromosomes.
B. The first meiotic division is preceded by duplication of DNA.
C. The first meiotic division produces cells with the haploid number of chromosomes.
D. There is exchange of genetic material between chromosomes during the second meiotic division.
E. The presence of an X chromosome will lead to a female phenotype.

10.2

During intrauterine development:

A. The female genital tract develops from the wolffian ducts.
B. Maturation of the male internal genital tract is dependent on fetal production of testosterone.
C. Maturation of the female internal genital tract is dependent on fetal production of oestrogens.
D. A lifetime's complement of spermatogonia are produced.
E. The external genitalia develop from bipotential primordial tissues.

10.3

Spermatogenesis:

A. Is promoted by the action of testosterone on Sertoli cells.
B. Is promoted by the action of follicle-stimulating hormone (FSH) on the Leydig cells.
C. Produces mature spermatozoa which contain hydrolytic enzymes within the acrosome.
D. Requires that the testes be at a temperature of 37°C.
E. Commences at puberty under the influence of rising levels of hypothalamic gonadotrophins.

10.4

Testosterone:

A. Is mainly protein bound in the plasma.
B. Stimulates closure of the epiphyses in bone.
C. Acts via receptors on the plasma membrane of target cells.
D. Is highly water soluble.
E. Is converted to the inactive metabolite dihydrotestosterone in peripheral tissues.

10.5

During the ovarian cycle:

A. Follicular development is stimulated by pituitary gonadotrophins.
B. Several follicles develop to the stage of secondary oocyte formation.
C. Follicle-stimulating hormone (FSH) stimulates androgen formation by follicular thecal cells.
D. The corpus luteum forms from the remains of the follicle after ovulation.
E. The length of the follicular phase is more variable than that of the luteal phase.

(Answers overleaf →)

10.6

With regard to the female reproductive cycle:

A. Plasma levels of oestrogens are highest in the week preceding ovulation.

B. The secretory phase of the uterine cycle is stimulated by high levels of follicle-stimulating hormone (FSH).

C. Menstruation occurs when plasma gonadotrophin levels are at their lowest.

D. Luteinizing hormone (LH) stimulates formation of the corpus luteum, thus causing a rise in progesterone levels.

E. High oestrogen levels favour the formation of very viscous cervical mucus.

10.7

During pregnancy:

A. The period from conception to birth normally lasts 40 weeks.

B. Secretion of progesterone increases steadily until parturition because human chorionic gonadotrophin (hCG) stimulates the corpus luteum.

C. Immune reactions against fetal tissues are rare because the placenta presents an impenetrable barrier to maternal immunoglobulins.

D. Prolactin levels rise.

E. Breast development is stimulated but milk production is inhibited.

10.8

Lactation:

A. Is stimulated by oestrogen.

B. Relies on reflex stimulation of hormone release from the anterior pituitary.

C. Relies on reflex stimulation of hormone release from the posterior pituitary.

D. Allows reinforcement of passive immunity by maternal secretion of type G immunoglobulins.

E. Helps inhibit ovulation.

10.9

During fetal development:

A. Deoxygenated blood is passed from the right to the left side of the heart through the foramen ovale.

B. The head and neck receive their blood supply from the right ventricle rather than the left.

C. Shunts bypass the hepatic portal and pulmonary circulations.

D. Fetal bilirubin levels are higher than those in the neonate.

E. Fetal haemoglobin has a higher affinity for O_2 than adult haemoglobin.

10.10

During sexual intercourse:

A. Erection of the penis is stimulated by vasodilator parasympathetic nerve.

B. Contraction of the vas deferens is stimulated by sympathetic nerves.

C. Ejaculation involves contraction of striated muscle.

D. Female orgasm involves rhythmic contractions of the vagina.

E. Vaginal secretion increases.

Answers

10.1

A. **True.** There are 44 pairs of autosomes and two sex chromosomes.

B. **True.** This doubles the amount of DNA, although the number of chromosomes remains diploid.

C. **True.** Each of these cells still contains the normal amount of DNA, however, since each chromosome still consists of two chromatids. The separation of these chromatids to form single chromosomes during the second meiotic division reduces the DNA content to half that in a normal cell, i.e. the chromosome number and the DNA content are now both haploid.

D. **False.** This exchange occurs during the first meiotic division.

E. **False.** The normal male karyotype is XY; it is the absence of a Y chromosome which leads to a female phenotype.

10.2

A. **False.** The female tract develops from the müllerian ducts.

B. **True.** This testosterone is produced by the developing testes.

C. **False.** Development of the internal female genital tract from the müllerian ducts will occur in the absence of testosterone without any need for female sex steroids.

D. **False.** Further multiplication of spermatogonia occurs throughout reproductive life from puberty onwards. This contrasts with the situation in the case of oogonia.

E. **True.** These tissues differ from the precursors of the internal genital tracts, the wolffian and müllerian tracts, which are unipotential.

10.3

A. **True.** Testosterone increases Sertoli cell sensitivity to FSH. It has other important actions in spermatogenesis, including direct stimulation of spermatogonia.

B. **False.** FSH acts on Sertoli cells, LH acts on the interstitial cells of Leydig.

C. **True.** These are released to allow digestion of the corona radiata and zona pellucida so that the sperm can reach and fertilize the oocyte.

D. **False.** This is too high a temperature for spermatogenesis; about 35°C is appropriate and this probably explains why the testes have to be located outside the abdominal cavity.

E. **False.** Rising levels of gonadotrophins are thought to be the key drive during puberty but these are produced by the anterior pituitary, not the hypothalamus. It is likely, however, that the hypothalamus is important since it produces gonadotrophin-releasing hormone which stimulates gonadotrophin release.

10.4

A. **True.** Approximately 98% is bound to sex steroid-binding globulin. Only the free form, however, is biologically active.

B. **True.** This is one of several actions related to somatic growth, including increased muscle growth and stimulation of long bone growth prior to epiphyseal closure.

C. **False.** Like other steroid hormones, testosterone, or rather its more active derivatives, acts intracellularly.

D. **False.** Steroid hormones are derived from cholesterol and are more soluble in lipid than water. This explains how they can cross the plasma membrane to act inside cells.

E. **False.** This metabolite is actually more active than testosterone.

10.5

A. **True.** FSH acts on the granulosa cells and luteinizing hormone (LH) acts primarily on theca cells.
B. **False.** Several primary follicles begin to develop but the secondary oocyte is only formed in the single follicle which matures to ovulation.
C. **False.** This is a function of LH.
D. **True.** It forms under the influence of LH.
E. **True.** This causes problems for natural family planning because it makes the time between menstruation and ovulation difficult to predict with security and so the risk of unplanned pregnancy is high during this period.

10.6

A. **True.** They rise as the antral follicle develops towards ovulation and fall again immediately afterwards.
B. **False.** The uterine cycle is controlled by ovarian hormones not gonadotrophins, except indirectly via their effects on the ovaries. The secretory phase of the uterine cycle is stimulated by high levels of progesterone from the corpus luteum.
C. **False.** Plasma gonadotrophin levels are at their lowest at the end of the secretory phase of the uterine cycle. They rise again during menstruation, stimulating the onset of the follicular phase of the next ovarian cycle. Oestrogen/progesterone levels are at their lowest during menstruation; these are the hormones which act on the endometrium.
D. **True.** The LH surge stimulates ovulation and the relatively high levels of LH in the luteal phase stimulate and support the corpus luteum.
E. **False.** The high oestrogen levels around ovulation stimulate a change in the cervical mucus to a less viscous, more alkaline form, reducing the resistance to the progress of spermatozoa should intercourse take place.

10.7

A. **False.** True gestation is normally 38 weeks but the duration of pregnancy is usually timed from the beginning of the last menstrual period. This adds approximately 2 weeks, i.e. the normal duration of the follicular phase of the ovarian cycle, to the length of pregnancy.
B. **False.** hCG levels rise up to about week 6 and then fall off again, with a concomitant decrease in size of the corpus luteum. Placental manufacture of progesterone, however, ensures that levels continue to rise throughout.
C. **False.** IgG can cross the placenta, providing passive immunity to infectious diseases. Immune reactions against fetal tissues, however, are generally cell mediated. In rare cases, IgG-mediated tissue damage can occur, e.g. red cell lysis in rhesus disease.
D. **True.** This helps stimulate breast development, particularly the functional maturation of milk-producing cells.
E. **True.** The rising levels of sex hormones promote growth of breast glands and ducts but inhibit milk production until after parturition.

10.8

A. **False.** Female sex steroids inhibit lactation.
B. **True.** The suckling reflex stimulates prolactin release which activates milk production.
C. **True.** Oxytocin is also released, causing contraction of myoepithelial cells and milk expulsion.
D. **False.** Milk contains IgA.
E. **True.** This seems to be a function of the elevated prolactin, which can inhibit gonadotrophin release.

10.9

A. **False.** The blood shunted through the foramen ovale is well oxygenated, consisting of a mix of oxygenated blood from the placental veins and deoxygenated blood from the abdomen and lower limbs. It is this blood which supplies the oxygen needs of the developing head, neck and upper limbs.

B. **False.** They receive it from the left ventricle via branches of the aorta.

C. **True.** These shunts are known as the ductus venosus and ductus arteriosus.

D. **False.** Fetal bilirubin levels are kept low by removal across the placenta. Levels rise markedly immediately after birth and take several weeks to come back to normal as hepatic function matures.

E. **True.** This helps ensure transfer of O_2 from maternal to fetal blood across the placenta.

10.10

A. **True.** This is one of the few examples of regulation of vascular tone by parasympathetic nerves. Most blood vessels are regulated by sympathetic constrictor nerves; indeed, these also supply penile vessels.

B. **True.** This is part of the emission phase where spermatozoa and seminal fluid are forced into the urethra.

C. **True.** Striated muscle, e.g. the bulbocavernosus muscle, rhythmically squeezes the urethra, forcing semen into the vagina.

D. **True.** These may assist movement of spermatozoa towards the opening of the uterine cervix but they are not essential for fertilization to occur.

E. **True.**

Index

963